Pathology of the Kidney

Volume I

Pathology of the Kidney

Fourth Edition

Robert H. Heptinstall, M.D.

Professor of Pathology, The Johns Hopkins University School of Medicine; Pathologist, The Johns Hopkins Hospital, Baltimore

Formerly Baxley Professor of Pathology and Director, Department of Pathology, The Johns Hopkins University School of Medicine; Formerly Pathologist-in-Chief, The Johns Hopkins Hospital, Baltimore

Little, Brown and Company
Boston/Toronto/London

NOTICE

The indications and dosages of all drugs in this book have been recommended in the medical literature and conform to the practices of the general medical community. The medications described do not necessarily have specific approval by the Food and Drug Administration for use in the diseases and dosages for which they are recommended. The package insert for each drug should be consulted for use and dosage as approved by the FDA. Because standards for usage change, it is advisable to keep abreast of revised recommendations, particularly those concerning new drugs.

Fourth Edition
Second Printing

Library of Congress Catalog Card No. 91-62350

ISBN 0-316-35800-2

Printed in the United States of America

To Ann

Contents

Volume III

Preface

This fourth edition of *Pathology of the Kidney* differs from previous ones in several respects.

There are important changes in the content of the book, including the introduction of new entities and new concepts, as well as an updating of our knowledge and understanding of already recognized conditions. Clearly, to address all this it was necessary to seek the help of new authors with specialized interests and to impose additional burdens on those who had contributed to previous editions. Almost without exception these various colleagues responded nobly to the task, delivered their manuscripts "close" to the deadlines imposed, and willingly accepted the suggestions I made to secure a more or less uniform style of presentation. By writing 15 of the 31 chapters they reduced the amount of my writing considerably, and I am most grateful to them for expending so much energy for so little reward.

The general arrangement of the book has been altered in several ways. It begins as before with a chapter on anatomy, which has been written by two new authors, Drs. Manjeri Venkatachalam and Wilhelm Kriz. It is larger and more profusely illustrated than before and the pictures are of exquisite quality. Chapter 2 is Development, Developmental Defects, and Cystic Diseases of the Kidney. It replaces Chapters 2 and 3 in the third edition. It is excellently written and illustrated by another newcomer, Dr. Anthony Risdon, who has drawn on his great experience and the wealth of material available at the Great Ormond Street Hospital for Sick Children in London. Dr. Robert McCluskey in Chapter 3 has expanded his chapter, Immunologic Mechanisms in Glomerular Disease in the third edition, to include immunologically mediated tubulointerstitial disease under the heading of Immunologic Aspects of Renal Disease. The new chapter provides much greater coverage of T cell mechanisms in renal disease, discusses recent discoveries on the safe disposal of circulating immune complexes by the erythrocyte complement receptor, and describes mechanisms of formation of immune deposits following interaction of antibodies with cell surface antigens.

Chapters 4 through 11 embrace the various types of primary glomerulonephritis. In Chapter 4, I describe contemporary classifications of glomerulonephritis as an introduction to the topic. In addition, the chapter contains a discussion of focal glomerulonephritis, mesangial proliferative glomerulonephritis, and other conditions causing recurrent hematuria. IgA nephritis, formerly discussed under focal glomerulonephritis, has been transferred to Chapter 6. Dr. Fred Silva, another new author, has utilized his wide experience and boundless energy to write Chapter 5, Acute Postinfectious Glomerulonephritis and Glomerulonephritis Complicating Persistent Bacterial Infection. This chapter brings together what was included in two separate chapters in the third edition. Chapter 6 is a new chapter entitled Primary and Secondary Forms of IgA Nephritis, Schönlein-Henoch Syndrome. I was fortunate in obtaining the services of Dr. Steven Emancipator, a recognized expert on these topics, to write this account and he has skillfully drawn together the various conditions that were discussed in scattered places in the third edition. Dr. Silva has written a comprehensive and authoritative account of the various forms of membranoproliferative glomerulonephritis in Chapter 7, and Dr. Melvin Schwartz has considerably improved Chapter 8, Membranous Glomerulonephritis. Dr. Schwartz has included in his new chapter the various secondary forms of membranous glomerulonephritis such as are seen with penicillamine and gold therapy, tumors, Sjögren syndrome, and sarcoidosis, which were scattered throughout the third edition. I wrote Chapter 9 on crescentic glomerulonephritis and Chapter 10 on anti-GBM antibody disease, the latter chapter including an account of pulmonary hemorrhage associated with glomerulonephritis of non-anti-GBM antibody pathogenesis. Chapter 11—formerly centered on chronic glomerulonephritis—has been expanded to include concepts of nonimmunologic glomerular injury and the pathologic changes seen in end-stage kidney disease. Renal osteodystrophy has been relocated in this chapter.

The chapter entitled The Nephrotic Syndrome (Chapter 12) has been extensively revised by a new author, Dr. Jean Olson, who has concentrated mainly on minimal change disease and focal segmental glomerular sclerosis. Her great experience with both experimental and human material has helped to make this an informative chapter. Certain conditions included in the comparable chapter in the third edition have been moved elsewhere (i.e., Chapters 8, 28, and 31). Dr. Gary Hill has again written Chapter 13, Systemic Lupus Erythematosus and Mixed Connective-Tissue Disease, and has made better an already excellent chapter. He has expanded on the pathogenesis of SLE, particularly the section devoted to murine models.

The pathology of hypertension is considered in Chapters 14 and 15. In Chapter 14 I have concentrated on essential hypertension and experimental studies on the pathogenesis of vascular and glomerular lesions, while in Chapter 15 the more important secondary forms of hypertension are discussed. Polyarteritis (Periarteritis) Nodosa, Wegener's Syndrome, and Other Forms of Vasculitis (Chapter 16) retains the same format as in the third edition. Our own experience is cited to discuss the classification of polyarteritis, and the significance of antineutrophil cytoplasmic antibodies, introduced in Chapter 3, is considered. I have retained the same format as in the third edition for Chapter 17, Hemolytic Uremic Syndrome, Thrombotic Thrombocytopenic Purpura, and Systemic Sclerosis (Systemic Scleroderma), and brought it up to date by describing such topics as the role of verotoxins and discussing the newer studies on pathogenesis.

Acute Renal Failure (Chapter 18) is again treated by Dr. Kim Solez, who as well as updating the chapter, has extended his treatment of the hepatorenal syndrome. Chapter 19, Interstitial Nephritis, contains an expanded section on infective causes, and discussion of the pathology of the tubulointerstitial changes in sarcoidosis is consolidated rather than being fragmented as in the third edition. Immunologic aspects of experimental disease are excluded but are discussed in Dr. McCluskey's expanded Chapter 3. Dr. Solez has taken over my old chapter dealing with renal complications of therapeutic and diagnostic agents (Chapter 20), but apart from adding sections on the adverse effects of immunosuppressive, antineoplastic, and nonsteroidal anti-inflammatory agents, has made few changes. The effects of cyclosporine and newer immunosuppressive agents are also described in Chapter 27, Renal Transplantation.

Chapters 21 and 22, on urinary tract infection, reflux, and pyelonephritis, have been revised in light of recent studies, but the basic structure of the chapters remains unchanged. Chapter 23 is a chapter by Dr. Hill, Calcium and the Kidney, Nephrolithiasis, and Hydronephrosis. It replaces the chapter entitled Calcium and the Kidney, Renal Osteodystrophy and Stone Formation in the third edition. Dr. Hill's chapter is completely new and his treatment of hydronephrosis is particularly enlightening. As noted earlier, renal osteodystrophy is now more appropriately dealt with in Chapter 11. Chapter 24, Dysproteinemias, Amyloidosis, and Immunotactoid Glomerulopathy, also by Dr. Hill, has been extensively revised and expanded by the addition of the newly described condition of immunotactoid glomerulopathy (fibrillary glomerulonephritis).

Chapter 25, Diabetes Mellitus, replaces the chapter in the third edition headed Diabetes Mellitus and Gout, and the topic of gout is removed and discussed along with other metabolic diseases in Chapter 29. Dr. Olson, the author of the new chapter, has treated diabetes mellitus more extensively than in the previous edition. In Chapter 26, Renal Disease in Pregnancy, I have added a new section on the effects of pregnancy on various forms of renal disease. Dr. Kendrick Porter has once again written the chapter Renal Transplantation (Chapter 27) and has increased its scope considerably. Greater emphasis is placed on the practical aspects of interpretation of biopsies from grafts, including a formal differential diagnosis for all the various forms of graft rejection and the use of monoclonal antibodies as specific cell markers. The pathogenesis of the different forms of renal injury in grafts is discussed in greater detail, and there is more extensive coverage of recurrent and *de novo* glomerulonephritis and of recurrence of systemic diseases in grafted kidneys.

Chapters 28 to 31, all of them my responsibility, are a mixed bag. Chapter 28, Renal Manifestations of Various Infective Conditions, is a new chapter that contains tuberculosis, cytomegalovirus infection, HIV infection, syphilis, fungal infections, malaria, and schistosomiasis. Several of these were scattered among various chapters in the third edition, but HIV infection and fungal infections are newcomers. Chapter 29, Tubular Disorders and Various Metabolic Diseases, consolidates the different tubular disorders, lysosomal storage and peroxisome disorders, LCAT deficiency, and gout. Chapter 30 comprises hereditary disorders such as Alport's syndrome, nail-patella syndrome, and sickling disorders. Newer concepts, such as lack of the so-called Goodpasture antigen in Alport's syndrome, are introduced. Finally, Chapter 31 contains irradiation injury and the adverse effects on the kidney of heavy metals such as cadmium, lead, and mercury.

There are also changes in the format of the book, and chief among them is an increase in the page size. This allows the adoption of double-columns and the inclusion of a list of contents at the beginning of each chapter. These lists contain the major topics to be discussed and provide the reader with an approximate idea of their location in the chapter. It must be clearly understood that minor headings are not included in these lists, which should not, therefore, be regarded as a substitute for the index located at the end of each volume. We have also completely altered the headings and subheadings throughout the chapters by making them bolder and more generously spaced. This restyling has greatly enhanced the clarity of presentation.

Apart from the various authors, many others played an important part in the production of this fourth edition. I am particularly indebted to Mr. Stanley Meyer and other members of the staff of the William H. Welch Library for their unfailing courtesy and help in retrieving references, and to Mr. Raymond Lund and Mr. Norman Barker for their unrivalled photomicrography. Three former residents, Drs. Lora Hedrick, Ralph Hruban, and Moira Larsen helped in the proofreading, and numerous colleagues provided material and illustrations; I should like to thank them all. It is impossible to praise too highly the efforts of my secretary Mrs. Ursula Jacob; suffice it to say that without her the edition would never have been completed.

Dr. Venkatachalam wishes to acknowledge the secretarial assistance of Ms. Sharon Cloer and Ms. Sue Clayton. His work was supported by grants DK 37139 and DK 17387 from the National Institutes of Health, and the work of Dr. Kriz by the Deutsche Forschungsgemeinschaft, grant Kr 546/5-3. Dr. Silva thanks Ms. Mary Greear, Donna Moreland, and Cheryl Ronck for their assistance, and all members of the Southwest Pediatric Nephrology Study (under the direction of Dr. Ron Hogg) for the renal biopsy material used in the preparation of his chapters.

Finally the devotion of my three friends, Jake, Emily, and Coconut should not go unnoticed. Their company sustained me over eighteen months of writing, and while their snoring often proved contagious, their barking at the mailman and sundry other visitors never failed to return me to the task in hand.

R.H.H.

Contributing Authors

Steven N. Emancipator, M.D.
Associate Professor of Pathology, Case Western Reserve University School of Medicine; Pathologist, University Hospitals of Cleveland, Cleveland

Robert H. Heptinstall, M.D.
Professor of Pathology, The Johns Hopkins University School of Medicine; Pathologist, The Johns Hopkins Hospital, Baltimore

Formerly Baxley Professor of Pathology and Director, Department of Pathology, The Johns Hopkins University School of Medicine; Formerly Pathologist-in-Chief, The Johns Hopkins Hospital, Baltimore

Gary S. Hill, M.D.
Associate Professor of Pathology, The Johns Hopkins University School of Medicine; Chief of Pathology, Francis Scott Key Medical Center, Baltimore

Wilhelm Kriz, M.D.
Professor and Chairman of Anatomy, University of Heidelberg, Heidelberg, Germany

Robert T. McCluskey, M.D.
Benjamin Castleman Professor of Pathology, Harvard Medical School; Chief, Department of Pathology, Massachusetts General Hospital, Boston

Jean L. Olson, M.D.
Associate Professor of Pathology, The Johns Hopkins University School of Medicine; Pathologist, The Johns Hopkins Hospital, Baltimore

Kendrick A. Porter, M.D., D.Sc., F.R.C.Path.
Professor of Pathology, St. Mary's Hospital Medical School, University of London; Honorary Consultant Pathologist, St. Mary's Hospital, London

R. Anthony Risdon, M.D., F.R.C.Path.
Professor of Histopathology, The Institute of Child Health; Consultant Pathologist, Department of Histopathology, The Hospital for Sick Children, London

Melvin M. Schwartz, M.D.
Professor of Pathology, Rush Medical College of Rush University; Associate Attending Pathologist, Rush-Presbyterian-St. Luke's Medical Center, Chicago

Fred G. Silva, M.D.
Lloyd R. Rader Professor and Chairman of Pathology, University of Oklahoma College of Medicine; Chief of Pathology Service, Oklahoma Medical Center, Oklahoma City

Kim Solez, M.D.
Professor and Chairman of Pathology, University of Alberta Faculty of Medicine; Director of Anatomical Pathology, University of Alberta Hospital, Edmonton, Alberta, Canada

Manjeri A. Venkatachalam, B.S., M.B.
Professor of Pathology and Medicine, University of Texas Medical School at San Antonio, San Antonio, Texas

Pathology of the Kidney

Manjeri A. Venkatachalam
Wilhelm Kriz

1
Anatomy

The object of this chapter is to present the state of understanding of the gross and microscopic structure of human kidneys. Studies in lower animals also have been essential to arrive at this understanding because of the lack of availability of normal human tissue fixed optimally for microscopy before postmortem autolytic changes have taken place. We have referred to some descriptions of nephron structure and vascular anatomy derived therefrom, particularly from work on rats, rabbits, and dogs. Among these species and human beings there are some generalities of structural features that are relevant to normal and altered renal function and to the changes observed in human pathologic states. When not specifically indicated, the provided descriptions may be considered appropriate for human beings, at least in a general sense.

GROSS ANATOMY

General Features

For details of the general anatomic features given here, the reader is referred elsewhere [73,228,335]. The kidneys are paired, bean-shaped organs that weigh 120 to 170 g in the normal adult human male and measure approximately 11 × 6 × 2.5 cm. In women, they are slightly smaller. The left kidney is slightly larger than the right. Total renal mass correlates best with body surface area [154]. Kidney size, determined in vivo, varies considerably with alterations of physiologic states, such as hydration and blood pressure [116]. They extend from the 12th thoracic to the 3rd lumbar vertebra, the left kidney being slightly higher in position than the right. Their positions vary with change of posture and with respiration. Situated in the retroperitoneum anterior to the transversalis fascia, the kidneys are enclosed in the so-called perirenal space, defined by the fascia of Gerota (renal fascia). The surgical anatomy of these fascial planes has been described elsewhere [73,252]. The superior poles are inclined slightly toward the midline and posteriorly, and the left kidney is nearer the midline. Their outer aspects are convex; the medial surface is concave and shows an elongated opening, or the hilus, which leads to a larger space

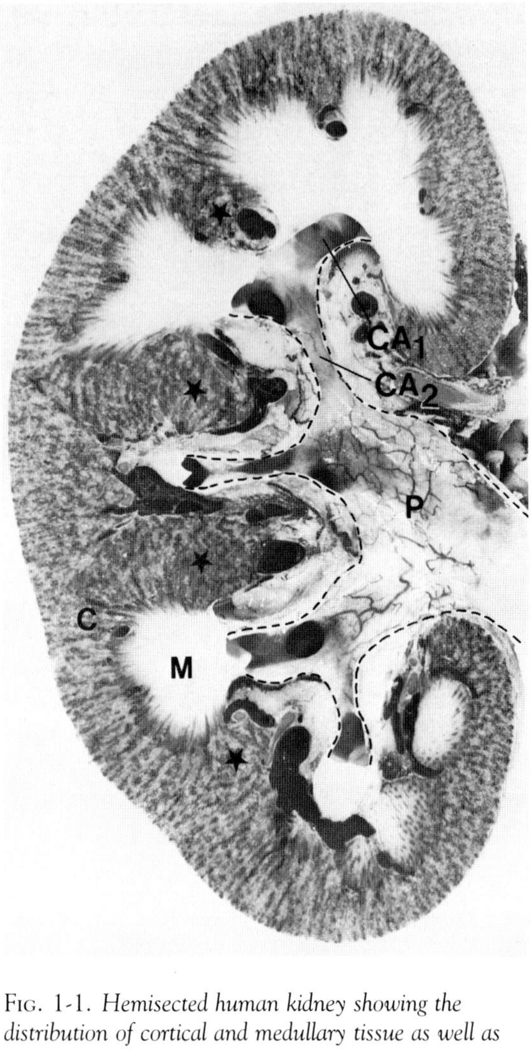

FIG. 1-1. *Hemisected human kidney showing the distribution of cortical and medullary tissue as well as the branching pattern of the renal pelvis (the borders are emphasized by dots). The cortex surrounds the individual medullary pyramids and reaches down to the renal sinus in between adjacent pyramids; these parts of the renal cortex are called septa or columns of Bertin (*). In the upper polar region, two compound papillae are seen each protruding into a calyx minor (CA_1), which then unite to form a calyx major (CA_2). C, cortex; M, medulla (pyramids); P, renal pelvis. Plastinated specimen; cortical vessels filled with dark-colored silicone rubber. (Prepared by G. von Hagens, Heidelberg.)*

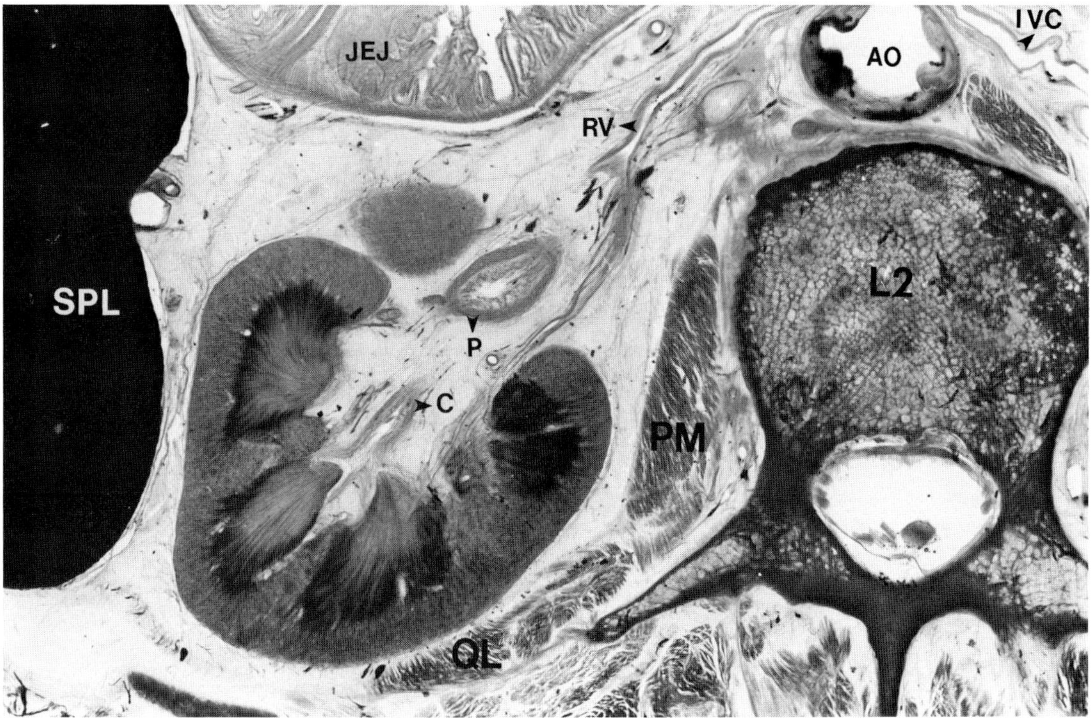

FIG. 1-2. *Cross section of a human cadaver at the level of body of 2nd lumbar vertebra, plastinated according to von Hagens [327a]. The section is seen from above and shows the topographic relationships of the left kidney. L2, 2nd lumbar vertebra; AO, aorta; PM, psoas major muscle; QL, quadratus lumborum muscle; SPL, spleen; JEJ, jejunum; C, calyx; P, pelvis; RV, renal vein; IVC, inferior vena cava.*

called the *renal sinus* (Fig. 1-1). The renal sinus, which is made up of fat and connective tissue, contains the pelvis, calyces, subdivisions of the renal artery and vein, lymphatics, and autonomic nerves. As will be described later, the calyces are cup-like structures that collect urine and transmit it to the pelvis. The pelvis is a muscular sac which, in turn, gives way to a narrow tube called the *ureter.* Kidneys are inclined with respect to the coronal plane of the body so that the renal hilus does not strictly face the midline but is disposed inwardly and toward the anterior (Fig. 1-2). The organ is covered by a thin fibrous capsule that is adherent at the hilus to the pelvis and to the vessels passing in or out of the kidney. The capsule is relatively smooth and may be stripped away with ease from the parenchyma. The renal parenchyma consists of an outer layer, called the *cortex,* and discrete conical inner portions known as the *pyramids,* which together constitute the medulla (see Fig. 1-1). The pyramidal tips are called *papillae,* and they protrude into the calyces. Adjacent pyramids may be fused; correspondingly, they have fused compound papillae.

Blood Vessels

The renal arteries arise perpendicularly from the aorta and show a characteristic but occasionally variable pattern of branching just before they enter into the hilus. The right renal artery arises a little lower than the left, and both take a slightly downward and lateral course toward the kidney. The renal artery divides most commonly into the anterior and posterior divisions (Fig. 1-3) and sometimes into an inferior division as well. Segmental arteries, which are branches of the anterior division, supply the upper, middle, and lower vascular segments of the kidney and very often the upper poles or apical segments as well [101, 109,119]. The posterior division runs behind the renal pelvis and continues on as the posterior segmental artery to supply the posterior segment, which consists of a large middle section of the posterior half of the kidney parenchyma. These patterns of vascular segmentation are shown in Figure 1-4. Other patterns of vascular segmentation of the kidney have been described [99,243]. Variant patterns occur and include the following: an inferior division that supplies the lower segment, a posterior division that supplies some or all of the apical and lower segments, accessory polar arteries that arise from the main renal artery, and aberrant accessory arteries that arise directly from the aorta [101,119,305]. Each of the segmental arteries is an end artery; that is, there is no significant collateral circulation between the vascular domains supplied by them. The segmental arteries divide within the renal sinus to form the interlobar arteries, which pierce the kidney between the renal pyramids. Corresponding interlobar veins accompany the arteries, but unlike the arteries, they anastomose with each other by means of lateral tributaries that encircle the renal calyces. The interlobar vessels are located in the space between the renal calyces and the adjacent cortical parenchyma. The interlobar veins are connected by anastomoses encircling individual calyces and join together in the renal sinus to form a variable number of venous trunks, which are disposed in front of the pelvis. At the hilus, they join together to form the renal vein, which is situated in front of the renal artery.

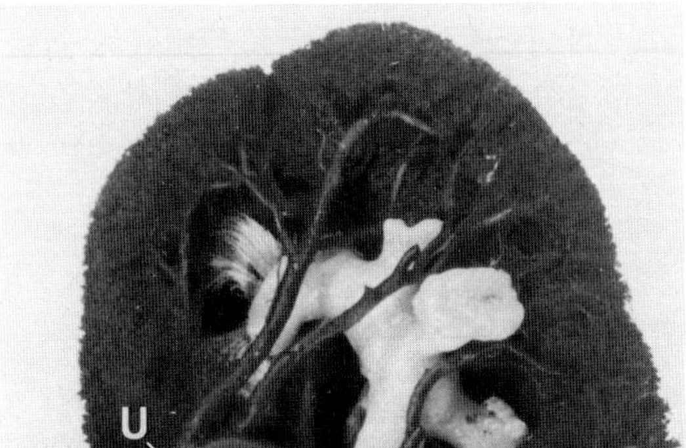

FIG. 1-3. *Corrosion cast of human kidney. The arterial vessels were filled with red silicone rubber (shown in dark shade), and the renal pelvis was filled with yellow silicone rubber (shown in light shade). The anterior parts of the injected vasculature were removed. The specimen shows the branching pattern of the renal artery, with an anterior division splitting into an upper (U) and a lower portion (L) and a posterior division (P). The renal pelvis (PE) is formed by the successive union of minor calyces (CA_1) and major calyces (CA_2). UR, ureter. Slightly smaller than normal size. (Prepared by R. Knebel, Heidelberg.)*

Nerves

The kidney is supplied by autonomic nerves derived from the renal plexus. The nerves continue into the kidney around the renal artery and its branches to supply the intrarenal vasculature, the

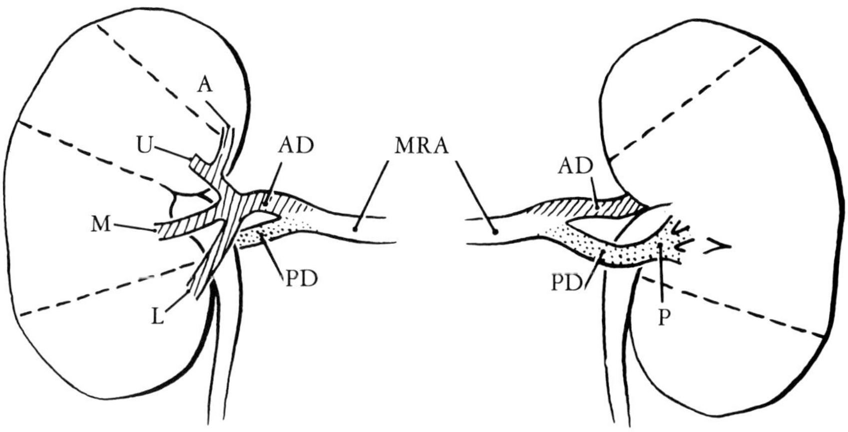

Fig. 1-4. *Main arterial divisions of kidney. MRA, main renal artery; PD, posterior division; AD, anterior division. Segmental arteries indicated by A (apical), U (upper), M (middle), L (lower), and P (posterior). (Modified from Graves, F. T.* Br. J. Surg. *42:132, 1954.)*

juxtaglomerular apparatus, and, to some extent, also the tubules [335].

Lymphatics

Lymph vessels from within the parenchyma of the kidney join together at the hilus to form four or five trunks that follow the renal vein to end in the lateral aortic nodes. As they emerge from the hilus, they are joined by tributaries from the subcapsular lymphatic plexus [335].

PARENCHYMA

General Architecture and the Lobes

The renal parenchyma consists of units known as *nephrons, blood vessels, lymphatics, nerves,* and the *interstitium.* The nephrons consist of glomeruli and the uriniferous tubules. The parenchyma of the human kidney is made up of approximately 14 units or subdivisions termed the *lobes.* The lobes consist of conical masses of medullary tissue, named the *pyramids,* that are invested on their basal surfaces and sides by the cortex (Fig. 1-5). The cortex is 1 cm thick. The basal surfaces of the pyramids face outward, while their truncated and rounded tips point inward toward the hilus. Together the pyramids constitute the medulla. Each pyramid shows distinct zonation. The outer two-thirds of the thickness from the base toward the apex constitutes the outer medulla; the inner one-third, at the tip of the pyramid, is the inner medulla (Fig. 1-6). The outer medulla is subdivided further. Immediately adjacent to the cortex, demarcated by the arcuate arteries (which curve laterally over the bases of the pyramids), there is a thin zone, the outer stripe of the outer medulla. The more voluminous part of the outer medulla is the inner stripe. The relative volumes of the cortex, outer medulla, and inner medulla of the human kidney have been computed to be 70, 27, and 3 percent, respectively [131]. There is much variation in the relative thicknesses of layers of the kidney in different species. For example, in the rat, the outer stripe makes up as much as one-third of the total thickness of the outer medulla, and the inner medulla is relatively elongated. In contrast,

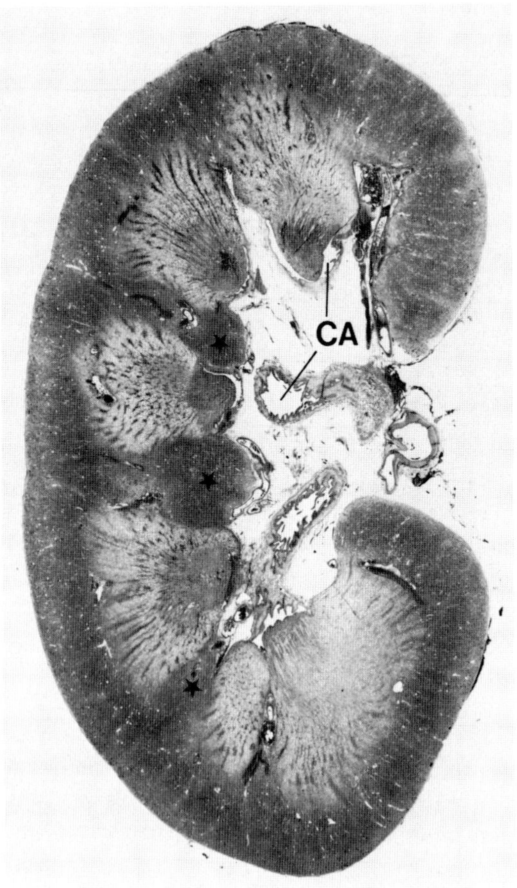

FIG. 1-5. *Longitudinal section through the human kidney showing the distribution of the cortical and medullary tissue. The medullary pyramids are surrounded by cortical tissue that reaches down to the renal sinus; these parts of cortical tissue (*) are called septa or columns of Bertin. In the lower polar region, a compound papilla is seen. CA, calyx. Paraffin section. (From Kriz [170].)*

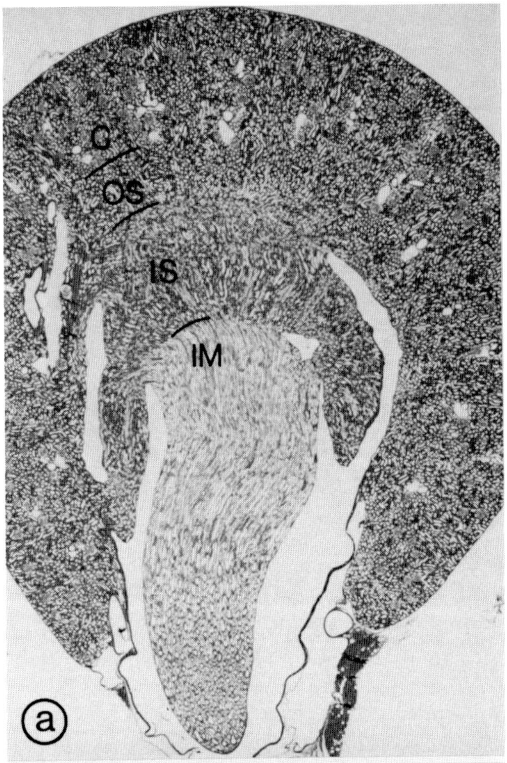

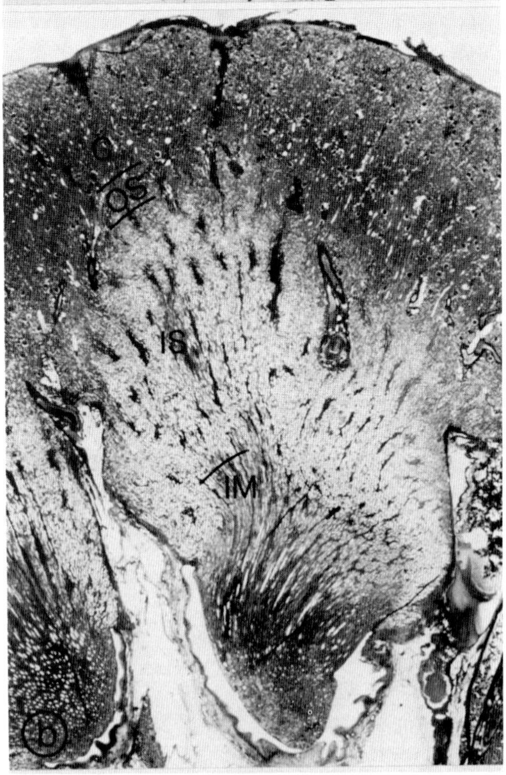

FIG. 1-6. *Longitudinal sections (longitudinal with respect to the papilla) through a unipapillary kidney (rat; A) and a single papilla of a multipapillary kidney (human; B). Note the different proportions of the individual zones. The outer stripe in the human kidney is very narrow; the inner stripe is thick. C, cortex; OS, outer stripe; IS, inner stripe; IM, inner medulla. Paraffin sections; (A) ×9; (B) ×3.*

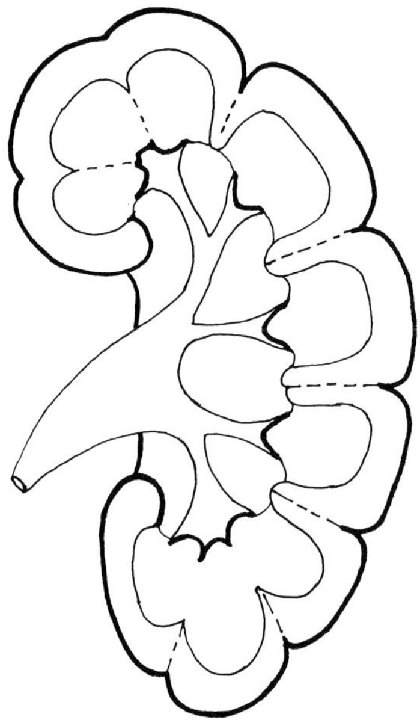

FIG. 1-7. *Diagram of arrangement of cortex and medulla in the human kidney. In the midzone, the double-layer interpyramidal cortical intrusions (septa of Bertin) reach down to the renal sinus. In the polar regions, they are smaller, owing to pyramidal fusion. Pyramidal fusion leads to the formation of compound papillae. (Reproduced with permission from Hodson, C. J. The Renal Parenchyma and Its Blood Supply. In R. D. Moseley, Jr., et al. (Eds.),* Current Problems in Diagnostic Radiology. *Copyright 1978 by Year Book Medical Publishers, Inc., Chicago.)*

in the human kidney, the outer stripe is attenuated, and the inner medulla is relatively shorter in proportion to the outer medulla [168]. The pointed tips of the inner medullary portions of the pyramids are the papillae. They project into cup-shaped calyces, which are extensions of the renal pelvis, and which drain into the pelvis in the form of tributary channels (Figs. 1-1, 1-3, 1-5, and 1-7). The tip of the papilla is called the *area cribrosa,* owing to the cribriform appearance given by the openings of the collecting ducts of Bellini, the terminal portions of the uriniferous tubules (see Anatomic Segments of the Nephron). There are an average of 44 openings in each papillary tip, with a range of 20 to 72 [227].

The cortex is about 1 cm thick, and it invests the pyramid on all sides, except the papillae, and extends downward between the pyramids in the form of the septa (or columns) of Bertin. The septa of Bertin extend inward all the way to the renal sinus, into which they protrude as ridges (Figs. 1-1, 1-5, and 1-7). The interlobar arteries are arranged along these ridges, and their branches, the arcuate arteries, penetrate the renal parenchyma in this area (Fig. 1-8). The septa of Bertin actually represent the fused cortices of adjoining pyramids and possess two distinct vascular domains supplied by arcuate arteries from the separate pyramids (see Fig. 1-8).

The human kidney is of multipapillary type, in which the cortex is continuous and undivided, while the medulla is discontinuous and consists of multiple, discrete, and divided pyramids [298] (Figs. 1-1, 1-5, 1-7, and 1-9). Each lobe in a multipapillary kidney may be regarded as the counterpart of an entire unipapillary kidney, the type that occurs in rats or rabbits (see Figs. 1-5, 1-6, and 1-9). The entire kidney may then be visualized as a series of unipapillary kidneys that have fused laterally [118,119]; the fused cortices in between each unipapillary kidney form the septa of Bertin (see Fig. 1-9). In certain animals, such as bears and whales, the kidneys consist of multiple unipapillary kidneys (or renculi) which, however, have not fused with each other and strictly retain their structural and functional autonomy [298]. During fetal life, the human kidney is extensively lobated, the lobes being separated by deep grooves, and endowed with separate calyces. The process of lobation is maximally manifest at 28 weeks of fetal life [98,197]. The lobes (~14 in number) are arranged in anterior and posterior sets, with 4 to 6 lobes each in the upper, middle, and lower portions of the kidney [197]. Each lobe, the counterpart of one pyramid, is associated with one calyx, into which the papilla projects. In subsequent phases of fetal development, the lobes of the kidney fuse with one another in a nonuniform manner. This results in a gradual reduction of the extent and depth of the furrows in between lobes on the surface and fusion of two or more papillae. As some of the papillae coalesce, the calyces are remodeled and decrease in number. Consequently, some calyces contain a single papilla, while others

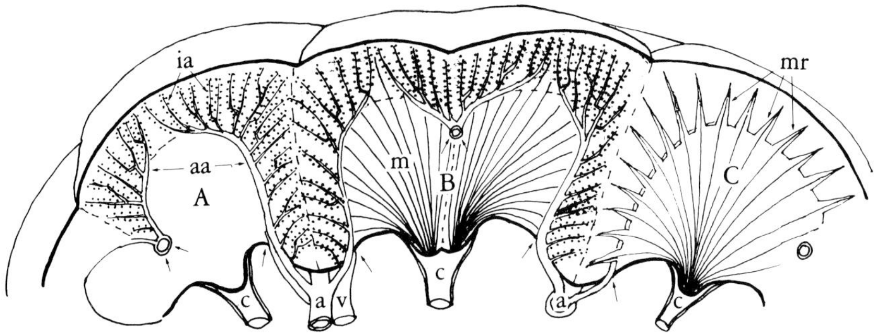

FIG. 1-8. *Diagram of three midzone lobes: (A) arcuate (aa) and interlobular (ia) arterial supply; (B) cortex and medulla drawn in, a double lobe with fused double papillae; and (C) lobe showing medullary rays (mr) with the courses of their central ducts leading to the papilla. (Small double arrows indicate subsidiary septal arteries. Single arrows indicate the points where arcuate vessels enter kidney tissue proper in the corticomedullary interphase. a, interlobar arteries; v, interlobar vein; c, calyces.) The double blood supply to the septum of Bertin between the pyramids of lobes A and B is clearly shown. (Reproduced with permission from Hodson, C. J. The Renal Parenchyma and Its Blood Supply. In R. D. Moseley, Jr. et al. (Eds.),* Current Problems in Diagnostic Radiology. *Copyright 1978 by Year Book Medical Publishers, Inc., Chicago.)*

harbor fused compound papillae. It seems that the process of lobar fusion may continue even after birth into adult life [306]. Thus, in mature, fully developed kidneys, calyces are fewer than papillae. In this fashion, one calyx may drain two and as many as four fused but previously separate lobes (see Figs. 1-1, 1-5, 1-7, and 1-9). In such fused lobes, the septa of Bertin do not extend all the way down toward the renal sinus, as is the case with separate, nonfused lobes, because they are obstructed by the fused papillae. Compound papillae occur predominantly in the poles of the kidney and are relatively uncommon in the middle region [73,306]. The description of the development of the human kidney starting with 14 individual anlagen (corresponding to 14 unipapillary kidneys) [197] is in debate. According to extensive studies by Inke [128], the human kidney develops from only four "protolobi" that later split in a variable fashion. Based on this hypothesis, the occurrence of kidneys with more than 14 papillae is understandable.

Although anatomic descriptions of compound papillae were provided early by Bertin [35], their significance in renal pathology has been recognized only recently [117,248,249,250,251]. Owing to the fusion of multiple papillae, the papillary tip, or the area cribrosa, is flattened or even concave. As mentioned earlier, the large terminal collecting ducts of Bellini open into the calyces in the area cribrosa; in compound papillae, the architectural feature of wide and gaping orifices of the ducts of Bellini apparently leaves them permanently open and unable to be compressed in the presence of vesicoureteral reflux (see Chap. 21). This can lead to backflow of urine by means of the gaping collecting duct openings into the renal tubular system, a phenomenon referred to as *calicotubular* or *intrarenal reflux.* In simple papillae, the ducts of Bellini open out in slit-like fashion on a sharply convex tip, and this configuration apparently favors closure of the ducts when pelvic pressure rises—a protective mechanism that prevents intrarenal reflux.

Kidneys in the newborn invariably show smooth lobes on their surfaces separated by sharp furrows

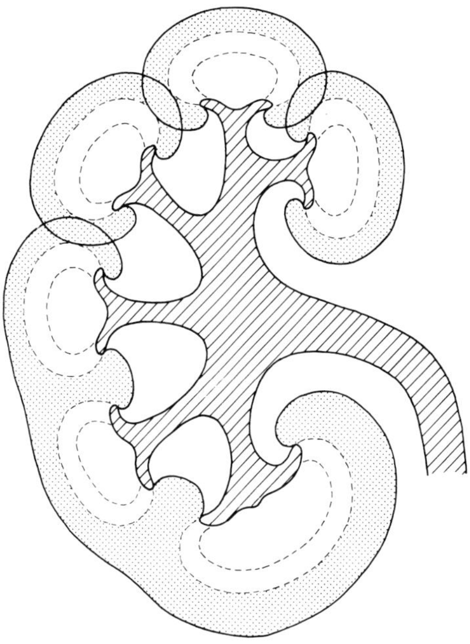

Fig. 1-9. *Diagram of the arrangement of cortex and medulla in the human kidney and of the manner of its possible development. Unipapillary kidney anlagen fuse to a multipapillary kidney (upper part of the drawing). The interpyramidal cortical intrusions (septa of Bertin) reach down to the renal sinus. In addition to the fusion of cortical tissue, pyramidal fusion occurs and is generally found in the polar regions (compound papilla, shown in the lower part).*

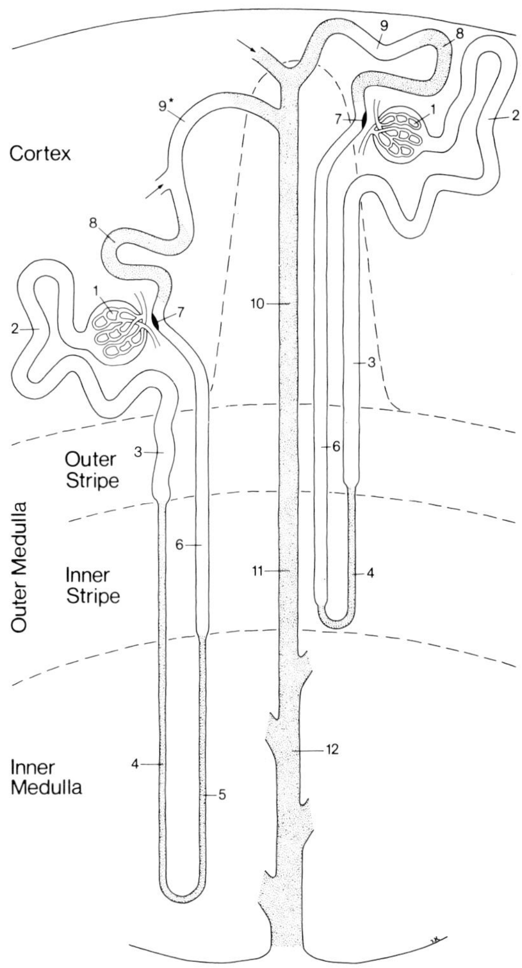

Fig. 1-10. *Scheme of the nephron. This scheme depicts a short-looped and a long-looped nephron together with the collecting system (not drawn to scale). Within the cortex, a medullary ray is delineated by a dashed line. 1, Renal corpuscle, including Bowman's capsule and the glomerulus (glomerular tuft); 2, proximal convoluted tubule; 3, proximal straight tubule; 4, descending thin limb; 5, ascending thin limb; 6, distal straight tubule (thick ascending limb); 7, macula densa, located within the final portion of the thick ascending limb; 8, distal convoluted tubule; 9, connecting tubule; 9*, connecting tubule of the juxtamedullary nephron that forms an arcade; 10, cortical collecting duct; 11, outer medullary collecting duct; 12, inner medullary collecting duct. (From Kriz et al. [173].)*

or grooves; this lobation persists through adult life in some people. In such cases, the phrase *persistence of fetal lobation* is employed.

Nephron Units

Before proceeding further with more detailed considerations of the architectural organization of the parenchyma, it is prudent to review the basic units of the kidney. Each human kidney consists of approximately 10^6 elongated structural and functional units, called *nephrons*. Each nephron consists of a glomerulus, or renal corpuscle, and the uriniferous tubule (Figs. 1-10 and 1-11). In rats and rabbits, nephrons are fewer in number

(~30,000 in each rat kidney). The glomerulus consists of a highly vascular glomerular tuft contained within a globoid epithelial sac, or Bowman's capsule. The glomerular tuft forms plasma ultrafiltrate. The space bounded by Bowman's capsule receives the ultrafiltrate and transmits it to the uriniferous tubule, where it is processed. The modified fluid flows into the pelvicalyceal system as urine. The uriniferous tubule is a long, cylindrical epithelial tube made up of many anatomically and cytologically distinct segments, each designed to perform specific and highly differentiated functions to modify the urine. The tubules have segments, some of which are disposed in randomly convoluted configurations (convoluted tubules) and others of which are arranged in straight and parallel loops (straight tubules; loops of Henle) (see Figs. 1-10 and 1-11). In a strict sense, the nephron does not include the system of collecting ducts, which form the terminal portion of the uriniferous tubule. This is so (1) because of the fact that many nephrons drain into a single collecting duct in the cortex and (2) because the nephron is derived from the metanephric blastema and the collecting ducts are formed from the ureteric bud. In mature kidneys, there is a transitional connecting segment or connecting tubule between the two. The origin of the connecting tubule is uncertain, but electron microscopic observations relate it to the ureteric bud [139]. On the other hand, nephron microdissection suggests derivation from the metanephric blastema [227,244]. Notwith-

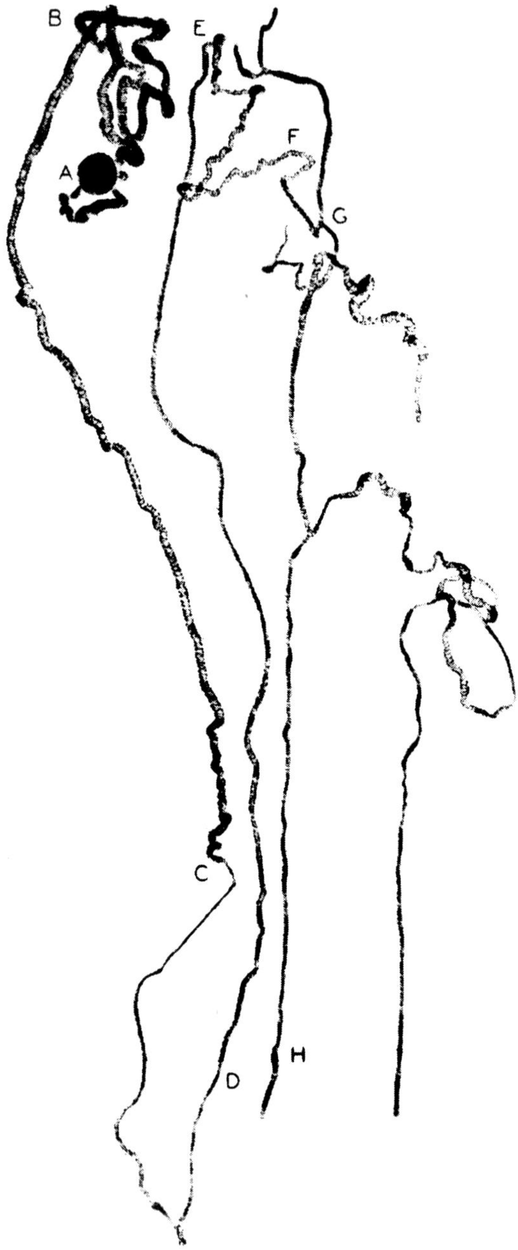

FIG. 1-11. *Isolated nephron of the human kidney. (A) Renal corpuscle. (B) Proximal tubule. (C) Transition of the proximal tubule to the thin descending limb. (D) Transition of the thin to the thick ascending limb (straight part of the distal tubule). (E) Transition to the convoluted part of distal tubule. (F) Transition to the connecting tubule. (G) Transition to the cortical collecting duct; below this point, three additional nephrons drain into the collecting duct. (H) Medullary collecting duct. The attachment of the thick ascending limb to the vascular pole of the parent glomerulus is detached as a result of the isolation procedure.* (*From Oliver, J.* Nephrons and Kidneys: A Quantitative Study of Development and Evolutionary Mammalian Renal Architectonics. *New York: Hoeber, 1968.*)

standing these considerations, the term *nephron* is commonly used to include the connecting segments and collecting ducts.

TYPES OF NEPHRONS

Nephrons may be characterized by the level of cortex at which they originate, that is, the cortical level where the parent glomeruli are situated [131,175] (see Fig. 1-10). Thus glomeruli may be superficial when they are located within a few millimeters deep to the cortical surface, juxtamedullary when they are situated immediately above the corticomedullary junction, or midcortical when they are intermediate in position. Glomeruli are usually absent in the outermost regions of the cortex (i.e., immediately below the capsule), except in particular species, such as the mutant Munich-Wistar rat.

Nephrons also may be characterized as short looped or long looped [131,175] (see Fig. 1-10). In the former, the parallel, looped portion of the tubule, or the loop of Henle, bends back in the outer medulla. Long-looped nephrons, as the name implies, are generally longer and bend back in the inner medulla. In the human kidney, some very superficial nephrons bend back to form short loops within the cortex itself. Superficial and most midcortical nephrons are of the short-looped type and bend back at various levels within the inner stripe of the outer medulla. Nephrons arising from some midcortical glomeruli and all juxtamedullary glomeruli are of the long-looped type; their Henle's loops penetrate the entire thickness of the outer medulla and enter the inner medulla, where they turn back at various levels. There are six to seven times as many nephrons with short loops as nephrons with long loops in the human kidney [237]. The relative occurrence of short and long loops among superficial, midcortical, and juxtamedullary nephrons varies considerably among species; in some species, such as the cat and the dog, all nephrons are long looped [131]. Urine-concentrating ability correlates better with extent and complexity of development of the medulla than with the number of nephrons with long loops. Some species have only short loops, do not have an inner medulla, and concentrate urine poorly [281,282].

ANATOMIC SEGMENTS OF THE NEPHRON

These are listed in Table 1-1. Correctly defined, a renal corpuscle consists of the glomerulus (glomerular tuft) and Bowman's capsule. The latter is lined by a flat epithelial monolayer; away from the vascular pole, the flat epithelium suddenly gives rise to a thick epithelium, indicating transition to the tubular portion of the nephron. There are several anatomically distinct segments and subtypes in the tubule [131,139,162,173,175]. In sequence, the segments are the proximal tubule, the intermediate tubule (descending and ascending thin limbs of Henle's loops), the distal tubule, the connecting tubule, and the collecting ducts (see Figs. 1-10 and 1-11).

The proximal tubule consists of two anatomic

TABLE 1-1. *Subdivisions of the nephron and collecting duct system*

- I. Nephron
  - A. Renal corpuscle
    1. Glomerulus (the most frequently used term to refer to the entire renal corpuscle)
    2. Bowman's capsule
  - B. Tubule
    1. Proximal tubule
       - a. Convoluted part
       - b. Straight part (pars recta) or descending thick limb of Henle's loop
    2. Intermediate tubule
       - a. Descending part or thin descending limb of Henle's loop
       - b. Ascending part or thin ascending limb of Henle's loop
    3. Distal tubule
       - a. Straight part or thick ascending limb of Henle's loop, subdivided into a medullary and a cortical part; the latter contains in its terminal portion the macula densa
       - b. Convoluted part
- II. Collecting duct system
  - A. Connecting tubule (including the arcades in most species)
  - B. Collecting duct
    1. Cortical collecting duct
    2. Outer medullary collecting duct subdivided into an outer- and inner-stripe portion
    3. Inner medullary collecting duct subdivided into a basal, middle, and papillary portion

segments, the proximal convoluted tubule (or pars convoluta), which follows a randomly tortuous course around the glomerulus of its origin, and the proximal straight tubule (or pars recta), which is relatively straighter, but twisted in a gentle, irregular spiral along its longitudinal axis. The proximal convoluted tubules are situated exclusively in the cortex. In nephrons derived from superficial and midcortical glomeruli, the initial portions of the proximal straight tubules are situated along elongated bundles of various nephron segments arranged in parallel and are oriented perpendicular to the cortical surface. These bundles are visible on the cut surfaces of the cortex as faint striae, known as the *medullary rays* (Fig. 1-12). The initial portions of the proximal straight tubules derived from juxtamedullary glomeruli join the outer aspects of the medullary rays near the corticomedullary junctions or enter directly the outer stripe of the outer medulla. Both types of straight tubules (i.e., from superficial and deep nephrons) course in parallel disposition through the entire thickness of the outer stripe of the outer medulla. At the junction of the outer stripe and inner stripe, they undergo sharp transition to relatively flat epithelium of the descending thin limb of Henle.

Descending thin limbs of long-looped nephrons penetrate the inner medulla, where they turn back as ascending thin limbs of Henle. More than half turn back in the upper half; as a consequence, the inner medulla becomes narrower and more tapered toward the tip. The ascending thin limbs run parallel to collecting ducts and descending limbs and undergo sudden change to a thick epithelium at the junction of the outer and inner medulla. This nephron segment, known as the *thick ascending limb of the Henle's loop* or the *pars recta (straight part) of the distal tubule,* courses through the entire thickness of the outer medulla as the medullary thick ascending limb and along variable distances through the medullary rays of the cortex and the cortical labyrinth (see below) as the cortical thick ascending limb. This segment makes contact with the vascular pole of the same glomerulus from which the nephron originated and, a little beyond this point of contact, undergoes transition to the distal convoluted tubule (see Fig. 1-10). In nephrons with short loops, the descending thin limbs

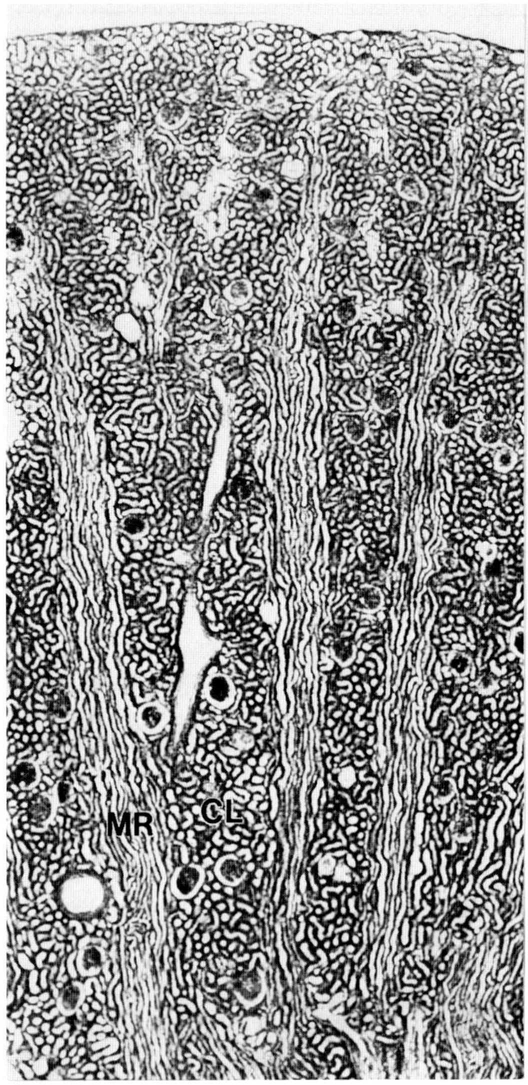

FIG. 1-12. *Longitudinal section through the cortex of a human kidney demonstrating the arrangement of the cortical labyrinth (CL) and the medullary rays (MR). The cortical labyrinth contains the interlobular vessels and the glomeruli together with the convoluted tubules; the medullary rays contain the straight tubular portions. Paraffin section; ×75 approx.*

turn back at various levels of the outer medulla directly as thick ascending limbs without an intervening ascending thin limb, unlike the situation in long-looped nephrons. The proximal straight tubule, the descending thin limb, the ascending thin limb (if long looped), and the thick ascending limbs together constitute the loop of Henle.

The distal convoluted tubule follows a tortuous course in the cortical labyrinth (see below) and undergoes a gradual transition to the connecting tubule. It is difficult to delineate the connecting tubule anatomically or cytologically except in some species (e.g., rabbit). As alluded to before, the connecting tubule may be a derivative of either the ureteric bud or the metanephric blastema, but in any case, it represents a structural and functional transitional segment connecting the tubular derivations of the two progenitors. Connecting tubules of nephrons draining juxtamedullary and midcortical glomeruli may join together as tributaries, ascend in the cortical labyrinth along with the interlobular vessels (known as *arcades*), and then continue on as the initial collecting tubules of the cortical collecting ducts. However, they also may continue individually as initial collecting tubules. In man, the majority of connecting tubules drain individually [227]. These tubules and the remaining tubular portions of the parenchyma make up the collecting duct system (see Figs. 1-10 and 1-11).

Embryologically derived from the ureteric bud, the collecting ducts include the cortical collecting duct, the outer medullary collecting duct, and the inner medullary collecting duct. In the human kidney, initial collecting tubules draining an average of 11 nephrons join in tributary fashion to form the cortical collecting duct. Soon after its origin, this duct takes a straight course inward through the medullary ray and enters the medulla. The outer medullary collecting duct may be subdivided into outer and inner stripe portions, and the inner medullary collecting duct may be subdivided into three equal portions between the outer, middle, and innermost parts of the inner medulla. In the inner medulla, the collecting ducts join together in succession at different levels to form ducts of larger caliber until the largest, the terminal papillary collecting ducts of Bellini, are formed. As discussed earlier, the ducts of Bellini open out into the renal calyces at the papillary tips in the area cribrosa. In addition to the anatomic types of nephron segments outlined here, cytologically distinct segments can be recognized (see the section entitled Tubules).

Structural Organization of Nephron Segments Within Defined Zones of the Kidney

Various nephron segments and vascular structures are arranged in distinctive patterns in different anatomic zones of the kidney (Figs. 1-13 through 1-18). This structural organization has important implications in understanding the mechanisms of renal function [162,167,168,175].

THE CORTEX

The glomeruli are located exclusively in the renal cortex. Two distinct architectural zones can be distinguished in the cortex: the cortical labyrinth, which is greater in volume, and the medullary rays (see Fig. 1-12). The glomeruli, proximal and distal convoluted tubules, connecting tubules, and initial collecting tubules are located within the cortical labyrinth (see Fig. 1-15). Also in these regions are the interlobular (cortical radial) blood vessels, the glomerular arterioles, and an anastomosing network of peritubular capillaries. Proximal convoluted tubules form the larger part of the nephron mass in these areas and bear no particular relationship to the other structures. Connecting tubules are usually in close association with the interlobular vessels. The medullary rays are well-knit bundles of relatively straight nephron segments arranged in parallel. They are oriented perpendicular to the surface of the kidney and occur in a regular distribution in between the larger tracts of cortical labyrinth. The medullary rays carry the straight segments of proximal and distal tubules, the cortical collecting ducts, and associated capillaries. Because the straight tubules of the more superficial nephrons enter or leave the medullary rays nearer the surface, they are located in a more central location within the medullary rays than those of the deeper nephrons. Although they are part of the cortex, the medullary rays are so named because they are anatomically composed like the outer stripe of the outer medulla. The renal cortex also has been divided into anatomic zones called the *lobules*. As more commonly understood, the lobules have cores of medullary rays located within areas of cortical labyrinth, their borders being demarcated by the interlobular vessels [227]. Another classification would place the interlobular artery at the core of the lobule, together with all surrounding nephron segments derived from or associated with that artery. The borders of the lobule in this classification are roughly formed by the collecting ducts in the medullary rays [131,328].

OUTER MEDULLA

The architectural organization of nephron segments in the medulla is related to the configuration of the microvasculature in this region [167,168,175,180,181]. In this context, an understanding of the arrangement of postglomerular blood vessels of the juxtamedullary glomeruli is necessary. As the section entitled The Microvasculature will illustrate, efferent glomerular arterioles of juxtamedullary glomeruli descend into the medulla and splay out into many branches. These descending vasa recta are arranged in close proximity, in parallel, and in countercurrent arrangement with their venous counterparts, the ascending vasa recta. Such arrangements result in the formation of spindle-shaped organoid structures called *vascular bundles* (see Figs. 1-16 and 1-17). From the corticomedullary junction where they begin to form, the girth of the vascular bundles increases progressively to reach a maximum within the inner stripe. The bundle size diminishes again,

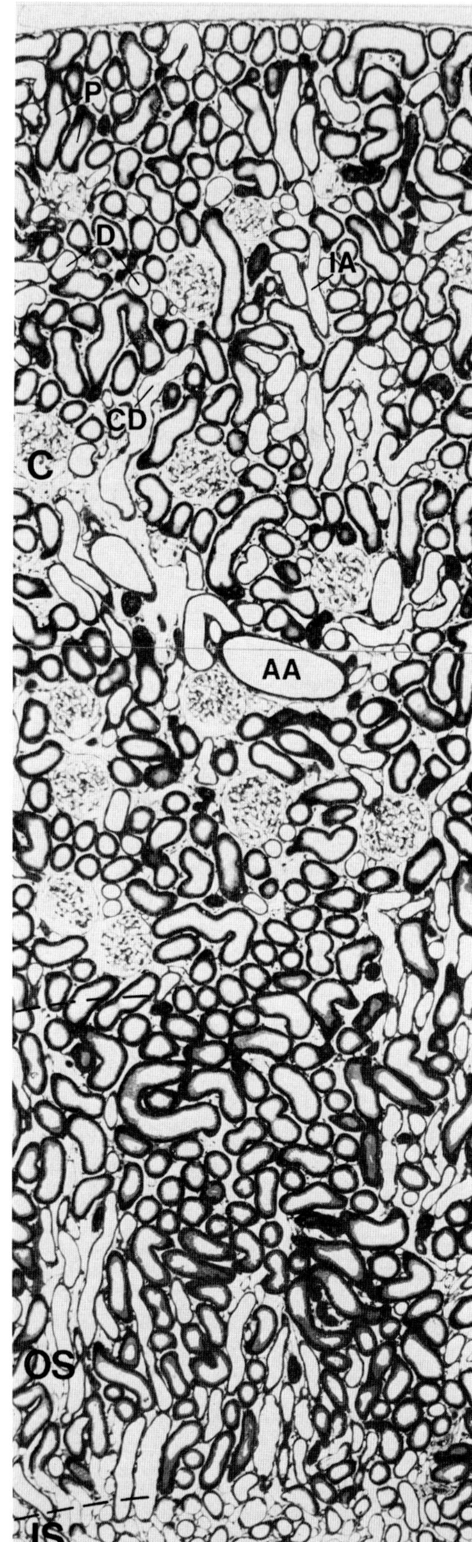

FIG. 1-13. *Longitudinal section through the rat kidney showing the cortex (C), the outer stripe (OS), and the beginning of the inner stripe (IS). Because of the plane of the section, only the cortical labyrinth is shown. P, proximal tubule; D, distal tubule; CD, collecting duct; AA, arcuate artery; IA, interlobular artery. 1-μm section of Epon-embedded tissue; ×72 approx.*

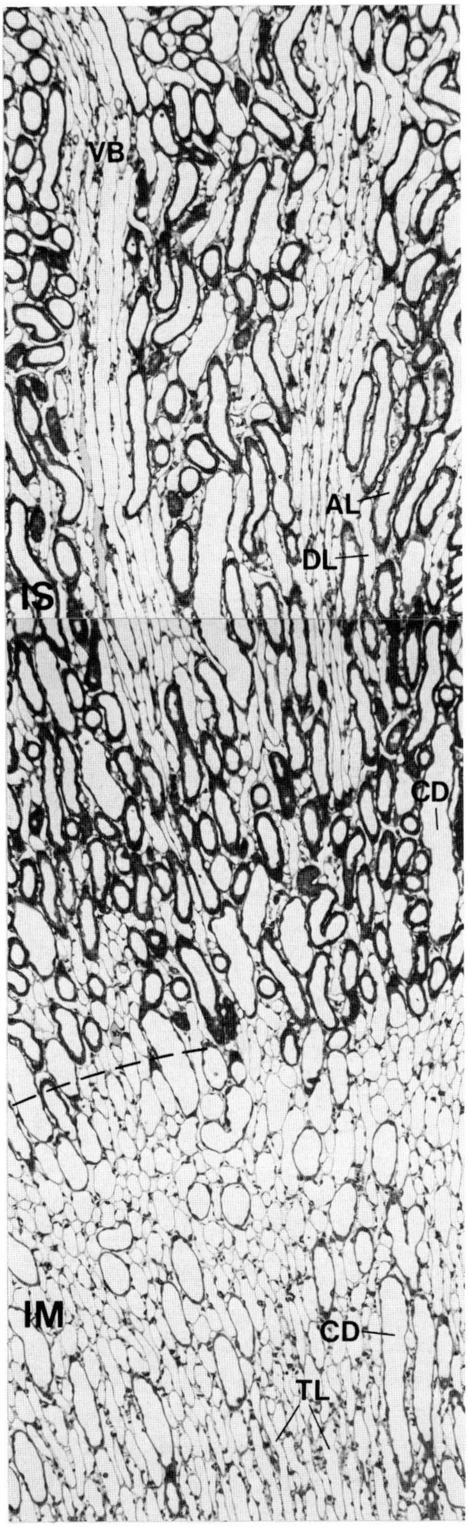

gradually in the lower part of the inner stripe, and more sharply in the inner medulla (see The Microvasculature and Figs. 1-22 and 1-28).

Nephron segments present in the outer stripe are the straight segments of the proximal tubules, straight segments of the distal tubules (ascending thick limbs) and collecting ducts (see Fig. 1-16). Tubules derived from juxtamedullary glomeruli are closely associated with the vascular bundles; those derived from the more superficial nephrons are more distantly located near the collecting ducts in the interbundle region. Here they are associated with ascending vasa recta coming up directly from the interbundle region of the inner stripe and carrying the venous blood from this region (see below). As mentioned earlier, straight segments of proximal tubules give rise to descending thin limbs at the outer stripe–inner stripe junction.

The following nephron segments are found in the inner stripe: descending thin limbs of short and long loops, ascending thick limbs of short and long loops, and the collecting ducts (see Fig. 1-17). As in the outer stripe, the histotopography of these segments is best considered in the context of the vascular bundles. In human kidneys and in other species such as rabbits, pigs, and monkeys, the vascular bundles are of the simple type and consist entirely of descending and ascending vasa recta. The descending thin limbs and ascending thick limbs of the long loops are situated close to and just outside the limits of the bundles. Descending thin limbs and ascending thick limbs of short-looped nephrons, as well as the collecting ducts, are situated in the interbundle region. As in the outer stripe, the collecting ducts are distant from the bundles. In species with high urine-concentrating ability, such as the rat, mouse, and

FIG. 1-14. *Longitudinal section through the rat kidney showing the inner stripe (IS) and the beginning of the inner medulla (IM). Within the inner stripe, the vascular bundles can clearly be separated from the interbundle regions. DL, descending thin limb; AL, ascending thick limb; CD, collecting duct; TL, thin limbs in the inner medulla. 1-μm section of Epon-embedded tissue; ×84 approx.*

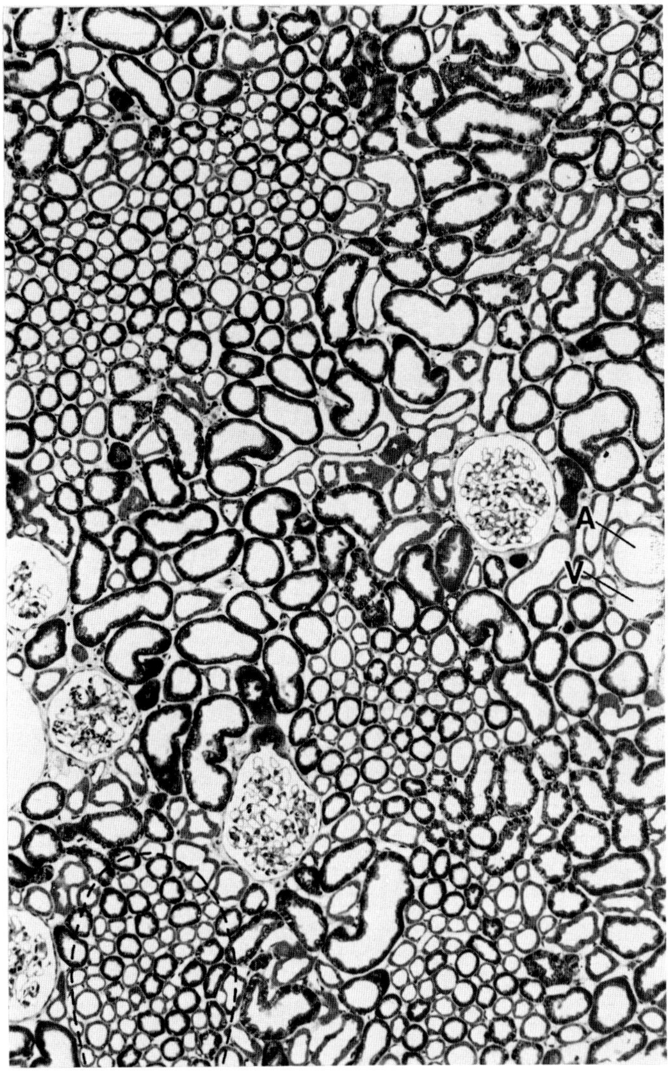

FIG. 1-15. *In a cross section of the cortex, the cortical labyrinth can clearly be delineated from the medullary rays (the cross section of one ray is marked by a dashed line). Within the labyrinth, the interlobular vessels (A, artery; V, vein), the glomeruli, and the convoluted tubular segments are found. The medullary rays contain the straight tubular segments. 1-μm section of Epon-embedded tissue; × 150 approx.*

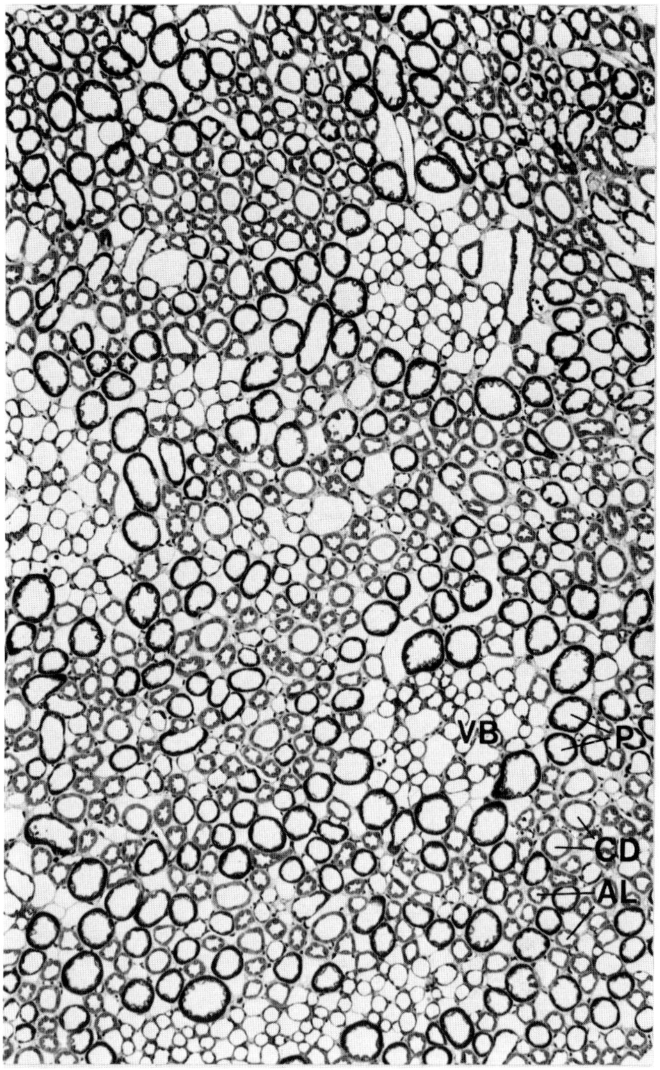

FIG. 1-16. *Cross section through the outer stripe in the outer medulla. The tubules are arranged around the vascular bundles (VB). In the vicinity of the bundles, the nearest segments are the straight proximal and distal tubules of the juxtamedullary nephrons. Outer to them are the straight proximal and distal tubules of midcortical and superficial nephrons; the collecting ducts are lying distant from the bundles. P, proximal tubule; AL, ascending limb (straight parts of distal tubule); CD, collecting duct. 1-μm section of Epon-embedded tissue;* × *150 approx.*

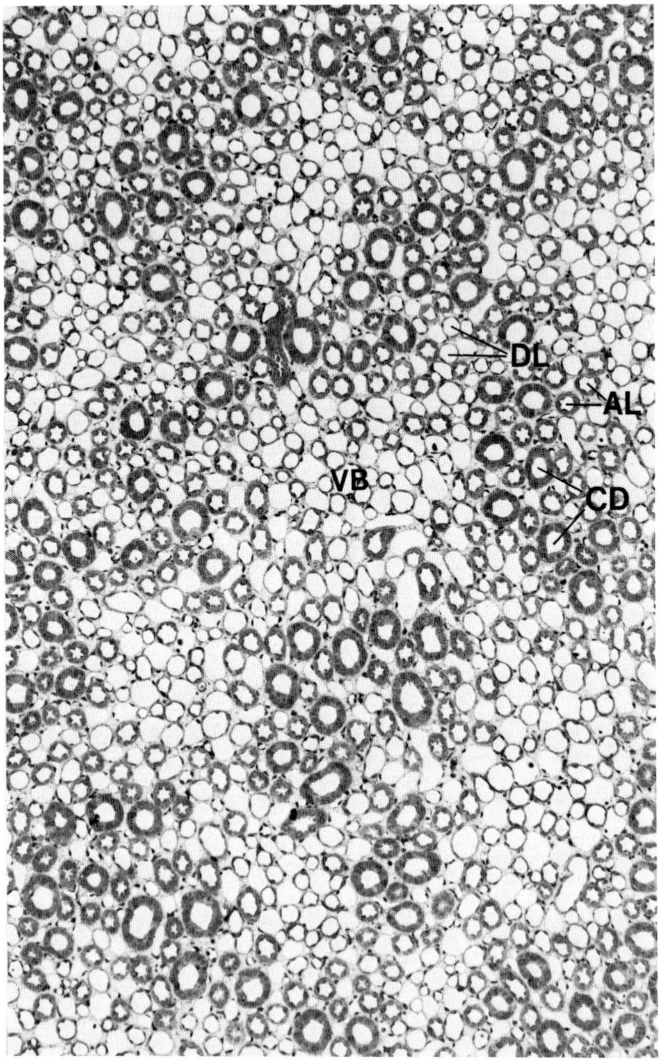

FIG. 1-17. *Cross section through the inner stripe of the outer medulla. The vascular bundles (VB) are well developed and surrounded by the limbs of short and long Henle's loops in an arrangement similar to that in the outer stripe. DL, descending thin limb; AL, ascending thick limb; CD, collecting duct. 1-μm section of Epon-embedded tissue; ×150 approx.*

desert rodents, the vascular bundles are of the so-called complex type. In this type, descending thin limbs of short-looped nephrons leave the inter-bundle region where they are formed, curve toward the vascular bundles, and course downward within the structure of the bundles intermingled predominantly with ascending vasa recta [175,181]. The thick limbs of both short and long loops and the thin limbs of long loops are present in the interbundle regions, with collecting ducts as de-

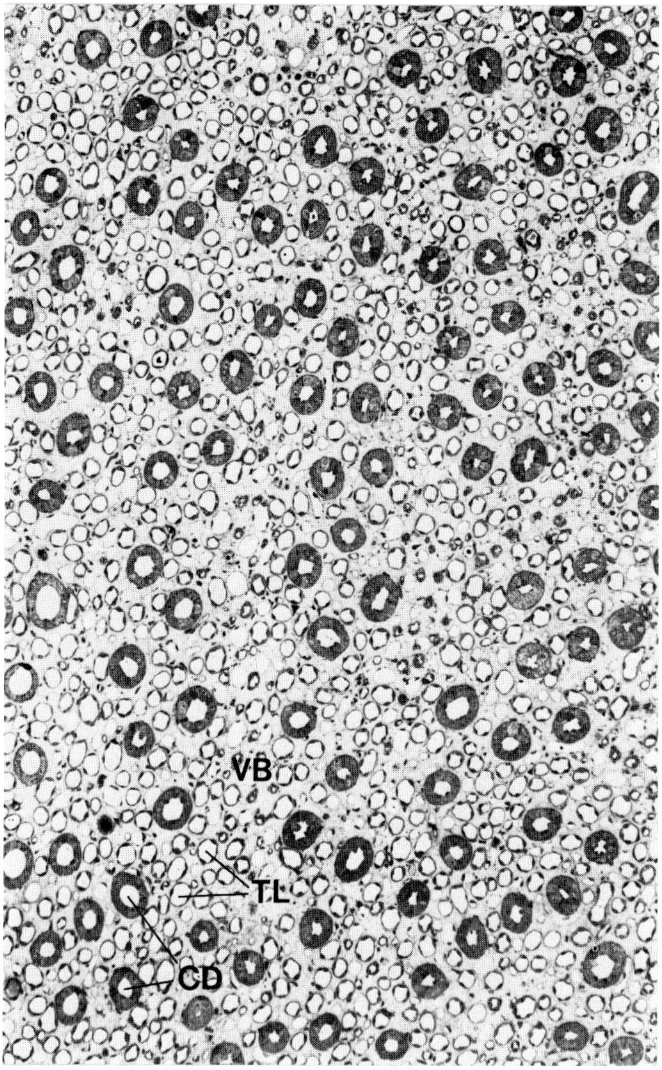

Fig. 1-18. *Cross section through the inner medulla. The vascular bundles (VB) are small and cannot clearly be separated from the surrounding thin limbs (TL). CD, collecting duct. 1-μm section of Epon-embedded tissue; × 120 approx.*

scribed previously. In the desert rodent *Psammomys obesus,* complex vascular bundles fuse with each other in the inner stripe to form giant vascular bundles.

These differences in the histotopography of vascular and tubular structures are generally correlated with the urine-concentrating ability of the species. However, notable individual exceptions occur, such as the presence of simple vascular bundles in some species with high urine-concentrating ability, such as the hamster. Notwithstanding these exceptions, it is clear that these unique vascular and tubular architectonics have mechanistic significance to the process of urine concentration. Discussion of these considerations is outside the scope of this chapter but is available elsewhere [195].

INNER MEDULLA

Nephron segments found in the inner medulla are the descending and ascending thin limbs of long loops and the collecting ducts (see Fig. 1-18). Notably, there are no thick ascending limbs. The length of the inner medulla, from its junction with the outer medulla to the papillary tip, is greater relative to kidney size in animals with higher urine-concentrating ability [281,298]. As alluded to previously, species without long-looped nephrons have poor urine-concentrating ability [282]. As a consequence of its tapering nature, tubular mass in the inner medulla is unevenly distributed. For example, in the rat, the first half of the inner medulla has approximately 80 percent of the total inner medullary volume and the papillary half has only approximately 20 percent. This is so because the thin limbs of Henle turn back at various levels of the inner medulla. As such, there is a decrease in the mass of both thin limbs and associated blood vessels. Moreover, there is progressive fusion of collecting ducts and a reduction in their total number toward the papillary tip.

A distinct architectural pattern is less apparent in the inner medulla than in the outer medulla (see Fig. 1-18). The vascular bundles are greatly attenuated as they leave the outer medulla and enter the inner medulla, because most descending vasa recta have already left the bundles in the inner stripe. In the inner medulla, there is a steady reduction in the numbers of descending and ascending vasa recta toward the papillary tip. Near the papillary tip, vasa recta are absent. In cross sections of the inner medulla, collecting ducts are generally away from the vascular bundles, and the thin segments occupy the space in between, along with a scant capillary plexus. The interstitial space, which contains lipid-laden interstitial cells, is prominent in the inner medulla and occupies a progressively greater fractional volume from the outer medullary boundary toward the papillary tip.

RENAL PELVIS AND CALYCES

The renal pelvis is a sac-like expansion of the upper end of the ureter. It occupies and is attached to the inside aspect of the renal sinus. Two or three large tributaries, the major calyces, extend from the pelvis toward the kidney. Each major calyx, in turn, is joined by smaller tributary channels, the minor calyces (Figs. 1-1, 1-7, 1-9, 1-19, and 1-

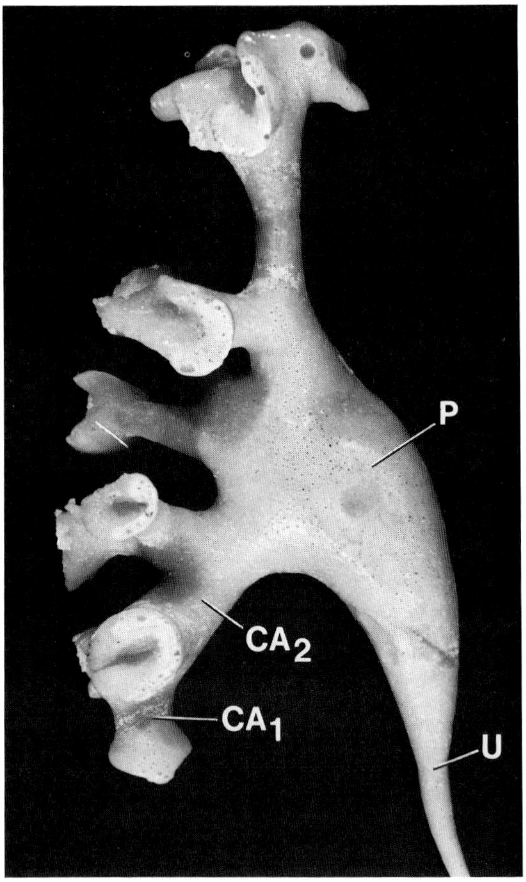

FIG. 1-19. *Corrosion cast of a human renal pelvis. Minor calyces (CA_1) fuse to major calyces, which finally empty into the renal pelvis (P). U, ureter.*

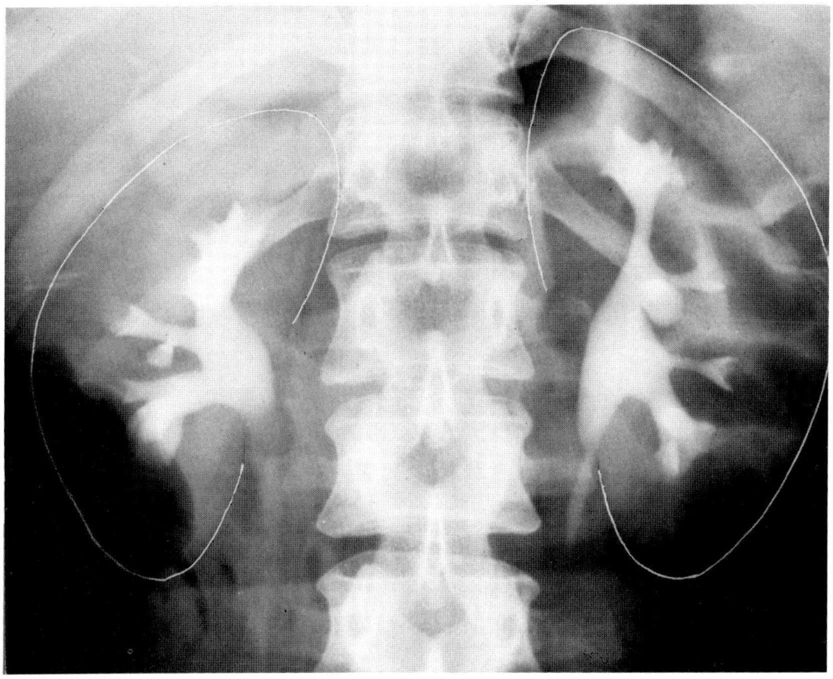

FIG. 1-20. *Intravenous pyelogram of healthy adult kidneys with renal outline marked in. The arrangement of the pelvis and calyces can be clearly seen; in particular, the way in which the papilla projects into the calyx and the delicate pattern of the fornices should be noted (Courtesy of Dr. C. J. Hodson.)*

20). In adult human kidneys, there are approximately nine minor calyces [306]. The parenchymal ends of the minor calyces are cup shaped, and the papillae protrude into them (see Figs. 1-1, 1-5, 1-6B, 1-7, 1-9, 1-19, and 1-20). As discussed previously, the number of papillae exceeds the number of calyces, and a single calyx may receive urine from more than one papilla or from compound papillae [73,306]. Compound papillae occur mainly in the polar regions of the kidneys and only uncommonly in the middle region [73] (see Figs. 1-1, 1-7, and 1-9). The protrusion of simple and compound papillae into the calyces results in distinctive radiographic images when radiopaque dye is present in the pelvicalyceal system during retrograde or excretory urography.

The walls of the calyces and the pelvis contain fibrous connective tissue and two layers of smooth muscle and are lined on their inner surfaces by transitional epithelium [79]. On all sides of the inner medulla, each minor calyx extends laterally toward the renal parenchyma, and at a point where the outer medulla is exposed to the urine, the cuboidal epithelium that lines the outer, urinary aspect of the medulla is reflected back onto the inner surface of the calyx. At this point it undergoes a change to transitional epithelium. Also in this region, the calyx sends leaf-like extensions into the parenchyma in the form of fornices and secondary pouches [183,240,280]. These extensions may be quite elaborate in some species, and it has been suggested that their function is to return concentrated solute from the urine to the medulla, thus conserving high concentrations of medullary solute. The pelvis and calyces exhibit rhythmic peristaltic movements, and these contractions are thought to aid the process of urinary concentration by agitating or temporarily retaining pelvic urine and thus returning urinary solute to the fornices. In addition, they are thought to affect fluid movements in inner medullary tubules and blood vessels [280]. However, a definitive relationship of pelvic-calyceal anatomy to the urine-concentrating process is not established [13]. Pelvic contractions travel in wave form to the ureter, and these contractions facilitate the onward passage of urine to the urinary bladder.

THE VASCULATURE

Arteries and Veins

We have seen how the interlobar arteries run within the renal sinus along ridges of cortical tissue between adjacent pyramids. They pierce the space in between the pyramids and the septa of Bertin (representing the fused cortices surrounding adjacent pyramids) and run toward the cortex lying adjacent to the calyceal walls. The interlobar arteries divide dichotomously into a spray of arcuate arteries at the junction of the cortex and medulla. This arrangement creates two sets of arcuate arteries between adjacent pyramids, each of the sets running between the septa of Bertin and the medullary tissue in the pyramids (see Fig. 1-8). Each one of the sets supplies a part of the septum proximate to it, consistent with the delineation of renal lobes according to distinct vascular domains supplied by the arcuate arteries on either side of one pyramid [119]. This pattern of vascular supply reinforces the concept that the septa of Bertin are derived by the process of lobar fusion, whereby the cortical cap of the pyramid in each lobe fuses with its neighbor during fetal development [118,119]. Each arcuate artery curves gently between the cortex and medulla as it ascends up the lateral surface of the pyramid and then bends over on its basal surface (Figs. 1-8 and 1-21). Because the arcuate arteries converge near the centers of the basal surfaces of the pyramids but do not anastomose with one another (being end arteries), the central parts of the renal lobes are farthest along the line of blood supply and therefore are most prone to suffer ischemic atrophy if small arteries are narrowed by disease [119]. The arcuate arteries give off branches, the interlobular (cortical radial) arteries, which are arranged obliquely in the septal part of the cortex and are radially disposed over the basal surface of the pyramids perpendicular to the surface of the kidney (Figs. 1-8 and 1-21 through 1-24).

It is important to note that there are no arteries that penetrate the renal medulla. The interlobular arteries branch dichotomously several times during their radial course toward the renal surface. The majority of interlobular arteries terminate within the cortex, and only a few reach the surface, where they anastomose with capsular branches of suprarenal, renal, and gonadal arteries. The interlobular arteries give off lateral branches at regular intervals—the afferent arterioles of the glomeruli. Depending on the level of the cortex at which they arise, afferent arterioles may continue in a radial direction toward the surface, be disposed at right angles to the parent artery, or curve back at acute angles toward juxtamedullary glomeruli [100].

The interlobular arteries are accompanied by interlobular (cortical radial) veins (see Figs. 1-21 and 1-22). A minority of these veins originate on the cortical surface as stellate veins, drain the most superficial parts of the cortex, and then run perpendicularly down the thickness of the cortex to join the arcuate veins (see Fig. 1-21). The remainder (which are the majority of interlobular veins) also take a similar course to join the arcuate veins (Figs. 1-21, 1-22, and 1-25) but originate within the cortex and drain the peritubular capillary plexus by means of thin-walled intermediary venules. Unlike the arcuate arteries, the arcuate veins anastomose freely across the basal surfaces of the pyramids in the form of arches. Also unlike the arcuate arteries, which do not send branches into the medulla, the arcuate veins accept venous tributaries from the medulla (see Figs. 1-21, 1-22, and 1-25). The arcuate veins leave the parenchyma along tracks corresponding to the arteries and join the interlobar veins. These, in turn, follow a course similar to the arteries, joining to-

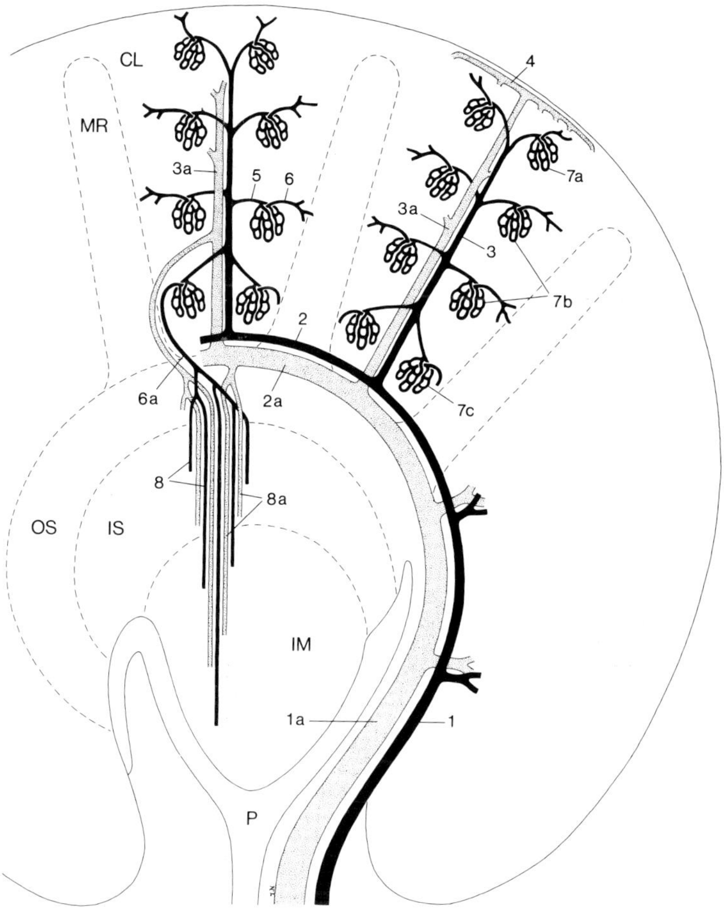

Fig. 1-21. *Scheme of renal vessels in a unipapillary kidney. This scheme depicts the course and distribution of the intrarenal blood vessels; peritubular capillaries are not shown (not drawn to scale). Within the cortex, the medullary rays of the cortex (MR) are delineated from the cortical labyrinth (CL) by a dashed line. OS, outer stripe; IS, inner stripe; IM, inner medulla; P, renal pelvis. 1/1a, interlobar artery and vein; 2/2a, arcuate artery and vein; 3/3a cortical radial (interlobular) artery and vein; 4, stellate vein; 5, afferent arteriole; 6, efferent arteriole; 6a, juxtamedullary efferent arteriole; 7a/7b/7c, superficial, midcortical, and juxtamedullary glomeruli; and 8/8a, descending vasa recta and ascending vasa recta in vascular bundle. (From Kriz et al. [173].)*

gether to form large venous trunks in front of the pelvis and then finally forming the renal vein.

The Microvasculature

Much of our knowledge of the microvasculature of the mammalian kidney has been obtained by the use of a variety of injection techniques. The injected materials include india ink, plastics such as methacrylates, silicone rubber, and radiopaque media. Tissue injected with india ink and silicone rubber can be studied either by microtomy and light microscopy or by clearing microslices in appropriate media to make them translucent. Plastic-injected specimens are usually studied by scanning electron microscopy following corrosion of

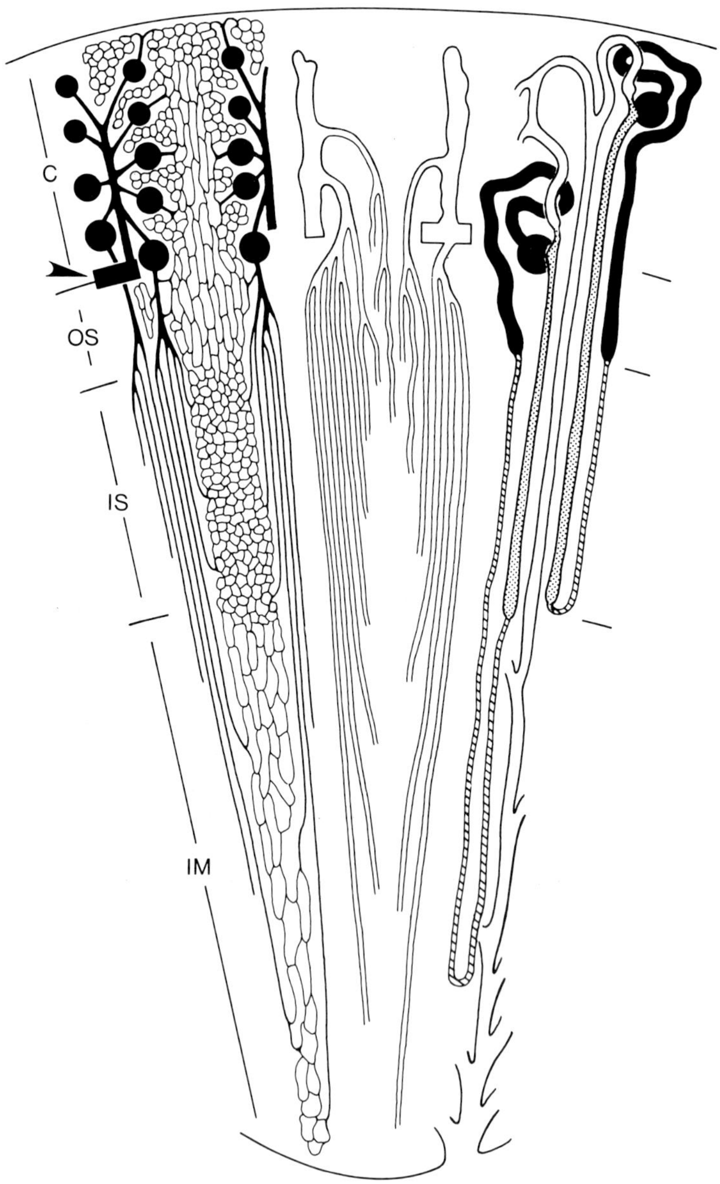

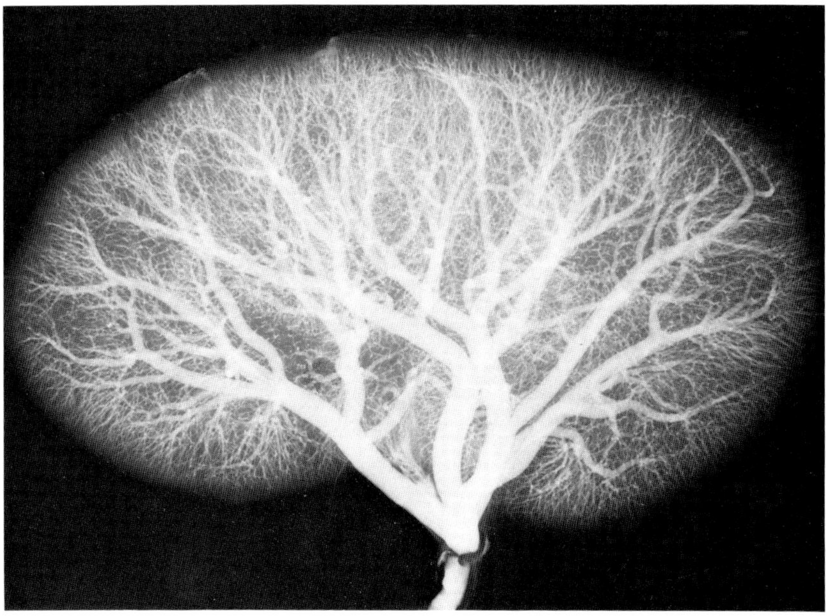

FIG. 1-23. *Angiogram of kidney prepared postmortem. The segmental and interlobar arteries give rise to the gently curving arcuate arteries, which in turn give rise to the interlobular arteries. The latter are arranged perpendicular to the surface of the kidney in radial fashion.*

FIG. 1-22. *Schematic diagram of microvasculature and nephrons (not drawn to scale). C, cortex; OS, outer stripe; IS, inner stripe; IM, inner medulla. (Left) Arterial vessels and capillaries. An arcuate artery (arrowhead) gives rise to an interlobular artery (cortical radial artery), from which afferent arterioles originate. Efferent arterioles from superficial and midcortical glomeruli split off into the cortical peritubular capillaries. Efferent arterioles of juxtamedullary glomeruli descend into the outer stripe and divide into the descending vasa recta, which supply the different capillary plexuses in the medulla. (Center) Venous vessels. Interlobular veins start in the superficial cortex. Stellate veins (characteristically found in human kidneys) that begin on the renal surface are not shown. The deep portions of interlobular veins and arcuate veins accept the ascending vasa recta, which drain the venous blood from the medulla. Ascending vasa recta and descending vasa recta together establish the vascular bundles. Note the dense pattern of ascending vasa recta traversing the outer stripe as wide tortuous channels. (Right) A short- and a long-looped nephron together with a collecting duct. Glomeruli and proximal tubules are drawn black; thin limbs, hatched; thick limbs, dotted; distal convoluted tubules, connecting tubules (including an arcade) and collecting ducts, white. This drawing allows correlation of the locations of tubules and vessels; the three panels should be imagined as being superimposed on each other.*

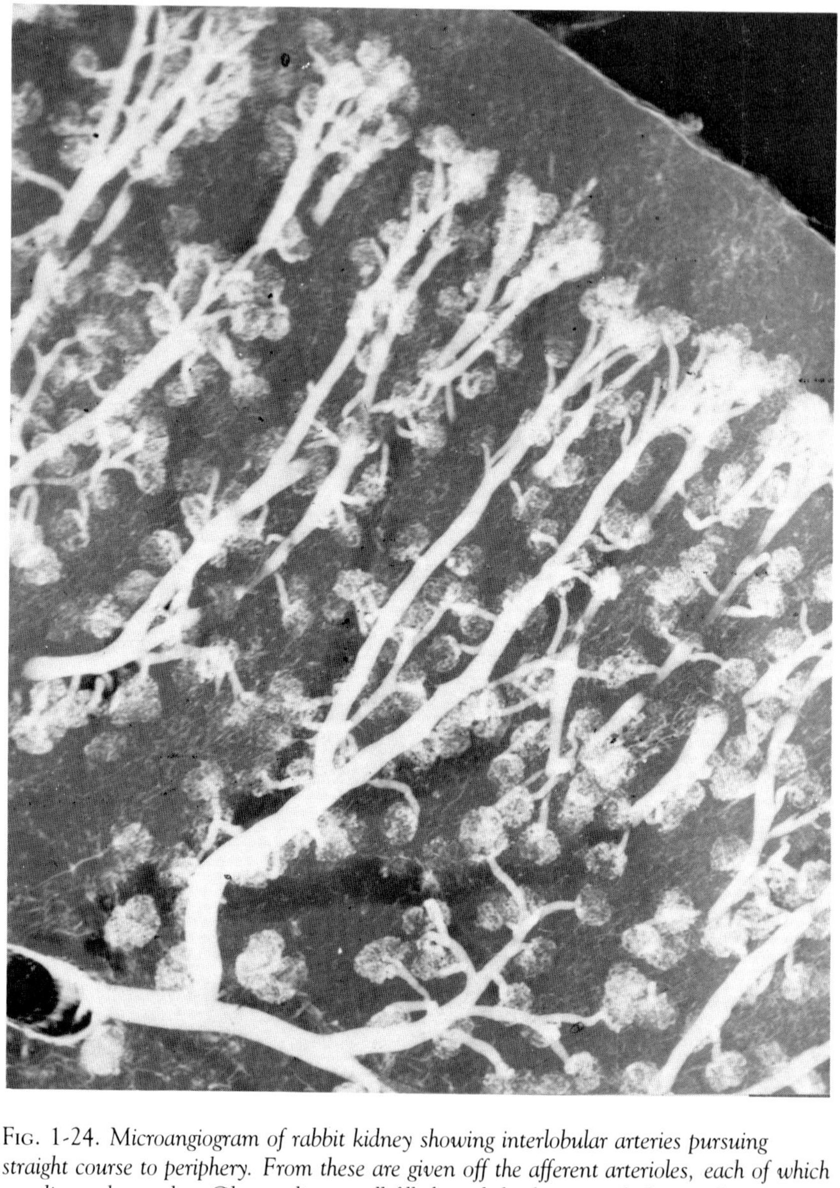

FIG. 1-24. *Microangiogram of rabbit kidney showing interlobular arteries pursuing straight course to periphery. From these are given off the afferent arterioles, each of which supplies a glomerulus. Glomeruli are well filled, and the fine peritubular capillary plexus can just be discerned.* ×30.

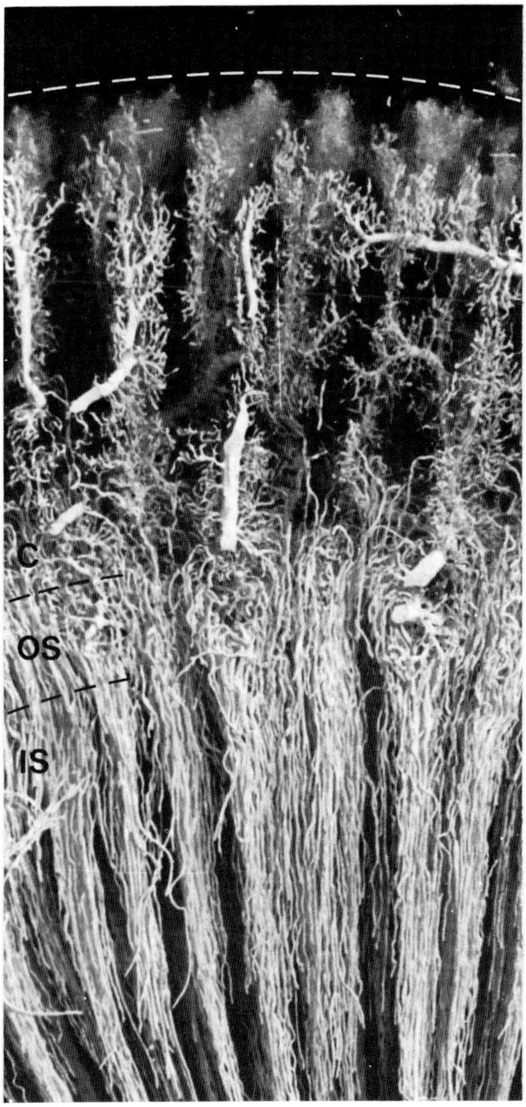

Fig. 1-25. *Venous vessels of rabbit kidney; venous injection with silicone rubber (Microfil). The interlobular veins of the cortex accept the blood from the cortical plexuses and descend to the corticomedullary border. The venous vessels of the medulla are the ascending vasa recta, which ascend within and in between the vascular bundles toward the corticomedullary border, where they empty into arcuate veins or the basal portions of interlobular veins. C, cortex; OS, outer stripe; IS, inner stripe. ×20 approx.*

the tissue. Kidneys injected with barium sulfate have been sliced and exposed to low-voltage x-ray radiography for long periods using high-resolution emulsions, and radiographs subjected to low-magnification microscopy. The results show a common vascular pattern in a number of species and no significant departures from this pattern in human kidneys [27–30,65,115,139,177,196,213,263]. This subject has been reviewed in considerable detail elsewhere [28,29,101,139,165,169].

Most afferent glomerular arterioles arise from the interlobular arteries and supply glomeruli in the midcortical and superficial cortical regions as well as some juxtamedullary glomeruli. Afferent arterioles also arise from the arcuate and even interlobar vessels. These vessels perfuse some juxtamedullary glomeruli situated in the adjacent parenchyma, including those in the septa of Bertin. Afferent arterioles from the interlobar arteries sometimes enter ectopic glomeruli near the pelvic wall. Except for branches that go toward the pelvic mucosa, all blood in the interlobar and arcuate arteries is directed into the glomerular capillary bed (see Figs. 1-21, 1-22, and 1-24). Aglomerular vessels are found sometimes, providing blood directly to the medullary circulation. Since these vessels are associated with sclerotic glomeruli, it is thought that these "shunts" occur as a result of disease rather than as true anatomic entities. The glomerular vasculature will be described in a later section. All glomeruli are drained by efferent arterioles (Figs. 1-21, 1-22, and 1-26).

EFFERENT VESSELS IN THE CORTEX

Cortical efferent arterioles enter the peritubular capillary plexus at short distances after they are formed or after running variable distances to the surface of the kidney or into the medullary rays. The capillary plexuses around convoluted tubules in the cortical labyrinth and straight tubules in the medullary rays receive branches of the efferent arterioles directly in parallel fashion. In the cortical labyrinth, the anastomosing capillaries assume a compact, round, meshed configuration, whereas in the medullary rays, the plexus is loose, with the anastomosing network oriented longitudinally along the axes of the straight tubules (Figs. 1-22 and 1-27). Blood from the medullary rays passes through the capillary plexus in the cortical labyrinth before emptying into the interlobular veins.

EFFERENT VESSELS IN THE MEDULLA

The medulla receives blood exclusively from the efferent arterioles of the juxtamedullary glomeruli. These arterioles take an inward course toward the medulla and commence branching in the outer stripe. While a few side branches supply the capillary plexus of the outer stripe, the majority are destined to enter the inner stripe. As mentioned in an earlier section, these branches of the juxtamedullary efferent arterioles are the descending vasa recta and, together with the ascending vasa recta, are organized in the form of vascular bundles (Figs. 1-21, 1-22, 1-25, and 1-28). In the bundles, descending and ascending vessels are arranged in close juxtaposition so that descending vessels are surrounded by ascending vessels and vice versa. At various levels of the inner stripe, descending vasa recta leave the bundles to enter the peritubular capillary plexus in the interbundle region (see Fig. 1-28). Most descending vasa recta leave the bundles in the inner stripe, and relatively few continue on to the inner medulla, accounting for attenuation of bundle size in this region (see Figs. 1-22 and 1-28). At various levels of the inner medulla, the descending vasa recta enter the capillary plexus, so progressively fewer reach the papilla.

Corresponding to the descending vasa recta, the inner medulla has ascending vasa recta. These are formed at various levels and ascend upward. Although vascular bundles in the inner medulla are

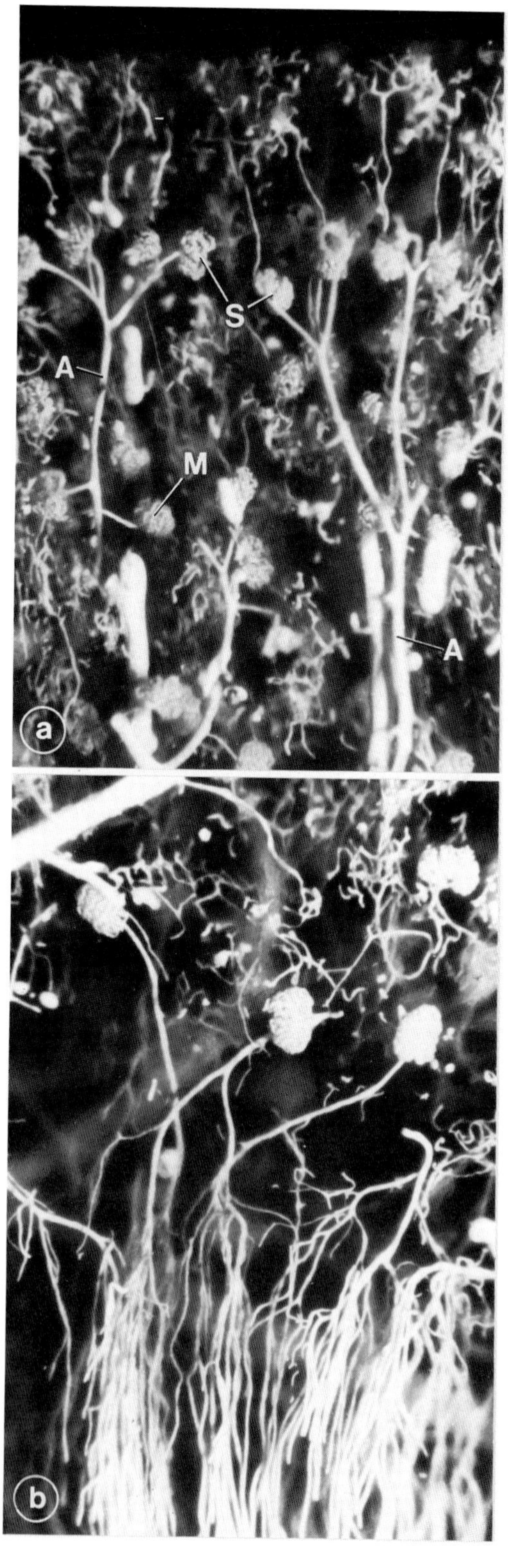

FIG. 1-26. *Arterial vessels of the rabbit kidney as seen after filling with silicone rubber. (A) Interlobular (corticoradial) arteries (A) with afferent arterioles to superficial (S) and midcortical (M) glomeruli. Note that the efferent arterioles of the superficial glomeruli ascend toward the surface of the kidney. (B) Juxtamedullary glomeruli, whose efferent arterioles turn toward the renal medulla and split off into the descending vasa recta. (A) ×47 approx.; (B) ×70 approx.*

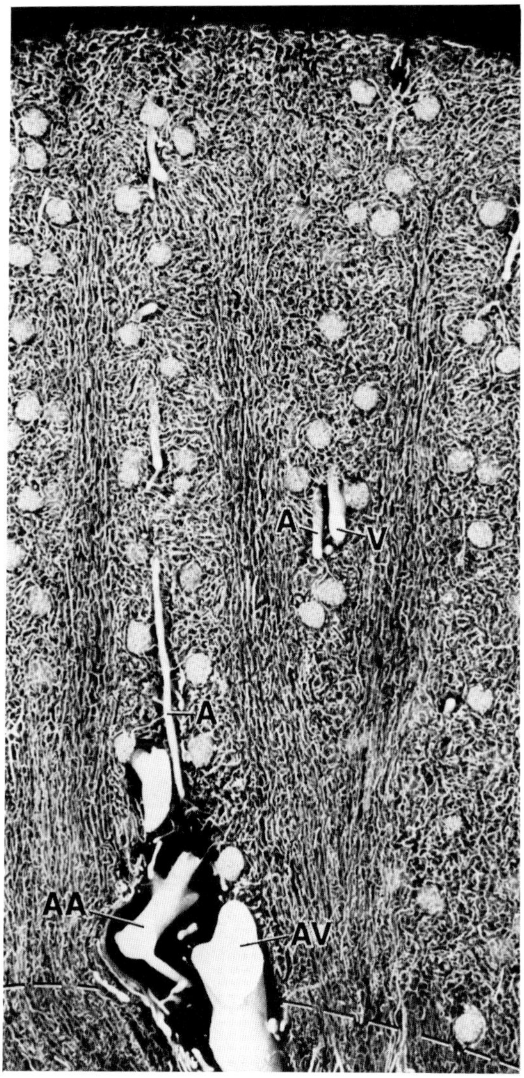

FIG. 1-27. *Longitudinal section through the cortex of a human kidney; arterial injection of silicone rubber (Microfil). The different capillary patterns of the cortical labyrinth and of the medullary rays are seen. Within the cortical labyrinth, the interlobular (corticoradial) arteries (A) and veins (V) as well as the glomeruli are found. Within the medullary rays, the capillary plexus consists of elongated meshes. AA and AV, arcuate artery and vein. ×70 approx.*

attenuated, the tendency for descending and ascending vessels to stay contiguous is preserved, so a countercurrent arrangement is present in this region also. The capillary plexuses of the medulla show distinctive patterns of arrangement. The plexus in the inner medulla is scant. In the papilla, there is a dense meshwork of capillaries; higher up, most of the vessels are in fact vasa recta, with a sparse, longitudinally disposed capillary network connecting them. At the junction of the inner and outer medulla, *all* the ascending vasa recta derived from the inner medulla enter the vascular bundles. Thus inner medullary venous outflow is exclusively by means of the vascular bundles (see Fig. 1-22). This arrangement contrasts with the geometry of capillary plexuses and venous outflow in the inner stripe. We noted earlier that descending vasa recta supplying the inner stripe peel away from the vascular bundles at different levels and enter the dense capillary plexus surrounding tubules in the interbundle region (see Fig. 1-28). Venules arising from this plexus unite to form ascending vasa recta that travel outward, away from the bundles, to enter the outer stripe (see Figs. 1-22 and 1-25). Ascending vasa recta derived from the inner medulla leave the upper ends of the fusiform vascular bundles in the outer stripe and course outward. Within the outer stripe, both sets of vessels take the form of wavy, thin-walled channels (see Fig. 1-22). These venous channels, like all ascending vasa recta, have a thin, attenuated, fenestrated endothelium and represent a large fraction of the vascular plexus in the outer stripe instead of true capillaries, which are sparse in this region. They have large lumens, course outward in a radial fashion, and empty directly into the arcuate veins or the basal aspects of the interlobular veins.

Vascular-Tubular Relations

Blood supply to the tubules is associated with or dissociated from the efferent arterioles of corresponding glomeruli in distinctive patterns in different regions of the kidney [27–30,195]. Cortical segments of tubules in superficial nephrons are perfused by capillaries derived from efferent arterioles of corresponding glomeruli. In midcortical

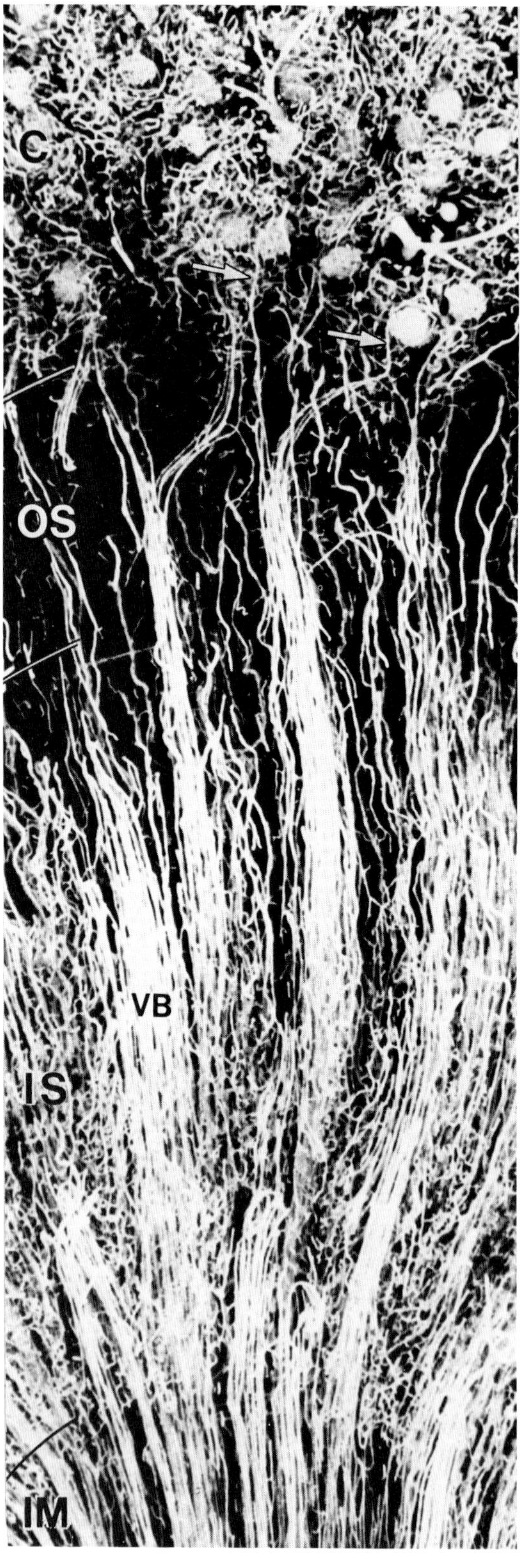

nephrons, this relationship is only partially true; efferent channels of one glomerulus may perfuse tubules of other nephrons too. Cortical segments of tubules in juxtamedullary nephrons are perfused entirely by efferent vessels from other nephrons, since juxtamedullary efferent arterioles perfuse the medulla exclusively (see Figs. 1-21, 1-22, and 1-26*B*). Also, there is complete dissociation of the perfusion of cortical nephron segments from that of the loops of Henle in the same nephrons (see Fig. 1-22). In the medulla, there is virtually complete separation of blood flow to the inner stripe of the outer medulla from that of the inner medulla (see Fig. 1-22). Descending vasa recta destined for the inner medulla do not provide branches for the outer medulla. Those heading for the inner stripe enter the capillary plexus of this zone separately; as we saw earlier, venous outflow from this zone is quite separate from that of the inner medulla. However, both venous outflows perfuse the outer-stripe capillary plexus (see Figs. 1-22 and 1-25). These distinctive vascular perfusion patterns and vascular-tubular relationships have implications for the complex mechanisms that concentrate urine [131,195]. Moreover, the complex geometry of the medullary circulation has relevance to renal pathology. For example, they help to explain the unique patterns of tubule injury during anoxia or ischemia [44,202,285,338].

Structure of Renal Blood Vessels

The structures of the arcuate and interlobular arteries and of the proximal portions of afferent arterioles are comparable with those of arterial vessels of similar caliber elsewhere in the body (Fig. 1-29). The structure of the terminal portions of

FIG. 1-28. *Arterial vessels of the medulla, mouse; arterial injection with Microfil. The juxtamedullary glomeruli give rise to efferent arterioles (arrows) that split into the descending vasa recta, establishing the arterial part of the vascular bundle (VB). The bundles are best developed in the inner stripe (IS) and decrease after the transition into the inner medulla (IM). C, cortex; OS, outer stripe. ×65 approx.*

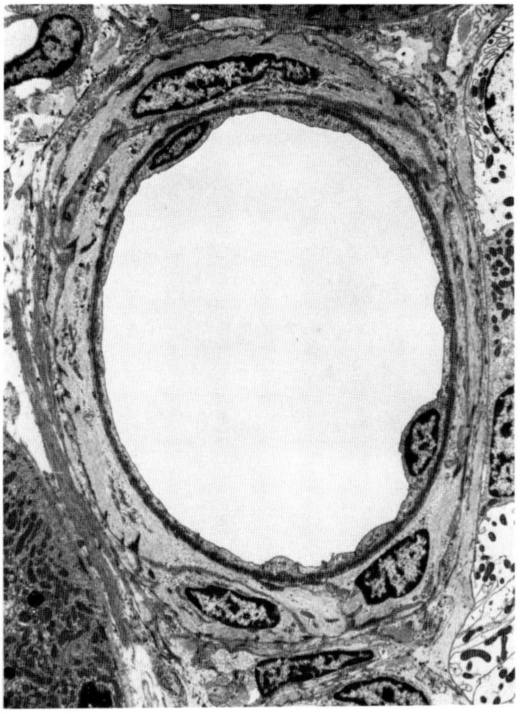

Fig. 1-29. *Glomerular afferent arteriole, proximal portion (a juxtaglomerular portion is shown later together with the JGA); rabbit. An internal elastic membrane surrounds the endothelium. The media consists of two to three layers of smooth-muscle cells. The periarteriolar tissue is collapsed.* ×*2300 approx.*

afferent arterioles will be described later under Juxtaglomerular Apparatus. Afferent arterioles are the main resistance vessels and regulate renal blood flow by contraction or relaxation of the one to three layers of smooth muscle in their walls [77,105,172]. The structure of glomerular capillaries is described in the next section. Efferent arterioles of juxtamedullary glomeruli show significant differences in their caliber and structure from corresponding arterioles derived from midcortical and superficial nephrons. In the latter group, efferent arterioles have diameters that are nearly half those of the afferent vessels; in contrast, juxtamedullary efferent arterioles are larger than their afferent counterparts [14,27,77,85]. Cortical efferent arterioles are thin walled and have no more than a single layer of smooth muscle (Fig. 1-30). Juxtamedullary efferent arterioles are not only larger, but have two to four layers of smooth muscle. Along their lengths, they become smaller in caliber with one layer of smooth muscle and have large numbers of longitudinally arranged endothelial cells [77] (see Fig. 1-30). In descending vasa recta, the smooth-muscle cells are gradually replaced by pericytes. The endothelium remains continuous and shows numerous longitudinally oriented cells separated by tight junctions [287]. Near their termination in the capillary plexuses, the descending vasa recta lose their layer of pericytes, and the endothelium becomes attenuated and fenestrated, as in the capillaries themselves. As described previously, descending and ascending vasa recta are arranged in countercurrent fashion in the vascular bundles. In cross section, they present a checkerboard pattern; the descending vasa recta with their thicker arteriolar walls contrast sharply with adjacent ascending vasa recta (Fig. 1-31). The ascending vasa recta have an attenuated, fenestrated endothelium of the type seen in peritubular capillaries [77,287] (see below and Fig. 1-32).

With the exception of glomerular capillaries, the structural features of the capillaries in the cortex and medulla are similar. The peritubular capillaries are of the fenestrated type (see Fig. 1-32). The capillary wall has a basement membrane and an endothelium that is attenuated in the nonnuclear regions. In these areas, the endothelium is punctured by numerous fenestrae that are arranged in clusters. The fenestrae measure between 500 and 800 Å in diameter and are bridged by approximately 40-Å-thick diaphragms. The complex structural features and functional significance of this type of capillary have been described in detail [295]. In contrast to fenestrated capillaries elsewhere, endothelial fenestrations of peritubular capillaries in the kidney allow large macromolecules to pass relatively freely across them into basement membranes and interstitium [322], accounting for the rich protein content of the renal interstitium [241]. Structurally, the interlobular and arcuate veins are not veins as usually understood. They are extremely thin walled, take the

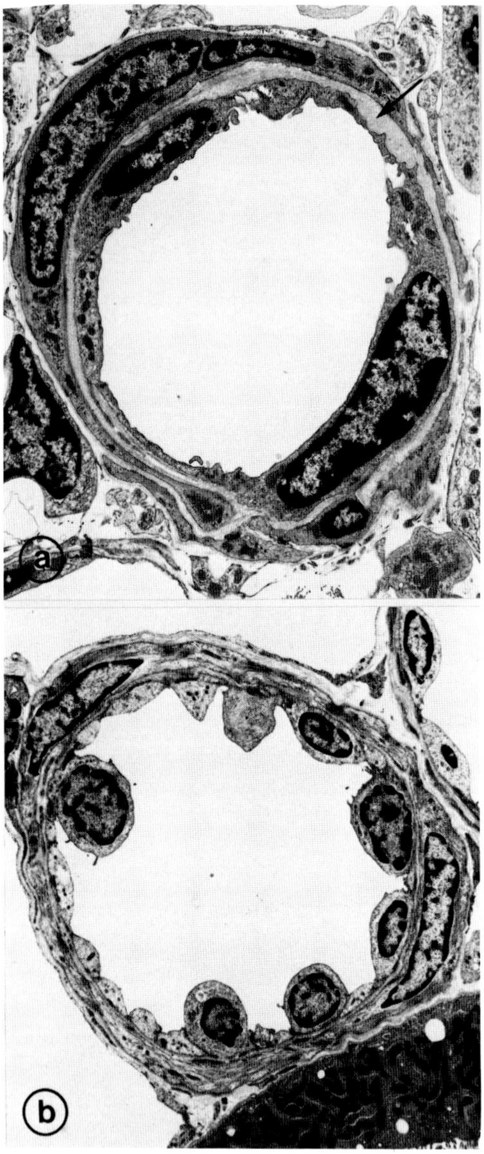

FIG. 1-30. *Glomerular efferent arterioles; rat. (A) Efferent arteriole of a midcortical glomerulus. The endothelial tube is encircled by a complete layer of smooth-muscle cells. Conspicuous basement-membrane–like material (arrow) lies beneath the endothelium, replacing a basement membrane proper. (B) Juxtamedullary efferent arteriole. The endothelium is conspicuously composed of very many endothelial cell profiles. A complete muscle layer encircles the endothelial tube. (A) ×4000 approx.; (B) ×3000 approx.*

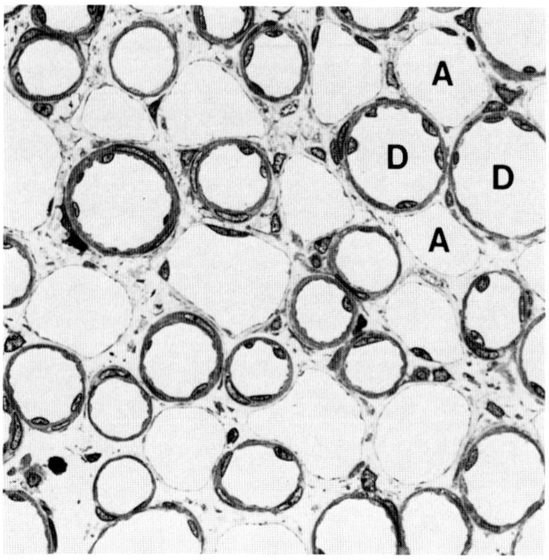

FIG. 1-31. *Cross section through a vascular bundle of the human kidney; light micrograph. The arteriolar character of the descending vasa recta (D) is clearly seen; the ascending vasa recta (A), in contrast, have a very thin wall consisting only of a fenestrated endothelium. Descending and ascending vasa recta are arranged in checkerboard pattern.*

shape of periarterial and peritubular spaces (Fig. 1-33), and, like capillaries, are lined by thin and fenestrated endothelium supported by a basement membrane. Also, like the capillaries, they are postulated to participate in the reabsorptive function by accepting interstitial fluid [133,171].

GLOMERULUS

The glomerulus is a vascular epithelial organ (Figs. 1-34 and 1-35). It consists of a tuft of capillaries arranged in lobules, a supporting framework of extracellular matrix and cells in so-called centrilobular locations called the *mesangium* (to which the capillaries are attached), a layer of visceral epithelium that invests the external surfaces of the capillaries, and Bowman's capsule, lined internally by the parietal epithelium. Bowman's capsule forms a pouch-like structure within which the glomerular capillary tuft is located. At the vascular pole, the

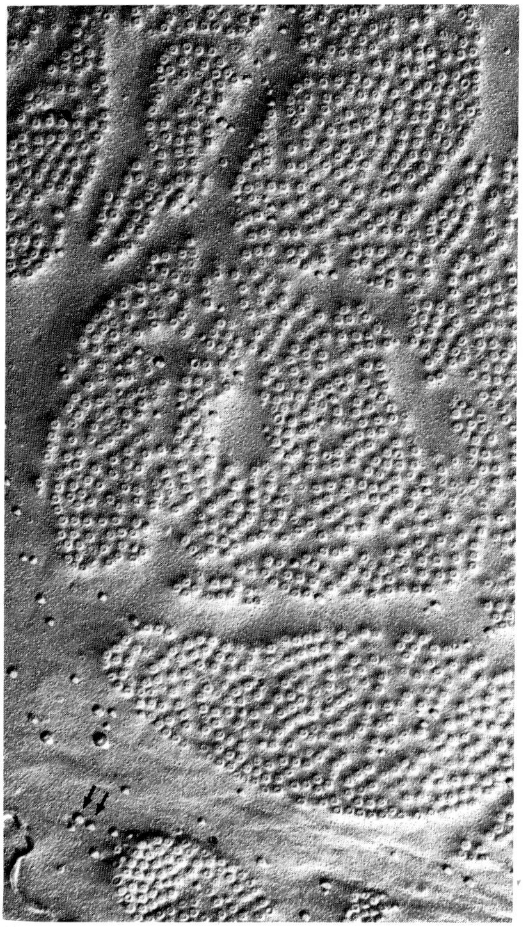

FIG. 1-32. *Freeze-fracture replica of a peritubular capillary; rat. The dense pattern of fenestrations in the capillary wall is seen. The thicker cytoplasmic strands of the endothelium contain pinocytotic vesicles (arrows). This type of endothelium is also found in cortical venules and veins and in ascending vasa recta.* $\times$ *12,500 approx.*

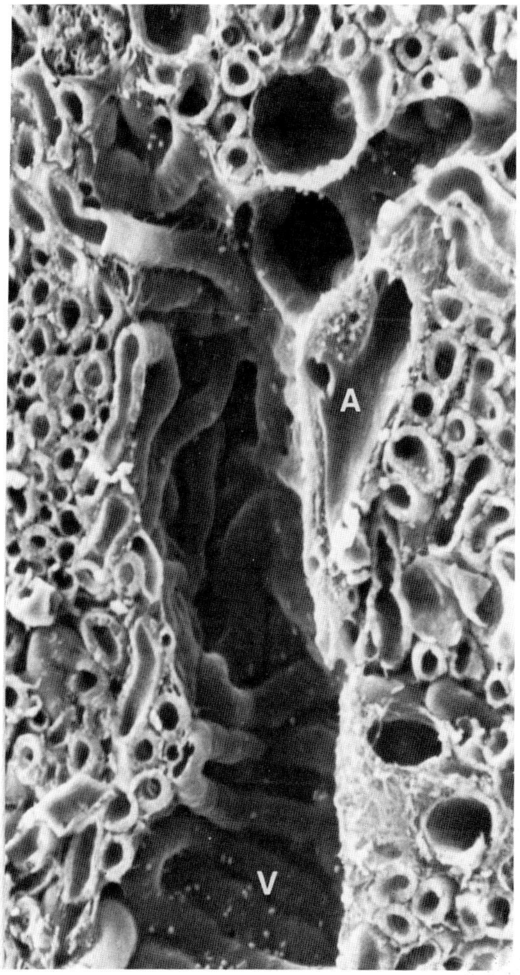

FIG. 1-33. *Scanning electron micrograph of the luminal aspect of an interlobular vein (V). Because of the thin wall of the vein, neighboring tubules invaginate into the vein, creating a striking tubular relief. A, interlobular artery.* $\times$ *180 approx.*

afferent and efferent arterioles enter and leave the glomerulus. The visceral epithelium, which covers the glomerular capillaries, is reflected back onto the inner surface of Bowman's capsule at the vascular pole; therefore, the visceral and parietal epithelia are anatomically in continuity and together enclose a space within the capsule, referred to as *Bowman's space* or the *capsular space*. It is in this space that plasma ultrafiltrate forms and then flows into the tubular portion of the nephron. Almost diametrically opposite the vascular pole, the parietal epithelium of the capsule is in continuity with and transforms abruptly into the epithelium of the proximal tubule. Thus, at the urinary pole of the glomerulus, Bowman's space is continuous with the lumen of the proximal tubule. As inferred

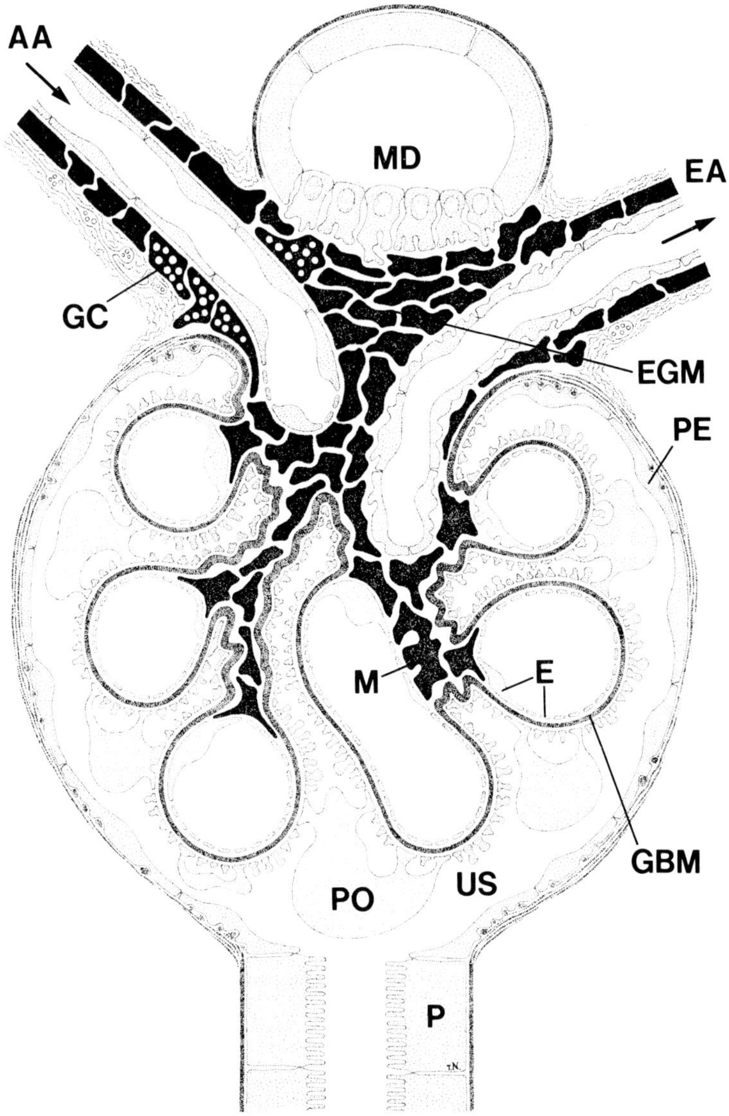

FIG. 1-34. *Schematic diagram of a longitudinal section through a glomerulus and the juxtaglomerular apparatus. At the vascular pole, an afferent arteriole (AA) enters and an efferent arteriole (EA) leaves the tuft. The glomerular capillary tuft is surrounded by Bowman's capsule. There are different epithelia, the visceral and the parietal. The visceral epithelium (podocytes; PO), reflects onto Bowman's capsule as the parietal epithelium (PE) at the vascular pole. Between both epithelia is the urinary space (US), which is continuous with the lumen of the proximal tubule (P). The endothelium (E) of glomerular capillaries is fenestrated. Between the endothelial cells and the podocytes, the glomerular basement membrane (GBM) is found. At the vascular pole, the GBM continues as the basement membrane of Bowman's capsule. Mesangial cells (M) are situated in the axis of glomerular lobules. At the vascular pole, mesangial cells are continuous with extraglomerular mesangial cells (EGM); together with the granular cells (GC) and the macula densa (MD), they make up the JGA. (Modified from Kriz et al. [179].)*

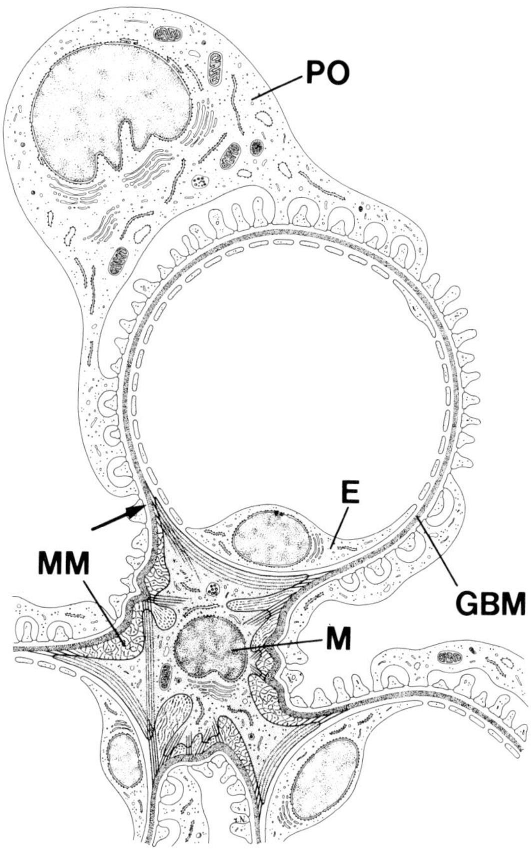

FIG. 1-35. *Schematic diagram to show the arrangement of structures in the glomerular tuft; part of a glomerular lobule is shown with three glomerular capillaries (two are incomplete) attached to a mesangial center. The glomerular capillary endothelium (E) is fenestrated. The peripheral part of the endothelial tube is surrounded by the GBM, which, at the mesangial angles (arrow), deviates from a pericapillary course and covers the mesangium. Interdigitating foot processes of the podocyte (PO) form the external layer of the filtration barrier. Podocyte foot processes are also found covering the paramesangial GBM. In the center, a mesangial cell (M) is shown. Its many processes contain microfilament bundles and run toward the GBM to which they are connected. The mesangial matrix (MM) contains an interwoven network of microfilaments. (Modified from Kriz [170].)*

from its embryology and ultrastructure, the glomerulus can be considered to be an invagination of a capillary network into a sac lined by epithelium. The epithelial layer that invests the capillaries is incorporated into and becomes an intrinsic part of the filtering membrane, whereas the remaining portion develops into the lining of the capsule.

The human glomerulus, including Bowman's capsule, is approximately 200 μm in diameter; the diameters of juxtamedullary glomeruli may be greater than those of more superficial glomeruli by up to 50 percent [14,227,237,297]. The mean filtration surface area per glomerulus has been measured by stereologic techniques to be 0.136 mm^2 in man and 0.184 mm^2 in the rat [235,292]. The published figure for human glomeruli seems low, however. More recent measurements in 33 normal human kidneys are closer to the figure reported for the rat (0.168 $\pm$ 0.065 mm^2 SD; Michael Steffes, University of Minnesota, personal communication).

Bowman's Capsule

Bowman's capsule consists of a spherical bag of basement membrane lined on its inner aspect by flat epithelial cells. Each cell shows a few microvilli and a central cilium. At the urinary pole, the flat epithelium undergoes sudden transition to the taller proximal tubule epithelium (see Fig. 1-34). The basement membrane is multilayered and forms specific structures such as microligaments that run around the vascular pole [206]. At the vascular pole, the basement membrane of Bowman's capsule transforms into the glomerular basement membrane (GBM); at the urinary pole, it transforms into the basement membrane of the proximal tubule.

Glomerular Capillary Tuft

The afferent arteriole divides dichotomously and gives rise to four to eight capillaries, each of which subdivides into an anastomosing network of capillaries called a *lobule* [2,24,220,291]. Within each lobule, capillaries anastomose freely, run toward the urinary pole, and then turn back to merge into

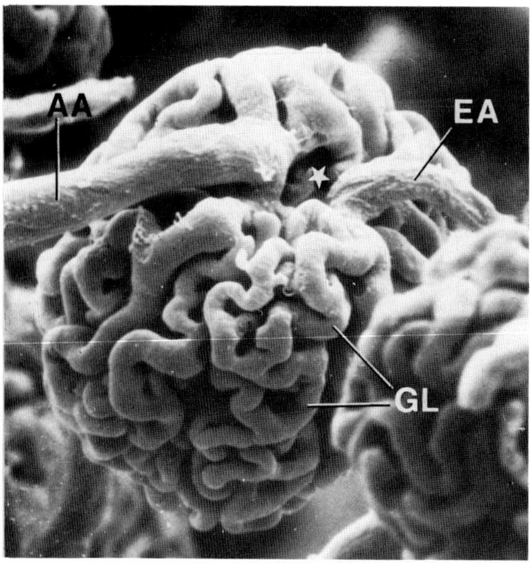

FIG. 1-36. *A scanning electron micrograph showing a vascular cast of a rat glomerulus with an afferent arteriole (AA) and an efferent arteriole (EA). In between both arterioles (*), an empty space is seen through which the extraglomerular mesangium continues into the stalk of the glomerular tuft. GL, glomerular capillaries.* ×*400 approx.*

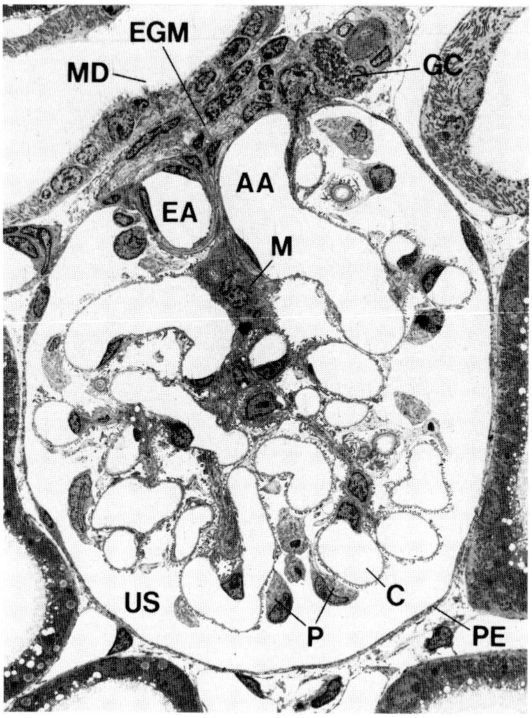

FIG. 1-37. *Electron micrograph of a section through a rat glomerulus. At the vascular pole, the afferent arteriole (AA) containing in its wall granular cells (GC), the efferent arteriole (EA), the extraglomerular mesangium (EGM), and the macula densa (MD) are seen. The glomerular tuft contains in its center the mesangium (M) surrounded by glomerular capillaries (C). P, podocytes; PE, parietal epithelium of Bowman's capsule; US, urinary space.*

efferent capillaries, which, in turn, merge together to form the efferent arteriole (Figs. 1-36 and 1-37). Anastomoses also may occur between capillaries of adjacent lobules in the center of the glomerular tuft [2,220,291]. At the vascular pole, the afferent and efferent arterioles are separated by a space that is packed with extracellular matrix and cells of the extraglomerular mesangium, also referred to as *lacis cells* (see Juxtaglomerular Apparatus) (see Figs. 1-36 and 1-37). The extraglomerular mesangium extends into the glomerulus in a tree-like fashion with branches and ramifications. These areas constitute the glomerular mesangium. Each of the branches forms the axis for a lobule and supports a network of capillaries around it (Figs. 1-34, 1-35, 1-37 through 1-39).

Glomerular Capillary Wall: Structure

The capillaries pursue a tortuous course around the mesangial areas (intercapillary areas, axial regions, centrilobular zones) so that in tissue sections, their profiles appear to be arranged in grape-like clusters around the mesangium (see Figs. 1-34, 1-35, 1-37 through 1-39). The capillaries are lined by a layer of endothelium. The nu-

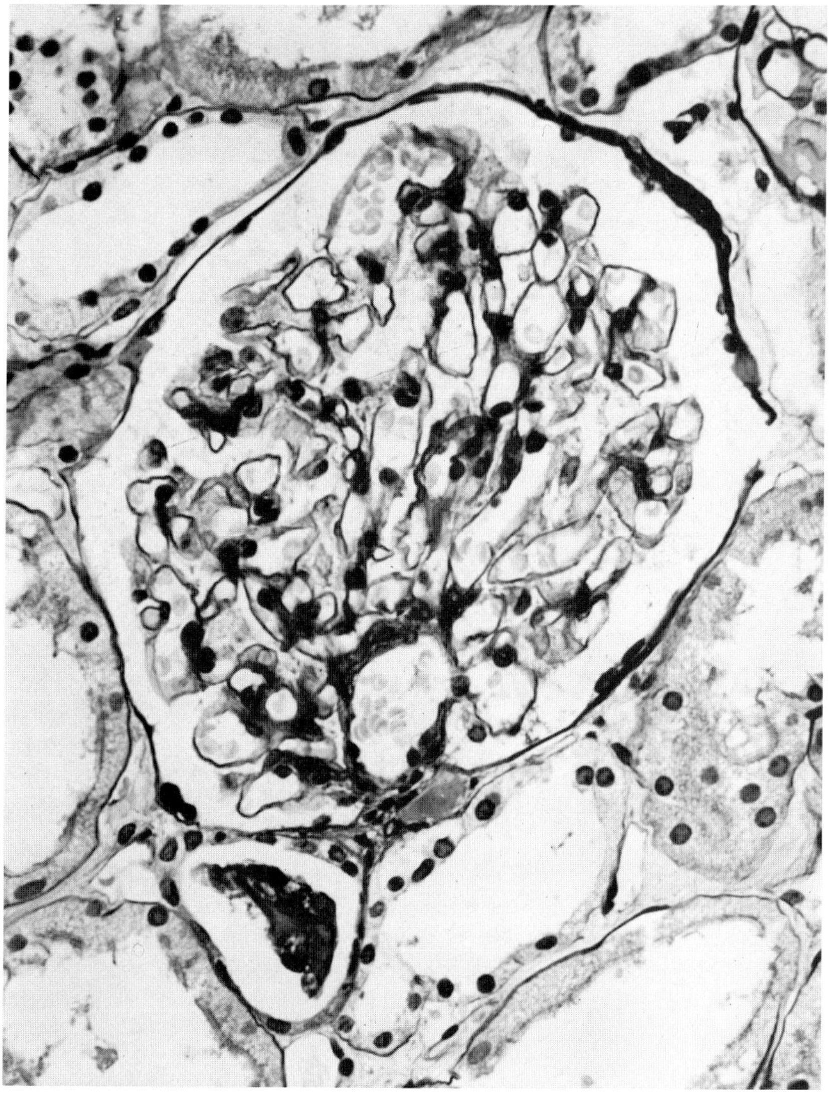

FIG. 1-38. *Normal glomerulus from renal biopsy on young man. Stained with silver to show delicate basement membrane, mesangial regions, and surrounding capillaries.* ×400.

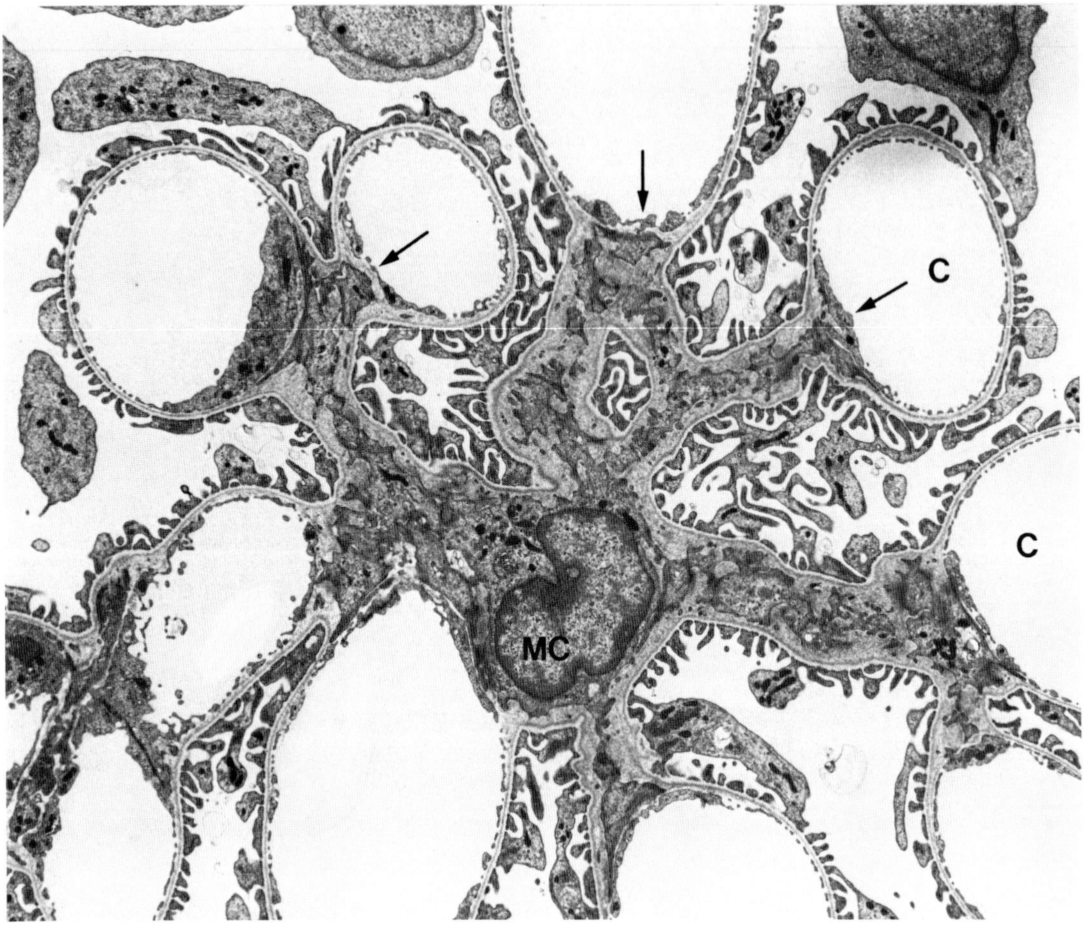

FIG. 1-39. *Overview of a glomerular lobule, rat; transmission electron micrograph. In the center, a mesangial cell (MC) is seen whose processes extend within the mesangial matrix toward the peripherally located glomerular capillaries (C). Note that the GBM envelops the entire glomerular lobule. Thus the juxtamesangial parts of the glomerular capillaries lack a basement membrane; at this site, the endothelium is directly exposed to the mesangium (arrows). The capillary endothelium is thin and fenestrated. Interdigitating foot processes of the podocytes abut the GBM on its outside surface. ×5000 approx.*

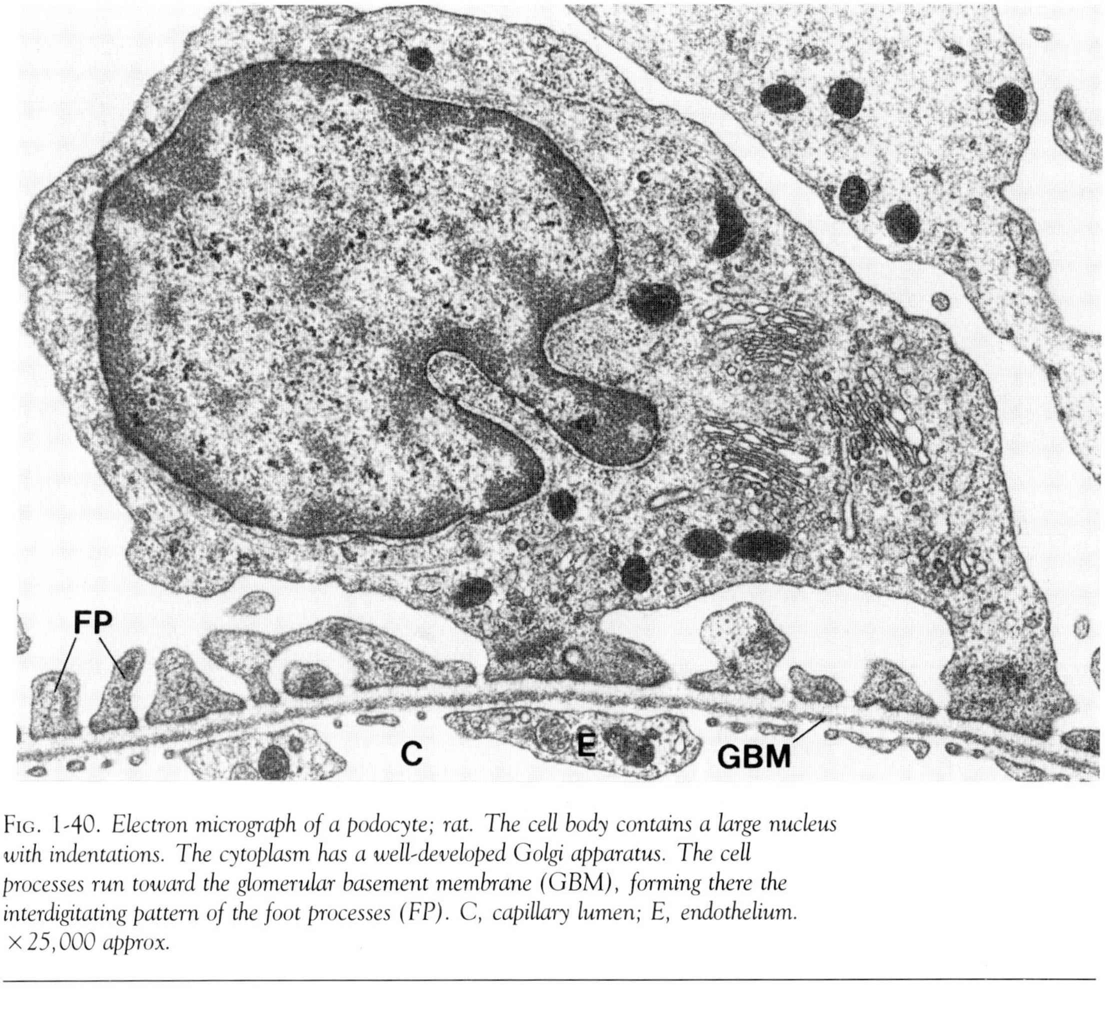

FIG. 1-40. *Electron micrograph of a podocyte; rat. The cell body contains a large nucleus with indentations. The cytoplasm has a well-developed Golgi apparatus. The cell processes run toward the glomerular basement membrane (GBM), forming there the interdigitating pattern of the foot processes (FP). C, capillary lumen; E, endothelium. ×25,000 approx.*

clei of the endothelial cells are disposed centrilobularly, toward the mesangium. Peripherally, the endothelium is considerably attenuated to approximately 40 nm in thickness and punctured by numerous fenestrations approximately 50 to 100 nm in diameter (Figs. 1-39 through 1-41). The majority of the fenestrae are devoid of diaphragms (unlike peritubular capillaries), and the total fenestral area is approximately 20 percent of the capillary surface [97,254]. The endothelial cells are attached to and line the internal surface of the glomerular basement membrane (GBM), which is 240 to 340 nm wide in the adult human kidney and slightly thicker in males than in females [134,135,234,301]. GBM thickness varies from species to species, being only 110 to 160 nm in the rat [253]. The GBM is a complex structure composed of three distinct layers; there is a central lamina densa and two peripheral relatively electron-lucent layers, the lamina rara interna and the lamina rara externa (see Fig. 1-41). The GBM appears to be made of a network of fine fibrils less than 10 nm in diameter (estimates of thickness vary). Fibrils are more tightly packed in the lamina densa than in the laminae rarae (see Fig. 1-41). The visceral epithelial cell, or podocyte,

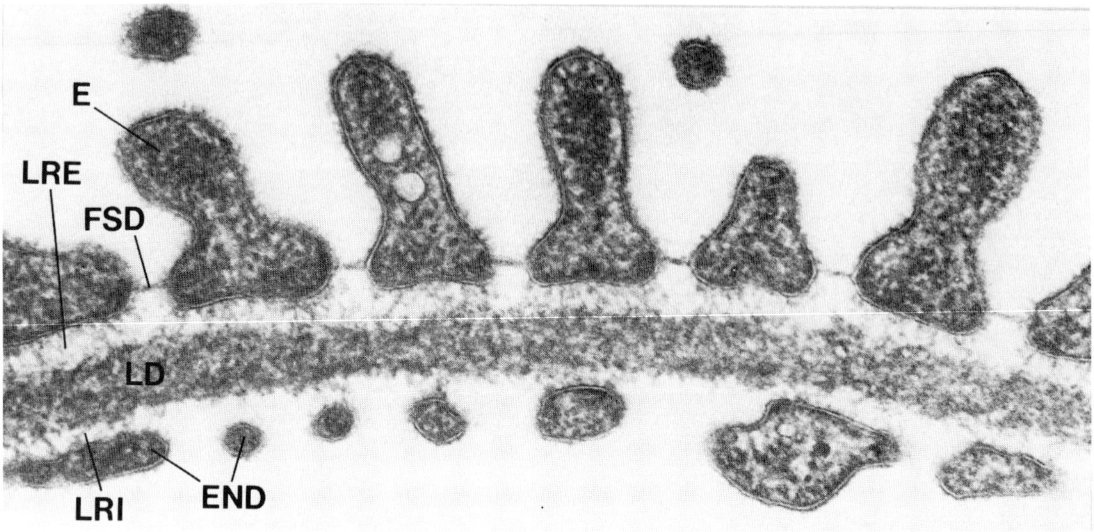

A

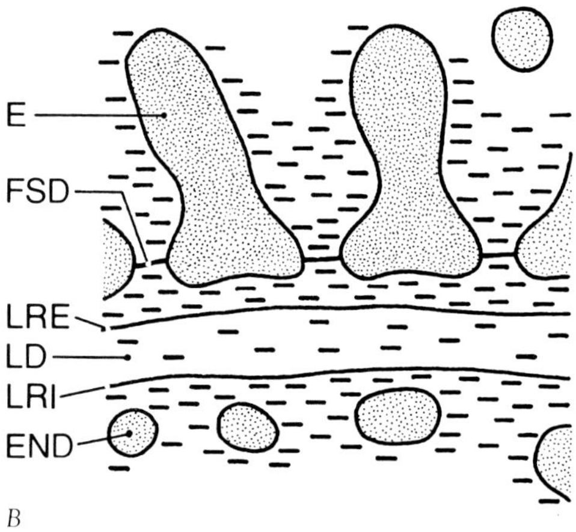

B

FIG. 1-41. *Filtration barrier. (A) Electron micrograph through the peripheral part of the glomerular capillary wall (rat) demonstrating the three layers, the endothelium, the basement membrane, and the layer of podocyte foot processes. (B) The accompanying drawing demonstrates the distribution of the negatively charged glycoproteins within the glomerular filtration barrier. END, endothelium; LRI, lamina rara interna; LD, lamina densa; LRE, lamina rara externa; FSD, filtration slit diaphragm; E, epithelium (podocyte foot process).* ×90,000 *approx.*

forms the outermost layer of the capillary wall and is attached to the lamina rara externa of the GBM [153,186] (see Fig. 1-40).

The podocyte is a complex cell with a large cell body or perikaryon and numerous branching cytoplasmic processes. The perikaryon bulges into the urinary space, and the indented nucleus is situated in this region. The cytoplasm shows large Golgi complexes, numerous profiles of rough and smooth endoplasmic reticulum, and a well-developed lysosomal system. The cytoplasm has abundant cytoskeletal elements, including numerous microtubules, actin and intermediate filaments, and coated vesicles with clathrin cages. The cell shows a number of blunt cytoplasmic extensions, the primary processes, that surround the capillary (Fig. 1-42). From these primary processes issue numerous secondary extensions of smaller caliber known as *foot processes,* or *pedicels.* Pedicels also may emerge from secondary and tertiary branches of the primary processes. The pedicels emerge at regular intervals much like the teeth of a comb and course in a direction longitudinal to the capillary axis. Pedicels from adjacent podo-

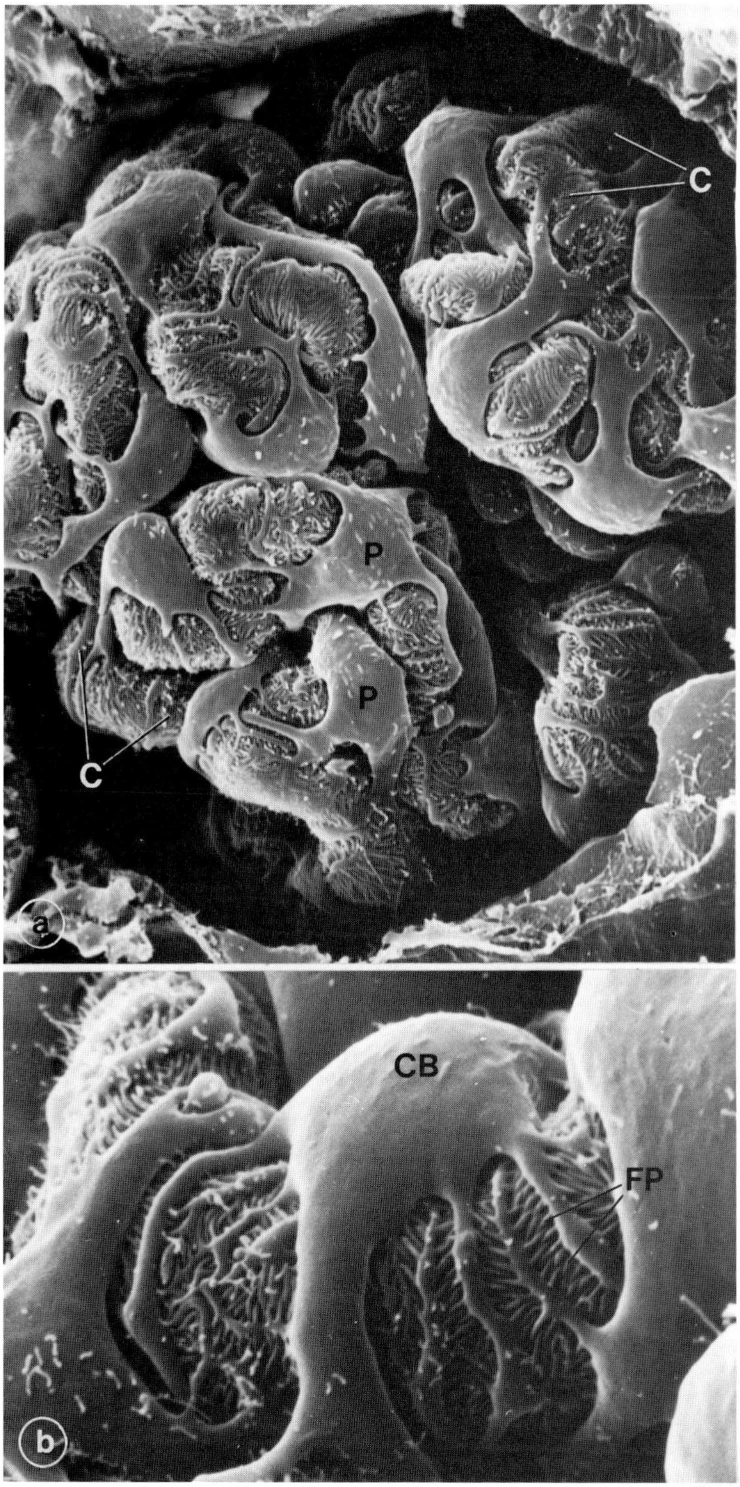

FIG. 1-42. *Scanning electron micrograph of a rat glomerular tuft seen from the urinary pole. (A) An overview with the cell bodies of podocytes (P) being attached to the outer surface of glomerular capillaries (C) by processes. (B) The branching pattern of podocytes on the surface of a glomerular capillary. The cell body (CB) gives rise to primary processes, which finally split into the interdigitating foot processes (FP). (A) ×800 approx.; (B) ×3000 approx.*

cytes interdigitate with one another in a regular and uniform pattern [9] (see Fig. 1-42) such that when the capillary wall is examined by transmission electron microscopy, profiles of adjacent foot processes seen in the two-dimensional images are derived from separate but adjacent podocytes. The pedicels are attached to the GBM by means of fine filaments that traverse the entire thickness of the lamina rara externa (see Fig. 1-41). The cytoplasm along the basal surfaces of the pedicels contains densely packed actin filaments [5,6,82], and the plasma membranes of the basal and lateral aspects of the pedicels often show the openings of clathrin-coated vesicles. Of much interest is gp330, a proximal tubule brush-border antigen related to the pathogenesis of membranous nephropathy, which has been shown to be present in coated vesicles in podocytes [157].

The spaces between adjacent pedicels form narrow channels called *filtration slits* that are 300 to 500 nm deep and 20 to 30 nm wide at their narrowest margins. In their narrowest parts, the filtration slits are bridged by approximately 4-nm-thick diaphanous membranes that are attached to the outer leaflets of the plasma membranes of adjacent pedicels (see Fig. 1-41). These membranes are known as *filtration slit diaphragms*. Recent studies show that the podocyte is a polarized cell and that the composition of the plasma membrane is markedly different in the foot processes above and below the sites of attachment of the diaphragms [158,230,231]. The filtration slit diaphragms are thought to be composed of protein, and they demonstrate a porous substructure when examined by electron microscopy after fixation with tannic acid–glutaraldehyde [258,283]. Visualized en face, the diaphragm shows a paired and staggered series of rod-like subunits extending from the pedicels to the center of the slit, where they apparently fuse with a bar that courses along the long axis of the diaphragm, forming a zipper-like structure. The rods define 4 × 14 nm rectangular spaces on both sides of the central bar, roughly corresponding to the dimensions of the albumin molecule (Fig. 1-43). The spaces have been calculated to account for 2 to 3 percent of the total surface area of the glomerular capillaries and have been considered to be potential barriers to the filtration of albumin and other proteins [153,258,283]. However, a barrier function for the filtration slits and structures contained within them has not yet been demonstrated with certainty [93,94]. In this regard, a recent study in rats has shown the existence of a distinctive antigenic epitope sharply localized to the filtration slit in the region of the diaphragms; intravenous injection of monoclonal antibodies against the epitope caused massive proteinuria [232].

A subsequent chapter in this book (Chap. 12) will discuss how proteinuria of glomerular origin is invariably associated with effacement of the normal architecture of the foot processes of podocytes. In this situation, interdigitations become simpler, the filtration slits become narrower, and electron microscopy reveals the appearance of masses of protoplasm covering the GBM instead of the delicate, alternating foot processes of adjacent cells. Similar anatomic lesions have been induced experimentally by maneuvers that reduce the negative surface charge of podocyte plasma membranes [290].

Glomerular Capillary Wall: Extracellular Matrix

The glomerulus allows the filtration of solutes with certain defined molecular characteristics, but not others. The pathway for ultrafiltration is strictly extracellular and consists of extracellular matrix components. Most of the water and small solutes—and all macromolecules—enter the capillary wall by means of the endothelial fenestrae, traverse the GBM, and exit into the urinary (Bowman's) space through the filtration slits. Therefore, aside from functional or hemodynamic factors, the composition and texture of the extracellular matrix in the filtration pathway must be determinants of the efficiency of ultrafiltration. In series, the extracellular filter matrix consists of the following elements: (1) glycocalyx of the endothelial cell, which partially fills the endothelial fenestrae, (2) lamina rara interna of the GBM, (3) lamina densa of the GBM, (4) lamina rara externa of the GBM, (5) filtration slit diaphragm, and (6) glycocalyx of the podocyte foot processes, which completely fills the filtration slit. The glycocalyx of the endothelial cells has a net negative charge (see Fig. 1-41) and possibly is composed of a num-

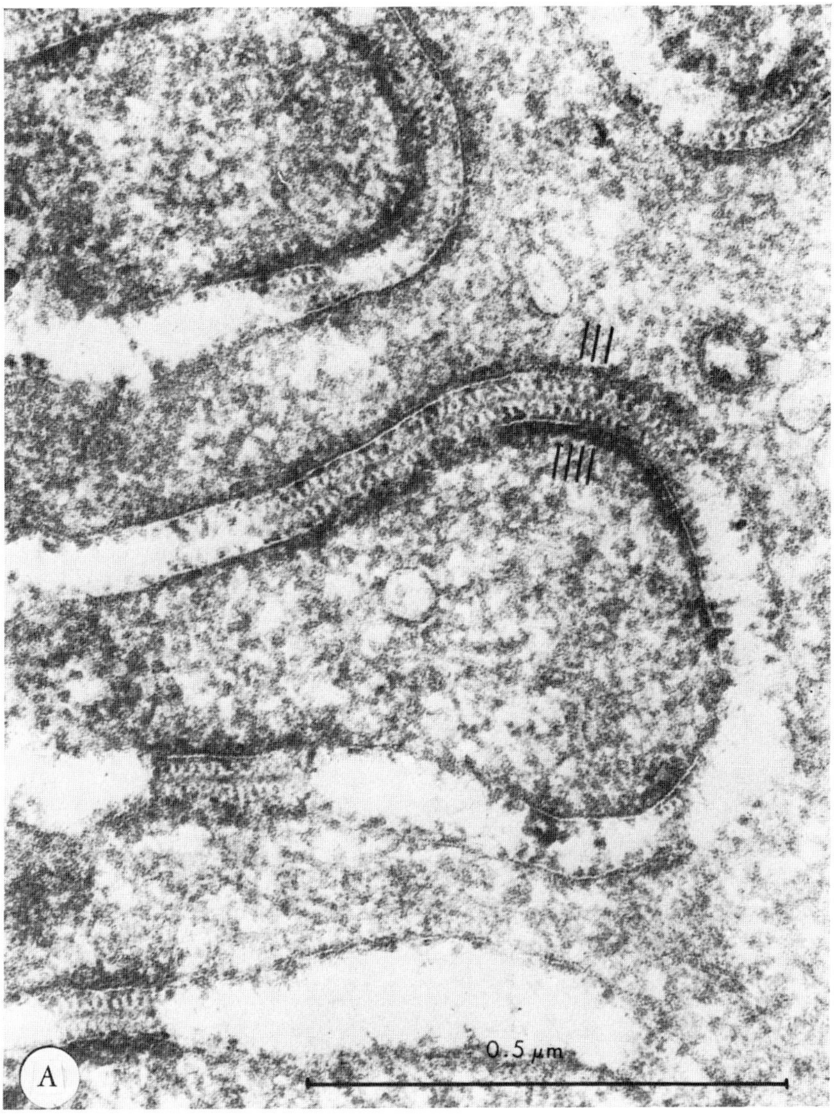

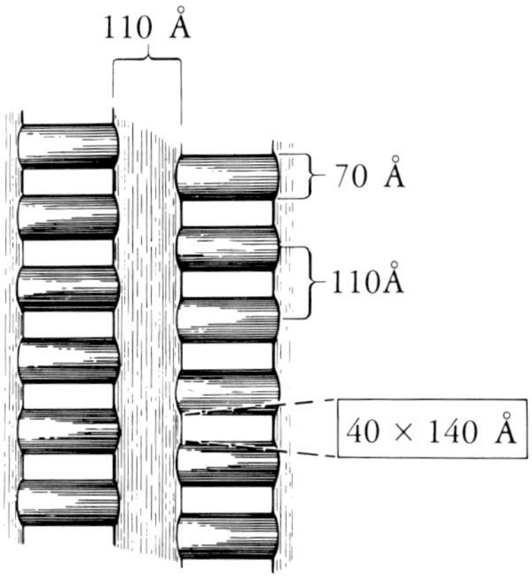

FIG. 1-43. *(A) Slit diaphragm from rat glomerulus. The central filament and cross-bridges are readily resolved in this micrograph. The marks indicate a region where cross-bridges appear to alternate on either side of the central filament. Also evident is the increased density of the cytoplasm opposite the points of attachment of the diaphragm to the epithelial-cell membranes. Apparent discontinuities in the diaphragm represent regions where this structure has left the plane of section (× 130,000). (B) Schematic drawing of the epithelial slit diaphragm. The average cross-sectional dimensions of the pores between cross-bridges are indicated within the rectangle. (From Rodewald, R., and Karnovsky, M. J.* Cell Biol. *60:423, 1974, by copyright permission of the Rockefeller University Press.)*

ber of glycoproteins and proteoglycans, including the major glomerular epithelial-cell sialoglycoprotein podocalyxin and heparan sulfate proteoglycan [120,132,146,187,214,303]. The GBM (and the mesangial matrix, described below) stains with the periodic acid–Schiff (PAS) stain, as well as with reagents that have an affinity for acidic glycoproteins and proteoglycans.

Biochemically, the GBM has collagen of type IV, the sialoglycoproteins laminin and fibronectin, the sulfated glycoprotein entactin, amyloid P component, heparan sulfate proteoglycan, and possibly other, as yet uncharacterized proteins [1, 64,71,74,84,121,144,150,151,156,189,198,200, 201,262,299,303]. Type IV collagen is the principal component and forms a highly ordered compact network of fibrils in the lamina densa, with a looser configuration in the laminae rarae. It has a triple-helical structure and has a noncollagenous domain, a collagenous domain, and a 7 S domain. A recently characterized sequence called the *NC1 domain* in the $\alpha 3$ chain has been identified as the antigen responsible for anti-GBM antibody disease [123] (see also Chap. 10). The so-called Goodpasture antigen has been localized by immunoelectronmicroscopy to the lamina rara interna of the GBM [296]. Laminin, fibronectin, and entactin are found in the more loosely interwoven fibrils of the laminae rarae, where heparan sulfate proteoglycan is also found [64,71,95,121,147,199,200]. The GBM is enriched with a newly discovered type of laminin that mediates tight attachment of apposing cells to the extracellular matrix between them [126]. In the lamina rara externa, where the basal membranes of the foot processes are attached to the GBM, there are clusters of *N*-acetyl-D-galactosamine residues that stain characteristically in a punctate manner with *Helix pomatia* lectin (HPL)–gold conjugates [267]. These residues are associated with a novel glycoprotein different from podocalyxin. In contrast to the HPL-stainable glycoprotein, podocalyxin is enriched in the podocyte plasma membranes above the level of the slit diaphragms [52,158].

The GBM has a net negative charge, and there is a concentration of polyanionic sites in the laminae rarae (see Fig. 1-41), indicated by staining with cationic reagents [32,36,112,132,145,255]. Amino acid and sialic acid carboxylic acids, as well as sulfate groups, are responsible for this electronegativity. Among these, carboxylic acids are thought to be the predominant negatively charged moieties [36]. Podocalyxin, a heavily sialylated, negatively charged integral membrane glycoprotein, is the major glycoprotein of the podocyte, and its carbohydrate residues form the large part of the 15- to 80-nm-thick glycocalyx that covers the podocyte plasma membrane and fills the filtration slits in their narrowest portions [158,159]. The glycocalyx also contains cell-associated proteoglycans [303] and can be stained with a number of lectins, indicating the presence of sugars other than *N*-acetylneuraminic acid or sialic acid [267]. The podocyte glycocalyx is strongly anionic (see Fig. 1-41), as revealed by its high affinity for cationic reagents, and sialic acid carboxyls are the dominant anionic moiety [32,112,132,214].

EXTRACELLULAR MATRIX: ROLE IN CELL ATTACHMENT

It has been shown that sialoglycoproteins in the capillary wall mediate the attachment of both epithelial and endothelial cells to the GBM; perfusion with neuraminidase leads to cell detachment [146]. In the adult, the GBM is a complex structure that is common to both epithelial and endothelial cells, but studies of its development suggest that it is formed separately by the epithelial and endothelial cells followed by fusion into one structure and that both cells also contribute to biosynthesis during adult life [1]. It has been postulated that fusion of the two components might be critically determined by the Goodpasture antigen [123].

EXTRACELLULAR MATRIX: ROLE IN ULTRAFILTRATION

Transit of macromolecules across the GBM is selective with respect to molecular size, electrical charge, and configuration [255,323]. The selectivity depends on interactions of the macromolecules with polyanionic gels of heterogeneous chemical composition. As determined by these interactions, the macromolecules are permitted entry or are excluded from the hydrated interstices of the gel by steric hindrance, electrical attraction or repulsion, and the ability of the molecules to undergo deformation during transit. The GBM is thought to be the major site for these types of interactions and therefore the prime determinant of selective restriction, although it is equally clear that optimal ultrafiltration characteristics depend on the concerted action of various elements in the filter from the endothelial fenestrae to the filtration slits. For example, the slit diaphragm and the polyanionic glycocalyx in the filtration slits might complete the process of selection restriction by retention and adsorption of molecules leaking through the GBM, thereby permitting endocytosis by the visceral epithelium. Thus, protein leakage might be induced by perturbation of the GBM anionic sites [25,125,148], but selective interference at the level of the filtration slit induces proteinuria as well [232]. By virtue of repulsion of negatively charged proteins, anionic sites in the GBM not only contribute to the selective permeability characteristics of the glomerulus, but also are thought to be important in preventing clogging of the filter mechanism that might result if large plasma proteins were permitted to enter the GBM in an unselective manner [149].

The Mesangium

The mesangium is the supporting framework on which the capillary network ramifies, and it consists of the mesangial matrix and mesangial cells (see Figs. 1-34, 1-35, and 1-37 through 1-39). A small juxtamesangial part of the outer circumference of each capillary abuts the mesangium, whereas the larger peripheral portion is covered by the GBM and podocytes (Fig. 1-44). Since the GBM and the podocytes invest the entire capillary tuft, they have a large pericapillary part and also a smaller perimesangial part (see Fig. 1-44). Consequently, the mesangium itself can be geographically defined as having a juxtacapillary region where it abuts against the capillary endothelium and more centrally located axial regions that are bound by the perimesangial GBM (see Figs. 1-34, 1-35, 1-39, and 1-44). The points where the pericapillary GBM deviates from a pericapillary

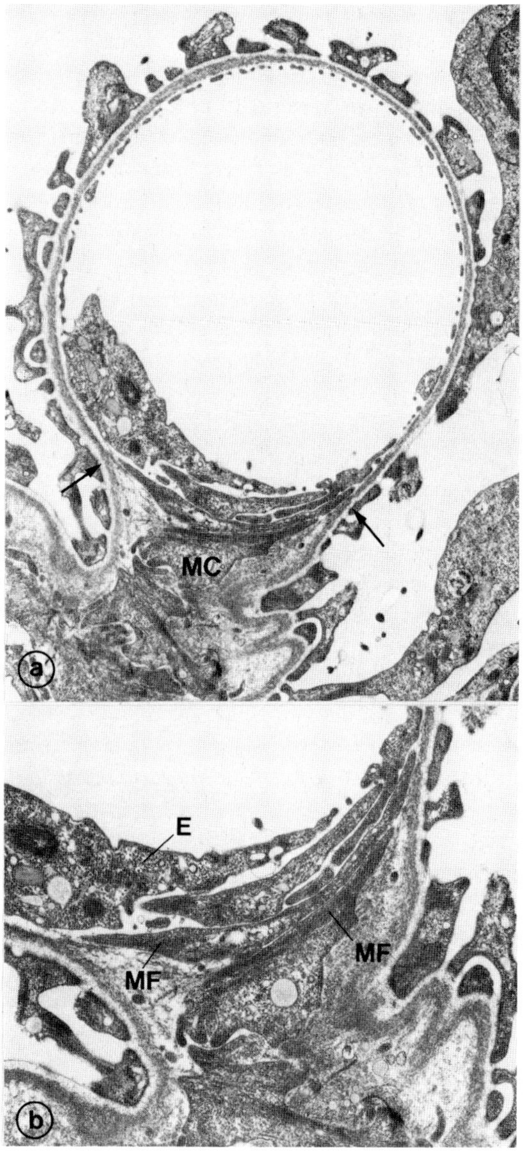

Fig. 1-44. *Glomerular capillary; rat. The peripheral wall of the glomerular capillary constitutes the filtration barrier. At the mesangial angles (arrows), the GBM deviates from a pericapillary course and covers the mesangium. The juxtamesangial part of the endothelium is underlain by mesangial-cell processes (MC, shown enlarged in the lower panel) that contain microfilament bundles (MF) and interconnect the GBM from two opposing mesangial angles. E, endothelium. (A) ×8,500 approx.; (B) ×14,000 approx.*

course and covers the mesangium are called *mesangial angles.* The perimesangial part of the GBM is thick and frequently wrinkled compared with the pericapillary GBM, and the podocyte foot processes over them are usually flattened. There are two cell types in the mesangium. A small minority (~2 percent of total glomerular cells) are phagocytic, Ia antigen–positive cells with Fc receptors, thought to be of monocytic lineage and functionally relevant in immune functions such as phagocytosis and antigen presentation to T-lymphocytes [61,284]. The remainder, which are more numerous, are the mesangial cells proper. They are irregular in shape and show numerous long extensions of their cytoplasm beyond the cell body [340]. These cytoplasmic extensions have abundant microfilaments (Fig. 1-45). In this and other respects they are similar to pericytes, which appear to be the counterparts of mesangial cells in other capillaries. The cytoplasm has actin and myosin filaments, consistent with a contractile function, by which mesangial cells are thought to control glomerular blood flow and, thereby, filtration [166,278].

Mesangial-cell processes are attached to the GBM at mesangial angles as well as to the more centrolibular portions of the perimesangial GBM either directly or indirectly through extracellular microfibrils in the mesangial matrix [218,271]. The mesangial cell–GBM connections are prominent in the juxtacapillary region of the mesangium. At this site, slender cytoplasmic processes (stuffed with microfilament bundles) run toward the mesangial angles, frequently continuing for some distance into the narrowing space between the endothelium and the GBM before finally attaching to the GBM. Thereby, the GBM from opposing mesangial angles is interconnected by processes that bridge the entire distance. This system apparently subserves a mechanical stabilizing function. The contractile apparatus of mesangial-cell processes, together with the GBM, appears capable of developing wall tension and thus counteracts the distending forces exerted on the capillary wall by the high transmural pressure difference. Occasionally, mesangial-cell processes may interpose through gaps in the endothelium and come in direct contact with the capillary lumens.

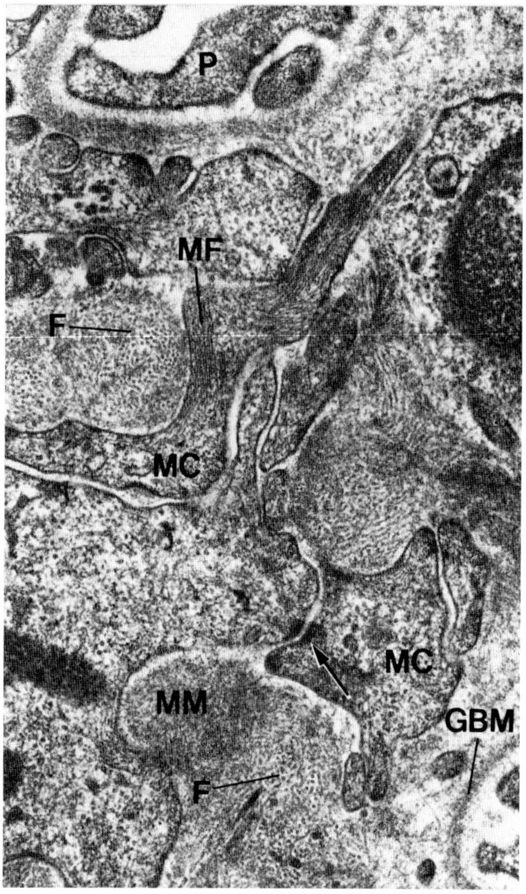

FIG. 1-45. *Mesangial region of the glomerular tuft; rat. Mesangial-cell processes (MC) contain microfilament bundles (MF). The mesangial matrix (MM) contains a network of extracellular microfibrils (F). Mesangial cells may be connected with each other by desmosomes (arrow). The mesangium is bounded by the GBM, which is seen in the upper and lower parts of the picture. P, podocyte.* × *30,500 approx.*

The mesangial cells are coupled by gap junctions with each other and in series with cells of the extraglomerular mesangium (Goormaghtigh cells) and the granular cells of the juxtaglomerular apparatus [246,308]. They are also attached to one another by means of desmosomes (see Fig. 1-45). They elaborate a diverse number of vasoactive agents and hormones, including prostanoids and platelet-activating factor, and are thought to respond by contraction or relaxation in vivo to a number of vasoactive hormones such as angiotensin II and atrial natriuretic peptide, for which they have receptors [166,209,233,278]. Contractile activity has been shown in cultured mesangial cells [166,278]. The mesangial cell is an important target cell in many glomerular immune and nonimmune diseases and characteristically responds by injury, repair, and proliferation. In this connection, it is being increasingly recognized that mesangial cells not only respond to a number of growth factors and inflammatory mediators, but also can produce them in an autocrine fashion. These processes are responsible for initiating and sustaining mesangial-cell proliferation following injury [209]. Although not a typical phagocyte, the mesangial cell can endocytose colloids, macromolecules, protein aggregates, and immune complexes and in this fashion clear extraneous material that finds its way into the mesangial matrix from the circulation [96,203,210,211]. It is possible that phagocytosed material may eventually find its way from cell to cell down the mesangial stalk to the vascular pole of the glomerulus [86]. In glomerular disease, the mesangial cell is thought to play a role in the sequestration and disposal of circulating immune complexes.

Mesangial cells are responsible for the production and degradation of the mesangial matrix, which is frequently increased in glomerular disease. The mesangial matrix surrounds the mesangial cells, is looser in texture than the GBM, and has been shown to have a fibrillar structure [218] (see Fig. 1-45). Biochemically, it contains types IV and VI collagen, heparan sulfate proteoglycan, chondroitin sulfate proteoglycan, laminin, and fibronectin [71,121,144,147,150,198,201,210,211, 262,327]. In comparison with the GBM, fibronectin is enriched in the mesangium [71].

TUBULES

Proximal Tubule

The proximal tubule is a heterogeneous structure with three or four cytologically distinct subdivisions, each with different cell types. In the rat, there are three cytologic types, S_1, S_2, and S_3 [204] (Figs. 1-46 and 1-47). The pars convoluta consists of the S_1 portion and the first part of the S_2; transition between the S_2 and S_3 occurs in the pars recta. Cytologic segmentation has not been well studied in the human kidney.

The typical features of proximal tubules [54,55, 87–90,204,313,315] are well developed in the S_1 portion. After first describing this type (Fig. 1-48), we will consider the differences among the three types. The epithelium is tall, and the apical plasma membrane is greatly expanded in the form of closely packed microvilli; these are visible by light microscopy as a brush border. The outer surfaces of the microvilli are covered by a cell coat or glycocalyx [112,265], which stains intensely with the periodic acid–Schiff (PAS) stain (Fig. 1-49). The microvilli expand the apical plasmalemma by a factor of 36 [332], which no doubt provides the anatomic basis for the high rates of reabsorption of a variety of substances by the proximal tubule. Consistent with this function, a number of membrane-bound enzymes and ion and solute transporters are found in the brush-border membrane [60,204]. Viewed by scanning electron microscopy, the apical surfaces of the cells invariably show one or more cilia protruding into the tubular lumen [7,58].

There is also a marked amplification of the basolateral plasma membrane. Viewed en face, proximal tubule cells are seen to interdigitate with each other by means of lateral cytoplasmic protrusions that extend as ridges from the apical surface to the base of the cells. Toward the basal surface, the ridges subdivide in the form of secondary and tertiary processes of progressively smaller size. These processes also interdigitate with their counterparts from adjacent cells; as a result of this unique configuration, the basolateral plasma membrane is amplified by a factor of 36 [331,332] (Fig. 1-50). This expansion of the basolateral membrane, together with the presence in this location of Na^+, K^+, and ATPase [91,160], is consistent with the high rates of active sodium transport shown by proximal tubules. The cells rest on an uninterrupted tubular basement membrane (TBM) that separates the basolateral intercellular

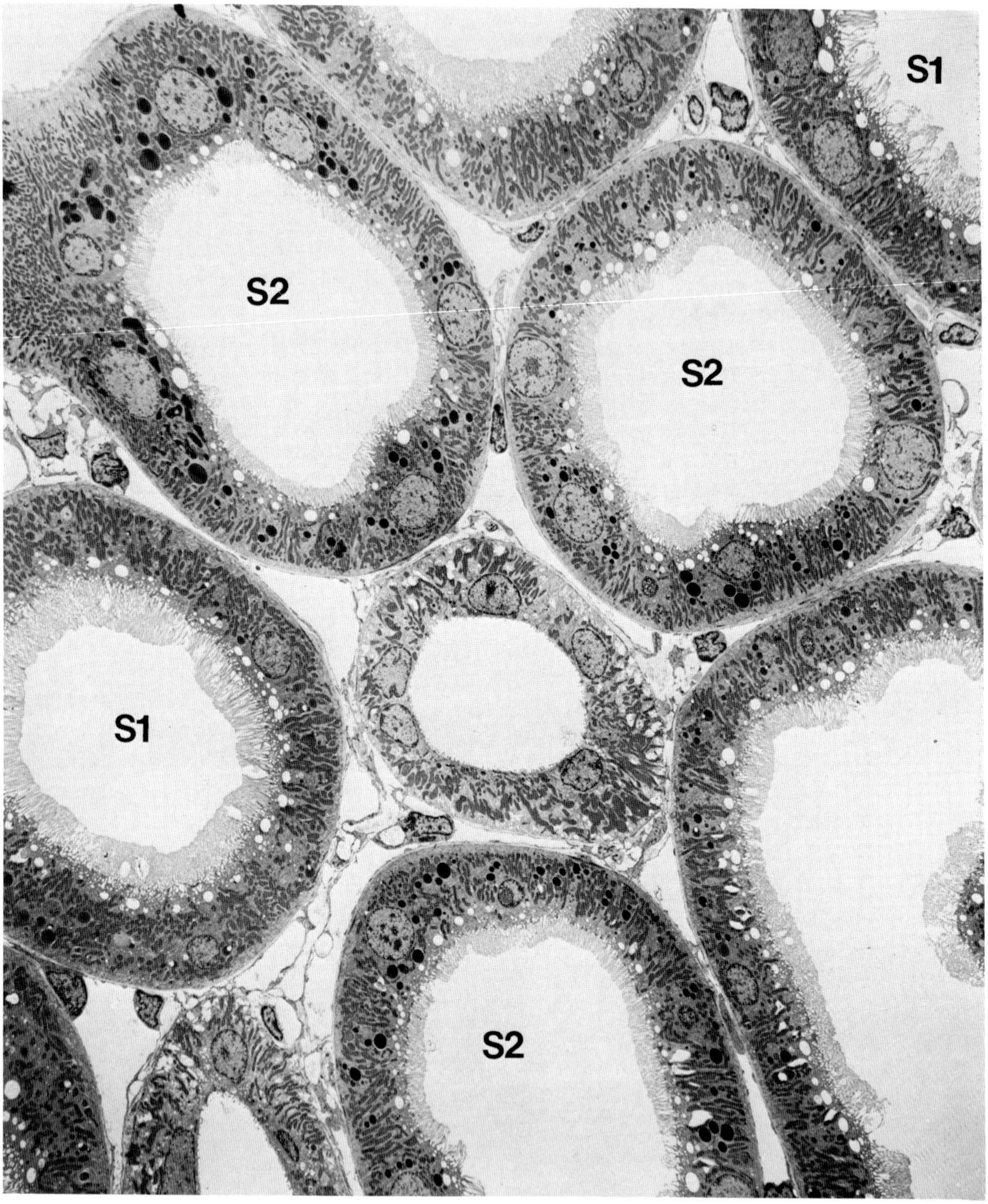

FIG. 1-46. *Electron micrograph of perfusion-fixed rat kidney to demonstrate proximal convoluted tubules. Brush borders are clearly visible and are longer in the S_1 segment than in the S_2 segment. Mitochondria are visible as elongated structures.* × 1968. (*From Maunsbach, A. B.* J. Ultrastruct. Res. *15:242, 1966.*)

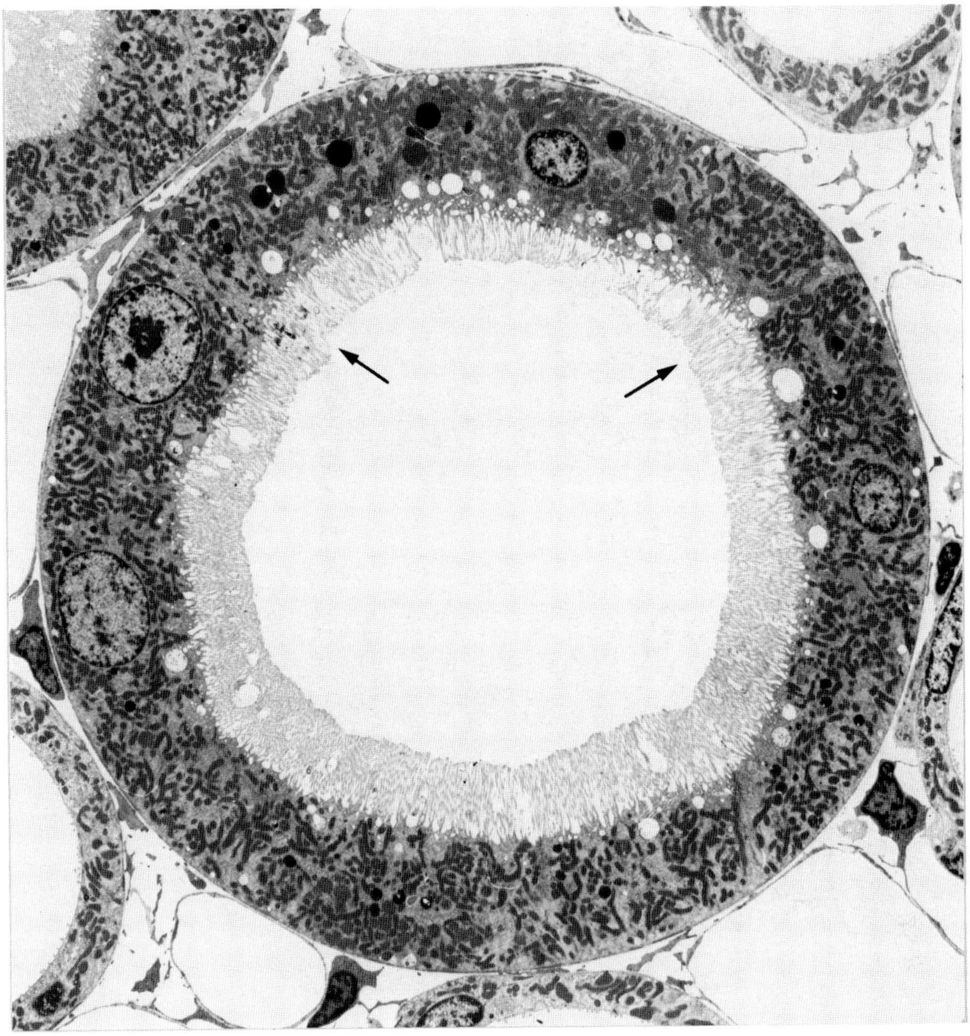

FIG. 1-47. *Cross-sectional profile of a proximal tubule at the transition from S_2 to S_3, rat; electron micrograph. In the upper part of the profile (arrows), the S_2 epithelium is seen; in the lower part, the S_3 epithelium is seen. Note that the brush border in S_3 is higher and more densely arranged. Lysosomal elements are prominent in S_2. × 1900 approx.*

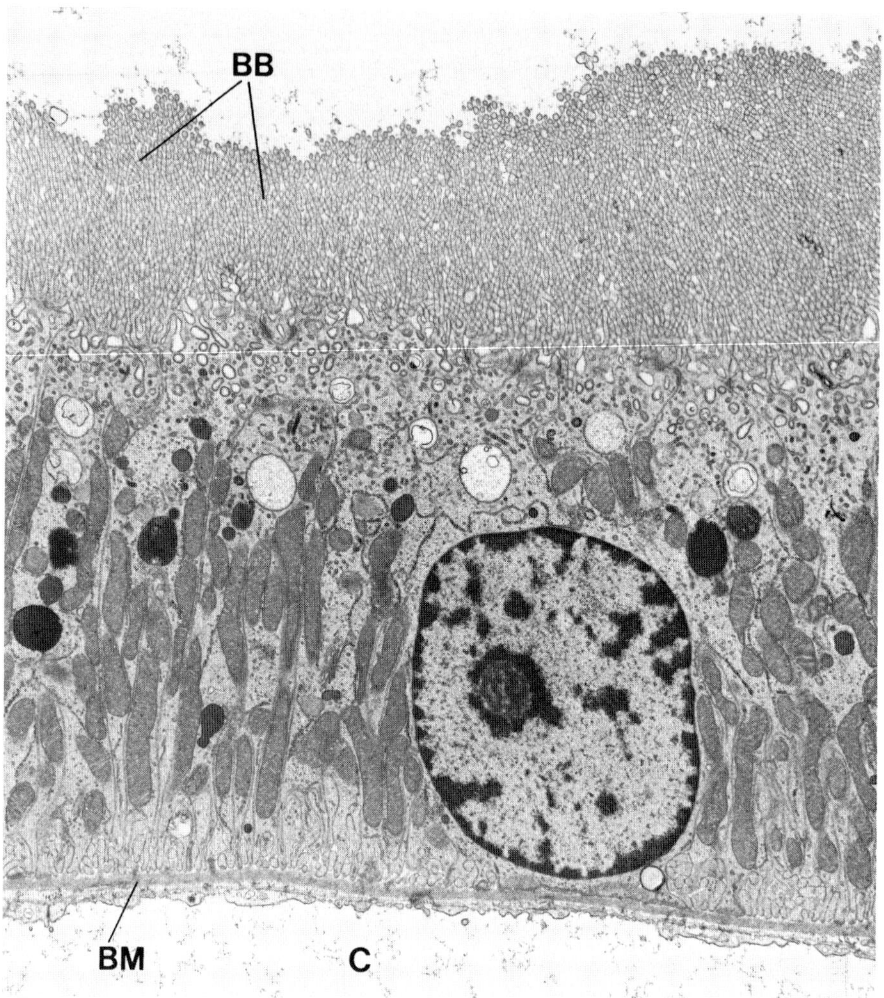

FIG. 1-48. *Proximal tubule epithelium, S_1 of rat kidney; transmission electron micrograph. The apical cytoplasmic zone contains a vacuolar apparatus with many small vesicles and larger lysosomal elements (either light- or dark-staining vacuoles); the latter are also found in deeper parts of the epithelium. Beneath the apical zone, the epithelium is made up of interdigitating cell processes that contain large mitochondria. BB, brush border; BM, basement membrane; C, peritubular capillary.* ×6500 *approx.*

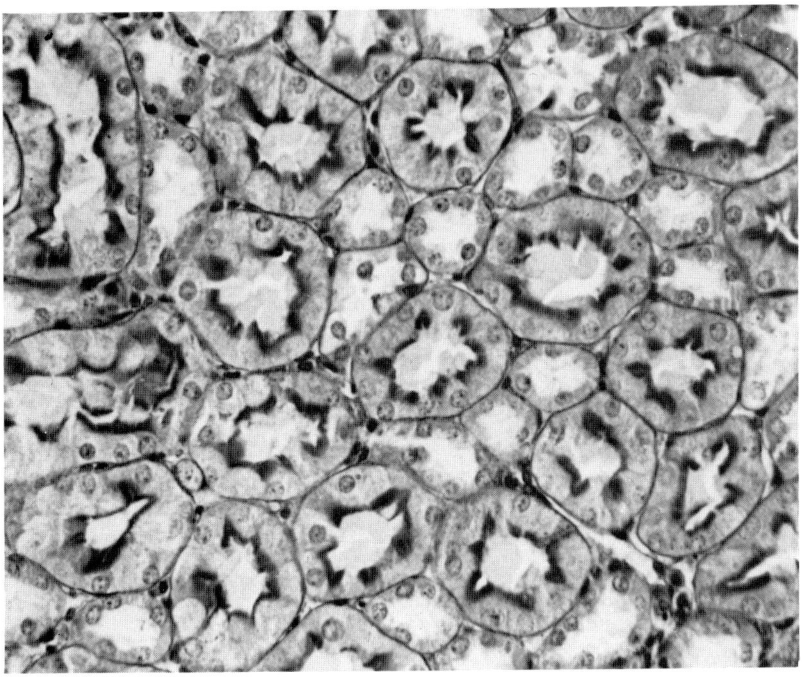

FIG. 1-49. *Periodic acid–Schiff stain of pars recta of proximal convoluted tubule to show brush border staining darker than the rest of the cell. The supporting basement membrane also stains darkly. From a normal rat.* ×400.

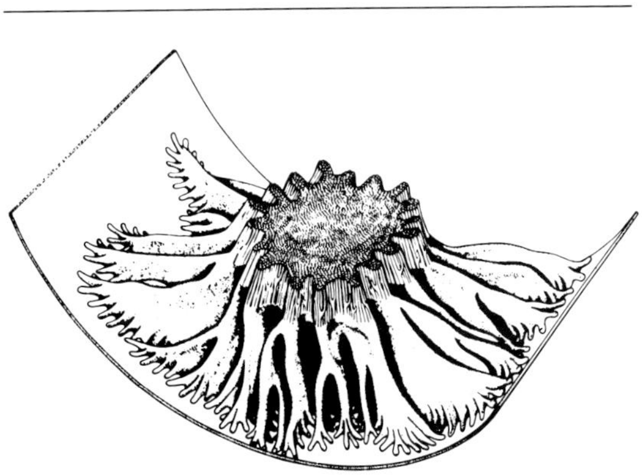

FIG. 1-50. *Three-dimensional model of a rabbit proximal tubule cell. The proximal tubular epithelium is made up of cells with complexly structured lateral cell processes that interdigitate intimately with each other. (From Welling and Welling [332].)*

spaces from the remainder of the renal interstitium.

Junctional complexes between proximal tubule cells consist of tight junctions near the apical surfaces, intermediate junctions immediately below them, and infrequently, desmosomes. The tight junctions are quite shallow in their zones of fusion and by the freeze-fracture technique show only one junctional strand that is often incomplete, consistent with a "leaky" epithelium with high rates of paracellular ion transport [182,261]. There are gap junctions between the lateral membranes, indicating the potential for electrotonic coupling [294].

Proximal tubules of the S_1 type have numerous large and elongated mitochondria that are situated quite close to the plasma membrane, generally within the basolateral cytoplasmic processes [33, 34] (see Fig. 1-48). More apically situated mitochondria are shorter. There is a well-developed Golgi apparatus, abundant rough and smooth endoplasmic reticulum, and numerous free cytoplasmic ribosomes [89,139,204,247,315]. The smooth endoplasmic reticulum is more abundant than the rough variety and includes specialized cisternae situated close to the lateral cell membranes and the mitochondria known as the *paramembranous cisternal system.* Also located in the cytoplasm are numerous peroxisomes or microbodies [26, 143,184] and a dense network of microtubules and other cytoskeletal fibrils.

The microvilli of the proximal tubules reveal a structure analogous to that of their counterparts in the intestine [70,83,265]. They show axial bundles of actin microfilaments that extend into the apical cytoplasm. In addition, they contain a host of associated cytoskeletal proteins, some of which link the actin filaments to the plasma membrane and others of which form a potentially contractile system in the apical cytoplasm and microvilli [70,83]. Distinct cytoskeletal arrangements suggesting actin-myosin–mediated contraction also occur in the basolateral aspects of the cells [319].

In between the basal portions of the microvilli, the apical plasmalemma invaginates inward in the form of an extensive system of pits and tubules; associated with them are numerous membrane-bound vesicles and larger vacuoles (see Fig. 1-48). The cytoplasmic aspects of the apical invaginations and probably the associated cuffs of plasma membrane are "coated" with protein structures typical of clathrin cages [259]. The membranes of the coated pits harbor gp330, one of the Heymann nephritis antigens [260]. Endocytic vesicles, or endosomes, are derived by the pinching of membrane from the coated pits; of note, the endosomes themselves lack clathrin but are lined internally by a material identical to the membrane glycocalyx [204,260]. Fusion of endosomes results in the formation of larger apical vacuoles, which may be as large as 1 to 2 μm in diameter. This system of coated pits, endosomes, and vacuoles forms an apparatus designed to perform the complex task of endocytosis of macromolecules, including proteins such as albumin from the filtrate into the cytoplasm [205,321]. Recent studies have suggested that there is a constant and rapid recycling of the membrane in endosomes back to the plasma membrane [321]. Endosomes and apical vacuoles fuse with primary lysosomes (derived from the Golgi apparatus) and form secondary lysosomes; these are larger, and in them, ingested material is digested by acid hydrolases derived from the primary lysosomes. Secondary lysosomes are bounded by membranes that are approximately 9 nm in thickness and have a variable morphology depending on the stage of digestion and the nature of material ingested. In addition to subserving a role in processing endocytosed material, secondary lysosomes participate in autophagocytosis and, as a consequence, may contain membrane-bound organelles in various stages of digestion. Thus secondary lysosomes may be large and have loose, amorphous material or may appear as smaller, dense bodies with condensed, indigestible material. They also may contain membrane-bound vesicles, myelin figures, or even recognizable organelles. The lysosomal apparatus is highly developed in the proximal tubule and is often the site of pathologic changes in diverse disease states.

Transition of S_1 epithelium to the S_2 occurs gradually and is accompanied by a decrease in structural complexity. In the S_2 segment, cells are flatter, and the microvilli are less numerous and shorter. Lateral interdigitation occurs only toward the base of the cells, and the mitochondria are shorter, less numerous, and more randomly distributed. However, peroxisomes increase in number, and secondary lysosomes are larger, despite a decrease in the number of endocytic vesicles. There are age-, sex-, and species-related variations in proximal tubules with respect to these features [24,67,339].

The S_3 segments have a relatively simple cuboidal shape with little lateral interdigitation or basal infoldings. The mitochondria are small and stubby and are randomly distributed [55]. In many species, such as the rabbit and dog, the height of the brush-border microvilli decreases progressively from S_1 through S_2 to S_3 [55,139]. In the rat, the brush border is tallest in S_3 (see Fig. 1-47). Interspecies differences are also seen in S_3 tight-junction architecture [261]. S_3 segments have the largest numbers of peroxisomes, the most abundant smooth endoplasmic reticulum, and the least developed endocytic apparatus. However, secondary lysosomes may be larger and more numerous than in S_1.

There are no differences among superficial, midcortical, and juxtamedullary nephrons with respect to cytologic segmentation of the proximal tubule. The S_1 segments are concentrated in the cortical labyrinth, whereas the S_2 segments are located partly in the cortical labyrinth and partly in the medullary rays. S_3 segments are present only in the medullary rays and in the outer stripe of the outer medulla. The S_1 segments in the cortical labyrinth are supplied by a rich anastomosing network of capillaries. In contrast, the capillary plexus around S_2 and S_3 segments is less well developed. In the basal parts of the medullary rays and in the outer stripe, S_3 segments are supplied predominantly by venous blood from the ascending vasa recta.

Thin Limbs of Henle

At the junction of the outer and inner stripes of the outer medulla, the proximal tubule gives rise to the descending thin limb and undergoes sharp transition to a flat type of epithelium devoid of a brush border. Cytologically, different types of epithelium may be distinguished in the thin limbs. There are many interspecies variations. In that the cytologic types of thin-limb epithelium may provide a basis for an understanding of how thin limbs participate in urine concentration, we provide a description of thin-limb epithelial structure in the rat, a species like other rodents with a high ability to concentrate urine. Pertinent differences seen in the rabbit, whose ability to concentrate urine is less than that of the rat, are also outlined [50,80,92,139,180,276,288,289]. Although the basic architecture of human thin limbs has been described [59], the information is scant and less reliable than that gleaned from studies in lower animals. For structure-function correlations and discussion of this complex subject, the reader is referred to other sources [60,131,139,168,169, 176,195].

In the rat, there are four types of thin-limb segments. They occur in the descending thin limbs of short loops, the upper portions of the descending thin limbs of long loops, the lower portions of the descending thin limbs of long loops, and the ascending thin limbs of long loops (Fig. 1-51).

Descending thin limbs of short loops represent the first type. They have a very simple, flat type of epithelium with no interdigitations among cells along their lateral borders (Fig. 1-52). There are few microvilli on their luminal surfaces, the plasma membranes have sparse intramembranous particles, and the interceullar tight junctions are deep, with multiple junctional strands and zones of membrane fusion. This type of epithelium is thought to be poorly permeable to solutes and may permit osmotic abstraction of water from the tubule lumen. In contrast, the upper parts of the descending thin limbs in long loops, which are of the second type, have a thicker epithelium that is quite complex in its configuration. The cells interdigitate with one another laterally, the tight junctions are shallow and "leaky" with only one junctional strand and zone of membrane fusion, and there are more numerous microvilli on the luminal surface. The basolateral plasma membranes are expanded owing to infoldings and cellular interdigitation. These characteristics result in a great expansion of the basolateral space to form an extracellular basal labyrinth (Fig. 1-53). Exclusively among the thin-limb types, this cell type has more numerous mitochondria and a high density of intramembranous particles in the luminal and basolateral membranes and, in addition, shows the presence of Na^+, K^+, ATPase, and carbonic anhydrase [50,92,139,276,288]. These characteristics suggest that the upper parts of the descending thin limbs of long loops are capable of active transport. As this nephron segment descends farther into the inner medulla, the epithelium becomes flatter and less complex while retaining its fundamental properties. At variable distances in the inner medulla, this epithelium undergoes an abrupt transition to a third type.

The epithelium of the third type is simple and flat and of the nature already described for descending thin limbs of short loops (Fig. 1-54). Therefore, functional properties of descending thin limbs of short loops and the lower portions of descending thin limbs of long loops may be expected to be similar. Shortly before the bend of

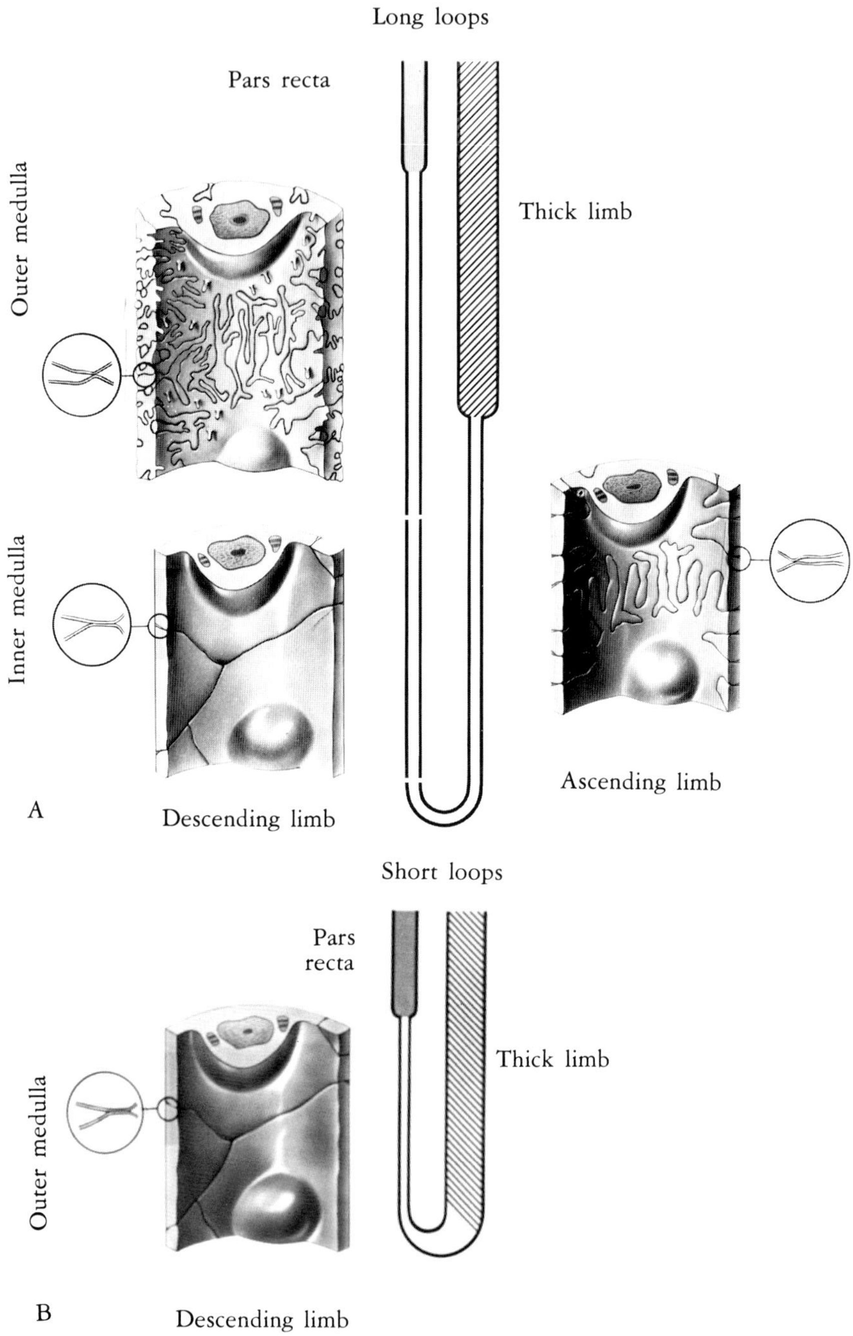
Long loops
Pars recta
Thick limb
Outer medulla
Inner medulla
Ascending limb
A
Descending limb
Short loops
Pars
recta
Thick limb
Outer medulla
B
Descending limb

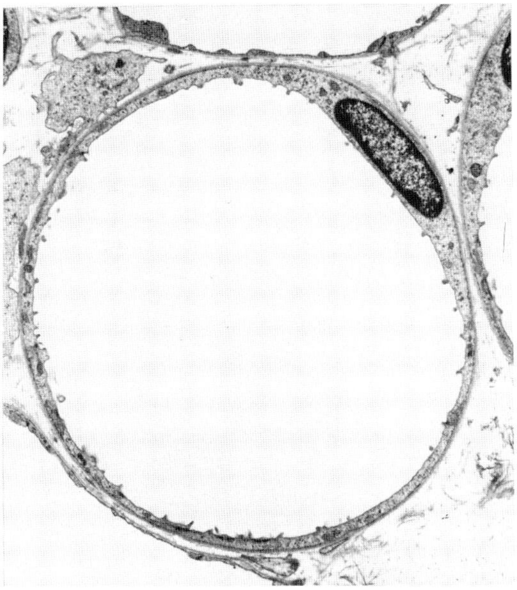

Fig. 1-52. *Cross-sectional profile of a thin descending limb of a short loop of Henle; rat. The simplicity of the epithelium is obvious.* ×4000 *approx.*

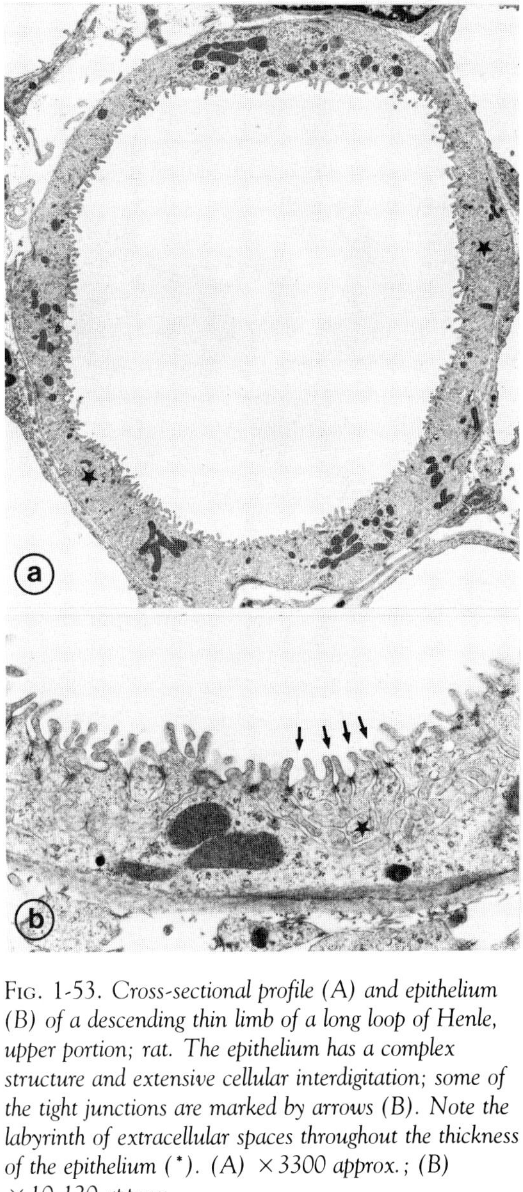

Fig. 1-53. *Cross-sectional profile (A) and epithelium (B) of a descending thin limb of a long loop of Henle, upper portion; rat. The epithelium has a complex structure and extensive cellular interdigitation; some of the tight junctions are marked by arrows (B). Note the labyrinth of extracellular spaces throughout the thickness of the epithelium (*). (A)* ×3300 *approx.; (B)* ×10,120 *approx.*

◄

Fig. 1-51. A, B. *Diagrammatic representation of thin limb structure in long and short loops showing the occurrence of the basic types in various segments and the morphology of occluding junctions (insets). The shapes of the constituent cells have been deduced from the electron microscopic images. Descending thin limbs of short loops (type 1) have simple, flat epithelium with deep tight junctions and extensive zones of membrane fusion. The upper parts of descending thin limbs in long loops (type 2) have complex epithelium with extensive lateral interdigitations with neighboring cells and shallow tight junctions. This type undergoes transition to an epithelium (type 3) very similar to that of descending thin limbs of short loops at variable distances along the upper half of the inner medulla. Just before the bend, this epithelium undergoes transition to yet another type, which characterizes the ascending thin limbs (type 4). This last type has lateral interdigitations with adjacent cells and shallow tight junctions. (Modified from Schwartz and Venkatachalam [289].)*

Henle's loops, the epithelium changes once more, to the fourth type found in the ascending thin limbs of Henle. The cells are very flat, and they interdigitate extensively with each other, although less than in the upper parts of the descending limbs of long loops (see Fig. 1-54). The tight junctions are shallow, with only one junctional strand and zone of membrane fusion, and plasma membranes have relatively sparse intramembranous particles. The basolateral spaces are of simple configuration, and the plasma membranes that bound the lateral spaces diverge from apex to base. By morphologic criteria, the epithelium is considered "leaky," and functional studies confirm this; however, they also indicate a high degree of impermeability to water, which must mean that both the tight junctions and plasma membranes impede water flow. The structural or molecular basis for this strikingly different passive permeability to water and ions remains to be unraveled.

The main difference in thin-limb epithelia between the rat, an efficient urine concentrator, and the rabbit, which concentrates urine to a lesser extent, is in the morphology of the upper parts of the thin limbs of the long loops. In this segment of the rabbit, the cells do not interdigitate, lack a prominent paracellular pathway, and have deeper tight junctions with multiple junctional strands and zones of fusion. However, the luminal microvilli are prominent, the plasma membranes are packed with intramembranous particles, and there are basal infoldings of the plasma membrane (as in rodents). The morphology of the tight junctions may explain functional studies that have shown relative solute impermeability in this segment of rabbit Henle's loops.

Although not well-studied, human thin limbs are probably similar to those of the lower animals. Concerning the upper part of the long descending thin limbs, the published data do not allow a final conclusion. In an older investigation of the human kidney [59] that was done at a time when it was not yet known that there are generally four different thin-limb epithelia, the epithelium of the descending thin limbs was described as being simply structured, but a picture of a thin limb was shown that had an interdigitating epithelium similar to that found in the rat.

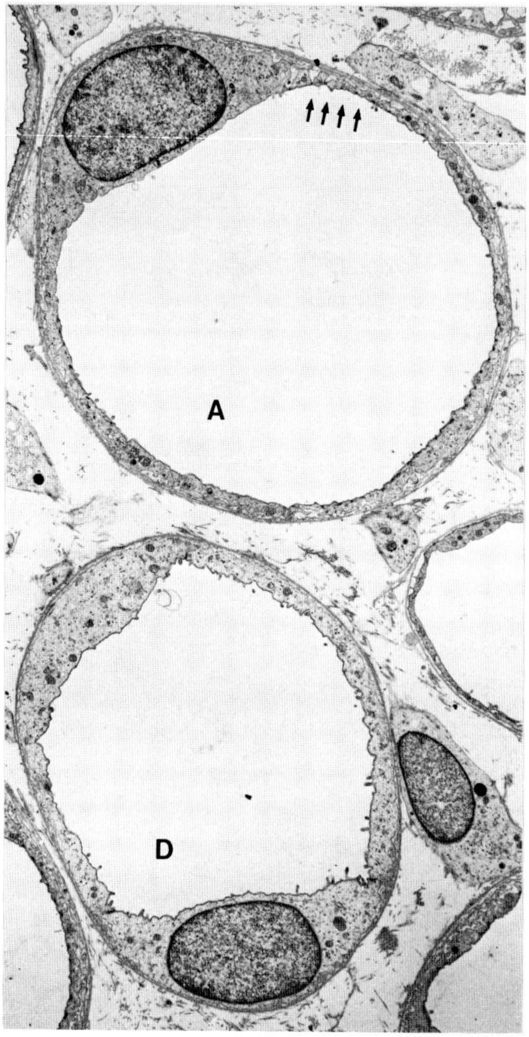

FIG. 1-54. *Cross-sectional profiles of a thin descending limb (D) and of a thin ascending limb (A) in the inner medulla; rabbit. The epithelium of the lower portion of the descending limb is simply structured, whereas the epithelium of the ascending thin limb is made of extensively interdigitating cells. Some of the shallow junctions between the cell profiles are marked by arrows. ×2600 approx.*

Distal Straight Tubule (Thick Ascending Limb of Henle's Loop)

This nephron segment takes its origin at the junction of the outer and inner medulla and terminates in the cortex shortly beyond the macula densa [139,237]. Transition between the thin limb and thick limb is gradual in the canine and human kidney [55,59] but sharp in the rat kidney. In short loops, transition from thin to thick segment occurs anywhere in the vicinity of the bend. As would be expected from their location, distal straight tubules of juxtamedullary nephrons have shorter cortical portions than those of more superficial nephrons [167,177]. Epithelium in the distal straight tubules of short loops is thicker than in the long loops [139]. The structure of the epithelium is without significant differences among species and has been well described on several occasions [4,12,54,55,58,139,164,316,333].

The epithelium is made up of tall cells that interdigitate with each other by means of basolateral cell processes. The interdigitated part of the epithelium comprises about three-quarters of the cell height. Therefore, viewed from the apical site, the cells are polygonal and lack interdigitations. The lateral cell processes harbor elongated mitochondria arranged regularly and perpendicularly to the basement membrane (Fig. 1-55). The cytoplasmic processes that contain the mitochondria subdivide into finer ramifications close to the basal lamina. Tight junctions between cells are of intermediate depth (i.e., between the "leaky" proximal tubule and the "tight" collecting duct) with several parallel and narrowly arranged junctional strands and zones of membrane fusion [277]. The cells have their usual complement of other organelles. Cell height decreases gradually from the inner-stripe portion of the thick limb to the outer stripe and the cortex. This occurs as a result of a decrease in the mass of the apical cytoplasm. Concurrently, there is amplification of the lateral surface area, because the basolateral cell processes extend up to the lumen. This results in a decrease in the ratio of mitochondrial mass to membrane surface area and expansion of the extent of the paracellular pathway.

The distal straight tubule is rich in Na^+-K^+-ATPase activity [92,104,155], which provides the energy for the reabsorption of sodium chloride by a Na^+-K^+-$2Cl^-$ cotransporter-mediated mechanism [60,110]. Na^+-K^+-ATPase activity—as well as net transport—declines concurrently with the morphologic changes undergone by the epithelium as the tubule courses toward the cortex. By scanning electron microscopy, the cells appear as two morphologic types judged by the configuration of the luminal membrane [4]. One type, with smooth luminal membrane, predominates in the inner stripe. The other type, with numerous stubby microvilli, appears in greater numbers toward the cortex. The smooth-surfaced cells are particularly rich in distinctive cytoplasmic vesicles and tubulovesicular profiles located near the luminal membrane. The significance of these morphologic types is unknown. The distal straight tubule is the site of production of Tamm-Horsfall glycoprotein (Fig. 1-56), the most abundant constituent of renal tubule casts that are shed in the urine in diverse diseases [10,122,293].

The macula densa, a plaque of specialized cells contained within the distal straight tubule at its point of contact with the vascular pole of the glomerulus (Fig. 1-57), will be described under Juxtaglomerular Apparatus.

Distal Convoluted Tubule, Connecting Tubules, and Cortical Collecting Duct: Problems of Definition and Terminology

Considerable difficulties are encountered in delineating these nephron segments anatomically and correlating the anatomic definitions with the occurrence of distinctive cell types unique to the segments. This is so because of variations in the distribution of diverse cell types in different segments, their intermingling within the same segment, and indistinct transition zones.

The distal convoluted tubule defines a nephron segment that begins shortly after the distal straight tubule makes contact with the vascular pole of the parent glomerulus (see Fig. 1-57) and terminates imperceptibly in a transitional nephron segment, the connecting tubule. Equally unobtrusively, the

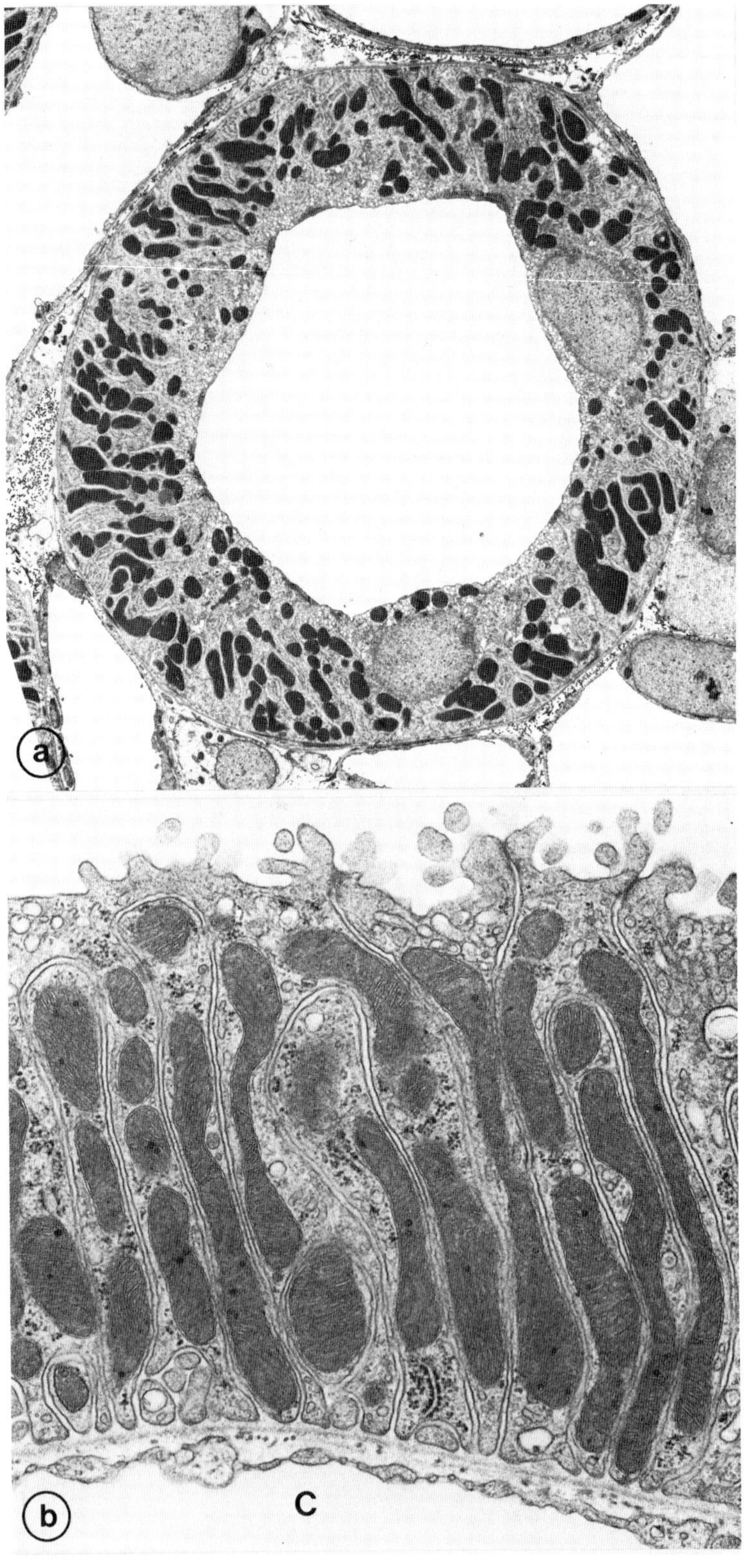

FIG. 1-55. *Thick ascending limb (distal straight tubule): (A) cross-sectional profile and (B) longitudinal section through the epithelium of the medullary part; rat. The epithelium is made up of cells that interdigitate with their neighbors (very similar to the interdigitation in the proximal tubule). The cell processes are filled with large mitochondria. Beneath the luminal cell membrane there are membrane-bound vacuoles. The luminal cell membrane bears some short, stubby microvilli. C, capillary. (A) ×2800 approx.; (B) ×16,000 approx.*

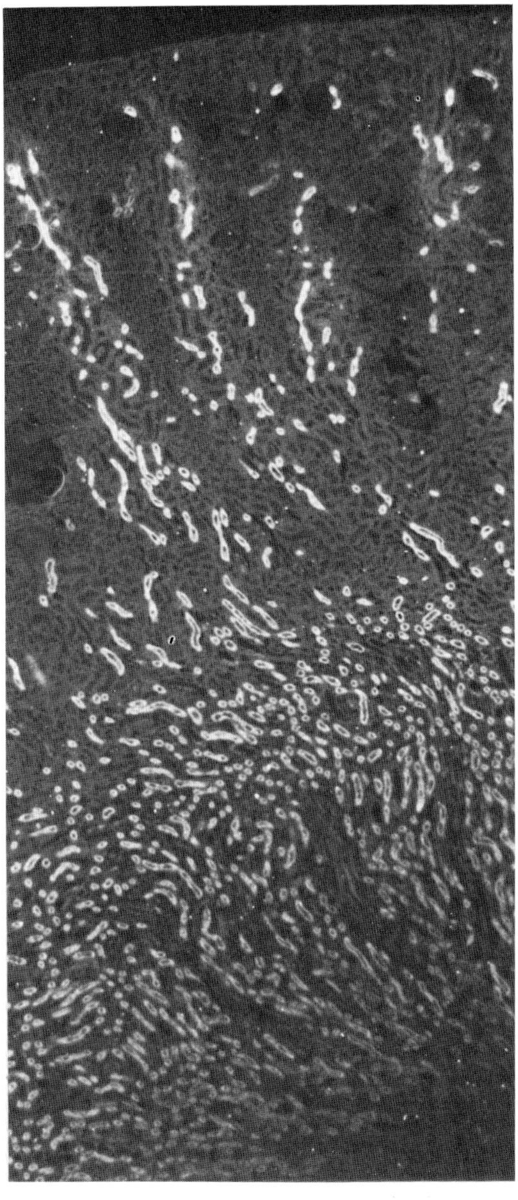

FIG. 1-56. *Low-magnification immunofluorescence micrograph showing the distribution of Tamm-Horsfall protein in the kidney. Thick ascending limbs of Henle (distal straight tubules) in the outer medulla are intensely reactive with a polyclonal antibody against the protein. In the cortex, toward the top, thick limbs in the medullary rays are also reactive. (Courtesy of S. Bachman, Heidelberg.)*

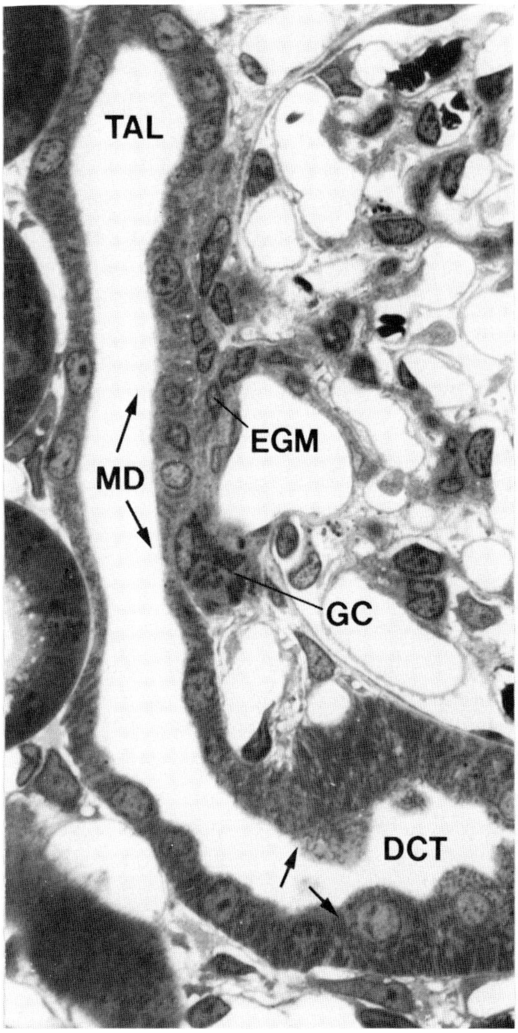

FIG. 1-57. *Transition of the thick ascending limb (TAL) into the convoluted part of the distal convoluted tubule (DCT); rat. The terminal portion of the thick ascending limb contains the macula densa (MD), which is attached to the vascular pole of the parent glomerulus. Shortly after this attachment, the transition to the convoluted part of the distal tubule is seen by the abrupt enlargement of the epithelial height (arrows). EGM, extraglomerular mesangium; GC, granular cells in the afferent arteriole × 1100 approx. (Courtesy B. Kaissling, Zurich.)*

connecting tubule terminates in the cortical collecting duct. There are four cell types in these three different segments that may be intermingled in patterns that show great variability among species. The four cell types are (1) the distal convoluted tubule cell, (2) the connecting tubule cell, (3) the principal cell or collecting duct cell, and (4) the intercalated cell. The specific patterns of distribution and the precise delineation of the three segments in individual species are of relevance to the interpretation of physiologic studies by micropuncture or microperfusion of tubules but will be ignored in the context of the purpose of this book. Only the characteristics of the specific cell types and the general pattern of their distribution will be outlined. The interested reader is referred to other sources that consider these issues [55,72,111,137–139,173,175,176,221,300,316].

Distal Convoluted Tubule

There is an abrupt increase of the height of epithelium at the point where this segment originates from the distal straight tubule [142,237] (see Fig. 1-57). The epithelium is homogeneously composed of one cell type, the distal convoluted tubule cell; in the terminal portion of this segment, intercalated cells may be found mixed up with distal convoluted tubule cells. The latter bear some resemblance to cells in the medullary part of the distal straight tubule (or thick ascending limb). They are characterized by extensive formation of lateral cell processes that interdigitate intimately with those of neighboring cells and extend over roughly two-thirds of the epithelial height. These processes account for a many-fold (20× in rabbit) amplification of the basolateral membrane. The cytoplasmic compartments of these interdigitating cell processes are occupied by elongated mitochondria that are situated close to the plasma membranes. The apical portion of the cytoplasm also has numerous shorter and randomly distributed mitochondria. The nucleus of the cell is characteristically located in the apical half of the cell, above the system of vertically oriented mitochondria (Fig. 1-58). Although the basal portions of the cells interdigitate with their neighbors, the cell outlines are polygonal on the luminal aspect

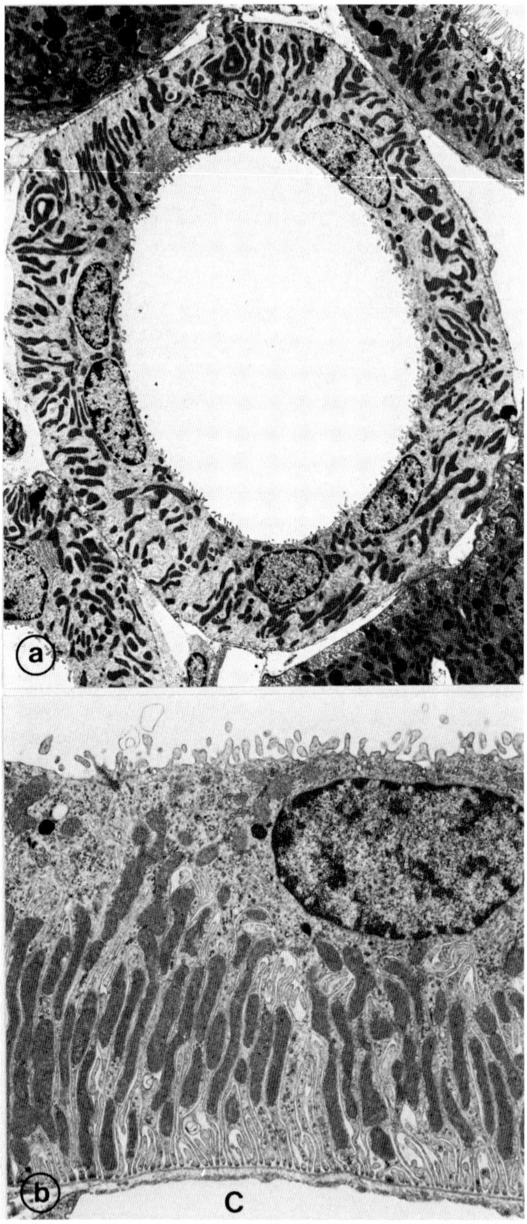

FIG. 1-58. *Distal convoluted tubule; rat. (A) Cross-sectional profile. (B) Longitudinal section through the epithelium. The epithelium is similarly structured as that of the distal straight tubule in the medulla. The nuclei are typically located in the apical region of the epithelium. In (B), the heavily interdigitating cell processes filled with mitochondria are seen. C, capillary. (A) ×19,400 approx.; (B) ×7000 approx.*

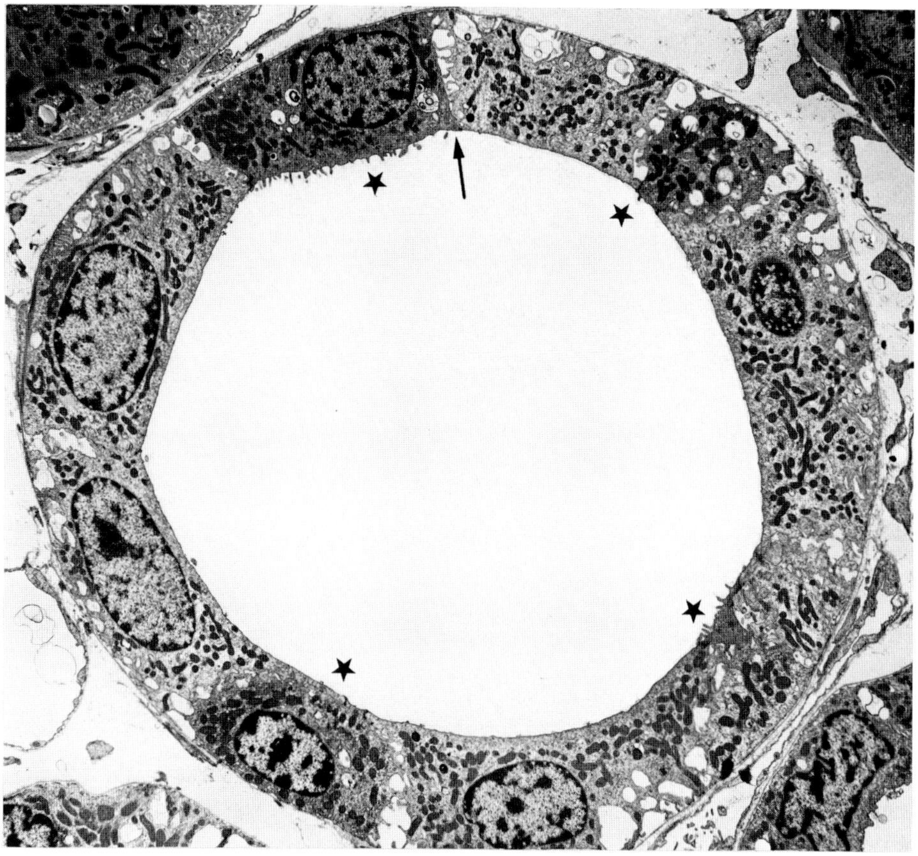

FIG. 1-59. *Cortical collecting duct, cross-sectional profile; rat. The epithelium is heterogeneously composed of collecting duct cells (principal cells) and intercalated cells (asterisks). The cells do not interdigitate with each other; in contrast, the lateral intercellular spaces are prominent (arrow) ×2800 approx. (From Kaissling and Kriz [139].)*

and lack lateral protrusions. The luminal membrane has short and stubby microvilli, and the cytoplasm immediately below the luminal plasmalemma contains numerous distinctive vesicles of unknown function. Tight junctions are of intermediate depth (~0.3 μm), indicating a potential paracellular pathway for the transport of solutes. Na^+-K^+-ATPase activity, located in the basolateral membranes, is the highest among all nephron segments [91,104,155,179] and is responsible for the transport of sodium chloride.

A vitamin D–dependent calcium-binding protein is present in the apical portion of the cells [266]. Tamm-Horsfall protein has been described to occur in the apical membrane of the human distal convoluted tubule [293], but not in the rat [122]. Intercalated cells (to be described later under Collecting Ducts) may be found in the second part of the distal convoluted tubule [111,316].

Connecting Tubule

This segment consists of connecting-tubule cells and intercalated cells. Connecting tubule cells

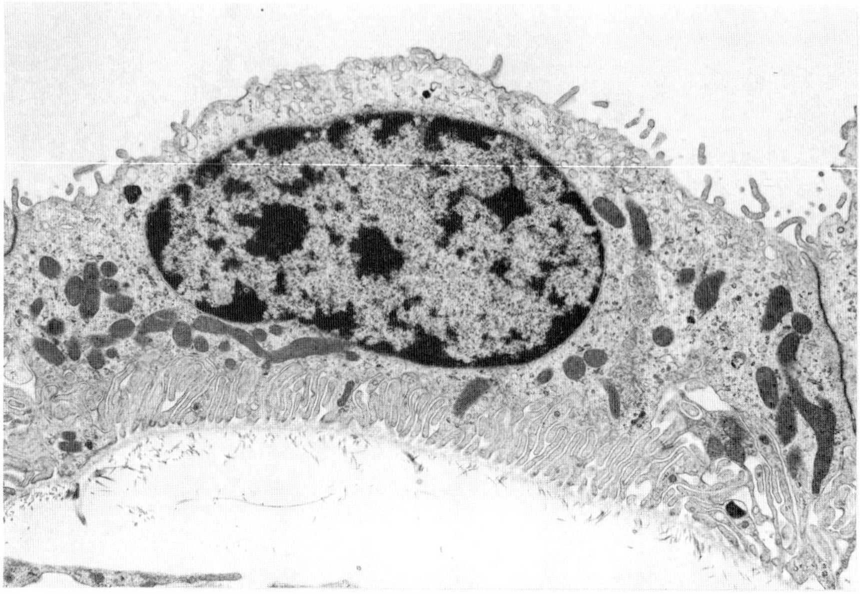

FIG. 1-60. *Cortical collecting duct, collecting duct cell (principal cell); rabbit. Note the characteristic basal labyrinth that is established by short basal infoldings. The cellular folds at this site generally do not contain mitochondria.* ×8000 *approx.*

have been defined as distinct entities with similarities and dissimilarities to distal convoluted tubule cells and to collecting duct cells in the rabbit [136,139], but are less easily distinguishable in other species, including man [175].

Collecting Ducts

Collecting ducts are composed of two cell types, principal cells (collecting duct cells) and intercalated cells (Fig. 1-59). Principal cells are found in all collecting ducts from the cortex to the inner medulla. Intercalated cells are found mostly in the cortical and outer medullary collecting ducts, and progressively decrease in number in the inner medulla. Along the middle and lower thirds of the inner medulla, they are totally absent. The ratio of intercalated cells to principal cells varies between species and in different segments of the collecting ducts. Furthermore, the morphology of the cell types shows subtle variations between different segments.

THE PRINCIPAL CELL (COLLECTING DUCT CELL)

The basic architecture of this type has been well described [139,191,221,330] (Fig. 1-60). The cell has a polygonal outline on its luminal aspect with no lateral interdigitations between cells. The basal surface shows numerous, regularly spaced basal infoldings arranged perpendicular to the basement membrane and extending up to the lower quarter or third of the height of the cell. There are no organelles in the cytoplasm within the folds. Mitochondria are few in number and are arrayed above the basal infolds; other major cell organelles show no special features. The luminal membrane shows a few short, stubby microvilli and a single cilium. Below the luminal membrane, there is a tight network of microfilaments and microtubules. The apical cytoplasm also contains many membrane-bound tubulovesicular profiles (Figs. 1-60 and 1-61). Laterally, the cells show narrow folds of cytoplasm that extend into the intercellular spaces and interlock with counterparts from adja-

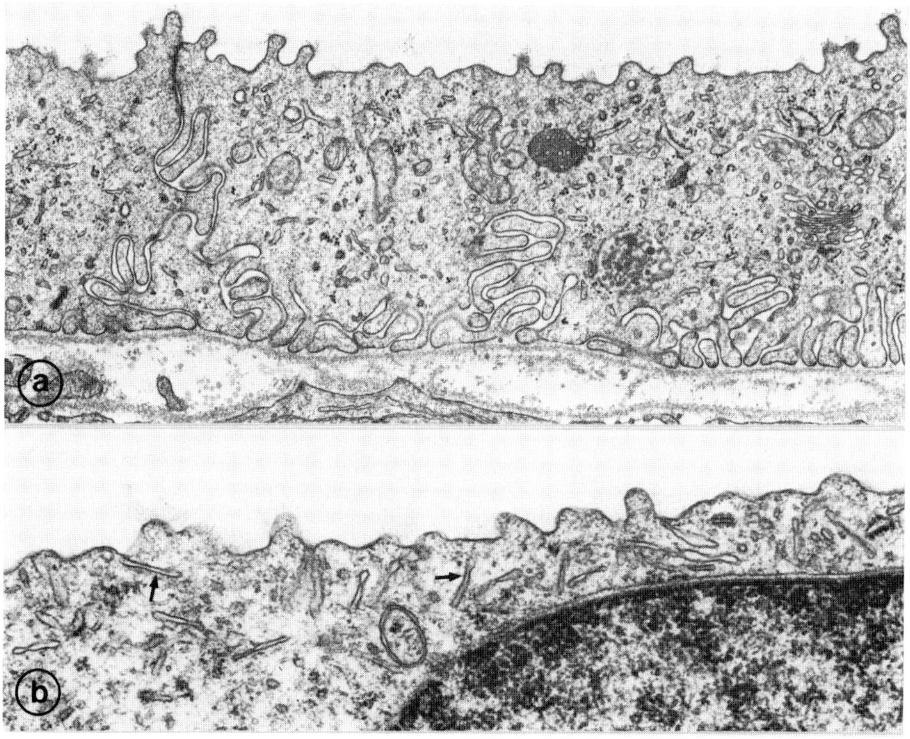

FIG. 1-61. *Epithelium of the inner medullary collecting duct (middle portion); rat. Within the epithelium, three zones may be described: a basal zone with basal infoldings; a middle zone containing profiles of Golgi apparatuses, mitochondria, and lysosomal elements; and a thin apical zone with tubular and vesicular profiles. In (B), the apical zone with many elongated tubular profiles (arrows) is shown. The membranes of these tubulovesicular profiles carry the water channels. Note the deep tight junction in (A). (A) ×14,000 approx.; (B) ×28,500 approx.*

cent cells. In these regions, adjacent cells are held together by numerous desmosomes [11,139]. Tight junctions between cells are deep—of the "tight" variety—(see Fig. 1-61) and show several anastomosing strands and zones of membrane fusion [182,245,273]. Under the influence of vasopressin, the water permeability of the luminal membrane is increased, and consequently, bulk flow of water across the basolateral membrane is also increased. Under these conditions, the lateral intracellular spaces have been shown to be enlarged [103,108,317,336] (see Fig. 1-59).

The structural and molecular basis for vasopressin-induced increase of water permeability has been investigated [46]. By the freeze-fracture technique, the luminal membrane shows patches of intramembranous particles. These particles are believed to be water channels. Vasopressin control of water permeability is achieved by rapid recycling of channels between intracellular vesicles and the apical plasma membrane. The endocytotic phase of recycling is mediated by clathrin-coated vesicles [46,324,325]. The clinical relevance of these exciting developments is suggested by the specific lack of intramembranous particle clusters in collecting ducts of mice with nephrogenic diabetes insipidus regardless of whether vasopressin is administered or not [51]. The principal cell also has an important salt-transporting function. This is reflected in the presence of Na^+-K^+-ATPase in the basolateral membrane and in the considerable amplification that this membrane undergoes in response to the state of salt balance (particularly K^+) and circulating mineralocorticoid levels [104,141,193,300,329].

The basal labyrinth of the principal cell undergoes progressive simplification from the cortex to the inner medulla, with a steep reduction occurring in the outer stripe [136,139,221]. Concurrently, cell organelles decrease in number, but the depth of the tight junctions increases. Toward the papillary tip, however, the depth of the tight junctions begins to decrease again, and the junction becomes "leakier" [275,318]. Although the basal labyrinth is sparsely developed in the inner medulla, the cell size increases substantially, and the cells look tall and columnar in the papillary collecting ducts of Bellini [139,221] (Fig. 1-62).

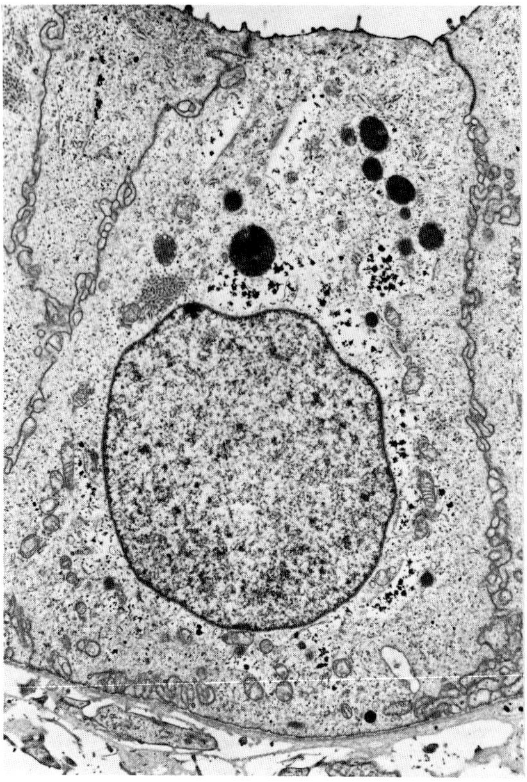

FIG. 1-62. *A papillary collecting duct cell of a human kidney. Longitudinal section through the epithelium. The epithelium is homogeneously composed of tall collecting duct cells.* ×*4500 approx.*

THE INTERCALATED CELL

The ratio of intercalated cells to principal cells in the cortical collecting duct is approximately 2 : 3 in the rat and rabbit [72,139,191,300]. Intercalated cells have a simple polygonal shape or may be rounded without lateral interdigitations; some basal infolds may be present. They have a dark cytoplasm, and in addition to the usual complement of organelles, including well-developed Golgi apparatuses and smooth endoplasmic reticulum, they possess numerous dark-staining mitochondria (Figs. 1-59 and 1-63). In the apical cytoplasm, numerous distinctive vesicles, tubulovesicular profiles, and flat cisternae are found (Fig. 1-64), whose membranes, as well as the apical plasma membranes, show numerous stud-shaped objects protruding into the cytoplasm [111,302] (see Fig. 1-64). By freeze-fracture techniques, both membranes show numerous arrays of densely arranged rod-shaped particles [124,302] (see Fig. 1-64). The luminal membrane has a prominent glycocalyx that has an affinity for cationic stains and, in the B subtype of rabbit intercalated cells, for peanut lectin [111,192,194]. By scanning electron microscopy, the luminal membrane shows a variable appearance [7,58,113,114,191] (Fig. 1-65). In some cells, there are numerous microplicae and microvilli; these particular cells have few vesicles and membrane profiles in their apical cytoplasm. Others have relatively few microplicae and microvilli, but numerous membrane-bound profiles are present in the apical cytoplasm. Yet others may present only a small fraction of their surface to the lumen, the larger part of their luminal surfaces being covered by adjacent cells. These "sunken" cells may be cells with opposite polarity in which tubulovesicular profiles and vesicles are found at the base. Considerable variability in morphologic appearance is encountered

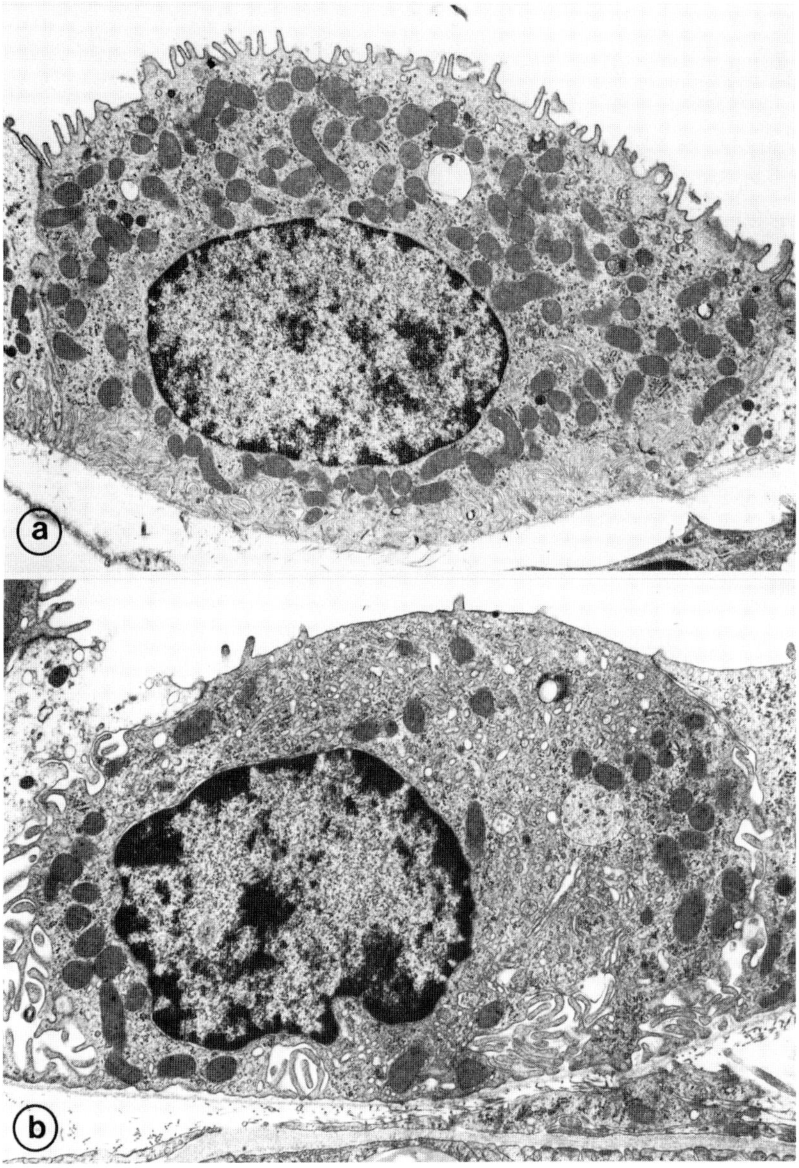

Fig. 1-63. *Cortical intercalated cells; rat. Two types are distinguished; The A type (A) contains luminal microfolds and a dense assembly of mitochondria predominantly in the apical cytoplasm. The B type (B) has a smooth luminal surface with few microvilli. The cytoplasm is densely filled with small vesicles reaching down to the basal aspect of the cell. Mitochondria are predominantly found in the lateral and basal parts of the cell. (A) ×7500 approx.; (B) ×9000 approx.*

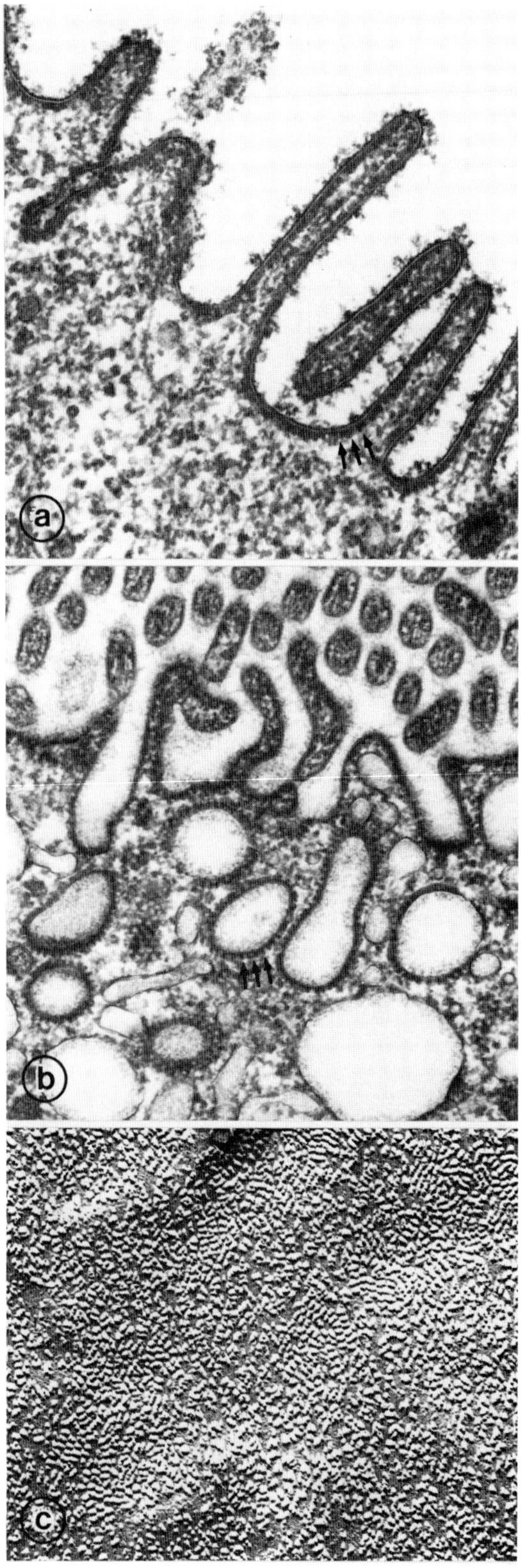

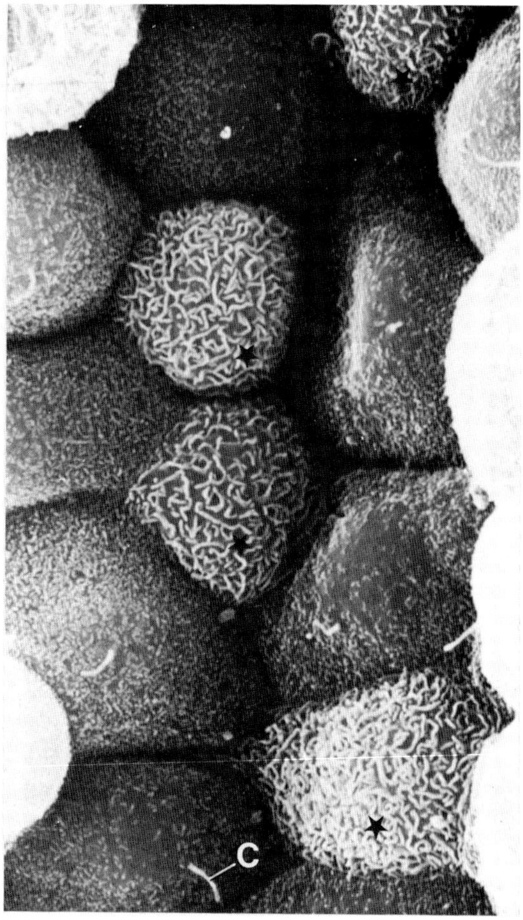

FIG. 1-65. *Scanning electron micrograph of a cortical collecting duct (rat) showing the luminal aspect of collecting duct cells and intercalated cells (stars), characteristically adorned by microfolds. The microfolds represent an amplification of the membrane. C, cilium on a collecting duct cell. ×6000 approx.*

FIG. 1-64. *Intercalated cell, type A; rat. (A) The luminal cell membrane is shown characteristically covered on its cytoplasmic side by "studs" (arrows). (B) Studs are also found on tubulovesicular profiles located in the apical cytoplasm. (C) In freeze-fracture replicas of the luminal membrane, characteristic rod-shaped particles are encountered that are generally believed to correspond to the studs seen in transmission electron microscopy. (A) ×58,000 approx.; (B) ×41,000 approx.; (C) ×54,000 approx.*

both between species and between different segments of the collecting duct system. Dramatic variations also can be accounted for by differences in mineralocorticoid status, salt and water balance, and acid-base balance. These apparently inexplicable and paradoxical observations are explained by the recent discovery that studs on the membrane-bound vesicles, flat cisternae, and plasma membrane represent the cytoplasmic portions of an H^+ ATPase responsible for proton secretion.

Two types of intercalated cells are presently distinguished based on the occurrence of the H^+ ATPase in the luminal or basolateral membrane (Fig. 1-66). The A type houses the proton pump in the luminal membrane and is responsible for proton secretion; the basolateral membrane of the A type contains an HCO_3^-/Cl^- exchanger known as the band 3 protein from red blood cells. The B type exhibits the H^+ ATPase in the basolateral membrane and is responsible for HCO_3^- secretion. The variability in the structural appearances of intercalated cells is complicated in that both types may be found in an active or an inactive state. In the active state, the proton pumps are largely incorporated into the respective plasma membranes; in the "inactive" (less active) state, the H^+ transporters are stored in the cytoplasm, within the membranes of the tubulovesicular profiles. In response to demand, the H^+ ATPase is shuttled back and forth from either the luminal or the basolateral membrane in vesicular form, changing the activity of the cells. Indeed, it has even been suggested that there is only one intercalated cell and that, depending on the metabolic status, cells may reverse polarity, cycling the pro-

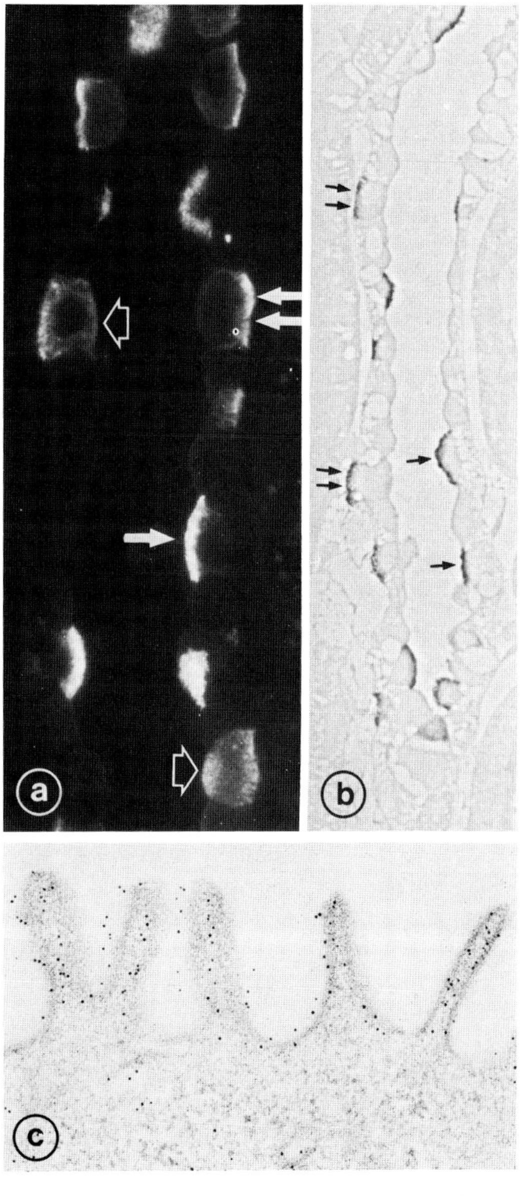

FIG. 1-66. *Immunocytochemical demonstration of the location of the proton pump in cortical intercalated cells; rat. (A) Semithin Epon-embedded section of rat renal cortex stained with affinity-purified antibodies against the 31-kD subunit of the proton pump. Intercalated cells are clearly distinguished as those which stain with the fluorescent marker apically (A type, one arrow) and those which stain basolaterally (B type, two arrows). Two cells (arrowheads) have a diffuse or bipolar distribution of the pumps. (B) The same finding is seen in a phase-contrast picture of 1-μm section after staining with peroxidase-labeled antibodies. Type A cells are marked with one arrow and type B cells are marked with two arrows, respectively. (C) Low-power electron micrograph of the apical part of a cortical A type intercalated cell from sections treated with the preceding antibody, followed by protein A gold staining. The luminal membrane and some vesicular profiles in the apical cytoplasm are stained. (Reprinted by permission from Brown et al.,* Nature *331:622. Copyright © 1988 Macmillan Magazines Ltd.)*

ton pump containing vesicles with either the luminal or the basolateral membrane. These important issues and the apparently bewildering but explainable variability in the morphology of intercalated cells have been discussed in detail in several recent papers [46–49,256,286,326].

Intercalated cells have less Na^+-K^+-ATPase activity than principal cells [91], but they show high carbonic anhydrase activity, as might be expected from their regulatory role in acid-base balance [50,80,264].

JUXTAGLOMERULAR APPARATUS

The juxtaglomerular apparatus (JGA) is a composite assembly of specialized structures situated at the vascular pole of the glomerulus. A critical point in this context is that the distal straight tubule of a nephron makes contact with the vascular pole of the parent glomerulus (i.e., the same glomerulus from which the nephron originated). At this point, there is a plaque of very specialized and differentiated cells in the distal straight tubule known as the *macula densa* (Figs. 1-34, 1-37, 1-57, and 1-67 through 1-70). The JGA consists of the terminal portion of the afferent arteriole, the first portion of the efferent arteriole, the extraglomerular mesangium between both arterioles, and the macula densa [16,19,20,21,68,106, 107,268,307] (see Figs. 1-34, 1-37, and 1-67 through 1-69). It has been suggested that the recently discovered peripolar cells [102,270] also should be included, but a functional role for these cells has not yet come to light, and not all species have these cells. Most prominent in sheep, these cells, which contain prominent granules, replace parietal cells of Bowman's capsule just at the transition of the parietal to the visceral epithelium of a renal corpuscle. In the context of this discussion, peripolar cells will be excluded.

The JGA is innervated by the sympathetic system, which controls its activity. As such, this neural component is considered to be a part of the apparatus [18,107]. The macula densa makes contact primarily with the extraglomerular mesangial cells, a collection of cells also known as *Goormaghtigh cells, lacis cells,* or the *polar cushion*; they are anatomically in continuity with the glomerular mesangium. In addition to the extraglomerular mesangium, the macula densa may or may not contact the afferent and/or the efferent arteriole. The extraglomerular mesangial cells show many branching processes and, like their counterparts within the glomerular tuft, the mesangial cells proper, are surrounded by prominent extracellular matrix. Many of the cells in the media of the afferent arteriole in this region are specialized and differentiated "granular" myoepithelioid cells; they contain membrane-bound granules of renin in their cytoplasm (Fig. 1-71). Occasionally, some cells in the polar cushion also show similar morphology and contain renin granules. The JGA regulates glomerular hemodynamics under the control of both systemic factors (blood pressure, autonomic nerves, hormones, salt balance) and local stimuli, particularly feedback control by the composition of tubular fluid at the macula densa [20,45,314,337]. The anatomic limits of the JGA are ill-defined and vary under the influence of different functional states in physiologic or pathologic conditions. Accordingly, the Goormaghtigh cells merge imperceptibly with cells of the glomerular mesangium at the glomerular stalk; the number and extent of granular cells varies considerably, and the agranular extraglomerular mesangial cells are able to undergo reversible metaplasia to granular cells [62].

The Macula Densa

This small plaque of cells has ultrastructural, histochemical, and functional features that are dramatically different from those of the surrounding cells of the ascending thick limb. The cells are cuboidal or even columnar, and although cell size is variable among species, these cells are generally taller than surrounding cells and protrude into the lumen [130]. The nucleus is apically located, while most cell organelles have a tendency to be located basally and laterally. The mitochondria are small and have no distinctive distribution, un-

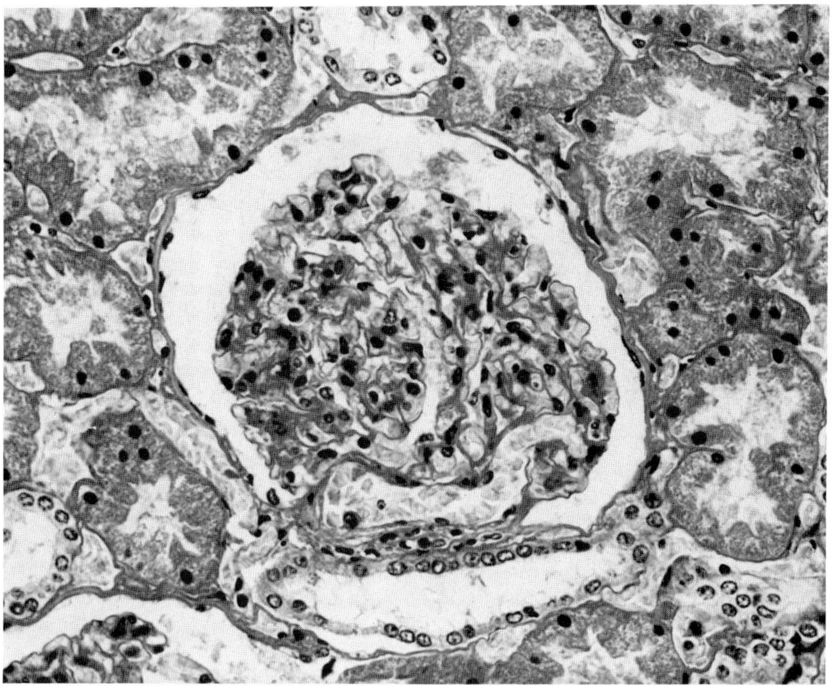

FIG. 1-67. *Glomerulus and surrounding tubules from autopsy specimen obtained from young man with no renal disease. The darkly staining tubules are proximal convoluted segments; the elongated tubule at the bottom is a distal tubule with a conspicuous macula densa. H&E; ×350.*

like the thick-limb cells. The luminal membrane is studded with slender microvilli; it lacks Tamm-Horsfall protein, which is present in thick limb cells [10,122,293]. The lateral membranes of adjacent cells do not interdigitate, but rather show small cytoplasmic projections that contact each other by means of desmosomes. Similar processes are present basally. The basement membrane of the macula densa is fused with the extracellular matrix and basement membranes of the extraglomerular mesangium. The cells lack epidermal growth factor and are poor in Na^+-K^+-ATPase activity, although both are plentiful in thick-limb cells [31,272]. The lateral interspaces expand and contract under different physiologic conditions; this is thought to be due to variations in paracellular water flow [140,161].

Granular Myoepithelioid Cells

Thought to be modified from smooth muscle, these endocrine cells elaborate renin mRNA [75] and harbor membrane-bound electron-dense granules containing renin [63,66,69,75,127,310] (Figs. 1-69 and 1-71). The cells have myofilaments, attachment bodies, and other features of smooth-muscle cells [139,188]. Renin is generally thought to be secreted by exocytosis into the interstitium surrounding the JGA. At this site, catalyzed by renin and locally present angiotensin-converting enzyme, angiotensin II, a vasoactive hormone is produced. In addition, there is evidence that angiotensin II also may be produced intracellularly within the granules [63,66,127,222, 257,269,307,310,312]. This renal production of angiotensin II is in addition to the substantial conversion of angiotensin I to angiotensin II in the lung. The cells occur in clusters of 4 or 5 (but up to 15) in the wall of the afferent arteriole and sometimes in the wall of the efferent arteriole or in the extraglomerular mesangium. In response to stimuli, additional smooth-muscle cells are recruited by metaplasia to granular cells [62,238]. Granular cells have many branching processes [107], and through gaps in the basement membrane matrix surrounding them they make gap-junction contacts with other smooth-muscle cells and granular cells, as well as with extraglomerular mesangial cells; junctions between granular cells and endothelial cells also have been described [37,107,139]. Granular cells have two types of granules. One contains lipofuscin. The other type, the specific granule, originates in the Golgi apparatus as protogranules and matures to large, amorphous granules that sometimes contain crystalline structures [15,17,37,53,188,226].

Extraglomerular Mesangium

The extraglomerular mesangial cells, also called *lacis cells* and *Goormaghtigh cells,* form a cone-shaped cluster with the base against the macula densa and the apex merging with the mesangial stalk (see Figs. 1-34, 1-37, and 1-69). This area is now called the *extraglomerular mesangium* (formerly the *lacis region*). Ultrastructurally, the cells are similar in appearance to glomerular mesangial cells [268]. The cells and their processes are surrounded and separated by an interlacing network of basement-membrane–like material. Through gaps in this matrix, cytoplasmic processes of extraglomerular mesangial cells contact each other, the cells of the mesangial stalk, and the granular cells by gap junctions [37,43,107,246,311], but not the macula densa cells. Although the mechanisms are not clear, it is generally considered that the extraglomerular mesangial cells mediate the signals received from the macula densa cells for transmission to both the granular cells and the glomerular mesangium [337]. The mechanism of transmission could be gap-junction mediated. From a biomechanical point of view, the extraglomerular mesangium serves as a closure device of the glomerular entrance [179].

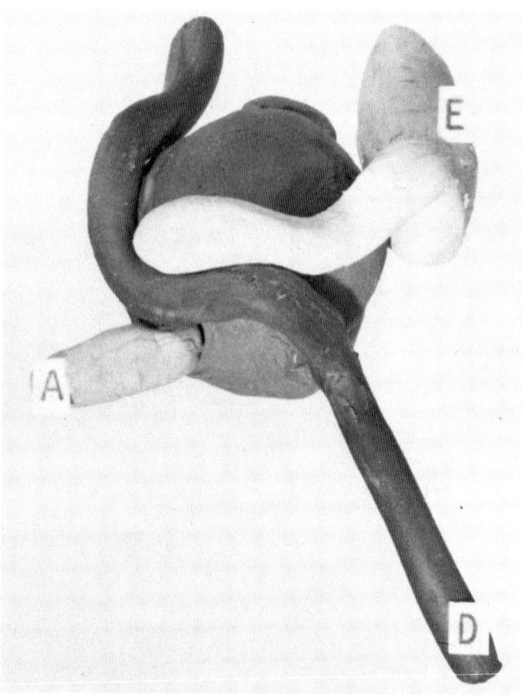

FIG. 1-68. *Reconstruction of the hilus of the glomerulus to show intimate relationships, in particular that of the efferent arteriole to the distal convoluted tubule. D, distal convoluted tubule; A, afferent arteriole; E, efferent arteriole. Grayish black solid structure is the glomerulus. (Modified from Barajas, L., and Latta, H.* Lab. Invest. *12: 257, 1963.)*

Innervation of the JGA

The JGA is richly innervated by "terminal axons" of the sympathetic system. Most of the nerves are monoaminergic and have been studied by fluorescence microscopy, histochemistry, autoradiography and serial-section analysis [18,21,23,37,107,308,309]. The nerve fibers course along arterioles and supply fine branches and terminals to granular cells and smooth-muscle cells in the afferent and efferent arterioles, peripherally located extraglomerular mesangial cells, and epithelial cells of surrounding tubules. Only peripheral cells of the macula densa may come into contact with

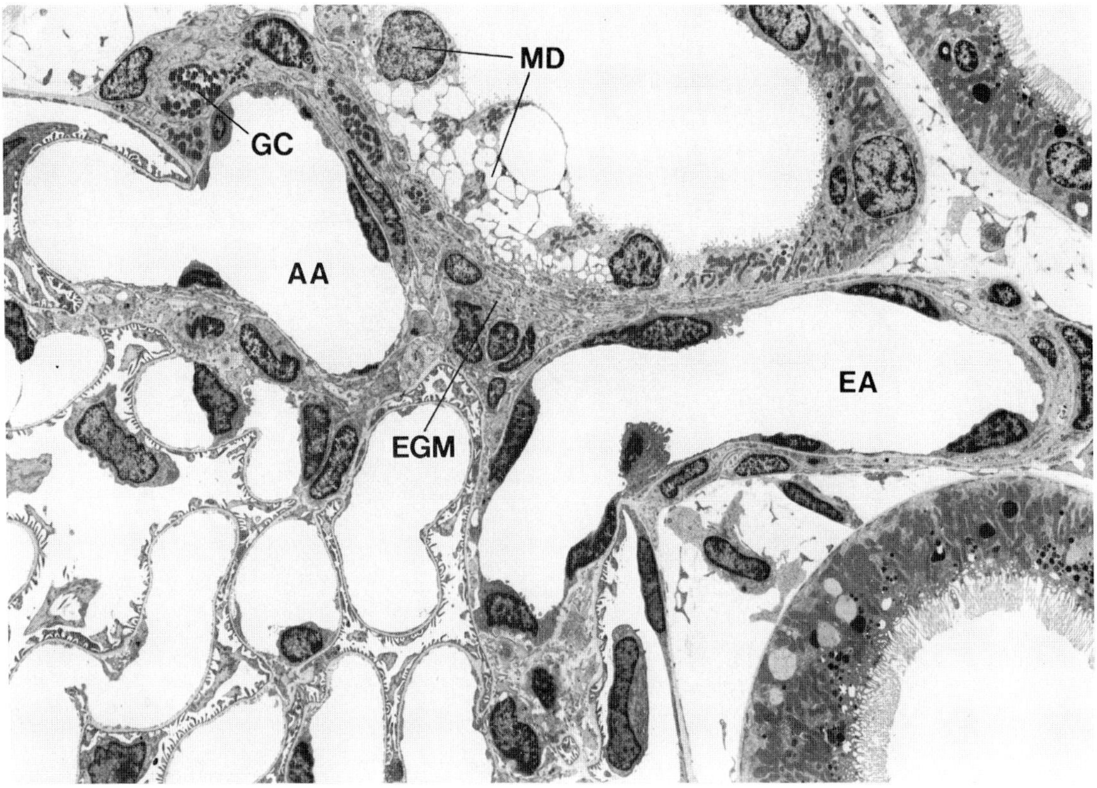

FIG. 1-69. *Vascular pole of a glomerulus; rat. The juxtaglomerular apparatus (JGA) is composed of the granular cells (GC) in the afferent arteriole (AA). Between the afferent and efferent arteriole (EA), the extraglomerular mesangium is found (EGM). The macula densa (MD) abuts the extraglomerular mesangium and, in this case, the afferent and efferent arterioles. The intercellular spaces between macula densa cells are extremely dilated. × 1700 approx.*

terminal axons. Nerves have not been observed within the extraglomerular mesangium.

INTERSTITIUM

The interstitium is scant in the cortex and outer stripe of the outer medulla, but it becomes more abundant in the inner stripe and inner medulla. In the cortex, the peritubular interstitium must be distinguished from the periarterial spaces, in which lymphatics are present (Fig. 1-72). In the rat renal cortex, the peritubular interstitium makes up some 7 to 9 percent of total volume [178, 236,239]. The interstitium is unevenly distributed. About 55 percent of the total capillary surface in the cortex is directly apposed to tubules, often with fused and shared basement membranes [178], indicating that much of the interstitium is in the irregular and angular spaces between tubules (Figs. 1-72 and 1-73). Thus reabsorbed fluid may go into capillaries almost directly, as well as indirectly by means of the interstitium. The periarte-

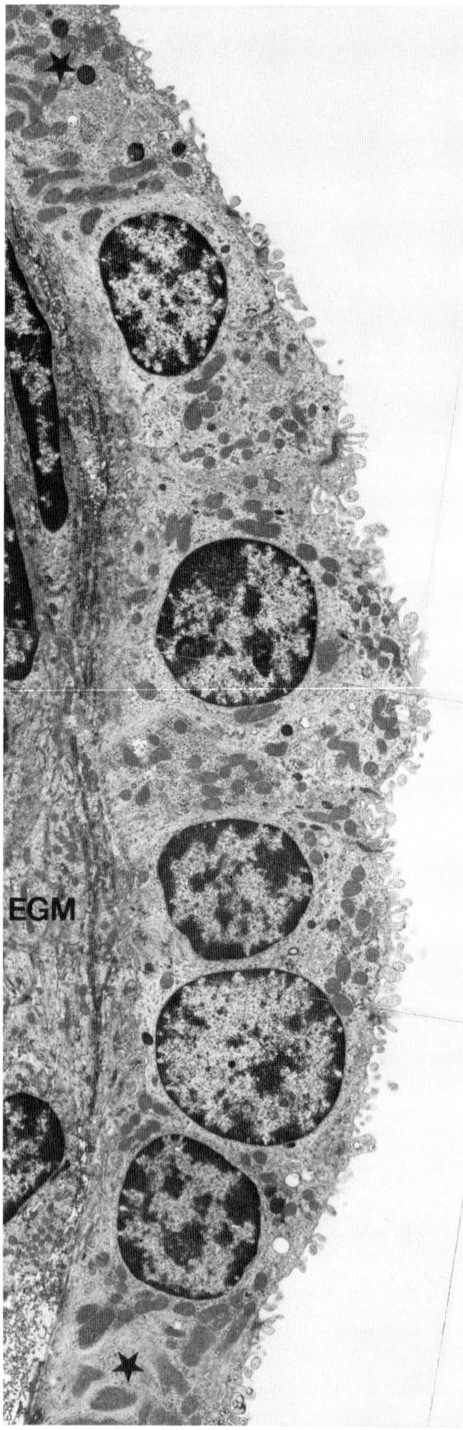

FIG. 1-70. *Macula densa; rat. The macula densa is a plaque of some 20 polygonal cells that peripherally are bordered by cells of the thick ascending limb (stars). The macula densa cells are characterized by large nuclei; the luminal cell membrane is densely covered by microvilli. The width of intercellular spaces between macula densa cells may change from narrow (as in this case) to dilated. The macula densa abuts the extraglomerular mesangium (EGM), separated by a tortuous basement membrane.* ×4500 *approx.*

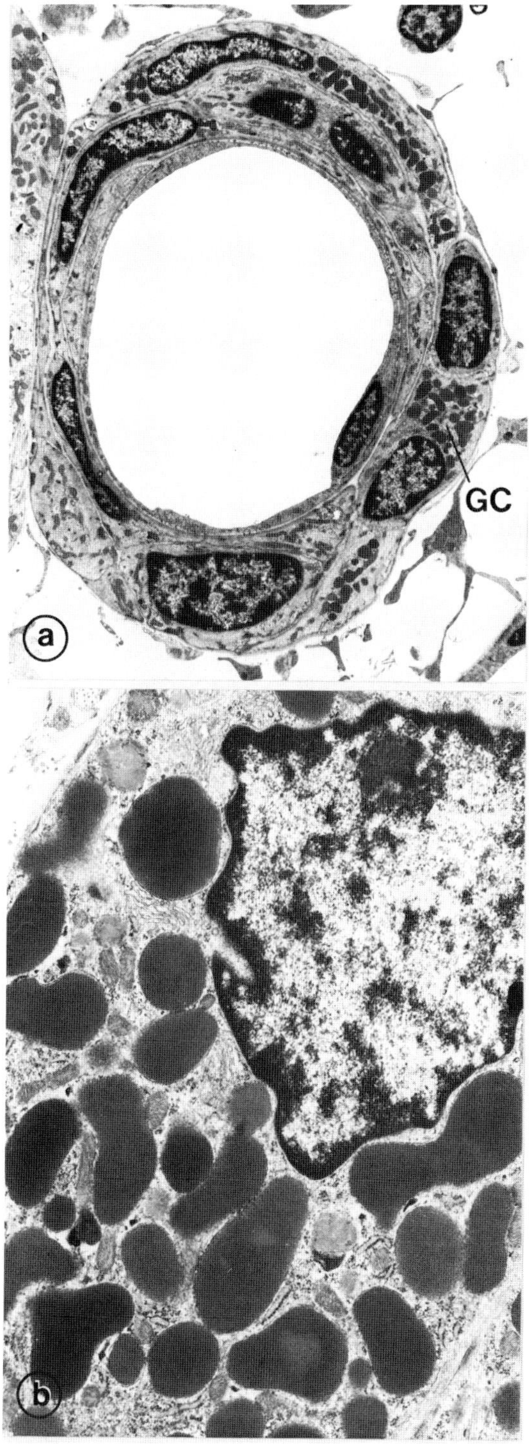

FIG. 1-71. *Juxtaglomerular portion of an afferent arteriole; rat. Some of the smooth-muscle cells of the media are replaced by granular cells (GC). In (B), part of a granular cell is shown, which contains a dense assembly of membrane-bound granules filled with an amorphous matrix (specific granules). (A) ×1900 approx.; (B) ×7800 approx.*

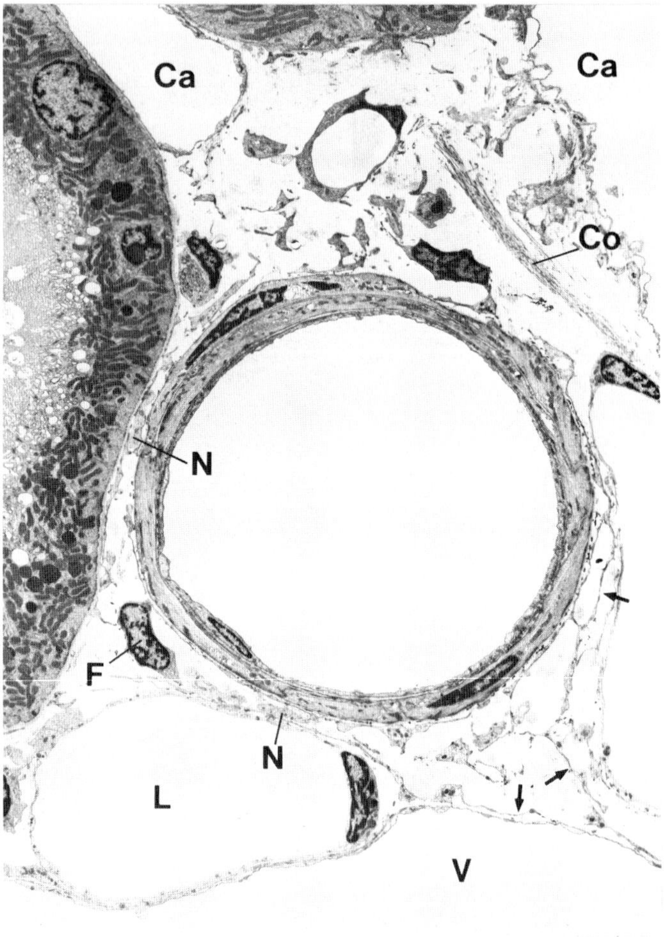

FIG. 1-72. *Cross section through an interlobular artery, electron micrograph; rat. The periarterial loose connective tissue surrounding the artery contains fibroblasts (F) with long, sheet-like processes (arrows) between which some sparse collagen bundles (Co) are found. L, lymphatic capillary; N, nerve; Ca, capillary, V, vein. × 1900 approx.*

rial interstitium is a loose layer of connective tissue surrounding the arteries and is continuous with the peritubular interstitium. Well shown only if kidneys are fixed following rapid freezing, these spaces are distended by interstitial fluid and contain lymphatics [174,304] (Fig. 1-74). The renal interstitium is composed of cells and extracellular fibrillar structures, proteoglycans, glycoproteins, and interstitial fluid. In the cortical interstitium, two types of interstitial cells are distinguished [39,57]. The majority, the type I interstitial cells of the cortical interstitium, are stellate in shape, have many processes that are often sheet-like, and resemble fibrocytes by morphologic characteristics (Figs. 1-73 and 1-75). Type II interstitial cells [39,57]—a round-shaped cell population—appear to be macrophages (see Fig. 1-73).

Several fibers make up the interstitial reticulum, among them typical interstitial collagenous fibers (types I, III, and VI) [152]. Type III fibers correspond to the classically described reticular fibers that form a network enveloping individual tubules [129]. In addition, microfibrils clearly identified by an electron-lucent core and a diameter of about 15 to 30 nm are found in the renal interstitium [185]. Proteoglycans are an important component of the interstitial matrix in the kidney, especially in the medulla. As elsewhere in the body,

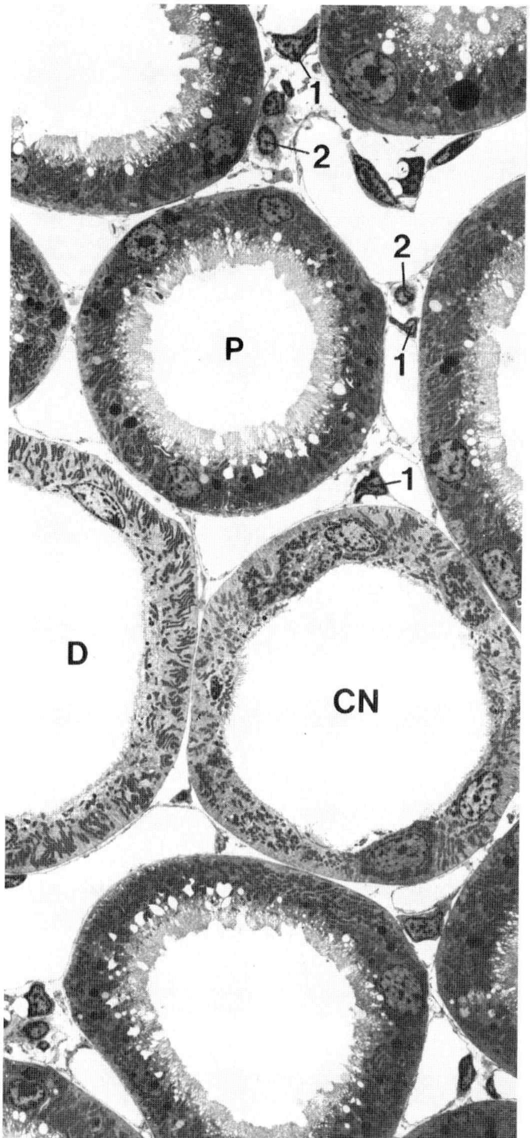

FIG. 1-73. *Peritubular interstitium in the renal cortex; rat. In the renal cortex, the peritubular interstitial spaces are sparse. Most of the spaces in between the tubules are occupied by capillaries. Two types of interstitial cells are seen: type I (1) are fibroblast-like cells, and type II (2) are rounded cells that often are macrophages. P, proximal tubule; D, distal convoluted tubule; CN, connecting tubule. ×570 approx.*

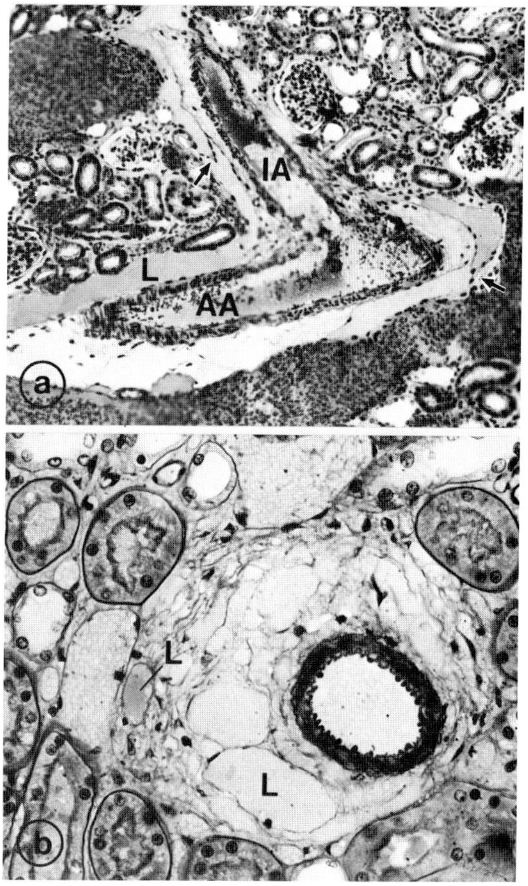

FIG. 1-74. *Lymphatic vessels of the kidney. (A) Lymphatics (L) pass from a course alongside an interlobular artery (IA) to a course alongside an arcuate artery (AA). Note the valves (arrows). (B) Cross section through a basal portion of an interlobular artery. Lymphatics (L) are embedded in the loose connective tissue surrounding the artery. (A) Paraffin section, feline kidney; ×120 approx. (From Kriz and Dieterich,* Z. Anat. Entwicklungsgesch. *131:111, 1970. Used by permission of Springer-Verlag.); (B) paraffin section, rat kidney; ×200 approx.*

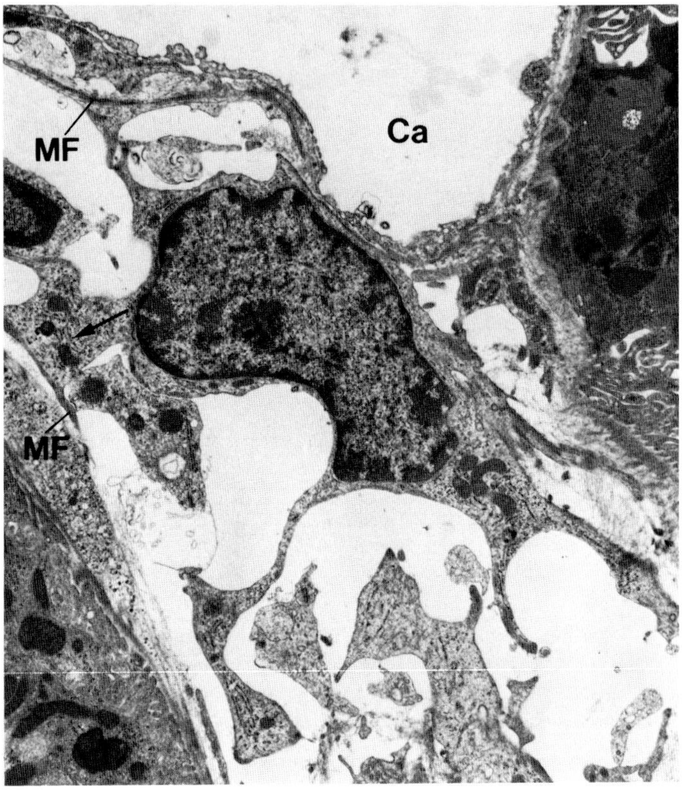

FIG. 1-75. *Peritubular interstitium, cortex; rat. Type I interstitial cell is a stellate-shaped fibroblast-like cell. The many cell processes contain abundant rough endoplasmic reticulum (arrows) as well as, in the most peripheral portions, microfilament bundles (MF). Ca, capillary.* ×*9700 approx.*

various glycoproteins (fibronectin, laminin, and others) are found associated with tubular basement membranes, connecting them to cell membranes as well as to fibrillar structures of the interstitial matrix.

In the outer stripe of the medulla, the interstitium constitutes only about 5 percent of total volume in the rat [163]; in this zone, capillaries are even more closely apposed and molded to the tubules than in the cortex. In the inner stripe, the interstitium is scant in the vascular bundles and more voluminous in the interbundle region (~10 percent in rat; ~20 percent in rabbit) [163]. In the inner medulla, the interstitium increases progressively from the base to the tip (base: 10 to 15 percent in rat, 20 to 25 percent in rabbit; tip: ~30 percent in rat, >40 percent in rabbit) [163]. The inner medullary interstitium is rich in acidic mucosubstances that stain with cationic dyes and lectins in a characteristic manner, with variations being observed in different states of hydration [334].

The inner medullary interstitium has interstitial cells of three types [38,39,40]. One occurs around the walls of the descending vasa recta; described as a type III interstitial cell, this type appears to

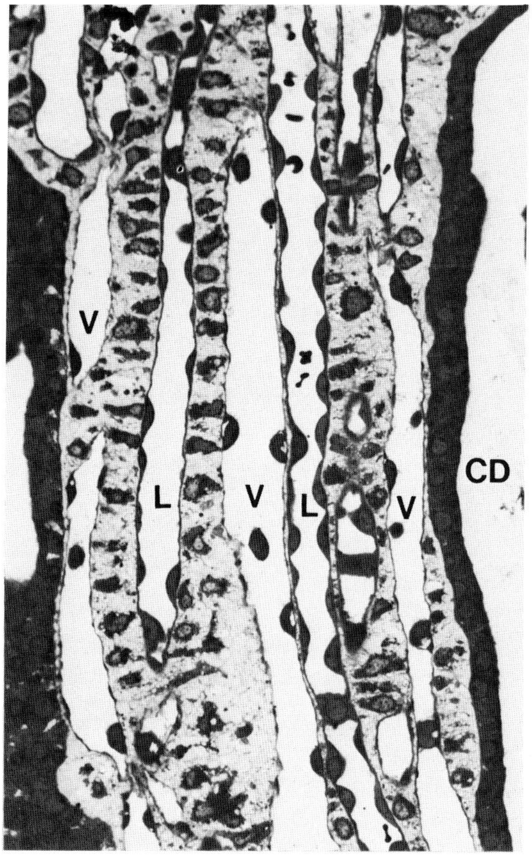

FIG. 1-76. *Longitudinal section through the inner medulla, light micrograph; rat. The interstitium in the inner medulla is well developed. The lipid-laden interstitial cells characteristically span the distance between parallel-running ascending vasa recta (V) and limbs (L) of Henle's loops like the rungs of a ladder. CD, collecting duct.* × *100 approx.*

be the pericyte of the vasa recta. The type I cells (corresponding to the fibrocyte-like cells in the renal cortex) are called *renal medullary granulated interstitial cells* or *lipid-laden interstitial cells* and are the dominant variety [38,39]. The cells are arranged in a characteristic manner like the rungs of a ladder, transversely interposed between longitudinally running loops of Henle and vessels (Fig. 1-76). They are irregular and stellate in shape with many microfilament-filled processes that anchor in the basement membranes of the loops of Henle and vessels. The cells are connected to each other by composite-type cell junctions, including gap junctions [274]. They also have electron-dense droplets in their cytoplasm (Fig. 1-77). The droplets contain neutral lipids rich in unsaturated fatty acids, small amounts of cholesterol ester and phospholipids, and other, as yet uncharacterized lipids [8,41,42]. The cells have abundant rough endoplasmic reticulum and distinctive cylindrical structures related to endoplasmic reticulum of unknown significance [56,190]. The lipid droplets may be surrounded by whorls of membranes but are not membrane bound.

A number of studies have attempted to correlate the number or size of the droplets with states of hydration, but the results have been inconclusive. However, their presence or absence, or relative numbers, has been reported to correlate with the hypertensive status of the animal in experimental models [242]. Some studies have suggested that one function of the cells may be to produce prostaglandins, particularly PGE_2 [217,341], but the primary biochemical function of the cells remains uncharacterized. However, there is compelling evidence that the granulated renomedullary interstitial cells produce an antihypertensive factor, most probably a lipid [215,216,217]. The type II interstitial cells in the medulla, as in the cortex, are mostly rounded cells; also as in the cortex, most of them appear to be histiocytes (macrophages).

INTRARENAL LYMPHATICS

The intrarenal lymphatics follow two systems: a periarterial hilar network and, clearly much less important for drainage of the renal parenchyma, a capsular (subcapsular) network [3,174,224,229] (Fig. 1-78). Within the cortex, lymphatic capillaries are typically found around interlobular arteries; smaller tributaries also may be present, located around glomeruli and the arterioles. These vessels drain along the periarterial connective tissue until

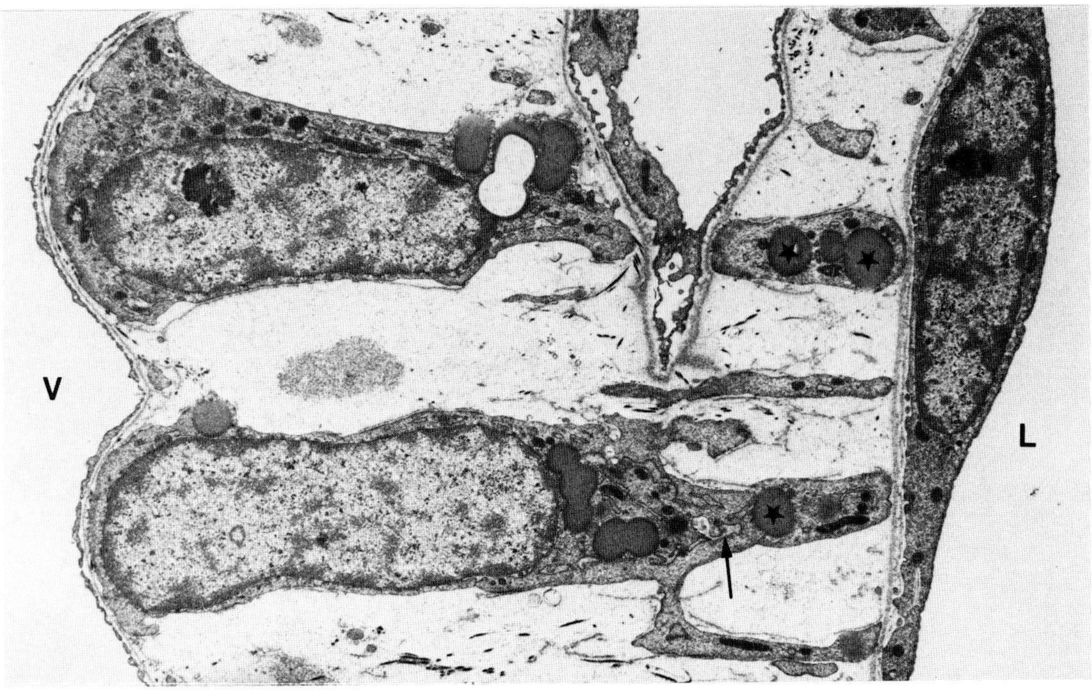

FIG. 1-77. *Lipid-laden interstitial cells; longitudinal section through the papilla, electron micrograph; rat. Two lipid-laden interstitial cells are shown spanning the distance between an ascending vas rectum (V) and a limb (L) of a loop of Henle. The lipid droplets (stars) as well as the characteristically dilated cisternae of the endoplasmic reticulum (arrow) are seen. Note the density of the interstitial matrix between the cells.* ×34,000 *approx.*

they form larger channels in the renal hilus. The other system is found as a plexus of anastomosing lymphatics in the capsular tissue; subcapsular lymphatics are generally sparse and are only found alongside perforating capsular arteries (which are rare) or alongside subcapsular superficial veins as they are found in the feline kidney [174]. The capsular lymphatic system may participate in draining the superficial cortex. There is general agreement that the medulla is devoid of lymphatics.

INTRARENAL NERVES

The nerve fiber distribution corresponds to the topography of arterial vessels in the cortex and outer stripe of the outer medulla. Nerves are found in the vicinity of smooth-muscle cells around arcuate and interlobular arteries and afferent arterioles [22,207,208,219,225] (Figs. 1-79 and 1-80). Nerve fibers are also richly supplied to the efferent vasculature of the juxtamedullary glomeruli, including the descending vasa recta [76,207,208, 212,219,223]. This nerve supply extends along the vasa recta as far as the level at which the smooth-muscle cells in their walls are replaced by pericytes. Nerve fibrils from the periarteriolar nerves branch out and are seen to supply terminal axons to proximal tubules and distal segments, *but only* in the vicinity of the juxtaglomerular apparatus and nearby arteries [18,107]. It is possible that neurotransmitters derived from these neural

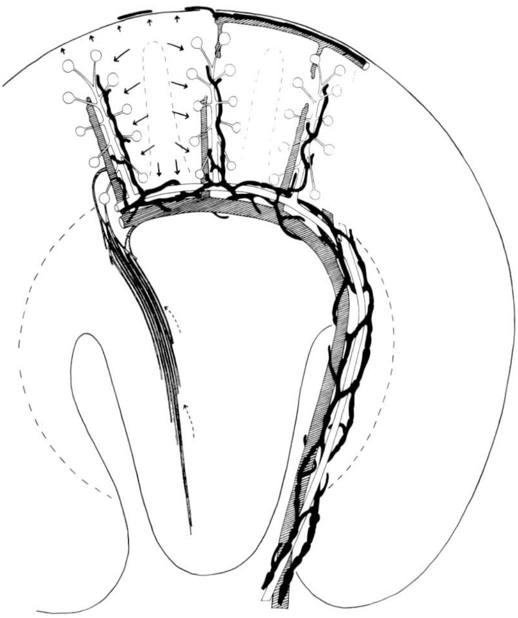

FIG. 1-78. *Schematic drawing to show the distribution of the intrarenal lymphatics. Arterial vessels and glomeruli are drawn in white, venous vessels are depicted by hatched marks, and lymphatics are drawn in black. Lymphatic capillaries begin alongside the interlobular arteries as well as afferent arterioles and join larger vessels that accompany the intrarenal arteries in a retrograde course leaving the kidney as hilar lymphatics. Subcapsular lymphatics, as shown here, are only found in species with a well-developed subcapsular venous system (cat, human beings); capsular lymphatics are commonly found. The arrows in the cortex indicate the possible flow of interstitial fluid toward the lymphatics. Note that the medulla is devoid of lymphatics. (Modified from Kriz and Dieterich,* Z. Anat. Entwicklungsgesch. *131:111, 1970. Used by permission of Springer-Verlag.)*

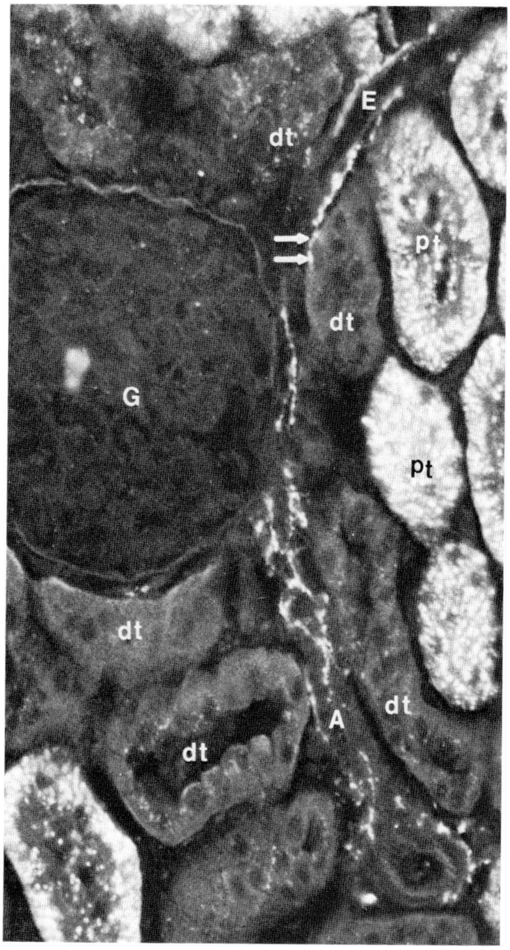

FIG. 1-79. *Nerve fibers demonstrated by catecholamine fluorescence histochemistry are seen along the afferent (A) and efferent (E) arterioles of rat kidney. A spot of fluorescence (arrows) appears adjacent to a distal tubule (dt). G, glomerulus; pt, proximal tubule. ×348. (From Barajas [18].)*

elements may be released into peritubular capillaries and affect tubular function downstream [139]. We have already seen that the JGA itself is richly innervated. Norepinephrine has been identified as an important transmitter in renal nerves; the occurrence of dopamine as a transmitter is in debate [23,78,81,107,308]. In addition, several neuropeptides are colocalized with norepinephrine in renal nerves [320].

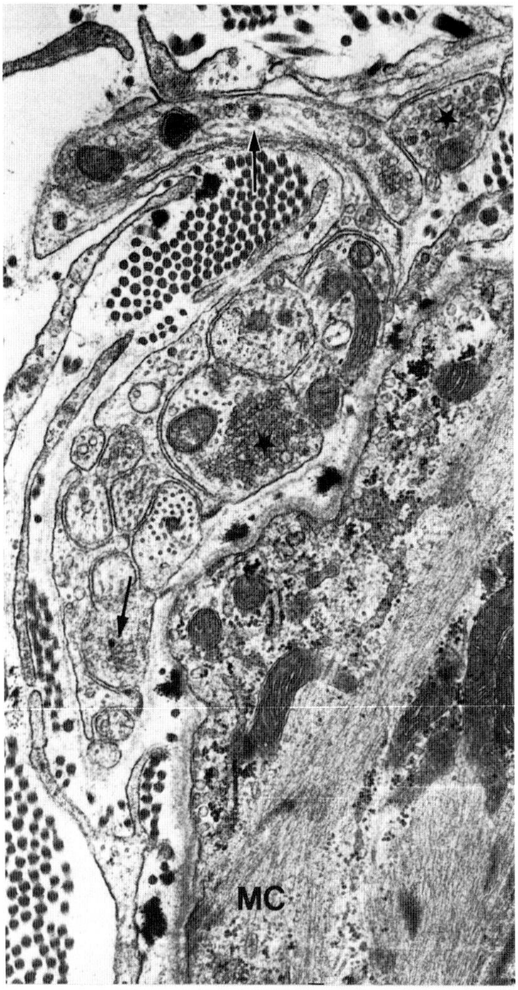

FIG. 1-80. *Nerve bundle alongside an afferent arteriole; rat. The bundle consists of several axons with varicosities containing clear vesicles (stars) and dense-core vesicles (arrow). MC, smooth-muscle cell of the afferent arteriole. ×22,500 approx.*

REFERENCES

1. Abrahamson, D. R. Structure and development of the glomerular capillary wall and basement membrane. *Am. J. Physiol.* 22:F783, 1987.
2. Aeikens, B., Eenboom, A., and Bohle, A. Untersuchungen zur Struktur des Glomerulum. Rekonstruktion eines Rattenglomerulum an 0.5 μ dicken Serienschnitten. *Virchows Arch.* [A] 381: 283, 1979.
3. Albertine, K. H., and O'Morchoe, C. C. C. Distribution and density of the canine renal cortical lymphatic system. *Kidney Int.* 16:470, 1979.
4. Allen, F., and Tisher, C. C. Morphology of the ascending thick limb of Henle. *Kidney Int.* 9:8, 1976.
5. Andrews, P. M. Investigations of cytoplasmic contractile and cytoskeletal elements in the kidney glomerulus. *Kidney Int.* 20:549, 1981.
6. Andrews, P. M., and Bates, S. B. Filamentous actin bundles in the kidney. *Anat. Rec.* 210:1, 1984.
7. Andrews, P. M., and Porter, K. R. A scanning electron microscopic study of the nephron. *Am. J. Anat.* 140:81, 1974.
8. Anggard, E., Bohman, S.-O., Griffin, J. E., III, Larsson, C., and Maunsbach, A. B. Subcellular localization of the prostaglandin system in the rabbit renal papilla. *Acta Physiol. Scand.* 84:231, 1972.
9. Arakawa, M. A scanning electron microscopy study of the human glomerulus. *Am. J. Pathol.* 64:457, 1971.
10. Bachmann, S., Koeppen-Hagemann, I., and Kriz, W. Ultrastructural localization of Tamm-Horsfall glycoprotein (THP) in rat kidney as revealed by protein A–gold immunocytochemistry. *Histochemistry* 83:531, 1985.
11. Bachmann, S., Kriz, W., Kuhn, C., and Franke, W. W. Differentiation of cell types in the mammalian kidney by immunofluorescence microscopy using antibodies to intermediate filament proteins and desmoplakins. *Histochemistry* 77:365, 1983.
12. Bankir, L., Bouby, N., Trinh-Trang-Tan, M. M., and Kaissling, B. The Thick Ascending Limb of Henle's Loop: Anatomical and Functional Characteristics and Role in the Urine Concentration Mechanism. In J. Crosnier, J. L. Funck-Brentano, J. F. Bach, and J. P. Gruenfeld (Eds.), *Current Topics in Nephrology from the Necker Hospital.* Paris: Flammarion Medicine Sciences, 1987.
13. Bankir, B., and de Rouffignac, C. Urinary concentrating ability: Insights from comparative anatomy. *Am. J. Physiol.* 249:R643, 1985.
14. Bankir, L., and Farman, N. Hétérogenéité des glomérules chez le lapin. *Arch. Anat. Microsci. Morphol. Exp.* 62:281, 1973.

15. Barajas, L. The development and ultrastructure of the juxtaglomerular cell granule. *J. Ultrastruct. Res.* 15:400, 1966.
16. Barajas, L. The ultrastructure of the juxtaglomerular apparatus as disclosed by three-dimensional reconstructions from serial sections: The anatomical relationship between tubular and vascular components. *J. Ultrastruct. Res.* 33:116, 1970.
17. Barajas, L. Renin secretion: An anatomical basis for tubular control. *Science* 172:485, 1971.
18. Barajas, L. The innervation of the renal cortex. *Fed. Proc.* 37:1192, 1978.
19. Barajas, L. The anatomy of the juxtaglomerular apparatus. *Am. J. Physiol.* 237:F333, 1979.
20. Barajas, L. The juxtaglomerular apparatus: Anatomical considerations in feedback control of glomerular filtration rate. *Fed. Proc.* 40:78, 1981.
21. Barajas, L., and Muller, J. The innervation of the juxtaglomerular apparatus and surrounding tubules: A quantitative analysis by serial section electron microscopy. *J. Ultrastruct. Res.* 43:107, 1973.
22. Barajas, L., and Wang, P. Myelinated nerves of the rat kidney: A light and electron microscopic autoradiographic study. *J. Ultrastruct. Res.* 65:148, 1978.
23. Barajas, L., and Wang, P. Simultaneous ultrastructural visualization of acetylcholinesterase activity and tritiated norepinephrine uptake in renal nerves. *Anat. Rec.* 205:185, 1983.
24. Bargmann, W. *Handbuch der mikroskopischen Anatomie des Menschen*, Bd. 7, Teil 5: *Niere und ableitende Harnwege.* Heidelberg: Springer-Verlag, 1978.
25. Barnes, J. L., Radnik, R. A., Gilchrist, E. P., and Venkatachalam, M. A. Size and charge selective permeability defects induced in glomerular basement membrane by a polycation. *Kidney Int.* 25:11, 1984.
26. Barrett, J. M., and Heidger, P. M. Microbodies of the rat renal proximal tubule: Ultrastructural and cytochemical investigations. *Cell Tissue Res.* 157:283, 1975.
27. Beeuwkes, R. Efferent vascular patterns and early vascular-tubular relations in the dog kidney. *Am. J. Physiol.* 221:1361, 1971.
28. Beeuwkes, R. The vascular organization of the kidney. *Annu. Rev. Physiol.* 42:531, 1980.
29. Beeuwkes, R. Vascular-Tubular Relationships in the Human Kidney. In A. Leaf, G. Giebisch, L. Bolis, and S. Gorini (Eds.), *Renal Pathophysiology.* New York: Raven Press, 1980. P. 155.
30. Beeuwkes, R., and Bonventre, J. V. Tubular organization and vascular-tubular relations in the dog kidney. *Am. J. Physiol.* 229:695, 1975.
31. Beeuwkes, R., Shabod, J., and Rosen, S. Macula densa: Absence of transport ATPase. *Kidney Int.* 8:467, 1975.
32. Behnke, O., and Zelander, T. Preservation of intracellular substances by the cationic dye alcian blue in preparative procedures for electron microscopy. *J. Ultrastruct. Res.* 31:424, 1970.
33. Bergeron, M., Guerette, D., Forget, J., and Thiéry, G. Three-dimensional characteristics of the mitochondria of the rat nephron. *Kidney Int.* 17:175, 1980.
34. Bergeron, M., and Thiéry, G. Three-dimensional characteristics of the endoplasmic reticulum of rat renal tubule cells: An electron microscopy study in thick sections. *Biol. Cell* 42:43, 1981.
35. Bertin, M. Memoire pour servir à l'histoire des reins. *In Histoire de l'Academie Royale des Sciences, Anneé MDCCXLIV.* Paris: Panckoucke, 1746. P. 77.
36. Bertolatus, J. A., and Hunsicker, L. G. Polycation binding to the glomerular basement membrane: Effect of biochemical modification. *Lab. Invest.* 56:170, 1987.
37. Biava, C. G., and West, M. Fine structure of normal human juxtaglomerular cells: I. General structure and intercellular relationships. *Am. J. Pathol.* 49:679, 1966.
38. Bohman, S.-O. The ultrastructure of the rat renal medulla as observed after improved fixation methods. *J. Ultrastruct. Res.* 47:329, 1974.
39. Bohman, S.-O. The Ultrastructure of the Renal Interstitium. In B. M. Brenner and J. H. Stein (Eds.), *Contemporary Issues in Nephrology.* New York: Churchill-Livingstone, 1983. P. 1.
40. Bohman, S.-O., and Jensen, P. K. A. The interstitial cells in the renal medulla of rat, rabbit, and gerbil in different states of diuresis. *Cell Tissue Res.* 189:1, 1978.
41. Bohman, S.-O., and Maunsbach, A. B. Ultrastructure and biochemical properties of subcellular fractions from rat renal medulla. *J. Ultrastruct. Res.* 38:225, 1972.
42. Bojesen, I. N. Fatty Acid Composition and Depot Function of Lipid Droplet Triacylglycerols in Renomedullary Interstitial Cells. In A. K. Mandal and S.-O. Bohman (Eds.), *The Renal Papilla and Hypertension.* New York: Plenum Press, 1980. P. 121.
43. Boll, H.-U., Forssmann, W. G., and Taugner, R. Studies on the juxtaglomerular apparatus: IV. Freeze-fracturing of membrane surfaces. *Cell Tissue Res.* 161:459, 1975.
44. Brezis, M., Rosen, S., Silva, P., and Epstein, F. H. Renal ischemia: A new perspective. *Kidney Int.* 26:375, 1984.
45. Briggs, J. P., and Schnermann, J. The tubulo-

glomerular feedback mechanism: Functional and biochemical aspects. *Annu. Rev. Physiol.* 49:251, 1987.
46. Brown, D. Membrane recycling and epithelial cell function. *Am. J. Physiol.* 256:F1, 1989.
47. Brown, D., Gluck, S., and Hartwig, J. Structure of the novel membrane-coating material in proton-secreting epithelial cells and identification as an H^+-ATPase. *J. Cell Biol.* 105:1637, 1987.
48. Brown, D., Hirsch, S., and Gluck, S. An H^+-ATPase in opposite plasma membrane domains in kidney epithelial cell subpopulations. *Nature* 331:622, 1988.
49. Brown, D., Hirsch, S., and Gluck, S. Localization of a proton-pumping ATPase in rat kidney. *J. Clin. Invest.* 82:2114, 1988.
50. Brown, D., Roth, J., Kumpulainen, T., and Orci, L. Ultrastructural immunocytochemical localization of carbonic anhydrase. *Histochemistry* 75:209, 1982.
51. Brown, D., Shields, G. I., Valtin, H., Morris, J. F., and Orci, L. Lack of intramembranous particle clusters in collecting ducts of mice with nephrogenic diabetes insipidus. *Am. J. Physiol.* 249:F582, 1985.
52. Brown, D., Vassalli, J. D., Kunz, A., Mulhauser, J., and Orci, L. Regional heterogeneity of glycoconjugate distribution in the glomerulus revealed by lectin-gold cytochemistry and SDS-PAGE. *Am. J. Pathol.* 125:601, 1986.
53. Bucher, O., and Kaissling, B. Morphologie des juxtaglomerulären Apparates. *Verh. Anat. Ges.* 67:109, 1973.
54. Bulger, R. E. The shape of rat kidney tubular cells. *Am. J. Anat.* 116:237, 1965.
55. Bulger, R. E., Cronin, R. E., and Dobyan, D. C. Survey of the morphology of the dog kidney. *Anat. Rec.* 194:41, 1979.
56. Bulger, R. E., Griffith, L. D., and Trump, B. F. Endoplasmic reticulum in rat renal interstitial cells: Molecular rearrangement after water deprivation. *Science* 151:83, 1966.
57. Bulger, R. E., and Nagle, R. B. Ultrastructure of the interstitium in the rabbit kidney. *Am. J. Anat.* 136:183, 1973.
58. Bulger, R. E., Siegel, F. L., and Pendergrass, R. Scanning and transmission electron microscopy of the rat kidney. *Am. J. Anat.* 139:483, 1974.
59. Bulger, R. E., Tisher, C. C., Myers, C. H., and Trump, B. F. Human renal ultrastructure: II. The thin limb of Henle's loop and the interstitium in healthy individuals. *Lab. Invest.* 16:124, 1967.
60. Burg, M. B. Renal Handling of Sodium, Chloride, Water, Amino Acids, and Glucose. In B. M. Brenner and F. C. Rector, Jr. (Eds.), *The Kidney,* 3rd Ed. Philadelphia: Saunders, 1986. Pp. 145–175.
61. Camazine, S. M., Ryan, G. B., Unanue, E. R., and Karnovsky, M. J. Isolation of phagocytic cells from the rat glomerulus. *Lab. Invest.* 35:315, 1976.
62. Cantin, M., Araujo-Nascimento, M. D., Benchimol, S., and Desormeaux, Y. Metaplasia of smooth muscle cells into juxtaglomerular cells in the juxtaglomerular apparatus, arteries, and arterioles of the ischemic (endocrine) kidney: An ultrastructural-cytochemical and autoradiographic study. *Am. J. Pathol.* 87:581, 1977.
63. Cantin, M., Gutkowska, J., Lacasse, J., Ballak, M., Ledoux, S., Inagami, T., Beuzeron, J., and Genest, J. Ultrastructural immunocytochemical localization of renin and angiotensin II in the juxtaglomerular cells of the ischemic kidney. *Am. J. Physiol.* 115:212, 1984.
64. Carlin, B., Jaffe, R., Bender, B., and Chung, A. E. Entactin, a novel basal lamina–associated sulfated glycoprotein. *J. Biol Chem.* 256:5209, 1981.
65. Casellas, D., and Mimran, A. Shunting in renal microvasculature of the rat: A scanning electron microscope study of corrosion casts. *Anat. Rec.* 201:237, 1981.
66. Celio, M. R. Angiotensin II immunoreactivity coexisting with renin in the human juxtaglomerular epithelioid cells. *Kidney Int.* 22:S30, 1982.
67. Christensen, E. I., and Madsen, K. M. Renal age changes: Observations on the rat kidney cortex with special reference to structure and function of the lysosomal system in the proximal tubule. *Lab. Invest.* 39:289, 1978.
68. Christensen, J. A., Meyer, D. S., and Bohle, A. The structure of the human juxtaglomerular apparatus: A morphometric, lightmicroscopic study on serial sections. *Virchows Arch.* [A] 367:83, 1975.
69. Corvol, P., Galen, F.-X., Devaux, C., Guyene, T. P., Menard, J., Bariety, J., Camilleri, J.-P., Phat, V. N., and Nochy, D. Human antirenin antibody: A new tool for studying the renin-angiotensin system. *Adv. Nephrol.* 12:3, 1983.
70. Coudrier, E., Kerjaschki, D., and Louvard, D. Cytoskeleton organization and submembranous interactions in intestinal and renal brush borders. *Kidney Int.* 34:309, 1988.
71. Courtoy, P. J., Timpl, R., and Farquhar, M. G. Comparative distribution of laminin, type IV collagen, and fibronectin in the rat glomerulus. *J. Histochem. Cytochem.* 30:874, 1982.
72. Crayen, M. L., and Thoenes, W. Architecture and cell structures in the distal nephron of the rat kidney. *Cytobiologie* 17:197, 1978.

73. Davidson, A. J. *Radiology of the Kidney.* Philadelphia: Saunders, 1985.
74. Dean, D. C., Barr, J. F., Freytag, J. W., and Hudson, B. G. Isolation of type IV procollagen-like polypeptides from glomerular basement membrane: Characterization of pro-alpha 1 (IV). *J. Biol. Chem.* 258:590, 1983.
75. Deschepper, C. F., Mellon, S. H., Cumin, F., Baxter, J. D., and Ganong, W. F. Analysis by immunocytochemistry and in situ hybridization of renin and its mRNA in kidney, testis, adrenal, and pituitary of the rat. *Proc. Natl. Acad. Sci. U.S.A.* 83:7552, 1986.
76. Dieterich, H. J. Electron microscopic studies of the innervation of the rat kidney. *Z. Anat. Entwicklungsgesch.* 145:169, 1974.
77. Dieterich, H. J. Die Struktur der Blutgefässe in der Rattenniere. *Norm. Pathol. Anat. (Stuttg.)* 35:1, 1978.
78. Dinerstein, R. J., Vannice, J., Henderson, R. C., Roth, L. J., Goldberg, L. I., and Hoffman, P. C. Histofluorescence techniques provide evidence for dopamine-containing neuronal elements in canine kidney. *Science* 205:497, 1979.
79. Dixon, J. S., and Gosling, J. A. The musculature of the human renal calyces, pelvis and upper ureter. *J. Anat.* 135:129, 1982.
80. Dobyan, D. C., Magill, L. S., Friedman, P. A., Hebert, S. C., and Bulger, R. E. Carbonic anhydrase histochemistry in rabbit and mouse kidneys. *Anat. Rec.* 204:185, 1982.
81. Dolezel, S., Edvinsson, L., Owman, C. H., and Owman, T. Fluorescence histochemistry and autoradiography of adrenergic nerves in the renal juxtaglomerular complex of mammals and man, with special regard to the efferent arteriole. *Cell Tissue Res.* 169:211, 1976.
82. Drenckhahn, D., and Franke, R. P. Ultrastructural organization of contractile and cytoskeletal proteins in glomerular podocytes of chicken, rat and man. *Lab. Invest.* 59:673, 1988.
83. Drenckhahn, D., and Gröschel-Stewart, U. Localization of myosin, actin, and tropomyosin in rat intestinal epithelium: Immunohistochemical studies at the light electron microscope levels. *J. Cell Biol.* 86:475, 1980.
84. Dyck, R. F., Lockwood, C. M., Kershaw, M., McHugh, N., Duance, V. C., Baltz, M. L., and Pepys, M. B. Amyloid P-component is a constituent of normal human glomerular basement membrane. *J. Exp. Med.* 152:1162, 1980.
85. Edwards, J. G. Efferent arterioles of glomeruli in the juxtamedullary zone of the human kidney. *Anat. Rec.* 125:521, 1956.
86. Elema, J. D., Hoyer, J. R., and Vernier, R. L. The glomerular mesangium: Uptake and transport of intrarenally injected colloidal carbon in rats. *Kidney Int.* 9:395, 1976.
87. Ericsson, J. L. E., Bergstrand, A., Andres, G., Bucht, H., and Cinotti, G. Morphology of the renal tubular epithelium in young, healthy humans. *Acta Pathol. Microbiol. Scand.* 63:361, 1965.
88. Ericsson, J. L. E., and Trump, B. F. Electron microscopic studies of the epithelium of the proximal tubule of the rat kidney, part I. *Lab. Invest.* 13:1427, 1964.
89. Ericsson, J. L. E., and Trump, B. F. Electron microscopic studies of the epithelium of the proximal tubule of the rat kidney: III. Microbodies, multivesicular bodies, and the golgi apparatus. *Lab. Invest.* 15:1610, 1966.
90. Ericsson, J. L. E., Trump, B. F., and Weibel, G. Electron microscopic studies of the proximal tubule of the rat kidney, part II. *Lab. Invest.* 14:1341, 1965.
91. Ernst, S. A. Transport ATPase cytochemistry: Ultrastructural localization of potassium-dependent and potassium-independent phosphatase activities in rat kidney cortex. *J. Cell Biol.* 66:586, 1975.
92. Ernst, S. A., and Schreiber, J. H. Ultrastructural localization of Na^+, K^+-ATPase in rat and rabbit kidney medulla. *J. Cell Biol.* 91:803, 1981.
93. Farquhar, M. G. The primary glomerular filtration barrier—Basement membrane or epithelial slits? *Kidney Int.* 8:197, 1975.
94. Farquhar, M. G. Structure and Function in Glomerular Capillary. In N. A. Kefalides (Ed.), *Biology and Chemistry of Basement Membranes.* New York: Academic Press, 1978. P. 43.
95. Farquhar, M. G., Lemkin, M. C., and Stow, J. L. Role of Proteoglycans in Glomerular Function and Pathology. In R. R. Robinson (Ed.), *Nephrology,* Vol. 1. New York: Springer-Verlag, 1984. P. 580.
96. Farquhar, M. G., and Palade, G. E. Functional evidence for the existence of a third cell type in the renal glomerulus: Phagocytosis of filtration residues by a distinctive "third" cell. *J. Cell Biol.* 13:55, 1962.
97. Farquhar, M. G., Wissig, S. L., and Palade, G. E. Glomerular permeability: I. Ferritin transfer across the normal glomerular capillary wall. *J. Exp. Med.* 113:47, 1961.
98. Fine, H. The development of the lobes of the metanephros and fetal kidney. *Acta Anat.* 113:93, 1982.
99. Fine, H., and Keen, E. N. The arteries of the human kidney. *J. Anat.* 100:881, 1966.
100. Fourman, J., and Moffat, D. B. Observations on the fine blood vessels of the kidney. *Symp. Zool. Soc. Lond.* 11:57, 1964.
101. Fourman, J., and Moffat, D. B. *The Blood Vessels*

of the Kidney. Oxford, England: Blackwell Scientific Publications, 1971.
102. Gall, J. A., Alcorn, D., Butkus, A., Coghlan, J. P., and Ryan, G. B. Distribution of glomerular peripolar cells in different mammalian species. *Cell Tissue Res.* 244:203, 1986.
103. Ganote, C. E., Grantham, J. J., Moses, H. L., Burg, M. B., and Orloff, J. Ultrastructural studies of vasopressin effect on isolated perfused renal collecting tubules of the rabbit. *J. Cell Biol.* 36:355, 1968.
104. Garg, L. C., Knepper, M. A., and Burg, M. B. Mineralocorticoid effects on Na-K-ATPase in individual nephron segments. *Am. J. Physiol.* 240:F536, 1981.
105. Gattone, V. H., II, Luft, F. C., and Evan, A. P. Renal afferent and efferent arterioles of the rabbit. *Am. J. Physiol.* 247:F219, 1984.
106. Goormaghtigh, N. Existence of an endocrine gland in the media of the renal arterioles. *Proc. Soc. Exp. Biol. Med.* 42:688, 1939.
107. Gorgas, K. Structure and innervation of the juxtaglomerular apparatus of the rat. *Adv. Anat. Embryol. Cell Biol.* 54:3, 1978.
108. Grantham, J. J. Mode of water transport in mammalian renal collecting tubules. *Fed. Proc.* 30:14, 1971.
109. Graves, F. T. *Anatomical Studies for Renal and Intrarenal Surgery*. Bristol, England: Wright, 1986.
110. Greger, R. Ion transport mechanisms in thick ascending limb of Henle's loop of mammalian kidney. *Physiol. Rev.* 65:760, 1985.
111. Griffith, L. D., Bulger, R. E., and Trump, B. F. Fine structure and staining of mucosubstance on "intercalated cells" from the rat distal convoluted tubule and collecting duct. *Anat. Rec.* 160:643, 1968.
112. Groniowsky, J., Biczyskowa, W., and Walski, M. Electron microscope studies on the surface coat of the nephron. *J. Cell Biol.* 40:585, 1969.
113. Hagege, J., Gabe, M., and Richet, G. Scanning of the apical pole of distal tubular cells under differing acid-base conditions. *Kidney Int.* 5:137, 1974.
114. Hansen, G. P., Tisher, C. C., and Robinson, R. R. Response of the collecting duct to disturbances of acid-base and potassium balance. *Kidney Int.* 17:326, 1980.
115. Hill, G. S. Experimental pyelonephritis: A microangiographic and histologic study of cortical vascular changes. *Bull. Johns Hopkins Hosp.* 119:79, 1966.
116. Hodson, C. J. Physiological changes in size of the human kidney. *Clin. Radiol.* 12:91, 1961.
117. Hodson, C. J. Reflux nephropathy: A personal historical review. *A.J.R.* 137:451, 1981.
118. Hodson, J. The lobar structure of the kidney. *Br. J. Urol.* 44:246, 1972.
119. Hodson, J. The renal parenchyma and its blood supply. *Curr. Probl. Diagn. Radiol.* 7:1, 1978.
120. Horvat, R., Hovorka, A., Dekan, G., Poczewski, H., and Kerjaschski, D. Endothelial cell membranes contain podocalyxin—The major sialoprotein of visceral glomerular epithelial cells. *J. Cell Biol.* 102:484, 1986.
121. Houser, M. T., Scheinman, J. I., Basgen, J., Steffes, M. W., and Michael, A. F. Preservation of mesangium and immunohistochemically defined antigens in glomerular basement membrane isolated by detergent extraction. *J. Clin. Invest.* 69:1169, 1982.
122. Hoyer, J. R., Sisson, S. P., and Vernier, R. L. Tamm-Horsfall glycoprotein: Ultrastructural immunoperoxidase localization in rat kidney. *Lab. Invest.* 41:168, 1979.
123. Hudson, B. G., Wieslander, J., Wisdom, B. J., and Noelken, M. E. Goodpasture syndrome: Molecular architecture and function of basement membrane antigen. *Lab. Invest.* 61:256, 1989.
124. Humbert, F., Pricam, C., Perrelet, A., and Orci, L. Specific plasma membrane differentiations in the cells of the kidney collecting tubule. *J. Ultrastruct. Res.* 52:13, 1975.
125. Hunsicker, L. G., Shearer, T. P., and Shaffer, S. J. Acute reversible proteinuria induced by infusion of the polycation hexadimethrine. *Kidney Int.* 20:7, 1981.
126. Hunter, D. D., Shah, V., Merlie, J. P., and Sanes, J. R. A laminin-like adhesive protein concentrated in the synaptic cleft of the neuromuscular junction. *Nature* 338:229, 1989.
127. Inagami, T., Kawamura, M., Naruse, K., and Okamura, T. Localization of components of the renin-angiotensin system in the kidney. *Fed. Proc.* 45:1414, 1986.
128. Inke, G. *The Protolobar Structure of the Human Kidney: Its Biologic and Clinical Significance*. New York: Alan R. Liss, 1988.
129. Ishii, T. Zur Darstellung der argyrophilen Fasern. *Mikroskopie* 20:1, 1965.
130. Isler, H., and Krstic, R. Scanning electron microscopy of the juxtaglomerular apparatus in the freeze-fractured rat kidney. *Arch. Histol. Jpn.* 44:15, 1981.
131. Jamison, R. L., and Kriz, W. *Urinary Concentrating Mechanism: Structure and Function*. New York: Oxford University Press, 1982.
132. Jones, D. B. Mucosubstances of the glomerulus. *Lab. Invest.* 21:119, 1969.
133. Jones, W. R., and O'Morchoe, C. C. C. Ultrastructural evidence for a reabsorptive role by intrarenal veins. *Anat. Rec.* 207:253, 1983.

134. Jorgensen, F. *The Ultrastructure of the Normal Human Glomerulus.* Copenhagen: Munksgaard, 1966.
135. Jorgensen, F., and Bentzon, M. W. The ultrastructure of the normal human glomerulus: Thickness of the glomerular basement membrane. *Lab. Invest.* 18:42, 1968.
136. Kaissling, B. Ultrastructural Characterization of the Connecting Tubule and the Different Segments of the Collecting Duct System in the Rabbit Kidney. In U. Schmidt and W. G. Guder (Eds.), *Current Problems in Clinical Biochemistry,* Vol. 8: *Biochemical Nephrology.* Bern: Huber, 1978. P. 435.
137. Kaissling, B. Ultrastructural organization of the transition from the distal nephron to the collecting duct in the desert rodent *Psammomys obesus. Cell Tissue Res.* 212:475, 1980.
138. Kaissling, B. Structural aspects of adaptive changes in renal electrolyte excretion. *Am. J. Physiol.* 243:F211, 1982.
139. Kaissling, B., and Kriz, W. Structural analysis of the rabbit kidney. *Adv. Anat. Embryol. Cell Biol.* 56:1, 1979.
140. Kaissling, B., and Kriz, W. Variability of intercellular spaces between macula densa cells: A transmission electron microscopic study in rabbits and rats. *Kidney Int.* 22:S9, 1982.
141. Kaissling, B., and Le Hir, M. Distal tubular segments in the rabbit kidney after adaptation to altered Na- and K-intake: I. Structural changes. *Cell Tissue Res.* 224:469, 1982.
142. Kaissling, B., Peter, S., and Kriz, W. The transition of the thick ascending limb of Henle's loop into the distal convoluted tubule in the nephron of the rat kidney. *Cell Tissue Res.* 182:111, 1977.
143. Kalmbach, B., and Fahimi, H. D. Peroxisomes: Identification in freeze-etch preparations of rat kidney. *Cell Biol. Int. Rep.* 2:389, 1978.
144. Kanwar, Y. S. Biophysiology of glomerular filtration and proteinuria. *Lab. Invest.* 51:7, 1984.
145. Kanwar, Y. S., and Farquhar, M. G. Anionic sites in the glomerular basement membrane: In vivo localization to laminia rarae by cationic probes. *J. Cell Biol.* 81:137, 1979.
146. Kanwar, Y. S., and Farquhar, M. G. Detachment of endothelium and epithelium from the glomerular basement membrane produced by kidney perfusion with neuraminidase. *Lab. Invest.* 42:375, 1980.
147. Kanwar, Y. S., Jakubowski, M. L., and Rosenzweig, L. J. Distribution of sulfated glycosaminoglycans in the glomerular basement membrane and mesangial matrix. *Eur. J. Cell. Biol.* 31:290, 1983.
148. Kanwar, Y. S., Linker, A., and Farquhar, M. G. Increased permeability of the glomerular basement membrane to ferritin after removal of glycosaminoglycans (heparan sulfate) by enzyme digestion. *J. Cell Biol.* 86:688, 1980.
149. Kanwar, Y. S., and Rosenzweig, L. J. Clogging of the glomerular basement membrane. *J. Cell Biol.* 93:489, 1982.
150. Kanwar, Y. S., Rosenzweig, L. J., and Jakubowski, M. L. Distribution of de novo synthesized sulfated glycosaminoglycans in the glomerular basement membrane and mesangial matrix. *Lab. Invest.* 49:216, 1983.
151. Kanwar, Y. S., Rosenzweig, L. J., and Kerjaschki, D. I. Glycosaminoglycans of the glomerular basement membrane in normal and nephrotic states. *Renal Physiol.* 4:121, 1981.
152. Karkavelas, G., and Kefalides, N. A. Comparative ultrastructural localization of collagen types III, IV, VI and laminin in rat uterus and kidney. *J. Ultrastruct. Mol. Struct. Res.* 100:137, 1988.
153. Karnovsky, M. J. The Structural Bases for Glomerular Filtration. In *Kidney Disease—Present Status* (IAP Monograph 20). Baltimore: Williams & Wilkins, 1979.
154. Kasiske, B. L., and Umen, A. J. The influence of age, sex, race and body habitus on kidney weight in humans. *Arch. Pathol. Lab. Med.* 110:55, 1986.
155. Katz, A. I., Doucet, A., and Morel, F. Na-K-ATPase activity along the rabbit, rat, and mouse nephron. *Am. J. Physiol.* 237:F114, 1979.
156. Kefalides, N. A. Structure and biosynthesis of basement membranes. *Int. Rev. Connect. Tissue Res.* 6:63, 1973.
157. Kerjaschki, D., and Farquhar, M. G. Immunocytochemical localization of the Heymann antigen (gp330) in glomerular epithelial cells of normal Lewis rats. *J. Exp. Med.* 157:667, 1983.
158. Kerjaschki, D., Sharkey, D. J., and Farquhar, M. G. Identification and characterization of podocalyxin—The major sialoprotein of the renal glomerular epithelial cell. *J. Cell Biol.* 98:1591, 1984.
159. Kerjaschki, D., Vernillo, A. T., and Farquhar, M. G. Reduced sialylation of podocalyxin—the major sialoprotein of the rat kidney glomerulus—in aminonucleoside nephrosis. *Am. J. Pathol.* 118:343, 1985.
160. Kinne, R., Schmitz, J. E., and Kinne-Saffran, E. The localization of the Na^+-K^+-ATPase in the cells of rat kidney cortex: A study on isolated plasma membranes. *Pflugers Arch.* 329:191, 1971.
161. Kirk, K. L., Bell, P. D., Barfuss, D. W., and Ribadeneira, M. Direct visualization of the isolated and perfused macula densa. *Am. J. Physiol.* 248: F890, 1985.

162. Knepper, M., and Burg, M. Organization of nephron function. *Am. J. Physiol.* 244:F579, 1983.
163. Knepper, M. A., Danielson, R. A., Saidel, G. M., and Post, R. S. Quantitative analysis of renal medullary anatomy in rats and rabbits. *Kidney Int.* 12:313, 1977.
164. Kone, B. C., Madsen, K. M., and Tisher, C. C. Ultrastructure of the thick ascending limb of Henle in the rat kidney. *Am. J. Anat.* 171:217, 1984.
165. Koushanpour, E., and Kriz, W. *Renal Physiology: Principles, Structure and Function*, 2nd Ed. New York: Springer-Verlag, 1986.
166. Kreisberg, J. I., Venkatachalam, M. A., and Troyer, D. Contractile properties of cultured glomerular mesangial cells. *Am. J. Physiol.* 249:F457, 1985.
167. Kriz, W. Der Architektonische und funktionelle Aufbau der Rattenniere. *Z. Zellforsch. Mikrosk. Anat.* 82:495, 1967.
168. Kriz, W. Structural organization of the renal medulla: Comparative and functional aspects. *Am. J. Physiol.* 241:R3, 1981.
169. Kriz, W. Structural organization of the renal medullary counterflow system. *Fed. Proc.* 42: 2379, 1983.
170. Kriz, W. 4.2 Die Nieren; 4.3 Die Harnableitenden Organe. In K. Fleischhauer (Ed.), *Benninghoff-Makroskopische und Mikroskopische Anatomie des Menschen*, Bd. 2: *Kreislauf und Eingeweide.* München: Urban & Schwarzenberg, 1985. Pp. 413–460.
171. Kriz, W. A periarterial pathway for intrarenal distribution of renin. *Kidney Int.* 31 (Suppl. 20):S51, 1987.
172. Kriz, W., and Bachmann, S. Pre- and postglomerular arterioles of the kidney. *J. Cardiovasc. Pharmacol.* 7(Suppl. 3): S24, 1985.
173. Kriz, W., Bankir, L., Bulger, R. E., Goncharevskaya, O. A., Imai, M., Kaissling, B., Maunsbach, A. B., Moffat, D. B., Morel, F., Morgan, T. O., Natochin, Y. V., Tisher, C. C., Venkatachalam, M. A., Whittembury, G., and Wright, F. S. A standard nomenclature for structures of the kidney (The Renal Commission of the International Union of Physiological Sciences). *Kidney Int.* 33:1, 1988.
174. Kriz, W., and Dieterich, H. J. Das Lymphgefässsystem der Niere bei einigen Säugetieren. Licht- und elektronenmikroskopische Untersuchungen. *Z. Anat. Entwicklungsgesch.* 131:111, 1970.
175. Kriz, W., and Kaissling, B. Structural Organization of the Mammalian Kidney. In D. W. Seldin and G. Giebisch (Eds.), *The Kidney: Physiology and Pathophysiology.* New York: Raven Press, 1985. P. 265.
176. Kriz, W., Kaissling, B., and Pszolla, M. Morphological Characterization of the Cells in Henle's Loop and the Distal Tubule. In H. G. Vogel and K. J. Ullrich (Eds.), *New Aspects of Renal Function*, Vol. 6. Amsterdam: Excerpta Medica, 1978. P. 67.
177. Kriz, W., and Koepsell, H. The structural organization of the mouse kidney. *Z. Anat. Entwicklungsgesch.* 144:137, 1974.
178. Kriz, W., and Napiwotzky, P. Structural and functional aspects of the renal interstitium. *Contrib. Nephrol.* 16:104, 1979.
179. Kriz, W., Sakai, T., and Hosser, H. Morphological Aspects of Glomerular Function. In A. M. Davison (Ed.), *Nephrology*, Vol. 1: *Proceedings of the Xth International Congress of Nephrology.* London: Baillière Tindall, 1988. P. 2.
180. Kriz, W., Schnermann, J., and Dieterich, H. J. Differences in the Morphology of the Descending Limbs of Short and Long Loops of Henle in the Rat Kidney. In H. Wirz and F. Spinelli (Eds.), *Recent Advances in Renal Physiology.* Basel: Karger, 1972. P. 140.
181. Kriz, W., Schnermann, J., and Koepsell, H. The position of short and long loops of Henle in the rat kidney. *Z. Anat. Entwicklungsgesch.* 138:301, 1972.
182. Kühn, K., and Reale, E. Junctional complexes of the tubular cells in the human kidney as revealed with freeze-fracture. *Cell Tissue Res.* 160: 193, 1975.
183. Lacy, E. R. The mammalian renal pelvis: Physiological implications from morphometric analysis. *Anat. Embryol.* 160:131, 1980.
184. Langer, K. H. Feinstrukturen der Mikrokörper (microbodies) des Proximalen Nieretubulus. *Z. Zellforsch. Mikrosk. Anat.* 90:432, 1968.
185. Langer, K. H. Renal Interstitium Ultrastructure and Capillary Permeability. In A. B. Maunsbach, T. S. Olsen, and E. I. Christensen (Eds.), *Functional Ultrastructure of the Kidney.* London: Academic Press, 1980. P. 431.
186. Latta, H. The glomerular capillary wall. *J. Ultrastruct. Res.* 32:526, 1970.
187. Latta, H., Johnston, W. H., and Stanley, T. M. Sialoglycoproteins and filtration barriers in the glomerular capillary wall. *J. Ultrastruct. Res.* 51: 354, 1975.
188. Latta, H., and Maunsbach, A. B. The juxtaglomerular apparatus as studied electron microscopically. *J. Ultrastruct. Res.* 6:547, 1962.
189. Laurie, G. W., Leblond, C. P., Inoue, S., Martin, G. R., and Chung, A. Fine structure of the GBM and immunolocalization of five basement membrane components to the lamina densa (basal lamina) and its extensions in both glomeruli and

tubules of the rat kidney. *Am. J. Anat.* 169:463, 1984.
190. Ledingham, J. M., and Simpson, F. O. Bundles of intracellular tubules in renal medullary interstitial cells. *J. Cell Biol.* 57:594, 1973.
191. LeFurgey, A., and Tisher, C. C. Morphology of rabbit collecting duct. *Am. J. Anat.* 155:111, 1979.
192. LeHir, M., and Dubach, U. C. The cellular specificity of lectin binding in the kidney: II. A light microscopical study in the rabbit. *Histochemistry* 74:531, 1982.
193. LeHir, M., Kaissling, B., and Dubach, U. C. Changes in Na-K-ATPase activity. *Cell Tissue Res.* 224:493, 1982.
194. LeHir, M., Kaissling, B., Koeppen, B. M., and Wade, J. B. Binding of peanut lectin to specific epithelial cell types in the kidney. *Am. J. Physiol.* 242:C117, 1982.
195. Lemley, K. V., and Kriz, W. Cycles and separations: The histotopography of the urinary concentrating process. *Kidney Int.* 31:538, 1987.
196. Ljungquist, A., and Lagergren, C. Normal intrarenal arterial pattern in adult and aging human kidney: A microangiographical and histological study. *J. Anat.* 96:285, 1962.
197. Löfgren, F. *Das topografische System der Malpighischen Pyramiden der Menschenniere.* Lund: Håkan Ohlssons Boktryckeri, 1949.
198. Madri, J. A., Ross, F. J., Furthmayr, H., and Foidart, J. M. Ultrastructural localization of fibronectin and laminin in the basement membranes of the murine kidney. *J. Cell Biol.* 86:682, 1980.
199. Martinez-Hernandez, A., and Amenta, P. S. The basement membrane in pathology. *Lab. Invest.* 48:656, 1983.
200. Martinez-Hernandez, A., and Chung, A. The ultrastructural localization of two basement membrane components: entactin and laminin in rat tissue. *J. Histochem. Cytochem.* 32:289, 1984.
201. Martinez-Hernandez, A., Gay, S., and Miller, E. J. Ultrastructural localization of type V collagen in rat kidney. *J. Cell Biol.* 92:343, 1982.
202. Mason, J., Torhorst, J ., and Welsch, J. Role of the medullary perfusion defect in the pathogenesis of ischemic renal failure. *Kidney Int.* 26:283, 1984.
203. Mauer, S. M., Fish, A. J., Blau, E. B., and Michael, A. F. The glomerular mesangium: I. Kinetic studies of macromolecular uptake in normal and nephrotic rats. *J. Clin. Invest.* 51:1092, 1972.
204. Maunsbach, A. B. Ultrastructure of the Proximal Tubule. In J. Orloff and R. W. Berliner (Eds.), *Handbook of Physiology,* Section 8. Washington: American Physiological Society, 1973. Pp. 31–79.
205. Maunsbach, A. B. Cellular mechanisms of tubular protein transport. *Int. Rev. Physiol.* 11:145, 1976.
206. Mbassa, G., Elger, M., and Kriz, W. The ultrastructural organization of the basement membrane of Bowman's capsule in the rat renal corpuscle. *Cell Tissue Res.* 253:151, 1988.
207. McKenna, O. C., and Angelakos, E. T. Acetylcholinesterase-containing nerve fibers in the canine kidney. *Circ. Res.* 23:645, 1968.
208. McKenna, O. C., and Angelakos, E. T. Adrenergic innervation of the canine kidney. *Circ. Res.* 22:345, 1968.
209. Mené, P., Simonson, M. S., and Dunn, M. J. Physiology of the mesangial cell. *Physiol. Rev.* 69:1347, 1989.
210. Michael, A. F. The glomerular mesangium. *Contrib. Nephrol.* 40:7, 1984.
211. Michael, A. F., Keane, W. F., Raij, L., Vernier, R. L., and Mauer, S. M. The glomerular mesangium. *Kidney Int.* 17:141, 1980.
212. Moffat, D. B. The fine structure of the blood vessels of the renal medulla with particular reference to the control of the medullary circulation. *J. Ultrastruct. Res.* 19:532, 1967.
213. Moffat, D. B., and Fourman, J. The vascular pattern of the rat kidney. *J. Anat.* 97:543, 1963.
214. Mohos, S. C., and Skoza, L. Glomerular sialoprotein. *Science* 164:1519, 1969.
215. Muirhead, E. E., Brooks, B., Pitcock, J. A., and Stephenson, P. Renomedullary antihypertensive function in accelerated (malignant) hypertension: Observations on renomedullary interstitial cells. *J. Clin. Invest.* 51:181, 1972.
216. Muirhead, E. E., Brooks, B., Pitcock, J. A., Stephenson, P., and Brosius, P. Role of the renal medulla in the sodium-sensitive component of renoprival hypertension. *Lab. Invest.* 27:192, 1972.
217. Muirhead, E. E., Germain, G. S., Armstrong, F. B., Brooks, B., Leach, B. E., Byers, L. W., Pitcock, J. A., and Brown, P. Endocrine-type antihypertensive function of renomedullary interstitial cells. *Kidney Int.* 8:S271, 1975.
218. Mundel, P., Elger, M., Sakai, T., and Kriz, W. Microfibrils are a major component of the mesangial matrix in the glomerulus of the rat kidney. *Cell Tissue Res.* 254:183, 1988.
219. Munkacsi, I. Distribution of the intrarenal monoaminergic nerves in the kidneys of the desert rat (*Dipodomys merriami*) and the white rat (*Rattus norvegicus*). *Acta Anat.* 73:56, 1969.
220. Murakami, T. Vascular arrangement of the rat renal glomerulus: A scanning electron microscope study of corrosion casts. *Arch. Histol. Jpn.* 34:87, 1972.
221. Myers, C. E., Bulger, R. E., Tisher, C. C., and

Trump, B. F. Human renal ultrastructure: IV. Collecting duct of healthy individuals. *Lab. Invest.* 15:1921, 1966.
222. Naruse, K., Inagami, T., Celio, M. R., Workman, R. J., and Takii, Y. Immunohistochemical evidence that angiotensins I and II are formed by intracellular mechanism in juxtaglomerular cells. *Hypertension* 4:70, 1982.
223. Newstead, J., and Munkacsi, I. Electron microscopic observations on the juxtamedullary efferent arterioles and arteriolae rectae in kidneys of rats. *Z. Zellforsch. Mikrosk. Anat.* 97:465, 1969.
224. Nordquist, R. E., Bell, R. D., Sinclair, R. J., and Keyl, M. J. The distribution and ultrastructural morphology of lymphatic vessels in the canine renal cortex. *Lymphology* 6:13, 1973.
225. Norvell, J. E. A histochemical study of the adrenergic and cholinergic innervation of the mammalian kidney. *Anat. Rec.* 163:236, 1969.
226. Oberling, C., and Hatt, P. Y. Etude de l'apparell juxtaglomérulaire du rat au microscope electronique. *Ann. Anat. Pathol.* 5:441, 1960.
227. Oliver, J. *Nephrons and Kidneys: A Quantitative Study of Development and Evolutionary Mammalian Renal Architectonics.* New York: Hoeber, 1968.
228. Olsson, C. A. Anatomy of the Upper Urinary Tract. In P. C. Walsh, R. F. Gittes, A. D. Perlmutter, and T. A. Stamey (Eds.), *Campbell's Urology,* 5th Ed. Philadelphia: Saunders, 1986. P. 12.
229. O'Morchoe, C. C., and Albertine, K. H. The renal cortical lymphatic system in dogs with unimpeded lymph and urine flow. *Anat. Rec.* 198: 427, 1980.
230. Orci, L., Brown, D., Amherdt, M., and Perrelet, A. Distribution of intramembrane particles and filipin-sterol complexes in plasma membranes of kidney: I. Corpuscle of Malpighi. *Lab. Invest.* 46:545, 1982.
231. Orci, L., Singh, A., Amherdt, M., Brown, D., and Perrelet, A. Microheterogeneity of protein and sterol content in kidney podocyte membrane. *Nature* 293:646, 1981.
232. Orikasa, M., Matsui, K., Oite, T., and Shimizu, F. Massive proteinuria induced in rats by a single intravenous injection of a monoclonal antibody. *J. Immunol.* 141:807, 1988.
233. Osborne, M. J., Droz, B., Meyer, P., and Morel, F. Angiotensin II: Renal localization in glomerular mesangial cells by autoradiography. *Kidney Int.* 8:245, 1975.
234. Østerby, R. Morphometric studies of the peripheral glomerular basement membrane in early juvenile diabetes: I. Development of initial basement membrane thickening. *Diabetologia* 8:84, 1972.
235. Østerby, R., Gundersen, H. J. G., Kroustrup, J. P., Mogensen, C. E., and Seyer-Hansen, K. Enlargement of the Glomerular Capillary Surface and Increased Glomerular Function in Early Diabetes. In A. B. Maunsbach, T. S. Olsen, and E. I. Christensen (Eds.), *Functional Ultrastructure of the Kidney.* New York: Academic Press, 1980. P. 143.
236. Pedersen, J. C., Persson, A. E. G., and Maunsbach, A. B. Ultrastructure and Quantitative Characterization of the Cortical Interstitium in the Rat Kidney. In A. B. Maunsbach, T. S. Olsen, and E. I. Christensen (Eds.), *Functional Ultrastructure of the Kidney.* New York: Academic Press, 1980. P. 443.
237. Peter, K. *Untersuchungen über Bau und Entwicklung der Niere.* Jena: Gustav Fischer, 1909.
238. Peter, S., Lazar, J., Gross, F., and Forssmann, W. G. Studies on the juxtaglomerular apparatus: II. Quantitative morphology after adrenalectomy. *Cell Tissue Res.* 151:457, 1974.
239. Pfaller, W. Structure function correlation on rat kidney: Quantitive correlation of structure and function in the normal and injured rat kidney. *Adv. Anat. Embryol. Cell Biol.* 70:1, 1981.
240. Pfeiffer, E. W. Comparative anatomical observations of the mammalian renal pelvis and medulla. *J. Anat.* 102:321, 1968.
241. Pinter, G. G., Wilson, P. D., Bell, D. R., Atkins, J. L., and Stork, J. E. Interstitial Albumin Pool in the Renal Cortex: Its Turnover and the Permeability of Peritubular Capillaries. In A. B. Maunsbach, T. S. Olsen, and E. I. Christensen (Eds.), *Functional Ultrastructure of the Kidney.* New York: Academic Press, 1980. P. 411.
242. Pitcock, J. A. Morphometric studies of the renomedullary interstitial cells. *Am. J. Med. Sci.* 295:246, 1988.
243. Poisel, S., and Spangler, H. P. Die Verästelungstypen der arteria renalis im Hinblick auf die arterielle Blutversorgung des Parenchyms der Niere: Ein Beitrag zum Problem der sogenannten Nierensegmente. *Acta Anat.* 76:516, 1970.
244. Potter, E. L. *Normal and Abnormal Development of the Kidney.* Chicago: Year Book Medical Publishers, 1972.
245. Pricam, C., Humbert, F., Perrelet, A., and Orci, L. A freeze-etch study of the tight junctions of the rat kidney tubules. *Lab. Invest.* 30:286, 1974.
246. Pricam, C., Humbert, F., Perrelet, A., and Orci, L. Gap junctions in mesangial and lacis cells. *J. Cell Biol.* 63:349, 1974.
247. Priestley, G. C., and Malt, R. A. Membrane-bound ribosomes in kidney: Methods of estimation and effect of compensatory renal growth. *J. Cell Biol.* 41:886, 1969.
248. Ransley, P. G. Intrarenal reflux: I. Anatomical, dynamic and radiological studies. *Urol. Res.* 5:61, 1977.
249. Ransley, P. G., and Risdon, R. A. Renal papil-

lary morphology and intrarenal reflux in the young pig. *Urol. Res.* 3:105, 1975.
250. Ransley, P. G., and Risdon, R. A. Renal papillary morphology in infants and young children. *Urol. Res.* 3:111, 1975.
251. Ransley, P. G., and Risdon, R. A. Reflux and renal scarring. *Br. J. Radiol.* [*Suppl.*] 14:1, 1978.
252. Raptopoulos, V., Kleinman, P. K., Marks, S., Synder, M., and Silverman, P. M. Renal fascial pathway: Posterior extension of pancreatic effusions within the anterior pararenal space. *Radiology* 158:367, 1986.
253. Rasch, R. Prevention of diabetic glomerulopathy in streptozotocin diabetic rats by insulin treatment: Glomerular basement membrane thickness. *Diabetologia* 16:319, 1979.
254. Reeves, W. H., Kanwar, Y. S., and Farquhar, M. G. Assembly of the glomerular filtration surface: Differentiation of anionic sites in glomerular capillaries of newborn rat kidney. *J. Cell Biol.* 85:735, 1980.
255. Rennke, H. G., Cotran, R. S., and Venkatachalam, M. A. Role of molecular charge in glomerular permeability: Tracer studies with cationized ferritins. *J. Cell Biol.* 67:638, 1975.
256. Ridderstrale, Y., Kashgarian, M., Koeppen, B., Giebisch, G., Stetson, D., Ardito, T., and Stanton, B. Morphological heterogeneity of the rabbit collecting duct. *Kidney Int.* 34:655, 1988.
257. Rightsel, W. A., Okamura, T., Inagami, T., Pitcock, J. A., Takaii, Y., Brooks, B., Brown, P., and Muirhead, E. E. Juxtaglomerular cells grown as monolayer cell culture contain renin, angiotensin I–converting enzyme, and angiotensins I and II/III. *Circ. Res.* 50:822, 1982.
258. Rodewald, R., and Karnovsky, M. J. Porous substructure of the glomerular slit diaphragm in the rat and mouse. *J. Cell Biol.* 60:423, 1974.
259. Rodman, J. S., Kerjaschski, D., Merisko, E., and Farquhar, M. G. Presence of an extensive clathrin coat on the apical plasmalemma of the rat kidney proximal tubule cell. *J. Cell Biol.* 98:1630, 1984.
260. Rodman, J. S., Seidman, L., and Farquhar, M. G. The membrane composition of coated pits, microvilli, endosomes, and lysosomes is distinctive in the rat kidney proximal tubule cell. *J. Cell Biol.* 102:77, 1986.
261. Roesinger, B., Schiller, A., and Taugner, R. A freeze-fracture study of tight junctions in the pars convoluta and pars recta of the renal proximal tubule. *Cell Tissue Res.* 186:121, 1978.
262. Roll, J. F., Madri, J. A., Albert J., and Furthmayr, H. Codistribution of collagen types IV and AB2 in basement membranes and mesangium of the kidney: An immunoferritin study of ultrathin frozen sections. *J. Cell Biol.* 85:597, 1980.
263. Rollhäuser, H., Kriz, W., and Heinke, W. Das Gefäss-System der Rattenniere. *Z. Zellforsch. Mikrosk. Anat.* 64:381, 1964.
264. Rosen, S. Localization of carbonic anhydrase activity in the vertebrate nephron. *Histochem. J.* 4:35, 1972.
265. Rostgaard, J., and Thuneberg, L. Electron microscopical observations on the brush border of proximal tubule cells of mammalian kidney. *Z. Zellforsch. Mikrosk. Anat.* 132:473, 1972.
266. Roth, J., Brown, D., Norman, A. W., and Orci, L. Localization of the vitamin D–dependent calcium-binding protein in mammalian kidney. *Am. J. Physiol.* 243:F243, 1982.
267. Roth, J., Brown, D., and Orci, L. Regional distribution of *N*-acetyl-D-galactosamine residues in the glycocalyx of glomerular podocytes. *J. Cell Biol.* 96:1189, 1983.
268. Rouiller, C., and Orci, L. The Structure of the Juxtaglomerular Complex. In C. Rouiller and A. F. Muller (Eds.), *The Kidney: Morphology, Biochemistry, Physiology,* Vol. 4. New York: Academic Press, 1971. P. 1.
269. Ryan, G. B., Alcorn, D., Coghlan, J. P., Hill, P. A., and Jacobs, R. Ultrastructural morphology of granule release from juxtaglomerular myoepithelioid and peripolar cells. *Kidney Int.* 22 (Suppl. 12):S3, 1982.
270. Ryan, G. B., Coghlan, J. P., and Scoggins, B. A. The granulated peripolar epithelial cell: A potential secretory component of the renal juxtaglomerular complex. *Nature* 277:655, 1979.
271. Sakai, T., and Kriz, W. The structural relationship between mesangial cells and basement membrane of the renal glomerulus. *Anat. Embryol.* 176:373, 1987.
272. Salido, E. C., Barajas, L., Lechago, J., Laborde, N. P., and Fisher, D. A. Immunocytochemical localization of epidermal growth factor in mouse kidney. *J. Histochem. Cytochem.* 34:1155, 1986.
273. Schiller, A., Forssmann, W. G., and Taugner, R. The tight junctions of renal tubules in the cortex and outer medulla: A quantitative study of the kidneys of six species. *Cell Tissue Res.* 212:395, 1980.
274. Schiller, A., and Taugner, R. Junctions between interstitial cells of the renal medulla: A freeze-fracture study. *Cell Tissue Res.* 203:231, 1979.
275. Schiller, A., and Taugner, R. Heterogeneity of tight junctions along the collecting duct in the renal medulla: A freeze-fracture study in rat and rabbit. *Cell Tissue Res.* 223:603, 1982.
276. Schiller, A., Taugner, R., and Kriz, W. The thin limbs of Henle's loop in the rabbit: A freeze-fracture study. *Cell Tissue Res.* 207:249, 1980.
277. Schiller, A., Taugner, R., and Roesinger, B. Vergleichende Morphologie der Zonulae occlu-

dentes am Nierentubulus. *Verh. Anat. Ges.* 72: 229, 1978.
278. Schlondorff, D. The glomerular mesangial cell: An expanding role for a specialized pericyte. *FASEB J.* 1:272, 1987.
279. Schmidt, U., Schmid, J., Schmid, H., and Dubach, U. C. Sodium- and potassium-activated ATPase: A possible target of aldosterone. *J. Clin. Invest.* 55:655, 1975.
280. Schmidt-Nielsen, B. The renal pelvis. *Kidney Int.* 31:621, 1987.
281. Schmidt-Nielsen, B., and O'Dell, R. Structure and concentrating mechanism in the mammalian kidney. *Am. J. Physiol.* 200:1119, 1961.
282. Schmidt-Nielsen, B., and Pfeiffer, E. W. Urea and urinary concentrating ability in the mountain beaver *Aplodontia rufa. Am J. Physiol.* 218:1370, 1970.
283. Schneeberger, E. E., Levey, R. H., McCluskey, R. T., and Karnovsky, M. J. The isoporous substructure of the human glomerular slit diaphragm. *Kidney Int.* 8:48, 1975.
284. Schreiner, G. F., and Cotran, R. S. Localization of an Ia-bearing glomerular cell in the mesangium. *J. Cell Biol.* 94:483, 1982.
285. Schurek, H. J., and Kriz, W. Morphologic and functional evidence for oxygen deficiency in the isolated perfused rat kidney. *Lab. Invest.* 53:145, 1985.
286. Schwartz, G. J., Barasch, J., and Al-Awqati, Q Plasticity of functional epithelial polarity. *Nature* 318:368, 1985.
287. Schwartz, M. M., Karnovsky, M. J., and Venkatachalam, M. A. Ultrastructural differences between rat inner medullary descending and ascending vasa recta. *Lab. Invest.* 35:161, 1976.
288. Schwartz, M. M., Karnovsky, M. J., and Venkatachalam, M. A. Regional membrane specialization in the thin limbs of Henle's loops as seen by freeze-fracture electron microscopy. *Kidney Int.* 16:577, 1979.
289. Schwartz, M. M., and Venkatachalam, M. A. Structural differences in thin limbs of Henle: Physiological implications. *Kidney Int.* 6:193, 1974.
290. Seiler, M. W., Venkatachalam, M. A., and Cotran, R. S. Glomerular epithelium: Structural alterations induced by polycations. *Science* 189: 390, 1975.
291. Shea, S. M. Glomerular hemodynamics and vascular structure: The pattern and dimensions of a single rat glomerular capillary network reconstructed from ultrathin sections. *Microvasc. Res.* 18:129, 1979.
292. Shea, S. M., and Morrison, A. B. A stereological study of the glomerular filter in the rat: Morphometry of the slit diaphragm and basement membrane. *J. Cell Biol.* 67:436, 1975.
293. Sikri, K. L., Foster, C. L., MacHugh, N., and Marshall, R. D. Localization of Tamm-Horsfall glycoprotein in the human kidney using immunofluorescence and immunoelectron microscopical techniques. *J. Anat.* 132:597, 1981.
294. Silverblatt, F. J., and Bulger, R. E. Gap junctions occur in vertebrate renal proximal tubule cells. *J. Cell Biol.* 47:513, 1970.
295. Simionescu, N. Cellular aspects of transcapillary exchange. *Physiol. Rev.* 63:1536, 1983.
296. Sisson, S., Dysart, N. K., Fish, A. J., and Vernier, R. L. Localization of Goodpasture antigen by immunoelectron microscopy. *Clin. Immunol. Immunopathol.* 23:414, 1982.
297. Smith. H. W. *The Kidney: Structure and Function in Health and Disease.* New York: Oxford University Press, 1951.
298. Sperber, J. Studies on the mammalian kidney. *Zool. Bidrag. Uppsala* 22:249, 1944.
299. Spiro, R. G. Basement Membranes and Collagens. In A. Gottschalk (Ed.), *Glycoproteins,* Part B. Amsterdam: Elsevier, 1972. P. 964.
300. Stanton, B. A., Biemesderfer, D., Wade, J. B., and Biebisch, G. Structural and functional study of the rat distal nephron: Effects of potassium adaptation and depletion. *Kidney Int.* 19:36, 1981.
301. Steffes, M. W., Barbosa, J., Basgen, J. M., Sutherland, D. E. R., Najarian, J. S., and Mauer, S. M. Quantitative glomerular morphology of the normal human kidney. *Lab. Invest.* 49:82, 1983.
302. Stetson, D. L., Wade, J. B., and Giebisch, G. Morphologic alterations in the rat medullary collecting duct following potassium depletion. *Kidney Int.* 17:45, 1980.
303. Stow, J. L., Sawada, H., and Farquhar, M. G. Basement membrane heparan sulfate proteoglycans are concentrated in the laminae rarae and in the podocytes of the rat renal glomerulus. *Proc. Natl. Acad. Sci. U.S.A.* 82:3296, 1985.
304. Swann, H. G., and Norman, R. J. The periarterial spaces of the kidney. *Tex. Rep. Biol. Med.* 28:317, 1970.
305. Sykes, D. The arterial supply of the human kidney with special reference to accessory renal arteries. *Br. J. Surg.* 50:368, 1963.
306. Sykes, D. The morphology of renal lobulations and calyces, and their relationships to partial nephrectomy. *Br. J. Surg.* 51:294, 1964.
307. Taugner, R., Buhrle, C. P., Hackenthal, E., Mannek, E., and Nobiling, R. Morphology of the juxtaglomerular apparatus and secretory mechanisms. *Contrib. Nephrol.* 43:76, 1984.
308. Taugner, R., Forssmann, W. G., Billich, H., Boll,

U., Ganten, D., and Seller, H. Innervation of the Juxtaglomerular Apparatus and the Effect of Renal Nerve Stimulation. In R. E. Coupland and W. G. Forssmann (Eds.), *Peripheral Neuroendocrine Interaction*. New York: Springer-Verlag, 1978. P. 153.

309. Taugner, R., Forssmann, W. G., Ganten, D., and Schiller, A. Studies on the juxtaglomerular apparatus: VI. Sympathetic innervation, catecholamines and the renin-angiotensin-system in rats and tree shrews (*Tupaia belangeri*). *Cell Tissue Res.* 212:375, 1980.
310. Taugner, R., and Hackenthal, E. Angiotensin II in epithelioid (renin-containing) cells of rat kidney. *Histochemistry* 72:499, 1981.
311. Taugner, R., Schiller, A., Kaissling, B., and Kriz, W. Gap junctional coupling between the JGA and the glomerular tuft. *Cell Tissue Res.* 186:279, 1978.
312. Taugner, R., Whalley, A., Angermuller, S., Buhrle, C. P., and Hackenthal, E. Are the renin-containing granules of juxtaglomerular epithelioid cells modified lysosomes? *Cell Tissue Res.* 239:575, 1985.
313. Thoenes, W. Transportwege in den Harnkanälchen der Säugerniere. In K. E. Wohlfarth-Bottermann (Ed.), *Organisation der Zelle: Sekretion und Exkretion*. Berlin: Springer, 1965. P. 315.
314. Thurau, K., Grüner, A., Mason, J., and Dahlheim, H. Tubular signal for the renin activity in the juxtaglomerular apparatus. *Kidney Int.* 22 (Suppl. 12):S55, 1982.
315. Tisher, C. C., Bulger, R. E., and Trump, B. F. Human renal ultrastructure: I. Proximal tubule of healthy individuals. *Lab. Invest.* 15:1357, 1966.
316. Tisher, C. C., Bulger, R. E., and Trump, B. F. Human renal ultrastructure: III. The distal tubule in healthv individuals. *Lab. Invest.* 18:655, 1968.
317. Tisher, C. C., Bulger, R. E., and Valtin, H. Morphology of the renal medulla in water diuresis and vasopressin-induced antidiuresis. *Am. J. Physiol.* 220:87, 1971.
318. Tisher, C. C., and Yarger, W. E. Lanthanum permeability of tight junctions along the collecting duct of the rat. *Kidney Int.* 7:35, 1975.
319. Trenchev, P., Dorling, J., Webb, J., and Holborow, E. J. Localization of smooth muscle–like contractile proteins in kidney by immunoelectron microscopy. *J. Anat.* 121:85, 1976.
320. Unwin, R. J., Ganz, M. D., and Sterzel, R. B. Brain-gut peptides, renal function and cell growth. *Kidney Int.* 37:1031, 1990.
321. van Deurs, B., and Christensen, E. I. Endocytosis in kidney proximal tubule cells and cultured fibroblasts: A review of the structural aspects of membrane recycling between the plasma membrane and endocytic vacuoles. *Eur. J. Cell Biol.* 33:163, 1984.
322. Venkatachalam, M. A., and Karnovsky, M. J. Extravascular protein in the kidney: An ultrastructural study of its relation to renal peritubular capillary permeability using protein tracers. *Lab. Invest.* 27:435, 1972.
323. Venkatachalam, M. A., and Rennke, H. G. Glomerular Filtration of Macromolecules: Structural, Molecular and Functional Determinants. In A. Leaf, G. Giebisch, L. Bolis, and S. Gorini (Eds.), *Renal Pathophysiology: Recent Advances*. New York: Raven Press, 1980. P. 43.
324. Verkman, A. S. Mechanisms and regulation of water permeability in renal epithelia. *Am. J. Physiol.* 257:C837, 1989.
325. Verkman, A. S., Lencer, W. I., and Brown, D. Endosomes from kidney collecting tubule cells contain the vasopressin-sensitive water channel. *Nature* 333:268, 1988.
326. Verlander, J. W., Madsen, K. M., and Tisher, C. C. Effect of acute respiratory acidosis on two populations of intercalated cells in rat cortical collecting duct. *Am. J. Physiol.* 253:F1142, 1988.
327. von der Mark, H., Aumailley, M., Wick, G., Fleischmajer, R., and Timpl, R. Immunochemistry, genuine size, and tissue localization of collagen VI. *Eur. J. Biochem.* 142:493, 1984.
327*a*. von Hagens, G., Tiedemann, K., and Kriz, W. The current potential of plastination. *Anat. Embryol. (Berl.)* 175:411, 1987.
328. von Möllendorff, W. Der Exkretionsapparat. In *Handbuch der Mikroskopischen Anatomie des Menschen*, Vol. 7. Berlin: Springer, 1930. P. 1.
329. Wade, J. B., O'Neil, R. G., Pryor, J. L., and Boulpaep, E. L. Modulation of cell membrane area in renal collecting tubules by corticosteroid hormones. *J. Cell Biol.* 81:439, 1979.
330. Welling, L. W., Evan, A. P., and Welling, D. J. Shape of cells and extracellular channels in rabbit cortical collecting ducts. *Kidney Int.* 20:211, 1981.
331. Welling, L. W., and Welling, D. J. Surface areas of brush border and lateral cell walls in the rabbit proximal nephron. *Kidney Int.* 8:343, 1975.
332. Welling, L. W., and Welling, D. J. Shape of epithelial cells and intercellular channels in the rabbit proximal nephron. *Kidney Int.* 9:385, 1976.
333. Welling, L. W., Welling, D. J., and Hill, J. J. Shape of cells and intercellular channels in rabbit thick ascending limb of Henle. *Kidney Int.* 13:144, 1978.
334. Weyer, P., Brown, D., and Orci, L. Lectin gold labeling of glycoconjugates in normal and Brattleboro rat papilla: Effect of vasopressin. *Am. J. Phys-*

iol. 254:C450, 1988.

335. Williams, P. L. (Ed.). *Gray's Anatomy,* 37th Ed. Edinburgh: Livingstone, 1989.

336. Woodhall, P. B., and Tisher, C. C. Response of the distal tubule and cortical collecting duct to vasopressin in the rat. *J. Clin. Invest.* 52:3095, 1973.

337. Wright, F. S., and Briggs, J. P. Feedback control of glomerular blood flow, pressure, and filtration rate. *Physiol. Rev.* 59:958, 1979.

338. Yamamoto, K., and Wilson, D. R. Outer medullary circulatory defect in ischemic acute renal failure. *Am. J. Pathol.* 116:253, 1984.

339. Zabel, M., and Schiebler, T. H. Histochemical, autoradiographic and electron microscopic investigations of the renal proximal tubule of male and female rats after castration. *Histochemistry* 69:255, 1980.

340. Zimmermann, K. W. Über den Bau des Glomerulus der Säugerniere. Weitere Mitteilungen. *Z. Mikroskop. Anat. Forsch.* 32:176, 1933.

341. Zusman, R. M., and Keiser, H. R. Prostaglandin biosynthesis by rabbit renomedullary interstitial cells in tissue culture: Stimulation by angiotensin II, bradykinin and arginine vasopressin. *J. Clin. Invest.* 60:215, 1977.

R. Anthony Risdon

2 Development, Developmental Defects, and Cystic Diseases of the Kidney

DEVELOPMENT OF THE KIDNEY

The human kidney develops from the nephrogenic cord, an intermediate mass of mesoderm located between the dorsal somites and the lateral plate mesoderm behind the embryonic coelom. Three successive excretory systems are formed, the pronephros from the most cranial (cervicodorsal) segments of the nephrogenic cord, the mesonephros from the intermediate (dorsolumbar) segments, and the pronephros from the most caudal (initially sacral) segments. The pronephros and mesonephros are transient organs, although both are essential to the formation of the definitive kidney from the metanephros. Mesonephric derivatives also form structures in the fully developed organism. While the pro-, meso-, and metanephros form sequentially in the developing embryo, there is some overlap so that the mesonephros begins to develop before the pronephros has disappeared, and likewise, the metanephros forms before the mesonephros has entirely regressed. Some authorities [333] have regarded a strict delineation of three kidneys as artificial, viewing the whole system as a single unit, the holonephros. However, in mammals, including man, the meso- and metanephros at least can be clearly recognized as separate organs.

The Pronephros

The most cranial portion of the nephrogenic cord between the 7th and 14th somites develops as the pronephros from the end of the third week after conception. The pronephros consists only of a few rudimentary tubules opening proximally to the coelomic cavity by nephrostomes and coalescing distally to form the pronephric duct, which grows caudally toward the cloaca. The pronephros does not function in the human embryo, and the most cephalic tubules regress before the more caudal tubules form; however, the pronephric duct survives as the mesonephric duct (see below).

The Mesonephros

The mesonephros begins to develop from the dorsolumbar segments of the nephrogenic cord below the pronephros and before the latter has entirely disappeared, growing to form a prominent (urogenital) ridge that bulges into the coelomic cavity (Fig. 2-1). A series of vesicles form, each of which develops into a nephron consisting of a glomerulus and a tubule with proximal, thicker-walled secretory and distal, thinner excretory segments. Capillaries forming each mesonephric glomerulus develop in situ, establishing connections with the primitive aorta by an afferent arteriole and with the posterior cardinal vein by an efferent arteriole. The tubules join an excretory duct (originally the pronephric duct, but now called the *mesonephric,* or *wolffian, duct*) that gradually extends caudally to communicate with the cloaca at the 26th to 28th somite stage (about 4 weeks postconception). From about the fifth week of gestation, the most cranial mesonephric nephrons begin to regress, while the more caudal nephrons are still forming; by the time the last nephrons are developing, about two-thirds have already disappeared. While it is possible that some excretory function is performed by the mesonephros in the human embryo, it is only transitory. Eventually, all the mesonephric glomeruli involute, but some mesonephric structures do persist. In the male, remnants of a number of caudal mesonephric tubules develop as the efferent ducts of the epididymis. The mesonephric duct forms the duct of the epididymis, the vas deferens, the seminal vesicle, and the ejaculatory duct. In the female, apart from a few vestigial and inconstant structures, such as the epoophoron, the paroophoron, and Gartner's duct, the whole mesonephros degenerates during the third month of gestation.

The Metanephros

The metanephros forms the definitive kidney and is developed in two parts: the renal parenchyma from the caudal end of the nephrogenic cord (called the *metanephric blastema*) and the excretory system (the collecting ducts, calyces, renal pelvis, and ureter) from the ureteric bud. This is a hollow, posteromedial offshoot arising during the fifth week (5-mm stage) from the caudal end of the mesonephric duct opposite the 28th somite, where it curves medially to join the cloaca. The proximal end of the ureteric bud grows dorsally and cranially

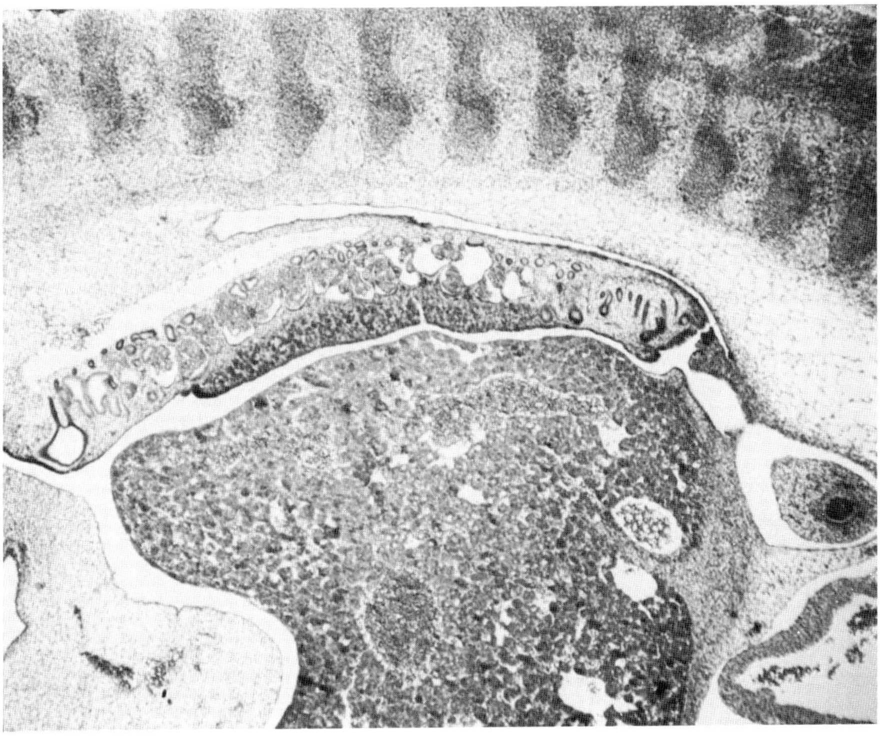

Fig. 2-1. *Longitudinal section of the mesonephros in a 14-mm human embryo. H&E; ×20.*

toward the metanephric blastema, while its distal end extends caudally as the embryo elongates. The ureteric bud develops a slightly swollen cranial tip, the ampulla, to be distinguished from the remaining tubular interstitial portion. When the ureteric bud impinges on the metanephric blastema, the latter is pushed upward to lie dorsal to the caudal end of the degenerating mesonephros. Here it is situated behind the peritoneum but ventral to the corresponding umbilical artery. As the ampulla of the ureteric bud contacts the metanephric blastema, which now forms a distinct cap of densely packed cells, it undergoes a process of rapid dichotomous branching, each branch forming a new ampulla. Each ampulla has the capacity for further dichotomous branching and ultimately to induce nephron formation from the mesenchyme of the metanephric blastema.

FORMATION OF THE RENAL PELVIS AND CALYCES

This process, together with the development of the nephrons and collecting ducts, has been studied by Osathanondh and Potter [233,235] by microdissection of fetal kidneys (Figs. 2-2 and 2-3). These authors showed that the renal pelvis and major calyces are formed from the first three to six generations of ureteric bud branches (branching occurs more rapidly at the poles than in the midzone) and the minor calyces from the subsequent generation of branches. Because branching is so rapid at this stage, the interstitial portions of the branches are very short, and indeed, sometimes a number of branches appear to arise from a single stem. Distention of the whole system, which is ascribed to the onset of urine production as neph-

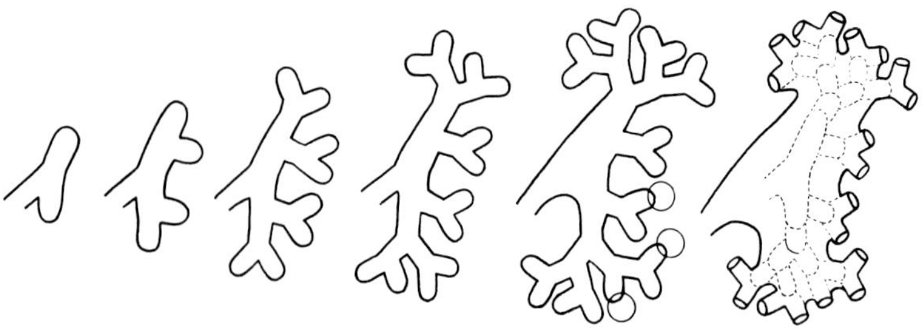

FIG. 2-2. *Development of the renal pelvis. Diagram represents coalescence of the third through fifth generations of branches (circled) of the ureteric bud to form the renal pelvis. (From Osathanondh, V., and Potter, E. L.* Arch. Pathol. *76: 277, 1963. Copyright 1963, American Medical Association.)*

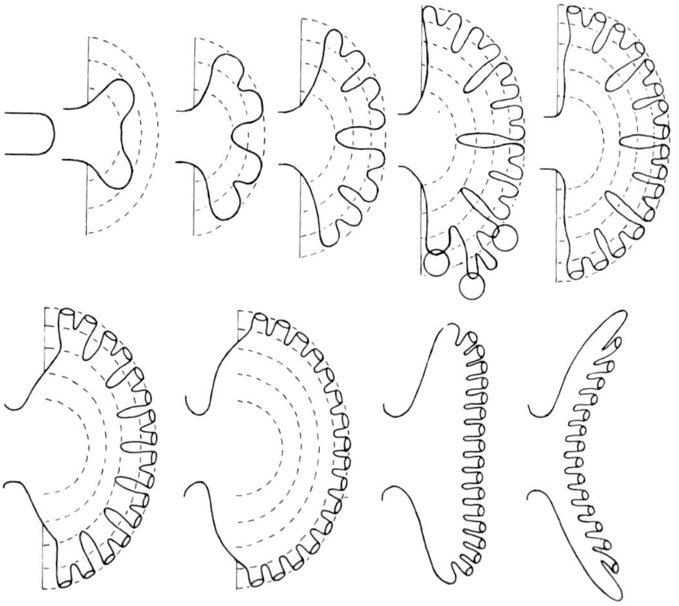

FIG. 2-3. *Development of renal calyces and papillae. Diagrams depict coalescence of the third through fifth generations of branches (circled) of the primordial calyx and inward prolapse of the renal papilla. (From Osathanondh, V., and Potter, E. L.* Arch. Pathol. *76: 277, 1963. Copyright 1963, American Medical Association.)*

rons start to function, results in the coalescence of the first generations of branches to give the more familiar appearance of the pelvicalyceal system seen postnatally. This is completed by about the tenth to twelfth week of gestation.

When the minor calyces are formed, some 20 or so ampullae are related to each minor calyx, and it is from these that the papillary collecting ducts originate. Further branchings of these ampullae are associated with nephron formation, and these branchings proceed more slowly with longer intervening periods of interstitial growth. From about the eleventh week, the spherical expansion of the calyces is limited by the development of nephrons associated with their own and surrounding collecting duct systems that form the developing renal papillae. The minor calyces are indented by the papillae and change from a spherical to a wineglass shape, with the cup-shaped portion around the developing papilla and a narrower stem-like infundibular portion connecting to the major calyx. This process is achieved by about the fourteenth week of gestation and can be appreciated in histologic sections of fetal kidneys at this gestational age.

FORMATION OF THE COLLECTING DUCT SYSTEM AND NEPHRONS

From the end of the seventh week (18- to 20-mm stage), the development of the collecting duct system and nephrons proceeds in parallel. The nephrons develop from oval condensations of metanephric blastemal cells that become related to the ampullary tip of each branch of the ureteric bud (Fig. 2-4). Some of the blastemal cells in each

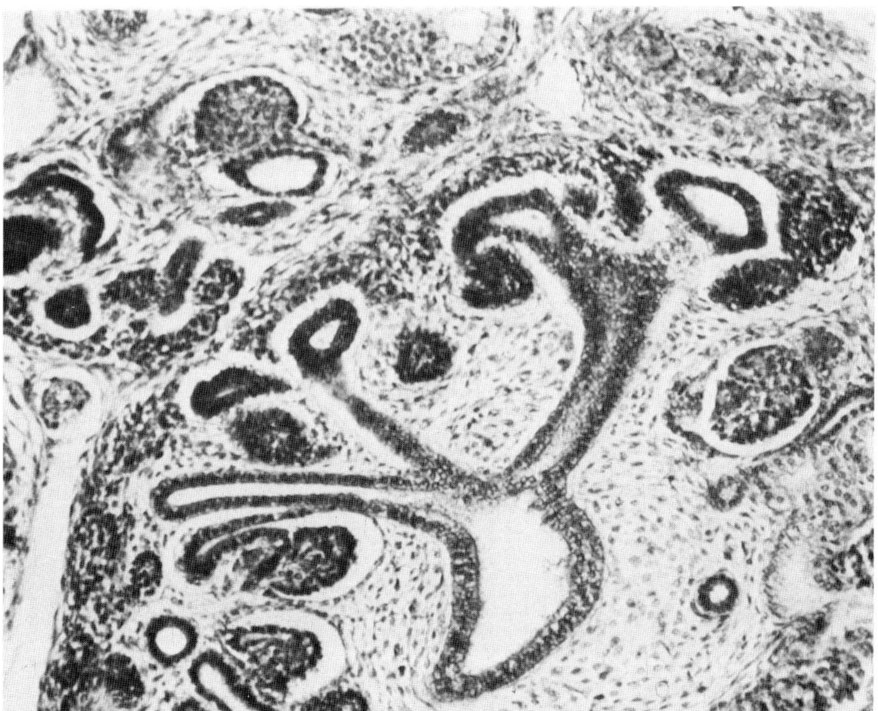

FIG. 2-4. *Metanephros from a 9-week human fetus. Branching of the ureteric bud with condensations of metanephric blastema from which nephrons form, related to the dilated ampullae. H&E; ×60.*

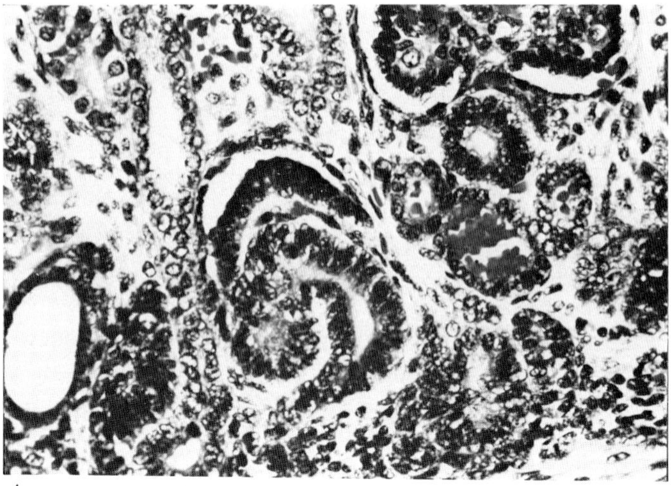

A

FIG. 2-5. *Glomerular differentiation (A–D) in a 24-week human fetus. (A) The S-shaped nephrogenic vesicle. H&E; × 170. (B) Early formation of glomerular tuft and Bowman's space. H&E; × 170. (C) Simple segmentation of the glomerular tuft; plump, cuboidal visceral epithelial cells. H&E; × 170. (D) Glomeruli from a term infant. H&E; × 170.*

condensation form a hollow (nephrogenic) vesicle, while others form a separate solid cap for the next subdivision of the ampulla.

Each hollow vesicle elongates and folds back on itself to become S-shaped (Fig. 2-5A). The proximal end of the upper limb joins and becomes continuous with the lumen of the related ureteric bud ampulla. The upper and middle limbs of the nephrogenic vesicle elongate further and differentiate to form the proximal and distal convoluted tubules and the loop of Henle. Adjacent to the lower limb of the vesicle a tuft of capillaries develops, and this forms the glomerular tuft (Fig. 2-5B–D). This invaginates the lower limb, which becomes concave. The outer-layer cells become flattened to form the parietal layer of Bowman's capsule, while the inner-layer cells remain columnar and stretch over the developing tuft capillaries to form the visceral epithelial cells of the glomerulus. Mesangial cells probably enter the glomerulus with the capillaries.

Since nephrons are attached to the growing tips of the ureteric bud branches at this stage, they advance progressively with the ampullae away from the future hilus of the kidney, the interstitial portions of the collecting ducts forming the future medullary collecting ducts.

After the fourteenth week of gestation, the first period of nephron induction ends and the second period commences. This second period of nephronogenesis, which lasts until about the twenty-second week of gestation, is characterized by the formation of nephron arcades. Each ampulla ceases to divide and becomes capable of inducing the formation of a further three to six nephrons. With the induction of further nephrons, the connecting tubule of the older nephron shifts the position of its point of attachment away from the ampulla to the connecting tubule of the next-formed nephron so that they are joined together in a string or arcade of between four and seven nephrons. The innermost and first-formed member of each nephron arcade is a nephron formed during the first period of nephronogenesis and becomes a juxtamedullary nephron in the fully developed organ. The loops of Henle are longest in these nephrons, extending almost to the papillary tip.

In the third period of nephronogenesis, from the twenty-second to the thirty-sixth week of gestation, the ampullae advance to the peripheral

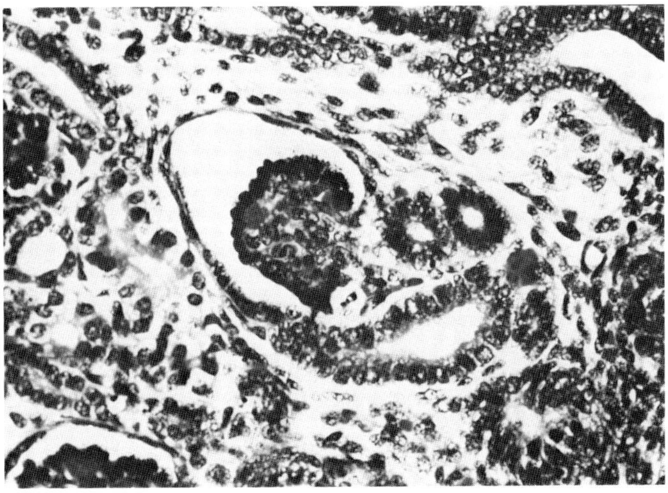

B

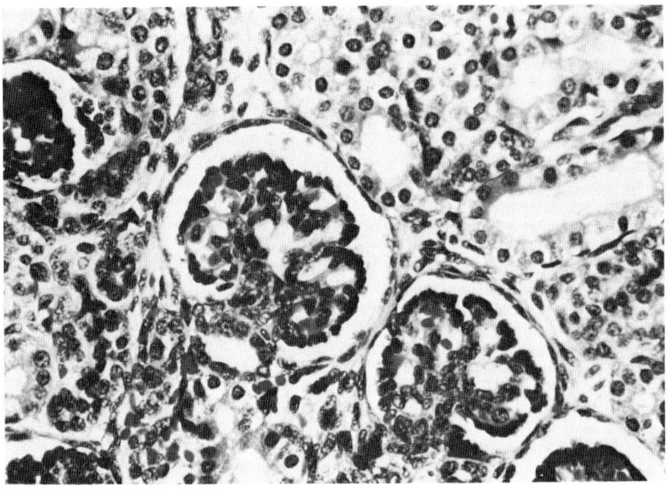

C

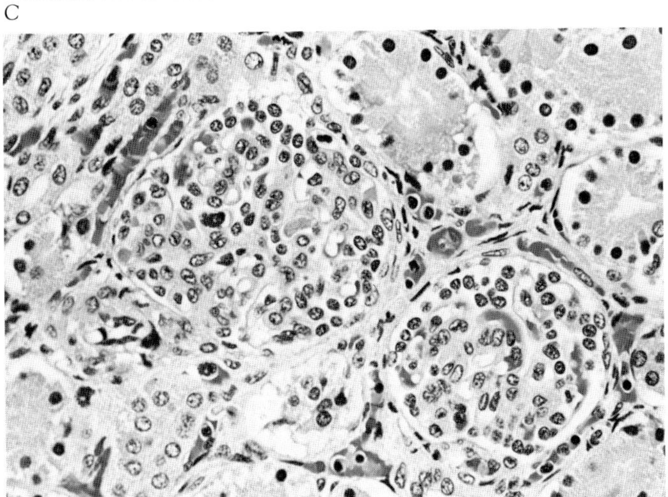

D

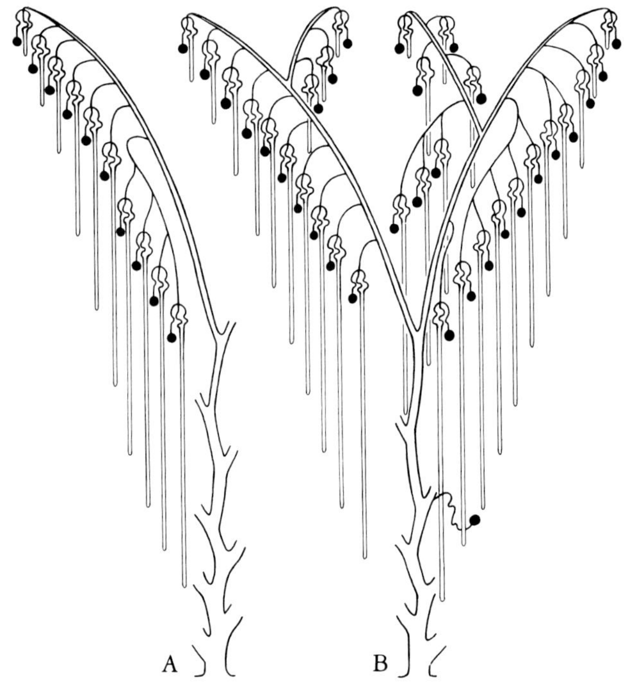

FIG. 2-6. *Arrangement of nephrons at birth as revealed by microdissection. (A) Usual pattern with, sequentially, an arcade of four nephrons that drain into a tributary of the collecting duct and six nephrons that drain individually into the collecting duct. (B) Possible variations. (From Osathanondh, V., and Potter, E. L.* Arch. Pathol. *76: 290, 1963. Copyright 1963, American Medical Association.)*

cortex beyond the region of nephron arcades. A further four to seven nephrons form and are attached separately just behind the ampullary tips. No further divisions of the ampullae occur, and as each new nephron is added, the ampullae advance further toward the surface. At about 36 weeks, the ampullae cease to function and disappear (Fig. 2-6). No new nephrons are then formed, the last to develop producing the subcapsular, so-called nephrogenic zone that can be seen in fetal kidneys up to 36 weeks and is useful in dating gestational age (Fig. 2-7).

In the fourth period of nephronogenesis, from 36 weeks to term, no new nephrons are formed, and this period is one purely of interstitial growth. Loops of Henle continue to increase in length, and the proximal and distal tubules become longer and more tortuous. In mature infants at birth, some 20 percent of the loops of Henle are still within the renal cortex [107].

Blood Supply of the Developing Kidney

When first formed, the metanephros is at the level of the upper sacral segments and receives its blood supply from the lateral sacral branches of the aorta. Largely as a result of differential growth of the caudal end of the embryo, the kidneys are found at a progressively higher level. This "ascent" of the kidney from its originally sacral to its ultimate lumbar position, which it reaches between the fifth and eighth week of gestation, is associated with its blood supply being derived from stem branches from the aorta at a progressively higher

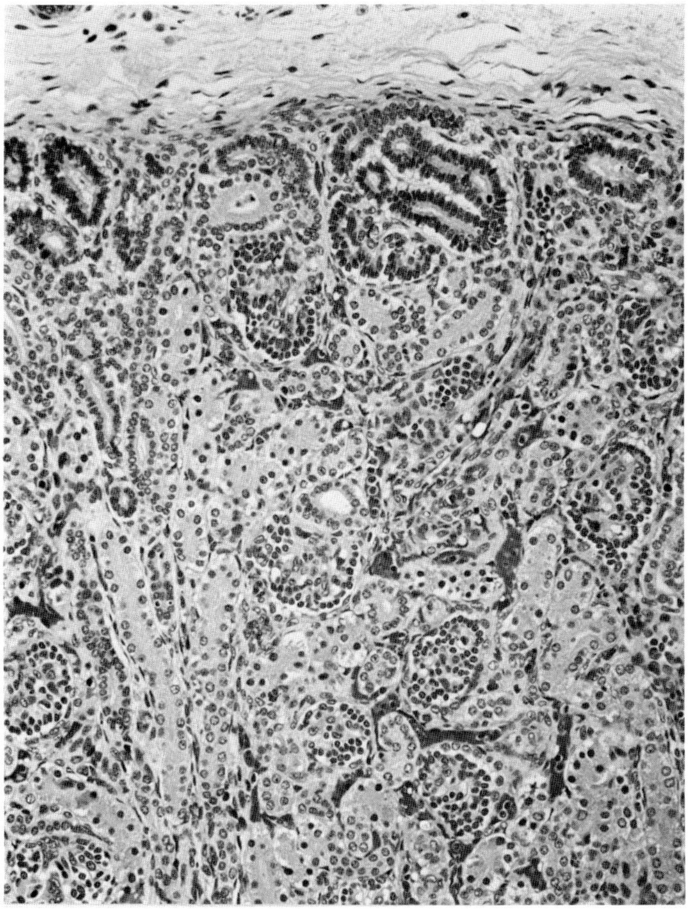

Fig. 2-7. *Subcapsular nephrogenic zone in the renal cortex of a 32-week human fetus. H&E;* ×60.

level, until the definitive renal arteries, arising from the aorta at about the level of the 2nd lumbar vertebra, are reached.

DEVELOPMENTAL DEFECTS OF THE KIDNEY

Malformations of the kidney and urinary tract are common, and if the full spectrum from minor, clinically insignificant lesions to severe, lethal abnormalities is considered, such malformations affect up to 10 percent of all births. Congenital malformations of the kidney are often associated with other anomalies in the urinary tract or other systems and are sometimes components of recognizable syndromes of multiple malformations. While some clues to the pathogenesis of individual anomalies can be gleaned from consideration of coexistent malformations and a knowledge of normal development, the exact causes are largely unknown.

In general, malformations of the kidney include abnormalities of size, number, position, form, or parenchymal differentiation. All are present at birth and broadly represent anomalies of metanephric induction and development. In this section, the categories of congenital renal anomalies to be considered are shown in Table 2-1; renal dysplasia is tabulated separately (see Table 2-2), and renal cystic diseases are considered in a later section of this chapter (see Table 2-3).

No attempt has been made to present a formal classification of congenital abnormalities of the kidneys because no satisfactory system exists. For example, dysplastic kidneys are often congenitally small and thus could be regarded as examples of a congenital deficiency of renal parenchyma as well as of anomalous metanephric differentiation. They also may be ectopic or part of a fused (horseshoe) kidney and thus could be categorized as congenital abnormalities of position and form.

Renal Agenesis

Renal agenesis is defined as complete absence of the kidney, which may be unilateral or bilateral. In the majority of affected individuals, the corresponding ureter and trigonal area of the bladder are also absent, although in 10 to 20 percent a short length of distal ureter can be recognized. Experimental studies of arsenate-induced renal agenesis in the rat [60] indicate that it results from a failure of the mesonephric duct to give rise to the ureteric bud with consequent failure to induce differentiation of the metanephric blastema.

TABLE 2-1. *Congenital abnormalities of the kidney*

I. Renal agenesis
   A. Unilateral renal agenesis
   B. Bilateral renal agenesis
   C. Hereditary renal adysplasia
II. Renal hypoplasia
   A. Oligonephronic hypoplasia (oligomeganephronia)
   B. Simple hypoplasia
III. Renal dysplasia (see Table 2-2)
IV. Congenital nephromegaly
V. Congenital hydronephrosis
VI. Renal ectopia and malrotation
VII. Renal fusion
VIII. Renal duplication
IX. Supernumerary kidney
X. Renal tubular dysgenesis

In a large study of over half a million consecutive births in British Columbia ending in 1982 [351], the incidence of unilateral agenesis was approximately 1 in 5000 and of bilateral agenesis 1 in 7000. These data were derived from the British Columbia Health Surveillance Registry, and the figure for bilateral agenesis, where the diagnosis is unlikely to be missed, is probably more accurate than that for unilateral agenesis, where particularly those cases in which the solitary kidney is an isolated anomaly may go unrecorded. Roodhooft et al. [276], basing the diagnosis of unilateral renal agenesis on abdominal ultrasonography, gave a much higher incidence of about 1 in 350 births. Other investigations, such as those of Longo and Thompson [198], based on hospital records, and Doroshow and Abeshouse [87], based on autopsy files, produce figures for unilateral agenesis of approximately 1 in 1000 births.

By analysis of the commonly associated anomalies in the lower end of the body, renal agenesis can be seen as part of a developmental field defect of varying extent [248]. This may be confined to the kidney, ureter, and usually mesonephric and paramesonephric duct derivatives; in this setting, renal agenesis is more commonly unilateral than bilateral. A more extensive field defect incorporates additional anomalies of the hindgut and cloacal membrane, when renal agenesis is usually bilateral. In the most extreme examples, the field defect involves the entire caudal end of the embryo (sirenomelia or the caudal regression syndrome), when renal agenesis is invariably bilateral.

Renal adysplasia is a condition in which unilateral renal agenesis accompanies dysplasia of the contralateral kidney. *Hereditary renal adysplasia* has a slightly different connotation and refers to the occurrence of renal dysplasia, renal adysplasia, and renal agenesis in any of its variations affecting different members of the same family. The genetic link between renal agenesis and some types of renal dysplasia (see p. 104) points to a common pathogenetic mechanism for these anomalies, and it may be that the distinction between them relates to the degree of failure of the ureteric bud in its inductive function on the metanephric blastema. Typically, the adrenal gland appears enlarged and disk-shaped in the presence of renal agenesis, the abnormal adrenal shape probably due to lack of the molding influence of the adjacent kidney. Occasionally, the adrenal gland is completely absent [221].

Severe congenital abnormalities of one or more other organ systems very frequently accompany both unilateral and bilateral renal agenesis. The most common of these are in the gastrointestinal tract (particularly esophageal atresia and tracheoesophageal fistula), in the heart (atrial and ventricular septal defect), and in the central nervous system (neural tube defects, particularly spina bifida with meningomyelocele). The association between renal agenesis and these other congenital anomalies probably reflects the action of some injurious agent operating between the third and sixth weeks of gestation when separation of the enteric and respiratory components of the foregut, cardiac septation, and neural tube closure are all occurring.

UNILATERAL RENAL AGENESIS

Unilateral renal agenesis is equally common in the two sexes. Following the concept that renal agenesis is part of a developmental field defect, unilateral agenesis represents the less severe end of the spectrum. Nevertheless, in about 70 percent of affected subjects there are accompanying anomalies of ipsilateral mesonephric or paramesonephric duct derivatives, and similar defects are seen in the rat model of arsenate-induced renal agenesis [60]. In males, these include absence, hypoplasia, or maldescent of the testis, absence or cystic malformation of the epididymis, and absence of the vas deferens, seminal vesicle, and ejaculatory ducts. In females, unicornuate or bicornuate uteri are the most common paramesonephric anomalies [331]. Absence or hypoplasia of the uterus, fallopian tubes, or ovaries and absence or aplasia of the vagina are also reported and constitute the so-called Rokitansky-Küster-Hauser syndrome. A double uterus (uterus didelphys) and an obstructed hemivagina also have been described [334].

Occasionally, imperforate anus, rectal atresia, and rectourethral or rectovaginal fistula accompany unilateral agenesis, but these anomalies are more common with bilateral agenesis. Hypospadias in boys also may occur with unilateral renal agenesis.

As an isolated anomaly, unilateral renal agenesis is generally asymptomatic, and it is the associated abnormalities that usually bring the condition to light. At autopsy in stillborn and newborn infants, unilateral agenesis is seen in conjunction with major gastrointestinal, cardiovascular, or neural tube defects that are generally responsible for death. In older infants and children, the condition is diagnosed more frequently in females because of obvious coexistent anomalies of the female genital tract.

Hypertrophy and compensatory growth of the contralateral kidney up to twice the normal size occurs, and this solitary kidney is occasionally ectopic and malrotated. In addition, there may be ureteric dilatation.

In older subjects, even isolated unilateral renal agenesis may be of practical significance. Because of its increased size, the solitary kidney may be more often subject to traumatic injury [89], and the inadvertent surgical removal of an injured solitary kidney has been reported [5]. Unilateral agenesis is sufficiently common to make it mandatory that the presence of two kidneys be clearly established before nephrectomy is contemplated, and most authorities regard the presence of both kidneys an essential prerequisite for percutaneous renal biopsy.

It also has been suggested that function of the solitary kidney in unilateral renal agenesis eventually may be compromised in a small minority of cases by the development of proteinuria, focal glomerular sclerosis, and renal failure, possibly because of hyperfiltration as a long-term consequence of a reduced nephron population from birth [174]. The suggestion that hyperfiltration in a solitary kidney can produce functional deterioration has obvious implications in live kidney donors for renal transplantation. However, recent publications suggest that although there is chronic hyperfiltration, a slight increase in urinary protein excretion, and sometimes an increase in systemic blood pressure in uninephrectomized kidney donors, renal failure has not been reported in follow-up studies that have ranged up to 20 years [113].

This matter is discussed in greater detail in Chapter 11.

BILATERAL RENAL AGENESIS

Bilateral renal agenesis (Fig. 2-8) is about twice as common in males as in females. It is incompatible with life, about 40 percent of affected infants being stillborn and the remainder dying in the immediate postnatal period, usually from respiratory insufficiency. As with unilateral renal agenesis, associated mesonephric and paramesonephric duct anomalies are frequent, as are major congenital malformations of the gastrointestinal, cardiac, and nervous systems. The developmental field defect of which renal agenesis is part is often more extensive with bilateral than with unilateral agenesis. The bladder is usually hypoplastic, atretic, or absent, and the urethra is generally atretic. Imperforate anus is more common with bilateral agenesis, and in a proportion of affected individuals, the caudal regression syndrome (absence of the hindgut, sacrum, urethra, and external genitalia) or sirenomelia (posterior limb bud fusion) is seen.

Since no urine is produced in utero in bilateral renal agenesis, oligohydramnios is a constant feature. This contributes to the abnormalities of the face (wide-set eyes, "parrot beak" nose, prominent epicanthic folds, receding chin, and low-set ears with deficient auricular cartilage; Fig. 2-9), spadelike hands, and lower limb deformities, collectively termed the *Potter sequence.* These deformities are thought to be due to pressure of the uterine wall on the developing fetus in the absence of adequate amniotic fluid. The Potter sequence is not confined to bilateral renal agenesis and also may occur with bilateral renal dysplasia or sometimes autosomal recessive polycystic kidney disease, in which intrauterine urine production is also deficient. Bilateral pulmonary hypoplasia, an almost invariable accompanying feature of bilateral agenesis, is usually responsible for early postnatal death. Pulmonary hypoplasia also has been attributed to the effects of oligohydramnios, although the fact that the amniotic fluid is largely derived from nonrenal sources in the first 12 weeks of gestation suggests that other factors also may interfere with early pulmonary development in bilateral renal agenesis.

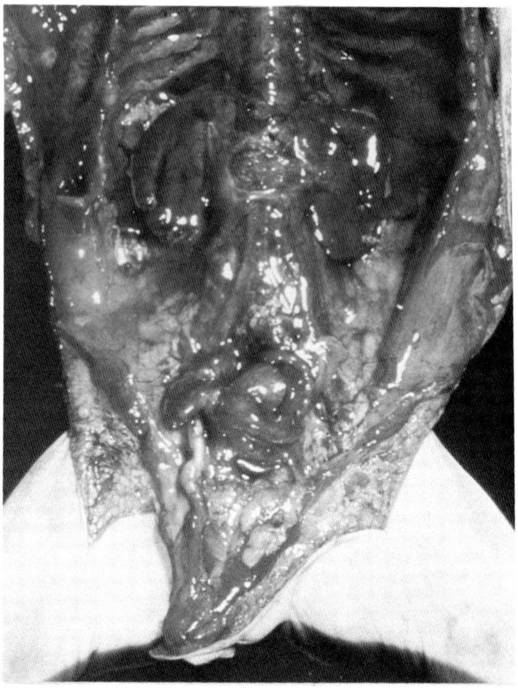

FIG. 2-8. *Bilateral renal agenesis. The kidneys are absent, the adrenals are disk-shaped, and there is a bicornuate uterus. (From Risdon, R. A. Diseases of the Kidney and Lower Urinary Tract. In C. L. Berry (Ed.),* Paediatric Pathology. *Heidelberg: Springer-Verlag, 1981.)*

HEREDITARY RENAL ADYSPLASIA

A familial tendency for bilateral renal agenesis has been recognized for some time [269,291]. More recently, the description of both bilateral and unilateral agenesis, renal dysplasia, and renal adysplasia in members of the same family has led to the concept of hereditary renal adysplasia. The dysplastic kidneys in this condition are usually tiny and rudimentary (renal aplasia) or occasionally multicystic [312]. Bilateral renal agenesis as part of hereditary adysplasia is not associated with si-

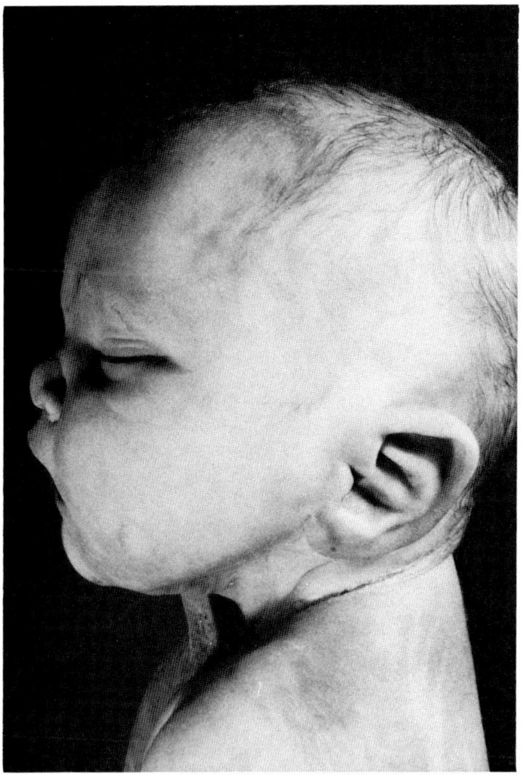

Fig. 2-9. *Potter facies. (From Risdon, R. A. Diseases of the Kidney and Lower Urinary Tract. In C. L. Berry (Ed.),* Paediatric Pathology. *Heidelberg: Springer-Verlag, 1981.)*

renomelia or caudal regression. In cases with unilateral involvement, ipsilateral genital anomalies are common. Bankier et al. [19] gave a recurrence risk of 8 percent for siblings of an index case of bilateral renal agenesis with urogenital anomalies alone. When there were accompanying multiple malformations, the recurrence risk for multiple malformations was 12.5 percent, but the risk of recurrent bilateral agenesis was not increased.

In hereditary renal adysplasia, index cases are usually recognized as perinatal deaths shown to have bilateral renal agenesis at autopsy. Family studies then reveal unilateral renal agenesis or dysplasia in parents or living siblings; other deaths from bilateral renal agenesis also may have occurred in siblings, and sometimes other generations of the family are shown to have been affected. Buchta et al. [59] have indicated good evidence of an autosomal dominant mode of inheritance in familial renal adysplasia, but the occasional cases of agenesis/dysplasia affecting siblings with normal parents suggests that other types of inheritance also may apply.

Renal Hypoplasia

The small kidney, especially when encountered in infancy and childhood, has presented a major problem in diagnosis and evaluation, particularly in the clinical setting where reduced renal size as a result of deficient postnatal growth or an inherent reduction in nephron mass may be difficult to distinguish from secondary atrophy as part of acquired disease [96,360]. These difficulties are compounded by the fact that anomalies of the urinary tract, especially those involving obstruction and vesicoureteral reflux, may not only be associated with acquired renal lesions such as hydronephrotic atrophy and segmental pyelonephritic scarring, but also may have effects in utero that interfere with renal development [266].

DISTINCTION FROM RENAL DYSPLASIA AND ACQUIRED DISEASE

Used correctly, the term *renal hypoplasia* describes a congenitally small kidney that lacks evidence of parenchymal maldifferentiation (renal dysplasia) or of acquired disease sufficient to explain the reduced size. Hypoplastic kidneys are significantly smaller than normal, and since they are often encountered in infancy and childhood, their size needs to be related to the expected mean for age and standard measurements of somatic growth. Most studies of normal renal growth are in the older literature. The work of Coppoletta and Wolbach [79], which compared body length and organ weights (including those of the kidneys) in infants and children, provides the usually accepted standards, and similar results were obtained by Emery and Mithal [95], Landing and Hughes [185], and

Oliver et al. [230]. The $\pm 2SD$ range generally falls between 50 and 150 percent of the expected mean kidney weight so that hypoplastic kidneys can be defined as weighing less than 50 percent of the expected mean.

The number of renal lobes (renunculi) is usually reduced in renal hypoplasia, and demonstration of this requires careful gross examination of the kidney, augmented when possible by radiologic examination after filling the pelvicalyceal system with contrast medium. This helps to exclude segmental scarring and atrophy with associated calyceal clubbing (a change almost diagnostic of acquired reflux-associated segmental scarring) as a reason for reduced renal size. The number of renal lobes is best established by opening the pelvicalyceal system and slicing the kidney to establish the numbers of lobes drained by each papilla. It is not sufficient to merely count the papillae, since compound papillae at the poles of the kidney frequently drain more than one lobe [254]. The traditional method of making a single slice through the long axis of the kidney is seldom sufficient for this assessment. Boissonnat [52] has shown that the normal kidney possesses 10 or more lobes, while hypoplastic kidneys usually have 5 or fewer and occasionally only 1 lobe (so-called unirenicular hypoplasia).

Another traditional criterion for ascribing small renal size to hypoplasia is that the main renal artery is narrow and hypoplastic. This is an unreliable sign in that atrophy of the renal artery can occur with any long-standing disease associated with atrophy of the kidney. However, Portsman [247] has suggested that in acquired renal disease the narrowed renal artery retains a wide, funnel-shaped segment at its origin from the aorta as an indication of its previously wider overall caliber.

Adequate histologic examination of the kidney is also required to exclude evidence of dysplasia or acquired disease sufficient in itself to explain the reduced renal size. It is clear that kidneys that are small entirely because of acquired disease are in no sense correctly described as hypoplastic. However, it is perhaps relevant at this point to mention the so-called Ask-Upmark kidney [9], a type of small kidney associated with hypertension in childhood. One or both kidneys may be affected, and the condition is characterized by reduced renal size and the presence of a transverse groove on the capsular surface, usually at or near the upper pole, overlying an area of parenchymal thinning and an elongated calyx-like recess arising from the renal pelvis (Fig. 2-10). Microscopy of the thinned area of parenchyma reveals sparse or absent glomeruli, atrophic tubules, and tortuous collections of thick-walled arteries and arterioles. Although Royer et al. [282] regarded this as a developmental defect which they termed *segmental renal hypoplasia,* current evidence shows that vesicoureteral reflux is present or has been present in the majority of cases so that the lesion is now regarded as a form of reflux-associated segmental atrophic scarring (reflux nephropathy) and thus an acquired disease [7]. It is further discussed in Chapter 22.

Clear separation of the hypoplastic from the small dysplastic (aplastic or hypodysplastic) kidney is perhaps less secure in that both may represent an intrinsic developmental abnormality of the renal parenchyma, which in both may reflect a primary deficiency of the metanephric blastema or an interference with the inductive capacity of the ureteric bud. The distinction lies in the fact that the small dysplastic kidney shows histologic evidence of parenchymal maldifferentiation that is lacking in the purely hypoplastic kidney. The validity of separating the two lies in the fact that recognizable patterns of ureteral and lower urinary tract anomalies very frequently accompany renal dysplasia, which is thus more properly seen as an abnormality of the whole urinary tract, while renal hypoplasia is generally an isolated anomaly affecting the kidney alone. Also, types of renal dysplasia other than aplasia and hypodysplasia may accompany particular urinary tract anomalies, indicating that renal dysplasia represents a spectrum of renal lesions that are quite separate from renal hypoplasia.

It is evident that much of the earlier literature, which often dealt with the unilateral small kidney in older children and young adults [52,93], failed to make the distinctions between acquired disease, dysplasia, and true hypoplasia discussed here, although the basic concepts had been formulated [16,21]. In particular, terms such as *miniature, dwarf,* or *doll's kidneys* [236,305], which imply only

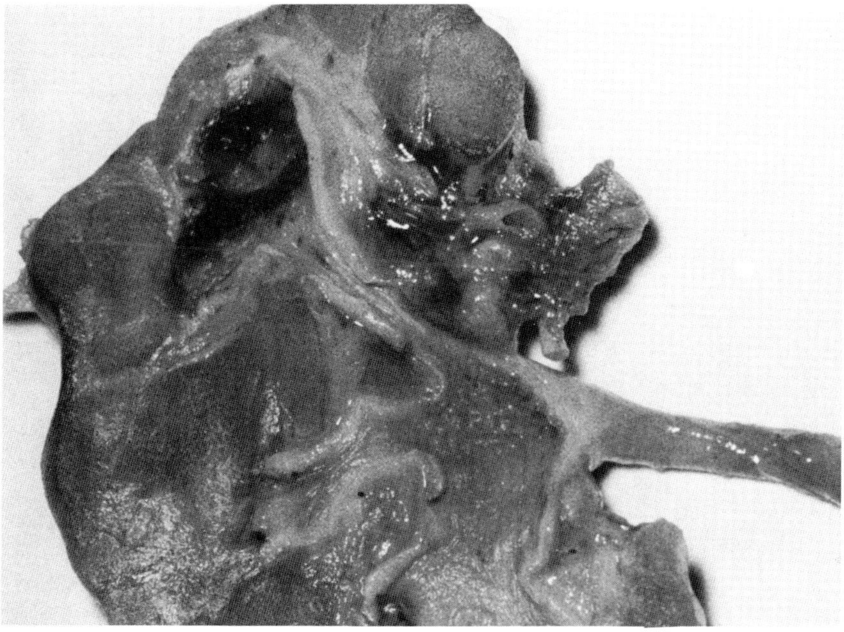

Fig. 2-10. *So-called Ask-Upmark kidney. A nephrectomy specimen from a 10-year-old girl with hypertension. This lesion is now regarded as a form of reflux-associated segmental scarring. (From Risdon et al. [268].)*

reduced renal size, were used to describe what were often clearly dysplastic kidneys.

While the true incidence of renal hypoplasia is difficult to establish, it is apparent that it is much rarer than formerly thought and that most cases are bilateral. Two main varieties can be distinguished, oligonephronic hypoplasia (*oligoméganéphronie*), first described by Royer et al. [281], and simple hypoplasia [40,283].

OLIGONEPHRONIC HYPOPLASIA OLIGOMEGANEPHRONIA)

This describes a distinctive form of nonfamilial bilateral renal hypoplasia in which the combined kidney weights are as low as 12 to 45 g and always less than 50 percent of the expected weight. The number of renal lobes is frequently reduced, and sometimes only one or two pyramids can be identified. The parenchyma is typically firm and pale, and the renal surfaces are smooth or finely granular.

Microscopically, the striking feature is a reduced number of glomeruli. The glomeruli are clearly enlarged by up to three times the normal diameter (Fig. 2-11A), and the tubules are dilated and lined by enlarged epithelial cells. Fetterman and Habib [106] performed microdissection of the kidneys of a 13-year-old with oligonephronic hypoplasia and found the glomerular cross-sectional area to be 5 times normal and the mean glomerular volume to be 12 times normal. The mean proximal tubular length showed a fourfold increase, and the proximal tubular volume was 17 times normal. Other workers [160,224] have demonstrated mesangial hypercellularity of the enlarged glomeruli.

Children with oligonephronic hypoplasia develop polyuria and polydipsia, a urine-concentrating defect, and often salt-wasting in the first 2 years of life. Dehydration, vomiting, unexplained

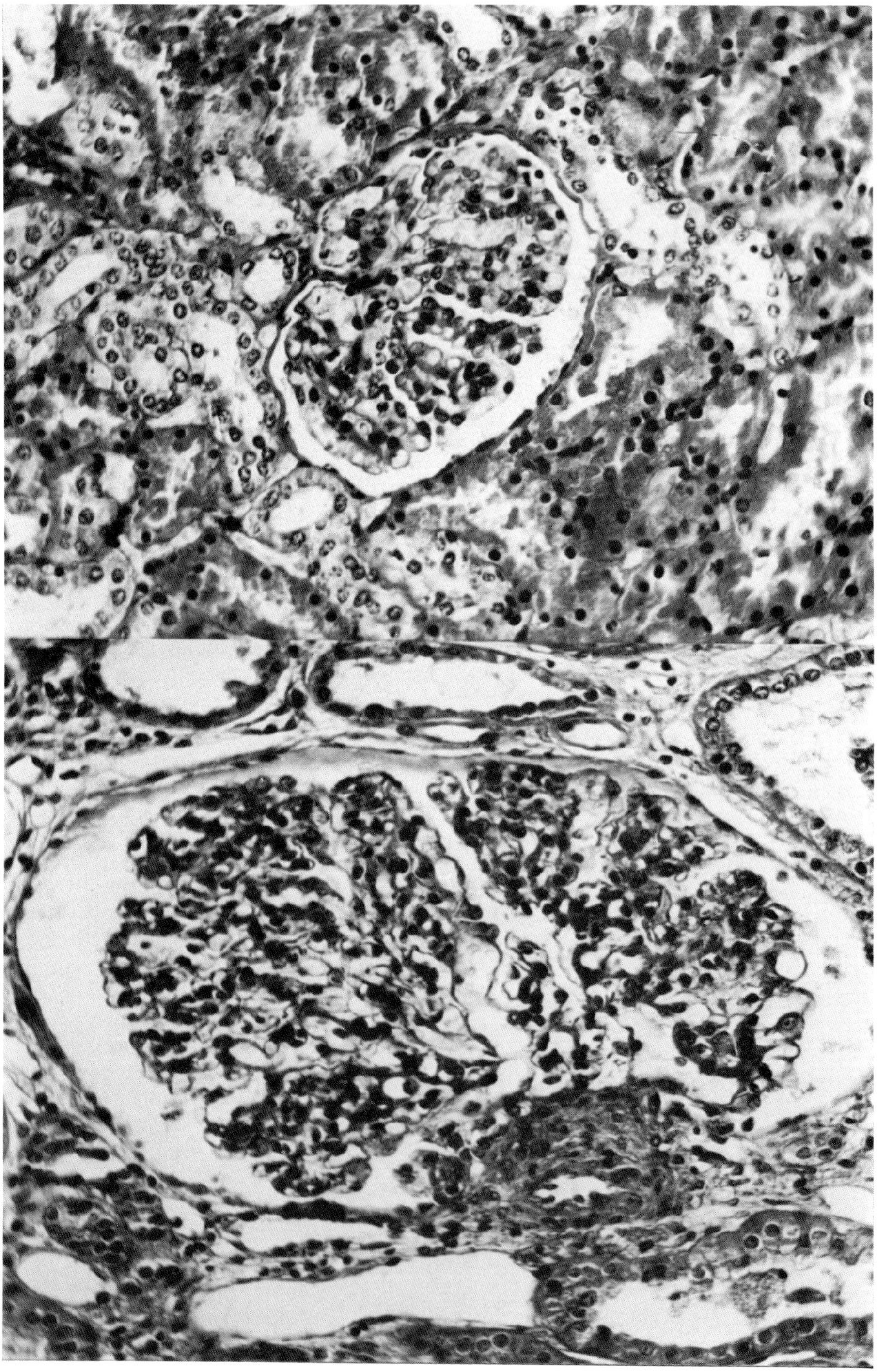

A

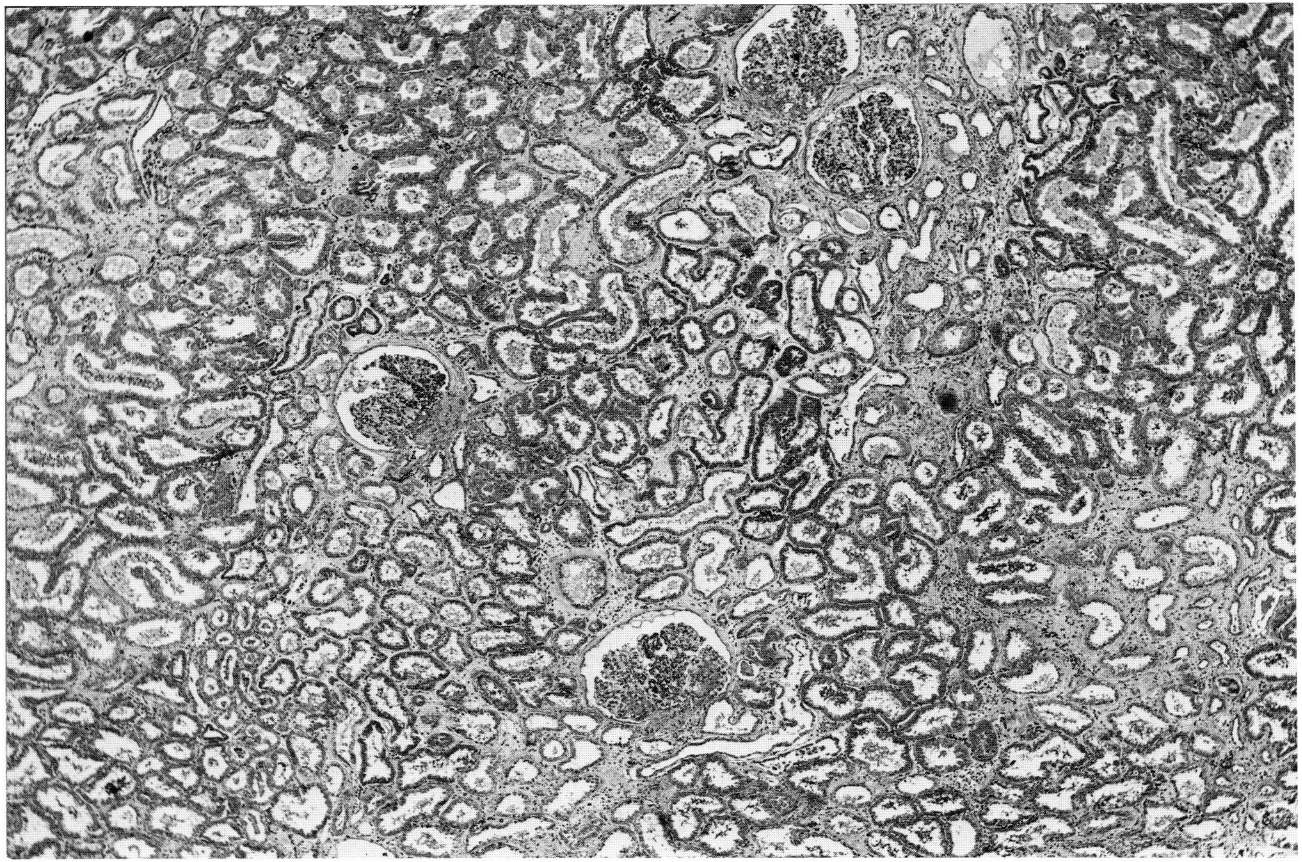

B

FIG. 2-11. (A) On the left, a markedly enlarged glomerulus from a child with oligonephronic hypoplasia. On the right, a glomerulus of normal size from an age-matched control. H&E; ×300. (B) Oligonephronic hypoplasia. Lower-power view showing enlarged glomeruli exhibiting focal glomerular sclerosis, hypertrophied tubules, and an increase in interstitial fibrous tissue. H&E; ×45. (Courtesy of Dr. Renée Habib.)

fever, and growth retardation are also common features, and the clinical picture may resemble closely that of juvenile nephronophthisis. However, significant proteinuria is more frequent with oligonephronic hypoplasia, and the absence of a family history may help to distinguish it from familial juvenile nephronophthisis, which is inherited as an autosomal recessive trait.

The glomerular filtration rate is diminished, but a relatively stable period of moderate azotemia usually persists through the first decade, later progressing to chronic renal failure. Royer et al. [281] described the gradual development of progressive segmental glomerular sclerosis, tubular atrophy, and interstitial fibrosis with time (Fig. 2-11*B*). McGraw et al. [203] noted that glomerular sclerosis was preceded by increasing proteinuria and that its presence was accompanied by the onset of chronic renal failure. Thus in many ways the clinical and microscopic findings in oligonephronic hypoplasia parallel those of the remnant kidney model [154,231,263,300]. This aspect is discussed in Chapter 11.

Broyer [58] reported that renal hypoplasia accounted for about one-fifth of the cases of chronic renal failure in children treated at the Hôpital des Enfants Malades in Paris. Although the figures for renal hypoplasia included renal dysplasia and segmental hypoplasia, *oligoméganéphronie* (oligonephronic hypoplasia) accounted for just over half the cases included.

SIMPLE HYPOPLASIA

Simple hypoplasia may be bilateral or, much less frequently, unilateral, and it differs from oligonephronic hypoplasia chiefly in that nephronic hypertrophy is not a feature. The number of renal lobes is generally reduced, and occasional unireniculate examples are encountered. Bernstein and Meyer [41] described bilateral simple hypoplasia with reduced numbers of renal lobes but without nephronic hypertrophy in a 5-month-old boy with hypokalemia and recurrent dehydration. Histologic examination reveals a reduced volume of normally differentiated renal parenchyma. Secondary glomerular sclerosis with focal tubulointerstitial damage may be apparent, particularly with more extreme reduction in renal size.

Bilateral small kidneys with less than 50 percent of the expected mean combined renal mass are sometimes encountered in children with multiple congenital malformations or with long-standing disease or anomalies of the central nervous system [40,277]. In this situation, the number of renal lobes is often normal, and it is possible that the reduced renal size represents a failure of normal postnatal growth rather than an intrinsic deficiency in renal parenchymal mass.

It is also true that some ectopic or malrotated kidneys may be smaller than expected even when histologic signs of dysplastic parenchymal differentiation are absent. The blood supply to such kidneys is often anomalous, and this may relate to their reduced size [268].

Renal Dysplasia

MORPHOLOGY

Renal dysplasia (Table 2-2) is defined as abnormal development of the renal parenchyma owing to anomalous differentiation of metanephric tissue [264]. The description encompasses both abnormality of renal organization in terms of its lobar architecture and dysgenetic differentiation of ductal and nephronic structures. The diagnosis re-

TABLE 2-2. *Renal dysplasia*

I. Multicystic and aplastic dysplasia
II. Hypoplastic dysplasia (hypodysplasia)
III. Dysplasia in duplex systems
  A. Ectopic ureterocele
  B. Lower-pole dysplasia
IV. Dysplasia associated with congenital lower urinary tract obstruction
  A. Posterior urethral valves
  B. Urethral atresia
  C. Prune belly and megacystis-megaureter syndromes
V. Diffuse cystic dysplasia
  A. In hereditary and multiple-anomaly syndromes
  B. Sporadic
VI. Hereditary renal adysplasia (see p. 104)
VII. Dysplasia with vesicoureteral reflux

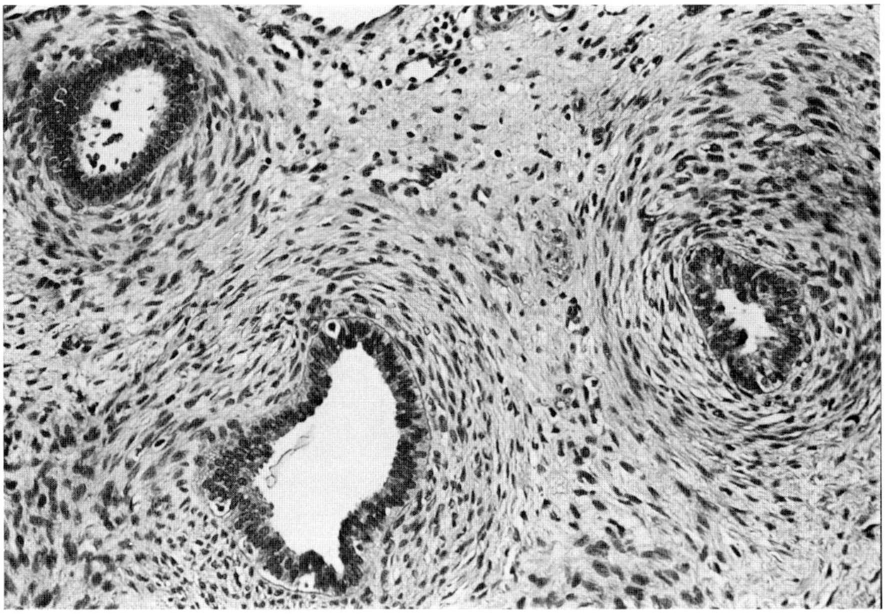

Fig. 2-12. *Renal dysplasia. Primitive ducts surrounded by mantles of concentrically arranged mesenchymal cells. H&E; ×60.*

quires careful evaluation of the gross as well as the microscopic appearances of the kidney and of the frequently coexisting abnormalities of the urinary tract. The fact that the latter occur in some 90 percent of patients with renal dysplasia [283] suggests that dysplasia should be regarded as an anomaly of the whole urinary tract and not solely of the kidney [268].

Dysplastic kidneys may be larger or smaller than expected and may be reniform or grossly misshapen; in addition, cyst formation is a variable but sometimes prominent feature. The distinction of the hypoplastic from the small dysplastic kidney has already been mentioned, and the differentiation of polycystic renal diseases from dysplasia with cyst formation will be discussed in the section entitled Cystic Diseases of the Kidney.

In general, dysplastic maldifferentiation may affect the cortex and medulla or principally the medulla alone and may involve part or all of the kidney.

Lobar disorganization in renal dysplasia is recognized by poor delineation of the renal pyramid, which lacks clear definition because of deficient development of the calyx and fornices. The pyramid is also deficient in vasa recta and loops of Henle and contains so-called primitive ducts [98] lined by undifferentiated columnar epithelium surrounded by collars of concentrically arranged fibroblastic and smooth-muscle cells (Fig. 2-12). These primitive ducts are fewer in number than collecting ducts in the normal papilla and are separated by varying amounts of collagenous connective tissue.

The associated renal cortex is usually thinned and may contain primitive ducts and ductules as well as immature tubular and nephronic structures, the morphology of which resembles that usually encountered only in the fetal kidney. These primitive tubules are lined by low cuboidal epithelium with darkly staining nuclei, and the glomeruli have prominent layers of epithelial cells

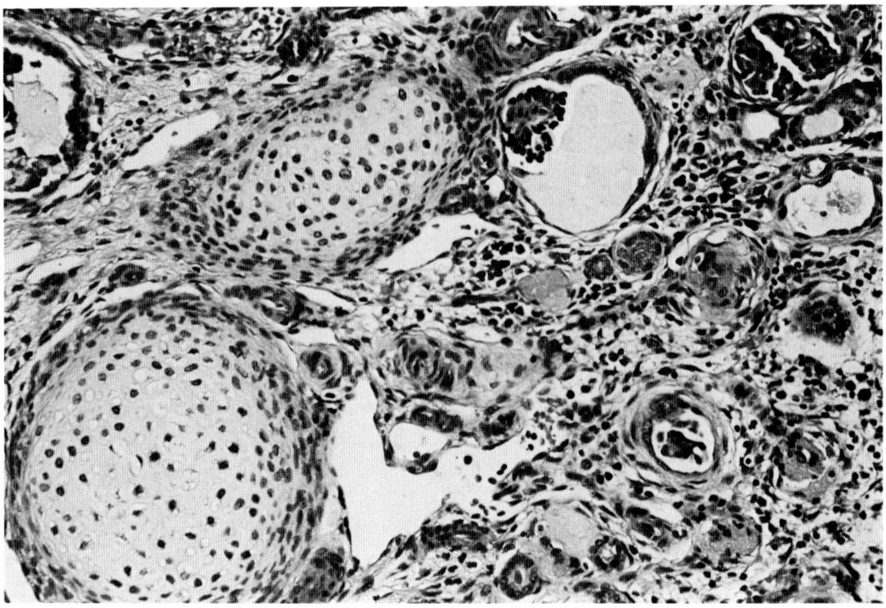

FIG. 2-13. *Renal dysplasia. Primitive glomeruli and tubules with bars of metaplastic cartilage. H&E;* ×60.

enveloping the tuft. Bars of hyalin cartilage may be present in the outer cortex [45] (Fig. 2-13). Cysts of varying size may be seen; the larger examples, with thin, fibrous walls lined by flattened and attenuated epithelial cells, occur principally in the outer cortex, while small cysts are seen as dilatations of tubular, ductular, and glomerular elements. There is a variable increase in loose and collagenous interstitial connective tissue, and regressive changes such as glomerular sclerosis and tubular atrophy may be present.

MORPHOGENESIS

Some explanation of the altered renal differentiation characterizing dysplastic development can be obtained from the microdissection studies of grossly cystic dysplastic kidneys performed by Osathanondh and Potter [234]. These revealed evidence of markedly diminished branching of the ureteric bud, often with failure of nephron induction and cystic dilatation of ureteric bud branches.

The primitive ducts in the medulla are thus seen to represent persistent, incompletely differentiated ureteric bud branches that are reduced in number compared with normal papillary collecting ducts; they are sometimes congregated together in nodular formations that suggest their derivation from single stems. The reduced cortical thickness is related to the diminished induction of cortical nephrons that are often of primitive morphology and may undergo cystic dilatation. Bars of cartilage indicate foci of altered, metaplastic differentiation of metanephric blastemal cells. Larger cysts appear to be dilated terminal portions of primitive duct branches, since communication between the duct and cyst can be demonstrated [288]. The most specific histologic markers of renal dysplasia are the primitive ducts, which are essential features for the diagnosis, and bars of metaplastic cartilage. The latter are not always present, but they do provide confirmation of dysplastic development when seen. Very occasionally, metaplastic cartilage can occur in the absence of dysplasia

[327] so that the combination of cartilaginous foci and primitive ducts is required to indicate dysplastic differentiation.

Cysts can, of course, occur in a variety of conditions other than dysplasia, and apparently immature glomeruli and tubules may be seen in renal scars and even in the tract of a previous needle biopsy of the kidney [30,39]. The morphologic alterations under these circumstances seem to be acquired rather than an expression of dysgenetic development. Thus the histopathologic diagnosis of dysplastic renal development requires intelligent interpretation of the overall structural disorganization as well as the recognition of particular microscopic features. The picture may well be complicated by regressive changes, particularly in longer-standing examples from older patients, and by secondary changes due to infective scarring. Pyelonephritis is a common complication in dysplastic kidneys because of the frequently coexistent urinary tract anomalies, which are usually obstructive and may be accompanied by vesicoureteral reflux.

PATHOGENESIS

With regard to the pathogenesis of renal dysplasia, it is clear from the involvement of the pelvicalyceal system, renal medulla, and renal cortical elements that the factors interfering with normal renal development act over a prolonged period starting from the earliest phase of nephrogenesis. Much evidence points to urinary obstruction and possibly vesicoureteral reflux occurring in utero as important elements in dysplastic development. The frequency of other, usually obstructive anomalies in the urinary tract has already been mentioned, and the pattern and severity of the dysplastic changes in the kidney relate in a fairly predictable fashion to the accompanying urinary tract abnormalities. Thus unilateral dysplasia is associated with ipsilateral ureteral anomalies, while bilateral dysplasia generally accompanies lower urinary tract obstruction. Segmental dysplasia, particularly in duplex systems, is associated with obstruction, and sometimes vesicoureteral reflux, in the system draining the dysplastic segment. In lower urinary tract obstruction, the most profound degrees of renal dysplasia occur when obstruction is complete, as in urethral atresia. In dysplasia accompanying posterior urethral valves, both the frequency and the severity of the dysplastic changes in the kidneys relate to the degree of obstruction produced by the valves. When the dysplastic changes are unequal on the two sides, their severity also correlates with the presence and degree of vesicoureteral reflux.

During normal development of the kidney, the remolding of the first-formed generations of branches of the ureteric bud probably depends on some temporary impedance to the flow of urine produced as the early generations of nephrons begin to secrete. If this impedance were prolonged or accentuated by mechanical obstruction, it is entirely conceivable that this would interfere with subsequent ureteric bud branching and nephron induction to produce the changes that characterize dysplastic renal development. It is also possible that vesicoureteral reflux operating in utero would similarly impede urine flow, particularly if reflux were accompanied by sustained abnormal detrusor contraction to simulate urinary obstruction.

It is clear, however, that severe corticomedullary dysplasia can occur in the absence of urinary obstruction, as seen, for example, in diffuse cystic dysplasia associated with syndromes of multiple congenital abnormalities. It is also possible that the ureteral atresia accompanying multicystic dysplasia might be a secondary consequence of absent urine flow from a nonfunctioning kidney rather than a primary obstructive event causing the dysplastic renal development. Thus, while it is generally accepted that urinary obstruction and possibly vesicoureteral reflux have a primary pathogenetic role in many cases of renal dysplasia, it is possible that they are coincidental, and certainly in some examples, other factors are evidently involved.

Stephens and colleagues [144,205,293] have proposed an alternative hypothesis that relates renal maldevelopment to the position of the ureteral orifice on the bladder trigone, indicating, in turn, the point of origin of the ureteric bud from the mesonephric duct. These authors maintain that only a limited portion of the metanephric blastema overlying the normal point of contact by the ureteric bud is capable of normal development, and should the ureteric bud arise too far cranially (laterally ectopic orifice within the bladder) or caudally (ectopic orifice in the bladder neck, urethra, or vagina), contact is made with blastema that lacks a capacity for normal differentiation so that a small dysplastic kidney results. These observations were supported by "hypodysplasia" counts that were correlated with the degree of ureteral ectopia. However, it is unclear whether "hypodysplasia" as used by Stephens is really the same as the dysplasia described by other authors. Certainly, many cases of renal dysplasia are not associated with ureteral ectopia.

MULTICYSTIC AND APLASTIC DYSPLASIA

The multicystic kidney is the clinically best recognized form of renal dysplasia. The affected kidney is enlarged and completely lacks a normal reniform shape owing to the presence of large peripheral cysts that give an appearance resembling a bunch of grapes (Fig. 2-14). There is generally a more solid central portion to which the ureter is attached. The pelvicalyceal system is severely attenuated and usually cannot be defined at all. The ureter is thin in its upper portion and is almost always atretic in the upper part and occasionally throughout its length. Sometimes there are multiple stenotic segments in the patent portion, and very occasionally, the ureter is completely absent for part or all of its course. In some cases, vesicoureteral reflux occurs into the distal patent part of the ureter, which can then appear dilated.

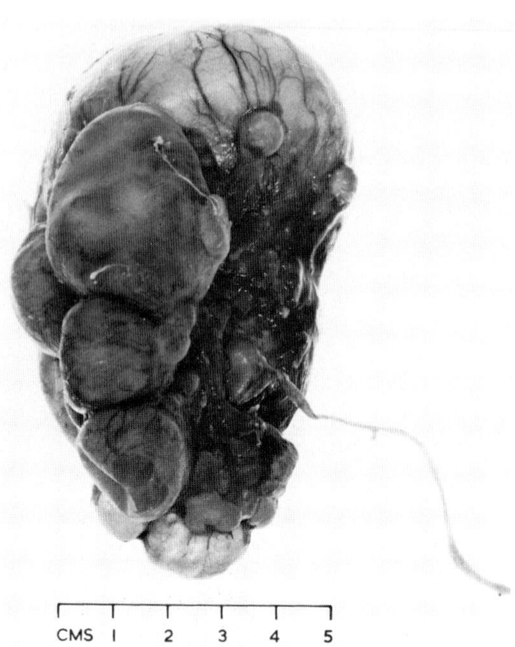

FIG. 2-14. *Multicystic dysplastic kidney with an atretic ureter. (From Risdon [264].)*

Histologically, the most obvious feature is the presence of peripheral cysts that vary in size from a few millimeters to several centimeters and account for the increased renal size. These have thin, fibrous walls and flattened epithelial linings and represent dilated terminal portions of primitive ducts that can be seen radiating from the hilus in the more solid central area. Some rudimentary lobar arrangement usually can be defined in the loose tissue between the cysts, where primitive glomerular and tubular structures and, in some examples, small areas of completely differentiated nephrons may be seen. Foci of hyalin cartilage are a variable but quite frequent finding in the periphery of the kidney. Parenchymal infection and scarring are not a feature of multicystic kidneys, which are protected from ascending infection by the atretic ureter [264]. In some examples, foci of extramedullary hemopoiesis are seen in the loose connective tissue, and rarely, small aggregates of primitive undifferentiated blastemal cells resembling nephroblastomatosis (nodular blastema) are present [118]. Currently, nodular blastema is regarded as a potential precursor of a Wilms tumor, and both nephroblastoma [139] and renal-cell carcinoma [46] have been reported as rare complications of multicystic dysplasia.

The aplastic kidney is perhaps the most extreme form of renal dysplasia and consists macroscopically of a barely recognizable, tiny nubbin of tissue that may contain a few cysts. Histologically, a few primitive ducts and immature nephronic structures and, sometimes, small, fibrous-walled cysts are seen. Ureteral anomalies of the same types observed in multicystic dysplasia accompany renal

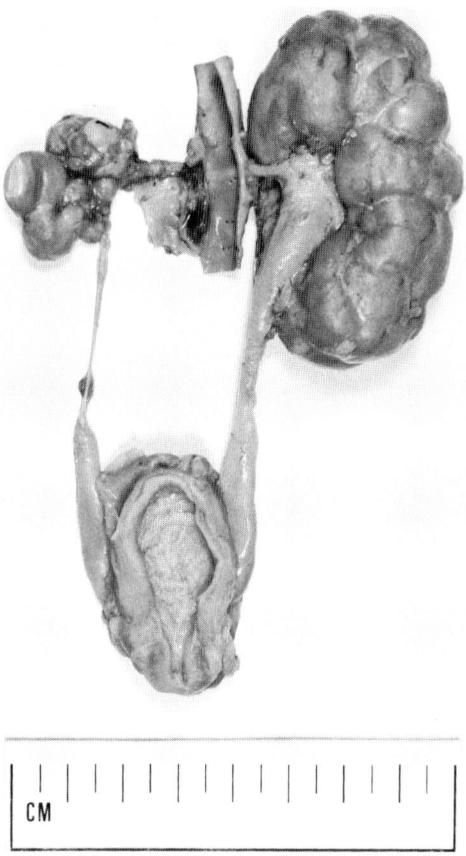

Fig. 2-15. *Right-sided aplastic kidney with an atretic upper ureter. The left ureter is stenosed, and there is hydronephrosis of the left kidney. (From Risdon, R. A. Cystic Diseases of the Kidney and Reflux Nephropathy. In P. P. Anthony and R. N. M. MacSween (Eds.),* Recent Advances in Histopathology, *Vol. 2. Edinburgh: Churchill-Livingtone, 1981.)*

aplasia, and indeed, the two conditions are basically very similar expressions of severe renal dysplasia, the enlargement of the multicystic kidney reflecting only the predominance of cysts rather than any increase in functional renal parenchyma.

The recent introduction of the technique of fetal ultrasonography as a means of diagnosis in utero has led to some interesting insights into these conditions. Serial examinations of fetuses harboring multicystic kidneys show that the size and configuration of the cysts may alter with time [10,140] and that occasionally the whole cystic mass may apparently disappear [242]. Since it is unlikely that the affected kidney would entirely regress, the intriguing possibility exists that what would be diagnosed as an aplastic kidney in postnatal life might, in some cases at least, have been a multicystic kidney in utero.

Multicystic and aplastic dysplasia can be unilateral or, much less frequently, bilateral. Since both types of dysplasia are associated with nonfunctioning kidneys, bilateral disease is incompatible with postnatal survival, and the clinical features resemble those of bilateral renal agenesis. Very occasionally, a multicystic kidney on one side may accompany an aplastic kidney on the other.

Both bilateral dysplasia and bilateral agenesis are associated with the Potter sequence, but they can be distinguished by ultrasonography [23,321].

Unilateral multicystic or aplastic dysplasia is more common in males than in females and affects the left kidney slightly more frequently than the right. Standard intravenous urography shows no excretion of contrast medium on the affected side, although occasionally the lower ureter is seen by reflux from the bladder. High-dose excretion urography may result in opacification of the more solid portions of the kidney with outlining of cysts [340]. In older individuals, particularly when diagnosis is delayed until adulthood, calcification of cyst walls may render them visible on plain radiographs of the abdomen.

With both unilateral and bilateral multicystic dysplasia, major malformations of other systems occur fairly commonly and may overshadow the renal anomaly clinically. These include isolated ventricular septal defect, coarctation of the aorta, duodenal and anal atresia, and meningomyelocele.

An important clinical aspect of unilateral multicystic and aplastic dysplasia is the high frequency of contralateral ureteral anomalies, which are said to occur in up to 10 percent [176]. Contralateral ureteral stenosis [239] is the most frequent finding (Fig. 2-15), but ureteral ectopia and duplication are also described [48]. Since these anomalies can be obstructive and may compromise the only remaining functioning kidney, their prompt diagnosis and correction are of obvious urgency.

HYPOPLASTIC DYSPLASIA

Small dysplastic (hypodysplastic) kidneys with patent ureters are more difficult to classify than multicystic or aplastic kidneys because of the wider range of changes within the kidneys and in the draining ureters. Such kidneys, at least initially, retain a degree of functional capacity and the ability to excrete urine. Renal weights are less than expected and commonly fall in the "hypoplastic" range of less than 2 SD below the mean. Dysplastic disorganization may involve part or all of the kidney but is generally less extreme than in multicystic or aplastic dysplasia. Some degree of normal lobation and corticomedullary demarcation is retained, and dysplastic development is usually more apparent in the medulla, which contains primitive ducts that radiate from a poorly differentiated papilla in a delta-like fashion. Cortical differentiation is variable, although cortical primitive ducts and occasionally a few cysts and foci of hyalin cartilage may be seen. Sometimes dysplastic cortical change may be minimal, although the cortex is usually thinner than expected, indicating a diminished number of nephrons.

A variety of ureteral anomalies occur; the ureter is frequently dilated and tortuous and may be subject to vesicoureteral reflux. The lower end of the ureter may be inserted ectopically, and sometimes a ureterocele is present. Infrequently, the ureter may appear normal. The pelvicalyceal system is often poorly formed but may be dilated.

Because the ureteral anomalies are often obstructive or associated with vesicoureteral reflux, hydronephrosis and chronic pyelonephritis are frequent complications, and the resultant inflammatory and regressive changes in the kidney may mask or completely overshadow evidence of dysplastic development. Primitive delta-like medullary ducts can usually be identified, although their distinction from dilated collecting ducts in the compressed papilla of a hydronephrotic kidney may pose problems. It may help that in pure hydronephrosis thinning of the medulla is usually more extreme than of the cortex, whereas in a hydronephrotic dysplastic kidney the reverse is more frequent.

Hypodysplasia may be unilateral or bilateral. Clinical presentation is usually related to the effects of ureteral obstruction or vesicoureteral reflux, particularly recurrent urinary infection, hypertension, or stone formation, or to the effects of chronic renal failure.

DYSPLASIA IN DUPLEX SYSTEMS

Ectopic Ureterocele

In this, the more common variety, the upper segment of a double (duplex) kidney is dysplastic. The pelvicalyceal system is completely duplicated, the lower-pole ureter being inserted orthotopically in the bladder trigone. The upper ureter draining the dysplastic pole is dilated and tortuous and is inserted ectopically below and medial to the nor-

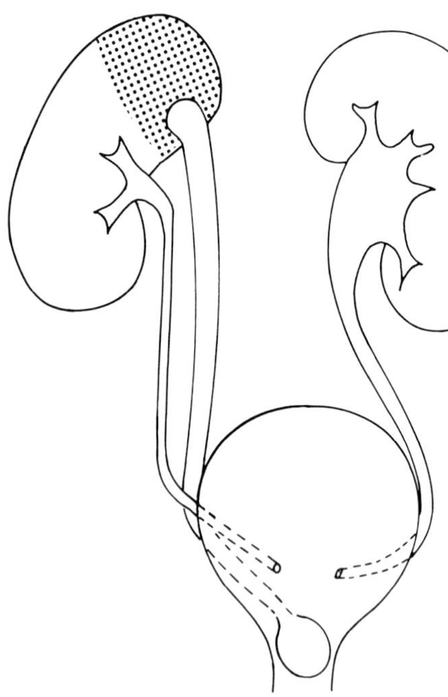

FIG. 2-16. *Diagram of ectopic ureterocele. The stippled upper pole of the right duplex kidney is dysplastic. The dilated right upper-pole ureter ends in a ureterocele and is inserted ectopically, medial to and below the orthotopic lower-pole ureter.*

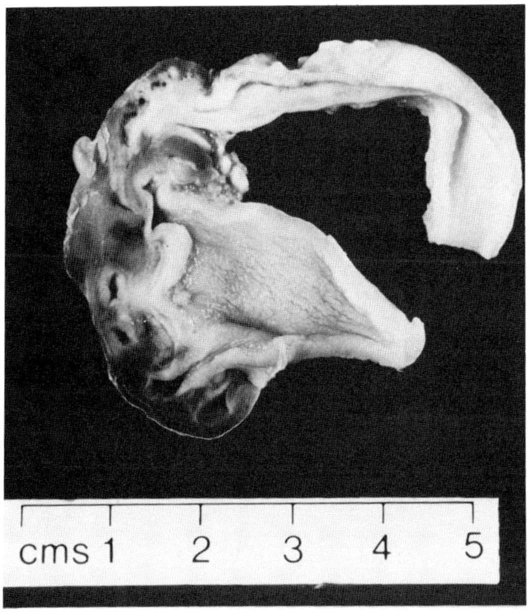

Fig. 2-17. *A duplex kidney with a dysplastic upper-pole moiety and dilated upper-pole ureter. The lower pole is hydronephrotic and was subjected to vesicoureteral reflux.*

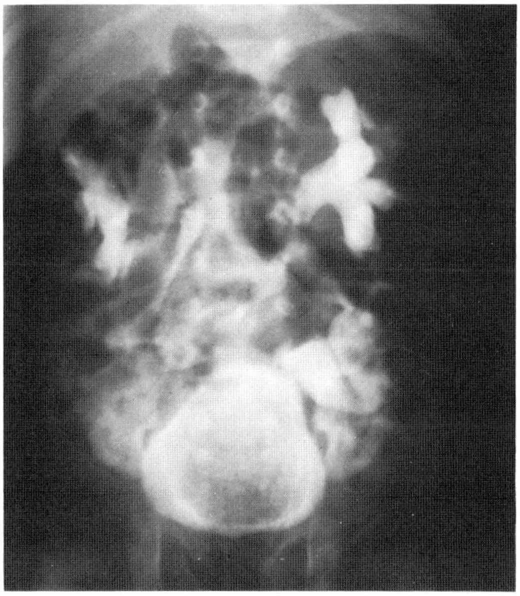

Fig. 2-18. *Ectopic ureterocele. Excretory urogram from a newborn male infant. The upper pole of a duplex right kidney and the upper-pole ureter are not visualized, but a large ureterocele is seen as a filling defect in the bladder. The left ureter and pelvicalyceal system are dilated as a result of obstruction by the ureterocele. (Courtesy of Dr. C. Dicks-Mireaux.)*

mal site in the bladder trigone, usually in the bladder neck but occasionally in the urethra. In most cases, the ectopic ureter ends in a cystic dilatation of the intravesical portion termed a *ureterocele* [316], and it is this feature that accounts for the term *ectopic ureterocele* (Fig. 2-16) used to describe the whole urinary tract anomaly [125,222, 349]. The ectopic ureteral anomaly is obstructive, and the upper pole of the kidney is dysplastic in up to 95 percent of cases [57], usually severely so. The upper pelvis is dilated, and the calyces are rudimentary. Medullary dysplasia is characterized by primitive ducts, and the cortex is usually markedly thinned. The latter contains dysplastic ductal and nephronic elements and, occasionally, cysts and metaplastic cartilage. Nodular renal blastema also has been described [81]. Pyelonephritic changes and scarring are usually prominent and may overshadow the dysplastic changes. The ureterocele in the bladder causes upward displacement of the lower-pole ureteral orifice, shortening its submucosal tunnel and rendering it subject to vesicoureteral reflux (Fig. 2-17); less commonly it may obstruct the lower-pole ureter or even the contralateral ureter (Fig. 2-18). These effects render the lower pole liable to hydronephrosis and ascending infection, although in most cases heminephrectomy of the dysplastic upper pole and surgical removal of the ectopic ureterocele give excellent results.

Ectopic ureterocele is a common anomaly and is much more frequent in girls, the female-to-male ratio being about 6 : 1. In about 10 percent of affected individuals the condition is bilateral. It is usually recognized in infancy and causes recurrent urinary infections and sometimes hematuria. Occasionally there is dribbling incontinence or acute retention due to the ureterocele, which in girls occasionally prolapses through the urethral orifice.

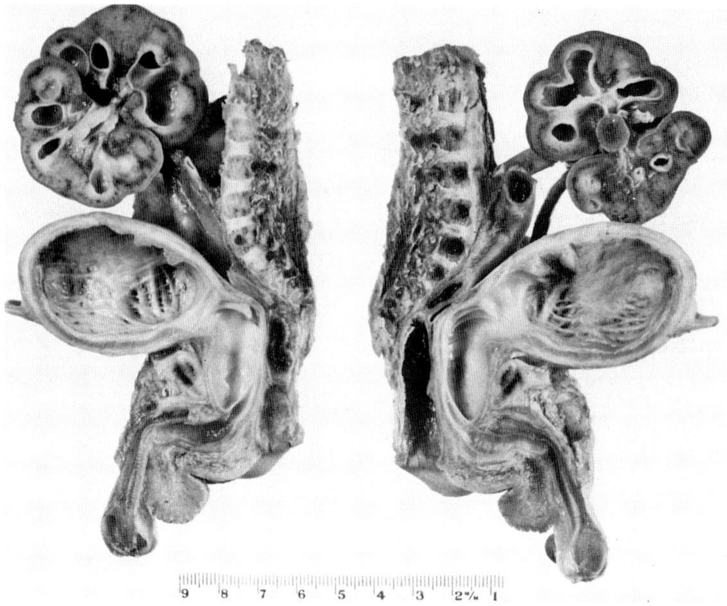

A

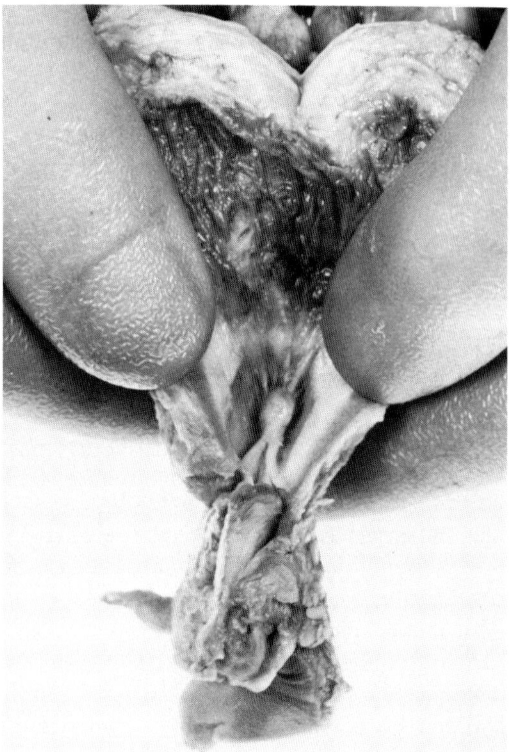

B

FIG. 2-19. *(A) Hemisected bladder and urethra from an autopsy on a male infant with posterior urethral valves demonstrating bilateral hydronephrosis, hypertrophied bladder, and dilated posterior urethra. (B) Dissection of the posterior urethra to demonstrate posterior urethral valves.*

Excretion urography demonstrates the ectopic ureterocele as a filling defect in the bladder. The dysplastic upper pole and its ureter fail to excrete contrast medium, but the lower segment is usually displaced downward and its calyces are arranged in a so-called drooping lily configuration.

Lower-Pole Dysplasia

Less commonly, complete duplication of the kidney and ureter is associated with ectopia of the lower-pole ureter. The upper-pole ureter is inserted normally in the trigone, and the lower-pole ureter is inserted above and lateral to it. In this anomaly, vesicoureteral reflux occurs into the lower-pole ureter, which is dilated. The lower pole of the kidney is hydronephrotic and frequently shows dysplasia as well as pyelonephritic scarring [103,125,347].

RENAL DYSPLASIA ASSOCIATED WITH CONGENITAL LOWER URINARY TRACT OBSTRUCTION

Posterior Urethral Valves

Renal dysplasia of this type is seen most commonly in infant boys with persistent posterior urethral valves (Fig. 2-19). Dysplastic renal development occurs in only a proportion of such patients and is particularly frequent in those presenting in the neonatal period with urinary retention and a large, distended, and trabeculated bladder in whom bladder outlet obstruction is most marked. The kidneys are often small and hydronephrotic, and the ureters are thick-walled, tortuous, and may have laterally displaced ureteral orifices that are subject to vesicoureteral reflux in about 80 percent of cases. Posterior urethral valves are now frequently diagnosed in utero by fetal ultrasonography. Bilateral hydronephrosis and bladder distention that persists in serial scans are demonstrated. When renal function is severely impaired in utero, oligohydramnios results, and in such cases, the kidneys are usually severely dysplastic as well as hydronephrotic.

The extent and severity of renal dysplasia complicating posterior urethral valves are variable, but this disorder usually involves cystic changes in the outer cortex and medullary dysplasia [258]. Medullary dysplasia with a delta-like, radiating configuration of primitive ducts is common, and cortical dysplasia is usually most evident in the outer cortex, where the last generations of nephrons form. The changes consist of dilated and sometimes cystic collecting ducts, primitive and often dilated nephronic structures, and occasionally bars of cartilage. In some examples, dysplastic changes are extreme with little lobar organization, marked cystic changes, and a paucity of nephrons mimicking diffuse cystic dysplasia.

Secondary regressive changes and pyelonephritic scarring are common [264] and reflect the frequency of ascending infection. The extent of the dysplastic alterations correlates with the severity of bladder outlet obstruction and the degree of vesicoureteral reflux. Henneberry and Stephens [144] and Schwarz et al. [293] also have related the severity of dysplasia to the degree of lateral displacement of the ureteral orifices. Often the extent of dysplasia and hydronephrotic atrophy varies on the two sides, and this seems to relate to the degree of vesicoureteral reflux, which can be asymmetrical. Hoover and Duckett [152] and Greenfield et al. [132] described patients with posterior urethral valves and unilateral vesicoureteral reflux in whom dysplasia was confined to the refluxing side.

Urethral Atresia and Prune Belly and Megacystis-Megaureter Syndromes

In complete urethral atresia, extreme degrees of bilateral dysplasia with cyst formation are usual. Patterns of renal dysplasia similar to those described for posterior urethral valves are seen in other forms of congenital urethral obstruction and in the prune belly [91,354] and megacystis-megaureter [237] syndromes, in which bilateral hydronephrosis, vesicoureteral reflux, and bladder distention occur usually in the absence of anatomic bladder outlet obstruction. As with posterior urethral valves, dysplastic changes in the kidneys may be unilateral or asymmetrical.

DIFFUSE CYSTIC DYSPLASIA

Sporadic and in Hereditary and Multiple-Anomaly Syndromes

This form of renal dysplasia involves enlarged kidneys with diffuse parenchymal cystic change and histologic evidence of dysplastic development. The condition is bilateral and requires distinction from multicystic dysplasia; it is rare, but it is important because it is frequently associated with hereditary syndromes of multiple congenital malformations.

On section, the kidneys show variable but usually extensive replacement of the cortex by small, rounded cysts, usually a few millimeters in diameter. Renal lobation is indistinct, and while the pelves are patent, the calyces are not defined and the medullary pyramids are poorly developed or absent. The ureter is thin but patent, and the bladder is often hypoplastic.

Histologically, the medulla contains scanty primitive ducts, and many of the cortical cysts appear to be dilated terminal portions of similar ductal structures. Nephronic structures are difficult to find, but some of the cysts appear to be dilated glomerular and tubular structures. There is an increased amount of loose connective tissue between cysts, but metaplastic cartilage is very unusual.

The gross cystic changes and bilateral involvement may suggest the possibility of autosomal recessive polycystic disease. However, important characteristics of this condition, such as the preserved reniform shape and corticomedullary demarcation of the kidneys and the tendency of the kidneys to collapse on sectioning as fluid drains from the cut surface, are lacking in diffuse cystic dysplasia. Microscopically, the conditions are easily distinguished. Separation of diffuse cystic from multicystic dysplasia is made by the usually unilateral involvement, the lack of any pelvicalyceal development, and the nonpatency of the ureter in the latter.

While diffuse cystic dysplasia is sometimes an isolated anomaly, it is often part of a hereditary syndrome of multiple congenital anomalies, of which the Meckel syndrome (Fig. 2-20) and its variants [31], the Zellweger [308], Jeune [31], oral-facial-digital [313], and trisomy D [217] syndromes, are the most notable [34].

RENAL DYSPLASIA AND VESICOURETERAL REFLUX

A close association between vesicoureteral reflux and renal disease, particularly segmental pyelonephritic scarring, is well recognized and is encompassed by the term *reflux nephropathy* [17]. While the direct role of vesicoureteral reflux in the pathogenesis of acquired renal damage has been the subject of considerable debate and research over the past 30 years [149,150,204,255,256,274,287,306], it is important to realize that vesicoureteral reflux and dysplastic renal differentiation may both represent aspects of abnormal development of the urinary tract and therefore not uncommonly coexist. It has, in fact, been estimated that some evidence of dysplastic development occurs in about 10 percent of scarred kidneys asso-

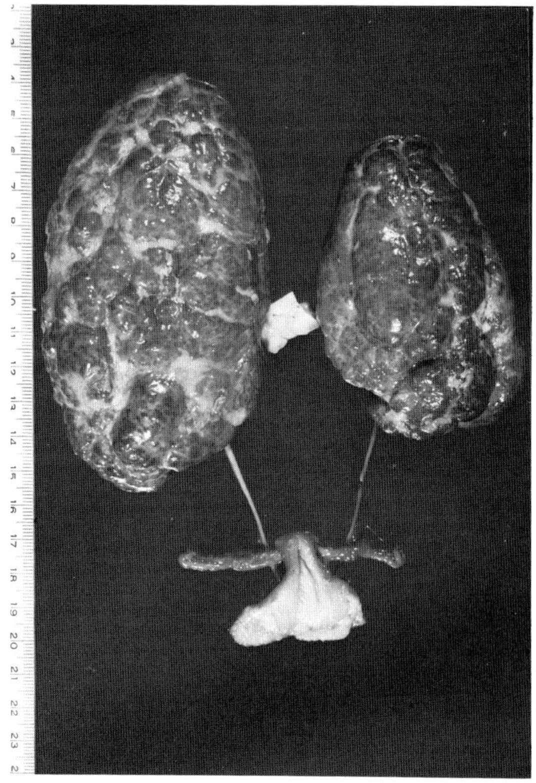

FIG. 2-20. *Kidneys from a newborn baby with Meckel's syndrome, characterized by microcephaly, a posterior encephalocele, congenital hepatic fibrosis, polydactyly, and bilateral diffuse cystic dysplasia. (From Risdon, R. A. The Urogenital System. In J. W. Keeling (Ed.),* Fetal and Neonatal Pathology. *Heidelberg: Springer-Verlag, 1987.)*

ciated with vesicoureteral reflux. The possibility that vesicoureteral reflux occurring in utero, perhaps coupled with abnormal detrusor activity, might simulate the effects of urinary obstruction to promote renal dysplasia has already been mentioned. Similarly, the theories of Stephens and colleagues [205] relating ectopia of the ureteral orifice to dysplastic development also may be relevant, since lateral displacement of the orifice is often associated with vesicoureteral reflux.

Congenital Nephromegaly

Compensatory growth and hypertrophy of one functioning kidney up to twice the normal size may occur when the contralateral kidney is totally dysplastic and nonfunctioning or congenitally absent (unilateral agenesis). Bilateral congenital renal enlargement due to increased renal mass is seen principally in the Wiedemann-Beckwith syndrome of visceromegaly, hyperinsulinemic hypoglycemia due to islet-cell hyperplasia, mild microcephaly, exomphalos, macroglossia, and adrenal cytomegaly [25,346] and the clinically similar but genetically distinct Perlman syndrome of visceromegaly, islet-cell hyperplasia, abnormal facies, nodular renal blastema, and nephroblastomata [131,244]. Wiedemann-Beckwith syndrome appears to have an autosomal dominant inheritance with incomplete penetrance [97], whereas Perlman syndrome is inherited as an autosomal recessive trait [244].

The kidneys in these conditions are enlarged to a variable degree and exhibit accentuated lobation. The medullary pyramids are frequently poorly demarcated and exhibit medullary dysplasia. Usually, in both Perlman and Wiedemann-Beckwith syndrome there is superficial nephroblastomatosis characterized by subcapsular nests and tumor-like nodules of primitive blastema cells, sometimes with focal epithelial tubule formation. Nephroblastomatosis has a malignant potential for the development of nephroblastoma [55] that is frequently associated with the syndromes cited and may be bilateral. In Wiedemann-Beckwith syndrome there is also an increased incidence of other tumors, including adrenal carcinoma, hepatoblastoma, and brainstem glioma [179].

Congenital Hydronephrosis

Obstruction at the level of the ureteropelvic junction occurring in utero is the usual cause of congenital hydronephrosis, which varies in degree from a mild pelvicalyceal dilatation with blunting of the medullary pyramids to severe dilatation with complete effacement of the pyramids and atrophy of the renal parenchyma. The condition is more commonly unilateral, with an unexplained predilection for the left side [170], but it is bilateral in about 20 percent of patients. It may be discovered clinically in infancy or in the first year of life [348], but often it is not diagnosed until later in childhood. In the very young, particularly in males, the condition is more likely to be bilateral. Furthermore, in infancy, the contralateral kidney may show multicystic dysplasia [239]. A familial occurrence has been reported [74].

Congenital ureteropelvic obstruction is usually due to an intrinsic abnormality of the muscle bundles with replacement of the normal spiral smooth-muscle bands by longitudinal fibers, often with an increase in interstitial fibrous connective tissue, to produce a narrow, aperistaltic segment [3,112,218,219]. Sometimes kinks, fibrous bands, or adhesions are found at the ureteropelvic junction that produce sharp angulation of the ureter against the lower margin of the pelvis to cause obstruction. Aberrant branches of the renal artery crossing the upper ureter or ureteropelvic junction, which are much more common in patients with ureteropelvic junction obstruction than in controls, also have been implicated, although there is usually an associated intrinsic abnormality of the muscle of the ureteric wall [3]. Very rarely, ureteropelvic junction obstruction may be due to mucosal folds or polypoid structures [208].

In infancy, congenital hydronephrosis is usually recognized as a palpable renal mass, the nature of which is confirmed by excretion urography and ultrasonography; fetal ultrasonography often allows a diagnosis in utero. In older children, abdominal pain and frank hematuria are frequent presenting symptoms.

Severe hydronephrosis (so-called congenital giant hydronephrosis) produces a cystic renal mass that is easily palpable in the abdomen. Histologic examination of such kidneys reveals extreme hydronephrotic parenchymal atrophy and sometimes evidence of dysplastic development, occasionally with cyst formation. With lesser degrees of hydronephrosis, dysplasia is not a feature, but its occasional presence in giant hydronephrosis suggests that, in these cases at least, obstruction is longstanding and probably occurred very early in fetal life.

Renal Ectopia and Malrotation

Permanent malposition of the kidney outside its normal lumbar site constitutes *renal ectopia*, which may affect one or both kidneys or a solitary kidney in unilateral agenesis. The condition is seen in about 1 in 800 radiologic examinations of the kidneys.

Ectopic kidneys need to be distinguished from abnormally mobile, so-called ptotic kidneys, which are less firmly anchored than normal to the posterior abdominal wall by their peritoneal covering and may, therefore, change position excessively with respiration. They are not, however, permanently displaced, and they have a normal blood supply.

During development, the kidneys are found at a progressively higher level, initially in the pelvis and ultimately in the lumbar region between the 12th dorsal and 3rd lumbar vertebral bodies. During the ascent, which is largely a result of differential growth of the caudal end of the embryo, the kidney rotates medially through 90 degrees so that the renal hilus and pelvis, which are at first located anteriorly, come to be on the medial aspect. Interference with this process results in renal ectopia below the normal position, usually in the pelvis or at the pelvic brim (Fig. 2-21). Such ectopic kidneys are almost always malrotated, with an anteriorly directed pelvis, and are discoid or lumpy rather than reniform in shape. Very rarely, reversed (lateral) rotation of the kidney occurs, with a laterally facing renal pelvis, and exceptionally, the kidney may rotate either way through 180 degrees so that the pelvis is posterior. Rarely, ectopic kidneys are at a higher level than normal and have even been located in the thorax in association with a diaphragmatic defect [148]. The blood supply to ectopic kidneys is generally anomalous and is derived from single or multiple branches from the common iliac artery or lower abdominal aorta.

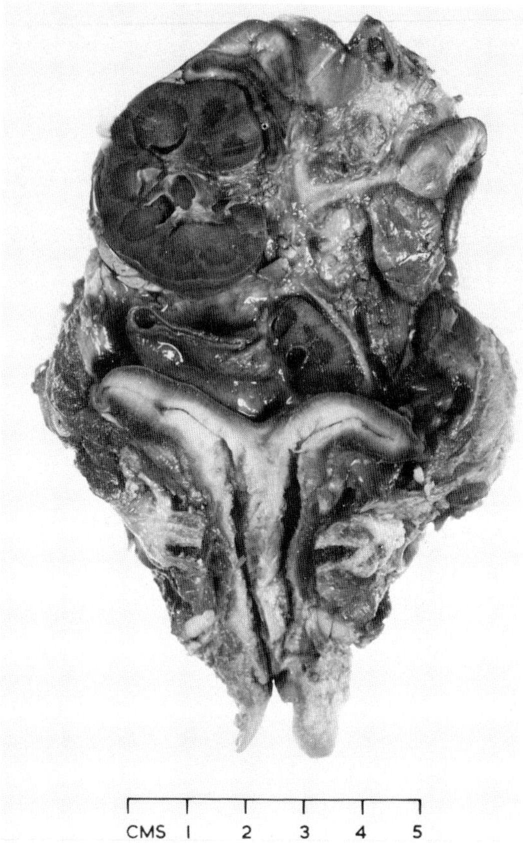

Fig. 2-21. *Simple renal ectopia. The left kidney is ectopic in the pelvis and is separated from the left adrenal. There is a bicornuate uterus.*

Renal ectopia may be simple or crossed. In simple ectopia, the kidney and ureter are on the correct side of the body. The ureter is short and may be inserted ectopically in the bladder neck, urethra, seminal vesicle, or vagina; sometimes it is subject to vesicoureteral reflux. In crossed ectopia, the kidney is situated on the opposite side of the body to the urethral orifice with the ureter crossing the midline (Fig. 2-22).

The two kidneys are thus located on the same side of the body, with the ectopic kidney generally

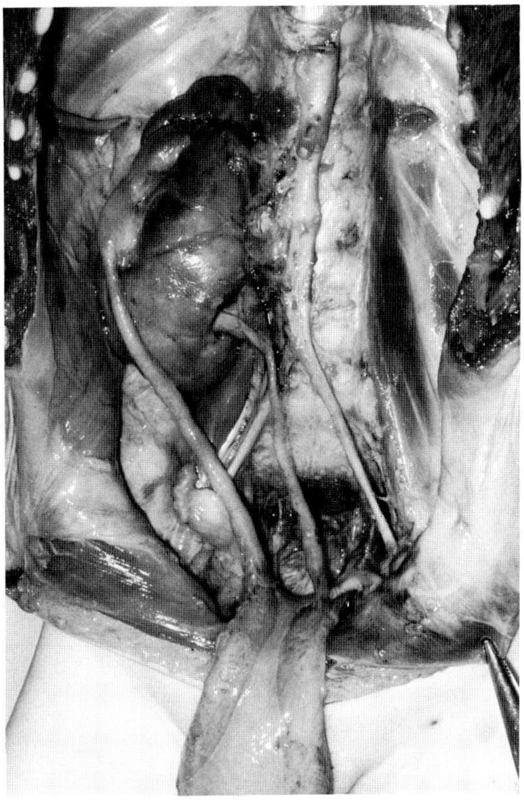

Fig. 2-22. *Crossed renal ectopia. The left kidney is situated on the right side below the small dysmorphic right kidney. The left ureter crosses the midline, and the two kidneys are fused together.*

below the orthotopic kidney. Usually the two kidneys are fused together (fused crossed ectopia [78]).

Quite often ectopic kidneys are dysplastic, and distortion or kinking of the renal pelvis or obstruction by blood vessels crossing anterior to the renal pelvis may lead to intermittent obstruction and hydronephrosis. This, particularly if accompanied by vesicoureteral reflux, predisposes to renal infection. In about 25 percent, renal calculi are present. Pelvic renal ectopia can be associated with anorectal anomalies, particularly rectal atresia, or with congenital absence or atresia of the vagina in females [90].

Renal Fusion

In renal fusion, the two kidneys are joined and the parenchyma is continuous between them. Each kidney has a separate collecting system and ureter that are inserted orthotopically on the two sides. Renal fusion should be distinguished from ureteral duplication, in which two ureters, even if completely separate, are inserted on the same side of the bladder.

Most commonly, the kidneys are fused by their lower poles across the midline, the so-called horseshoe kidney, which is seen in approximately 1 in 600 radiologic examinations. Horseshoe kidneys are often situated lower than normal and so can be regarded as ectopic as well as fused. The renal pelves are usually located anteriorly, and hydronephrosis due to a high ureteropelvic junction or compression by aberrent renal arteries is not uncommon. Occasionally, there is accompanying ureteral duplication and ectopia, and sometimes part or all of a horseshoe kidney is dysplastic (Fig. 2-23). Much less commonly, the upper poles of the kidney are fused across the midline, and exceptionally, both poles are fused to give the so-called ring or doughnut kidney [127].

Midline fusion is about twice as common in males as in females. It is not infrequently associated with other congenital malformations and is common in Turner's syndrome. Although usually asymptomatic, the presence of hydronephrosis predisposes to renal infection and calculus formation. Occasionally, the fused renal tissue may be palpable as an apparently pulsatile midline mass that has been mistaken for an aortic aneurysm.

Renal Duplication

Some degree of duplication of the renal pelvis and ureter (duplex kidney) is very common, occurring in about 5 percent of unselected autopsies. The extent of the duplication varies from mere bifurcation of the extrarenal renal pelvis to complete duplication of the whole system with two completely separate ureters with separate orifices. Complete ureteral duplication is rare (1 percent of all duplications) and may be associated with segmental renal dysplasia, ectopia of one of the ure-

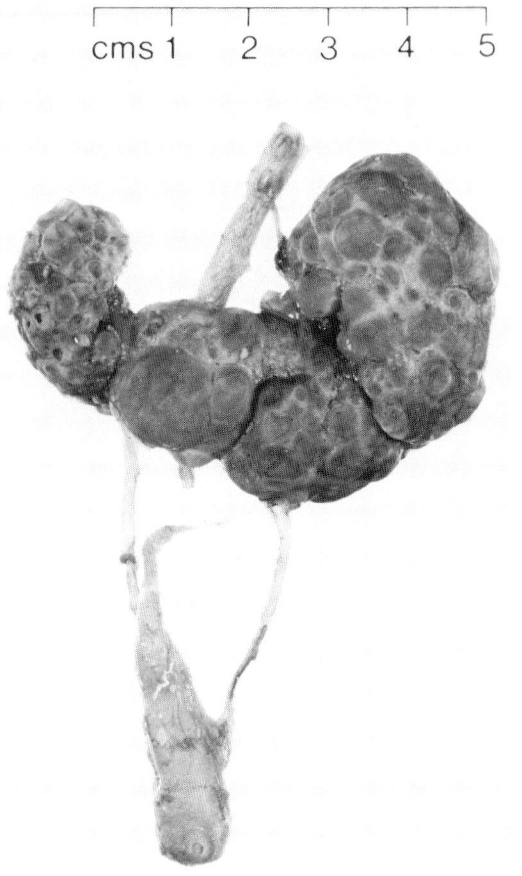

FIG. 2-23. *Fused (horseshoe) kidney exhibiting cystic dysplasia.*

ters, and ureterocele. The conjoint ureter, in which separate renal pelves and upper ureters join to form a single lower ureter, is relatively common. Very rarely, triplication and even quadruplication of the ureter occurs.

Supernumerary Kidney

This extremely rare anomaly is characterized by the presence of a third kidney morphologically separate from the other two, with its own pelvicalyceal system and blood supply. The extra kidney is ectopic, usually situated beneath the lower pole of a normal kidney, and its ureter may join one of the other two or drain separately. Sometimes it is inserted ectopically. Exceptionally, multiple supernumerary kidneys have been described. The condition is usually asymptomatic, but renal infection, obstruction, and stone formation may occur.

Renal Tubular Dysgenesis

Recently, a new syndrome has been described that is characterized clinically by oligohydramnios, the Potter sequence and premature stillbirth or neonatal death from respiratory insufficiency, and pathologically by kidneys that exhibit glomerular crowding and renal tubular dysgenesis [2,292,323, 337]. The condition occurs in siblings and appears to be hereditary. Voland et al. [337] described two affected male siblings and suggested an X-linked recessive inheritance, but other reports include female siblings and consanguineous parents, indicating an autosomal recessive trait [323].

Grossly, the kidneys have been apparently normal or enlarged. The glomeruli appear crowded together, and the tubules are lined by small, rather darkly staining cells that cannot be differentiated histologically into proximal and distal convoluted tubules (Fig. 2-24A). Immunochemical staining for epithelial membrane antigen (EMA) shows uniform positive staining of tubules (proximal tubules are normally negative) (Fig. 2-24B), and lectin-binding studies with *Arachis hypogaea* (peanut) lectin show uniform apical staining of tubular cells, a characteristic of distal tubules and collecting ducts. Microdissections [337] indicate that the tubules are shorter than normal and relatively straight.

CYSTIC DISEASES OF THE KIDNEY

The presence of fluid-filled cysts within or immediately adjacent to the kidney is a feature of many renal diseases. In some it is the predominant abnormality, and it is these that are generally classified as cystic diseases of the kidney. However, they are a widely heterogeneous group of largely

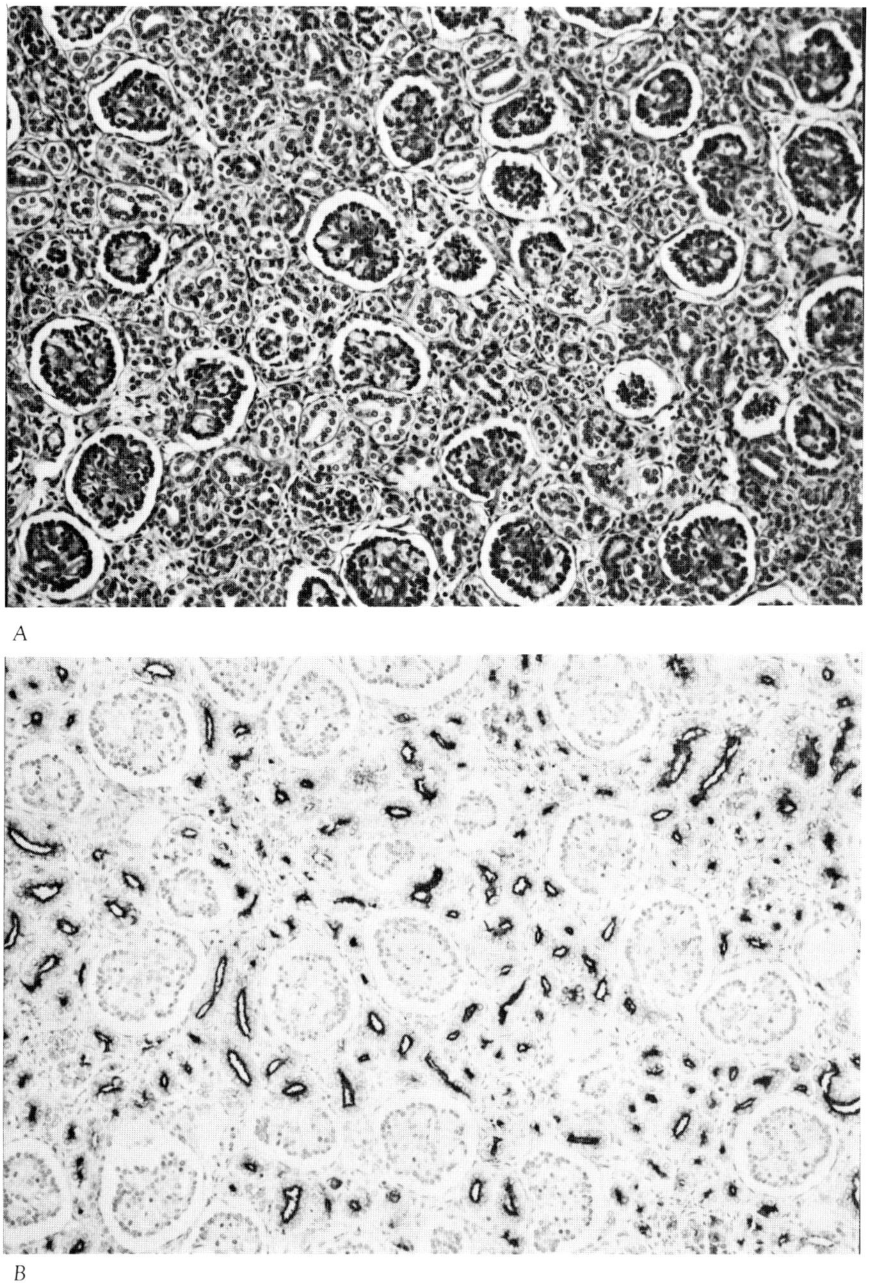

FIG. 2-24. *Renal tubular dysgenesis. (A) Section of kidney from a female infant with the Potter sequence who died of respiratory insufficiency after 27 hours. The glomeruli appear crowded together, and the tubules are lined by darkly staining cells with no differentiation into proximal and distal tubules. H&E; ×60. (B) Immunochemical staining for epithelial membrane antigen (EMA) shows positive staining of all tubular epithelial cells. ×80.*

unrelated conditions, and cystic changes may affect part or all of the kidney, may be unilateral or bilateral, and may involve the renal cortex, medulla, or both. In addition, the cysts may be unilocular or multilocular, they may be congenital or acquired, and the condition may be sporadic or genetically determined. Renal cysts may be the only anomaly, or there may be other associated renal or systemic anomalies. The clinical significance may be trivial or grave, and an understanding of this group of disorders is clearly important both for the individual patient and in terms of genetic counseling. However, this understanding has been greatly hampered by confused nomenclature, particularly the indiscriminate use of such terms as *polycystic* and *multicystic* kidneys and the application of a variety of different descriptions to the same entity and of similar or identical terms to quite different ones. A notable problem in the past has been the classification of renal cystic diseases purely on the basis of their morphologic characteristics.

Still much used is the system of Osathanondh and Potter [234], who recognized four varieties of cystic disease (Potter types 1, 2, 3, and 4) defined by morphologic characteristics revealed by microdissection. While this valuable study did clarify some of the structural abnormalities present, not all varieties of cystic disease were covered, and the Potter type 3 clearly lumped together a number of genetically and clinically diverse conditions [267].

More recently there has been a much better understanding that the classification of renal cystic disease requires detailed clinical, genetic, and radiologic in addition to morphologic criteria, and this has resulted in more satisfactory listings [31,36]. The classification used here (Table 2-3) is derived from these, and the text is set out in the same sequence as the table. Cystic renal dysplasia has already been covered in this chapter (p. 110), and acquired cystic disease is discussed in Chapter 11. An entirely satisfactory classification, however, would require a more complete understanding of the pathogenesis of the different forms of renal cystic disease.

Renal cysts can be produced in animal models by the administration of drugs such as alloxan [336], diphenylamine [284], aminodiphenylthiazole [64], tetrahydrocarbazole [202], and corticosteroids [110], as well as other chemicals such as biphenyl [53], dihydrotrimethylquinolone [352], and the defoliant 2,4,5-T [80]. While the implications of these experiments in terms of human disease are unclear, they do confirm that cysts may be produced in previously normal nephrons, thus showing that cystic change is by no means always an indication of abnormal development or a genetically determined predisposition. At the same time, some cysts, notably those in cystic renal dysplasia, clearly are an expression of altered renal development. Equally, extraneous factors, such as drugs and chemicals ingested during pregnancy, and endogenous genetic influences may operate to produce cystic changes in the developing fetal kidney, just as they may in postnatal life in fully developed nephrons and tubules.

While the precise pathogenetic mechanisms are obscure, on theoretical grounds, cystic transformation of nephronic or ductal elements in the renal parenchyma could be due to (1) obstruction

TABLE 2-3. *Classification of renal cystic diseases*

I. Polycystic disease
    A. Autosomal recessive polycystic kidney disease (ARPKD)
        1. In newborn and young infants (classic infantile polycystic disease)
        2. In older children and adults with congenital hepatic fibrosis
    B. Autosomal dominant polycystic kidney disease (ADPKD)
        1. In adults and older children (classic adult polycystic disease)
        2. In infants (glomerulocystic disease)
II. Simple cysts
III. Acquired renal cystic disease (see Chap. 11)
IV. Localized cystic disease
V. Medullary cystic disease
    A. Medullary sponge kidney
    B. The familial nephronophthisis–medullary cystic disease (FN-MCD) complex
VI. Renal dysplasia (see Table 2-2)
VII. Glomerulocystic disease
VIII. Renal cysts in hereditary syndromes:
    A. Tuberous sclerosis
    B. von Hippel-Lindau
    C. Diffuse cystic dysplasia (see p. 119)
IX. Multilocular renal cysts
X. Miscellaneous
    A. Pyelocalyceal diverticula and cysts
    B. Pericalyceal lymphangiectasis
    C. Perinephric pseudocysts

followed by increased intraluminal pressure and tubular stretching, (2) abnormally increased compliance of the tubular basement membrane allowing tubular dilatation with normal intraluminal pressure, or (3) hyperplasia of the lining tubular epithelial cells that generates increased amounts of tubular basement membrane with enlargement of tubular dimensions. Welling and Grantham [344] argue persuasively that the third possibility (i.e., proliferation of cells lining tubules) is central to cystic dilatation, since stretching alone, whether due to increased pressure behind an obstruction or to increased basement-membrane compliance, would result in an impossibly attenuated and stretched wall and lining [345].

That the tubular basement membrane and cells lining renal cysts are of more or less normal dimensions is evidence in itself that cellular proliferation has occurred. In addition, the presence of polypoid ingrowths of lining epithelial cells, which may be observed in both animal models [100] and human renal cystic disease [99], is further indication of hyperplasia, and these structures may be in a position to obstruct egress of fluid from the cyst. Indeed, while tubular obstruction and abnormal tubular compliance are not necessarily the primary causes of cyst dilatation, they could well be additional factors.

Polycystic Diseases

Polycystic diseases are characterized as hereditary disorders with diffuse cystic changes involving both kidneys. They include at least two genetically distinct disorders. One, inherited as an autosomal recessive condition, typically occurs in infancy (*infantile polycystic disease*); the other, inherited as an autosomal dominant condition, generally affects adults (*adult polycystic disease*). In fact, these older terms are unsatisfactory in that both diseases are diagnosed in children and adults, and the terms *autosomal recessive* and *autosomal dominant polycystic kidney disease* are now preferred.

AUTOSOMAL RECESSIVE POLYCYSTIC KIDNEY DISEASE (ARPKD)

This is a rare condition occurring in 1 in 6000 to 14,000 live births [54]. Until the 1970s, this type of polycystic disease was recognized almost exclusively in the perinatal period, affecting infants who were stillborn or died soon after birth, and this accounted for the term *infantile polycystic disease*. The recognition of a hepatic lesion described as *congenital hepatic fibrosis* [171] that almost invariably accompanies infantile polycystic disease and the fact that other, usually less diffuse forms of cystic renal disease may be associated with congenital hepatic fibrosis in older children and adults have now widened the spectrum of ARPKD.

Classic Form of ARPKD

In the classic infantile form, the kidneys are variably enlarged, sometimes to an extent that may interfere with delivery. The renal enlargement is symmetrical and bilateral, with retention of a normal reniform shape complete with fetal lobation (Fig. 2-25). The surface of the kidney is smooth but studded with innumerable cysts 1 to 2 mm in diameter that, on sectioning of the kidney, are seen as fusiform dilatations running radially

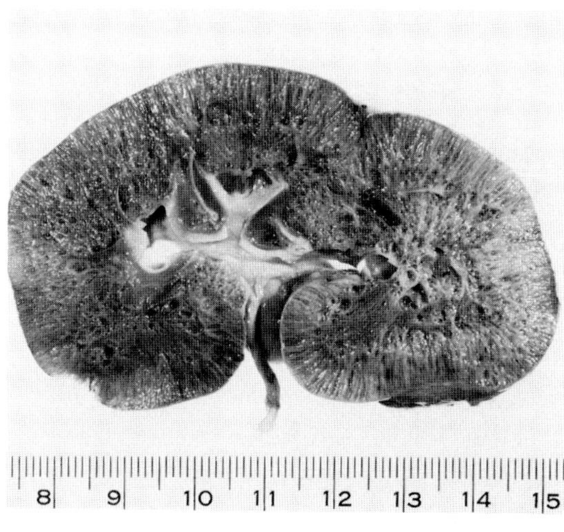

FIG. 2-25. *Autosomal recessive polycystic kidney disease (ARPKD) in a newborn infant. There are radially aligned fusiform cysts in the cortex and more rounded cysts in the medulla. (From Risdon, R. A. Diseases of the Kidney and Lower Urinary Tract. In C. L. Berry (Ed.),* Paediatric Pathology. *Heidelberg: Springer-Verlag, 1981.)*

through the cortex. Similar cystic dilatations, usually rounded in contour, are present in the medulla. Demarcation of the renal cortex from the medulla is apparent but somewhat obscured. On cutting the kidney, it tends to collapse as fluid drains from the cysts. The pelvicalyceal system is enlarged commensurate with the size of the kidney but is normal in shape and configuration; the ureter is normally sited and undilated.

Microscopically, diffuse involvement of the kidney is confirmed. The cysts are seen as uniformly dilated ducts lined by cuboidal epithelium (Fig. 2-26A), and their derivation from collecting ducts has been confirmed by microdissection studies [234] and by staining of their lining epithelial cells with *Arachis hypogaea* (peanut) lectin [102].

The microdissections also demonstrated saccular or fusiform dilatations of papillary collecting ducts; occasionally, more proximal connecting ducts, distal convoluted tubules, and ascending limbs of the loop of Henle also were slightly dilated, and not uncommonly, small cysts (up to 0.5 cm in diameter) were located in the hairpin bend of the loops of Henle. In histologic sections, the cysts may occasionally be seen to branch in the plane of the section, which is further evidence of their collecting duct origin. Between the cysts are groups of histologically normal glomeruli and tubules that are usually crowded together by the dilated collecting ducts and sometimes form wedges beneath the capsular surface. The microdissections of Osathanondh and Potter [234] in this variety of cystic disease, which they termed *Potter type 1,* confirmed normal numbers of nephrons with normal attachments to the dilated and hyperplastic collecting ducts. In the infantile form of ARPKD there is no increase in interstitial fibrous tissue, and no dysplastic elements are evident.

The hepatic lesion of congenital hepatic fibrosis is, in my experience, an invariable feature of ARPKD, although there are rare reports of cases in which it is absent [338]. The lesion involves portal tracts and consists of a variable increase in fibrous connective tissue together with an apparent increase in bile ducts (Fig. 2-26B). Jørgensen [164] has described the bile ductal abnormality as a ductal plate malformation. The bile ducts are slightly dilated, frequently appear to be seen in the plane of the section, often exhibit a curious angulated branching, and may encircle portal venous radicals. Reconstructions from serial sections [161–163] show that the bile ducts form a ring of interconnecting sacs and cisterns in the portal zones rather than separate tubules, and this explains the two-dimensional appearances in sections of the liver. This arrangement is a feature of normal bile duct development that precedes the differentiation of tubular bile ducts, and for this reason, the appearances seen in ARPKD are regarded as an arrest of normal differentiation.

ARPKD Associated with Congenital Hepatic Fibrosis

Since the 1970s, forms of ARPKD associated with congenital hepatic fibrosis occurring in older children and even adults have been recognized. The spectrum of renal and hepatic changes varies with age [49]. With increasing age at presentation, the degree of renal enlargement tends to be less and cystic changes less diffuse (Fig. 2-27A); the hepatic lesion is characterized by more extensive portal fibrosis (Fig. 2-27B), sometimes accompanied by the formation of incomplete fibrous septa and occasionally by regenerative nodules, although true cirrhosis is not a feature. Bile plugs are seen occasionally, but jaundice is very unusual. Portal hypertension accompanied by splenomegaly, symptoms and signs of hypersplenism, and sometimes ascites or esophageal varices, bleeding from which can be fatal, are the clinical expressions of congenital hepatic fibrosis in older individuals. Sometimes there is nonobstructive cystic dilatation of the bile duct elements (so-called Caroli's disease), which may be complicated by ascending suppurative cholangeitis [4,63,209].

The significance of this spectrum of hepatorenal involvement in ARPKD remains controversial. One interpretation is that extensive renal cystic changes produce early death from renal failure so that the hepatic lesion is of little significance. Less diffuse cystic involvement of the kidneys, on the other hand, may be associated with progressive portal fibrosis. This may itself cause portal hypertension, although the possibility that this complication reflects an associated anomaly of portal ve-

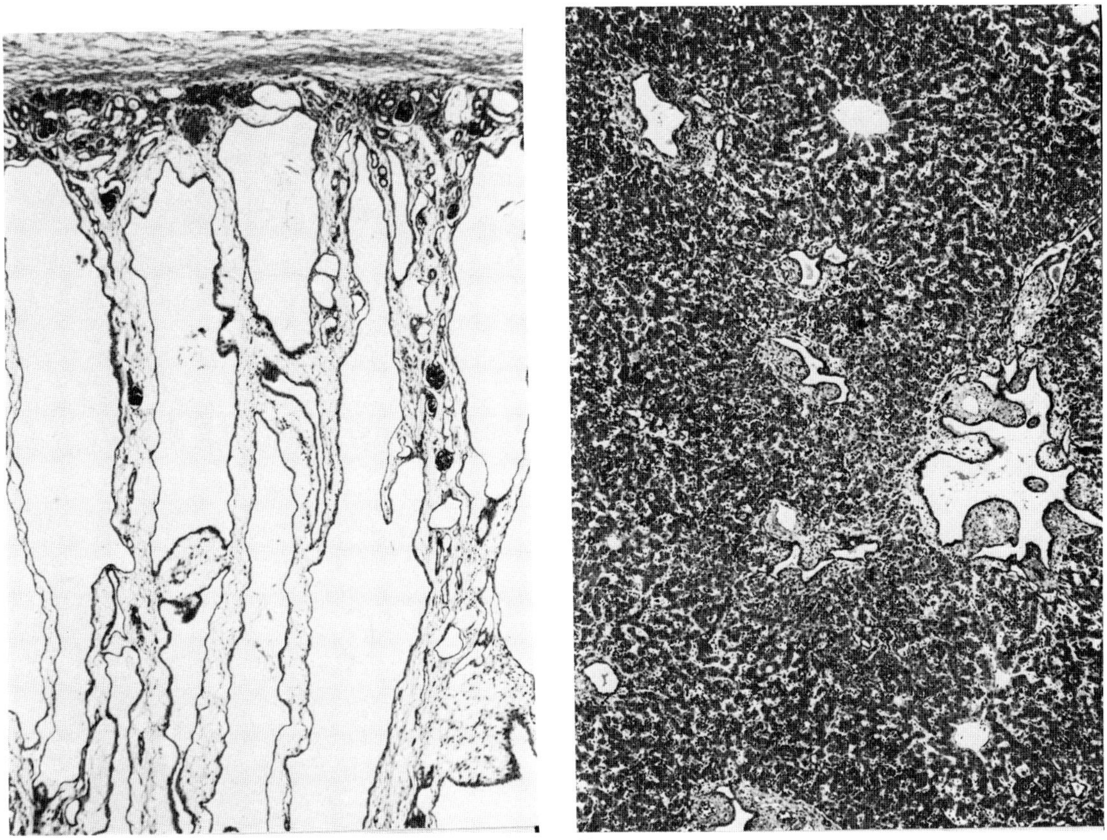

A B

Fig. 2-26. *Microscopic appearances of ARPKD. (A) Kidney from an infant who died in the neonatal period. The cysts are fusiform dilatations of collecting ducts. H&E; ×18. (B) Liver from the same infant. Note the angulated branching of bile ducts in the portal tracts, many of which appear to run in the plane section. H&E; ×36.*

nous radicals causing increased vascular resistance [1,227,330] also has been suggested.

In their 1971 publication, Blyth and Ockenden [49] showed that within a particular family the relative degree of renal and hepatic involvement appeared to breed true. They suggested that a number of mutant genes may operate in ARPKD and divided the spectrum of polycystic disease with hepatic fibrosis into four types (perinatal, neonatal, infantile, and juvenile). Later studies, however, indicate that the separation is less clear and that siblings do not necessarily present at the same age nor with the same relative degrees of hepatic and renal involvement [69,120,168,194,304]. Presentation in the first month of life does not necessarily result in early death; in one series [186], 3 of 13 patients diagnosed at birth survived to between 11.3 and 14.2 years, while 3 of 6 patients identified under 1 month of age were still alive 6.5 to 17.5 years later.

Current concepts of ARPKD present the disease as a continuum of phenotypic expressions, the extremes of which are characterized by younger children with typical infantile polycystic kidney dis-

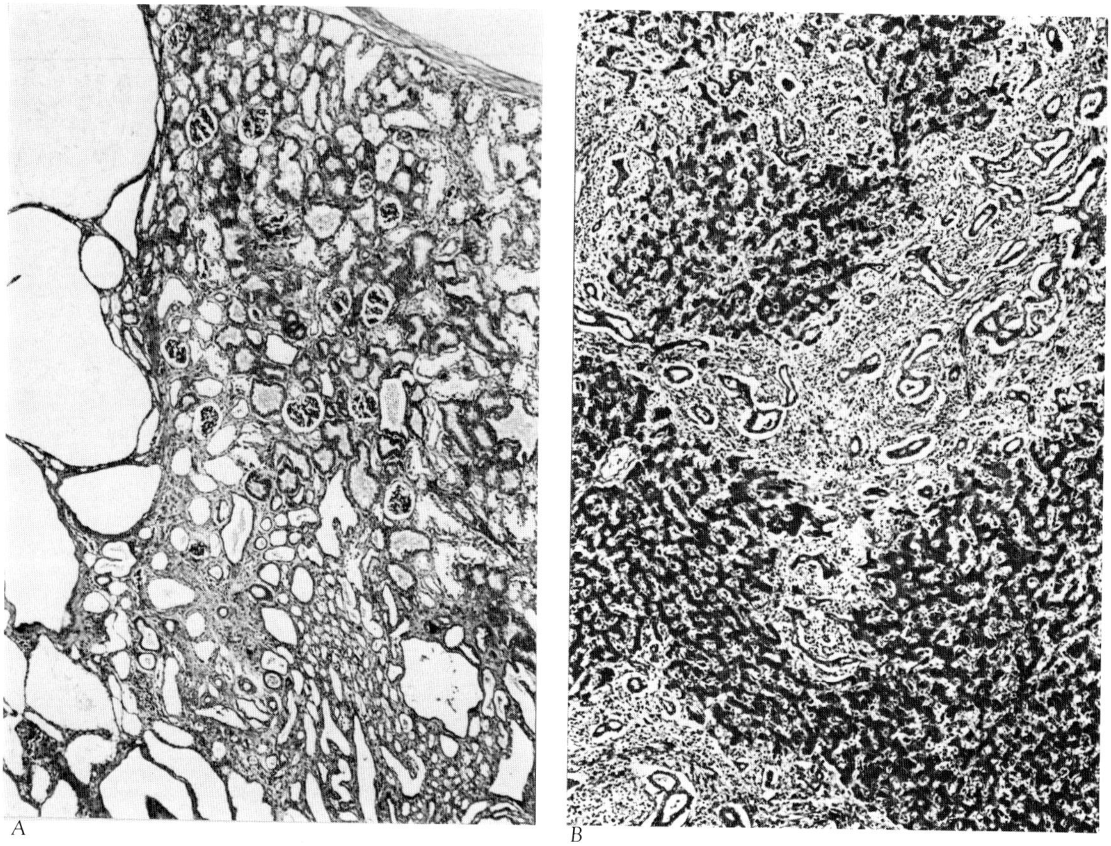

A B

FIG. 2-27. *Microscopic appearances of ARPKD. (A) Kidney from an older child. Cystic changes are less diffuse than those shown in Fig. 2-26A. H&E; ×36. (B) Liver from the same child. Portal fibrosis is more marked than in Fig. 2-26B. H&E; ×36.*

ease and older children or adults with portal hypertension and only mild renal involvement [33,194]. This interpretation has been supported by morphometric studies of the liver in ARPKD that demonstrate that portal fibrosis is nearly twice as severe in patients presenting after the first year [142,186]. Whether or not these differences reflect genetic distinctions or whether incomplete renal expression of the disease allows development of a progressive hepatic involvement until portal hypertension supervenes remains unclear. However, two of the patients reported by Landing et al. [186] showed no increase in portal fibrosis between biopsy and postmortem examinations over intervals of 4.4 and 7.4 years. In any case, portal hypertension is not an invariable consequence of congenital hepatic fibrosis, as exemplified by the case of an elderly woman without evidence of hepatic or renal dysfunction who was discovered to have medullary ectasia and hepatic fibrosis during the investigation of renal calculi [265].

Renal involvement in patients with congenital hepatic fibrosis is variable. Only a small proportion of collecting ducts may be cystically dilated, although these tend to be larger (up to 2 cm in diameter) and more spherical than in classic infantile polycystic kidney disease. However, papillary and medullary duct ectasia is a fairly constant feature, and the radiologic appearances in intravenous urograms are indistinguishable from the medullary sponge kidney (see p. 143) [172,261,341]. This has led to some confusion over nomenclature, and descriptions of medullary cystic kidneys associated with congenital hepatic fibrosis are almost certainly examples of ARPKD [341].

When renal cystic changes are confined to medullary duct ectasia, renal functional impairment is likely to be mild and may be confined to a urine-concentrating defect. With more extensive but subtotal cystic change, the dilated collecting ducts are irregularly distributed in the cortex; they are often rounded in shape and may have fibrous walls. There is an accompanying variable degree of interstitial fibrosis, glomerular obsolescence, and tubular atrophy. The kidneys are generally palpably enlarged, although the enlargement is relatively less gross than in classic infantile polycystic kidney disease. They may even decrease in size with time, possibly as a result of cyst regression [194].

Because of the irregular distribution of cysts and the scarring of the intervening parenchyma, the renal contour tends to be irregular and lumpy and could be confused with the appearance in autosomal dominant polycystic kidney disease (see p. 132), particularly in biopsy specimens. The presence of prominent medullary duct ectasia seen radiologically is a useful distinction, and when a biopsy of the kidney is made during the diagnosis of polycystic kidney disease, it is very important to biopsy the liver at the same time to seek evidence of congenital hepatic fibrosis.

It should be emphasized that ARPKD is not the only condition that may be accompanied by congenital hepatic fibrosis. Certain hereditary syndromes with renal cystic or dysplastic changes (notably Meckel, Jeune, and Zellweger syndromes) may be associated with hepatic lesions indistinguishable from congenital hepatic fibrosis, and the concurrence of this liver disease in some examples of juvenile nephronophthisis has been reported [85,353]. In addition, congenital hepatic fibrosis can exist as an isolated, though probably familial entity in the absence of renal disease. How often this occurs is difficult to establish, since minor degrees of kidney involvement in the absence of significant renal functional impairment may be overlooked. However, Kissane [175] suggests that congenital hepatic fibrosis as an isolated abnormality occurs in about half the patients with this anomaly.

Cystic lesions in other organs are described in ARPKD, although in my experience these are rare and have been confined to pancreatic ducts. Berry aneurysms also have been described but are very much less common than in autosomal dominant polycystic kidney disease [194].

Clinical Features

Clinical manifestations in ARPKD vary with the age at presentation. In classic infantile polycystic kidney disease, children are either stillborn or die in the early postnatal period, usually from pulmonary insufficiency. Although oliguric renal failure is present, this is usually of secondary importance. The Potter sequence is often apparent, and pulmonary insufficiency is related either to this or to mechanical difficulty with breathing due to renal enlargement. Problems with delivery may be related to renal size or oligohydramnios. The increasing use of fetal ultrasonography makes prenatal diagnosis more frequent, although the sonographic appearances in utero may be difficult or impossible to distinguish from other forms of bilateral renal cystic disease [137,207,298]. This is obviously easier when other siblings have been affected.

Patients who survive the neonatal period may have little evidence of renal insufficiency, but progressive renal failure usually develops unless renal involvement is slight. In most cases, the kidneys are enlarged, and although occasionally the degree of renomegaly lessens with time, the kidneys generally remain palpable. Urinalysis reveals a low specific gravity and mild proteinuria, a urine-concentrating defect is characteristic, and a normochronic, normocytic anemia commensurate with the degree of renal failure is usual.

Systemic hypertension is very common and may lead to congestive cardiac failure. In older subjects, renal insufficiency is generally slight or absent, and presentation is usually with the effects of portal hypertension, particularly splenomegaly, hypersplenism, and bleeding esophageal varices.

AUTOSOMAL DOMINANT POLYCYSTIC KIDNEY DISEASE (ADPKD)

This form of polycystic kidney disease is encountered much more frequently than ARPKD. Its true incidence is about 1 in 1000 in the general population [158], and its distribution is worldwide, although it is suggested to be less common in blacks than in Caucasians [332]. About 6 percent of patients entering renal dialysis and transplantation programs have ADPKD [262], and the condition is the third most common cause of end-stage renal failure.

ADPKD has been designated *adult polycystic kidney disease* because clinical presentation with symptoms of renal failure and systemic hypertension is usually delayed until the third or fourth decade. However, given that the disease may rarely present earlier, occasionally in childhood or even infancy, and that improved diagnostic imaging techniques may allow its recognition at a presymptomatic stage, the term *autosomal dominant polycystic kidney disease (ADPKD)* is more appropriate and emphasizes its genetic transmission.

Inheritance

The description of this form of renal polycystic disease as an autosomal dominant trait has been attributed to Cairns [61] and was amply confirmed by the study of Dalgaard [83] that included 284 patients and their families. This latter investigation also showed that while there was considerable variation in the age of onset of clinical symptoms, the age at which clinical disease developed in affected members within a particular kindred was remarkably constant, showing a standard deviation around the mean of only 4 years.

With an autosomal dominant inheritance, it might be expected that affected individuals would be equally likely to be male or female, to have a parent with the disease, and to have a 50 percent risk of transmission to their offspring. While the sex ratio is generally regarded to be equal, the study of Gabow et al. [117] showed a slight excess of males in a ratio of 1.4 : 1. It also has been reported by Rall and Odel [253] and Hatfield and Pfister [141] that the expected family history was not obtained in something over 25 percent of cases diagnosed as ADPKD. Various possible explanations exist for this apparent discrepancy, and these include inadequate communication between family members, failure to diagnose the condition in asymptomatic individuals, the variable expressivity of the disease, and the possibility of a new mutation being responsible for the disease in some individuals. Dalgaard [83] considered the rate of spontaneous mutation to be fairly high and estimated it to be between 6 and 12 per 10,000 mutations/gene/generation. On the other hand, Shemke [297] concluded that sporadic mutations in ADPKD are highly unlikely, and according to this view, cases apparently lacking an appropriate family history would reflect the extreme variability of the disease.

The degree of expressivity is clearly wider than first conceived, as shown not only by the occasional cases presenting in childhood, but also by individuals who remain asymptomatic or have only mild renal impairment even into old age. Although Dalgaard [83] stated that gene penetrance approaches 100 percent in affected individuals surviving to 80 years, it is clear from recent studies, such as that of Cam et al. [62], that asymptomatic patients represent a significant proportion of those with ADPKD, in many of whom lifespan may be normal.

With regard to the diagnosis of ADPKD in presymptomatic and asymptomatic subjects, deformities of the pelvicalyceal system may be apparent on simple intravenous urography, but in a study comparing various imaging techniques [193], computed tomographic (CT) scanning was found to be most effective in delineating the less obvious cases, particularly in children and young adults. In patients older than 20 years, a completely normal ultrasonographic evaluation of the kidneys has been regarded as very strong evidence that they do not have ADPKD [22,151,286].

The abnormal gene associated with ADPKD has been found to be closely linked with the alpha-globin gene cluster and the phosphoglycolate phosphatase gene on the short arm of chromosome 16 [56,259,260]. However, in some families with ADPKD, linkage of the mutant gene to chromosome 16 cannot be identified [173,275], so at least two different mutant genes exist for ADPKD, that on chromosome 16 being designated PCK-1 and the less frequent one unlinked to chromosome 16 as PCK-2.

Pathologic Changes

In its typical form, exemplified by specimens obtained from adult patients after death in renal failure or following bilateral nephrectomy prior to renal transplantation, ADPKD is characterized by marked enlargement of both kidneys with diffuse cystic changes.

Gross examination reveals that the normal reniform shape is variably obscured by cysts that are usually spherical and unilocular and range in size from a few millimeters to several centimeters (Fig. 2-28A). The cysts are distributed throughout the whole kidney and range from numerous to innumerable; more extensive cystic changes and the presence of cysts greater than 3 cm in diameter are said to be more common when the disease is clinically symptomatic [141]. Viewed through the intact capsule, the fluid cyst contents may be clear yellow, turbid, dark brown, or black (the latter colors reflecting hemorrhage into a cyst). When cystic changes are less complete, distinction of ADPKD from multiple simple cysts may be difficult. Not uncommonly, there may be asynchronous involvement of the two kidneys, Hatfield and Pfister [141], for example, recording a difference in kidney weights on the two sides of more than 30 percent in a quarter of their patients (Fig. 2-29). Occasionally, the discrepancy may be so great as to suggest unilateral involvement [180, 188,295], but this point is discussed further in the section entitled Localized Cystic Disease (p. 139).

On cutting the kidney, pressure within the cysts may cause their contents to be forcefully ejected. The cysts are seen in both the cortex and medulla, and corticomedullary demarcation is completely obscured in most cases. The renal papillae are often impossible to identify, and there is considerable distortion of the pelvicalyceal system that is reflected in the radiologic appearances during intravenous urography. Most of the cysts contain clear amber fluid that resembles urine, but particularly in larger examples, some of the cysts may contain fluid or clotted blood or purulent debris of an often putty-like consistency.

In the series of Bennett et al. [29], single kidney weights ranged from 2000 to 4000 g, with a mean of 2600 g, compared with a normal adult kidney weight of about 150 g. However, increased renal size is obviously variable, depending on such factors as age and severity of renal impairment. In the series of Gregoire et al. [133], combined renal weights (mean ± SD) were 943 ± 664 g in 19 patients with no azotemia (serum creatinine <1.3 mg/dl), 1143 ± 733 g in 11 patients with mild azotemia (serum creatinine 1.3–3.0 mg/dl), and 3665 ± 1847 g in 57 patients with moderate azotemia or end-stage chronic renal failure (serum creatinine >3.0 mg/dl). The implication is that the kidneys gradually enlarge throughout life until, at a stage that varies between individuals, renal failure supervenes [115]. The mechanisms responsible for the gradual deterioration in renal function remain controversial. Even at an advanced stage, considerable amounts of noncystic renal parenchyma are evident on histopathologic examination of the kidneys in ADPKD. It seems likely that gradual enlargement of the cysts over many years causes the increase in kidney size and compression atrophy of the residual, initially normal parenchyma with consequent functional deterioration.

The development of systemic hypertension, which occurs in at least half the patients with ADPKD [83], also may be a factor in the genesis of renal failure. The development of new cysts as opposed to enlargement of those already present seems unlikely, and quantitative studies such as those of Grantham et al. [129] counting the numbers of cysts in 5-mm cross sections of a number of kidneys affected by ADPKD suggest that only 1 to 2 percent of nephrons are cystic. The general phenotypic variability between affected individuals and the fact that only a small minority of nephrons are involved by cystic changes may seem curious in a genetically mediated disease but probably reflect a diversity of epigenetic and environmental influences operating on the background of a genetic defect.

Microdissection studies [11,234] have shown that the cysts in ADPKD arise in any part of the nephron or collecting duct and usually retain luminal continuity with their tubules of origin. However, examination of the cysts by scanning

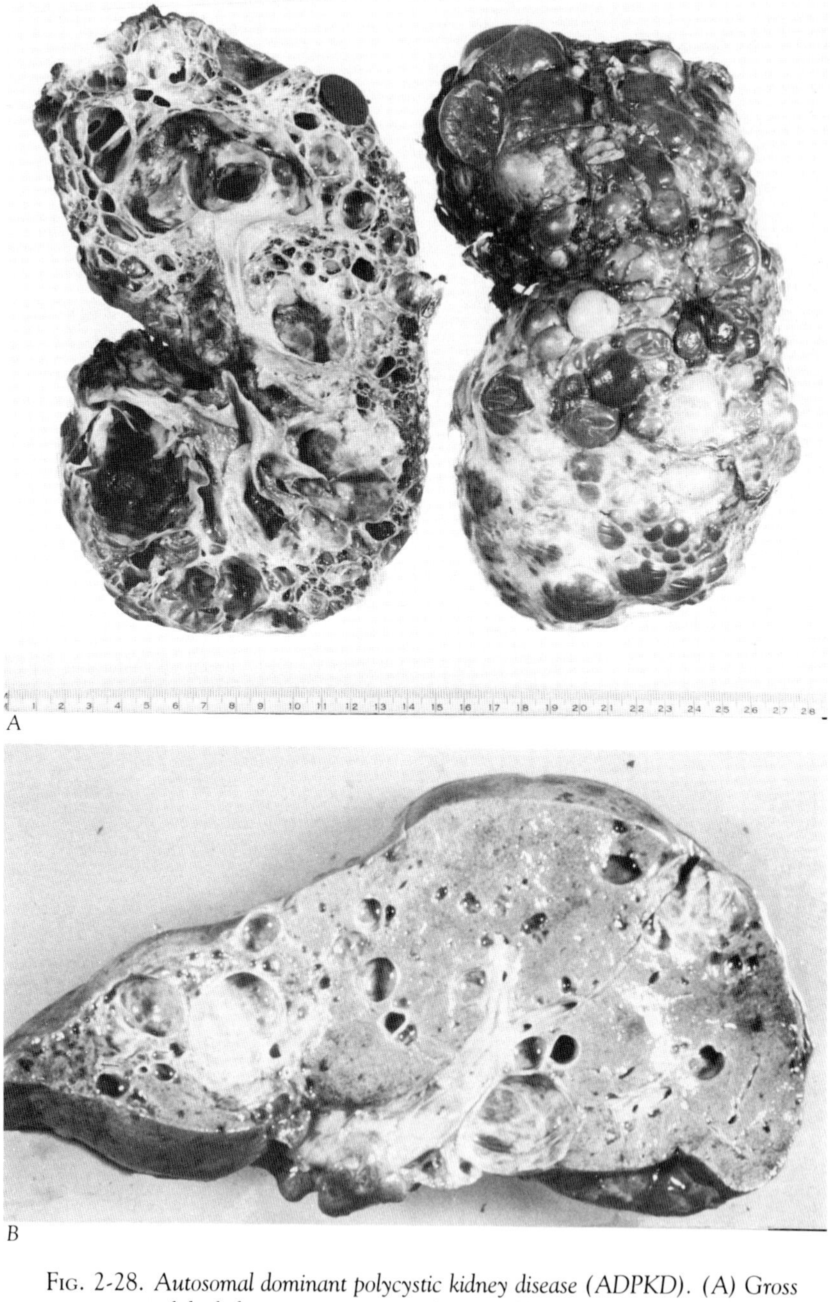

FIG. 2-28. *Autosomal dominant polycystic kidney disease (ADPKD). (A) Gross appearance of the kidney at autopsy in a 50-year-old man. (B) Liver from the same patient. (From Risdon, R. A. Cystic Diseases of the Kidney and Reflux Neuropathy. In P. P. Anthony and R. N. M. MacSween (Eds.),* Recent Advances in Histopathology, *Vol. 2. Edinburgh: Churchill-Livingstone, 1981.)*

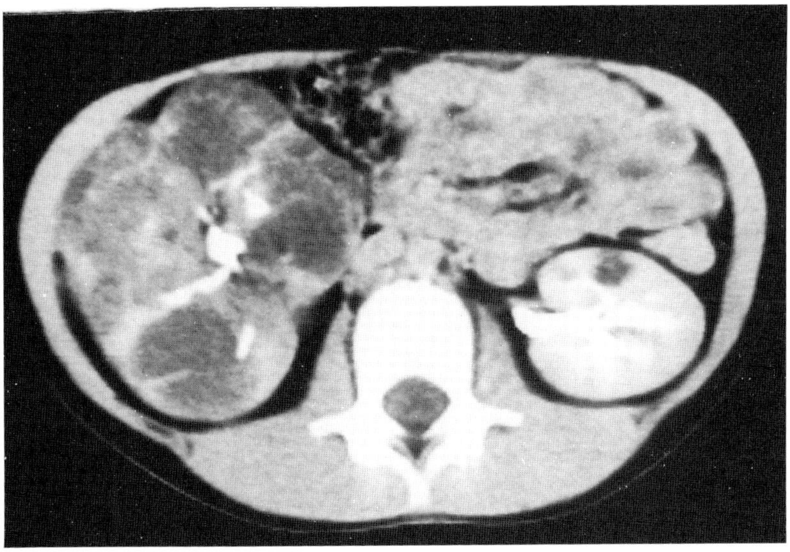

Fig. 2-29. *Computed tomographic scan of the kidneys in a patient with ADPKD showing asymmetrical involvement that is more marked on the left side. (Courtesy of Dr. C. Dicks-Mireaux.)*

electron microscopy [129] demonstrated tubular openings to the cysts in only about a quarter. This discrepancy may reflect different sizes of cysts examined, perhaps indicating that tubular connections are obscured or lost in larger cysts while remaining obvious in the smaller cysts included in the microdissections. In any case, analysis of the cyst fluid shows evidence both of retained tubular function and of cyst origin from proximal or distal nephron segments [82,121,157]. The generally smaller "proximal" cysts had sodium, potassium, chloride, hydrogen ion, and urea concentrations equal to those of serum, while in the usually larger, "distal" cysts these concentrations are lower than in serum.

The mechanisms by which cyst formation and enlargement might occur are incompletely understood. Epithelial hyperplasia is clearly a key element, since covering the increased surface area of a cyst compared with that of a parent tubule evidently requires an increased complement of lining epithelial cells. Evidence of active epithelial hyperplasia in the form of flattened or polypoid proliferations of cyst lining cells is a recently emphasized feature of ADPKD [133] and is present to some extent in the vast majority (over 90 percent) of affected kidneys, particularly those from patients with advanced disease. Cellular proliferation might be important in cyst dilatation as the parent tubule expands in volume to accommodate an increasing number of lining cells and might actually initiate the process by causing partial or complete tubular blockage [35,99]. However, cellular proliferation alone would simply fill the tubular lumens with cells, unless the intracystic fluid volume continued to accumulate through fluid transport across the cyst wall [245] or persistent glomerular filtration into an obstructed nephron. In the latter event, increased hydrostatic pressure would be required. Although this can be demonstrated directly in only a proportion of cysts [47,157], it might be that obstruction in relation to the cysts is often only partial or intermittent. It is also conceivable that increased hydrostatic pressure might be important only in the initial phase of cyst formation, although this is not supported by the observation of Huseman et al. [157] that intracystic pressure is not related to cyst size.

With regard to the actual location of cysts within nephrons, it is possible that this might be related to abnormalities in basement-membrane compliance. While no such abnormality has been demonstrated, the occurrence in some patients with ADPKD of cysts in other organs, intracranial berry aneurysms, colonic diverticula, aortic root dilatation, and mitral valve prolapse suggests that defects of basement-membrane elasticity may be a feature of the condition.

Lectin-binding studies in ADPKD [102] showed some cysts to stain with *Arachis hypogaea* (peanut) lectin, indicating their origin from collecting ducts, and others to stain with *Tetragonolobus lotus* lectin, suggesting their derivation from proximal tubules, while the remainder failed to stain with either lectin.

Histologic examination reveals that most of the cysts are lined by a single layer of cuboidal epithelium, although in some cysts there may be foci of epithelial hyperplasia, sometimes with polypoid projections [133]. The origin of individual cysts is usually difficult to identify by simple microscopy, although the fortuitous inclusion of a glomerular tuft may sometimes indicate a cystic glomerular space formed by expansion of Bowman's capsule. The largest cysts tend to be subcapsular and are usually of collecting duct origin. These often have thickened walls formed by condensation of dense fibrotic connective tissue. Some normal or atrophic renal parenchyma adjacent to the cysts is invariably present on microscopic examination, even in the most floridly cystic examples, a feature that may be difficult to appreciate macroscopically (Fig. 2-30).

Scanning electron microscopy of the cyst walls [129] shows them to be lined for the most part by a single layer of epithelial cells with occasional polypoid hyperplastic foci. The area covered by individual epithelial cells approximates to that occupied in normal renal tubules, indicating that epithelial cell numbers increase in proportion to the increased surface area of the cysts. The surface morphology of the cyst lining cells allows their identification as glomerular parietal, proximal tubular, or collecting duct epithelium in only a minority of cysts, the remainder being lined by undefined or undifferentiated cells.

By transmission electron microscopy [32,82], most cyst lining cells contain a variable number of mitochondria and other organelles and have a basement membrane that may be thickened or even laminated; apical microvilli and significant lateral cellular interdigitations are generally lacking. Cuppage et al. [82] showed that the cysts defined as "proximal" in type by the constitution of their fluid contents were lined by cuboidal cells with smooth surfaces and undilated intercellular channels. "Distal" cysts, on the other hand, were taller and columnar, with a cobblestoned surface, distinct margins, and dilated intercellular channels.

ADPKD in Infancy and Childhood

In the unusual cases of ADPKD presenting clinically at birth or in the first few months of life, the kidneys vary in size and range from normal to considerably enlarged. Cortical and medullary cysts up to 3 cm in diameter are seen, and histologically, cysts of the glomerular space often dominate the picture [250,257]. In addition, there may be evidence of impaired nephrogenesis [104,301]. ADPKD accounts for about half the cases of so-called glomerulocystic disease (see p. 147) occurring in this age group.

Neoplastic Change in ADPKD

Although uncommon, there are a number of reports of renal neoplasms arising in ADPKD [141,155,201,223,270,318]. While many such neoplasms are benign (single or multiple renal adenomas were identified in 19 patients in the series of Gregoire et al. [133]), others have been renal-cell carcinomas. The fact that these malignant tumors occur at a younger age in patients with ADPKD than in those without cystic disease, as well as the fact that many are bilateral, argue that there is a real increased risk of malignancy in ADPKD.

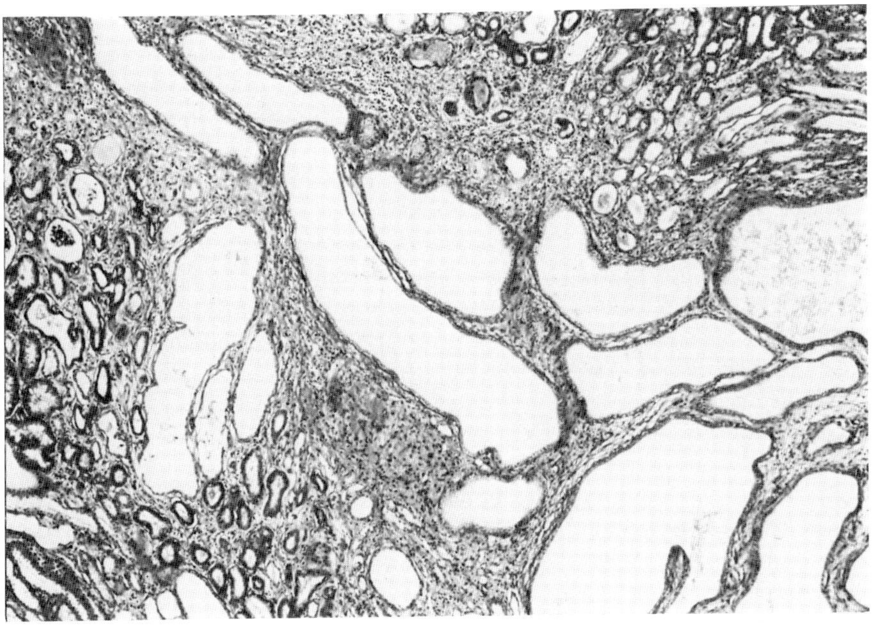

Fig. 2-30. *ADPKD. Microscopic appearance of the cysts with intervening cortex. H&E; ×20.*

Abnormalities in the Liver and Other Organs in ADPKD

Changes in organs other than the kidneys occur to variable extents in ADPKD. Cysts in the liver are the most frequent and were demonstrated by CT scanning in just over half of 44 patients at risk in a recent study [192]. Liver cysts are rare in affected children and are uncommon in young adults, but there is evidence that their prevalence increases with age [135], and they are present in the great majority of patients given renal transplants for ADPKD [294].

The hepatic cysts in this condition are usually numerous and scattered throughout the liver (Fig. 2-28B). The latter is occasionally enlarged, but its function is not impaired [192]. The cysts are usually only a few millimeters in diameter, but occasionally, larger examples are encountered. They arise in portal tracts, have thin, fibrous walls, and are lined by a single layer of apparent biliary epithelium, although they do not contain bile and do not communicate with the normal bile ducts [241]. Diffuse portal fibrosis is not a usual feature in ADPKD as it is in ARPKD, although it has been described [329]. Infection of these cysts is rare [192], and cholangiocarcinoma arising in them also has been reported [183].

Cysts may occur in organs other than the liver and kidneys in ADPKD. In the pancreas, ductal proliferation with fibrosis and cyst formation is seen in about 10 percent of cases, and rarely, cysts in the spleen, thyroid, and seminal vesicles are recorded. Diverticular disease of the colon occurs in up to 80 percent of patients with ADPKD [289].

Vascular anomalies are also associated with ADPKD. Berry aneurysms of the cerebral arteries have been noted in up to one-third of patients [44,190], and their rupture, particularly in hypertensive patients, is a frequent cause of death. Abdominal aortic aneurysms [66], sometimes dissecting in type [332], aortic root dilatation, and mitral valve disease [189] all have been documented in ADPKD.

Clinical Features

ADPKD seldom causes difficulty in clinical diagnosis in typical patients presenting in the third, fourth, or fifth decade with dull loin pain worsened by activity, azotemia, palpable flank masses, and a positive family history. The diagnosis can be confirmed by the radiologic demonstration of renal enlargement with distortion of the pelvicalyceal system by cysts on intravenous urography, by the ultrasonographic delineation of echo-free zones in both kidneys, or by radionuclide or CT imaging [130,193,214,278].

Gross or microscopic hematuria is common, and renal colic due to blood clots or renal calculi occurs in about one-fifth of patients. Some degree of proteinuria is common, but heavy proteinuria is rare. Hypertension occurs in half the patients with ADPKD. Rupture of a berry aneurysm is frequently fatal, and this may occasionally be the presenting event.

Progressive renal failure with the development of a normocytic, normochromic anemia is the usual course of the disease and is characterized by gradual diminution of the glomerular filtration rate with rising serum creatinine and urea levels. The first sign of renal failure may be a diminished urine-concentrating ability [210]. A complicating renal infection is common, particularly in women [28,303] and may be difficult to eradicate.

Problems in diagnosis are likely to arise in the very young or in older patients with normal or near-normal renal function. Although rare, neonatal and childhood cases (Fig. 2-31) are increasingly recognized [6,27,104,169,250,317,326,359] but ideally require a positive family history for confirmation, and this has now been achieved in a number of kindreds.

Ultrasonographic prenatal diagnosis [359] has been reported, and DNA analysis of a sample of chorionic villi has allowed the diagnosis to be made in a 9-week fetus by demonstrating the same gene linkage as in older affected members of the same family [260].

Simple Cysts

Simple renal cysts are an extremely common finding in adult autopsy examinations. Their frequency increases with age [187], and although rare in childhood [302], about half of all subjects over 40 years of age have renal cysts of this type. They appear to be more common in arteriosclerotic kidneys and those scarred for other reasons [13,84]. Increasing use of ultrasonography and, in particular, CT scanning has allowed their frequent identification as an incidental finding in the middle-aged and elderly [325].

Simple cysts may be solitary or just as often multiple and bilateral. They are generally unilocular but occasionally bi- or multilocular; they are usually round or oval in shape and range in size from the barely visible up to several centimeters in diameter. Large cysts are often accompanied by small cysts in the same kidney and are distributed in the renal cortex and occasionally in the medulla. They are said to be more common in males than in females and on the left rather than on the right side [309], although these observations are not universally accepted and the distribution is probably entirely random. Larger examples may project above the renal surface. Usually, they have thin, often translucent, fibrous walls sometimes containing smooth-muscle elements [114] and occasionally a scattering of chronic inflammatory cells. The cysts appear to arise as dilated tubules or collecting ducts and are lined by a flattened and sometimes discontinuous epithelium. When cysts are located deeper in the cortex, the surrounding parenchyma may be compressed and atrophic. Simple cysts normally contain clear, amber-colored serous fluid but rarely contain altered blood. Cysts subject to hemorrhage or past infection may have thicker and occasionally calcified walls [24] in which brown hemosiderin deposits may be seen.

The pathogenesis of simple cysts is incompletely understood. Their rarity in children [215] and their increasing frequency with advancing age argue strongly that they are acquired rather than developmental lesions. Their high incidence in arteriosclerotic or otherwise scarred kidneys has been taken to suggest that ischemia and local obstruction of nephrons with subsequent proximal nephron dilatation are important [143]. More recently, small diverticula on renal tubules have been noted to occur increasingly with advancing age [105]; Baert and Steg [12,14,15] suggest that simple cysts may arise by closure of the connection between a diverticulum and its parent tubule, followed by gradual accumulation of fluid within the diverticulum and progressive expansion with thinning of the lining epithelium and cyst formation.

From a clinical standpoint, the vast majority of simple cysts are entirely asymptomatic and, even when multiple, have no effect on renal function. The rare, very large cyst may give rise to loin pain and be palpable in the abdomen. Bleeding into a cyst also may cause loin pain and sometimes gross or microscopic hematuria [225], and even fatal perirenal hemorrhage has been reported [310]. Rarely, simple cysts may be infected and even rupture [111,195]. There are also reports of hypertension [72,272] and polycythemia [178,280] attributed to the presence of simple renal cysts.

Because cysts of this type only rarely produce clinical disease, their main significance lies in their distinction from other, more relevant conditions. Solitary cystic lesions may need to be differentiated from cystic renal neoplasms. This can nearly always be achieved by modern ultrasonography or CT scanning [200,285], even in the very rare event of a tumor actually arising within a cyst [226]. In addition, cytologic examination of the aspirated cyst content may be helpful in this respect [134,342].

Multiple diffuse simple cysts, particularly when bilateral, must be differentiated from ADPKD, and this has actually become more of a problem with the recognition that the latter condition may produce markedly asymmetrical cystic changes in the two kidneys and be associated with little or no renal impairment in some cases. In contrast to ADPKD, multiple simple cysts are generally irregularly distributed with extensive intervening solid parenchyma. In ADPKD, a family history is usual, and hepatic cysts—detectable by ultrasonography or CT scanning—are commonly present. Advances in the development of markers for the ADPKD gene indicate that this problem may soon be solved.

Localized Cystic Disease

In 1979, Cho et al. [70] described three patients with a form of unilateral renal cystic disease localized to part of one kidney. Two of the patients were middle-aged males, and the other was a 3-year-old girl; all presented with gross or microscopic hematuria and hypertension. Pathologic examination of the kidneys revealed cystic changes microscopically indistinguishable from ADPKD but confined to only part of one kidney, with no clear demarcation or capsule separating the cystic from the normally differentiated portions. In none of the patients described was there a family history of renal cystic disease. The pathologic features can be distinguished from segmental renal dysplasia by the lack of lobular disorganization or dysgenetic elements such as metaplastic cartilage or primitive ducts. Distinction from a multilocular cyst (see p. 151) can be made by the fact that the lesion is unencapsulated and contains normally differentiated parenchyma between the cysts.

Unilateral localized cystic disease of this nature is probably more common than the literature would suggest, and I have seen three cases in the last few years in male children, all of whom lacked a family history. One of these was a neonate, suggesting that the condition may well be developmental in nature (Fig. 2-32).

The recognition of localized cystic disease is also relevant to descriptions of apparently unilateral renal involvement in ADPKD [180,188,295]. Better appreciation that cystic changes in ADPKD may be deceptively asymmetrical invites the suggestion that they may be wholly unilateral or appear so during life, when detailed pathologic examination is impossible. Equally, if localized cystic disease is recognized as involving part of one kidney, it is logical to suppose that it might sometimes affect most of or even the whole of one kidney. From a practical point of view, it is hard to accept a diagnosis of unilateral ADPKD in the absence of, at least, thorough diagnostic imaging procedures to demonstrate a normal contralateral kidney and, perhaps most important, a positive family history. The demonstration of typical hepatic cysts would be useful additional evidence. In the absence of this evidence, localized cystic disease involving

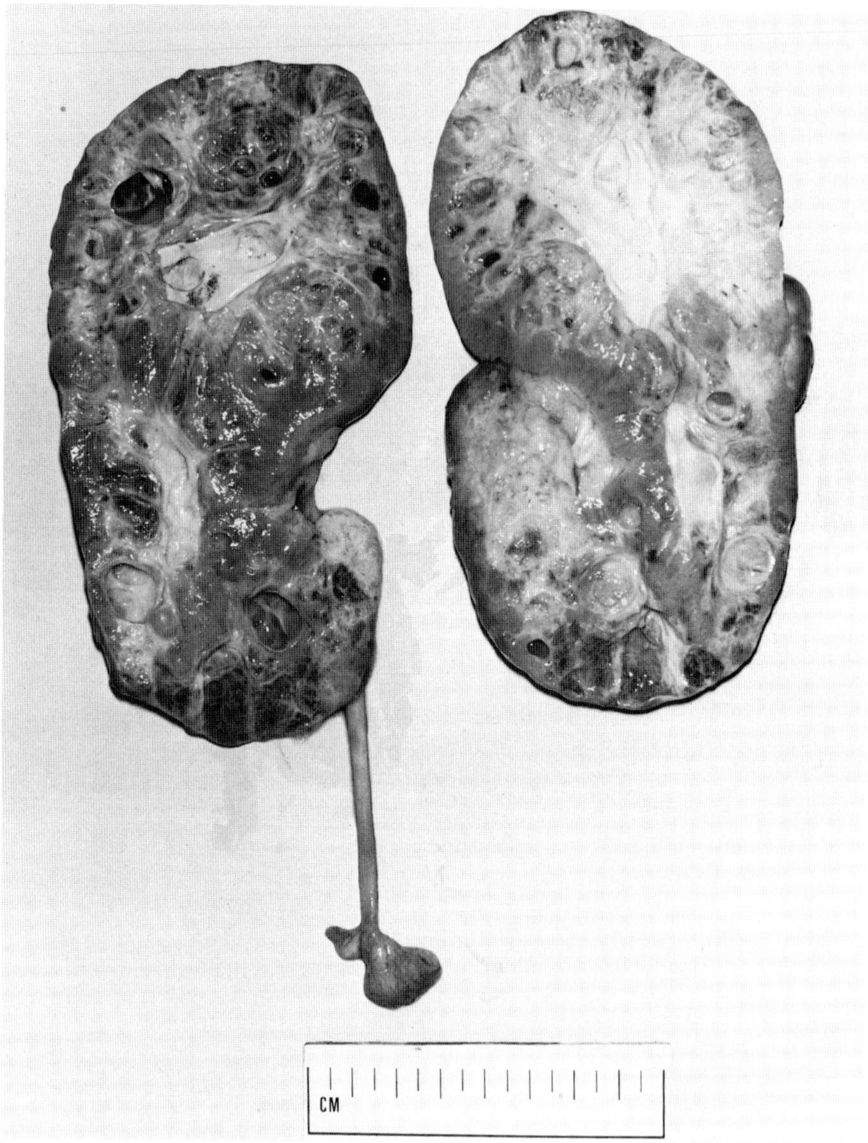

A

Fig. 2-31. *Clinically unsuspected ADPKD in an 11-year-old boy who died suddenly from subarachnoid hemorrhage from a ruptured berry aneurysm. (A) Kidneys. (B) Brain.*

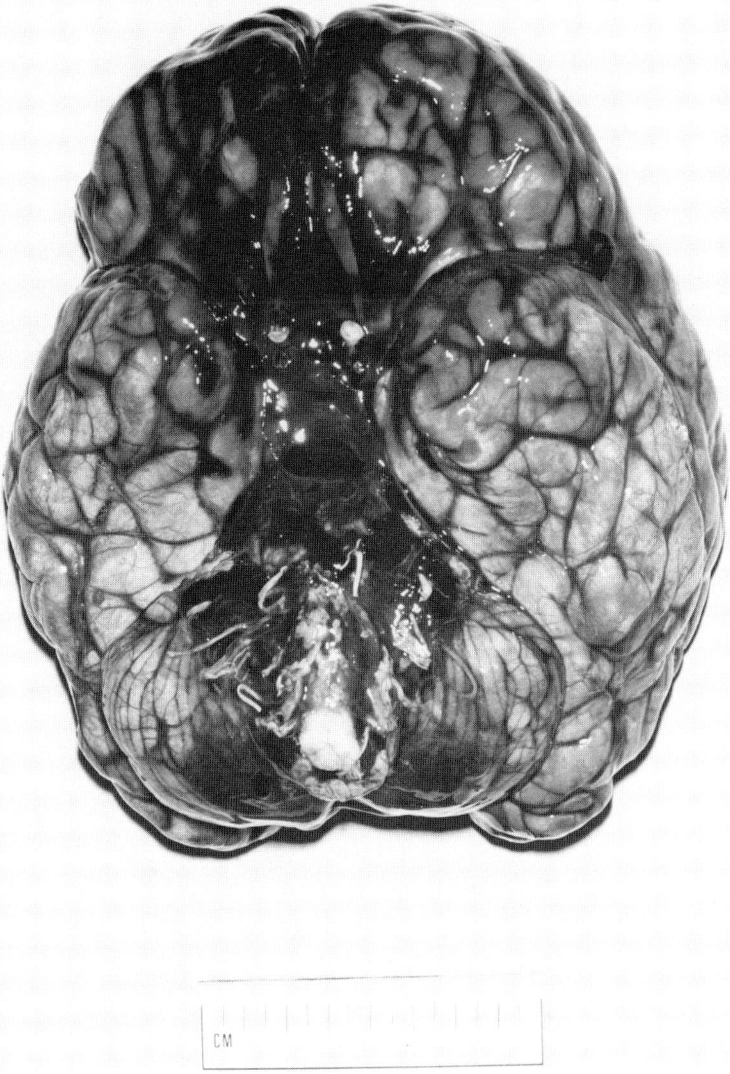

B

Fig. 2-31. (continued)

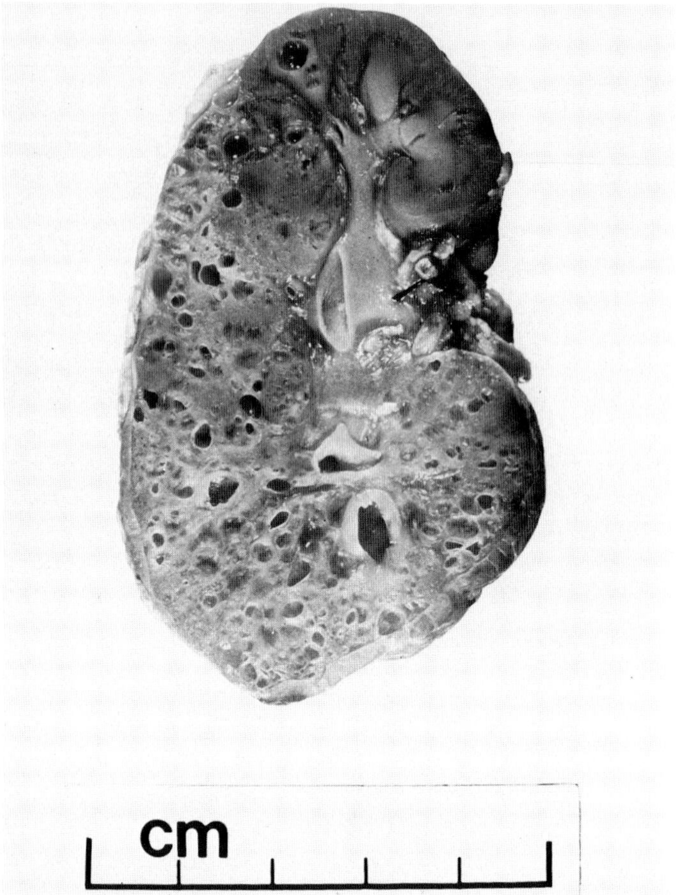

A

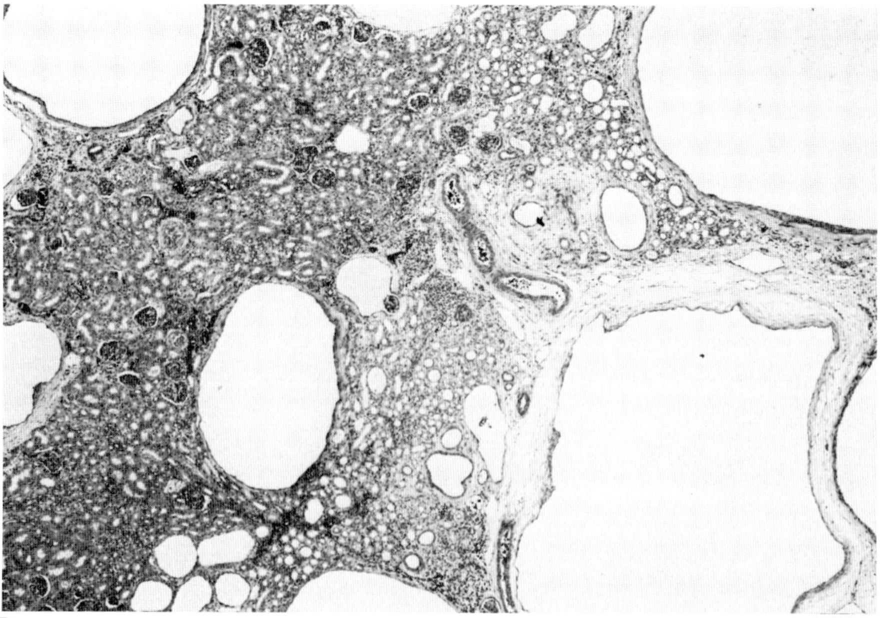

B

most or all of one kidney provides an alternative diagnosis. Resolution of this problem, like that of distinguishing bilateral multiple simple cysts from ADPKD, will probably lie in the application of genetic probes for the diagnosis of ADPKD.

Medullary Cystic Disease

Renal cystic diseases with cysts confined to or predominating in the medulla are of two quite distinct types—the medullary sponge kidney and familial nephronophthisis–medullary cystic disease. The latter is also referred to as *uremic medullary sponge kidney,* but this is not a good description because it invites confusion with medullary sponge kidney.

MEDULLARY SPONGE KIDNEY

This quite common condition is characterized by ectasia of papillary collecting ducts, usually affecting all the pyramids of both kidneys, but occasionally only affecting one or two pyramids or only one kidney [147]. In itself, the medullary sponge kidney is usually asymptomatic and does not give rise to significant renal functional impairment unless complicated by infection or stone formation.

It is recognized radiologically by intravenous urography, which shows characteristic radial linear streaking in the renal papillae as contrast medium collects in the ectatic or cystic papillary collecting ducts (Fig. 2-33). Calcium deposits are frequently present in the ectatic ducts and need to be distinguished from contrast medium.

The exact incidence of medullary sponge kidney, particularly in asymptomatic patients, is unclear. Incidence figures of approximately 1 in 5000 for the general population have been suggested [124]; the higher incidence of about 1 in 1000 among urologic patients [182] probably reflects the increased frequency of complications, such as urolithiasis and urinary infection, and the greater probability of intravenous urography being performed in such patients. Similarly, the rarity with which medullary sponge kidney is diagnosed during childhood [240] is probably explained by the lack of symptoms in these young subjects and does not conflict with the concept that the papillary duct ectasia is a congenital anomaly usually recognized only when complications lead to clinical manifestations. Medullary sponge kidney is rarely diagnosed by pathologists because nephrectomy for this condition per se would almost never be indicated, except perhaps for advanced nephrolithiasis, and it could be easily overlooked at autopsy unless specifically looked for.

The condition is equally common in males and females and is usually sporadic, although its occurrence in siblings and even in three consecutive generations of the same family has been reported [177,181].

Associations with the Ehlers-Danlos [191], Marfan [290], and Wiedemann-Beckwith syndromes [67], as well as with congenital hemihypertrophy [138,311], are described. The two latter associations have been particularly emphasized, although there is some suggestion that the renal abnormality observed is a form of medullary dysplasia with medullary ductal dilatation rather than medullary sponge kidney. Although medullary sponge kidney is reported in association with congenital hepatic fibrosis, these cases are almost certainly examples of ARPKD.

Grossly, the medullary sponge kidney is usually normal in size, but in about 30 percent of cases, it is slightly enlarged by the presence of medullary cysts. In the absence of infection or obstruction, the renal surfaces are smooth, and the renal cortices are of normal appearance. The medulla, on cut section, consists of ectatic ducts and cysts of varying size, usually small but occasionally up to 7.5 mm in diameter [182], most prominent near

Fig. 2-32. *Unilateral localized cystic disease of the kidney. (A) Right nephrectomy specimen from a 4-day-old female infant. Cysts are scattered throughout the lower pole and midzone but spare the upper pole. (B) Microscopy shows thin-walled cysts separated by normal or compressed renal parenchyma. H&E; ×20.*

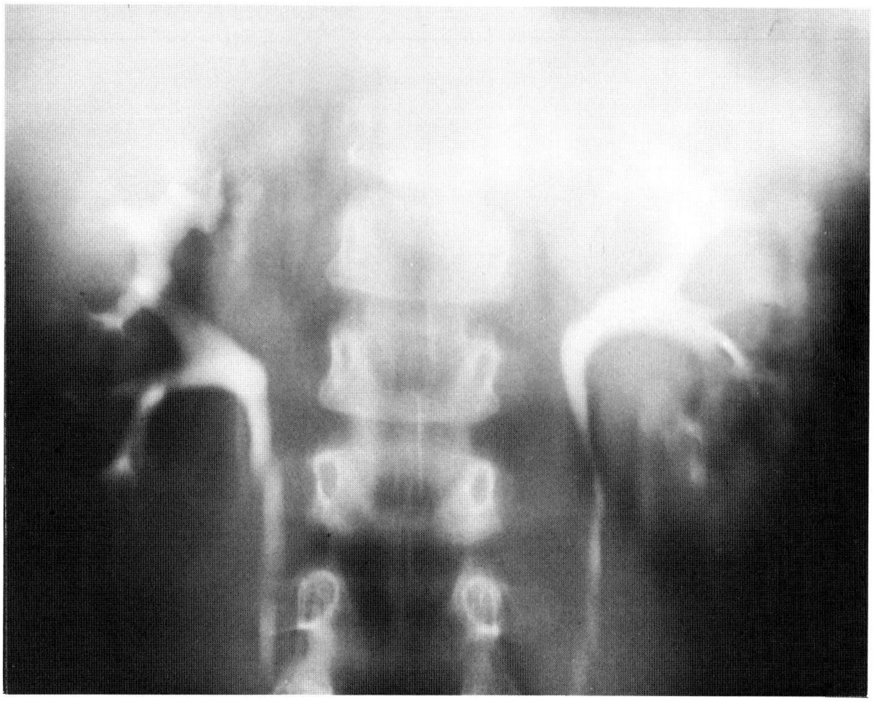

FIG. 2-33. *Medullary sponge kidney. An excretory urogram with tomography showing radial linear streaking in the renal papillae due to contrast medium in the ectatic papillary ducts. (Courtesy of Dr. R. de Bruyn.)*

the papillary tips, which appear flattened and enlarge the associated calyces [94,252]. The medullary cysts sometimes contain inspissated material and small calculi. Microscopically, the cysts are lined by columnar, transitional, or sometimes metaplastic squamous epithelium. They may be denuded of epithelium or ulcerated, particularly in the presence of calculi, which occasionally erode through the cyst wall to produce intercystic communications. Proximal communications with medullary collecting ducts and distal communications with the minor calyces may be seen depending on the plane of section. A prominent inflammatory infiltrate, maximal near the papillary tips, is almost always seen.

Clinically, the condition is often discovered as an incidental finding during intravenous urography, and in most instances, long-term follow-up shows neither deterioration in renal function nor progression of the radiologic abnormalities [181]. Hematuria and renal colic due to stone formation may be presenting symptoms, and nephrolithiasis is a common complication of medullary sponge kidney, occurring in up to 50 percent of affected patients [356]. Chemical analysis shows the stones to be composed of calcium phosphate or, less commonly, calcium oxalate or magnesium ammonium phosphate. Although stone formation has been attributed to stasis within the dilated and cystic papillary ducts, it is noteworthy that a significant number of patients with medullary cystic disease have hypercalciuria [94,232], and some have a defective urinary acidification capacity [147]. In addition, a majority (over two-thirds) of affected subjects have impaired maximal urine-concentrating ability [94,128].

Urinary infections also may complicate medullary sponge kidney, although it is unclear whether this is a direct complication or a consequence of nephrolithiasis [156].

THE FAMILIAL NEPHRONOPHTHISIS–MEDULLARY CYSTIC DISEASE (FN-MCD) COMPLEX

Medullary cystic disease and so-called juvenile nephronophthisis were originally described as separate entities [101,307]. The former was characterized as a type of renal cystic disease with a mainly medullary distribution, and the latter was described as an autosomally recessive familial nephropathy causing polyuria and progressive renal failure in childhood. However, the recognition of common clinical and pathologic features both with and without medullary cysts [320] and the occurrence of cases with and without medullary cysts in the same family [324] have blurred the pathologic differentiation between the two. While the pathologic features may be indistinguishable, it is clear that there is genetic heterogeneity with the existence of apparent autosomal recessive, autosomal dominant, and sporadic forms. These considerations have led to the concept of the FN-MCD complex to cover all these eventualities together with the ocular and skeletal anomalies that coexist in some cases.

The renal lesions in the FN-MCD are similar whatever the genetic background or associated abnormalities [238,343,361]. The kidneys are diffusely shrunken, often to less than half the expected weight, firm, and pale in color. Both cortex and medulla are thinned, and in the majority of cases, thin-walled, fluid-filled cysts in variable numbers are located near the corticomedullary junction (Fig. 2-34), although in about 25 percent the cysts are very sparse or absent [123] (Fig. 2-35). The cysts vary from barely visible to up to about 1 cm in diameter. Microdissection studies [299] have demonstrated a marked increase in tubular diverticula, most prominent in the loops of Henle, distal convoluted tubules, and collecting ducts. These may well be relevant to the formation of medullary cysts by mechanisms similar to those responsible for simple cysts.

Microscopically, the changes are usually severe but essentially nonspecific (Fig. 2-36). Many glomeruli are globally sclerotic and converted to hyalin balls. Others may be segmentally sclerosed, while in the remainder, the tufts may be morphologically normal, although both in sclerosed glomeruli and apparently normal ones there is often marked thickening of the basement membrane of Bowman's capsule that is accompanied by periglomerular fibrosis. Widespread tubular atrophy is generally a prominent feature, particularly of distal tubular segments, and this is accompanied by marked thickening of the tubular basement membranes. This is best seen in PAS or PA–methenamine silver stains, where the tubular basement membranes often exhibit lamination to produce a net-like or "flaky pastry" effect. This appearance also can be seen with the electron microscope, and occasionally, abrupt transitions from thin to thick tubular basement membranes are present [73]. As well as atrophic tubules, hypertrophied and microcystically dilated tubules are usually evident, as in any end-stage kidney.

Diffuse interstitial fibrosis, particularly in areas of tubular atrophy, is a constant finding, and often there is a pronounced nodular chronic inflammatory cell infiltrate with sometimes homogeneous, PAS-positive interstitial masses identified as Tamm-Horsfall protein [358].

Cystically dilated tubules and larger cysts are mostly located at the corticomedullary junction and occasionally deeper in the medulla, although not at the papillary tips, as in the medullary sponge kidney. Also, unlike medullary sponge kidney, calcification of the cyst walls and intracystic calculi are not seen.

The cysts are lined by flattened epithelium, which by scanning electron microscopy is shown to be continuous with that of collecting ducts, and near the points of connection with the collecting ducts it is morphologically similar to the duct lining cells [238].

In renal biopsy specimens taken early in the disease, the microscopic abnormalities are less severe, and their nonspecific nature may make diagnosis difficult without a typical clinical history and evidence of genetic transmission. The clinical features of patients with FN-MCD vary somewhat

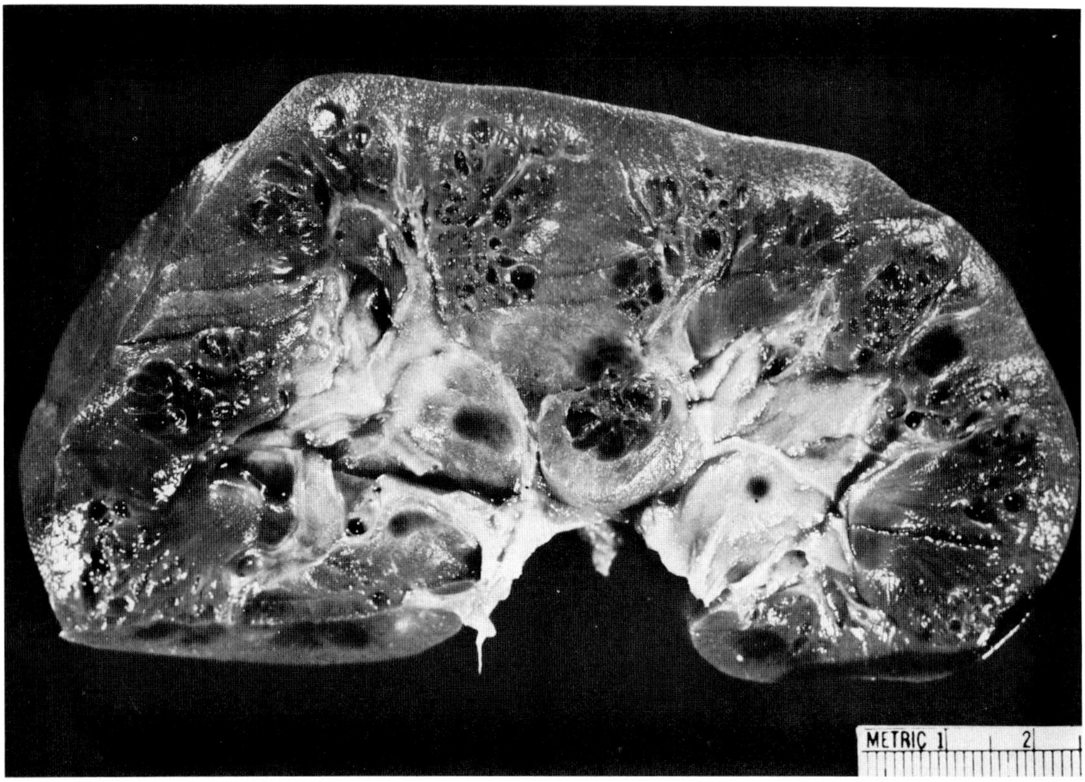

FIG. 2-34. *Familial nephronophthisis–medullary cystic disease (FN-MCD) complex. Gross specimen of a kidney showing collections of cysts at the corticomedullary junction.*

according to the particular genetic variant and the age at presentation. In about half the patients, the disease is inherited as an autosomal recessive trait. Such patients are usually children with progressive azotemia ending in terminal renal failure, usually in the second decade. Males and females are equally affected. The disease is an important cause of chronic renal failure in childhood and accounts for between a quarter and a fifth of children entering chronic dialysis programs [43].

There is often a normochromic, normocytic anemia and delayed growth with small stature. Polydipsia and polyuria are common and are related to an impaired urine-concentrating capacity that may be evident before renal failure is present. Urinalysis is usually unrewarding, with no red or white cells present in the urinary deposit. Proteinuria is generally mild or absent. Heavy proteinuria has been reported [92], but normally this finding would suggest a diagnosis other than FN-MCD. Renal salt wasting, which may be severe, has been regarded as characteristic, but it is present in only about 70 percent of cases [123]. Salt wasting apparently protects against hypertension complicating chronic renal failure. Particularly in children, renal osteodystrophy and secondary hyperparathyroidism are common as renal failure progresses.

Associated nonrenal anomalies are usually noted with autosomal recessive disease. Most commonly, these anomalies are ocular, particularly

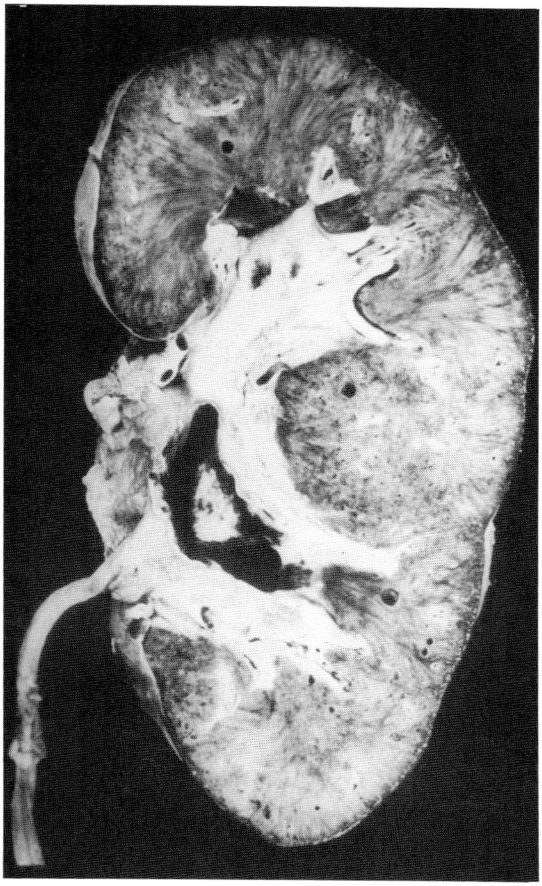

Fig. 2-35. *FN-MCD complex. Kidney from a 6-year-old girl with juvenile nephronophthisis, who died in renal failure. The kidney is uniformly contracted, and only one or two tiny cysts are visible at the corticomedullary junction. (From Jones, D. N., Risdon, R. A., Hayden, K., et al.,* Paediatr. Radiol. *1: 164, 1973.)*

tapetoretinal degeneration and retinitis pigmentosa [51,109,197,296,339,361]. However, other anomalies are also reported, and they include congenital hepatic fibrosis [50,85,251] and skeletal abnormalities, particularly phalangeal cone-shaped epiphyses [246,271,315]. In addition, apparently similar renal changes to those in FN-MCD have been described in the Bardet-Biedl (obesity, hypogonadism, polydactyly, mental retardation, retinitis pigmentosa) and the Alström (obesity, blindness, diabetes mellitus, nerve deafness) syndromes.

In about a third of patients with FN-MCD, the disease appears to be inherited as an autosomal dominant trait [76,77,122,177]. An X-linked chromosomal inheritance also has been suggested, although this seems unlikely, since no sex predilection is apparent. Patients with autosomal dominant FN-MCD are usually adults rather than children, and there are no accompanying extrarenal anomalies. The clinical characteristics are otherwise similar and progression of renal failure following diagnosis equally rapid.

Patients without an apparent family history form a significant proportion of both childhood and adult cases.

Glomerulocystic Disease

Glomerulocystic disease, first coined by Taxy and Filmer [328], is now used to describe a heterogeneous group of disorders rather than a specific entity, the common link being a variable degree of cystic dilatation of Bowman's spaces [38,167]. Glomerular cysts may occur in a bewildering number of genetic and sporadic disorders, including early-onset ADPKD [27,104,250], the Zellweger cerebral-renal-hepatic syndrome [167], tuberous sclerosis [273,314], trisomy 13 syndrome, Majewski type short rib–polydactyl syndrome [167], oral-facial-digital syndrome [38,313], brachymesomelia-renal syndrome [184], and some types of sporadic and familial renal dysplasia.

From a practical viewpoint, the term *glomerulocystic disease* should only be applied when this is the predominant histopathologic change, and should not be used when a few cystically dilated glomeruli are seen against a background of, for example, obvious renal dysplasia. This distinction may, of course, be more difficult in biopsy specimens.

In infancy, about half the examples of glomerulocystic disease described appear to be an expression of ADPKD with unusually early clinical onset. This is supported by the presence of other

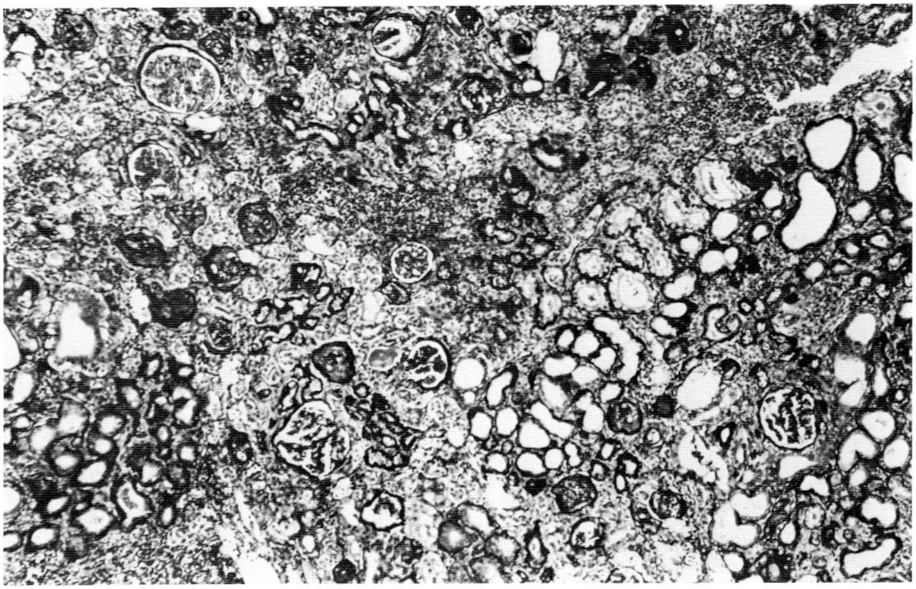

FIG. 2-36. *FN-MCD complex. Histologic appearance of the kidney shown in Fig. 2-35. PAS; ×40.*

family members with more typical features of the disease [27,104,250,279] and, more specifically, by the demonstration using DNA probe analysis of the ADPKD-associated gene linkage on chromosome 16 in both a mother with ADPKD and her fetus with glomerulocystic disease [260]. Although glomerulocystic disease appears to be the most common change associated with ADPKD in the very young, not all cases of infantile-onset ADPKD have predominantly glomerular cysts, and the exact significance of this morphologic expression in relation to ADPKD is not yet established. Perhaps it merely represents one way in which, for reasons unknown, the genetic anomaly affects the immature kidney [38]. To further complicate the issue, dominantly inherited glomerulocystic disease has been reported in an adult male and his three children (two boys and a girl) [211]. It thus remains possible that dominantly inherited glomerulocystic disease may be a separate entity rather than a variant of ADPKD.

As well as the associations already noted, glomerulocystic disease may be encountered, particularly in infants and young children, as an apparently sporadic condition (Fig. 2-37). Although many patients present in renal failure, the prognosis is extremely variable, and both adult cases and long-term survivors are reported [65,88,228]. This probably points to the essentially nonspecific nature of glomerulocystic change.

From a practical point of view, the presence of glomerular cysts should prompt examination of the histologic sections for other markers such as dysplastic elements or evidence of tuberous sclerosis. Obtaining a detailed family history and a careful review of the clinical findings to discover syndromal associations are also important. In the absence of other clinical findings or a positive family history, the condition should be regarded as sporadic. However, the report by Bernstein et al. [42] of a patient with severe glomerulocystic disease who was later found to have skin le-

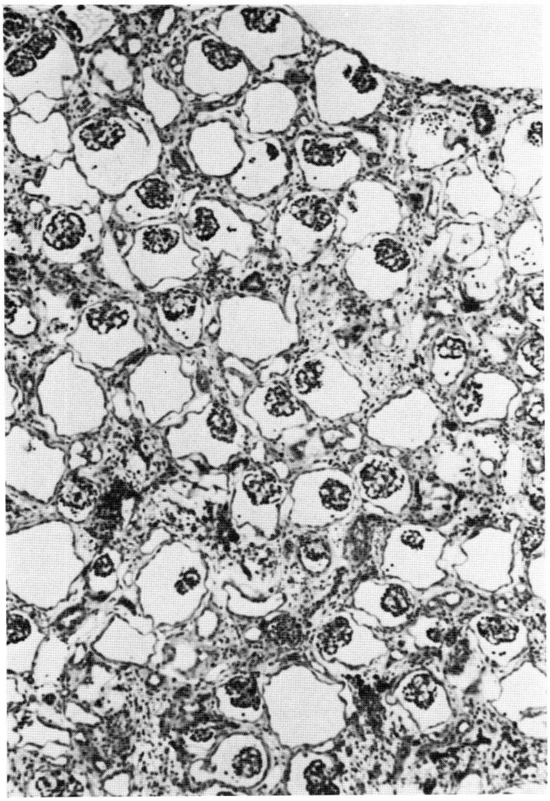

Fig. 2-37. *Glomerulocystic disease. Renal biopsy from a 1-month-old girl in renal failure. No family history was obtained. H&E; ×36.*

sions of tuberous sclerosis prompts caution in this respect.

Renal Cysts in Hereditary Syndromes

TUBEROUS SCLEROSIS

Tuberous sclerosis is a systemic disorder inherited as an autosomal dominant trait and characterized by hamartomatous malformations affecting, singly or in combination, the skin, kidney, brain, eye, bone, liver, and lung. Its expression is variable, so small lesions, particularly those affecting single organs, may be overlooked. Penetrance is equally variable, so involvement of other family members may be demonstrated in only about half the index cases [26].

Renal involvement is common, affecting about 50 percent of patients [319]. The most frequently described renal lesions are angiomyolipomas, which are tumor-like nodules of varying size composed of mature adipose tissue, smooth muscle, and thick-walled blood vessels. They are often multiple and bilateral.

Renal cysts are also common, although this was less well appreciated before modern diagnostic imaging techniques allowed the demonstration of even quite small cysts [216,357]. The combination of angiomyolipomas and renal cysts is particularly suggestive of tuberous sclerosis [243], although renal cystic changes can occur in the absence of angiomyolipomata [314] (Fig. 2-38).

The cysts occur in both the renal cortex and the medulla and vary greatly in size. Microscopically, the epithelial lining is distinctive; it is composed of large, hyperplastic cells with acidophilic or clear cytoplasm (Fig. 2-39) that are focally multilayered or thrown into papillary excrescences that sometimes fill the cyst lumen. Despite the apparent resemblance to proximal tubular epithelial cells, microdissection studies indicate their origin from all portions of the nephron [248]. Occasionally, glomerular cysts may predominate, so tuberous sclerosis constitutes one form of so-called glomerulocystic disease. Sometimes renal cystic changes are sufficiently diffuse as to cause renal failure [229]. In addition, many patients with tuberous sclerosis and renal involvement develop systemic hypertension. There are also several reports of renal-cell carcinoma in patients with tuberous sclerosis, these tumors apparently arising de novo or in combination with angiomyolipomas or cystic change [20,136,199].

As well as renal cysts and angiomyolipomas, curious, apparently microhamartomatous glomerular lesions have recently been described in tuberous sclerosis [220]. These are characterized by compact collections of large, clear polygonal or cuboidal cells containing lipid-filled vacuoles confined within the glomerular tufts and bounded by the glomerular basement membrane (Fig. 2-40).

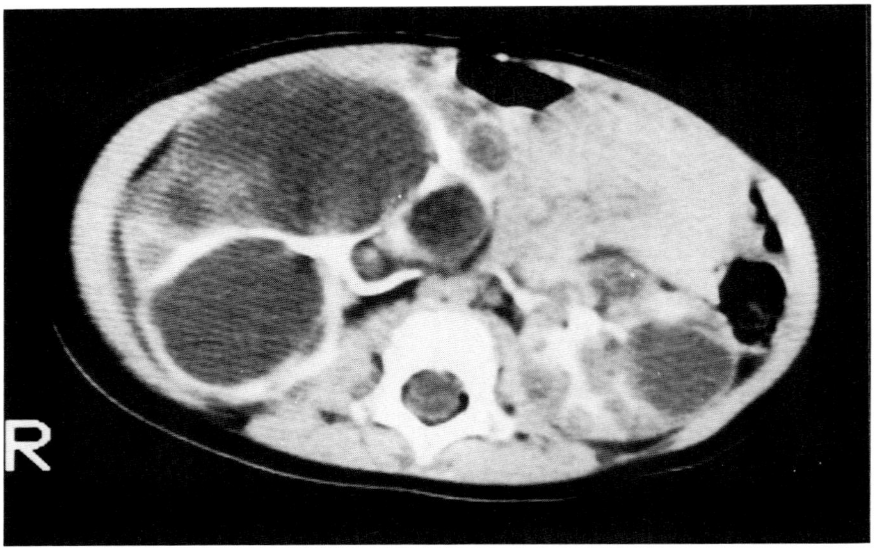

FIG. 2-38. *CT scan of the kidneys showing diffuse cystic changes in a child with tuberous sclerosis. (Courtesy of Dr. C. Dicks-Mireaux.)*

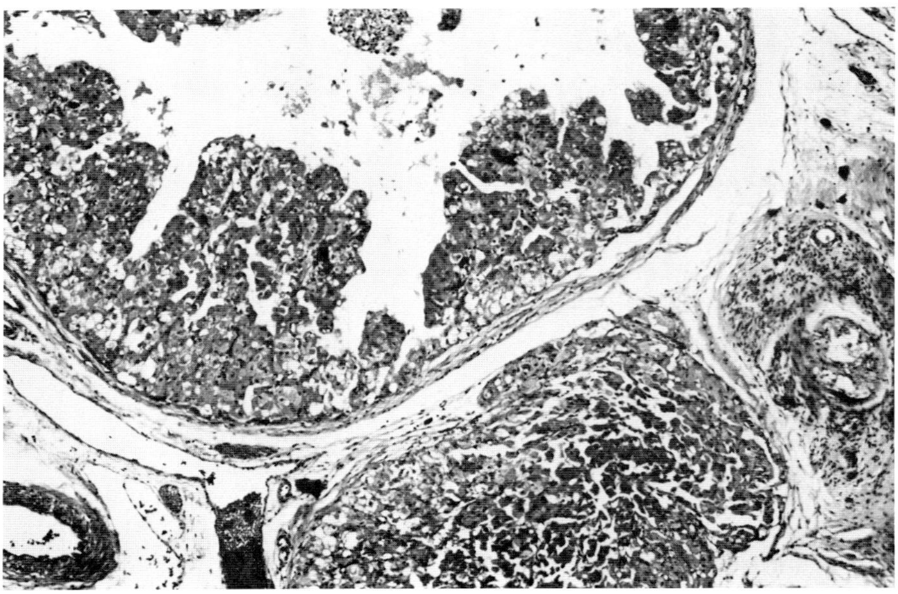

FIG. 2-39. *Tuberous sclerosis. Large hyperplastic cells with clear cytoplasm line a cyst. A nodule of similar cells is seen adjacent to the cyst. H&E; ×100.*

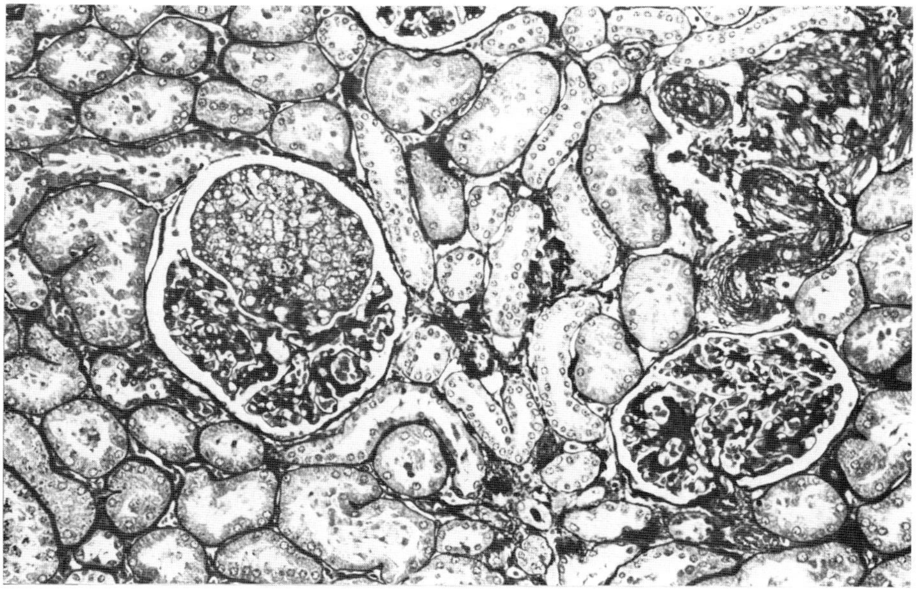

Fig. 2-40. *Tuberous sclerosis. Microhamartomatous glomerular lesion. PA–methenamine silver;* × *100.*

VON HIPPEL-LINDAU DISEASE

Von Hippel-Lindau disease is inherited as an autosomal dominant trait and is characterized by a variable combination of angiomatous cysts of the cerebellum, retinal angiomatosis, and cysts or tumors of abdominal organs, principally the pancreas and kidneys. Although the condition is said to show variable penetrance, this is questionable because the lesions are often not apparent until middle or old age, and with time, probably most, if not all, patients at risk show some manifestation of the disease [108].

Renal lesions occur in about two-thirds of patients and include renal-cell carcinomas and cysts which, like simple cysts, vary in size and may be solitary or multiple; they are often bilateral and occasionally sufficiently numerous as to simulate ADPKD [116]. The epithelial lining of the often fibrous-walled cysts is usually flattened and attenuated but is from time to time hyperplastic. Occasionally, small nodules of apparent renal-cell carcinoma arise within the cysts [37, 71]. This fact, together with the observation that the renal-cell carcinomas that complicate von Hippel-Lindau disease in about 25 percent of patients [153] are often multiple, suggests that an association between cystic changes and malignant transformation in this condition is more than a chance occurrence [35].

Multilocular Renal Cysts

Multilocular renal cysts are regarded as cystic neoplasms and are not in the strict sense related to the other cystic disorders included in this chapter. They are described here only because they are part of the differential diagnosis of these conditions.

The multilocular cyst has been called by a number of other names, including *multilocular cystic nephroma, renal cystadenoma, cystic mesoblastic nephroma, polycystic nephroblastoma,* and *cystic differentiated nephroblastoma.* The last two synonyms in particular reflect the current concept of a spectrum of related tumors ranging from the classic

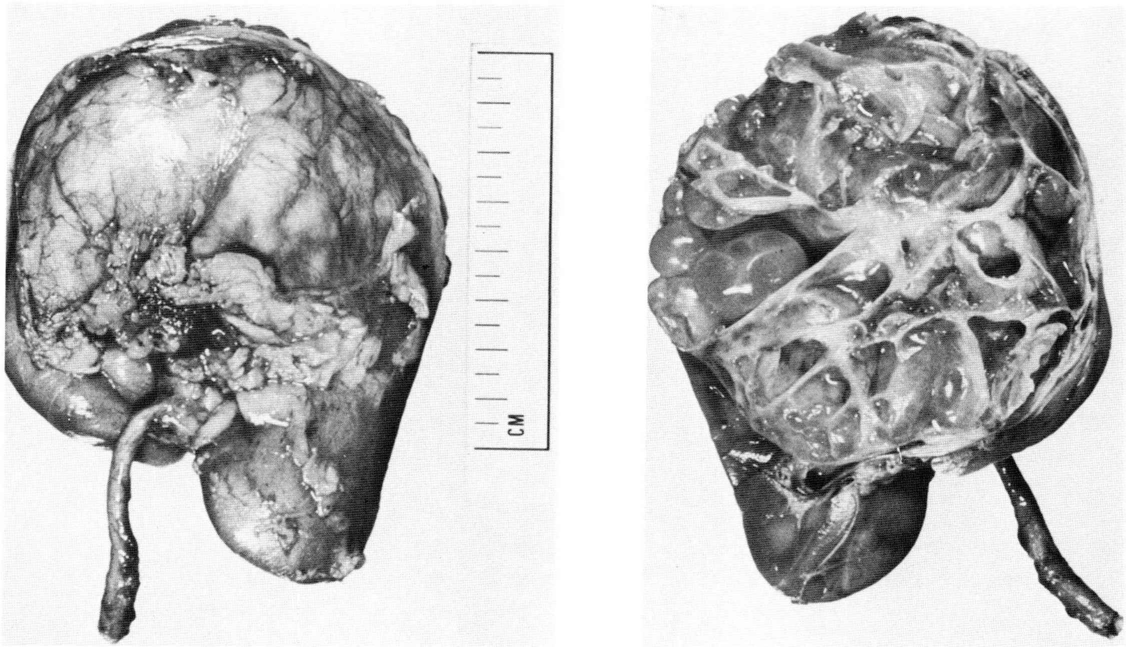

FIG. 2-41. *Multilocular cyst (multilocular cystic nephroma). The lesion is encapsulated and confined within the kidney.*

solid nephroblastoma (Wilms tumor) at one end to the multilocular cyst at the other, with intervening intermediate forms usually referred to as *cystic partially differentiated nephroblastoma* [165].

Multilocular cysts are rare, with only about 150 cases described in the literature. The age distribution is biphasic. There is an early peak at under 2 years in which the sexes are about equally represented and a second peak in middle-aged adults with a marked female predominance [18]. About two-thirds of reported cases are in children, and very few examples are seen between 5 and 20 years of age.

The vast majority of multilocular cysts are unilateral, with the left and right kidneys equally affected, although the lower poles appear to be more frequently involved than the upper poles. Clinical presentation is usually with an abdominal mass, occasionally giving rise to abdominal pain or hematuria. Both affected children and adults may have hypertension, which is sometimes relieved by nephrectomy. There are no reports of familial incidence or associated extrarenal anomalies. Occasionally, rapid growth of the tumor has been seen in childhood, but slow enlargement is more usual. Excretory urography is less useful for diagnosis than more modern imaging techniques. Ultrasonography demonstrates the cystic nature of the lesion and CT scanning or magnetic resonance imaging (MRI) is particularly helpful in delineating its circumscribed, multilocular morphology.

Powell et al. [249] defined a number of criteria that distinguish the multilocular cyst. These were that it is unilateral, solitary, and multilocular, with no communications between the "daughter" cysts or the renal pelvis. The cysts possess an epithelial lining but no differentiated elements in the cyst septa. Some of these stipulations have required subsequent modification in that multilocular cysts are rarely bilateral [68], and particularly in children, the cyst septa may occasionally contain tubular structures, mesenchymal tissue, smooth muscle, or even skeletal muscle, and exceptionally, cartilage and bone [75,119,126].

Grossly, the multilocular cyst is generally large, spherical, sharply demarcated, and encapsulated (Fig. 2-41). It is usually confined within the kidney, which may be up to three times the expected weight, but occasionally, the tumor may expand through the renal capsule to protrude into the perinephric fat. The adjacent kidney is normal apart from the effects of compression. Cysts often prolapse through the tumor capsule into the renal pelvis, which may become obstructed. On cross section, the lesion is bounded by a thick white capsule from which delicate, pale, fibrous trabeculae extend to subdivide the tumor into multiple, spherical, noncommunicating, clear fluid-filled locules that vary from a few millimeters up to several centimeters in diameter.

Microscopically (Fig. 2-42), the cysts are lined for the most part by nondescript cuboidal or occasionally pegged epithelial cells. Sometimes the lining cells are heaped up or form papillary structures. Occasionally, aggregates of clear cells occur, and transformation to renal-cell carcinoma is claimed [104A], although metastases have not been described. The cells lining the multilocular cyst are said to have the ultrastructural characteristics of collecting duct epithelium [75], but our own unpublished immunocytochemical findings conflict with this conclusion. The cells stain with CAM 5.2 but not with epithelial membrane antigen (EMA), as would be usual for collecting ducts. Furthermore, staining with *Arachis hypogaea* (peanut) and *Tetragonolobus lotus* lectins shows positive results with both lectins in some cysts and negative results in others. If the cyst linings were of collecting duct origin, uniformly positive results would be expected with *Tetragonolobus lotus* lectin alone [102].

The thin septa between the cysts consist of fibrovascular tissue, but particularly in children, they may contain more cellular mesenchyme, occasional tubules and microcysts, as well as smooth-muscle or even striated-muscle cells and foci of cartilage and bone [119,126,206]. The thick tumor capsule not infrequently contains smooth muscle and occasionally compressed renal parenchymal elements and focal calcification.

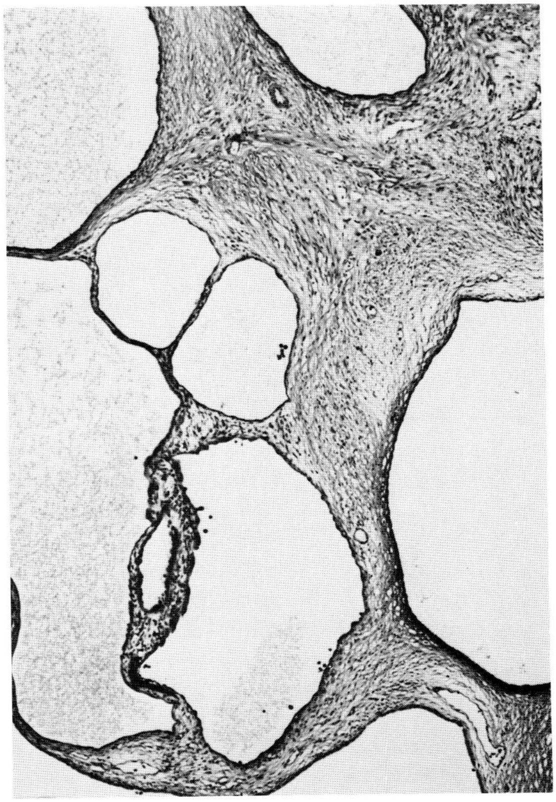

Fig. 2-42. *Multilocular cyst. Microscopic appearance showing cysts lined by nondescript epithelial cells. Septa between the cysts are composed of mesenchymal tissue but contain no differential nephronic elements. H&E;* ×36.

The suggestion that the multilocular cyst constitutes the "benign" end of a continuum of tumors originating from metanephric blastema and related to nephroblastoma (Wilms tumor) is derived from the recognition of various intermediate forms between these two extremes. The most notable is the so-called cystic partially differentiated nephroblastoma [165,166], which macroscopically is indistinguishable from the multilocular cyst, but on microscopic examination contains within the cyst trabeculae tubular elements and areas of blastema indistinguishable from that in nephroblastoma (Fig. 2-43). The latter occasionally form nodules projecting into the cyst lumens [166]. We have recently encountered a renal tumor in a 2-year-old child in which different areas displayed the appearances of multilocular cyst, cystic partially differentiated nephroblastoma, and classical triphasic Wilms tumor, adding further to the suggested relationship between these entities.

A typical multilocular cyst occurring in a child or an adult can be regarded as a wholly benign neoplasm requiring no treatment beyond nephrectomy or even partial nephrectomy if this is technically feasible. The presence of foci of blastemal tissue is the hallmark of the cystic partially differentiated nephroblastoma. Although this lesion is considered to be at least potentially malignant, there are no reports of metastases, so nephrectomy and follow-up seem to be appropriate therapy. The one clear exception from the otherwise excellent prognosis is the very rare multilocular cyst of adult patients in which histologically malignant and mitotically active spindle-celled sarcomatous elements are seen in the cyst walls [206].

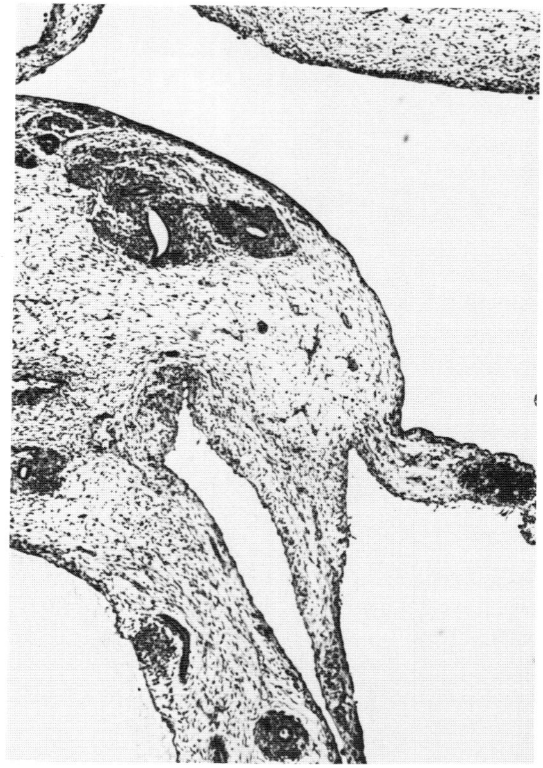

Fig. 2-43. *Cystic partially differentiated nephroblastoma. Note the tubules and focal condensations of blastemal cells in the cyst septa. H&E; ×70.*

Miscellaneous Cystic Conditions

PYELOCALYCEAL DIVERTICULA AND CYSTS

Pyelocalyceal diverticula and cysts are saccular outpouchings from the renal pelvis or minor calyces, with which they communicate by a narrow isthmus. They are usually solitary and occur most frequently in the upper pole of the kidneys. Both sexes and both kidneys are equally affected, and rarely, bilateral examples are encountered.

Pyelocalyceal diverticula are usually discovered incidentally during excretory urography and are seen in 3.3 per 1000 of these examinations during childhood [355]. The diverticulum is visualized by retrograde flow of contrast medium from the renal pelvis, and emptying of contrast medium from the diverticulum is usually delayed.

The diverticula appear to be equally common from the newborn period throughout life, which supports an embryologic origin. This is considered to be either from a coalescence of branches of the ureteric bud that has failed to induce nephron formation [213] or from earlier ureteric bud branches that have failed to become incorporated normally in the pelvicalyceal system [355].

Approximately one-third of children with pyelocalyceal diverticula develop symptoms of loin pain and urinary infection, occasionally with gross hematuria. In later life, up to 40 percent develop diverticular calculi [213,350].

Pyelocalyceal diverticula are lined by attenuated transitional epithelium, and there may be a thin submucosal layer of smooth muscle. Inflammation of the wall may be a feature, and squamous metaplasia of the lining epithelium may occur, particularly with recurrent infection or stone formation. Most cases require no treatment, but if symptoms are persistent, partial or total nephrectomy may be indicated.

PERICALYCEAL LYMPHANGIECTASIS (HYGROMA RENALIS)

Pericalyceal lymphangiectasis describes a circumscribed cystic mass representing dilated lymphatic channels that invests the renal pelvis [86]. The lesion may consist of single or multiple cysts and may be unilateral or bilateral [145]. It has been variously considered to be either a hamartomatous malformation analagous to the cystic hygromas of the head, neck, and mediastinum or to be an acquired lesion resulting from lymphatic obstruction. Occasionally, lymphatics in the renal capsule are also involved so that the whole kidney is covered by cysts to give an appearance superficially reminiscent of polycystic disease [196]. Microscopically, the cysts have thin, fibrous walls; they are lined by endothelial cells and contain eosinophilic proteinaceous material.

Pericalyceal lymphangiectasis is usually asymptomatic, but it may be associated with urinary obstruction. It is generally discovered in adults and diagnosed either at laparotomy or by ultrasonography or CT scan [146].

PERINEPHRIC PSEUDOCYSTS

Perinephric pseudocysts are uncommon and are due to extravasation of urine into the perinephric fat as a result of blunt trauma to the kidney or following surgical procedures where the renal pelvis or calyces are damaged or the renal capsule is torn. Often there is some degree of accompanying urinary obstruction [8,159,322], and occasionally, the lesion may occur with urinary obstruction alone [335].

Macroscopically, perinephric pseudocysts consist of a cavity containing urine and sometimes altered blood and fatty material, and they are usually confined within the layers or renal fascia [212]. There is no epithelial lining, and the wall consists of reactive fibrous tissue and chronically inflamed adipose connective tissue, often with evidence of fat necrosis. In long-standing examples, the wall of the pseudocyst may become calcified.

Clinically, the condition is characterized by a flank mass and abdominal pain that may be recognized only some considerable time after an episode of abdominal trauma or surgery. Radiologically, the findings are of a perinephric mass confined within the renal fascia, and often the kidney is displaced.

REFERENCES

1. Albukerk, J., and Duffy, J. L. Fibrogenesis in congenital hepatic fibrosis: An electron and light microscopic study. *Arch. Pathol.* 92:126, 1971.
2. Allanson, J. E., Pantzar, J. T., and MacLeod, P. M. Possible new autosomal recessive syndrome with unusual renal histopathological changes. *Am. J. Med. Genet.* 16:56, 1983.
3. Allen, T. D. Congenital ureteral strictures. *J. Urol.* 104:196, 1970.
4. Alvarez, F., Hadchouel, M., and Bernard, O. Latent chronic cholangitis in congenital hepatic fibrosis. *Eur. J. Pediatr.* 139:203, 1982.
5. Anderson, E. E., and Harrison, J. H. Surgical importance of the solitary kidney. *N. Engl. J. Med.* 273:683, 1965.
6. Anton, P. A., and Abramowsky, C. R. Adult polycystic renal disease presenting in infancy. *J. Urol.* 128:1290, 1982.
7. Arant, B. S., Sotelo-Avila, C., and Bernstein, J. Segmental "hypoplasia" of the kidney (Ask-Upmark). *J. Pediatr.* 95:931, 1979.
8. Arnold, E. P. Pararenal pseudocyst. *Br. J. Urol.* 44:40, 1972.
9. Ask-Upmark, E. Über juvenile maligne Nephrosklerose und ihr Verhältnis zu Störungen in der Nierenentwicklung. *Acta Pathol. Microbiol. Scand.* 6:383, 1929.
10. Avni, E. F., Thoua, Y., Lalmand, B., Didier, F., Droulle, P., and Schulman, C. C. Multicystic dysplastic kidney: Natural history from in utero diagnosis and postnatal follow-up. *J. Urol.* 138: 1420, 1987.
11. Baert, L. Hereditary polycystic kidney disease (adult form): A microdissection study of two cases at an early stage of the disease. *Kidney Int.* 13:519, 1978.
12. Baert, L., and Steg, A. Cystic changes in adult human kidneys after ureteral obstruction: Microdissection studies. *Urology* 7:526, 1976.
13. Baert, L., and Steg, A. On the pathogenesis of simple renal cysts in the adult. A microdissection study. *Urol. Res.* 5:103, 1977.

14. Baert, L., and Steg, A. Is the diverticulum of the distal and collecting tubules a preliminary stage of the simple cyst in the adult? *J. Urol.* 118:707, 1977.
15. Baert, L., and Steg, A. Diverticula on distal tubule, simple renal cysts, and ureteral obstruction: Causal relationship. *Urology* 11:221, 1978.
16. Baggenstoss, A. H. Congenital anomalies of the kidney. *Med. Clin. North Am.* 35:987, 1951.
17. Bailey, R. R. The relationship of vesicoureteric reflux to urinary tract infection and chronic pyelonephritis: Reflux nephropathy. *Clin. Nephrol.* 1: 132, 1973.
18. Baldauff, M. C., and Shulz, D. M. Multilocular cyst of the kidney: Report of three cases with review of the literature. *Am. J. Clin. Pathol.* 65:93, 1976.
19. Bankier, A., DeCampo, M., Newell, R., Rogers, J. G., and Danks, D. M. A pedigree study of perinatally lethal renal disease. *J. Med. Genet.* 22:104, 1985.
20. Barbour, G. L., and Casali, R. E. Bilateral angiomyolipomas and renal cell carcinoma in polycystic kidney. *Urology* 12:694, 1978.
21. Batzenschlager, A., Blum, E., and Weill-Bousson, M. Le petit rein unilatéral (Étude anatomo-clinique). *Ann. Pathol.* 7:427, 1962.
22. Bear, J. C., McManamon, P., Morgan, J., Payne, R. H., Lewis, H., Gault, M. H., and Churchill, D. N. Age at clinical onset and at ultrasonographic detection of adult polycystic kidney disease: Data for genetic counselling. *Am. J. Med. Genet.* 18:45, 1984.
23. Bearman, S. B., Hine, P. L., and Sanders, R. C. Multicystic kidney: A sonographic pattern. *Radiology* 118:685, 1976.
24. Becker, J. A., and Schneider, M. Simple cyst of the kidney. *Semin. Roentgenol.* 10:103, 1975.
25. Beckwith, J. B. Macroglossia, omphalocele, adrenal cytomegaly, giantism, and hyperplastic visceromegaly. *Birth Defects* 5:188, 1969.
26. Bender, B. L., and Yunis, E. J. The pathology of tuberous sclerosis. *Pathol. Annu.* 17:339, 1982.
27. Bengtsson, U., Hedman, L., and Svalander, C. Adult type of polycystic kidney disease in a newborn child. *Acta Med. Scand.* 197:447, 1975.
28. Bennett, W. M. General Features of Autosomal Dominant Polycystic Kidney Disease: F. Evaluation and Management of Renal Infection. In J. J. Grantham and K. D. Gardner (Eds.), *Problems in the Diagnosis and Management of Polycystic Kidney Disease. Proceedings of the First International Workshop on Polycystic Kidney Disease.* Kansas City: PRK Foundation, 1985. P. 98.
29. Bennett, A. H., Stewart, W., and Lazarus, J. M. Bilateral nephrectomy in patients with polycystic renal disease. *Surg. Gynecol. Obstet.* 137:918, 1973.
30. Bernstein, J. Developmental abnormalities of the renal parenchyma: Renal hypoplasia and dysplasia. *Pathol. Annu.* 3:213, 1968.
31. Bernstein, J. A Classification of Renal Cysts. In K. D. Gardner, Jr. (Ed.), *Cystic Diseases of the Kidney.* New York: Wiley, 1976. P. 7.
32. Bernstein, J. Morphology of Human Renal Cystic Disease. In N. B. Cummings and S. Klahr (Eds.), *Chronic Renal Disease: Causes, Complications, and Treatment.* New York: Plenum Press, 1985. P. 47.
33. Bernstein, J. Hepatic involvement in hereditary renal syndromes. *Birth Defects* 23:115, 1987.
34. Bernstein, J., Brough, A. J., and McAdams, A. J. The renal lesion in syndromes of multiple congenital malformations. *Birth Defects* 10:35, 1974.
35. Bernstein, J., Evan, A. P., and Gardner, K. D., Jr. Epithelial hyperplasia in polycystic kidney diseases: Its role in pathogenesis and risk of neoplasia. *Am. J. Pathol.* 129:92, 1987.
36. Bernstein, J., and Gardner, K. D., Jr. Renal Cystic Disease and Renal Dysplasia. In P. C. Walsh, R. F. Gittes, A. D. Perlmutter, and T. A. Stamey (Eds.), *Campbell's Urology,* 5th Ed. Philadelphia: Saunders, 1986. P. 1760.
37. Bernstein, J., and Kissane, J. M. Hereditary Disorders of the Kidney. In H. Rosenberg and R. P. Bolande (Eds.), *Perspectives in Pediatric Pathology,* Vol. 1. Chicago: Year Book Medical Publishers, 1973. P. 435.
38. Bernstein, J., and Landing, B. H. Glomerulocystic kidney diseases. *Prog. Clin. Biol. Res.* 305: 27, 1989.
39. Bernstein, J., and Meyer, R. Congenital abnormalities of the urinary system: II. Renal cortical and medullary necrosis. *J. Pediatr.* 59:657, 1961.
40. Bernstein, J., and Meyer, R. Some speculations on the nature and significance of developmentally small kidneys (renal hypoplasia). *Nephron* 1:137, 1964.
41. Bernstein, J., and Meyer, R. Parenchymal Maldevelopment of the Kidney. In V. Kelly (Ed.), *Brennemann-Kelley Practice of Pediatrics,* Vol. 3. Hagerstown, Md.: Harper & Row, 1967. P. 4.
42. Bernstein, J., Robbins, T. O., and Kissane, J. M. The renal lesions of tuberous sclerosis. *Semin. Diagn. Pathol.* 3:97, 1986.
43. Betts, P., and Forrest-Hay, I. Juvenile nephronophthisis. *Lancet* 2:475, 1973.
44. Bigelow, N. H. The association of polycystic kidneys with intracranial aneurysms and other related disorders. *Am. J. Med. Sci.* 225:485, 1953.
45. Bigler, J. A., and Killingworth, W. P. Cartilage in the kidney. *Arch. Pathol.* 47:487, 1949.
46. Birken, G., King, D., Vane, D., and Lloyd, T.

Renal cell carcinoma arising in a multicystic dysplastic kidney. *J. Pediatr. Surg.* 20:619, 1985.
47. Bjerle, P., Lindqvist, B., and Michaelson, G. Pressure measurements in renal cysts. *Scand. J. Clin. Lab. Invest.* 27:135, 1971.
48. Bloom, D. A., and Brosman, S. The multicystic kidney. *J. Urol.* 120:211, 1978.
49. Blyth, H., and Ockenden, B. G. Polycystic disease of kidneys and liver presenting in childhood. *J. Med. Genet.* 8:257, 1971.
50. Boichis, H., Passwell, J., David, R., and Miller, H. Congenital hepatic fibrosis and nephronophthisis: A family study. *Q. J. Med.* 42:221, 1973.
51. Bois, E., and Royer, P. Association de néphropathie tubulo-interstitielle chronique et de dégénérescence tapéto-rétinienne: Etude génétique. *Arch. Fr. Pediatr.* 27:471, 1970.
52. Boissonnat, P. What to call hypoplastic kidney? *Arch. Dis. Child.* 37:142, 1962.
53. Booth, A. N., Ambrose, A. M., DeEds, F., and Cox, A., Jr. The reversible nephrotoxic effects of biphenyl, a citrus fungistat. *Toxicol. Appl. Pharmacol.* 3:560, 1961.
54. Bosniak, M. A., and Ambos, M. A. Polycystic kidney disease. *Semin. Roentgenol.* 10:133, 1975.
55. Bove, K. E., and McAdams, A. J. The nephroblastomatosis complex and its relationship to Wilms' tumor: A clinicopathologic treatise. *Perspect. Pediatr. Pathol.* 3:185, 1976.
56. Breuning, M. H., Reeders, S. T., and Brunner, H. Improved early diagnosis of adult polycystic kidney disease with flanking DNA markers. *Lancet* 2:1359, 1987.
57. Brock, W. A., and Kaplan, W. G. Ectopic ureteroceles in children. *J. Urol.* 119:800, 1978.
58. Broyer, M. Chronic Renal Failure. In P. Royer, R. Habib, H. Mathieu, and M. Broyer (Eds.), *Pediatric Nephrology.* Philadelphia: Saunders, 1974. P. 363.
59. Buchta, R. M., Viseskul, C., Gilbert, E. F., Sarto, G. E., and Opitz, J. M. Familial bilateral renal agenesis and hereditary renal adysplasia. *Z. Kinderheilk.* 115:111, 1973.
60. Burk, D., and Beaudoin, A. R. Arsenate-induced renal agenesis in rats. *Teratology* 16:247, 1977.
61. Cairns, H. W. B. Heredity in polycystic disease of the kidney. *Q. J. Med.* 18:359, 1925.
62. Cam, G., Simon, P., and Ang, K. S. Prevalence of symptomatic forms of adult polycystic kidney disease (APKD). (Abstract). *Kidney Int.* 37:247, 1990.
63. Caroli, J., Couinaud, C., Soupault, R., Porcher, P., and Etévé, J. Une affection nouvelle, sans doute congénitale, des voies biliaires: La dilatation kystique unilobaire des canaux hépatiques. *Sem. Hop. Paris* 34:496, 1958.
64. Carone, F. A., Rowland, R. G., Perlman, S. G., and Ganote, C. E. The pathogenesis of drug-induced renal cystic disease. *Kidney Int.* 5:411, 1974.
65. Carson, R. W., Bedi, D., Cavallo, T., and DuBose, T. D., Jr. Familial adult glomerulocystic kidney disease. *Am. J. Kidney Dis.* 9:154, 1987.
66. Chapman, J. R., and Hilson, A. J. W. Polycystic kidneys and abdominal aortic aneurysms. *Lancet* 1:646, 1980.
67. Charro Salgado, A. L., Lopez Marcia, A., Freire, A., Paramo, P., and Fernandez-Cruz, A. Beckwith-Wiedemann syndrome with medullary sponge kidneys, agonadism and persistent testosterone production. *Eur. Urol.* 3:108, 1977.
68. Chatten, J., and Bishop, H. C. Bilateral multilocular cysts of the kidney. *J. Pediatr. Surg.* 12:749, 1977.
69. Chilton, S. J., and Cremin, B. J. The spectrum of polycystic disease in children. *Pediatr. Radiol.* 11:9, 1981.
70. Cho, K. J., Thornbury, J. R., Bernstein, J., Heidelberger, K. P., and Walter, J. F. Localized cystic disease of the kidney: Angiographic-pathologic correlation. *Am. J. Radiol.* 132:891, 1979.
71. Christenson, P. J., Craig, J. P., Bibro, M. C., and O'Connell, K. J. Cysts containing renal cell carcinoma in von Hippel-Lindau disease. *J. Urol.* 128:798, 1982.
72. Churchill, D., Kimoff, R., Pinsky, M., and Gault, M. H. Solitary intrarenal cyst: Correctable cause of hypertension. *Urology* 6:485, 1975.
73. Cohen, A. H., and Hoyer, J. R. Nephronophthisis: A primary tubular basement membrane defect. *Lab. Invest.* 55:564, 1986.
74. Cohen, B., Goldman, S. M., Kopilnick, M., Khurana, A. V., and Salik, J. O. Ureteropelvic junction obstruction: Its occurrence in three members of a single family. *J. Urol.* 120:361, 1978.
75. Coleman, M. Multilocular renal cyst: Case report, ultrastructure and review of the literature. *Virchows Arch.* [*Pathol. Anat.*] 387:207, 1980.
76. Coles, G. A., and Branch, R. A. Familial interstitial nephritis. *Clin. Nephrol.* 6:513, 1976.
77. Collan, Y., Sipponen, P., Haapanen, E., Lindahl, J., Jokinen, E. J., and Hjelt, L. Hereditary nephronophthisis with a life span of three decades. *Virch. Arch.* [*Pathol. Anat.*] 376:195, 1977.
78. Cook, W. A., and Stephens, F. D. Fused kidneys: Morphologic study and theory of embryogenesis. *Birth Defects* 13:327, 1977.
79. Coppoletta, J. M., and Wolbach, S. B. Body length and organ weights of infants and children: Study of body length and normal weights of more important organs of body between birth and 12

years of age. *Am. J. Pathol.* 9:55, 1933.
80. Courtney, K. D., Gaylor, D. W., Hogan, M. D., and Falk, H. L. Teratogenic evaluation of 2,4,5-T. *Science* 168:864, 1970.
81. Cromie, W. J., Engelstein, M. S., and Duckett, J. W., Jr. Nodular renal blastema, renal dysplasia and duplicated collecting systems. *J. Urol.* 123:100, 1980.
82. Cuppage, F. E., Huseman, R. A., Chapman, A., and Grantham, J. J. Ultrastructure and function of cysts from human adult polycystic kidneys. *Kidney Int.* 17:372, 1980.
83. Dalgaard, O. Z. Bilateral polycystic disease of the kidneys: A follow-up study of 284 patients and their families. *Acta Med. Scand.* 158(Suppl. 328): 1, 1957.
84. Dalton, D., Neiman, H., and Grayhack, J. T. The natural history of simple renal cysts: A preliminary study. *J. Urol.* 135:905, 1986.
85. Delaney, V., Mullaney, J., and Bourke, E. Juvenile nephronophthisis, congenital hepatic fibrosis and retinal hypoplasia in twins. *Q. J. Med.* 47:281, 1978.
86. Deliveliotis, A., and Kavadis, C. Parapelvic cysts of the kidney: Report of seven cases. *Br. J. Urol.* 41:386, 1969.
87. Doroshow, L. W., and Abeshouse, B. S. Congenital unilateral solitary kidney: Report of 37 cases and a review of the literature. *Urol. Surv.* 11:219, 1961.
88. Dosa, S., Thompson, A. M., and Abraham, A. Glomerulocystic kidney disease: Report of an adult case. *Am. J. Clin. Pathol.* 82:619, 1984.
89. Dowse, J. L. A., and Kihn, R. B. Renal injuries: Diagnosis, management and sequelae in 67 cases. *Br. J. Surg.* 50:353, 1963.
90. Dretler, S. P., Olsson, C., and Pfister, R. C. The anatomic, radiologic and clinical characteristics of the pelvic kidney: An analysis of 86 cases. *J. Urol.* 105:623, 1971.
91. Duckett, J. W., Jr. The Prune Belly Syndrome. In T. M. Holder and K. W. Ashcroft (Eds.), *The Surgery of Infants and Children.* Philadelphia: Saunders, 1980. P. 802.
92. Eiser, A. R., Grishman, E., Neff, M. S., Allerhand, J., and Slifkin, R. F. Nephronophthisis with massive proteinuria. *Am. J. Kidney Dis.* 11:640, 1983.
93. Ekström, T. Renal hypoplasia: A clinical study of 179 cases. *Acta Chir. Scand.* Suppl. 203:1, 1955.
94. Ekström, T., Engfeldt, B., Lagergren, C., and Lindvall, N. *Medullary Sponge Kidney: A Roentgenologic, Clinical, Histopathologic and Biophysical Study.* Stockholm: Almqvist and Wiksell, 1959.
95. Emery, J. L., and Mithal, A. The weights of kidneys in late uterine life and childhood. *J. Clin. Pathol.* 13:490, 1960.
96. Emmett, J. L., Alvarez-Ierena, J. J., and McDonald, J. R. Atrophic pyelonephritis versus congenital renal hypoplasia. *JAMA* 148:1470, 1952.
97. Engström, W., Lindham, S., and Schofield, P. Wiedemann-Beckwith syndrome. *Eur. J. Pediatr.* 147:450, 1988.
98. Ericsson, N. O., and Ivemark, B. I. Renal dysplasia and pyelonephritis in infants and children: Primitive ductules and abnormal glomeruli, I and II. *Arch. Pathol.* 66:255, 264, 1958.
99. Evan, A. P., Gardner, K. D., Jr., and Bernstein, J. Polypoid and papillary epithelial hyperplasia: A potential cause of ductal obstruction in adult polycystic disease. *Kidney Int.* 16:743, 1979.
100. Evan, A. P., Hong, S. K., Gardner, K. D., Jr., Park, Y. S., and Itagaki, R. Evolution of the collecting tubular lesion in diphenylamine-induced renal disease. *Lab. Invest.* 38:242, 1978.
101. Fanconi, G., Hanhart, E., von Albertini, A., Uhlinger, R., Dolivo, E., and Prader, A. Die familiäre juvenile Nephronophthise. *Helv. Paediatr. Acta* 6:1, 1951.
102. Faraggiana, T., Bernstein, J., Strauss, L., and Churg, J. Use of lectins in the study of histogenesis of renal cysts. *Lab. Invest.* 53:575, 1985.
103. Fehrenbaker, L. G., Kelalis, P. P., and Stickler, G. B. Vesicoureteral reflux and ureteral duplication in children. *J. Urol.* 107:862, 1972.
104. Fellows, R. A., Leonidas, J. C., and Beatty, E. C., Jr. Radiologic features of "adult type" polycystic kidney disease in the neonate. *Pediatr. Radiol.* 4:87, 1976.
104*a*. Ferrer-Roca, O., and Fernandez-Cruz, L. Papillary adenocarcinomatous degeneration occurring in a multilocular renal cyst. *Br. J. Urol.* 52:13, 1981.
105. Fetterman, G. H. Microdissection in the study of normal and abnormal renal structure and function. *Pathol. Annu.* 5:173, 1970.
106. Fetterman, G. H., and Habib, R. Congenital bilateral oligonephronic renal hypoplasia with hypertrophy of nephrons (oligoméganéphronie): Studies by microdissection. *Am. J. Clin. Pathol.* 52:199, 1969.
107. Fetterman, G. H., Shuplock, N. A., Philipp, F. J., and Gregg, H. S. The growth and maturation of human glomeruli and proximal convolutions from term to adulthood. *Pediatrics* 35:602, 1965.
108. Fill, W. L., Lamiell, J. M., and Polk, N. O. The radiographic manifestations of von Hippel-Lindau disease. *Radiology* 133:289, 1979.
109. Fillastre, J. P., Gruenel, J., Riberi, P., Marx, P., Whitworth, J. A., and Kuhn, M. J. Senior-Løken syndrome (nephronophthisis and tapeto-

retinal degeneration): A study of eight cases from five families. *Clin. Nephrol.* 5:14, 1976.
110. Filmer, R. B., Carone, F. A., Rowland, R. G., and Babcock, J. R. Adrenal corticosteroid induced renal cystic disease in the newborn hamster. *Am. J. Pathol.* 72:461, 1973.
111. Finlay, D. B., Lowe, J. S., and Kaur, K. Perforation of a suppurative solitary renal cyst. *Br. J. Surg.* 68:585, 1981.
112. Foote, J. W., Blennerhassett, J. B., Wigglesworth, F. W., and Mackinnon, K. J. Observations on the ureteropelvic junction. *J. Urol.* 104: 252, 1970.
113. Fotino, S. The solitary kidney: A model of chronic hyperfiltration in humans. *Am. J. Kidney Dis.* 13:88, 1989.
114. Franc, B., Steg, A., Galian, P., and Baert, L. Simple renal cysts in the adult: Anatomical study. *J. Urol. Nephrol. (Paris)* 83:185, 1977.
115. Franz, K. A., and Reubi, F. C. Rate of functional deterioration in polycystic kidney disease. *Kidney Int.* 23:526, 1983.
116. Frimodt-Moller, P. C., Nissen, H. M., and Dyreborg, U. Polycystic kidneys as the renal lesion in Lindau's disease. *J. Urol.* 125:868, 1981.
117. Gabow, P. A., Ikle, D. W., and Holmes, J. H. Polycystic kidney disease: Prospective analysis of nonazotemic patients and family members. *Ann. Intern. Med.* 101:238, 1984.
118. Gaddy, C. D., Gibbons, M. D., Gonzales, E. T., Jr., and Finegold, M. J. Obstructive uropathy, renal dysplasia and nodular renal blastema: Is there a relationship to Wilms' tumor? *J. Urol.* 134:330, 1985.
119. Gallo, G. E., and Penchansky, L. Cystic nephroma. *Cancer* 39:1322, 1977.
120. Gang, D. L., and Herrin, J. T. Infantile polycystic disease of the liver and kidneys. *Clin. Nephrol.* 25:28, 1986.
121. Gardner, K. D., Jr. Composition of fluid in 12 cysts of a polycystic kidney. *N. Engl. J. Med.* 281:985, 1969.
122. Gardner, K. D., Jr. Evolution of clinical signs in adult-onset cystic disease of the renal medulla. *Ann. Intern. Med.* 74:47, 1971.
123. Gardner, K. D., Jr. Juvenile Nephronophthisis and Renal Medullary Cystic Disease. In K. D. Gardner, Jr. (Ed.), *Cystic Diseases of the Kidney.* New York: Wiley, 1976. P. 173.
124. Gardner, K. D., Jr. The Medullary Cystic Diseases: The Nephronophthisis–Cystic Renal Medulla Complex and Medullary Sponge Kidney. In L. E. Earley, and C. W. Gottschalk (Eds.), *Strauss and Welt's Diseases of the Kidney,* 3rd Ed. Boston: Little, Brown, 1979. P. 1147.
125. Gartell, P. C., MacIver, A. G., and Atwell, J. D. Renal dysplasia and duplex kidneys. *Eur. Urol.* 9:65, 1983.
126. Gonzalez-Crussi, F., Kidd, J. M., and Hernandez, R. J. Cystic nephroma. Morphologic spectrum and implications. *Urology* 20:88, 1982.
127. Gordon-Taylor, G. On horseshoes and on horseshoe kidney concave downwards. *Br. J. Urol.* 8:112, 1936.
128. Granberg, P. O., Lanergren, C., and Theve, N. O. Renal function studies in medullary sponge kidney. *Scand. J. Urol. Nephrol.* 5:177, 1971.
129. Grantham, J. J., Geiser, J. L., and Evan, A. P. Cyst formation and growth in autosomal dominant polycystic kidney disease. *Kidney Int.* 31: 1145, 1987.
130. Green, L. F., and Barrett, D. M. Renal Cystic Disease: Radiologic Appearances. In K. D. Gardner, Jr. (Ed.), *Cystic Diseases of the Kidney.* New York: Wiley, 1976. P. 91.
131. Greenberg, F., Stein, F., Gresik, M. V., Finegold, M. J., Carpenter, R. J., Riccardi, V. M., and Beaudet, A. L. The Perlman familial nephroblastomatosis syndrome. *Am. J. Med. Genet.* 24: 101, 1986.
132. Greenfield, S. P., Hensle, T. W., Berdon, W. E., and Wigger, H. J. Unilateral vesicoureteral reflux and unilateral nonfunctioning kidney associated with posterior urethral valves: A syndrome? *J. Urol.* 130:733, 1983.
133. Gregoire, J. R., Torres, V. E., Holley, K. E., and Farrow, G. M. Renal epithelial hyperplastic and neoplastic proliferation in autosomal dominant polycystic kidney disease (ADPKD). *Am. J. Kidney Dis.* 9:27, 1987.
134. Gross, M., and Beach, P. D. The simultaneous occurrence of renal carcinoma and cyst: Problems in management. *South. Med. J.* 64:1059, 1971.
135. Grunefeld, J.-P., Albouze, G., Jungers, P., Landais, P., Dana, A., Droz, D., Moynot, A., Lafforgue, B., and Boursztyn, F. D. Liver changes and complications in adult polycystic disease. *Adv. Nephrol.* 141:1, 1984.
136. Gutierrez, O. H., Burgener, F. A., and Schwartz, S. Coincident renal cell carcinoma and renal angiomyolipoma in tuberous sclerosis. *Am. J. Radiol.* 132:848, 1979.
137. Habif, D. V., Jr., Berdon, W. E., and Yeh, M.-N. Infantile polycystic disease: In utero sonographic diagnosis. *Radiology* 142:475, 1982.
138. Harrison, A. R., and Rose, G. A. Medullary sponge kidney. *Urol. Res.* 7:197, 1979.
139. Hartman, G. E., Smolik, L. M., and Shochat, S. J. The dilemma of the multicystic kidney. *Urology* 15:152, 1980.
140. Hashimoto, B. E., Filly, R. A., and Callen, P. W. Multicystic dysplastic kidney in utero: Changing

appearance on US. *Radiology* 159:107, 1986.
141. Hatfield, P. M., and Pfister, R. C. Adult polycystic disease of the kidneys (Potter type 3). *JAMA* 222:1527, 1972.
142. Helczynski, L., Wells, T. R., Landing, B. H., and Lipsey, A. I. The renal lesion of congenital hepatic fibrosis: Pathologic and morphometric analysis with comparison to the renal lesion of infantile polycystic disease. *Pediatr. Pathol.* 2:441, 1984.
143. Hepler, A. B. Solitary cysts of kidney: Report of seven cases and observations on the pathogenesis of these cysts. *Surg. Gynecol. Obstet.* 50:668, 1930.
144. Henneberry, M. O., and Stephens, F. D. Renal hypoplasia and dysplasia in infants with posterior urethral valves. *J. Urol.* 123:912, 1980.
145. Henthorne, J. Peripelvic lymphatic cysts of the kidney: A review of the literature on perinephric cysts. *Am. J. Clin. Pathol.* 8:28, 1983.
146. Hidalgo, H., Dunnick, N. R., Rosenberg, E. R., Ramm, P. C., and Korbin, M. Parapelvic cysts: Appearances on CT and sonography. *Am. J. Radiol.* 138:677, 1982.
147. Higashihara, E., Nutahara, K., Tago, K., Ueno, A., and Niijima, T. Unilateral and segmental medullary sponge kidney: Renal function and calcium excretion. *J. Urol.* 132:743, 1984.
148. Hill, J. E., and Bunts, R. C. Thoracic kidney: Case reports. *J. Urol.* 84:460, 1960.
149. Hodson, C. J., and Edwards, D. Chronic pyelonephritis and vesicoureteric reflux. *Clin. Radiol.* 11:219, 1960.
150. Hodson, C. J., Maling, T. M., McManamon, P. J., and Lewis, M. G. The pathogenesis of reflux nephropathy (chronic atrophic pyelonephritis). *Br. J. Radiol. Suppl.* 13:1, 1975.
151. Hogewind, B. L., Veltkamp, J. J., Koch, C. W., and De Graeff, J. Genetic counselling for adult polycystic kidney disease: Ultrasound, a useful tool in presymptomatic diagnosis? *Clin. Genet.* 18:168, 1980.
152. Hoover, D. L., and Duckett, J. W., Jr. Posterior urethral valves, unilateral reflux and renal dysplasia: A syndrome. *J. Urol.* 128:994, 1982.
153. Horton, W. A., Wong, V., and Eldridge, R. von Hippel-Lindau disease: Clinical and pathological manifestations in nine families with 50 affected members. *Arch. Intern. Med.* 136:769, 1976.
154. Hostetter, T. H., Olson, J. L., Rennke, H. G., Venkatachalam, M. A., and Brenner, B. M. Hyperfiltration in remnant nephrons: A potential adverse response to renal ablation. *Am. J. Physiol.* 241:F85, 1981.
155. Howard, R. M., and Young, J. D., Jr. Two malignant tumors in a polycystic kidney. *J. Urol.* 102:162, 1969.
156. Huland, H., Lewin, K., and Stamey, T. A. Unilateral medullary sponge kidney: Cause of persistent bacteriuria. *Urology* 8:373, 1976.
157. Huseman, R., Grady, A., Welling, D., and Grantham, J. Micropuncture study of polycystic disease in adult human kidneys. *Kidney Int.* 18:375, 1980.
158. Iglesias, C. G., Torres, V. E., Offord, K. P., Holley, K. E., Beard, C. M., and Kurland, L. T. Epidemiology of adult polycystic kidney disease, Olmstead county, Minnesota: 1935–1980. *Am. J. Kidney Dis.* 2:630, 1983.
159. Jalundhwala, J. M., and Shah, R. C. Traumatic perinephric cyst. *Br. J. Urol.* 35:133, 1963.
160. Janin-Mercier, A., Palcoux, J. B., Gubler, M. C., de Latour, M., Dalens, H., and Fonck, Y. Oligomeganephronic renal hypoplasia with tapetoretinal degeneration: Report of one case with ultrastructural study of the renal biopsy. *Virchows Arch.* [A] 407:477, 1985.
161. Jørgensen, M. Three-dimensional reconstruction of intrahepatic bile ducts in a case of polycystic disease of the liver in an infant. *Acta Pathol. Microbiol. Scand.* 80:201, 1972.
162. Jørgensen, M. A stereological study of intrahepatic bile ducts: 3. Infantile polycystic disease. *Acta Pathol. Microbiol. Scand.* 81:670, 1973.
163. Jørgensen, M. A stereological study of intrahepatic bile ducts: 4. Congenital hepatic fibrosis. *Acta Pathol. Microbiol. Scand.* 82:21, 1974.
164. Jørgensen, M. The ductal plate malformation. *Acta Pathol. Microbiol. Scand. Suppl.* 257:1, 1977.
165. Joshi, V. V., Bannerjee, A. K., Yardar, K., and Pathak, I. C. Cystic partially differentiated nephroblastoma. *Cancer* 40:789, 1977.
166. Joshi, V. V., and Beckwith, J. B. Multilocular cyst of the kidney (cystic nephroma) and cystic partially differentiated nephroblastoma: Terminology and criteria for diagnosis. *Cancer* 64:466, 1989.
167. Joshi, V. V., and Kaszina, J. Clinicopathologic spectrum of glomerulocystic kidneys: Report of two cases and a brief review of literature. *Pediatr. Pathol.* 2:171, 1984.
168. Kaplan, B. S., Kaplan, P., de Chadarevian, J.-P., Jequier, S., O'Regan, S., and Russo, P. Variable expression of autosomal recessive polycystic kidney disease and congenital hepatic fibrosis within a family. *Am. J. Med. Genet.* 29:639, 1988.
169. Kaplan, B. S., Rabin, I., Nogrady, M. B., and Drummond, K. N. Autosomal dominant polycystic renal disease in children. *J. Pediatr.* 90:782, 1977.
170. Kelalis, P. P., Culp, O. S., Stickler, G. B., and Burke, E. C. Ureteropelvic obstruction in children: Experiences with 109 cases. *J. Urol.* 106:418, 1971.

171. Kerr, D. N. S., Harrison, C. V., Sherlock, S., and Waler, R. M. Congenital hepatic fibrosis. *Q. J. Med.* 30:91, 1961.
172. Kerr, D. N. S., Warrick, C. K., and Hart-Mercer, J. A lesion resembling medullary sponge kidney in patients with congenital hepatic fibrosis. *Clin. Pathol.* 13:85, 1962.
173. Kimberling, W. J., Fain, P. R., Kenyon, J. B., Goldgar, D., Sujansky, E., and Gabow, P. A. Linkage heterogeneity of autosomal dominant polycystic kidney disease. *N. Engl. J. Med.* 319:913, 1988.
174. Kiprov, D. D., Colvin, R. B., and McCluskey, R. T. Focal and segmental glomerulosclerosis and proteinuria associated with unilateral renal agenesis. *Lab. Invest.* 46:275, 1982.
175. Kissane, J. M. The Morphology of Renal Cystic Disease. In K. D. Gardner, Jr. (Ed.), *Cystic Diseases of the Kidney.* New York: Wiley, 1976.
176. Kleiner, B., Filly, R. A., Mack, L., and Callen, P. W. Multicystic dysplastic kidney: Observations of contralateral disease in the fetal population. *Radiology* 161:27, 1986.
177. Kliger, A. S., and Scheer, R. L. Familial disease of the renal medulla: A study of the progeny in a family with medullary cystic disease. *Ann. Intern. Med.* 85:190, 1976.
178. Koplan, J. P., Sprayregan, S., Ossias, A. L., and Zanjani, E. D. Erythropoietin-producing renal cyst and polycythemia vera: Clarification of their relationship. *Am. J. Med.* 54:819, 1973.
179. Kosseff, A. L., Herrmann, J., Gilbert, E. F., Viseskul, C., Lubinsky, M., and Opitz, J. M. Studies of malformation syndromes of man XXIX: The Wiedemann-Beckwith syndrome. Clinical, genetic and pathogenetic studies of 12 cases. *Eur. J. Pediatr.* 123:139, 1976.
180. Kossow, A. S., and Meek, J. M. Unilateral adult polycystic kidney disease. *J. Urol.* 127:297, 1982.
181. Kuiper, J. J. Medullary sponge kidney in three generations. *N.Y. State J. Med.* 71:2665, 1971.
182. Kuiper, J. J. Medullary Sponge Kidney. In K. D. Gardner, Jr. (Ed.), *Cystic Diseases of the Kidney.* New York: Wiley, 1976. P. 151.
183. Landais, P., Grunfeld, J.-P., Droz, D., Drueke, T., Albouze, G., Goguser, J., Chauveau, D., and Moynot, A. Cholangiocellular carcinoma in polycystic kidney and liver disease. *Arch. Intern. Med.* 144:2274, 1984.
184. Langer, L. O., Jr., Nishino, R., Yamaguchi, A., Ito, Y., Ueke, T., Togari, H., Kato, T., Opitz, J. M., and Gilbert, E. F. Brachymesomelia-renal syndrome. *Am. J. Med. Genet.* 15:57, 1983.
185. Landing, B. H., and Hughes, M. L. Analysis of weight of kidneys of children. *Lab. Invest.* 11:452, 1962.
186. Landing, B. H., Wells, T. R., and Claireaux, A. E. Morphometric analysis of liver lesions in cystic diseases of childhood. *Hum. Pathol.* 11:549, 1980.
187. Laucks, S. P., Jr., and McLachlan, M. S. F. Aging and simple cysts of the kidney. *Br. J. Radiol.* 54:12, 1981.
188. Lee, J. K. T., McClennan, B. L., and Kissane, J. M. Unilateral polycystic kidney disease. *Am. J. Radiol.* 130:1165, 1978.
189. Leier, C. V., Baker, P. B., Kilman, J. W., and Wooley, C. F. Cardiovascular abnormalities associated with adult polycystic kidney disease. *Ann. Intern. Med.* 100:683, 1984.
190. Levey, A. S. General Features of Autosomal Dominant Polycystic Kidney Disease: K. Cerebral Aneurysms. In J. J. Grantham and K. D. Gardner (Eds.), *Problems in Diagnosis and Management of Polycystic Kidney Disease. Proceedings of the First International Workshop on Polycystic Kidney Disease.* Kansas City: PKR Foundation, 1985. P. 135.
191. Levine, A. S., and Michael, A. F. Ehlers-Danlos syndrome with renal tubular acidosis and medullary sponge kidney. *J. Pediatr.* 71:107, 1967.
192. Levine, E., Cook, L. T., and Grantham, J. J. Liver cysts in autosomal-dominant polycystic kidney disease: Clinical and computed tomographic study. *Am. J. Radiol.* 145:229, 1985.
193. Levine, E., and Grantham, J. E. The role of computed tomography in the evaluation of adult polycystic kidney disease. *Am. J. Kidney Dis.* 1:99, 1981.
194. Lieberman, E., Salinas-Madrigal, L., Gwinn, J. L., Brennan, L. P., Fine, R. N., and Landing, B. H. Infantile polycystic disease of the kidneys and liver: Clinical, pathological, and radiological correlations and comparison with congenital hepatic fibrosis. *Medicine* 50:277, 1971.
195. Limjoco, U. R., and Stranch, A. E. Infected solitary cyst of the kidney: Report of a case and review of the literature. *J. Urol.* 96:625, 1966.
196. Lindsey, J. R. Lymphangiectasia simulating polycystic disease. *J. Urol.* 104:658, 1970.
197. Løken, A. C., Hanssen, O., Halvorsen, S., and Jølster, N. J. Hereditary renal dysplasia and blindness. *Acta Paediatr. Scand.* 50:177, 1961.
198. Longo, V. J., and Thompson, G. J. Congenital solitary kidney. *J. Urol.* 68:63, 1952.
199. Lynne, C. M., Carrion, H. M., and Bakshandeh, K. Renal angiomyolipoma: Polycystic kidney and renal cell carcinoma in a patient with tuberous sclerosis. *Urology* 14:174, 1979.
200. McClennan, B. L., Stanley, R. J., Melson, G. L., Levitt, R. G., and Sagel, S. S. CT of the renal cyst: Is cyst aspiration necessary? *Am. J. Radiol.* 133:671, 1979.
201. McFarland, W. L., Wallace, S., and Johnson, D. E. Renal carcinoma and polycystic disease. *J.*

Urol. 107:530, 1972.
202. McGeoch, J. E. M., Woodhouse, M. A., and Darmady, E. M. Experimental infantile polycystic disease in rats: The influence of age and sex. *Br. J. Exp. Pathol.* 53:322, 1972.
203. McGraw, M., Poucell, S., Sweet, J., and Baumal, R. The significance of focal glomerulosclerosis in oligomeganephronia. *Int. J. Pediatr. Nephrol.* 5:67, 1984.
204. McLachlan, M. S. F., Meller, S. T., Verrier Jones, E. R., Asscher, A. W., Fletcher, E. W. L., Mayon-White, R. T., Ledingham, J. G. G., Smith, J. C., and Johnson, H. H. Urinary tract in schoolgirls with covert bacteriuria. *Arch. Dis. Child.* 50:253, 1975.
205. Mackie, G. G., and Stephens, F. D. A correlation of renal dysplasia with position of ureteral orifice. *J. Urol.* 114:274, 1975.
206. Madewell, J. E., Goldman, S. M., Davis, C. J., Jr., Hartman, D. S., and Lichtenstein, J. E. Multilocular cystic nephroma: A radiologic-pathologic correlation of 58 patients. *Radiology* 146:309, 1983.
207. Mahony, B. S., Callen, P. W., Filley, R. A., and Golbus, M. S. Progressions of infantile polycystic disease in early pregnancy. *J. Ultrasound Med.* 3:277, 1984.
208. Maizels, M., and Stephens, F. D. Valves of the ureter as a cause of primary obstruction of the ureter: Anatomic, embryologic and clinical aspects. *J. Urol.* 123:742, 1980.
209. Mall, J. C., Ghahremani, G. G., and Boyer, J. L. Caroli's disease associated with congenital hepatic fibrosis and renal tubular ectasia. *Gastroenterology* 66:1029, 1974.
210. Martinez-Maldonado, M., Yium, J. J., Eknoyan, G., and Suki, W. N. Adult polycystic disease: Studies of the defect in urine concentration. *Kidney Int.* 2:107, 1972.
211. Melnick, S. C., Brewer, D. B., and Oldham, J. S. Cortical microcystic disease of the kidney with dominant inheritance: A previously undescribed syndrome. *J. Clin. Pathol.* 37:494, 1984.
212. Meyers, M. A. Uriniferous perirenal pseudocyst: New observations. *Radiology* 117:539, 1975.
213. Middleton, A. W., Jr., and Pfister, R. C. Stone-containing pyelocaliceal diverticulum: Embryogenic, anatomic, radiologic and clinical characteristics. *J. Urol.* 111:2, 1974.
214. Milutinovic, J., Agodoa, L. C. Y., Cubler, R. E., and Striker, G. E. Autosomal dominant polycystic kidney disease: Early diagnosis and consideration of pathogenesis. *Am. J. Clin. Pathol.* 73: 740, 1980.
215. Mir, S., Rapola, J., and Koskimies, O. Renal cysts in pediatric autopsy material. *Nephron* 33: 189, 1983.
216. Mitnick, J. S., Bosniak, M. A., Hilton, S., Raghavendra, B. N., Subramanyam, B. R., and Genieser, N. B. Cystic renal diseases in tuberous sclerosis. *Radiology* 147:85, 1983.
217. Mottet, N. K., and Jensen, H. The anomalous embryonic development associated with trisomy 13–15. *Am. J. Clin. Pathol.* 43:334, 1965.
218. Murnaghan, G. F. The dynamics of the renal pelvis and ureter with reference to congenital hydronephrosis. *Br. J. Urol.* 30:321, 1958.
219. Murnaghan, G. F. The mechanism of congenital hydronephrosis with reference to the factors influencing surgical treatment. *Ann. R. Coll. Surg. Engl.* 23:25, 1958.
220. Nagashima, Y., Yoshihara, O., Tanaka, Y., Misugi, K., and Horiuchi, M. A case of renal angiomyolipomas associated with multiple and various hamartomatous microlesions. *Virchows Arch. [A]* 413:177, 1988.
221. Nakada, T., Furuta, H., Kazama, T., and Katayama, T. Unilateral renal agenesis with and without ipsilateral adrenal agenesis. *J. Urol.* 140: 933, 1988.
222. Newman, L. B., McAlister, W. H., and Kissane, J. Segmental renal dysplasia associated with ectopic ureteroceles in childhood. *Urology* 3:23, 1974.
223. Ng, R. C. K., and Suki, W. N. Renal cell carcinoma occurring in a polycystic kidney of a transplant recipient. *J. Urol.* 124:710, 1980.
224. Ng, W. L., Cheung, M. F., Chan, C. W., and Yu, C. L. Oligomeganephronic renal hypoplasia. *Pathology* 12:639, 1980.
225. Notley, R. G., and Williams, J. P. Renal cysts and haematuria. *Br. J. Urol.* 41:535, 1969.
226. Novetsky, G. J., Berlin, L., Epstein, A. J., Lobo, N., and Miller, S. H. CT diagnosis of renal cyst wall tumor. *J. Comput. Assist. Tomogr.* 7:539, 1983.
227. Odiévre, M., Chaumont, P., Montagne, J. P., and Alagille, D. Anomalies of the intrahepatic portal venous system in congenital hepatic fibrosis. *Radiology* 122:427, 1977.
228. Oh, Y., Onoyama, K., Kobayashi, K., Nanishi, F., Mitsuoka, W., Ohchi, N., Tsuruda, H., and Fujiishima, M. Glomerulocystic kidneys. Report of an adult case. *Nephron* 43:299, 1986.
229. Okada, R. D., Platt, M. A., and Fleishman, J. Chronic renal failure in patients with tuberous sclerosis: Association with renal cysts. *Nephron* 30:85, 1982.
230. Oliver, J. T., Rubenstein, M., Meyer, R., and Bernstein, J. Congenital abnormalities of the urinary system: III. Growth of the kidney in childhood—Determination of normal weight. *J. Pediatr.* 61:256, 1962.
231. Olson, J. L., Hostetter, T. H., Rennke, H. G.,

Brenner, B. M., and Venkatachalam, M. A. Altered glomerular permselectivity and progressive sclerosis following extreme ablation of renal mass. *Kidney Int.* 22:112, 1982.
232. O'Neill, M., Breslau, N. A., and Pak, C. Y. C. Metabolic evaluation of nephrolithiasis in patients with medullary sponge kidney. *JAMA* 245:1233, 1981.
233. Osathanondh, V., and Potter, E. L. Development of human kidney as shown by microdissection: I, II, III. *Arch. Pathol.* 76:271, 277, 290, 1963.
234. Osathanondh, V., and Potter, E. L. Pathogenesis of polycystic kidneys: Historical survey; type 1 due to hyperplasia of interstitial portions of collecting tubules; type 2 due to inhibition of ampullary activity; type 3 due to multiple abnormalities of development; type 4 due to urethral obstruction; survey of results of microdissection. *Arch. Pathol.* 77:459, 1964.
235. Osathanondh, V., and Potter, E. L. Development of human kidney as shown by microdissection: IV, V. *Arch. Pathol.* 82:391, 403, 1966.
236. Paelzel, W. Zwergnieren. *Chirurgie* 27:444, 1956.
237. Paquin, A., Marshall, V. F., and McGovern, J. H. The megacystis syndrome. *J. Urol.* 83:634, 1960.
238. Pascall, R. R. Medullary cystic disease of the kidney: Study of a case with scanning and transmission electron microscopy and light microscopy. *Am. J. Clin. Pathol.* 59:659, 1973.
239. Pathak, I. G., and Williams, D. I. Multicystic and cystic dysplastic kidneys. *Br. J. Urol.* 36:318, 1964.
240. Patriquin, H. B., and O'Regan, S. Medullary sponge kidney in childhood. *Am. J. Radiol.* 145: 315, 1964.
241. Patterson, M., Gonzales-Vitale, J. C., and Fagan, C. J. Polycystic liver disease: A study of cyst fluid constituents. *Hepatology* 2:475, 1982.
242. Pedicelli, G., Jequier, S., Bowen, A., and Boisvert, J. Multicystic dysplastic kidneys: Spontaneous regression demonstrated with US. *Radiology* 160:23, 1986.
243. Perez-Atayde, A. R., Iwaya, S., and Lack, E. E. Angiomyolipomas and polycystic renal disease in tuberous sclerosis: Ultrastructural observations. *Urology* 17:607, 1981.
244. Perlman, M., Levin, M., and Wittels, B. Syndrome of fetal giantism, renal hamartomas, and nephroblastomatosis with Wilms' tumor. *Cancer* 35:1212, 1975.
245. Perrone, R. D. In vitro function of cyst epithelium from human polycystic kidney. *J. Clin. Invest.* 76:1688, 1985.
246. Popovic-Rolovic, M., Calic-Perisic, N., Bunje-Racki, G., and Negovanovic, D. Juvenile nephronophthisis associated with retinal pigmentary dystrophy, cerebellar ataxia, and skeletal abnormalities. *Arch. Dis. Child.* 51:801, 1976.
247. Portsman, W. Renal angiography in children. *Prog. Pediatr. Radiol.* 3:51, 1970.
248. Potter, E. L. *Normal and Abnormal Development of the Kidney.* Chicago: Year Book Medical Publishers, 1972.
249. Powell, T., Shackman, R., and Johnson, H. D. Multilocular cysts of the kidney. *Br. J. Urol.* 23:142, 1951.
250. Proesmans, W., van Damme, B., Caeser, P., and Marchal, G. Autosomal dominant polycystic kidney disease in the neonatal period: Association with cerebral arteriovenous malformation. *Pediatrics* 70:971, 1982.
251. Proesmans, W., van Damme, B., and Macken, J. Nephronophthisis and tapetoretinal degeneration associated with liver fibrosis. *Clin. Nephrol.* 3:160, 1975.
252. Pyrah, L. N. Medullary sponge kidney. *J. Urol.* 95:274, 1966.
253. Rall, J. E., and Odel, H. M. Congenital polycystic disease of the kidney: Review of the literature and data on 207 cases. *Am. J. Med. Sci.* 218:399, 1949.
254. Ransley, P. G., and Risdon, R. A. Renal papillary morphology in infants and young children. *Urol. Res.* 3:111, 1975.
255. Ransley, P. G., and Risdon, R. A. Reflux and renal scarring. *Br. J. Radiol. Suppl.* 14:1, 1978.
256. Ransley, P. G., and Risdon, R. A. Reflux nephropathy: Effects of antimicrobial therapy on the evolution of the early pyelonephritic scar. *Kidney Int.* 20:733, 1981.
257. Rapola, J., and Kääriäinen, H. Morphologic diagnosis of recessive and dominant polycystic kidney disease in infancy and childhood. *Acta Pathol. Microbiol. Scand.* 96:68, 1988.
258. Rattner, W. H., Meyer, R., and Bernstein, J. Congenital abnormalities of the urinary system: IV. Valvular obstruction of the posterior urethra. *J. Pediatr.* 63:84, 1963.
259. Reeders, S. T., Breuning, M. H., Davies, K. E., Nicholls, R. D., Jarman, A. P., Higgs, D. R., Pearson, P. L., and Weatherall, D. J. A highly polymorphic DNA marker linked to adult polycystic kidney disease on chromosome 16. *Nature* 317:542, 1985.
260. Reeders, S. T., Gal, A., Propping, P., Waldherr, R., Davies, K. E., Zerres, K., Hogenkamp, T., Schmidt, W., Dolata, M. M., and Weatherall, D. J. Prenatal diagnosis of autosomal dominant polycystic kidney disease with a DNA probe. *Lancet* 2:6, 1986.
261. Reilly, B. J., and Neuhauser, E. B. D. Renal tubular ectasia in cystic disease of the kidneys and liver. *Am. J. Radiol.* 84:546, 1960.

262. Renal Transplantation Registry, Advisory Committee. The 12th Report of the Human Renal Transplant Registry. *JAMA* 233:787, 1975.
263. Rennke, H. G. Hemodynamically Mediated Glomerular Damage Following Reduction of Functioning Nephron Units. In H. Losse, A. W. Asscher, A. E. Lison, and V. T. Andriole (Eds.), *Pyelonephritis,* Vol. 5: *Urinary Tract Infections.* Stuttgart: Thieme-Verlag, 1984. P. 66.
264. Risdon, R. A. Renal dysplasia: 1. A clinicopathological study of 76 cases. 2. A necropsy study of 41 cases. *J. Clin. Pathol.* 24:57, 65, 1971.
265. Risdon, R. A. Cystic Diseases of the Kidney and Reflux Nephropathy. In P. P. Anthony and N. M. MacSween (Eds.), *Recent Advances in Histopathology,* Vol. 2. Edinburgh: Churchill-Livingstone, 1981. P. 163.
266. Risdon, R. A. The small scarred kidney of childhood: A congenital or an acquired lesion? *Pediatr. Nephrol.* 1:632, 1987.
267. Risdon, R. A. Polycystic Disease: A Reevaluation of the Potter Classification. In E. V. Cosmi and G. C. de Renzo (Eds.), *Proceedings of the XI European Congress of Perinatal Medicine.* Chur: Harwood Academic, 1989. P. 409.
268. Risdon, R. A., Young, L. W., and Chrispin, A. R. Renal hypoplasia and dysplasia: A radiological and pathological correlation. *Pediatr. Radiol.* 3:213, 1975.
269. Rizza, J. M., and Dowling, S. E. Bilateral renal agenesis in two female siblings. *Am. J. Dis. Child.* 121:60, 1971.
270. Roberts, P. F. Bilateral renal carcinoma associated with polycystic kidneys. *Br. Med. J.* 3:272, 1973.
271. Robins, D. C., French, T. A., and Chakera, T. M. H. Juvenile nephronophthisis associated with skeletal abnormalities and hepatic fibrosis. *Arch. Dis. Child.* 51:799, 1976.
272. Rockson, S. G., Stone, R. A., and Gunnells, J. C. Solitary renal cyst with segmental ischemia and hypertension. *J. Urol.* 112:550, 1974.
273. Rolfes, D. B., Towbin, R., and Bove, K. E. Vascular dysplasia in a child with tuberous sclerosis. *Pediatr. Pathol.* 3:359, 1985.
274. Rolleston, G. L., Maling, T. M. J., and Hodson, C. J. Intrarenal reflux and the scarred kidney. *Arch. Dis. Child.* 49:531, 1974.
275. Romeo, G., Devoto, M., Costa, G., Roncuzzi, L., Catizone, L., Succhelli, P., Germino, G. G., Keith, T., Weatherall, D. J., and Reeders, S. T. A second genetic locus for autosomal dominant polycystic kidney disease. *Lancet* 2:8, 1988.
276. Roodhooft, A. M., Birnholz, J. C., and Holmes, L. B. Familial nature of congenital absence and severe dysgenesis of both kidneys. *N. Engl. J. Med.* 310:1341, 1984.
277. Roosen-Runge, E. C. Retardation of postnatal development of kidneys in persons with early cerebral lesions. *Am. J. Dis. Child.* 77:185, 1949.
278. Rosenfield, A. T., Curtis, A. McB., Putnam, C. E., Taylor, K. J. W., Allen, W. E., Siegel, N. J., and Hsia, Y. E. Gray scale ultrasonography, computerized tomography, and nephrotomography in evaluation of polycystic kidney and liver disease. *Urology* 9:436, 1977.
279. Ross, D. G., and Travers, H. Infantile presentation of adult-type polycystic kidney disease in a large kindred. *J. Pediatr.* 87:760, 1975.
280. Rosse, W. F., Waldmann, T. A. C., and Cohen, P. Renal cysts, erythropoietin and polycythemia. *Am. J. Med.* 34:76, 1963.
281. Royer, P., Habib, R., Mathieu, M., and Courtecuisse, V. L'hypoplasie rénal bilatérale congénitale avec reduction du nombre et hypertrophie des néphrons chez l'enfant. *Sem. Hop. Paris* 38:753, 1962.
282. Royer, P., Habib, R., Broyer, M., and Nanaille, Y. Segmental Hypoplasia of the Kidney in Children. In J. Hamburger, J. Crosnier, and M. H. Maxwell (Eds.), *Advances in Nephrology,* Vol. 1. Chicago: Year Book Medical Publishers, 1971. P. 145.
283. Rubenstein, M., Meyer, R., and Bernstein, J. Congenital abnormalities of the urinary system: 1. A postmortem survey of developmental abnormalities and acquired congenital lesions in a children's hospital. *J. Pediatr.* 58:356, 1961.
284. Safouh, M., Crocker, J. F. S., and Vernier, R. L. Experimental cystic disease of the kidney: Sequential, functional and morphologic studies. *Lab. Invest.* 23:392, 1970.
285. Sagel, S. S., Stanley, R. J., Levitt, R. G., and Geisser, G. Computed tomography of the kidney. *Radiology* 124:359, 1977.
286. Sahney, S., Sandler, M. A., Weiss, L., Hricak, H., and Madrazo, B. L. Adult polycystic kidney disease: Presymptomatic diagnosis for genetic counselling. *Clin. Nephrol.* 20:89, 1983.
287. Savage, D. C. L., Wilson, M. I., McHardy, M., Dewar, D. A. E., and Fee, W. M. Covert bacteriuria of childhood: A clinical and epidemiological study. *Arch. Dis. Child.* 48:8, 1973.
288. Saxton, H. M., Golding, S. J., Chantler, C., and Haycock, G. D. Diagnostic puncture in renal cystic dysplasia (multicystic kidney): Evidence on the aetiology of the cysts. *Br. J. Radiol.* 54:555, 1981.
289. Scheff, R. T., Zuckerman, G., Harter, H., Delmez, J., and Koehler, R. Diverticular disease in patients with chronic renal failure due to polycystic kidney disease. *Ann. Intern. Med.* 92:202, 1980.
290. Schoeneman, M. J., Plewinska, M., Mucha, M.,

and Mieza, M. Marfan syndrome and medullary sponge kidney: Case report and speculation of pathogenesis. *Int. J. Pediatr. Nephrol.* 5:103, 1984.
291. Schmidt, E. C. H., Hartley, A. A., and Bower, R. Renal aplasia in sisters. *Arch. Pathol.* 54:403, 1952.
292. Schwartz, B. R., Lage, J. M., Pober, B. R., and Driscoll, S. G. Isolated congenital renal tubular immaturity in siblings. *Hum. Pathol.* 17:1259 1986.
293. Schwarz, R. D., Stephens, F. D., and Cussen, L. J. The pathogenesis of renal dysplasia: III. Complete and incomplete urinary obstruction. *Invest. Urol.* 19:101, 1981.
294. Segal, A. J., and Spataro, R. F. Computed tomography of adult polycystic disease. *J. Comput. Assist. Tomogr.* 6:777, 1982.
295. Sellers, A. L., Winfield, A., and Rosen, V. Unilateral polycystic kidney disease. *J. Urol.* 107:527, 1972.
296. Senior, B. Familial renal-retinal dystrophy. *Am. J. Dis. Child.* 125:442, 1973.
297. Shemke, R. N. Hereditary Features of Autosomal Dominant Polycystic Kidney Disease: A. A Genetic Approach. In J. J. Grantham and K. D. Gardner, Jr. (Eds.), *Problems in Diagnosis and Management of Polycystic Kidney Disease. Proceedings of the First International Workshop on Polycystic Kidney Disease.* Kansas City: PRK Foundation, 1984. P. 187.
298. Shenker, L., and Anderson, C. Intrauterine diagnosis and management of fetal polycystic kidney disease. *Obstet. Gynecol.* 59:385, 1982.
299. Sherman, F. M., Studnicki, F. M., and Felterman, G. H. Renal lesions of familial juvenile nephronophthisis examined by microdissection. *Am. J. Clin. Pathol.* 55:391, 1971.
300. Shimamura, T., and Morrison, A. B. A progressive glomerulosclerosis occurring in partial five-sixths nephrectomy. *Am. J. Pathol.* 79:95, 1975.
301. Shokeir, M. H. K. Expression of "adult" polycystic renal disease in the fetus and newborn. *Am. J. Clin. Pathol.* 55:391, 1971.
302. Siegel, M. J., and McAlister, W. H. Simple cysts of the kidney in children. *J. Urol.* 123:75, 1980.
303. Simon, H. B., and Thompson, G. J. Congenital renal polycystic disease: A clinical and therapeutic study of 366 cases. *JAMA* 159:657, 1955.
304. Six, R., Oliphant, M., and Grossman, H. A spectrum of renal tubule ectasia and hepatic fibrosis. *Radiology* 117:117, 1975.
305. Slungaard, R. K., and Jaeck, J. L. Bilateral dwarfed kidneys. *Am. J. Dis. Child.* 97:575, 1959.
306. Smellie, J. M., Hodson, C. J., Edwards, D., and Normand, I. C. S. Clinical and radiological features of urinary tract infection in childhood. *Br. Med. J.* 2:1222, 1964.
307. Smith, C. H., and Graham, J. B. Congenital medullary cysts of the kidney in severe refractory anemia. *Am. J. Dis. Child.* 69:367, 1945.
308. Smith, D. W., Opitz, J. M., and Inhorn, S. L. A syndrome of multiple developmental defects including polycystic kidneys and intrahepatic biliary dysgenesis in two siblings. *J. Pediatr.* 67:617, 1976.
309. Sommerkamp, H. Nierencysten: Diagnostik und Operationbefunde. *Urologe* [A] 9:314, 1970.
310. Spires, S. M., Gaede, J. T., and Glenn, J. F. Death from a renal cyst. *Urology* 16:606, 1980.
311. Sprayrengen, S., Strasberg, A., and Naidich, T. P. Medullary sponge kidney and congenital total hemihypertrophy. *N.Y. State J. Med.* 73:2768, 1973.
312. Squiers, E. C., Morden, R. S., and Bernstein, J. Renal multicystic dysplasia: An occasional manifestation of the hereditary renal adysplasia syndrome. *Am. J. Med. Genet. Suppl.* 3:279, 1987.
313. Stapleton, F. B., Bernstein, J., Koh, G., Roy, S., III, and Wilroy, R. S. Cystic kidneys in a patient with oral-facial-digital syndrome type I. *Am. J. Kidney Dis.* 1: 288, 1982.
314. Stapleton, F. B., Johnson, D., Kaplan, G. W., and Griswold, W. The cystic renal lesion in tuberous sclerosis. *J. Pediatr.* 97:574, 1980.
315. Steele, B. T., Lirenman, D. S., and Battie, C. W. Nephronophthisis. *Am. J. Med.* 68:531, 1980.
316. Stephens, D. Caecoureterocele and concepts on the embryology and aetiology of ureteroceles. *Aust. N.Z. J. Surg.* 40:239, 1971.
317. Stickler, G. B., and Kelalis, P. P. Polycystic kidney disease: Recognition of the "adult form" (autosomal dominant) in infancy. *Mayo Clin. Proc.* 50:547, 1975.
318. Stigsson, L., Ekelund, L., and Karp, W. Bilateral concurrent renal neoplasms: Report of 11 cases. *Am. J. Radiol.* 132:37, 1979.
319. Stillwell, T., Gomez, M. R., and Kelalis, P. P. Renal lesions in tuberous sclerosis. *J. Urol.* 138: 477, 1987.
320. Strauss, M. B., and Sommers, S. C. Medullary cystic disease and familial juvenile nephronophthisis. *N. Engl. J. Med.* 277:863, 1967.
321. Stuck, K. J., Koff, S. A., and Silver, T. M. Ultrasonic features of multicystic dysplastic kidney: Expanded diagnostic criteria. *Radiology* 143:217, 1982.
322. Sturdy, D. E., and Magell, J. Traumatic perinephric cyst (pseudohydronephrosis). *Br. J. Surg.* 48:315, 1960.
323. Swinford, A. E., Bernstein, J., Toriello, H. V., and Higgins, J. V. Renal tubular dysgenesis: Delayed onset of oligohydramnios. *Am. J. Med. Genet.* 32:127, 1989.

324. Sworn, M. J., and Eisinger, A. Medullary cystic disease and juvenile nephronophthisis in separate members of the same family. *Arch. Dis. Child.* 47:278, 1972.
325. Tada, S., Yamagishi, J., Kobayashi, H., Hata, Y., and Kobari, T. The incidence of simple cysts by computed tomography. *Clin. Radiol.* 34:437, 1983.
326. Taitz, L. S., Brown, C. B., Blank, C. E., and Steiner, G. M. Screening for polycystic kidney disease: Importance of clinical presentation in the newborn. *Arch. Dis. Child.* 62:45, 1987.
327. Taxy, J. B., and Filmer, R. B. Metaplastic cartilage in nondysplastic kidneys. *Arch. Pathol.* 99: 101, 1975.
328. Taxy, J. B., and Filmer, R. B. Glomerulocystic disease: Report of a case. *Arch. Pathol. Lab. Med.* 100:186, 1976.
329. Tazelaar, H. D., Payne, J. A., and Patel, H. S. Congenital hepatic fibrosis and asymptomatic familial adult-type polycystic kidney disease in a 19-year-old woman. *Gastroenterology* 86:757, 1984.
330. Thaler, M. M., Ogata, E. S., Goodman, J. R., Piel, C. F., and Korobkin, M. T. Congenital fibrosis and polycystic disease of liver and kidneys. *Am. J. Dis. Child.* 126:374, 1973.
331. Thompson, D. P., and Lynn, H. B. Genital anomalies associated with solitary kidney. *Mayo Clin. Proc.* 41:538, 1966.
332. Torres, V. E., Holley, K. E., and Offord, K. P. General Features of Autosomal Dominant Polycystic Kidney Disease: A. Epidemiology. In J. J. Grantham and K. D. Gardner (Eds.), *Problems in the Diagnosis and Management of Polycystic Kidney Disease. Proceedings of the First International Workshop on Polycystic Kidney Disease.* Kansas City: PKR Foundation, 1985. P. 49.
333. Torrey, T. W. The early development of the human nephros. *Contrib. Embryol. Carnegie Inst.* 35:175, 1954.
334. Tridenti, G., Armanetti, M., Flisi, M., and Benassi, L. Uterus didelphys with an obstructed hemivagina and ipsilateral renal agenesis in teenagers: Report of three cases. *Am. J. Obstet. Gynecol.* 159:882, 1988.
335. Twersky, J., Twersky, N., Phillips, G., and Coppersmith, H. Peripelvic extravasation, urinoma formation and tumor obstruction of the ureter. *J. Urol.* 116:305, 1976.
336. Vargas, L., Friederici, H. H. R., and Maibenco, H. C. Cortical sponge kidney induced in rats by alloxan. *Diabetes* 19:33, 1970.
337. Voland, J. R., Hawkins, E. P., Wells, T. R., Saunders, B., Jones, M., and Venirschke, K. Congenital hypernephronic nephromegaly with tubular dysgenesis: A distinctive inherited renal anomaly. *Pediatr. Pathol.* 4:231, 1985.
338. Vuthibhagdee, A., and Singleton, E. B. Infantile polycystic disease of the kidney. *Am. J. Dis. Child.* 125:167, 1973.
339. Waldherr, R., Lennert, T., Weber, H.-P., Födisch, H. J., and Schärer, K. The nephronophthisis complex: A clinicopathologic study in children. *Virchows Arch.* [A] 394:235, 1982.
340. Warshawsky, A. B., Miller, K. E., and Kaplan, G. W. Urographic visualization of multicystic kidneys. *J. Urol.* 117:94, 1977.
341. Weiss, L., Reynolds, W. A., Saeed, S. M., and Cabal, L. Congenital hepatic fibrosis and polycystic disease of the kidneys with roentgen appearance of medullary sponge kidney. *Birth Defects* 10:22, 1974.
342. Weitzner, S. Clear cell carcinoma of the free wall of a simple renal cyst. *J. Urol.* 106:515, 1971.
343. Welling, L. W., and Grantham, J. J. Cystic and Developmental Diseases of the Kidney. In B. M. Brenner and F. D. Rector, Jr. (Eds.), *The Kidney,* 3rd Ed. Philadelphia: Saunders, 1986. P. 1341.
344. Welling, L. W., and Grantham, J. J. Cystic Diseases of the Kidney. In C. C. Tisher and B. M. Brenner (Eds.), *Renal Pathology with Clinical and Functional Correlations.* Philadelphia: Lippincott, 1989. P. 1233.
345. Welling, L. W., and Welling, D. J. Kinetics of Cyst Development in Cystic Renal Disease. In N. B. Cummings and S. Klahr (Eds.), *Chronic Renal Disease: Causes, Complications, and Treatment.* New York: Plenum Press, 1987. P. 95.
346. Wiedemann, H. R. Complexe malformatif familiale avec hernie ombilicale et macroglossie, un syndrome nouveau? *J. Genet. Hum.* 13:223, 1964.
347. Williams, D. I. Reflux in double ureters. *Proc. R. Soc. Med.* 55:423, 1962.
348. Williams, D. I., and Karlaftis, C. M. Hydronephrosis due to pelvi-ureteric obstruction in the newborn. *Br. J. Urol.* 38:138, 1966.
349. Williams, D. I., and Woodward, J. R. Problems in the management of ectopic ureteroceles. *J. Urol.* 92:635, 1964.
350. Williams, G., Blandy, J. P., and Tresidder, G. G. Communicating cysts and diverticula of the renal pelvis. *Br. J. Urol.* 41:163, 1969.
351. Wilson, R. D., and Baird, P. A. Renal agenesis in British Columbia. *Am. J. Med. Genet.* 21:153, 1985.
352. Wilson, R. H., and DeEds, F. Feedstuff antioxidants: Toxicology studies on the antioxidant 6-ethoxy-1,2-dihydro-2,2,4-trimethylquinolone. *J. Agric. Food Chem.* 7:206, 1959.
353. Witzleben, C. L., and Sharp, A. R. Nephronophthisis—Congenital hepatic fibrosis: An additional hepatorenal disorder. *Hum. Pathol.* 13: 728, 1982.
354. Woodard, J. R. Prune-Belly Syndrome. In P. P.

Keladis, B. L. R. King, and A. B. Belman (Eds.), *Clinical Pediatric Urology,* 2nd Ed. Philadelphia: Saunders, 1985. P. 805.
355. Wulfsohn, M. A. Pyelocaliceal diverticula. *J. Urol.* 123:1, 1980.
356. Yendt, E. R. Medullary sponge kidney and nephrolithiasis. *N. Engl. J. Med.* 306:1106, 1982.
357. Yu, D. T., and Sheth, J. K. Cystic renal involvement in tuberous sclerosis. *Clin. Pediatr.* 24:36, 1985.
358. Zager, R. A., Cotran, R. S., and Hoyer, J. R. Pathologic localization of Tamm-Horsfall protein in interstitial deposits in renal disease. *Lab. Invest.* 38:52, 1978.
359. Zerres, K., Weiss, H., Bulla, M., and Roth, B. Prenatal diagnosis of an early manifestation of autosomal dominant adult-type polycystic kidney disease. *Lancet* 2:988, 1982.
360. Zollinger, H. U. Pathogenese und Folgen einseitiger Zwergnieren bei Jugendlichen: Frühinfantile Pyelonephritis oder Hypogenese? *Schweiz. Med. Wochenschr.* 87:990, 1957.
361. Zollinger, H. U., Mihatsch, M. J., Edefonti, A., Gaboardi, F., Imbasciati, E., and Lennert, T. Nephronophthisis (medullary cystic disease of the kidney): A study using electron microscopy, immunofluorescence, and a review of the morphological findings. *Helv. Paediatr. Acta* 35:509, 1980.

Robert T. McCluskey

3

Immunologic Aspects of Renal Disease

The belief that many forms of human glomerulonephritis and some types of tubulointerstitial nephritis are immunologically mediated is supported by clinical, serologic, and pathologic studies in man and by investigation of animal models.

In the previous edition of this book I described in considerable detail major experimental models with respect to methods of induction, pathologic features, and immunologic mechanisms [352]. In the present chapter I will place most emphasis on the immunologic mechanisms that have been shown to produce renal injury and draw on individual models principally in attempts to illustrate the mechanisms. To some extent I will review the subject from an historical perspective, not in an attempt to identify priorities of discoveries, but rather to trace the development of thinking about immunopathogenetic mechanisms. The relevance of experimental models to human renal diseases will be considered at the end of the chapter; however, some comments will be interspersed with discussion of models for the sake of continuity.

THE ROLES OF ANTIBODIES AND T CELLS IN IMMUNOLOGICALLY MEDIATED RENAL INJURY

For a long time it was believed that all forms of immunologic renal injury result from humoral antibodies. However, there is now no question that T cells also can produce glomerular or tubulointerstitial damage. Furthermore, in some models, both T cell– and antibody-mediated mechanisms participate in the renal injury. Nevertheless, I will

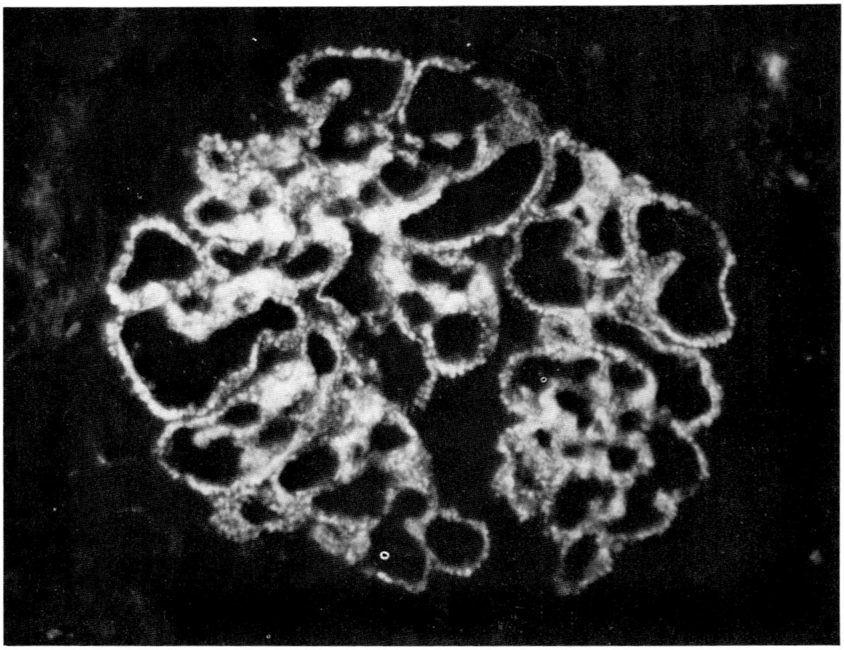

FIG. 3-1. *Granular deposits of immunoglobulin are seen all along the glomerular basement membrane. Electron microscopy showed corresponding subepithelial deposits. From a case of membranous lupus nephritis. (From Baldwin, D. S., and McCluskey, R. T. In E. L. Becker (Ed.),* Structural Basis of Renal Disease. *New York. Harper & Row, 1968.)*

discuss these two major types of immune damage separately. I will begin with a review of models in which antibody-mediated mechanisms have been considered to play a dominant or exclusive role. In the section on T cell–mediated renal injury, I will discuss how both mechanisms may operate simultaneously.

ROLE OF IMMUNE COMPLEXES IN RENAL DISEASE

Most forms of human glomerulonephritis in which antibodies are believed to play a dominant pathogenetic role are classified as *immune complex glomerulonephritis.* There are numerous models, both experimentally induced and naturally occurring, that more or less resemble the human diseases.

Immune complex glomerulonephritis can be defined as a heterogeneous group of diseases characterized by extracellular accumulation within glomeruli of immune complexes, which are also known as antigen-antibody (Ag-Ab) complexes. Anti-glomerular basement membrane (GBM) nephritis is generally excluded from this category and will be considered separately. Immune complexes are usually identified by immunofluorescence as irregular or granular deposits containing immunoglobulins, complement components, and antigen (when known); these are often referred to as *immune deposits.* Generally, corresponding granular dense deposits are found by electron microscopy. Complexes accumulate in various sites within glomeruli, and as has been learned from experimental models [459] and human diseases, their location is of importance in determining the type of damage that results. The major patterns are subepithelial, mesangial, and subendothelial (Figs. 3-1 through 3-3), which can be seen alone or in various combinations. In contrast, in anti-GBM nephritis, im-

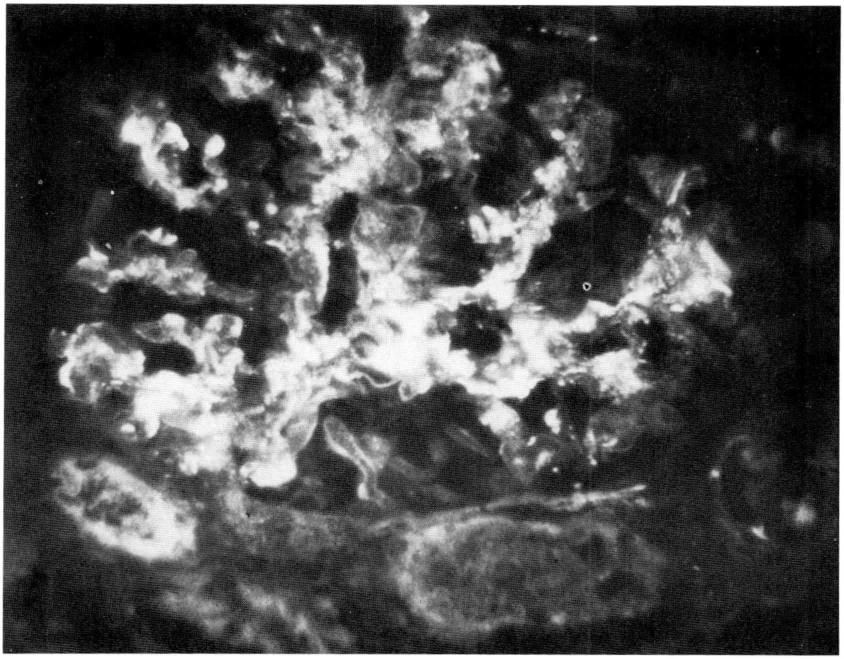

Fig. 3-2. *Irregular deposits of IgA are seen almost entirely in mesangial regions. From a patient with IgA nephritis. (From McCluskey, R. T.* J. Exp. Med. *134: 242S, 1971, Fig. 6, by copyright permission of the Rockefeller University Press.)*

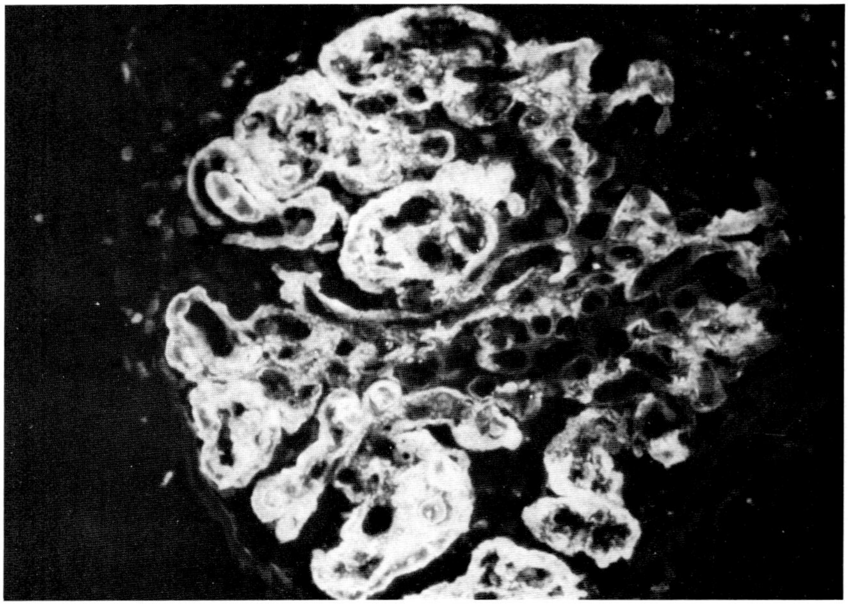

Fig. 3-3. *Broad, irregular deposits of immunoglobulin are seen along the basement membrane and in mesangial regions. From a case of severe (diffuse) proliferative lupus nephritis. (From McCluskey, R. T. In N. R. Rose and F. Milgrom (Eds.),* The First International Convocation on Immunology. *Basel: Karger, 1969.)*

munoglobulins are distributed uniformly along the GBM in a so-called linear pattern (Fig. 3-4).

A variety of antigens can participate in the formation of immune deposits in glomeruli, including heterologous materials, such as foreign proteins, products derived from viruses, bacteria, or parasites, as well as certain autologous antigens.

Experimental Studies on Immune Complex Glomerulonephritis and Factors Leading to Accumulation of Immune Complexes in Glomeruli

Experimental studies have shown that immune complexes can accumulate in glomeruli either through deposition of circulating immune complexes or through combination of antibodies and antigens within glomeruli (in situ formation). The two mechanisms are not entirely mutually exclusive, since following the initial accumulation of complexes, either through deposition from the circulation or by in situ formation, free antibodies or antigens and even circulating complexes [161] can combine with the reactants in the glomeruli.

Glomerular Deposition of Circulating Immune Complexes

For many years it was believed that arrest of circulating complexes was the major, if not the only, mechanism leading to glomerular deposits. Accordingly, factors favoring such deposition have been investigated extensively. Nevertheless, a number of important questions remain unanswered. It is obvious that most types of circulating immune complexes do not accumulate appreciably in glomeruli or other vulnerable sites. In fact, immune-complex formation is usually beneficial,

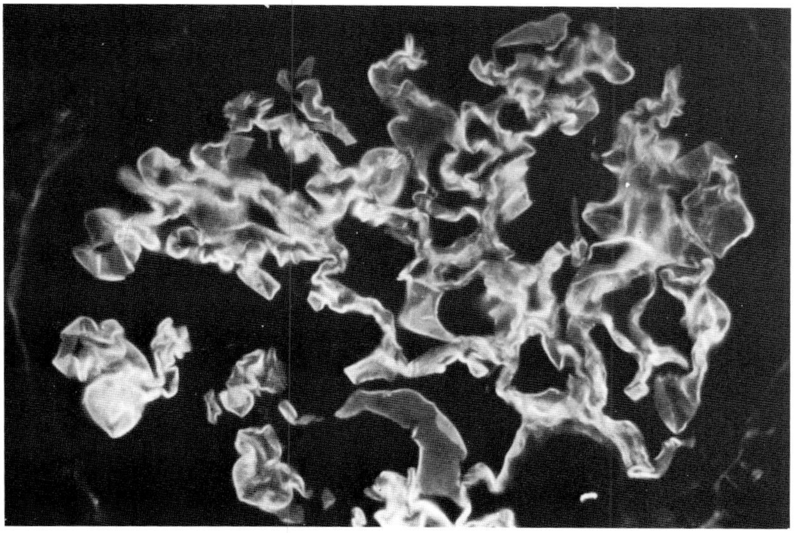

Fig. 3-4. *IgG is present continuously along the GBM in a so-called linear pattern. From a patient with anti-GBM nephritis. (Courtesy of Mr. A. B. Collins.)*

since it leads to the rapid removal of foreign substances from the circulation. Both the intrinsic properties of complexes and host factors influence the fate of circulating complexes. It is important to understand not only why immune complexes localize in glomeruli, but also why they accumulate in certain sites within glomeruli. I will not discuss factors that promote vascular localization of circulating immune complexes, but I do note that they appear to be different from those causing glomerular deposition [301].

EVIDENCE FOR GLOMERULAR DEPOSITION OF CIRCULATING IMMUNE COMPLEXES DERIVED FROM SERUM SICKNESS MODELS

Acute Serum Sickness

Evidence that immune complexes formed in the circulation can deposit in glomeruli was first obtained in studies of acute (one-shot) serum sickness in rabbits. Following a single injection of a large amount (250–500 mg/kg) of a high-molecular-weight foreign-serum protein, commonly bovine serum albumin (BSA), rabbits often develop acute glomerulonephritis, endocarditis, and necrotizing arteritis, generally in about 8 to 14 days. The fully developed glomerular lesions are usually characterized by diffuse hypercellularity, due mainly to an influx of monocytes, and generally by scattered immune deposits, especially in subepithelial locations. When first seen, the deposits stain for antigen, IgG, and C3; a few days later, only C3 may be found [158]. The lesions are rapidly and completely reversible.

The conclusion that immune complexes formed in the circulation initiate tissue damage was based on analysis of the temporal relationship between the concentrations of antigen and antibodies in the circulation and the appearance of lesions. Following intravenous injection, the concentration of circulating antigen is found to decline in three phases [135,179,186]. The first lasts 1 to 2 days, during which a fairly sharp drop in the level of circulating antigen occurs, principally as the result of equilibration with the extravascular space. Thereafter, the level declines more slowly for several days, at an exponential rate that reflects catabolism of the protein. In the third phase, which usually begins during the second week, there is increasingly rapid elimination of antigen, which results from combination with antibody; this phase is therefore referred to as the *immune phase* of antigen elimination. Since high levels of circulating antigen are still present when antibody is first produced, the first complexes formed in the circulation are in extreme antigen excess and are therefore small and soluble. During the next several days, as more antibody is produced and more antigen is removed from the circulation, larger, aggregated complexes are formed, and these are cleared with increasing efficiency by the mononuclear phagocyte system. After antigen has disappeared, free antibody appears in the circulation, rises rapidly for a few days, and then falls off.

In a very important study, Germuth [179] demonstrated that the lesions of acute serum sickness appear during the immune phase of antigen elimination. He therefore suggested that soluble complexes formed in the circulation deposit in the sites where lesions develop. Dixon and associates [135] confirmed and extended these findings and reported that antigen was not detectable by immunofluorescence within glomeruli in the first few days after injection but could be found when lesions appeared, in association with rabbit gamma globulin, in the form of granular deposits. These findings provided evidence against the possibility that free antigen first localized in glomeruli and subsequently combined with antibody, as had been postulated earlier by Hawn and Janeway [211]. Further evidence that circulating immune complexes can deposit in glomeruli and induce acute injury was provided by experiments in which mice were injected intravenously with preformed immune complexes [356,358,359]. It was assumed that complexes are passively trapped in glomeruli, primarily because of their size and because of the filtering function of the glomerulus.

Chronic Serum Sickness

Additional support for the interpretation that soluble circulating immune complexes are important in glomerulonephritis came from studies of chronic serum sickness. Models of chronic serum sickness have been produced in rabbits, rats, or mice by repeated (usually daily) intravenous injections of a foreign-serum protein (commonly BSA) over prolonged periods, often 2 to 3 months. Chronic serum sickness is characterized by abundant immune deposits in glomeruli [133,180] and often in other sites [72]. The glomerular deposits are found in different patterns and may predominate in mesangial regions or along capillary loops, where they are often found in a subepithelial location. In some studies, a transition from an early phase with predominantly mesangial pattern to a later phase with peripheral loop deposits has been described [20,564]. The histologic features vary widely and correlate to some extent with the location of deposits. In contrast with acute serum sickness, the deposits and lesions are only slowly, if at all, reversible.

In 1961, Dixon and associates [133] performed a careful study of the relationship between the intensity of the antibody response and the development of lesions in rabbits injected repeatedly with BSA. The initial daily dose of BSA was 12.5 mg, and the dose was adjusted upward in animals that produced large amounts of antibodies in an attempt to achieve slight antigen excess in the circulation following each injection. The rabbits fell into three roughly defined groups on the basis of their antibody response. *One group* failed to produce antibody and developed no lesions despite the presence of large amounts of foreign protein in the circulation and tissues for long periods. A *second group* had very high amounts of circulating antibodies; it was assumed that following each daily injection of antigen, large, aggregated complexes were formed, which are known to be rapidly removed from the circulation. Some of these animals developed evidence of acute glomerulonephritis within the first 2 weeks, but this usually resolved quickly, and in most animals, no further glomerular disease developed. A *third group* produced an intermediate amount of antibody, and in these animals the daily injected antigen was cleared fairly slowly. It was assumed that soluble, small to intermediate-sized immune complexes were present in the circulation throughout much of each day. Most rabbits in this group eventually developed chronic glomerular lesions.

Extensive studies of experimental chronic serum

sickness also have been performed by Germuth and associates [180–183]. Their usual protocol differed from that just described in that no attempt was made to adjust the antigen dose once the experiment was underway. Nevertheless, as in the experiments of Dixon et al. [133], it was found that only rabbits with relatively low levels of antibodies and evidence of small to intermediate-sized soluble complexes in the circulation were the ones that usually developed severe chronic glomerular lesions, often with predominantly peripheral loop deposits.

REEVALUATION OF THE ROLE OF SOLUBLE CIRCULATING COMPLEXES IN SERUM SICKNESS MODELS

The experiments just reviewed on acute and chronic serum sickness provide compelling evidence that arrest of circulating immune complexes can produce glomerular deposits and disease. Moreover, it was concluded that relatively small soluble complexes, especially those formed in antigen excess, are responsible; this interpretation has not gone unchallenged. *A major problem in serum sickness models is that the exact relationship between the immune complexes detected in the circulation and those which produce glomerular deposits cannot be determined.* The assumption that the type of complex that predominates in the circulation accounts for the deposits may not be valid, since complexes that localize in glomeruli may quickly disappear from the circulation, leaving only irrelevant complexes. Clearly, even in animals with conspicuous deposits, only very small fractions of the circulating complexes arrest in glomeruli. Even if one could recover and examine the composition of complexes within glomeruli, the nature of the earliest complexes that accumulate would not be clarified, because the deposits are extensively modified by addition of free antibodies, antigens, complement, or anti-idiotypes.

As noted earlier, a pathogenic role of very large, insoluble complexes formed in the circulation in chronic serum sickness had been dismissed because rabbits with high levels of antibodies, in which such complexes should form after each antigen injection, usually failed to develop severe glomerular injury. However, the composition of circulating complexes in animals injected repeatedly with antigen is constantly changing, and with most experimental protocols may swing each day from moderate antigen excess to moderate antibody excess, thus transversing equivalence. Cameron and Clark [84] reexamined the data in the Dixon et al. and Germuth et al. studies on chronic serum sickness and have provided arguments favoring a role of insoluble immune complexes. Other experiments [168,481] had shown that if insoluble complexes can be delivered to or be caused to form within glomeruli, as occurs after injection of antigen into the aorta or renal artery of immunized rabbits, severe glomerular lesions can be produced. As discussed later, experiments in which preformed immune complexes are injected into normal animals also have provided evidence that relatively large latticed complexes ($>Ag_2 Ab_2$) localize in glomeruli.

An important study bearing on the role of soluble immune complexes in chronic serum sickness was performed by Boyns and Hardwicke [70]. They injected rabbits daily for prolonged periods with trace-labeled BSA and measured antigen and immune complex levels daily. Each daily dose of antigen was carefully selected to prevent the appearance at any time of free circulating antibodies, with the result that soluble complexes were continuously circulating, generally in high levels, for periods up to 90 days. Despite this, none of the rabbits developed evidence of severe glomerulonephritis, and only scanty electron-dense deposits were found. *The observations provide impressive evidence that soluble immune complexes do not necessarily produce serious glomerular damage, even when present in the circulation in high concentrations and for long periods.* However, the conditions in these experiments were very carefully controlled so as to avoid at any time the formation of large-latticed complexes; in naturally occurring chronic antigenemia—such as viremia or bacteremia—complexes of varying composition are certain to be formed.

Based on consideration of the studies just described, as well as on other studies on serum sickness performed in rabbits, rats, and mice [129, 130,180,410,431,498,499], it is reasonable to conclude that both relatively large complexes composed of high-avidity, or precipitating, antibodies and smaller complexes containing low-avidity antibodies can produce glomerular disease, but with different time courses and different features. In particular, among animals injected daily with antigen for prolonged periods, those forming high levels of precipitating antibodies often develop mild acute glomerular disease with predominantly mesangial deposits, whereas those with lower levels of complexes containing nonprecipitating or low-avidity complexes often develop more serious chronic glomerular disease with proteinuria, renal functional impairment, and predominantly peripheral loop deposits. As discussed later, certain experiments performed with preformed complexes indicate that combinations of complexes with different properties may be necessary to produce immune deposits.

ROLE OF ANTIBODY CLASS IN SERUM SICKNESS MODELS

The importance of the *class* of antibodies forming the complexes in determining glomerular localization and injury also has been examined. In virtually all models, IgG has been identified in the glomerular deposits, but it is not clear how often other immunoglobulin classes were looked for, especially in early studies. Germuth and Rodriguez [180] reported that an occasional rabbit among a group given a single injection of 500 mg of BSA responded with a predominantly IgM response. The sera contained complexes of about 1×10^6 daltons. Glomerular lesions developed that were characterized by focal and segmental tuft necrosis and hypercellularity rather than by diffuse hypercellularity, as is usually seen in rabbits with acute serum sickness. It was assumed that the changes resulted from extremely large complexes. Necrotizing lesions are also seen in sensitized rabbits that receive intraaortic injections of antigens, with the formation of large, poorly soluble complexes [168,481]. It may be noted in passing that IgM (usually in addition to IgG or other immunoglobulins) is present in glomerular deposits in a variety of forms of human glomerulonephritis, only a few of which show focal necrotizing lesions. Models in which IgA predominates in the complexes are usually characterized by mesangial deposits, as reviewed in Chapter 6.

THE FATE AND DISTRIBUTION OF PREFORMED IMMUNE COMPLEXES FOLLOWING INTRAVENOUS INJECTION

In view of the difficulties in interpretation of active serum-sickness models, it is useful to review experiments in which preformed immune complexes have been injected intravenously [174,175,336, 338,339,341,356,358,359]. This approach makes it possible to examine critically the importance of a variety of properties of immune complexes that influence their fate and distribution, including antibody class, precipitability, charge, lattice structure, nature of the antigen, and ability to bind Fc or complement receptors. There are, nevertheless, problems with the use of preformed complexes. For one thing, almost all preparations contain mixtures of complexes, and the small amounts that accumulate in glomeruli may not be the same as the major constituents. Furthermore, the experiments are designed to be of short duration (usually less than 2 days) to avoid an immune response by the recipient against the injected reactants. Thus, certain kinds of modifications of deposits that occur in chronic immune complex disease, as through addition of rheumatoid factor or anti-idiotypes, do not occur. Moreover, because of the short duration of the experiments, only acute glomerular damage can be produced. Finally, most types of complexes may dissociate in vivo, making possible independent deposition of antigen and antibody with local recombination.

Studies employing preformed complexes have been carried out in mice, rats, rabbits, or nonhuman primates, often with complexes composed of BSA or human serum albumin (HSA) and rabbit antibodies. The rate of clearance has generally been studied by the use of complexes containing ^{131}I or ^{125}I trace-labeled antibodies, and the distribution of the complexes has been examined by determining radioactive content of various tissues or by immunofluorescence and electron microscopy. A large number of such studies has been performed; only the salient findings will be summarized here. I will first discuss intrinsic properties of complexes that favor glomerular deposition and then host factors that influence the fate of circulating complexes; it is obvious that these two subjects are interrelated.

Effect of Concentration and Composition of Preformed Immune Complexes on Glomerular Localization

Following injection into mice of preformed soluble complexes prepared at moderate antigen excess with IgG antibodies and native serum proteins (5× in the HSA–anti-HSA system), glomerular accumulation develops rapidly [203,339,341]. However, this occurs only if fairly large doses are given (>1.0 mg ab). Only a very small fraction of the injected complexes accumulates in glomeruli, with most being removed from the circulation by the mononuclear phagocyte system and in particular by Kupffer cells. With most kinds of complexes, prepared with unmodified protein antigens and antibodies, glomerular deposits are found principally in mesangial regions, although early subendothelial accumulation also may be seen. The accumulation of complexes in subendothelial regions probably results from their entrance through endothelial fenestrae, followed by trapping along the glomerular basement membranes. Some subendothelial complexes may subsequently move into mesangial regions. Complexes also may enter the mesagnium directly, through fenestrae overlying mesangial regions.

Haakenstad and Mannik [203] concluded that only relatively large latticed complexes (>Ag_2 Ab_2) localize in glomeruli, since deposits appear when large-latticed complexes are present in the circulation and disappear within a few days, even though smaller complexes (<Ag_2 Ab_2) continue to circulate. Furthermore, administration of a large dose of free antigen caused a rapid disappearance of existing deposits, presumably because the excess antigen converted the deposited complexes into small, soluble complexes that were released from glomeruli [343].

Although predominantly mesangial deposits are seen following injection of most types of immune complexes, with certain preparations peripheral loop accumulation is seen. Complexes prepared with antibodies of moderate or low avidity localize predominantly along the peripheral loops, often as subepithelial deposits [181,291]. Lew and colleages [311] performed studies with immune complexes prepared with monoclonal antibodies of defined affinity and showed that complexes containing high-affinity IgG antibodies produced predominantly mesangial localization, whereas complexes containing low-affinity antibodies produced subepithelial deposits. It has been argued that complexes composed of low-avidity antibodies are particularly likely to dissociate, which raises the possibility that subepithelial deposits are formed by recombination of antigens and antibodies within glomeruli. However, Lew et al. [312] reported that covalent (i.e., nondissociable) immune complexes of 500,000 MW (but not 800,000 MW) prepared with a monoclonal antibody and an anionic haptenated antigen, 4-azido-2 nitrophenylated BSA, localized along the outerside of the basement membranes, as well as in mesangial and subendothelial regions. Once complexes with low-affinity antibodies localize along capillary walls, complexes containing high-affinity antibodies of the same specificity can combine with them; in contrast in animals without complexes bound to capillary walls, circulating complexes with high-affinity antibodies localize preferentially in mesangial regions [381].

Effect of Charge of Preformed Immune Complexes on Glomerular Localization

Following the demonstration of fixed negatively charged sites in glomeruli [93,260], several groups investigated the effects of alteration of charge of immune complexes on their ability to accumulate in glomeruli [169,170,174–176,259]. [As discussed later, localization of free cationic antigens in glomeruli ("planted antigens") has provided a basis for in situ formation of complexes in several models.] Complexes prepared with cationic antigens or antibodies show a much greater capacity to deposit in glomeruli than do unmodified complexes [169,170,339,340]. Furthermore, cationic complexes accumulate much more effectively than do cationic antibodies alone [340]. Moreover, in contrast with unmodified complexes, cationic complexes generally localize preferentially along the basement membranes, where the concentration of fixed anionic sites is highest [259]. Shortly after injection, cationic complexes accumulate at the sites of fixed anionic charges of the lamina rarae interna and externa. However, later the complexes may condense into larger subendothelial or subepithelial deposits.

A key question is whether charge plays a role in the glomerular localization of naturally occurring immune complexes. Certain observations of Gallo et al. [170] are relevant to this question. One method they employed to prepare cationic complexes was to separate immunoglobulins obtained from immunized rabbits by isoelectric focusing. It was not possible by this means to prepare immune complexes that were sufficiently cationic to deposit in the glomerular basement membrane, and chemical modifications were required to achieve this result. These findings do not preclude the possibility that in other situations sufficiently cationic antibodies may be produced. Circulating IgG in man or animals can reach an isolectric point as high as 9. Furthermore, evidence has been obtained that antibodies eluted from glomeruli of mice with lupus-like nephritis contain slightly more cationic antibodies than circulating antibodies [122,139]. However, there is a wide range of charge among eluted antibodies, and it appears that charge has only a minor role in determining which antibodies localize in glomeruli in murine lupus nephritis.

Glomerular Lesions Produced by Injections of Preformed Immune Complexes

Although glomerular localization of appropriately prepared preformed immune complexes is regularly observed following intravenous injection, the production of glomerular lesions is variable. In some experiments in mice, moderately severe abnormalities have been found histologically, characterized by accumulation of neutrophils and monocytes [291,356,359]. The most severe lesions were produced by repeated injections over periods of 2 or 3 days [359]. In contrast, in other studies, including some performed in rabbits, glomerular abnormalities have been absent or minimal [98]. Part of the variability may be due to differences in immune complex preparations or in the dose of complexes, the schedule of their administration, or the species studied. Furthermore, the type of lesions produced can only be compared with those of acute serum sickness because of the short duration of experiments with preformed complexes. Nevertheless, it seems clear that lesions produced by passive administration of immune complexes are not as severe as those sometimes seen following active immunization, even in acute serum sickness. A possible explanation for this is the necessity for combined effects of cellular mechanisms, as discussed later.

ROLE OF THE MONONUCLEAR PHAGOCYTE SYSTEM IN THE REMOVAL OF CIRCULATING IMMUNE COMPLEXES

The concentration of immune complexes in the circulation depends on their relative rates of formation and removal. The most important mechanism for elimination of circulating immune complexes is uptake by cells of the mononuclear phagocyte system [48], which usually follows attachment of complexes to red blood cells or platelets by means of the complement receptor CR1. The efficient removal of circulating complexes by the cells of the mononuclear phagocyte system, within which they are degraded without harmful effects, reduces or eliminates the possibility that the complexes will localize in vulnerable sites, including glomeruli.

Particularly informative studies on the clearance function of the mononuclear phagocyte system have been performed by Mannik and associates, employing preformed complexes of varying composition [203,342]. Large-latticed, soluble complexes (those with more than two antibody molecules) are quickly removed from the circulation. In contrast, very small complexes ($Ag_1 Ab_1$) are cleared very slowly, with a half-life approaching that of the immunoglobulin itself. Among cells of the mononuclear phagocyte sytem, Kupffer cells are largely responsible for removal of circulating soluble complexes, and only a small fraction are taken up by the spleen. In contrast, the spleen plays an important role in the clearance of particles, such as red cells coated with IgG antibodies.

The uptake of immune complexes by cells of the mononuclear phagocyte system is apparently mediated principally by means of their Fc and C3 receptors. Complexes prepared in ways that render them ineffective in interacting with Fc and C3 receptors (i.e., with alkylated and reduced antibodies) are cleared more slowly and accumulate in glomeruli to a greater extent than unmodified complexes [204]. High levels of circulating complexes can lead to saturation of the mononuclear phagocyte system, and this results in prolonged circulation and increased glomerular deposition [202]. The saturation of the mononuclear phagocyte system is associated with loss of Fc and C3 receptor activity on Kupffer cells [408].

Defective clearance of preformed immune complexes by the mononuclear phagocyte system has been documented in MRL-lpr/lpr mice, a strain that develops a lupus-like syndrome with immune complex nephritis [254]. This defect may result not only from saturation by circulating complexes, but also from autoantibodies against Fc receptors, which have been described in NZB/W and MRL-lpr/lpr mice [62].

Although most types of immune complexes are taken up by mononuclear phagocytes by means of Fc or C3 receptors, there is evidence that certain complexes are removed because of recognition of the antigen component of the complex; in particular, evidence of antigen-mediated clearance has been described for complexes containing carbohydrates and DNA [156].

ROLE OF THE COMPLEMENT SYSTEM IN THE PREVENTION OF IMMUNE COMPLEX DISEASE

Among the most important advances in recent years in the field of immune complex diseases has been the recognition of the role of the complement system in the clearance of circulating immune complexes and in the prevention of the formation of immune deposits. Evidence for the protective role of complement has come from observations on the association of human immune complex diseases with inherited complement deficiencies, as well as from experimental studies. Excellent reviews have appeared on these subjects [213,466,469,549].

Role of Complement Receptor 1 (CR1) in the Clearance of Circulating Immune Complexes

In 1953, Nelson [401] reported that microorganisms coated with specific antibodies bind to human erythrocytes, a process he referred to as *immune adherence.* Subsequently, it was shown that soluble immune complexes also exhibit immune adherence. It is now known that the phenomenon depends on the complement receptor CR1 (CD35).

CR1 is a membrane glycoprotein found on a variety of cells, including primate erythrocytes, neutrophils, monocytes, B cells, some T cells, and human podocytes [21,213,466]. Although CR1 is present in lower concentrations on primate erythrocytes than on leukocytes, erythrocytes are so much more numerous that they account for over 80 percent of CR1 on circulating cells.

The major ligand for CR1 is C3b, the main fragment of the activated third component of complement. Accordingly, in order to attach to erythrocytes, immune complexes must be capable of activating and fixing C3b. Large complexes bind to CR1 more effectively than small complexes. Complexes composed of IgA antibodies bind C3b relatively poorly and therefore do not exhibit immune adherence [554].

Following intravascular injection of complement-fixing immune complexes, they rapidly bind to cells with CR1 receptors [213]. Erythrocytes account for most of the binding in primates, but in rodents, platelets appear to be mainly responsible. Most of the erythrocytes are not noticeably affected by the binding and merely serve as transport vehicles. Immune complexes bound to erythrocytes are largely prevented from accumulating in vulnerable sites, such as glomeruli or blood vessels, perhaps because in most tissues red cells circulate in the central part of the stream or because there is no mechanism for transfer to endothelial cells. However, within the liver and spleen, the complexes are transferred to fixed mononuclear phagocytic cells, possibly because of their higher concentration and affinity of Fc and C3 receptors. The transfer process is apparently not accompanied by loss of CR1 from most of the erythrocytes, which can therefore participate again in immune adherence.

Evidence has been obtained for an important role in vivo of the erythrocyte CR1 transport system in the handling of circulating complexes in primates [213,553]. In complement-depleted animals, preformed complexes failed to bind to erythrocytes and were thus free in the plasma; in contrast with what was found in normal animals, complexes accumulated not only in the liver and spleen but also in the lung and kidneys [553]. Paradoxically, complement depletion resulted in slighly *accelerated clearance* of immune complexes from the circulation. These results indicate that the erythrocyte transport system prolongs the presence of immune complexes in the circulation, but only slightly and in a way that permits their safe disposal [553].

In addition to the transport function of erythrocytes for immune complexes, there is evidence that complexes may be "processed" on red blood cells in ways that lead to the formation of generally smaller and less pathogenic complexes, which may be released into the circulation [213].

Modification of Immune Complex Solubility by Complement

The complement system also may protect against immune complex diseases by inhibition of the formation of insoluble complexes. Heidelberger [214] noted in 1941 that precipitation of antigen-antibody complexes is partially inhibited in the presence of complement. It is now known that this requires activation of the classical pathway, as shown by the failure of serum lacking C4 or C2 to mediate the effect [224,465–470], as well as by lack of complement-mediated inhibition of precipitation by IgA-containing complexes. The complexes that are kept in solution by complement are large (>19 S) and contain C1, C4, and C3b. The incorporation of C3b prevents cross-linking of complexes, possibly by interfering with Fc-Fc interactions, which account for rapid aggregation of immune complexes.

The complement system not only can inhibit precipitation but also can solubilize immune complex precipitates, although this process is less effective than prevention. Solubilization is critically dependent on the alternative pathway [371,507–510] but is also enhanced by activation of the classical pathway. The solubilized complexes are small and have reduced capacity to bind to cells with Fc and C3 receptors or to activate the complement system.

ROLE OF VASOACTIVE AMINES IN THE LOCALIZATION OF CIRCULATING IMMUNE COMPLEXES

Under certain circumstances, release of vasoactive amines promotes accumulation of circulating complexes in glomeruli (and more important, in blood vessels). The first evidence of this was obtained in studies by Benacerraf et al. [47], who showed that the injection of vasoactive amines into mice increased the glomerular accumulation of circulating colloidal carbon. Moreover, injections of preformed immune complexes had a similar effect, and it was postulated that when complexes form in the circulation, they bring about release of amines, which favor the deposition of the complexes themselves in glomeruli [356]. In support of this, Kniker and Cochrane [287] found that antagonists of serotinin and histamine largely prevented glomerular deposition of complexes and glomerulonephritis in acute serum sickness in rabbits. The release of vasoactive amines in acute serum sickness apparently depends on IgE antibodies that coat basophils. Upon contact with antigen, the basophils degranulate and release phospholipid factors (platelet-activating factor, PAF) that bring about liberation of amines from platelets [88,216]. Whether similar mechanisms operate in chronic immune complex diseases is unknown.

In Situ Formation of Glomerular Immune Complex Deposits

For the past 15 years or so, the importance of circulating immune complexes in the formation of glomerular immune deposits has been under question, and increasing attention has been given to the role of in situ formation. This term should be restricted to conditions in which the interactions of antibodies and antigens *initiate* the formation of immune deposits within glomeruli, since free antibodies or antigens can combine with complexes that have been trapped from the circulation. In many situations, it is not clear how glomerular accumulation of immune complexes is initiated.

There are two general ways in which circulating antibodies can initiate in situ formation: (1) by interaction with native constituents of the glomerulus, and (2) by combination with nonglomerular antigens that have been "planted" in glomeruli.

The concept of in situ formation of immune complex deposits is not new. The Arthus reaction, which was described in the first decade of this century, results from the local combination of injected antigens with circulating antibodies, with the formation of insoluble deposits. Furthermore, nephrotoxic serum nephritis, which also was described around the beginning of the century, results from the combination of circulating antibodies with components of the GBM. When models of serum sickness were found to be characterized by discrete granular immune deposits and anti-GBM nephritis by continuous accumulation of IgG, these patterns were considered to be evidence of two distinct mechanisms. In particular, granular deposits were thought to result only from deposition of circulating complexes; it is now known, however, that granular deposits also can result from in situ formation.

IN SITU FORMATION OF IMMUNE DEPOSITS WITH INTRINSIC GLOMERULAR ANTIGENS

Heymann Nephritis

It was largely through studies of Heymann nephritis that the mechanism of in situ formation of glomerular deposits came to the forefront. In view of this, and because Heymann nephritis has been studied extensively as a model of human membranous glomerulonephritis, I shall review the model in some detail.

In 1959, Heymann and associates [217] reported that intraperitoneal injections of rats with homologous kidney homogenates in Freund's adjuvant resulted in a chronic glomerular disease that was manifested by heavy proteinuria. The experimental design was similar to that employed in the production of other autoimmune organ-specific diseases, such as thyroiditis, and the investigators correctly concluded that they had induced a form of autoimmune glomerulonephritis. Subsequent studies showed that the lesions bear a striking resemblance to human membranous glomerulonephritis [10]. In histologic preparations, the glomeruli appear normal or show only slight capillary wall thickening. Immunofluorescence shows granular deposits of IgG along the glomerular basement membrane (Fig. 3-5), and electron microscopy reveals corresponding dense deposits on the epithelial side of the basement membrane (Fig. 3-6).

In most studies, Heymann nephritis is induced in Lewis rats by immunization with a crude fraction (designated Fx1A) of rat renal cortical tissue, in complete Freund's adjuvant, often with an added injection of *Bordetella pertussis* [281].

Primary Immunologic Mechanisms in Heymann Nephritis. Studies in the late 1960s [143,144,188,198,199] provided evidence that the glomerular deposits were composed of autoantibodies and of antigens normally found in the brush-border regions of proximal convoluted tubules. Thus the sera of rats with Heymann nephritis and, more important, eluates obtained from diseased glomeruli were found by immunofluorescence to contain antibodies reactive with antigens in the brush-border regions of proximal tubules of normal rat kidneys. Furthermore, the glomerular deposits contained antigens that could be detected with heteroantisera prepared against renal tubular antigens.

Since the deposits are composed of autoantibodies and autologous antigens, the term *autologous immune complex (AIC) nephritis* was coined and is sometimes used as a synonym for Heymann nephritis [143].

The first widely accepted explanation for the formation of glomerular deposits in Heymann nephritis was that they resulted from the deposition of autologous immune complexes formed in the circulation [143,188]. The reasons for this conclusion were as follows: (1) serum sickness models had provided evidence that arrest of circulating complexes is a mechanism for the formation of glomerular deposits, including epimembranous de-

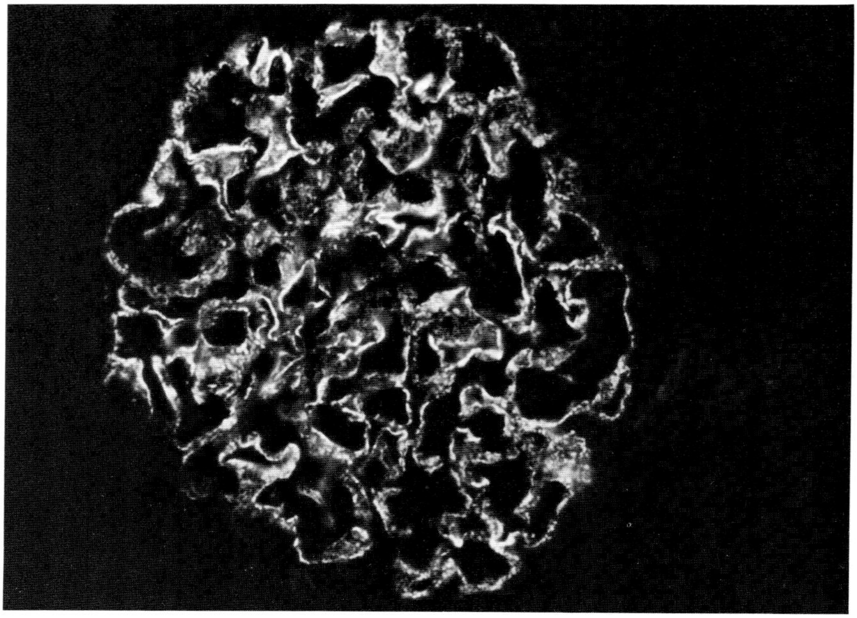

FIG. 3-5. *Finely granular deposits of IgG are seen along the glomerular capillary walls. From a rat with Heymann nephritis.*

posits; (2) evidence had been obtained that renal tubular antigens are normally present in the circulation in small amounts; and (3) most important, neither circulating antibodies nor antibodies eluted from glomeruli of rats with Heymann nephritis appeared to react with normal glomeruli, as far as could be determined by immunofluorescence, which argued against the possibility that the glomerulus is a direct target of the autoantibodies.

In the past several years, however, compelling evidence has been obtained that the glomerular deposits result principally or exclusively from the combination of antibodies with antigens normally present in glomeruli. Evidence for in situ formation was first obtained in studies of passive Heymann nephritis produced by the administration to rats of heteroantisera prepared against rat Fx1A [31,152]. Shortly after administration, heterologous IgG is demonstrable by immunofluorescence in the form of granular deposits along the GBM. Corresponding epimembranous dense deposits are seen by electron microscopy. Van Damme et al. [534] showed by immunofluorescence that rabbit anti-rat Fx1A antisera can bind to normal glomeruli in tissue sections in a granular pattern along the GBM. In other studies involving perfusion in vivo and in vitro under conditions where the formation of circulating complexes could be eliminated, it was shown that the heterologous antibodies themselves can accumulate in glomeruli and form epimembranous deposits [113].

It is known that the heteroantisera used in these experiments contain antibodies that react with determinants other than those recognized by the autoantibodies present in actively immunized rats, and the possibility that these additional antibodies accounted for the deposits had to be considered [219,457]. However, other studies provided evidence that even in active Heymann nephritis, deposits form in situ. IgG eluted from the kidneys of rats with active Heymann nephritis [159] was

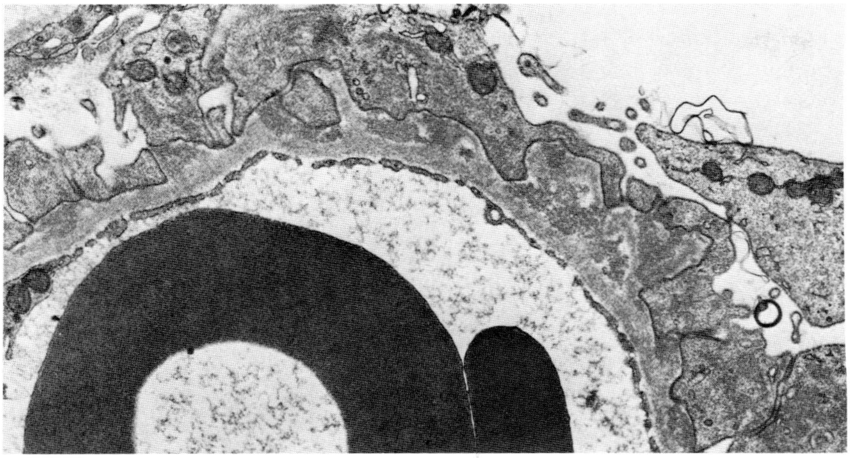

Fig. 3-6. *Electron micrograph of glomerular capillary wall from a rat with Heymann nephritis. Scattered dense deposits are seen along the outer side of the basement membrane.* × *12,800. (Courtesy of Dr. Eveline E. Schneeberger.)*

found to produce typical glomerular deposits following perfusion of kidneys in vivo during short periods. Furthermore, Neale and Wilson [388] reported that antibodies obtained in eluates from large pools of kidneys from rats with Heymann nephritis can bind to normal rat glomeruli, as shown by immunofluorescence. The titer of antibodies reactive with glomeruli was only about one-tenth that of antibodies reactive with brush-border antigens. By immunoelectron microscopy, binding of the antibodies was described in a scattered granular pattern on the epithelial side of the GBM, at the site where deposits develop [388]. The failure of other investigators to detect glomerular reactivity of sera or glomerular eluates from rats with Heymann nephritis is due to the low concentration of the antigen in normal glomeruli.

Although the evidence is overwhelming that in situ formation is the major mechanism of immune deposit formation in Heymann nephritis, some recent evidence continues to support a contributory role of circulating complexes. Hori and Abrass [227] isolated circulating complexes from rats with Heymann nephritis induced by Fx1A and obtained evidence that the complexes contain a tubular antigen with a mass estimated to be between 60 and 65 kD. The antigen reacted with antibodies eluted from the glomeruli of rats with Heymann nephritis and was capable of inducing active disease.

Identification of gp330, the Major Pathogenic Antigen of Heymann Nephritis. Additional and more conclusive evidence for in situ combination of autoantibodies with glomerular antigens, as well as further elucidation of the mechanism of formation of the glomerular deposits, was obtained following the identification by Kerjaschki and Farquhar [268,269,270] of the main pathogenic antigen of Heymann nephritis—gp330. The gp330, so called because it is a glycoprotein with an estimated mass of 330 kD, was purified from isolated microvillar membranes of rat kidney cortex. The membranes were solubilized in detergent, the soluble components were fractionated by gel filtration, and gp330 was isolated by affinity chromatography on lentil lectin columns.

Normally, gp330 is found on the apical plasmalemmal domain of some epithelial cells, in particular proximal renal tubules, glomerular podocytes, lung (type II pneumocytes), epididymis, and yolk sac [94,137,273]. Because of its location on absorptive epithelial cells, and because it is generally concentrated in coated pits, it is possible that gp330 is a receptor. Evidence has been reported that a 76-kD serum protein may be a ligand for gp330 [258], but further work is needed to confirm this study.

Raychowdhury et al. [440] have recently partially characterized the primary structure of gp330. Partial cDNAs coding for gp330 were isolated and sequenced. The deduced amino acid sequence of gp330 contained regions with homology to the human low-density-lipoprotein (LDL) receptor, which indicates that gp330 and the LDL receptor may be members of the same gene family. The deduced protein sequences of gp330 contained a 29 amino acid transmembrane sequence and a 188 amino acid cytoplasmic tail.

Evidence that gp330 is the major pathogenic antigen responsible for Heymann nephritis induced by Fx1A can be summarized as follows [270]: First, antibodies *eluted* from the glomeruli of rats with Heymann nephritis recognize principally or exclusively gp330. In contrast, the *sera* of rats immunized with Fx1A react with multiple proteins. Second, immunization of rats with purified gp330 results in characteristic glomerular deposits (although proteinuria is produced only in some rats and is generally not severe). Third, immunization with renal microvillar membrane preparations selectively depleted of gp330 (by gel filtration) results in the production of anti-brush border antibodies but not of glomerular deposits. Fourth, the administration to normal rats of rabbit antibodies prepared against purified rat gp330 results in the rapid formation of glomerular subepithelial deposits.

Thus there is no doubt that gp330 is a major pathogenic antigen in Heymann nephritis. However, the disease induced by immunization with Fx1A is usually considerably more severe than that induced with purified gp330, as measured by the size and abundance of the deposits and the severity of proteinuria [257]. Furthermore, eluates from the glomeruli of rats with Heymann nephritis induced with Fx1A sometimes contain antibodies not only against gp330 (which are by far the most abundant) but also against a 95-kD protein [257] or a 60- to 65-kD tubular antigen [227]. Despite this and other evidence that Fx1A may contain additional nephritogenic antigens, they have not been well characterized [51,71]. Candidates include dipeptidyl peptidase IV [386], intrinsic GBM antigens and the 60- to 65-kD tubular antigen [227]. As noted earlier, the 60- to 65-kD tubular antigen may form circulating complexes that contribute to glomerular deposits [227].

Immune Deposits in Heymann Nephritis Form from Cell-Surface Antigens. The availability of specific antibodies against gp330, including monoclonal antibodies, made it possible to explore the early interactions between antibodies and glomerular antigens that lead to the formation of immune deposits in Heymann nephritis. With the use of immunoultrastructural techniques, gp330 has been found within normal glomeruli in association with epithelial cells, but not in basement membranes, endothelium, or mesangium [51,269]. In podocytes, gp330 is found in the endoplasmic reticulum, occasional Golgi elements, multivesicular bodies, and coated pits at the cell surface.

The finding that gp330 in glomeruli is restricted to podocytes argues against earlier suggestions that the deposits form initially within the GBM [388]. Kerjaschki and Farquhar postulated that the coated pits on the soles of foot processes are the sites where the antibodies meet gp330 [269]. In support of this, they showed that shortly after intravenous injection of rabbit anti-gp330 antibodies, rabbit IgG is first demonstrable in podocyte coated pits and that deposits, which form quickly in the lamina rara externa, remain in contact with coated pits [272]. They postulated that the deposits result from shedding of the complexes into the lamina rara interna.

The concept that immune complex deposits can develop as the result of interaction of antibodies with cell-surface components is fairly new and is based in large part on the work of Andres and associates [13,14,71]. Their first studies were carried out in vivo. They injected rabbits with heterologous antibodies to angiotensin-converting enzyme, which is expressed in high concentrations on the surface of pulmonary endothelial cells [32]. Shortly after injection, aggregation of the enzyme on the pulmonary endothelium was seen, followed by its disappearance. Immune deposits were not produced in this model, presumably because immune complexes were formed on the plasma membrane of cells facing the bloodstream and were either endocytosed or shed into the circulation. Similarly, the interaction of antibodies with gp330 on the apical surface of proximal tubule cells, which occurs in proteinuric rats with circulating anti-gp330 antibodies, may produce shedding of complexes into the tubular lumens [201].

Andres and associates [14] postulated that the interaction of antibodies with surface antigens on domains of cells facing basement membranes might result in the formation of insoluble immune deposits in these structures. This prediction was borne out in experiments in which the effects of interaction of antibodies with angiotensin-converting enzyme in rabbit ovaries were examined [344]. Ovaries were studied because the enzyme was found to be present on the oolemma of mature oocytes, which are surrounded by the zona pellucida, a basement membrane-like structure. In rabbits injected with goat antibodies to angiotensin-converting enzyme, patching of the antigen on oocytes rapidly occurred, and this was followed by the formation of large immune aggregates in the zona pellucida. Aggregation and shedding required cross-linking of complexes, as indicated by the requirement for divalent antibodies. The findings provided direct evidence that in situ formation of immune deposits may occur in vivo when immune complexes containing cell-surface antigens are shed into basement membranes.

Camussi et al. [85,86] also performed in vitro experiments with cultured rat glomerular epithelial cells and anti-gp330 or anti-Fx1A antibodies in attempts to elucidate mechanisms of immune complex formation in Heymann nephritis. Following incubation of living cells with polyclonal antibodies at 4°C, gp330 was found diffusely distributed over the cell surface in a granular pattern. At 37°C, a rapid clustering of immune complexes occurred, with the formation of patches and caps and then the disappearance of complexes from the cells, through either shedding or endocytosis. Redistribution was not produced by monovalent antibodies, unless they were cross-linked. Furthermore, drugs that block energy production or inhibit cytoskeletal function prevented redistribution of immune complexes at the cell surface. Camussi et al. [86] also showed that anti-gp330 antibodies were less effective in causing redistribution and shedding of antigens than antibodies prepared against renal tubular brush-border vesicles. These results may help explain why immunization with Fx1A, which induces multiple autoantibodies, results in more severe disease than does immunization with gp330.

In other experiments using cultured glomerular epithelial cells, Cybulsky et al. [116] showed that anti-Fx1A antibodies, most of which were directed at gp330, converted Heymann antigens from a detergent-soluble membrane-associated form to an insoluble cytoskeletal-bound form.

Formation of Immune Deposits with Podocyte Cell-Surface Antigens Other than gp330

As far as is known, gp330 is not normally expressed on glomerular podocytes in species other than the rat (although proteins analogous to gp330 are present in brush-border regions of proximal tubules in all species that have been examined, including man) [271]. It is therefore not surprising that a glomerular disease involving gp330 has been produced only in rats. However, similar glomerular deposits have been produced with antibodies against a different cell-surface antigen, a 90-kD protein (apparently dipeptidyl peptidase IV) [23–25]. Unlike gp330, the 90-kD antigen is not concentrated in coated pits but is diffusely distributed on the surface of glomerular epithelial cells and, to a lesser degree, on endothelial cells. Following intravenous injection of rabbit antibodies against the 90-kD protein, rabbit IgG was seen on mouse podocytes. However, subepithelial deposits did not form unless mouse antibodies against rabbit Ig were produced and combined with the rabbit immunoglobulin on the surface of podocytes [24]. In some mice, subepithelial deposits persisted for at least a year. This study is important because it shows that podocyte cell-surface antigens other than gp330 can participate in the formation of subepithelial deposits. As discussed later, dipeptidyl peptidase IV also may participate in the formation of glomerular immune deposits in murine models of graft-versus-host (GVH) disease.

Formation of Subepithelial Immune Deposits with Antibodies Against Angiotensin-Converting Enzyme

Matsuo et al. [345] have made the surprising observation that the interaction of antibodies with an endothelial cell-surface antigen, angiotensin-converting enzyme, may lead to subepithelial glomerular deposits. Rabbits were injected intravenously with goat antibodies against angiotensin-converting enzyme, and the distribution of goat IgG within glomeruli was studied sequentially. At day 1, goat IgG was seen exclusively on glomerular endothelial cells, whereas after day 3, subepithelial deposits containing goat and rabbit IgG developed. It was suggested that complexes were shed from the endothelium and then driven to the epithelial side of the basement membrane by hydrodynamic forces. If this interpretation is correct, it would lengthen the list of mechanisms by which subepithelial deposits containing glomerular antigens may form.

Anti-endothelial antibodies may play a role in passive Heymann nephritis induced with heterologous antiserum against tubular antigens, which contain a variety of antibody specificities [219]. Following injection of such antibodies, an early reaction with endothelial cells has been seen, with disappearance of endothelial antigens and subsequent formation of subepithelial deposits [247]. The presence of multiple antibody specificities in heterologous antitubular antisera may explain why they are generally more effective than antisera prepared against gp330 in the production of passive Heymann nephritis.

Formation of Subepithelial Immune Deposits with Intrinsic Glomerular Basement Membrane Antigens

Although the interaction of most types of anti-GBM antibodies with glomerular antigens results in continuous ("linear") accumulation along the GBM, evidence has been obtained in a model induced by mercuric chloride that certain anti-GBM antibodies also can result in granular subepithelial deposits [167]. The administration of mercuric chloride to rabbits or rats induces a biphasic autoimmune glomerular disease characterized in the early weeks by linear deposition of IgG along the GBM and later by subepithelial deposits. The serum and glomerular eluates contain antibodies to laminin and type IV collagen [331], which are major components of the GBM. Fukatsu et al. [167] have provided evidence that these antigens are produced and secreted by cultured glomerular epithelial cells. Thus, antibodies eluted from the kidneys of animals with mercuric chloride–induced nephritis reacted with the secreted antigens, but unlike anti-Fx1A antibodies, they did not interact with the surface of cultured glomerular epithelial cells. The findings are consistent with the interpretation that combination of antibodies with basement membrane antigens secreted by podocytes can produce subepithelial immune deposits.

Makino et al. [330] have obtained evidence that antibodies against another basement constituent, heparan sulfate–proteoglycan (HS-PG), also can lead to the formation of subepithelial immune deposits, as seen following administration of rabbit antibodies to rats that had been preimmunized with rabbit IgG. Shortly after injection, heterologous IgG was found in both the lamina rara interna and externa, sites where HS-PG is concentrated in the GBM [500]. Later, the antibodies disappeared from the lamina rara interna, but persisted in the outer layer, where they combined with rat anti-rabbit IgG antibodies to form subepithelial deposits. The clearance of antibodies from the lamina rara interna was attributed to "lateral sweeping plasma water currents," causing their displacement into the mesangium. These observations indicate that differential clearance or penetration of reactants within the glomerulus may influence the site of accumulation of immune complexes, as apparently occurs with complexes containing endothelial antigens such as angiotensin-converting enzyme (see above).

In Situ Formation of Glomerular Immune Deposits in Murine Chronic Graft-Versus-Host (GVH) Disease

Although immune complex glomerulonephritis was described in models of GVH disease many years ago [313], only recently has evidence been obtained that intrinsic glomerular antigens are involved in the formation of glomerular deposits.

Graft-versus-host disease can arise when lymphocytes are transferred into recipients incapable of rejecting them. The models of GVH disease associated with glomerulonephritis are generally induced in F_1 hybrids derived from two inbred strains of mice by injections of parenteral lymphocytes of one strain that are not rejected by F_1 recipients [75]. Various strain combinations have been used, including BALB/c × A/JAX and C57Bl/10 × DBA/2 F_1 hybrids. It is thought that parenteral alloreactive T cells react with H2-incompatible structures of the host and generate excessive help, which activates host B cells to produce a variety of autoantibodies. With certain strain combinations, chronic GVH disease has similarities to systemic lupus erythematosus (SLE), with the production of antinuclear antibodies, including anti-DNA and antihistone antibodies, and severe immune complex glomerulonephritis [75]. However, in addition, certain organ-specific autoantibodies are formed, some of which appear to be involved in glomerular immune-deposit formation.

Bruijn et al. [76] have studied the specificities of antibodies eluted from isolated glomeruli of C57Bl10 × DBA F_1 hybrids in which GVH disease was induced by injection of DBA/2 lymphocytes. Antibodies eluted early in the disease were directed against renal brush-border antigens, including dipeptidyl peptidase IV and GBM components, notably laminin, although later antinuclear antibodies also were recovered. Transfer of the anti-brush-border antibodies to normal mice resulted in the formation of subepithelial glomerular deposits, probably as the result of the interaction of antibodies with dipeptidyl peptidase IV on podocytes. These results show that antibodies against nephritogenic antigens can be induced by means other than immunization with homologous or heterologous antigens in complete Freund's adjuvant.

IN SITU FORMATION OF GLOMERULAR IMMUNE DEPOSITS WITH PLANTED ANTIGENS

Over the past two decades or so, a variety of models have been described in which formation of glomerular deposits and injury are produced by interaction of antibodies with nonglomerular antigens that were previously fixed ("planted") in glomeruli. Apparently the first description of such a model was that of Mauer et al. [346], who showed that intravenously injected aggregated human IgG accumulated in mesangial regions of rabbits and that subsequent administration of anti-human IgG antibodies resulted in the formation of immune complexes within glomeruli and in severe acute glomerular injury. Recently, Cosio et al. [107] described another model in which mesangial deposits are produced in situ. The planted antigen was phenylated gelatin (DNP-GL), which binds to mesangial fibronectin by the gelatin portion; the DNP is the antigenic site. These authors showed that precipitating anti-DNP antibodies were retained longer in the mesangium that nonprecipitating antibodies.

Most other models produced with planted antigens are characterized by the formation of deposits along the glomerular capillary wall. Several kinds of antigens have been used: cationic antigens, which interact with fixed anionic sites in glomeruli [544,545,562], predominantly in the GBM; lectins, which have an affinity for the GBM [189] or endothelial cells; and DNA, which binds to the GBM [239].

The combination of antibodies with certain cationic antigens may result in subendothelial deposits, especially with large antigens, such as ferritin [545], but such complexes generally rapidly redistribute to the subepithelial space. With small cationic antigens, subepithelial deposits form directly. Kagami et al. [256] have described experiments in which high-valency cationic antigens (i.e, with numerous determinants) were effective in inducing subepithelial deposits, whereas low-valency antigens were relatively ineffective. Agodoa et al. [6] reported that precipitating antibodies are required to produce subepithelial immune deposits in a model that involved a planted cationic antigen. Although certain cationic immune complexes also may directly traverse the GBM and produce subepithelial deposits, planting of free antigen followed by in situ formation is a more likely explanation for most subepithelial deposits.

The demonstration that glomerular deposits, and especially subepithelial deposits, can result from in situ formation with planted exogenous antigens has led to the resurrection of the interpretation [211] that this is the way deposits form in serum sickness models induced with BSA [544]. In support of this, Fleuren et al. [160] have found that perfusion of rat kidneys alternately with BSA and anti-BSA antibodies resulted in the formation of subepithelial deposits, whereas preformed complexes did not. Although the conditions of perfusion were clearly not physiologic, the experiments provide evidence for the postulated mechanism. However, arguing against in situ formation in serum sickness is the absence of glomerular-bound antigen in animals without corresponding antibodies. As discussed earlier, it is impossible to determine precisely how immune complexes first accumulate in vivo in active serum sickness models.

Modification of Immune Complex Deposits

It is clear that no matter how immune complexes first accumulate in tissues, they are subject to extensive modification in ways that can lead to their aggregation and enlargement or to their partial or complete elimination [350]. Immune complexes within glomeruli can be altered by the combination of reactants derived from the circulation, including free antibodies, antigens, immune complexes, complement components, and autoantibodies against immunoglobulin or complement components. In addition, immune complexes can be phagocytosed by infiltrating leukocytes or mesangial cells, or redistributed by hemodynamic forces within glomeruli.

The development of large deposits recognizable by immunofluoresence or electron microscopy requires local rearrangements following the initial accumulation of immune complexes. Mannik et al. [337] provided direct evidence for this conclusion in experiments in which mice were injected intravenously with preformed complexes that were either covalently cross-linked or non-cross-linked. The cross-linked complexes were unable to rearrange in vitro, as shown by their lack of precipitation and absence of changes in lattice following purification and concentration. At 1 hour, comparable (and generally small) amounts of complexes were detected within glomeruli by immunofluorescence in groups of mice given either type of complexes. At later times, mice given the non-cross-linked complexes showed increasing glomerular deposits by immunofluorescence and increasing electron-dense deposits, whereas in mice injected with cross-linked complexes, the complexes detected by immunofluorescence diminished and electron-dense deposits did not develop. The interactions among non-cross-linked complexes may be either immunologically specific or nonspecific, notably through Fc-Fc interactions that can cause aggregation of complexes [376].

The addition of free antigen to immune complexes can have different effects depending on the composition of the complexes. If a small amount is added to complexes in antibody excess, increased lattice formation may occur. In contrast, the addition of a large excess of antigen can lead to the formation of soluble complexes, with dissolution of existing deposits [205].

Important modifications of immune complexes can result from the addition of anti-immunoglobulin antibodies, namely rheumatoid factors and anti-idiotypes. Rheumatoid factors are autoantibodies against IgG, most of which react with antigenic determinants in the Fc region, although some are said to recognize Fab determinants [90]. Anti-idiotypes react with variable region determinants (idiotopes) in the Fab portion of specific antibodies; idiotopes may be related to antigen-binding sites or framework regions. Both rheumatoid factors and anti-idiotypes can combine with antibodies present in complexes, either in the circulation or within deposits [162,486]. Evidence has been obtained that anti-IgG antibodies are important components of the glomerular deposits in the late stages of experimental chronic serum sickness induced with BSA in rabbits [428]. In early stages, BSA was readily detectable within deposits, and these could be solubilized in tissue sections by incubation with excess antigen. Later in the disease, deposits often could not be solubilized by antigen, but they could be removed with rabbit gamma globulin, probably through an effect on IgG–anti-IgG complexes.

In addition, rheumatoid factors have been shown to potentiate nephrotoxic serum nephritis [365] or to combine with IgG in immune complexes passively trapped in mouse glomeruli [162]. Lambert et al. [299] have obtained evidence that idiotype–anti-idiotype immune complexes may have pathogenetic significance in the glomerular immune complexes that can be produced in mice by injection of bacterial lipopolysaccharide, presumably as the result of polyclonal B cell activation.

Thus, even at a time when there is no further formation of complexes through combinations of the original antigen and antibodies, complexes may continue to enlarge through additions of autoanti-immunoglobulin antibodies, and probably by antibodies against complement components. Nevertheless, complexes do, of course, disappear from glomeruli after limited exposure to antigens. The mechanisms responsible for elimination of complexes vary, in part depending on their location in glomeruli.

Considerable attention has been directed at mechanisms for disposal of mesangial immune deposits. In addition to solubilization by excess antigen or by a complement-mediated effect, the following mechanisms have been considered [350]: phagocytosis by infiltrating leukocytes or mesangial cells, passage through mesangial channels leading to egress at the vascular pole (as has been shown to occur with colloidal carbon), excretion across the mesangial waist region, and degradation within the mesangial matrix, possibly by locally released proteases.

Disposal of subendothelial deposits may result from dissolution by excess antigen, extracellular degradation by proteases, complement solubilization, and in particular, phagocytosis by leukocytes. Subepithelial deposits cannot ordinarily be attacked by phagocytes, but they may be internalized and degraded by podocytes or solubilized by excess antigen, complement, or proteolytic enzymes. In man, internalization of C3b-containing complexes may be facilitated by CR1 receptors on podocytes, although direct evidence for this is lacking [429].

MODELS OF IMMUNE COMPLEX GLOMERULONEPHRITIS ASSOCIATED WITH INFECTIONS

Although models of serum sickness induced by foreign-serum proteins may provide basic information about how glomerular immune deposits can develop, they do not directly provide insight into how foreign antigens may participate in human immune complex glomerulonephritis. The most likely sources of exogenous antigens in human glomerulonephritis are bacteria, viruses, and parasites.

Virus-Induced Immune Complex Glomerulonephritis

Several models of immune complex glomerulonephritis associated with viral infection have been described [379,418,420,448]. Some are seen in animals with laboratory-induced infections, whereas others are seen in the course of naturally occurring infections. In the previous edition of this book, I reviewed several models in detail. Here I will merely summarize salient points.

Viruses can apparently induce immune complexes by three general mechanisms [418,419]. First, and most important, complexes may be formed by combination of specific antibodies with viral antigens, either in solution or on the surface of infected cells. Second, viruses may cause polyclonal B cell activation or enhance nonspecific T cell helper activity, which may result in the production of a variety of antibodies that can participate in immune complex formation. Third, viral antigens may stimulate the formation of specific autoantibodies as the result of shared amino acid sequences with host antigens (molecular mimicry).

Immune complexes containing viral antigens have been implicated in glomerulonephritis associated with several chronic viral infections in animals. The viruses are generally not cytopathic and do not produce glomerular (or other tissue) injury in the absence of an immune response. The most thoroughly studied models are lymphocytic choriomeningitis (LCM), Aleutian disease of mink, leukemia virus infections in mice, and equine infectious anemia [379,448].

In each of these infections, immunofluorescence studies have shown granular glomerular deposits of immunoglobulins, complement components, and viral antigens. In some cases, demonstration of antigen requires partial elution of immunoglobulins to free up antigenic sites [420]. In most of these models, the deposits are found predominantly in mesangial regions, particularly early in the disease. However, deposits are also seen along glomerular capillary walls, especially with severe disease. By electron microscopy, varying combinations of mesangial, subendothelial, and subepithelial deposits have been described. In Aleutian disease of mink, unusually severe lesions develop with prominent subendothelial deposits.

Circulating immune complexes containing infectious viruses or viral products have been found in several models, and antiviral antibodies have been demonstrated in eluates of renal tissue. In Aleutian disease of mink and in equine infectious anemia, free circulating antibodies against viral products are found as well.

Although it was first assumed that the glomerular deposits associated with viral infections result entirely from deposition of circulating complexes, it is highly likely that local formation occurs as well. In situ formation was apparently first proposed by Pascal et al. [427], who observed a good correlation between the presence of viral particles in mesangial and endothelial cells and the presence of glomerular deposits in AKR mice infected with Gross leukemia virus.

Several features of virus-induced chronic immune complex glomerulonephritis deserve emphasis because they are relevant to evaluation of the role of viruses in human glomerulonephritis. For one thing, glomerular lesions may develop in the course of an inapparent chronic viral infection, and the glomerular disease may be the most serious manifestation of the infection. In addition, in some infections, such as LCM, free antibody is not demonstrable in the circulation (at least not by ordinary techniques). In these cases, eluates of renal tissue may provide the best source of antiviral antibodies in studies designed to detect causative agents. Finally, glomerular deposits usually do not contain identifiable viral particles, so electron microscopic studies may not help identify the causative agent.

Obviously, persistence of the viral infection is required for the production of chronic immune complex disease; this is generally attributed to an inadequate (although clearly not absent) immune response. In most of the viral infections that have been associated with immune complex glomerulonephritis, the antibodies are incapable of virus neutralization. Both environmental and genetic factors that control the intensity of the immune response are important in determining whether a viral infection will be eradicated or persist.

At least one model of virus-induced acute immune complex glomerulonephritis has been described. Wright et al. [567] reported that some dogs infected with canine adenovirus develop acute glomerular abnormalities, which are characterized by hypercellularity and neutrophil infiltration. The lesions begin at 5 or 6 days after virus inoculation and gradually resolve after about 10 days as the animals recover from the systemic infection. By immunofluorescence, conspicuous granular deposits of IgG, IgM, C3, and viral antigens are found in mesangial regions. Eluates from affected kidneys have been shown to contain antiviral antibodies. Ultrastructural findings include electron-dense deposits in the mesangial matrix and virions in the nuclei of swollen endothelial and mesangial cells.

Bacteria-Induced Immune Complex Glomerulonephritis

Despite numerous attempts to induce experimental glomerular disease with group A streptococci or products of these organisms, no entirely satisfactory model of human poststreptococcal glomerulonephritis has been described [43,317,547]. Becker and Murphy [43] described a variety of glomerular lesions in rabbits repeatedly inoculated with group A streptococci, including hypercellularity of tufts, crescents, and sclerosis. However, immunofluorescence studies were not reported, and the underlying immunologic mechanisms were not elucidated.

Albini and associates [7] have reported induction of glomerulonephritis in rabbits by repeated injections of disrupted *Streptococcus mutans*, an organism that has been implicated in human dental caries (but not in glomerulonephritis). The glomerular lesions, which developed over a period of several weeks, were characterized by infiltration with granulocytes and monocytes, and by glomerular deposits, many of which had the electron microscopic appearance of "humps"—distinctive subepithelial deposits that are characteristic of human poststreptococcal glomerulonephritis. *S. mutans* antigens were demonstrable in the deposits early in the experimental disease. Glomerular eluates contained antibodies against streptococcal products, as well as against basement membrane constituents. The results indicate that immune complexes containing bacterial antigens as well as autoantibodies against basement membrane antigens are important. The relevance of this model to human poststreptococcal glomerulonephritis is unclear. Other attempts to produce models of poststreptococcal glomerulonephritis are reviewed in Chapter 5.

MURINE MODELS OF SYSTEMIC LUPUS ERYTHEMATOSUS (SLE)

Most of the models I have described so far are induced by highly artificial methods, such as injections of very large amounts of foreign proteins or of tissue antigens in adjuvants, or by passive administration of antibodies or immune complexes. Even when microbial agents have been used, the methods of infection have generally been contrived. Available forms of naturally occurring glomerulonephritis in laboratory animals are largely limited to some viral diseases and to models of SLE. Three strains of mice, NZB/W, BXSB, and MRL-lpr/lpr, spontaneously develop a disease that resembles SLE. A large amount of research has been performed to elucidate the immunologic derangements that underlie these disorders [124,283,284,286,515,516]. The main abnormalities are generalized B cell hyperactivity with hypergammaglobulinemia and production of a variety of autoantibodies and, in particular, antibodies against nuclear antigens, including double-stranded (ds) and single-stranded (ss) DNA, and histones.

The causes of the B cell hyperactivity are not fully understood and probably differ from one strain to another. It is clear that multiple genetic backgrounds are associated with B cell hyperactivity. Explanations for the abnormality that have been suggested include impaired T cell suppressor function, hyperresponsiveness of B cells to interleukins, dysregulation of idiotype–anti-idiotype interactions [483], or excessive production of B cell activators. A fundamental and unanswered question is whether the autoantibodies in SLE are antigen driven or the result of antigen-independent polyclonal B cell activation. These mechanisms are not entirely mutually exclusive; for example, antigen-independent polyclonal activation could increase the number of B cell clones with specific immunoglobulin receptors for various autoantigens [478]. In support of this view are data obtained by Klinman et al. [285] in studies on MRL-lpr/lpr mice. They found that the early B cell repertoire was dominated by IgM-secreting B cells, with no bias toward production of specific autoantibodies, whereas later the repertoire was dominated by IgG-secreting B cells, with reactivity against a limited number of autoantigens.

The development of disease appears to depend not only on the underlying immunologic defect, but also on so-called accelerating factors, which include endogenous factors such as genes or hormones and exogenous factors such as viral infection. I will restrict the rest of the discussion of murine models of SLE to the features and pathogenesis of the renal disease.

Glomerulonephritis in Murine SLE

Glomerulonephritis is a major cause of death in all strains, but there are differences among strains in the time of onset and severity of the renal lesions and in the relative severity in males and females [18]. In NZB/W mice, the glomerular disease appears first in females at around 5 months. In contrast, in the BXSB strain, males are affected first, and severe glomerular abnormalities are observed by 3 months. MRL-lpr/lpr mice manifest severe early disease in both males and females.

Histologically, the glomerular lesions in all strains are characterized by hypercellularity, due to infiltrates of monocytes and proliferation of mesangial cells, accumulation of mesangial matrix, varying degrees of capillary wall thickening, and occasional crescent formation. In BXSB mice, neutrophils are often found in appreciable numbers in glomeruli. Interstitial infiltrates of lymphocytes and plasma cells are common in all strains, and these are often intense around glomeruli. By immunofluorescence, conspicuous granular deposits of IgG and C3 are seen in glomeruli and occasionally in tubulointerstitial sites [18]. In NZB/W and MRL-lpr/lpr mice, the glomerular deposits have been observed to be first confined to mesangial regions; with progressiosn of the disease, the mesangial deposits increase in size and capillary wall deposits also develop [61,265]. Electron microscopic studies of the lesions in NZB/W and MRL-lpr/lpr mice have shown dense deposits in mesangial regions and along both sides of the basement membrane, but especially on the epithelial side [265].

Several investigators have attempted to identify antigens and determine the specificity of antibodies in the deposits. Immunofluorescence studies have revealed evidence of DNA [298] and of glycoprotein (gp70), an envelope antigen of murine retrovirus, in the deposits in some mice [134]. Studies of IgG eluted from the kidneys of SLE mice have revealed antinuclear antibodies, including antibodies against ds and ss DNA, in higher concentrations than in the serum [515]. Although gp70-containing complexes were once thought to be important in the pathogenesis of the glomerular lesions [134], later studies have shown that mice without gp70 develop equally severe glomerulonephritis [19]. As noted earlier, anti-DNA antibodies eluted from the kidneys of MRL-lpr/lpr and NZB/W mice are enriched for antibodies with high isoelectric points, which probably reflects the propensity of cationic serum proteins to penetrate the GBM [122,139].

It was first proposed that glomerular immune deposits in SLE mice resulted from the deposition of circulating complexes, in keeping with serum-sickness models. And although evidence of circulating complexes has been obtained in some studies, DNA-containing complexes have not been convincingly demonstrated. Moreover, it has been shown that DNA or most types of preformed complexes containing DNA are very rapidly cleared in the liver, apparently through recognition of DNA, as well as through the usual mechanisms for removal of circulating complexes [108,141]. However, small complexes containing DNA are cleared more slowly and may have the opportunity to accumulate to some extent in glomeruli [146].

Recently, increasing attention has been given to the possibility that autoantibodies, and in particular anti-DNA antibodies, interact directly with antigens in glomeruli, producing complexes in situ [145]. One way this could happen is by combination of anti-DNA antibodies with DNA planted in glomeruli. It has been reported that DNA has an affinity for collagen, types I and III, and for isolated GBM in vitro [239]. The binding of DNA to glomeruli may require the formation of complexes with histones, a set of highly cationic proteins [471].

Another way in which anti-DNA antibodies might produce glomerular deposits in situ is by combination with intrinsic glomerular antigens other than DNA. Suggestions for this mechanism stemmed from the finding that many monoclonal anti-DNA antibodies interact with a wide range of antigens, including multiple polynucleotides, heparan sulfate, cytoskeletal, and cell-membrane proteins [17,149,241,242,297,555]. However, it has been reported that much of the cross-reactivity is caused by contaminating DNA–anti-DNA immune complexes produced in culture [74]. Furthermore, most of the data on cross-reacting of anti-DNA antibodies have come from studies employing monoclonal antibodies, which may differ from most naturally occurring autoantibodies. If, nevertheless, certain anti-DNA autoantibodies do react with cell-surface antigens or with heparan sulfate, they might initiate immune complex formation within glomeruli. Pankewycz et al. [423] reported that immunoglobulins eluted from nephritic kidneys of MLR-lpr/lpr mice showed a high degree of polyreactivity. In addition, Madaio et al. [328] reported that two monoclonal anti-DNA antibodies, derived from MRL-lpr/lpr mice, directly bound to isolated normal glomeruli and that one of these antibodies interacted with glomeruli in vivo to produce immune deposits. The nature of the antigens within the glomerular deposits was not determined. The authors presented evidence against the possibility that DNA was the antigen, but this was not excluded. Dang and Harbeck [123] reported on similar experiments that failed to provide evidence that anti-DNA antibodies can interact directly with normal glomerular components. Anti-ds-DNA antibodies were isolated from the sera of old NZB/W mice labeled and injected into NZB/W mice of different ages. Glomerular accumulation of the injected antibodies occurred in old mice (with glomerular deposits), but not in young mice. The findings indicate that free anti-ds-DNA antibodies interact with immune complexes in glomeruli (presumably DNA-containing complexes) but not with normal glomeruli.

It has been shown in several studies that renal eluates from SLE mice are enriched for anti-DNA antibodies [145]. The key question concerning this finding is whether the anti-DNA antibodies are combined with DNA or with some cross-reacting antigen. Evidence for the presence of DNA in the immune deposits of mice (or human beings) with lupus nephritis has come largely from immunofluorescence studies. Using serum with anti-DNA antibodies obtained from a patient with SLE, Lambert and Dixon [298] showed by immunofluorescence that human IgG bound to the glomeruli of nephritic mice in tissue sections in the same sites where mouse IgG and C3 were found. Eilat [145] has questioned the evidence that DNA was demonstrated, because the studies failed to eliminate the possibility that the anti-DNA antibodies bound to cross-reactive glomerular antigens.

In summary, in murine lupus nephritis there is evidence both for glomerular accumulation of DNA–anti-DNA complexes and for formation of complexes by interaction of anti-DNA antibodies with cross-reacting antigens in glomeruli. Further studies are needed to characterize the antigens that participate in glomerular deposits in murine lupus nephritis and to clarify the mechanisms by which immune deposits develop.

Summary of Factors Leading to the Formation of Glomerular Immune Deposits

Despite an enormous amount of research on mechanisms of formation of glomerular immune deposits, a number of important questions remain unanswered. Nevertheless, a few conclusions appear warranted.

1. The *initial* event in immune deposit formation can be either deposition of circulating immune complexes or in situ formation. In either case, secondary events are necessary for the formation of aggregates that are recognized by immunofluorescence and electron microscopy as immune deposits; these include redistribution of complexes or addition of free antibodies or other reactants.

2. One mechanism of in situ formation is through combination of autoantibodies with native glomerular antigens. If the antigen can be identified and localized, the initial event can be clarified, as in Heymann nephritis. However, the secondary events, which may include shedding, aggregation, or redistribution by hemodynamic forces, are more difficult to elucidate.

3. Another mechanism of in situ formation is through combination of antibodies with planted antigens. Such deposits generally form along peripheral loops and especially in subepithelial regions. In most experimental models, the antigen is first planted in glomeruli, followed by administration of antibodies; under these circumstances, the initial event in immune deposit formation clearly occurs in situ. However, in naturally occurring diseases, it is possible that complexes containing antigens with an affinity for the glomerulus form in the circulation and that these circulating complexes initiate or contribute to the development of immune deposits.

4. The ways in which circulating complexes lead to glomerular immune deposits are diverse and not completely understood. In several models it is clear that the complexes that initially localize in glomeruli must subsequently be modified by complexes or antibodies with different properties in order to form deposits recognizable by immunofluorescence or electron microscopy. For example, complexes with antibodies of low avidity may localize along the GBM, but in order to aggregate and persist, they must combine with antibodies or complexes of high avidity. Similarly, following initial localization of cationic complexes, neutral complexes may interact with those in glomeruli to produce deposits. Thus it is often futile to look for nephritogenic complexes; only certain combinations of complexes may be effective in producing immune deposits.

Despite these comments, studies on active serum sickness models suggest that high levels of complexes, especially those containing precipitating, or high-avidity, antibodies, often result in

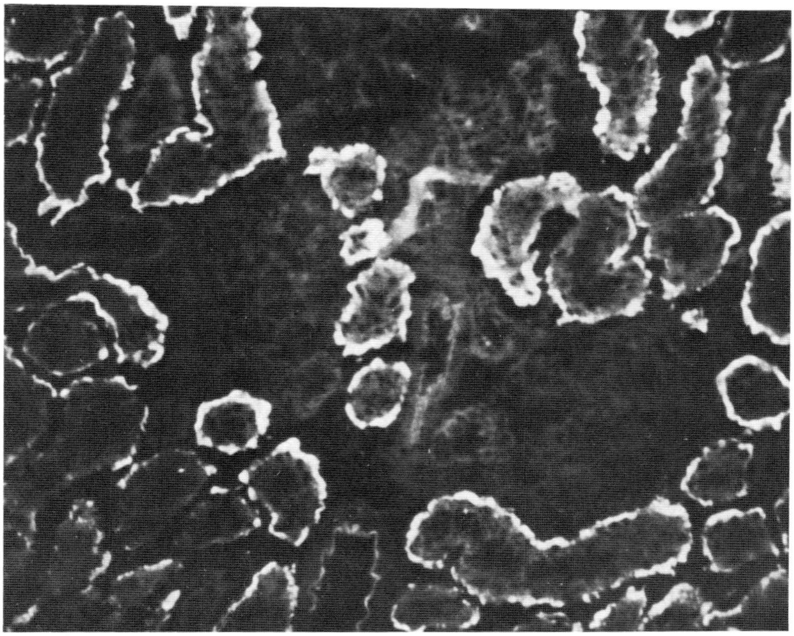

FIG. 3-7. *Granular deposits of IgG are seen along the basement membranes of proximal tubules. The glomeruli contain no deposits. From a rabbit immunized with homologous kidney and Freund's adjuvant. (From McCluskey, R. T. J. Exp. Med. 134: 242S, 1971, by copyright permission of the Rockefeller University Press.)*

mesangial deposits and mild disease, whereas lower levels of complexes composed of antibodies of low avidity or with positive charge often produce more serious diseases with peripheral loop deposits.

5. Certain host factors promote the glomerular deposition of circulating complexes, including reduced clearance capacity of the CR1 transport or mononuclear phagocyte system and defective complement-mediated inhibition of precipitation or solubilization of complexes.

Experimental Studies on Tubulointerstitial Immune Complex Nephritis

Until about 1970, models of immunologically mediated renal disease were studied almost entirely with respect to glomerular injury, and any observed tubulointerstitial damage was often labeled "secondary." Since then, numerous studies have shown that immunologic mechanisms can produce tubulointerstitial renal disease either through humoral antibodies—by immune complex formation or anti-tubular basement membrane (TBM)—or through cell-mediated mechanisms.

The first reported models with tubulointerstitial immune deposits were in rabbits given renal allografts or immunized with homologous crude renal extracts in complete Freund's adjuvant [278—280]. After repeated injections over several weeks, many of the rabbits developed granular deposits of IgG and C3 along the tubular basement membranes of proximal tubules (Fig. 3-7) and often tubular atrophy, interstitial fibrosis, and irregular, generally sparse interstitial mononuclear cell infiltrates. Evidence was obtained that the deposits contained autoantibodies and autologous antigens of proximal tubular-cell origin. Thus circulating antibodies, as well as antibodies eluted from kidneys, were found by immunofluorescence to react with the deposits and with the cytoplasm of proximal tubules, but not with other parts of the kidney [280]. The deposits appear to form locally as antigens escape from tubular cells and encounter autoantibodies derived from the circulation. Similar mechanisms may account for tubulointerstitial deposits seen in some rats with Heymann nephritis [281] or in rats injected with Tamm-Horsfall protein [165].

Renal tubulointerstitial immune deposits (as well as extrarenal deposits) also have been described in chronic serum sickness in rabbits, especially in a model induced by multiple intradaily injections of relatively large doses of BSA [72], a protocol that results in the production of very high levels of precipitating antibodies. In the kidney, extraglomerular deposits containing BSA, IgG, IgM, and C3 were found along the tubular basement membrane and in the interstitium. It is not clear whether the complexes form in situ or are deposited from the circulation. However, it is possible that circulating complexes adhere to Fc-binding sites in the interstitium [177].

ROLE OF ANTI-BASEMENT MEMBRANE ANTIBODIES IN RENAL DISEASE

The traditional classification of antibody-mediated glomerular disease includes two major categories: immune complex glomerulonephritis and anti-GBM nephritis. Both forms involve combination of antigens and antibodies, and the distinction between them is based largely on immunofluorescence findings of granular immune deposits in the first category and of continuous (linear) accumulation of IgG in the second. The reason certain anti-GBM antibodies do not form granular deposits is that they do not cause redistribution and aggregation of the target antigens. However, as described earlier, antibodies against certain components of the GBM can cause deposit formation. Thus the distinction between anti-GBM nephritis and immune complex nephritis is somewhat arbitrary. Nevertheless, the best defined and most serious form of anti-GBM nephritis—that associated with autoantibodies against the Goodpasture antigen—is always characterized by linear accumulation of IgG and continues to be classified separately from immune complex glomerulonephritis.

Experimental Studies on Anti-Basement Membrane Nephritis

Experimental models of anti-basement membrane nephritis were first produced with glomerular basement membrane antigens (anti-GBM nephritis) and later with tubular basement membrane antigens (anti-TBM nephritis).

ANTI-GLOMERULAR BASEMENT MEMBRANE (GBM) NEPHRITIS

There are two main ways in which anti-GBM nephritis can be produced experimentally: (1) by intravenous injection of heterologous anti-GBM antibodies into nonimmunized recipients [532] (nephrotoxic serum or Masugi nephritis), and (2) by immunization with basement-membrane preparations, with the production of autoimmune glomerulonephritis (Steblay nephritis) [493].

Nephrotoxic Serum Nephritis (Masugi Nephritis)

Nephrotoxic serum nephritis has been produced in a number of species, but models have been most extensively investigated in rabbits and rats [532]. The disease has two phases. The first (heterologous phase), which begins shortly after injection, results from the fixation of the injected antibodies in the GBM. The second (autologous phase) begins several days later, when host antibodies combine with the heterologous immunoglobulin in the glomerular basement membrane. In both, the heterologous- and autologous-phase immunoglobulins can be demonstrated within glomeruli by immunofluorescence in a highly characteristic pattern of completely continuous (linear) accumulation along the basement membrane (Fig. 3-8).

A modification of the basic model of nephrotoxic serum nephritis was described by Unanue

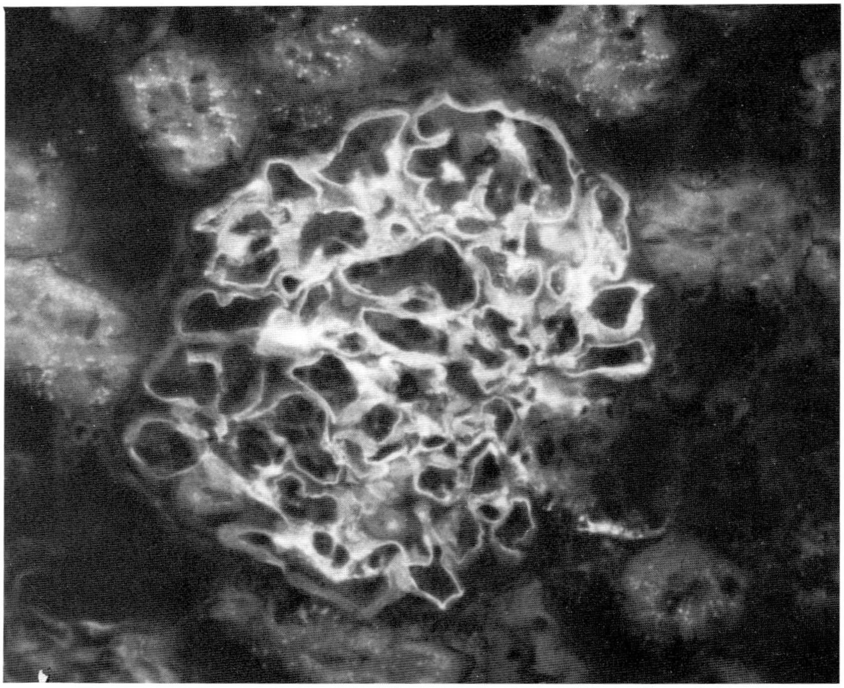

FIG. 3-8. *Immunoglobulins are seen in a completely continuous, linear pattern along the glomerular basement membrane. From a rabbit with nephrotoxic serum nephritis. (From McCluskey, R. T., and Vassalli, P. In C. Rouiller and A. E. Muller (Eds.),* The Kidney, *Vol. 2. New York: Academic Press, 1969.)*

and Dixon in 1965 [531]; rats were preimmunized with rabbit IgG in complete Freund's adjuvant and then given rabbit anti-rat kidney serum. Because of the preimmunization, the autologous phase begins early and the glomerular disease is accelerated and intensified. The model is sometimes referred to as *accelerated* or *telescoped nephrotoxic serum nephritis*. In other models, accelerated disease is produced not by active immunization, but by passive administration of antibodies against the heterologous immunoglobulin shortly after the administration of nephrotoxic serum.

The glomerular changes in the second (autologous) phase of nephrotoxic serum nephritis are more severe than those in the first, and are generally characterized by marked hypercellularity of the tufts and exuberant crescent formation [538,539]. The tuft hypercellularity appears to result principally from infiltration of mononuclear cells [290], although some increase in mesangial and endothelial cells also occurs. With severe disease, deposits of fibrin appear in Bowman's space, often in association with breaks in the GBM, and this is generally followed by crescent formation [538,539].

The second phase may be characterized by severe glomerular damage even though the amount of heterologous immunoglobulin fixed in glomeruli is far below that required to produce detectable damage in the first phase. This may be explained in part by the continuing production of host antibodies, which results in repeated and multiple combinations with the heterologous immunoglobulin. However, it is also possible that cell-

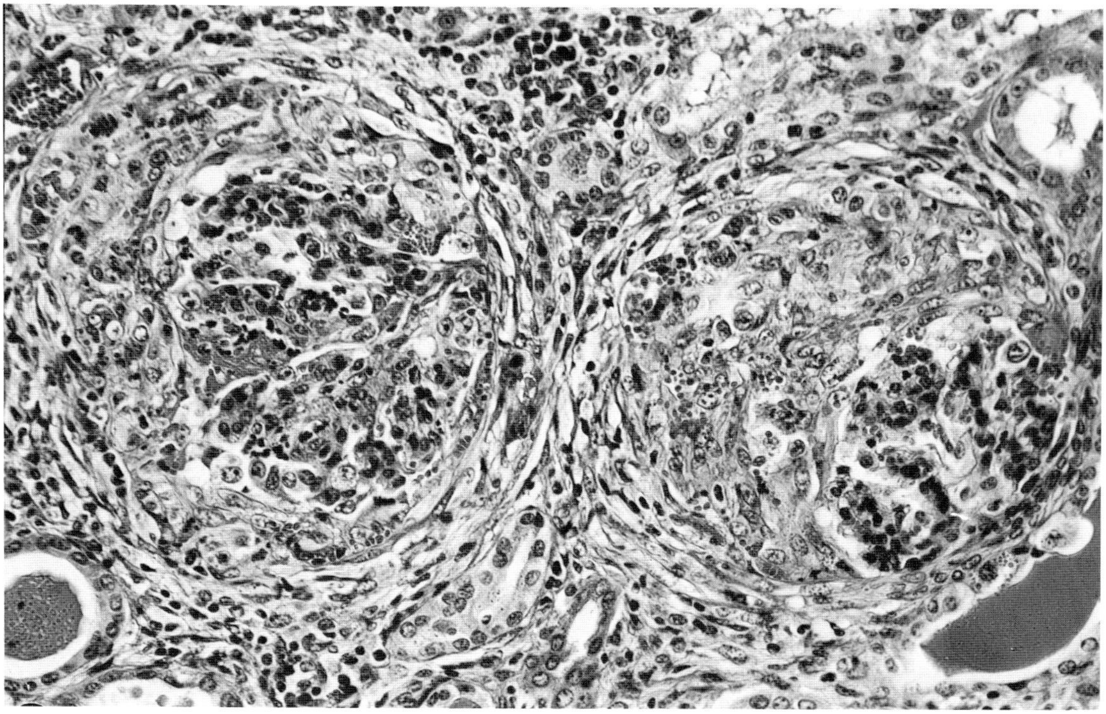

Fig. 3-9. *Sheep with autoimmune glomerulonephritis. The sheep received four injections of human glomerular basement membrane and was killed on day 50, at which time the blood urea nitrogen was 300 mg/100 ml. Large crescents are seen. There is hypercellularity of glomerular tufts. H&E; ×291. (From Steblay, R. W.* J. Exp. Med. *116: 253, 1962, by copyright permission of the Rockefeller University Press.)*

mediated reactivity against the heterologous immunoglobulin contributes to the damage, as discussed below. It also has been suggested that an autoimmune response against the GBM is triggered in Masugi nephritis [300], but this has not been substantiated [532].

In the accelerated model of nephrotoxic serum nephritis, neutrophils are seen to infiltrate the glomeruli transiently shortly after injection, but within 4 days, monocyte infiltration and some degree of proliferation of intrinsic cells lead to severe hypercellular glomerular lesions [473].

Although nephrotoxic serum nephritis is produced in a highly contrived fashion, studies of the model have been useful in elucidating secondary mechanisms of glomerular injury, as discussed later.

Autoimmune Anti-GBM Glomerulonephritis (Steblay Nephritis)

In 1962, Steblay [493] reported that sheep given injections of heterologous GBM preparations developed severe glomerulonephritis. Following repeated injections of human, monkey, rabbit, rat, or dog glomerular basement membrane preparations in complete Freund's adjuvant, the sheep died within 38 to 90 days in renal failure and were found to have severe glomerulonephritis with hypercellularity and extensive crescent formation (Fig. 3-9).

The evidence that autoantibodies to glomerular basement membrane play a pathogenic role in Steblay nephritis is compelling. Immunofluorescence typically shows continuous (linear) accumulation of immunoglobulin and complement along the GBM in a pattern indistinguishable from that seen in nephrotoxic serum nephritis. In addition, circulating antibodies reactive with normal sheep GBM are found [308,455,495], as shown by indirect immunofluorescence. The fact that the levels of circulating anti-GBM antibodies often increase following removal of both kidneys [308] indicates that some of the antibodies, presumably those of highest avidity, are rapidly removed from the circulation by fixation in glomeruli. Finally, it has been possible to produce transient glomerular lesions in nonimmunized sheep by transfer of serum [308,455]. The capacity of the serum to produce lesions was eliminated by absorption in vitro with isolated sheep glomerular basement membranes. Evidence that cell-mediated mechanisms also play a role in autoimmune anti-GBM nephritis is discussed later.

The major antigen of the basement membrane involved in Steblay nephritis is in the NC1 domain of type IV collagen, as shown by the reactivity of glomerular eluates [81]. The characterization of this antigen (the Goodpasture antigen) came from studies on human anti-GBM nephritis, as reviewed later.

ANTI-TUBULAR BASEMENT MEMBRANE (TBM) NEPHRITIS: DESCRIPTION OF THE MODELS

Several models of autoimmune tubulointerstitial nephritis have been described in which the target antigens are in tubular basement membranes (TBM) [16]. The first description of renal disease associated with anti-TBM antibodies was that of Steblay and Rudofsky [496], who reported that guinea pigs injected with rabbit TBM preparations in adjuvant developed severe tubulointerstitial nephritis. Others subsequently showed that similar lesions could be induced by immunizing guinea pigs with bovine TBM preparations [304,536] or by immunizing certain strains of rats with homologous or heterologous TBM or GBM preparations [294,306,443,504]. In guinea pigs, the lesions are usually fully developed within 2 weeks and are characterized by cortical infiltrates of mononuclear and multinuclear cells, as well as by tubular-cell damage and disruption of tubular basement membranes; mononuclear cells are often seen invading tubules. In rats, the lesions are similar but develop more slowly and often exhibit numerous neutrophils, especially early. In both species, immunofluorescence reveals a highly characteristic picture, with a continuous (linear) accumulation of IgG along the basement membranes of proximal tubules (Fig. 3-10). Anti-TBM antibodies are found in the circulation, as shown by indirect immunofluorescence.

Several investigators have described the development of circulating or renal-bound anti-TBM antibodies, or both, in certain strains of mice following immunization with heterologous basement-membrane preparations in complete Freund's adjuvant [55,209,451,452]. However, in contrast with guinea pigs or rats, tubulointerstitial damage in mice is usually mild or absent and develops only weeks after the appearance of anti-TBM antibodies. Anti-TBM antibodies also have been observed to develop "spontaneously" in some NZB/W mice [451].

Nephritogenic TBM Antigens

Although some basement-membrane antigens capable of inducing renal disease are present in both the GBM and the TBM, the nephritogenic antigens involved in most models of anti-TBM nephritis are apparently confined to tubules.

Clayman et al. [96] isolated a nephritogenic TBM antigen from rabbit kidneys by collagenase digestion and showed it to be a 48-kD glycoprotein (3M-1). Immunization of guinea pigs with 3M-1 in complete Freund's adjuvant induced anti-TBM nephritis in guinea pigs, whereas TBM preparations depleted of 3M-1 were ineffective. These findings indicate that 3M-1 is a major nephritogenic antigen in experimental anti-TBM nephritis. Moreover, 3M-1 is apparently similar to the TBM antigen associated with the very rare forms of isolated anti-TBM nephritis in man [97]. How-

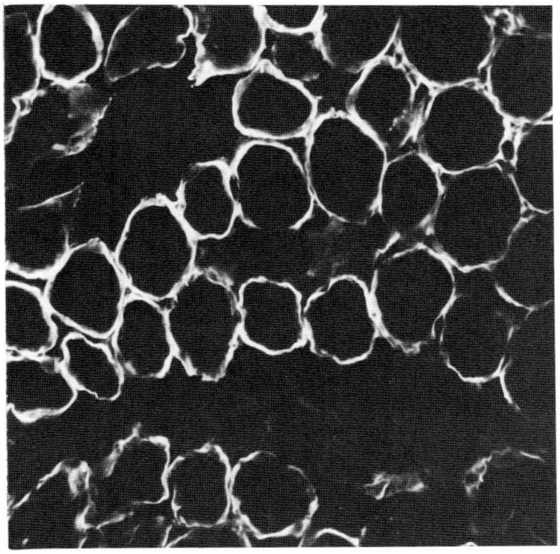

Fig. 3-10. *Smooth, linear staining of IgG is seen along the basement membrane of proximal tubules. From a Brown Norway rat immunized with rat kidney. (From McCluskey, R. T., and Klassen, J.* N. Engl. J. Med. *288: 564, 1973. Reprinted by permission of the* New England Journal of Medicine.*)*

ever, other TBM antigens may be involved in anti-TBM nephritis, especially forms associated with anti-GBM nephritis [563].

The Role of Antibodies in Anti-TBM Nephritis

Both antibodies and T cells have been shown to participate in the renal damage, although the relative importance of these two mechanisms varies from one model to another. In this section I will review the evidence that supports the pathogenic role of anti-TBM antibodies. The transfer of serum IgG fractions from guinea pigs with actively induced anti-TBM nephritis to outbred or strain-13 guinea pigs leads to the development in the recipients of histologic and immunofluorescence findings that are indistinguishable from those seen in the donors [494,496,536]. Thus the evidence that anti-TBM antibodies can initiate renal damage seems incontrovertible, at least in susceptible strains of guinea pigs.

Transfer experiments with serum in rat anti-TBM nephritis have yielded variable results. Early attempts to transfer lesions with serum were largely or entirely unsuccessful [504]. More recently, however, Bannister and Wilson [30] reported that transfer of anti-TBM alloantibodies to BN rats resulted in fixation of antibodies along the TBM and focal tubulointerstitial infiltrates. The failure of earlier transfer experiments may be due to the fact that the most pathogenic antibodies are fixed to the TBM and are not available in the serum. Passive transfer of anti-TBM antibodies in mice has been reported to produce mild lesions [571].

T CELL MECHANISMS IN RENAL DISEASE

So far I have discussed ways in which humoral antibodies can participate in the production of renal injury. I will now consider the role of the other major branch of the immune response, that of T cells.

A pathogenic role of T cells in renal disease was not appreciated until relatively recently. This belated recognition was due in part to the lack of knowledge of T cells and in part to overinterpretation of the importance of antibodies in experimental models. It is now known that T cells can play a role in renal disease either indirectly, through helper-cell function for antibody production, or directly, through T cell mechanisms of tissue injury, which can cause either tubulointerstitial or glomerular injury.

Following the discovery in the late 1960s that T cells are required for most antibody responses, an essential role of the helper function of T cells in most immunologically mediated renal diseases was readily accepted. (Probably only under exceptional circumstances can T cell–*independent* antibody responses lead to renal disease, such as, for example, through polyclonal B cell activation by bacterial lipopolysaccharide [190].) However, acceptance of the importance of direct renal injury by T cell mechanisms has been slow in coming, especially with respect to glomerular injury [132]. The main reasons for this are as follows: For one thing, when immunofluorescence studies of renal tissue were performed, it was learned that glomerular deposits of immunoglobulins and complement are present in most forms of human and experimental glomerulonephritis in which there is reason to suspect immunologic mechanisms. In addition, in some models, notably in anti-GBM nephritis and Heymann nephritis, it was shown that lesions can be readily induced by passive transfer of antibodies. Furthermore, in anti-GBM nephritis, quantitative studies showed a correlation between the amount of antibodies transferred and their severity of injury. However, in acute serum sickness models, it was obvious that there was a poor correlation between the abundance of glomerular deposits and the severity of lesions [138]. Nevertheless, the belief in the role of antibodies was so firmly held that even in a model of acute glomerulonephritis that virtually lacked immunoglobulin deposits, induced in rabbits by injections of ovalbumin, the lesions were attributed to immune complexes [184]. An important reason why cellular mechanisms were not considered was that a key histologic feature of delayed-type hypersensitivity, namely the accumulation of mononuclear cells, was not fully appreciated in glomerular lesions until recently. And although interstitial lymphocyte infiltrates were long known to be present in many renal diseases, their significance was not understood—they were often considered to be "secondary," although this clearly did not explain their presence.

In the past decade or so, several models of T cell–mediated glomerular and tubulointerstitial injury have been described. In addition, evidence of T cell–mediated mechanisms has been obtained in experimental and human renal diseases by identification of T cells and other mononuclear cells in tissue sections. Before I discuss the results of these studies, I will review some basic aspects of the T cell response, the role of T cells in autoimmune disease, and salient features of T cell–mediated reactions.

T Cell Recognition of Antigen

Almost all immune responses begin with the interaction of antigen with T cells. An enormous amount has been learned in recent years about how T cells recognize antigen. A thorough discussion of this subject is beyond the scope of this chapter, but because of its importance to the understanding of the origins of immunologic disease, especially of autoimmune diseases, I will review some aspects (for key articles, see refs. 45, 46, 80, 163, 178, 200, 319, 321, 323, and 482).

Unlike B cells, T cells do not react with antigens directly, but rather with peptide fragments of antigens bound to class I or class II (Ia or HL-DR) major histocompatibility complex (MHC) molecules on the surface of antigen-presenting cells (such as macrophages, B cells, or dendritic cells). The requirement for binding of antigen fragments to MHC molecules is referred to as *MHC restriction.* The recent elucidation of the complete three-dimensional structure of a class I MHC molecule has revealed a single potential antigen-binding site formed by a groove on the outer surface of the molecule [54]. Each MHC molecule can bind multiple peptides, and different peptides can compete for the binding site; this offers a theoretical approach for prevention of a specific immune response [2,4,195].

Among T cell subsets, $CD4^+$ (T4) cells recognize antigen bound to class II molecules and $CD8^+$ (T8) cells react with antigens bound to class I molecules. There is evidence that CD4 and CD8 molecules interact with nonpolymorphic regions on class II or class I molecules, which may promote cellular adhesion.

In order to react with T cells, most antigens must first be "processed" by antigen-presenting cells through incompletely understood mechanisms that involve internalization and degradation of the antigen with combination of peptide fragments with MHC molecules, which are delivered to the cell surface for presentation. The antigenic peptide fragments (sometimes referred to as *sequential epitopes*) must contain at least seven amino acids.

T cells recognize the peptide-MHC complex by means of T cell antigen receptors (usually $\alpha\beta$ receptors), which are heterodimeric glycoproteins expressed on the surface of T cells in association with the CD3 complex [126]. The T cell antigen receptors are composed of variable and constant regions, and the variable regions are encoded by distinct germline gene elements that rearrange during differentiation to form continuous functional genes in a manner similar to the rearrangement of immunoglobulin genes. The process of rearrangement largely accounts for the enormous diversity of the T cell repertoire, with the generation of clones bearing unique T cell receptors, each with its own antigen specificity [126].

Autoimmune Diseases

The origins of autoimmunity and autoimmune diseases are extraordinarily complex and incompletely understood. Because T cells are pivotal to most autoimmune responses, it is convenient to consider the subject here. Several reviews and key articles have appeared recently on this rapidly developing topic [2,3,208,212,332,421,521]. Here I will discuss general concepts of autoimmunity, with emphasis on aspects that may be relevant to the development and potentially the prevention or treatment of autoimmune diseases.

An *autoimmune disease* can be defined as one in which cell or tissue injury results from an immunologically specific reaction against an autologous antigen. Not all autoimmune responses lead to disease [449]; certain types of autoantibodies are commonly found in apparently normal individuals, and autoreactive B and T cells also may be demonstrated [59]. However, differences between the fine specificity of pathogenic and nonpathogenic autoantibodies have been demonstrated in some cases. Moreover, certain types of autoantibodies are almost never found in normal individuals—in particular, anti-GBM antibodies against the Goodpasture antigen, or anti-neutrophil cytoplasmic antibodies (ANCA), which are associated with necrotizing and crescentic glomerulonephritis, as discussed later.

Autoimmune injury may be mediated by antibodies, by effector T cells, or by a combination of antibody and T cell mechanisms. Most pathogenic autoantibodies are IgG antibodies, and their production is T cell dependent. Autoimmune diseases can be classified as organ-specific or systemic, although there are overlapping forms. Examples of clearly defined experimental autoimmune renal diseases are listed in Table 3-1.

Table 3-1. *Experimental autoimmune renal diseases*

Disease	Major autoantigens	Primary immunopathogenetic mechanisms
Anti-GBM nephritis	NC1 domain of type IV collagen [81]	Antibodies and/or T cells interact with autoantigens in GBM
Heymann nephritis	Gp330 on podocytes [268,269]	Shedding of complexes from podocyte surface into GBM
Mercuric chloride–induced glomerulonephritis	Laminin; type IV collagen [167]	Antibodies combine with fixed and secreted GBM antigens
Nephritis in graft-versus-host disease	Dipeptidyl peptidase IV on podocytes [76]	Shedding of complexes from podocyte surface into GBM
Murine lupus nephritis	DNA? Histones? Intrinsic glomerular antigens? [145]	Deposition of circulating immune complexes and in situ formation
Anti-TBM nephritis	TBM Ag 3M-1 [96]	Antibodies and/or T cells interact with TBM antigens
Tubulointerstitial immune complex nephritis	Proximal tubular cytoplasmic antigen [280]	Combination of antibodies with antigens released from tubules

MAINTENANCE OF TOLERANCE TO SELF ANTIGENS

The mechanisms that are normally responsible for tolerance to self antigens are not entirely understood. Two general mechanisms are often considered: (1) deletion of autoreactive clones of lymphocytes, and (2) suppression of autoreactive cells, in one of several ways. There is evidence that both mechanisms play a role in maintaining tolerance.

Deletion of Autoreactive Clones

Burnet [79] proposed that autoreactive clones of lymphocytes are eliminated during ontogeny by an undefined intrathymic process. Belief in this mechanism was shaken by the finding that precursors of autoreactive clones are present in normal individuals in the T and especially the B cell compartment [59]. However, recent experiments have provided compelling evidence that most thymocytes with T cell receptors for self antigens are deleted or rendered inactive (anergic) in the thymus [261,322,439*a*]. Nevertheless, some self-reactive T cells escape and reach the peripheral lymphoid tissue or perhaps develop in the periphery.

Suppression of Autoreactive Clones

There is evidence that self-reactive T cells that escape deletion in the thymus are held in check by suppressor cells (Ts) [121,246,506,522]. Antigen-specific suppressor cells have been convincingly demonstrated in a number of systems, both in vitro and in vivo (mainly through transfer experiments), but have fallen out of favor in recent years because there are no entirely specific markers for such cells and because genes and gene products accounting for their actions have not been isolated. Anti-idiotypes may explain some T cell suppressor function [400]. Of relevance to renal disease, there is evidence that antigen-specific suppressor cells or their products can ameliorate tubulointerstitial nephritis in mice [334,394,398,526].

Another mechanism of tolerance that has been proposed consists of functional elimination of autoreactive peripheral T cells by "veto cells," which include not only lymphocytes, but other cell types. When a T cell recognizes and binds to a self antigen on the surface of a veto cell, the T cell is rendered nonfunctional, probably mainly through cytolysis [157].

INITIATION OF THE AUTOIMMUNE RESPONSE THROUGH BREAKING OF TOLERANCE

The mechanisms accounting for naturally occurring autoimmune responses are not understood. Both genetic and environmental factors appear to be important. Models of organ-specific autoimmune diseases are generally induced by immunization with homologous or heterologous antigens in adjuvants; autologous antigens are generally less effective or ineffective. In a general way, it is thought that such immunization procedures break T cell tolerance because the immunogens closely resemble the corresponding autologous antigens, yet are sufficiently different to be recognized as foreign. Similarly, infection with certain microorganisms may break tolerance because the microbes bear epitopes like those on target autoantigens (molecular mimicry) [419]. Many viral proteins share epitopes with mammalian proteins [166].

Precisely how a cross-reacting antigen breaks tolerance is unknown. In order to induce a T cell–dependent response, the antigen must be bound to MHC molecules on antigen-presenting cells, as described earlier. Susceptibility to most of the models of autoimmune renal disease is under MHC control [233,234,294,390,392,497]. Furthermore, there is abundant evidence for a strong MHC linkage of many human autoimmune diseases [402,521]. The MHC association of autoimmune diseases may result *in part* from the ability of MHC products in susceptible, but not other, individuals to bind and present relevant autologous peptide fragments. In support of this, recent evidence shows an association of certain nucleotide sequences, even in different MHC molecules, with susceptibility to rheumatoid arthritis [193,194]. Since most autoreactive T cell clones are eliminated in ontogeny, and because binding of self peptides can occur with only some MHC molecules, one might expect that only a very limited number of epitopes would be recognized by autoreactive T cells [200]. Indeed, several studies have provided evidence that T cells involved in autoimmune disease have limited heterogeneity [1,572]. This raises the possibility that selective elimination of specific autoreactive T cells or of specific MHC products can prevent autoimmune disease [1], and this has been achieved in certain models [1,572]. However, these experiments have involved inbred strains and well-defined autoantigens; the complexity of human diseases and populations makes this approach a distant hope for mankind.

INITIATION OF THE AUTOIMMUNE RESPONSE THROUGH RELEASE OF SEQUESTERED ANTIGENS

If an autologous antigen normally does not have any contact with lymphocytes, it should behave as a foreign antigen upon release from its "sequestered" site [421]. The number of antigens that are entirely hidden is probably very small and is certainly smaller than once believed. However, some antigens in the brain, eye, testis, and basement membrane may be effectively sequestered. It is possible that release of hidden antigens from basement membranes may initiate an autoimmune response, although the evidence for this is not compelling and rests largely on the observation that anti-GBM antibodies sometimes arise in the course of other glomerular diseases in which basement-membrane damage occurs [277].

INAPPROPRIATE (ABERRANT) EXPRESSION OF CLASS II MHC MOLECULES: POSSIBLE ROLE IN INITIATION OF AUTOIMMUNE RESPONSE

It has been postulated that expression of class II MHC antigens on cells that normally lack such antigens may induce autoimmunity. This hypothesis has received considerable attention in recent years [65]. Aberrant class II MHC expression has been observed in epithelial or endothelial cells in several autoimmune diseases [65], as well as in other inflammatory conditions, including interstitial nephritis in man [67] and in MRL-lpr/lpr mice [568]. Interferon γ is a potent inducer of aberrant MHC antigen expression on many types of cells, including renal tubule cells [209]. The hypothesis that aberrant MHC expression can induce autoimmune disease depends on the following assumptions: T cells normally fail to recognize certain organ-specific antigens not because self-reactive clones have been eliminated, but rather because potential autoantigens cannot be recognized by T cells in the absence of MHC molecules on the parenchymal cells. With the acquisition of MHC class II molecules (perhaps as the result of a viral infection, with release of interferon γ), the parenchymal cells can present their own antigens and induce autoimmunity. Although this hypothesis is attractive, there is no direct evidence to support it. Thus induction of expression of class II MHC usually does not by itself initiate autoimmune disease [424]. And even in autoimmune diseases in which aberrant MHC expression occurs, it is possible that locally released autoantigens are processed and presented by conventional antigen-presenting cells [546]. Nevertheless, increased expression of MHC antigens on epithelial cells may render them more susceptible to cytotoxic injury, and this could perpetuate or intensify certain autoimmune diseases. In this regard, Haverty et al. [209] showed that increased expression of class II MHC products on proximal tubule cells, induced by interferon γ, is associated with heightened susceptibility to anti-TBM nephritis in mice.

Functional Roles of T Cells

Our ability to analyze cellular interactions and functions in cell-mediated reactions has increased considerably in recent years in part because of the acquisition of knowledge of the heterogeneity of T cells. T cells can be classified on the basis of phenotypic markers, especially clusters of differentiation (CD) surface antigens, on the basis of function, or on profiles of lymphokine production. On a functional basis, T cells are commonly divided into effector or regulatory cells, although there is overlap between the two categories. Cells with the following functional roles are generally considered: (1) cells with helper or inducer function for B cell or T cell differentiation (Th), (2) cells that mediate delayed-type hypersensitivity reactions (Tdth), (3) cells with suppressor function (Ts), or (4) cells with cytolytic function (Tc). There is only an imperfect correlation between phenotype and function, and the widely used designations of $CD4^+$ T cells as helper/inducer or of $CD8^+$ T cells as cytotoxic/suppressor cells, although generally valid, is not entirely correct [293].

Classification and Analysis of T Cell–Mediated Reactions inVivo

The term *cellular,* or *cell-mediated, immunity* is sometimes used in reference to reactions in which mononuclear phagocytes play a role, irrespective of whether these cells are recruited by T cells, as occurs in DTH reactions, or through other mechanisms, such as Fc receptor adherence or chemotactic attraction. In this section I will deal with reactions that are initiated by interaction of T cells with antigens. Two prototypic T cell–mediated reactions are recognized: delayed-type hypersensitivity (DTH) and cytotoxic T cell reactions.

DELAYED-TYPE HYPERSENSITIVITY (DTH)

The development of DTH depends on proliferation of sensitized T cells in lymphoid tissue following exposure to certain antigens [295]. The sensitized cells enter the circulation, making it possible for them to interact with antigen virtually anywhere in the host. Reactions are triggered by interaction of a few sensitized T cells with antigen presented on accessory cells—such as macrophages, B cells, or dendritic cells—bound to major histocompatibility complex (MHC) products. Most of the T cells that initiate DTH reactions have the $CD4^+$ (T4) phenotype; however, since $CD8^+$ (T8) cells also can sometimes trigger DTH reactions [574], and since it may be that not all $CD4^+$ T cells mediate DTH reactions, the functional designation Tdh is useful. Following contact with antigen, the Tdh cells are stimulated to produce and release lymphokines, which result in a slowly developing inflammatory reaction with recruitment of various leukocytes [357,360,362]. Prominent among the cells that emigrate at sites of DTH reactions are monocytes and recently formed lymphocytes with various antigen specificities and phenotypes.

The infiltrates in DTH reactions vary considerably and may be characterized by diffuse or perivascular collections of lymphocytes and mononuclear phagocytes, by granulomas with relatively few lymphocytes, or even by granulocyte-rich infiltrates. Similar infiltrates can be induced by mechanisms that are independent of T cells. Thus histologic features do not provide a reliable guide to the identification of DTH reactions.

CYTOLYTIC T CELL REACTIONS

The second major prototypic T cell reaction, T cell–mediated cytolysis has been studied mainly in vitro; however, evidence for cytolytic T cell killing in vivo also has been obtained, especially in experimental viral infections [573], in allografts undergoing rejection, and possibly in tumors or autoimmune diseases. The killing of a target cell by a cytolytic T cell requires close contact between the two cells. The binding of a cytolytic T cell to its target (an MHC-restricted event) stimulates the cell's cytolytic activity. Although the mechanism of lysis has not been fully elucidated, there is evidence that the cytolytic cells secrete factors that damage cell membranes [569]. Most human T cells that exert cytolytic effects belong to the $CD8^+$ subset and recognize target cells bearing class I MHC antigens [369]. However, $CD4^+$ T cells also can function as cytolytic T cells against targets bearing class II MHC antigens [293].

Analysis of the Role of Infiltrating Cells by Immunohistochemical Techniques

The development of monoclonal antibodies against antigens on lymphoid cells has made it possible to identify various cell types in tissue sections by immunohistochemical methods. Despite a number of problems in interpretation [362], characterization of subsets of mononuclear cells in inflammatory infiltrates can provide evidence for certain cellular mechanisms. Thus the finding of large numbers of T cells in a lesion, especially cells with activation markers, notably transferrin receptors [439], and class II MHC antigens, especially HLA-DR [82,380], indicates that T cells are playing an active role, probably in response to an antigen present at the site. In addition, a preponderance of $CD4^+$ T cells (especially in association with mononuclear phagocytes) is indicative of DTH reaction. Furthermore, since most nucleated cells bear class I MHC antigens and are targets for $CD8^+$ cell cytolysis, lesions with $CD8^+$ cells in juxtaposition to parenchymal cells undergoing necrosis may be interpreted as cytolytic T cell reactions. Studies of human viral infections [425], autoimmune diseases [49], and allografts undergoing rejection support this view.

Although these interpretations are probably valid in general, they are not definitive and do not provide a complete picture of cellular events in an inflammatory reaction, largely because of the complexity and changing composition of infiltrating cells and the imperfect correlation between phenotype and function. Another problem with the analysis of infiltrating mononuclear cells through immunohistochemical methods is that no information is gained about the antigen specificity of the lymphocytes. However, recently developed methods employing IL-2–containing media make it possible to propagate activated T cells from lesions, and this permits assessment of antigen reactivity of at least some of the infiltrating cells [295,295*a*].

Analysis of Cell-Mediated Reactions in Experimental Studies by Cell Transfer

Evidence for the role of T cells or of T cell subsets in the production of immunologic disease can best be obtained in transfer experiments, which obviously can be performed only in experimental models. *The most reliable evidence for a primary role of T cells is provided by the demonstration that the systemic transfer of T cells, but not of serum, from an affected donor to a normal syngeneic recipient results in lesions within a few days at sites where antigen is present.*

Local transfer experiments that involve the direct introduction into tissue of large numbers of cells are difficult to interpret unless appropriate controls are entirely negative.

T Cell Mechanisms in Experimental Tubulointerstitial Nephritis

T cell–mediated mechanisms have been shown to be largely or partially responsible for injury in several forms of experimentally induced tubulointerstitial nephritis.

TUBULOINTERSTITIAL LESIONS DUE TO DTH REACTIONS ELICITED BY EXOGENOUS ANTIGENS

It has been shown that local DTH reactions can be elicited in the renal cortex by the injection into the kidney of an exogenous antigen, bovine gamma globulin (BGG), in sensitized guinea pigs or rats [537]. The lesions contained mononuclear-cell infiltrates with focal tubular destruction. The transfer of lymphocytes, but not of serum, resulted in the ability of normal recipients to develop lesions following local injection of antigen. Lesions were regularly produced with heat-aggregated BGG, whereas soluble BGG was generally ineffective, although this was as effective as aggregated material in eliciting DTH reactions in the skin. The findings suggest that in the renal interstitium only antigens that are aggregated (such as antigens in immune complexes), particulate (such as bacteria), or fixed (such as drugs covalently bound to structural components or structural components themselves) can elicit DTH reactions.

Eddy [142] has reported that daily intraperitoneal administration of large amounts of BSA to rats resulted in accumulation of macrophages and T cells in the renal interstitium. Although the infiltrates were considered to be somehow the result of protein-overload proteinuria, immunologic mechanisms were not entirely excluded.

In experimental pyelonephritis induced in the rat by *Escherichia coli,* numerous T cells appear in the renal infiltrate after several days [295*a*]. Most of the cells were shown to have the inducer/helper phenotype (W3/25). Furthermore, T cells propagated from the infiltrates showed an MHC-restricted proliferative response to *E. coli,* but not to unrelated organisms. The MHC restriction indicates that the T cells recognized antigens by means of their antigen receptors and were not stimulated nonspecifically through bacterial products, such as lipopolysaccharide. The bacterial antigens responsible for the proliferative response have not been characterized. It is possible that the *E. coli*–reactive T cells trigger a DTH reaction in the kidney, which could have harmful effects, although they also may function to facilitate local antibody production, which would facilitate elimination of the bacteria.

T CELL–MEDIATED TUBULOINTERSTITIAL LESIONS DUE TO AUTOLOGOUS ANTIGENS

A model of cell-mediated tubulointerstitial lesions produced by autologous renal antigens has been described by Sugisaki et al. [505]. Lewis rats immunized with homogenates of syngeneic kidney tissue in adjuvant often developed tubulointerstitial nephritis, which was most intense at 10 to 14 days (Fig. 3-11). The kidneys were irregularly infiltrated by mononuclear cells. Most of the infiltrating cells appeared to be large lymphocytes, but they were not characterized phenotypically because the lack of availability at the time of appropriate monoclonal antibodies. By immunofluorescence, no deposits of immunoglobulins or C3 were detected. The transfer of lymph node or spleen cells, but not of serum, from kidney-injected donors to normal rats resulted in focal interstitial infiltrates and tubular cell damage at 24 to 48 hours. The responsible autologous antigens were not identified, but since lesions could not be induced by immunization with liver tissue, it is possible that the antigens were restricted to or concentrated in the kidney. Macrophage inhibitory factor (MIF) activity was observed when lymph node or spleen cells were incubated with kidney antigens, which provides evidence of DTH reactivity. However, the possible participation of cytolytic T cells with specificity toward renal-cell surface antigens was not excluded.

THE ROLE OF T CELLS IN ANTI-TBM NEPHRITIS

The methods of induction and the evidence favoring a pathogenic role of humoral antibodies in models of anti-TBM nephritis were described earlier. In this section I will review evidence that T cells also can participate in the production of renal damage.

Anti-TBM Nephritis in Rats

Immunization of Brown Norway rats with homologous or heterologous TBM preparations results in severe tubulointerstitial nephritis. Early in the disease (8–10 days), the lesions appear to be mediated largely or entirely by antibodies; IgG and C3 are found along the TBM, and the infiltrates consist predominantly of neutrophils. Several days later, however, the infiltrates are composed almost entirely of mononuclear cells. A study of infiltrating cells in tissue sections or in suspension showed that most of the cells at day 13 were reactive with monoclonal antibodies against pan T cells (W3/13). The majority of T cells were Ia^+ (indicating activation) and $CD4^+$ (W3/25). $CD8^+$ T cells ($OX8^+$), B cells (Ig^+), and macrophages (esterase positive) were present in smaller numbers [333, 527]. Although the early infiltration by neutrophils could be largely prevented by decomplementation, this had less effect on the later influx of mononuclear cells [528].

The presence of large numbers of activated $CD4^+$ T-infiltrating cells suggests that a T cell–mediated reaction, probably a DTH reaction directed against TBM antigens, develops in the kidneys in the later stages of rat anti-TBM nephritis. This conclusion would be supported by the demonstration of infiltrating T cells with reactivity to autologous TBM antigens. Attempts to demonstrate such cells by in vitro assays have so far been unsuccessful. Ulich et al. [527] reported that lymphocytes isolated from renal infiltrates were reactive with the immunizing antigen preparation (bovine TBM), but not with several autologous renal antigen preparations. These findings do not, how-

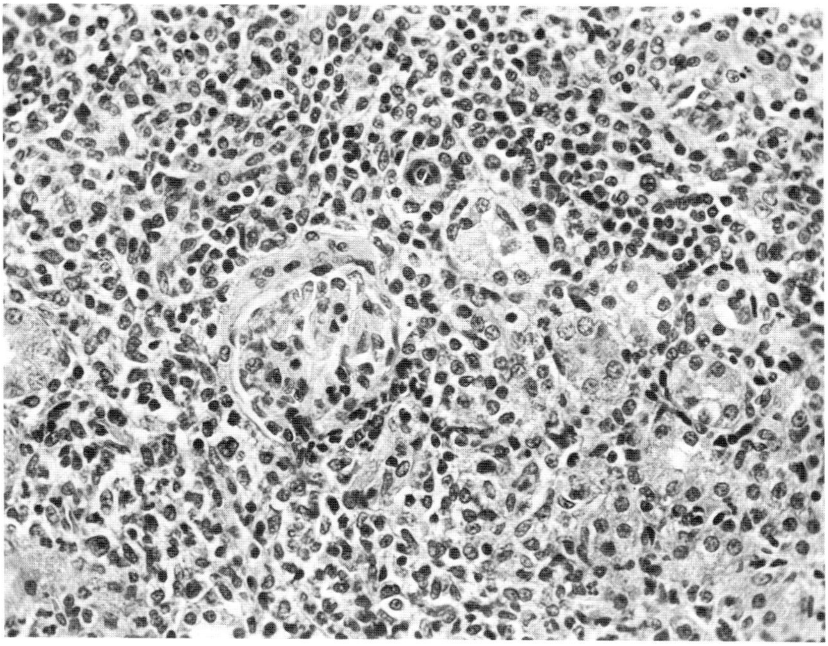

Fig. 3-11. *Mononuclear cells are seen in the renal interstitium and invading tubules. From a rat injected 10 days earlier with a renal preparation and adjuvant (see text). H&E; ×313.*

ever, exclude the presence of autologous TBM-reactive T cells, since the infiltrates of cell-mediated reactions are known to contain only a very small percentage of specifically sensitized cells [357,558]. Moreover, the concomitant presence of suppressor cells might make their detection difficult.

Cell-transfer experiments in rat anti-TBM nephritis have yielded variable results. Lehman and Wilson [305] described the production of mild inflammatory lesions by subcapsular renal injections of lymph node or peritoneal exudate cells from donors immunized with bovine TBM preparations. Early attempts to produce rat anti-TBM nephritis by systemic transfer of cells failed [504]. Recently, however, Ulich and associates [527] reported that lymph node cells obtained from TBM-immunized rats and cultivated in vitro for 5 days in the presence of the immunizing preparation or concanavalin A were capable of producing severe tubulointerstitial nephritis in syngeneic recipients, as seen at 9 and 14 days. However, since the recipients developed anti-TBM antibodies and had TBM-bound IgG, it cannot be concluded that cellular mechanisms were entirely responsible for the lesions.

Taken together, studies on the composition of the renal infiltrates, the direct immunofluorescence findings, and the results of transfer studies strongly support the participation of both humoral and cell-mediated mechanisms in most models of rat anti-TBM nephritis.

Pure T Cell–Mediated Anti-TBM Nephritis in Rats

An interesting model of rat tubulointerstitial nephritis in Lewis rats has been described by Bannister and associates [29]. Lewis rats are known to lack the TBM antigen(s) with which rat anti-TBM antibodies react, as detected by immunofluorescence [504]. In the experiments of Bannister et al. [29], Lewis rats were immunized with a TBM antigen preparation from Brown Norway (BN) rats, a strain that possesses the TBM antigen. Severe tubulointerstitial nephritis developed by 10 to 14 days and was characterized by focal mononuclear infiltrates with a granulomatous appearance. There were numerous activated T (Ia^+ $OX19^+$) cells in the lesions. Although the Lewis rats had high titers of circulating anti-BN-TBM antibodies, they had, as expected, no antibodies bound to the TBM. Transfer of lymphoid cells from immunized to normal Lewis rats resulted in tubulointerstitial lesions that were indistinguishable from those of actively immunized rats. The model of Bannister et al. indicates that cell-mediated tubulointerstitial nephritis can be induced in rats by TBM antigens and provide indirect evidence that T cells participate in those models in which anti-TBM antibodies are also present. Moreover, the results indicate that the determinants recognized by the TBM-reactive T cells are different from those recognized by anti-TBM antibodies.

Recently, Rennke and colleagues [442] have described another model of cell-mediated tubulointerstitial nephritis. Brown Norway rats were immunized with azobenzenarsonate (ABA) coupled to keyhole limpet hemocyanin. Ten days later, the rats exhibited DTH reactivity to ABA. The left kidney was perfused with ABA, which resulted in fixation of ABA to renal structures. This was followed by the development of massive granulomatous interstitial nephritis, with periglomerular granulomas and crescent formation (Fig. 3-12). Immunoglobulins did not accumulate in the kidneys. Lesions were produced by transfer of T cells, but not by antibodies. The results indicate that if a hapten is bound to renal tissue in a host that exhibits DTH reactivity to the hapten, cell-mediated interstitial nephritis can develop. The model is relevant to drug-induced acute interstitial nephritis, which is discussed later.

Anti-TBM Nephritis in Mice

Anti-TBM nephritis can be induced in mice by immunization with heterologous TBM preparations in adjuvants. Although anti-TBM antibodies appear within a week or so after immunization, interstitial nephritis is first found several weeks later. The lesions are characterized by mononuclear cell infiltrates with occasional giant cells. In one study, transfer of $Ly2^+$ (CD8) lymphocytes resulted in lesions in normal recipients after several weeks; although transfer of a $L3T4^+$ (CD4) cell line also produced disease, the development of lesions was even more delayed [335]. Administration of interferon γ, which results in increased expression of MHC class II products on tubular cells, increased the effect of transferred $CD4^+$ cells [209]. Evidence was obtained that the transferred $CD4^+$ T cells induced $CD8^+$ effector cells in the recipients [335]. These findings suggest that cytolytic T cells, possibly directed against TBM antigens expressed on tubular cells, are major effectors in mouse anti-TBM nephritis. Serum transfer also has produced lesions, but these were generally not severe [571]. The infiltrates in recipients of either cells or serum were found to contain T cells, natural killer (NK) cells, macrophages, and B cells. It is difficult to evaluate the relative importance of humoral and cellular immunity in mouse anti-TBM nephritis, but the evidence favors a predominant role of T cells, especially of cytolytic T cells.

Neilson and associates [390,391,395,396,400] have conducted a large number of studies on the complex interrelationship between effector and regulatory cells in anti-TBM nephritis in mice, rats, and guinea pigs. The results parallel and extend those obtained in other studies employing exogenous antigens.

Anti-TBM Nephritis in Guinea Pigs

As noted earlier, transfer of serum from TBM-immunized strain 13 guinea pigs to syngeneic recipients results in severe tubulointerstitial nephritis, which provides convincing evidence for a primary pathogenic role of antibodies. Nevertheless, there are certain puzzling aspects of the transfer, which leave open the possibility that T cell mechanisms also may be involved. For one thing, transfer of heterologous anti-TBM antibodies appears to be ineffective. In addition, although antibodies accumulate along the TBM in strain 2 guinea pigs [234] following transfer of isologous

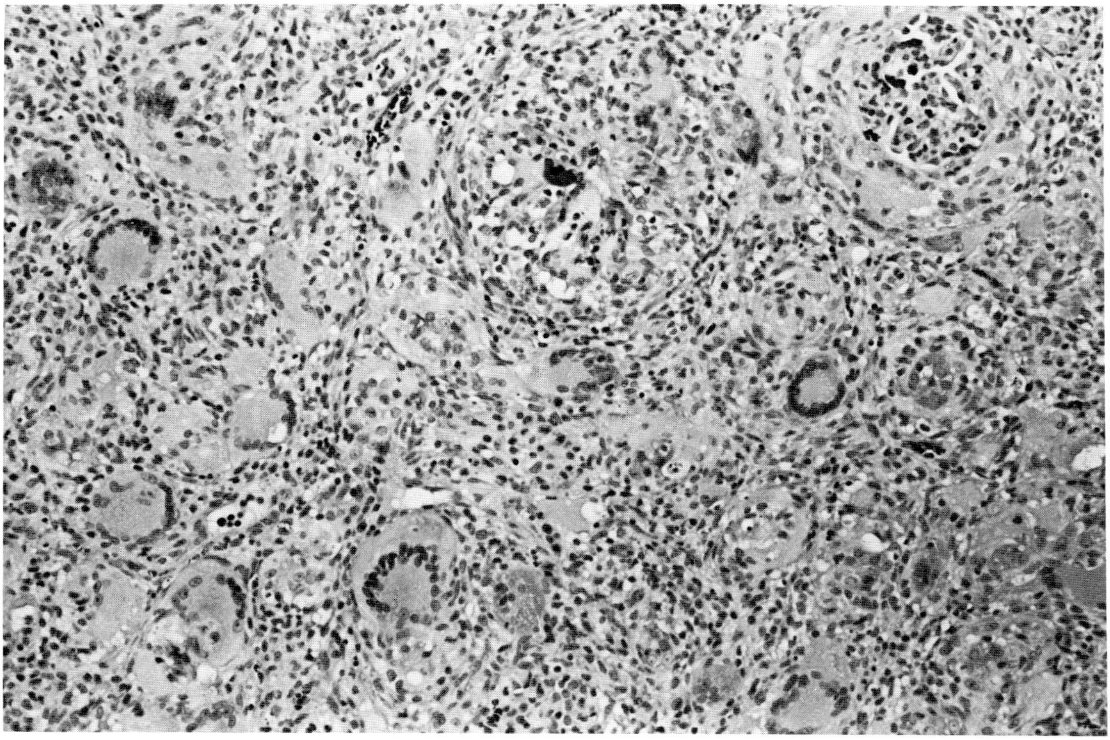

Fig. 3-12. *Section of kidney from a rat sensitized with ABA keyhole limpet hemocyanin and challenged at day 10 with ABA (see text). There is intense interstitial accumulation of mononuclear and multinuclear cells, with invasion of tubules and Bowman's space. H&E; ×191. (Courtesty of Dr. Helmut G. Rennke.)*

antibodies, only mild histologic abnormalities are found.

Furthermore, even in susceptible guinea pigs, an unexpectedly long time is required for the full development of lesions; thus, although small mononuclear cell infiltrates can be seen as early as 3 days after the transfer of serum or IgG, the abnormalities in some animals continue to progress in severity for 2 weeks or more [536]. Possible explanations for the slow development of disease include the time required for accumulation of sufficient antibodies along the TBM, the induction of autoantibodies against the TBM in the recipient (autoimmune amplification) [206], or the induction of T cell–mediated reactivity against TBM antigens.

A possible role of T cells in guinea pig anti-TBM nephritis is supported by the finding that the renal infiltrate is predominantly mononuclear and includes numerous T cells [363,536]. Furthermore, lymph node cells from TBM-immunized guinea pigs were shown to be cytotoxic to fetal kidney monolayers [396]. However, attempts to produce guinea pig anti-TBM nephritis by systemic transfer of lymphocytes have not been successful [536]; it is possible that failure has resulted from the concomitant transfer of suppressor cells or from the use of inadequate numbers of TBM-reactive T cells. The latter possibility is suggested by observations in rat and mouse anti-TBM nephritis, and in several other models of autoimmune disease in which successful transfer has required or is facilitated by the use of cell preparations expanded by in vitro cultivation with antigen [527]. Moreover, it is conceivable that the transfer of serum containing anti-TBM antibodies stimulates the proliferation of TBM-reactive T cells in the recipients, possibly through anti-idiotypic antibodies, and that these cells infiltrate the kidney and contribute to renal injury. That this hypothesis is not entirely fanciful is suggested by the finding that the transfer of anti-TBM antibodies in guinea pigs can stimulate the production of additional autoantibodies; this may depend on stimulation of TBM-reactive T cells by anti-idiotypes [206]. Nevertheless, the most direct explanation at present for the successful transfer of guinea pig anti-TBM nephritis with serum is that antibodies can initiate damage following combination with the TBM, possibly through the generation of chemotactic factors [267] or through ADCC mechanisms [397].

T Cell–Mediated Glomerular Injury

Although a role of T cells in the initiation of glomerular injury was established more than a decade ago in several models, acceptance of this mechanism has been slow in coming. Early skepticism stemmed in part from the failure to recognize that mononuclear cells can accumulate in glomeruli in immunologically mediated glomerulonephritis. Hypercellularity was generally attributed to proliferation of intrinsic glomerular cells. A number of studies have shown that mononuclear phagocytes infiltrate glomeruli in models of serum sickness and anti-GBM nephritis [221,223,230, 462]. However, mononuclear phagocytes can accumulate not only through T cell mechanisms, but through interaction with Fc portions of glomerular-bound antibodies by means of Fc receptors [220] or as a result of chemotactic attraction.

Until recently, there was no conclusive evidence for the presence of lymphocytes within glomeruli in experimental glomerulonephritis, although histologic and ultrastructural studies had revealed cells with the appearance of lymphocytes in acute serum sickness nephritis in rabbits [230] and in models of anti-GBM nephritis. More recently, Tipping et al. [520] reported that small numbers of T cells, especially of the helper phenotype, can be detected by monoclonal antibodies in the glomeruli of rats with an accelerated form of autologous anti-GBM nephritis, a model in which Schreiner et al. [473] had previously demonstrated an injurious role for macrophages. Of interest was the finding that lymphocyte accumulation in glomeruli preceded the peak influx of macrophages, with the numbers of lymphocytes declining in later stages of the disease. The results are consistent with a role for T cells in the influx of mononuclear phagocytes in a model of anti-GBM nephritis. The findings also suggest that even when few, if any, T cells can be demonstrated in glomeruli, a pathogenic role for these cells cannot be excluded.

Noble et al. [409] have described the appearance of T cells in glomeruli in a model of chronic serum sickness in rats induced by repeated intravenous injections of BSA. T cells and macrophages accumulated at the onset of proteinuria. However, T cells were present only in small numbers and only for a brief period of time, and their pathogenic role was not established. In addition, Camussi et al. [87] have reported that unusually severe glomerular injury can be produced by administration of phytohemagglutinin to rabbits developing acute BSA-induced serum sickness. The lesions are characterized by glomerular infiltration of activated lymphocytes. It is possible that the infiltrating lymphocytes included cells sensitized against BSA, which was present in small amounts in glomeruli.

Unlike antibodies, T cells cannot easily be recovered from glomeruli and studied for antigen specificity. Documentation of a pathogenetic role of T cells has therefore depended on models produced by transfer of lymph node cells or on the use of bursectomized chickens, as described in the following sections.

MODELS OF T CELL–MEDIATED GLOMERULAR INJURY

Bhan et al. [50,52] obtained direct evidence that T cell–mediated mechanisms can induce glomerular injury in rats in the following experiments:

Small amounts of exogenous antigens were fixed in glomeruli, following which lymphocytes were transferred from syngeneic donors that had been sensitized against that antigen. In experiments of one type, Lewis rats were injected intravenously with small doses of rabbit anti-rat GBM antiserum; rabbit gamma globulin (RGG) was thus fixed in glomeruli without producing histologically detectable injury [52]. Subsequently, the animals received lymph node cells, T cell–enriched preparations, or serum from syngeneic donors that had been immunized with RGG or ovalbumin. Only the rats injected with anti-GBM antiserum plus lymph node cells or T cells from RGG-immunized donors showed histologic glomerular abnormalities, in the form of segmental hypercellular and necrotizing lesions. Electron microscopic observations indicated that the glomerular hypercellularity resulted to some extent from infiltration by monocytes; occasional lymphocytes also were seen. In other studies of similar design, Bhan et al. [50] obtained evidence that cell-mediated reactivity directed against antigens deposited in mesangial regions in the form of immune complexes also can lead to glomerular reactions. Although most of the damage in these models probably resulted from delayed hypersensitivity reactions locally triggered in glomeruli, some of the glomerular accumulation of mononuclear cells may have resulted from systemic release of lymphokines, following interaction of sensitized cells with antigen in the circulation [53].

Bolton et al. [58] showed that in neonatally bursectomized chickens with severely depressed humoral immunity, but with unimpaired cellular immunity, proliferative glomerulonephritis developed following immunization with GBM preparations, often in the absence of anti-GBM antibodies. The glomerular lesions were as severe as those in nonbursectomized animals immunized with GBM preparations. Lesions could be produced by transfer of lymphocytes, but not of serum [56]. These studies provide impressive evidence that T cell mechanisms can produce glomerular injury without the participation of humoral antibodies. Of interest was the finding that the glomerular hypercellularity was due in large part to proliferation of intrinsic cells, presumably as a result of an effect of lymphocyte or monocyte products [525]. Macrophages and a few lymphocytes also were seen in glomeruli by electron microscopy [525].

ROLE OF T CELLS IN SERUM SICKNESS GLOMERULONEPHRITIS

The experiments of Bhan et al. [50] show that antigens localized in glomeruli in the form of immune complexes can trigger DTH reactions. Several lines of evidence suggest that this is an important factor in acute serum sickness in rabbits. First, lymphocytes have been described in glomeruli [230]. Second, the glomeruli show accumulation of monocytes and not of neutrophils – the characteristic inflammatory cell seen in known immune complex–mediated lesions (Arthus reactions) in rabbits. Third, cyclosporine treatment can inhibit the glomerular lesions, which suggests that T cells may contribute to the accumulation of monocytes [389]. In these experiments, the rabbits were given endotoxin, which bypasses the requirement for helper T cells in antibody production; thus the effect of cyclosporine was probably not due to prevention of antibody production. Fourth, passive administration of preformed immune complexes has not produced acute glomerulonephritis in rabbits [98]. Finally, fully developed glomerular lesions may be seen with few, if any, glomerular immune deposits [138].

SECONDARY PATHOGENETIC MECHANISMS (MEDIATORS) IN EXPERIMENTAL IMMUNOLOGIC RENAL DISEASES

So far I have discussed mainly the immunologic mechanisms that initiate renal injury (primary mechanisms). In the present section I will review briefly what is known about how these mechanisms bring about tissue damage through activation or release of mediators. There is overlap between primary and secondary mechanisms. For example, systemic release of vasoactive amines resulting from the formation of circulating immune complexes may produce tissue injury and also promote the glomerular deposition of circulating complexes [287]. Most studies on mediators in renal disease have dealt with glomerular injury, and the following discussion therefore deals largely with this topic rather than tubulointerstitial damage.

A major approach to the study of secondary mechanisms is to deplete the factors or block the pathways thought to be important in pathogenesis, and to determine how these procedures affect a particular model as assessed by proteinuria, renal function, immunofluorescence findings, or structural glomerular damage. Obviously, such maneuvers are most easily performed in short-term experiments, so there is more evidence concerning models of acute disease than of chronic disease. Because of these considerations, and because of the complexity and overlapping effects of mediators of tissue injury, many important questions remain unanswered. Nevertheless, experimental evidence has implicated the complement system, leukocytes, platelets, the coagulation system, eicosanoids, cytokines, and other factors released by infiltrating leukocytes or mesangial cells in various models of immunologically mediated glomerular injury.

Role of the Complement System

A pathogenic role of the complement system in some forms of immunologically mediated diseases is well established. An injurious role has been inferred from the presence of complement components in most immune deposits; however, direct evidence of pathogenicity has been obtained in only a few models. The earliest evidence of complement-dependent renal injury was obtained in studies on nephrotoxic serum nephritis. Animals depleted of complement by cobra venom factor developed less proteinuria and less neutrophil infiltration than normal animals in the heterologous phase of nephrotoxic serum nephritis [100, 530]. This effect of complement depends on the accumulation of neutrophils. The complement-dependent leukocyte accumulation may involve chemotactic attraction by C5a and immune adherence to glomerular-bound C3b by means of leukocyte C3b receptors.

There is also evidence that complement is involved in renal injury in guinea pig and rat anti-TBM nephritis [456]. When guinea pig recipients of anti-TBM antibodies are pretreated with cobra venom factor, renal lesions are largely prevented or greatly delayed. However, anti-TBM nephritis can be induced in guinea pigs with a total genetic deficiency of C4 [453], which indicates that classical pathway activation is not required. The early neutrophil infiltration in rats with anti-TBM nephritis can be markedly reduced by decomplementation [528].

A complement mechanism of glomerular injury that is independent of neutrophils has been demonstrated in studies on passive Heymann nephritis [27,112,127,460]. Proteinuria can be abrogated by procedures that prevent formation of the C5b-9 membrane attack complex in the glomerular deposits [27]. The mechanism by which C5b-9 produces damage to the filtration barrier has not been elucidated, but the podocyte appears to be the primary target [461].

Because of the attention paid to the injurious role of complement, it is important to note that in some models, complement is either not required for injury or even serves a protective role through mechanisms described earlier. In a model of accelerated anti-GBM nephritis, immunoglobulin deposits and glomerular injury, although slightly delayed in onset, were greater in C6-deficient rabbits than in normocomplementemic rabbits [197], apparently because of impaired removal of deposits. Moreover, complement depletion of rabbits fails to interfere with the development of the glomerular lesions of acute serum sickness, although the necrotizing arteritis is prevented [216]. Indeed, complement depletion retards removal of renal-bound complexes in rabbits with acute serum sickness [39].

Direct evidence concerning a pathogenic role of the complement system in chronic serum sickness or other models of chronic immune complex disease is lacking because of the difficulty in producing protracted depletion, but is suspected in view of the heavy glomerular deposits of complement.

Role of Neutrophils

Neutrophil infiltration is seen in some models of immunologically mediated glomerulonephritis, including early nephrotoxic serum nephritis and some forms of immune complex glomerulonephritis. Depletion of neutrophils in the heterologous phase of nephrotoxic serum nephritis reduces proteinura [100,561], and sometimes prevents histologic abnormalities and preserves renal function [384,485,487]. However, some anti-GBM antibodies produce proteinuria by mechanisms that are not dependent on neutrophils [114].

Neutrophils also have been shown to exert injurious effects in a rat model of acute glomerulonephritis produced by in situ formation of immune complexes [253]. The model is produced by infusion of concanavalin A (ConA) into the renal artery, which results in glomerular binding, followed by administration of anti-ConA antibodies. The glomeruli quickly exhibit endothelial-cell damage, subendothelial immune deposits, fibrin deposition, and infiltration by neutrophils and platelets. Rats rendered neutropenic by anti-neutrophil antibodies developed significantly less proteinuria than untreated rats.

MECHANISMS OF GLOMERULAR ACCUMULATION OF NEUTROPHILS

A number of factors undoubtedly contribute to neutrophil accumulation in glomerulonephritis, as in other forms of inflammation. Particular interest is being focused on the role of adhesion molecules on endothelial cells, some of which are upregulated by cytokines [110]. Another mechanism that is assumed to be important in neutrophil accumulation in glomeruli is chemotactic attraction, through factors produced by complement activation, principally C5a, or by factors released from intrinsic glomerular cells, infiltrating leukocytes, or platelets. However, direct evidence of the importance of chemotactic factors is lacking. West [559] has argued that an effective concentration gradient of a chemoattractant could not be readily established in glomeruli.

Neutrophils can probably accumulate in glomeruli that contain immunoglobulin deposits through neutrophil Fc or C3b receptors on their surface. Direct evidence for a role of Fc receptors in promoting adherence to glomerular-bound antibodies was obtained in a model of accelerated nephrotoxic serum nephritis [487]. Rabbits were given sheep nephrotoxic serum and 48 hours later rabbit anti-sheep IgG, either as intact antibodies or as F(ab')2 fragments. The recipients of F(ab')2 fragments had appreciably fewer neutrophils in glomeruli than recipients of intact antibodies.

MECHANISMS OF PRODUCTION OF GLOMERULAR INJURY BY NEUTROPHILS

Two major ways in which neutrophils cause tissue damage are (1) generation of oxygen metabolites (reactive oxygen species) through the membrane-associated NADPH oxidase system, and (2) release of intracellular proteases [215]. There is increasing evidence that these two pathways operate in a synergistic fashion [556]. Neutrophils can be caused to produce reactive oxygen species and release proteases by contact with immune complexes [550,551].

Neutrophil granules contain numerous enzymes, but three proteolytic enzymes, elastase (a serine protease), collagenase, and gelatinase, appear to be particularly important. Their damaging effects derive mainly from their ability to degrade components of the extracellular matrix [99,556].

Neutrophil proteases have been implicated in damage to the GBM through both in vitro and in vivo experiments. Several neutrophil proteases are capable of digesting GBM in vitro, including acidic proteases and neutral serine proteases [248,252]. In vitro experiments performed by Vissers et al. [542,543] probably reflect in vivo events in anti-GBM nephritis. Isolated GBM fragments were coated with anti-GBM antibodies and then incubated with neutrophils or monocytes. The leukocytes adhered and spread on the surface of the GBM, underwent a respiratory burst, and released lysosomal enzymes. Neutrophils produced rapid degradation of the GBM, as measured by solubilization of collagenous and noncollagenous proteins, an effect that was due mainly to serine proteases.

Electron microscopic observations in models of anti-GBM nephritis and chronic serum sickness have shown that neutrophils can similarly be in close contact with the GBM in vivo [564]. The release of proteases directly onto the GBM apparently makes it possible for the enzymes to avoid inactivation by circulating inhibitors. In addition, oxidants may inactivate antiproteases [556]. Fragments of basement-membrane material have been found in the urine in the heterologous phase of nephrotoxic serum nephritis [99,210].

ROLE OF REACTIVE OXYGEN SPECIES IN NEUTROPHIL-MEDIATED GLOMERULAR INJURY

Evidence obtained in the last decade or so indicates that superoxide anion, hydrogen peroxide, the hydroxyl radical, and hypochlorous acid are involved in neutrophil-mediated tissue injury [252,480,556]. Following activation, neutrophils undergo a respiratory burst with the formation of powerful oxidants. A major product involved in neutrophil-mediated glomerular injury appears to be hydrogen peroxide, which may interact with halides in the presence of myeloperoxidase (MPO) to form long-lived oxidants [253]. MPO is a cationic protein that can therefore bind to fixed anionic sites in glomeruli. The infusion of MPO into the renal artery of rats, followed by nontoxic concentrations of H_2O_2 and a halide, resulted in mild histologic damage and proteinuria. Inhibitors of reactive oxygen species have been shown to reduce injury in experimental anti-GBM nephritis [26,480]. In addition to their direct injurious effects, oxygen metabolites may potentiate the effects of proteases by activation of the enzymes or inhibition of antiproteases [556].

Role of Mononuclear Phagocytes (Monocytes and Macrophages)

As noted earlier, monocyte accumulation is now recognized as a major cause of glomerular hypercellularity in several immunologically mediated disorders, including acute and chronic serum sickness in rabbits [221,230,462], passive serum sickness [417], nephrotoxic serum nephritis [290], murine SLE, and certain forms of human glomerulonephritis, as discussed later. Mononuclear phagocytes have been identified by electron microscopic and immunohistochemical techniques. Within the glomerular tufts, monocytes can accumulate not only in capillaries, but also within mesangial regions, where they have been shown to be responsible for the phagocytosis of colloidal material or immune complexes [502]. Mononuclear phagocytes also have been detected in crescents in models of nephrotoxic serum nephritis in rabbits both by ultrastructural studies [290] and by examination of cells cultured from isolated glomeruli [223]. As discussed later, macrophages play an important role in crescent formation.

Direct evidence for an injurious role of macrophages has been obtained in several models of immunologic glomerulonephritis. Schreiner et al. [473] showed that irradiation of rats with an accelerated form of nephrotoxic serum nephritis resulted in diminished glomerular accumulation of monocytes and reduced proteinuria. Depletion of mononuclear phagocytes by anti-macrophage serum largely prevented the glomerular lesions and proteinuria in acute serum sickness or in accelerated nephrotoxic serum nephritis in rabbits [222]. Thaiss et al. [513] have shown that monocytes (as well as neutrophils and complement) participate in glomerular injury in a model of in situ immune complex glomerulonephritis. In addition, monocytes appear to contribute to renal damage in guinea pig anti-TBM nephritis [454].

Mononuclear phagocytes (and neutrophils) may not only participate in the production of renal damage, but also may serve a protective function through phagocytosis and degradation of immune complexes [502]. The mechanisms that lead to glomerular or tubulointerstitial accumulation of monocytes are not entirely understood. In a model of in situ immune complex glomerulonephritis in rabbits, monocyte accumulation was shown to be Fc dependent, and the degree of monocyte accumulation correlated with the affinity for Fc receptors of the antibodies used to induce disease [68]. As noted earlier, DTH reactions triggered by glomerular-bound antigens also can bring about an influx of monocyte infiltration in glomeruli.

Clearly, other mechanisms that operate in a variety of inflammatory reactions are involved as well.

MECHANISMS OF GLOMERULAR INJURY BY MACROPHAGES

Production of tissue injury by monocytes probably depends on their local activation to macrophages. As with neutrophils, reactive oxygen species [69] and proteases are important. However, Vissers et al. [542] have shown that human peripheral blood monocytes are less efficient in degrading GBM than neutrophils because of lower proteolytic activity. In addition to proteases and oxidants, macrophages produce eicosanoids and a variety of cytokines that may be involved in injury, as discussed later [385]. Moreover, macrophages may be involved in the production of DTH reactions within glomeruli by presenting antigen to sensitized T cells. This function could be performed by infiltrating cells, as well as by resident macrophages in the mesangium [474].

Role of Platelets

There is evidence that platelets produce injury in some forms of glomerulonephritis [36,83]. Platelets have been shown to accumulate in glomeruli in several models [250,251]. In a form of in situ immune complex nephritis in rats produced with concanavalin A, platelet depletion resulted in reduction in proteinuria [249]. In another rat model induced by antibodies against an antigen present on mesangial cells, Thy-1, platelet depletion reduced mesangial-cell proliferation [251]. The effect of platelets in promoting proliferation appears to be independent of leukocytes or complement.

There are numerous mechanisms by which platelets can induce inflammation and injury, including procoagulant activity, release of vasoactive amines (which favors immune complex deposition), and production of oxygen species, growth factors, and proteases [34]. In vitro and in vivo evidence suggests that platelets may enhance neutrophil effects, including adherence and release of proteases and reactive oxygen species [250]. In addition, platelet factor 4 and other cationic proteins released from activated platelets can combine with fixed anionic sites in the GBM and result in increased glomerular permeability [33,35].

Role of the Coagulation System

There is clear evidence that coagulation contributes to certain forms of glomerular injury, and in particular to crescent formation. Fibrin deposition in Bowman's space is found in early crescents both in experimental models and in human disease, and prevention of fibrin deposits has been shown to eliminate or reduce crescent formation in several models. Most studies on crescent formation have been carried out in models of nephrotoxic serum nephritis [355].

The accumulation of fibrin in Bowman's space appears to involve activation of the intrinsic pathway, as evidenced by the presence in the deposits of factor VIII and factor XII (Hageman factor) [484,519,560]. It is likely that factor XII (an 80kD protein) passes through the damaged capillary wall and is activated to factor XIIa in Bowman's space by fragments of basement membrane, which are known to be released from damaged glomeruli in nephrotoxic serum nephritis [210]. Activation of the extrinsic pathway of coagulation through tissue factor (factor III) also may participate in the formation of fibrin in Bowman's space. Thus monocytes and macrophages, cells that are known to produce tissue factor (tissue thromboplastin), accumulate in developing crescents [26], as discussed below.

Although fibrin may provide a matrix on which crescent formation occurs, it is probable that substances and products of cells within the clot, such as growth and chemotactic factors, provide the stimuli for the full development of the crescent. There is compelling evidence that monocytes and macrophages play a critical role [26]. The mechanisms that cause emigration of monocytes into Bowman's space are only partially understood. Monocytes accumulate in glomerular capillaries and sometimes in periglomerular infiltrates in nephrotoxic serum nephritis and other glomerular diseases with crescents. Chemotactic factors in the fibrin deposits, such as thrombin or fibronectin fragments [37,430], may attract monocytes into

Bowman's space, and this may be facilitated by breaks in the glomerular capillary wall or Bowman's capsule. Delayed-type hypersensitivity directed against glomerular-bound antigens (heterologous immunoglobulins in the case of nephrotoxic serum nephritis) also may contribute to monocyte accumulation in some forms of glomerulonephritis [387]. Monocytes or macrophages may play a role in crescent formation in several ways: through increasing fibrin deposition as a result of production of tissue factor and other procoagulants, by contributing to the mass of cells that comprise crescents (in addition to neutrophils, epithelial cells, and later fibroblasts), and by their ability to stimulate proliferation of epithelial cells or fibroblasts [26]. On the other hand, monocytes may serve to reduce crescent formation by phagocytosis and degradation of fibrin or by plasminogen activation. Other factors in the fibrin deposits, such as fibrinopeptides, fibronectin, or thrombin, may contribute to cell proliferation in crescents or to fibrosis of crescents in ways that are not entirely understood but which may be similar to those occurring in wound healing [104].

The most direct evidence for the crucial role of fibrin in crescent formation comes from experiments in which fibrin deposits have been prevented or eliminated. Vassalli and McCluskey [538,539] reported that the anticoagulant warfarin entirely prevented crescent formation in nephrotoxic serum nephritis in rabbits when given in very high doses before and after an injection of anti-GBM antiserum. However, fatal hemorrhage was quite common in the warfarin-treated group. Heparin has had variable effects on crescent formation, with beneficial effects in some studies and none in others [355]. However, treatment with ancrod, a defibrinating agent, markedly reduced glomerular fibrin deposition and inhibited the development of crescents and renal functional impairment in rabbit nephrotoxic serum nephritis without causing hemorrhagic complications [383, 517]. Thompson et al. [518] also showed that ancrod was effective in preventing crescent formation in experimental chronic serum sickness. This indicates that even with different underlying immunologic mechanisms, crescent formation depends on coagulation and may follow a final common pathway.

In other experiments, warfarin and ancrod were shown to have a beneficial effect in rabbit nephrotoxic serum nephritis even when treatment was started a few days after crescent formation had begun, provided severe renal failure was not already present [63,517]. The therapeutic effect presumably occurred because intrinsic fibrinolytic mechanisms cleared existing fibrin deposits [185] while the treatment prevented further fibrin accumulation.

Zoja et al. [575] recently reported that recombinant tissue plasminogen activator (t-PA) can ameliorate crescent formation and prevent deterioration of renal function in rabbit nephrotoxic serum nephritis. Although the rabbits had prolonged bleeding times, there were no hemorrhagic complications. Like other thrombolytic agents, such as streptokinase and urokinase, t-PA leads to lysis of fibrin clots by activating plasminogen to plasmin. t-PA bound to fibrin has a considerably higher affinity for plasminogen than does t-PA in the absence of fibrin. Thus t-PA, in contrast to streptokinase, activates plasminogen to plasmin mainly within clots; this accounts for the relative specificity of fibrin clot lysis by t-PA without degradation of circulating fibrinogen.

Although the pathogenic role of coagulation has been most convincingly documented in crescent formation, there is also evidence that abnormalities in glomerular tufts can result from coagulation. Vassalli et al. [540] showed that induction of intravascular coagulation can produce a variety of glomerular abnormalities, including damage to endothelial cells, hypercellularity, and sclerosis. Moreover, warfarin treatment of rabbits with nephrotoxic serum nephritis greatly reduced intracapillary hypercellularity and sclerosis of tufts [538,539]. Recently, ancrod therapy has been shown to reduce glomerular fibrin deposition and retard progression of glomerular tuft lesions in BXSB mice [102].

Role of Eicosanoids

Eicosanoids are known to mediate a variety of effects in inflammatory reactions and have been implicated in several models of immunologically mediated renal disease [314,438]. Eicosanoids are products of arachidonic acid, which is a 20-carbon polyunsaturated fatty acid present in cell membranes. Unlike certain other mediators of inflammation, such as histamine or lysosomal enzymes, eicosanoids are not preformed but are synthesized following cell stimulation. Within glomeruli, eicosanoids can be generated by infiltrating leukocytes, as well as by mesangial cells. Eicosanoids can be synthesized by two pathways: the cyclooxygenase pathway, which generates prostaglandins and thromboxanes, and the lipoxygenase pathway, which leads to hydroxyeicosatetraenoic acids (HETEs) and leukotrienes. As stated by Lianos [314], "Eicosanoids exhibit a bewildering and often widely differing spectrum of biological activities with frequently opposing biological effects which may further depend on the species studied." In addition to inflammatory and vasoactive effects, eicosanoids may modify the immune response [192]. Although at present it is impossible to present a complete account of the role of eicosanoids in renal disease, it has been shown that alterations in eicosanoid synthesis occur in various models with either protective or injurious effects [438]. A few examples follow.

Lianos et al. [315] demonstrated enhanced glomerular production of thromboxane A_2 (TxA_2) shortly after administration of nephrotoxic serum nephritis and showed that this was responsible for reduction in the glomerular filtration rate. Rahman et al. [438] reported enhanced glomerular synthesis of PGE_2 and TxA_2 in a rat model of immune complex glomerulonephritis.

Administration of PGE_1 to NZB/W or MRL-lpr/lpr mice can lessen the severity and slow the progression of the glomerular lesions that spontaneously develop in these strains [264,366,576]. Glomerular immune deposits were reduced, even though PGE_1 treatment apparently did not change the serum level of antibodies to single- or double-stranded DNA. However, there was reduction in the formation of circulating immune complexes containing gp70, a retrovirus product [238], which may play a role in the glomerular disease (although, as noted earlier, there is evidence that gp70-containing complexes are not required). Rahman et al. [438] have suggested that the beneficial effects of PGE therapy may be secondary to inhibition of endogenous eicosanoid synthesis. Kelley et al. [265] showed that PGE_1 treatment of MRL-lpr/lpr mice reduced the proliferation of T cells characteristically seen in this strain, an effect that might lead to reduction of helper function and thereby of immune complex formation.

It also has been shown that administration of PGE_1 prevents the development of anti-TBM nephritis in Brown Norway rats induced by immunization with heterologous tubular basement membrane antigens [529]. Levels of anti-TBM antibodies were not affected or were only slightly reduced by PGE_1 treatment. Kelly et al. [266] showed that in vitro reactivity of lymphocytes to TBM and other antigens was suppressed in murine interstitial nephritis by PGE_1 treatment.

Another way in which the role of eicosanoid synthesis in experimental immunologic glomerular disease has been studied is through dietary-induced essential fatty acid (EFA) deficiency, which results in suppression of eicosanoid synthesis. EFA deficiency has been shown to ameliorate murine lupus nephritis [231,475]. In addition, EFA deficiency was associated with reduction in the glomerular influx of monocytes that characterize the heterologous phase of nephrotoxic serum in rats [475]. In contrast, the infiltration of neutrophils was unaffected. In rats with normal diets, there was a marked increase in glomerular thromboxane and leukotriene B_4 (LTB_4) production in the heterologous phase, and EFA deficiency largely eliminated this change. Resident macrophages are the principal sources of LTB_4 in normal rat glomeruli, and EFA deficiency causes a depletion of these cells [302,303].

Although the effects of EFA deficiency on glomerulonephritis provide some insight into pathogenetic mechanisms, this approach appears to offer little hope for treatment of human renal diseases because of the potentially serious dangers of achieving such dietary deficiency.

Because marine lipids are known to reduce cyclooxygenase products derived from arachidonic acid, Robinson and colleagues [444,445] performed experiments to determine the effects of dietary fish oil on murine lupus nephritis. They showed that renal disease was appreciably ameliorated in NZB/W, BXSB, and MRL-lpr/lpr mice. However, the mechanism was not clearly attributable to effects of eicosanoids, since marine lipids alter the synthesis of other mediators, including platelet-activating factor.

Role of Cytokines

In the past decade or so there has been a remarkable growth of knowledge of cytokines, and information is beginning to be gathered about their participation in renal disease. Cytokines are a group of biologically active polypeptides, some of which have other names, including lymphokines, monokines, lymphotoxin (LT), interleukins (IL), and interferons (IFN). In addition, certain growth factors, mainly epidermal growth factor, platelet-derived growth factor, and transforming growth factor α, have similar structural properties and could be considered cytokines. Cytokines play important roles in the immune response and in inflammation, necrosis, and repair [28,263,432, 552]. The main sources of cytokines are monocytes/macrophages and lymphocytes, but some are produced by a variety of other cells, including endothelial cells and mesangial cells. The effects of cytokines are generally mediated by binding to cell-surface receptors. Different cytokines may have synergistic or antagonistic effects.

Much of the recent growth in knowledge of cytokines stems from the availability of pure recombinant cytokines and molecular probes for their genes. However, many of the studies on cytokine effects have been performed in vitro, and as discussed by diGiovine and Duff [131], "the conditions under which they are tested in vitro are unlikely to occur in vivo. For example, cells in vivo probably never see a sudden change in the concentration of a single cytokine." And even many of the in vivo experiments conducted with cytokines are of dubious relevance to naturally occurring events. In the following sections I will cite a few observations concerning cytokines that appear pertinent to immunologically mediated renal disease.

Certain cytokines, especially IL-1, IL-2, and IL-6, are crucial in T cell activation and proliferation following interaction of specific T cells with antigen [503]. Methods that can impair the function of these cytokines, such as antibodies to their receptors, might therefore dampen undesirable immune responses. High-affinity IL-2 receptors are found principally on activated proliferating T cells, as well as on some newly activated B cells. Thus the major effects of anti-IL-2 receptor antibodies in immunologically mediated diseases would probably be restricted to stages characterized by intense T cell proliferation [173,503]. Although the effects of anti-IL-2 antibodies might therefore be somewhat restricted, the selectivity would fall far short of that resulting from elimination of antigen-specific clones.

Several cytokines, especially IL-1, interferon γ, and tumor necrosis factor (TNF), are important in the mediation of DTH reactions [243], which, as discussed earlier, produce certain forms of glomerular and tubulointerstitial injury.

There is evidence that infiltrating macrophages in glomeruli may produce IL-1 and TNF. Boswell et al. [64] reported that the kidneys of MRL-lpr/lpr mice contain TNF mRNA and IL-1 mRNA, and that isolated glomeruli secrete detectable levels of TNF. They presented evidence that macrophages were the source of the increased cytokine production. In addition, Vissers et al. [541] have reported that monocytes produce TNF and IL-1 in vitro following contact with GBM fragments that have been coated with anti-GBM antibodies.

Several cytokines, notably IL-1, TNF, LT, and interferon γ, can produce profound changes in endothelial cells. IL-1, TNF, and LT can induce increased expression of adhesion molecules, which are important in leukocyte binding in the inflammatory response, and can induce changes that reduce the anticoagulant properties of endothelial cells [110]. Furthermore, interferon γ induces class I and II MHC antigen expression on endothelial cells, which may heighten the susceptibility of these cells to immunologic injury and possibly result in their ability to present antigen to T cells.

It is reasonable to assume that many of the effects of cytokines just described are involved in renal injury, but direct evidence is for the most part lacking. Recently, however, Camussi et al. [87] reported that if rabbits developing acute serum sickness are injected with IL-1 or TNF, the glomeruli exhibit unusually severe lesions, with endothelial-cell damage and lymphoblast and neutrophil infiltration. Similar effects were seen following phytohemagglutinin injection, which increased production of IL-1 and TNF. It seems likely that the phytohemagglutinin or cytokines caused intensification of glomerular damage through effects on endothelial and mesangial cells and on infiltrating mononuclear cells. There is also evidence that cytokines contribute to interstitial fibrosis in interstitial nephritis [393,399].

Cytokines also may play an important role in the pulmonary manifestations of anti-GBM nephritis. Although the GBM is normally accessible to circulating antibodies, because of the endothelial fenestrations, the alveolar basement membrane is not. The administration to mice of IL-2 and IFN-α leads to the fixation of circulating anti-basement membrane antibodies to alveolar basement membranes associated with lung hemorrhage [435]. The liberation of cytokines may similarly be required for pulmonary hemorrhage in patients with anti-GBM nephritis.

Role of Mesangial Cells

There is increasing evidence that mesangial cells may not only be targets of immunologic injury, but also may function as effectors of glomerular damage. Mesangial cells can produce certain cytokines, notably IL and IL-6, as well as other mediators, including reactive oxygen species [436], platelet-activating factors, IL-1 [324,325] and IL-6 [228], prostaglandins, and proteases [557]. In addition, it has been shown that transforming growth factor β regulates production of proteoglycans by mesangial cells, which may be important in the accumulation of mesangial matrix seen in many glomerular diseases [60].

IMMUNOLOGIC MECHANISMS IN HUMAN RENAL DISEASES

Although it was postulated early in this century that some human renal diseases are immunologically mediated, direct evidence for this hypothesis was not obtained until the 1950s [367,479], when immunofluorescence studies showed that forms of human glomerulonephritis are characterized by granular deposits of immunoglobulins and complement components. Later, similar deposits were found in some forms of tubulointerstitial nephritis. The patterns of glomerular and tubulointerstitial immune deposits found in human diseases have more or less faithful counterparts in experimental models of immune complex disease (Tables 3-2 and 3-3). Furthermore, immunofluorescence and serologic studies have provided evidence that rare forms of glomerulonephritis and tubulointerstitial nephritis are associated with anti-basement-membrane antibodies. More recently, immunohistochemical studies with monoclonal antibodies

Table 3-2. *Major human glomerular diseases with immunologic mechanisms*

- I. Immune complex glomerulonephritis
  - A. Associated with infections
    1. Poststreptoccocal glomerulonephritis[a,b]
    2. Glomerulonephritis associated with bacterial endocarditis, infected atrioventricular shunt[c]
    3. Glomerulonephritis associated with chronic hepatitis B infection[d]
  - B. Associated with systemic diseases
    1. Lupus nephritis[e]
    2. Nephritis with Schönlein-Henoch syndrome
    3. Nephritis with idiopathic mixed cryoglobulinemia[f]
  - C. Primary glomerular diseases
    1. Membranous glomerulonephritis
    2. Membranoproliferative glomerulonephritis, type I
    3. IgA nephritis
- II. Anti-GBM Nephritis[a]
- III. Glomerulonephritis with anti-neutrophil cytoplasmic antibodies (ANCA)[g]
  - Necrotizing and crescentic glomerulonephritis, primary or associated with Wegener's granulomatosis or systemic vasculitis

[a]T-cell mechanisms may participate.
[b]Streptococcal antigens may have been identified in glomerular deposits.
[c]Bacterial antigens have been identified in glomerular deposits.
[d]Hepatitis B antigens (HB_s, HB_e) have been identified in glomerular deposits.
[e]DNA or intrinsic glomerular antigens may be involved.
[f]Antigen is IgG, combined with anti-IgG antibodies.
[g]Nature of immunologic mechanisms is obscure.

Table 3-3. *Immunologic mechanisms in human tubulointerstitial nephritis and possible responsible antigens*

- I. Predominantly antibody-mediated
  - A. Immune complex–mediated
    1. Lupus nephritis—DNA probably most important antigen [73]
    2. Sjögren syndrome—autologous antigen(s)?
    3. Mixed cryoglobulinemia—IgG (in IgM-IgG complexes)
    4. With glomerulonephritis—antigens unknown
  - B. Anti-tubular basement membrane (TBM) nephritis
    1. With anti-glomerular basement membrane antibodies [15]
    2. In renal allograft recipients—H3M-1 [97]
    3. Idiopathic—H3M-1 [97]
    4. In drug-induced interstitial nephritis [363]
- II. Predominantly cell-mediated
  - A. Drug-induced—antigens probably drug hapten-host conjugates [361]
  - B. Interstitial nephritis with uveitis—probably autologous antigens [275]
  - C. Idiopathic interstitial nephritis—antigens unknown

have provided evidence that T cell mechanisms operate in some forms of tubulointerstitial and glomerular diseases.

It is not possible to provide a thorough review here of the evidence concerning immunologic mechanisms in individual forms of human renal disease. Much of this information is reviewed in other chapters of this book. Instead, I will provide highlights of the evidence for immunologic mechanisms in major forms of human renal disease, discuss some unresolved issues, and review some diseases that appear to be immunologically mediated and for which there are no exact experimental counterparts (drug-induced acute interstitial nephritis, necrotizing and crescentic glomerulonephritis as seen in Wegener's granulomatosis).

A thorough understanding of immunologic renal disease would involve knowledge of predisposing host factors, etiologic agents, primary immunopathogenetic mechanisms, and secondary mediators. Unfortunately, we have too little knowledge concerning these areas in most diseases on which to base a meaningful discussion. I will place most emphasis on primary immunologic mechanisms and on efforts to identify relevant antigens in individual diseases.

Immune Complex Glomerulonephritis

EVIDENCE THAT GLOMERULAR DEPOSITS REPRESENT IMMUNE COMPLEXES

The close resemblance of glomerular deposits in many forms of human glomerulonephritis to those of established experimental models strongly supports the interpretation that they are immune complexes rather than deposits of abnormal or nonspecifically trapped immunoglobulins, which have been offered as alternative explanations. However, conclusive proof would require the demonstration of specific antibodies and corresponding antigens in the deposits. The specificities of the immunoglobulins can best be examined in eluates prepared from renal tissue. Various methods have been used to dissociate immune complexes in homogenates of renal tissue or isolated glomeruli [38]. There are several problems in elution studies, including loss of eluted antibodies through combination with eluted antigens, incomplete dissociation, and denaturation. Furthermore, to detect specific antibodies, it is necessary to have the corresponding antigens—in most disease there is no clue to the identity of antigens. Moreover, elution studies generally require a substantial amount of tissue, such as specimens obtained at nephrectomy or autopsy. In a few cases, however, antibody activity has allegedly been identified in material eluted from biopsy specimens [171,255].

DEMONSTRATION OF ANTIGENS IN GLOMERULAR DEPOSITS

The interpretation that immunoglobulin-containing deposits in glomeruli are immune complexes can be strengthened by the demonstration of antigens in the deposits through immunofluoresence. However, in view of problems inherent in the immunofluorescence technique, the claim that an antigen has been demonstrated should be carefully examined. In particular, nonspecific staining, the presence of multiple antibodies in the conjugates, and the reaction of conjugated antibodies by means of Fc fragments with rheumatoid factor in the deposits can give false-positive results. Certainly, a number of reports do not provide evidence of adequate controls or convincing photographic documentation that antigen is present in the deposits. To substantiate specificity, it should be shown that the antigen is not detected in glomerular deposits of unrelated conditions and that staining can be prevented by absorption of the antibodies with a purified preparation of the antigen. Even if all these criteria are met, the possibility exists that demonstrated antigens are merely secondarily trapped in immune deposits; however, experimental studies suggest that such trapping is transient [44,472].

Numerous antigens and etiologic agents have been implicated in several forms of presumed immune complex glomerulonephritis. Despite the number of antigens supposedly identified, the number of cases accounted for remains quite small. Why have attempts to identify antigens in glomerular deposits proved so unsuccessful? One explanation may be that in most cases there is no clue concerning the nature of the postulated antigen and therefore no feasible way of searching for it. In addition, if endogenous proteins, such as IgG or complement components, are present as antigens in immune deposits, they would not ordinarily be recognized as such.

In the following sections, evidence of immune complexes and studies concerning the nature of antigens in several forms of glomerulonephritis will be reviewed.

DETECTION OF CIRCULATING IMMUNE COMPLEXES

There has been considerable discussion in recent years concerning the relative importance of deposition of circulating complexes and in situ formation in human immune complex glomerulonephritis. As discussed earlier, these mechanisms are not necessarily mutually exclusive. Nevertheless, as learned from experimental studies, in situ formation clearly initiates deposit formation in some models, whereas in others circulating complexes are responsible. Conclusive proof of in situ formation in human disease could be provided by the demonstration that a glomerular antigen is involved, but this evidence has not been obtained in immune complex glomerulonephritis (although a glomerular antigen is clearly the target in anti-GBM nephritis). Another way in which evidence concerning the origin of glomerular deposits has been sought is through tests for circulating immune complexes.

In the 1970s, a number of methods were developed to detect and measure immune complexes in the blood or other fluids [207,514]. It was hoped that the assays would not only strengthen the evidence for a pathogenic role of circulating immune complexes, but also would provide material in which the offending antigens could be detected and would offer ways of diagnosing and monitoring "immune complex diseases." These hopes have not been realized. In fact, the tests are rarely used today for diagnostic purposes. An important reason for their demise is that the validity of most of the methods is open to question. Thus different methods often produce different results in the same serum [274]. Virtually all detect aggregated immunoglobulins. In addition, Uwatoko et al. [533] have shown that positive results obtained with the widely used C1q solid-phase radioimmunoassay often result from monomeric IgG, much of which represents autoantibodies to collagen-like regions of C1q. Newer immune complex assays are being developed through the use of monoclonal antibodies against complement components that bind to immune complexes [274]. Another problem with tests for circulating immune complexes arises because erythrocyte-bound complexes are released into the serum in variable amounts after collection of the specimens [466].

Nevertheless, it is likely that many of the results that have been obtained with assays for immune complexes are valid. Thus positive tests are often found in conditions in which there are other reasons to suspect a role of circulating complexes, in particular those with chronic antigenemia, such as hepatitis B infection and bacterial endocarditis. Further, positive tests occur in conditions in which the location of deposits (subendothelial, intraluminal, or mesangial) is consistent with a role of circulating complexes—MPGN type I, lupus nephritis, IgA nephritis, and mixed cryoglobulinemia. Such findings provide evidence for a primary role of circulating complexes in the formation of deposits. However, not all circulating complexes are pathogenic; for example, evidence of circulating immune complexes is found in several conditions without glomerulonephritis, such as in primary biliary cirrhosis or malignancies [514].

SPECIFIC FORMS OF IMMUNE COMPLEX GLOMERULONEPHRITIS

Poststreptococcal Glomerulonephritis

The evidence for the role of immune complexes in poststreptococcal glomerulonephritis and studies designed to identify the relevant antigens are extensively reviewed in Chapter 5. Based on my own studies [347] and review of the literature, I do not believe that pathogenic antigens have been convincingly identified. It seems likely that a streptococcal product(s) is the nephritogenic antigen rather than an autologous antigen, but even this is not certain [292]. Thus, although three groups have reported finding streptococcal antigens within glomeruli through the use of fluorescein-labeled antisera against streptococci or streptococcal products [12,370,524], at least two other groups have been unable to detect such material [153,364]. Furthermore, even among those who have reported positive results, there is disagreement concerning the nature of the streptococcal antigen, which reinforces doubts about the specificity of the findings.

A possible explanation for the difficulty in detection of streptococcal antigens in glomeruli is that they are present only in very small amounts, since in some cases immune deposits are scanty. It may be that the antigens serve not so much to produce immune complex injury, but rather to trigger T cell–mediated reactions, as suggested by considerations of acute serum sickness in rabbits (see p. 211) and by the findings of glomerular T cells and monocytes in the human disease [426].

Glomerulonephritis Associated with Bacterial Diseases Other than Group A Streptococcal Infections

The finding of abundant granular deposits of immunoglobulins and complement components in glomerulonephritis associated with bacterial endocarditis and atrioventricular shunt infections strongly supports an immune complex pathogenesis. The bacteria most often responsible are *Staphylococcus aureus* and those of the streptococcus viridans group. Because of the persistent presence of large numbers of bacteria in infected heart valves or shunts, it is likely that bacterial products are continuously or intermittently released into the circulation for prolonged periods in a manner that parallels protocols used to induce experimental chronic serum sickness. Furthermore, evidence of circulating immune complexes is found in many of these patients [40,226,262,375,403,404]. Studies have revealed evidence of bacterial antigens in glomeruli by direct immunofluorescence or of antibacterial antibodies in renal eluates [310]. However, the bacterial antigens present in the deposits have not been characterized. Bacterial antigens also have been identified in circulating cryoglobulins [501]. Successful treatment of the infections, which eliminates the source of bacterial antigens, is generally followed by disappearance of urinary abnormalities and improvement of renal function.

There is also evidence that visceral abscesses resulting from a variety of bacteria may be associated with immune complex glomerulonephritis, and in a few instances, bacterial antigens may have been demonstrated in glomeruli [41,42].

Syphilitic Nephritis

It is fairly well established that syphilis can produce an immune complex–mediated glomerular disease. Renal biopsies in some patients with secondary or congenital syphilis have shown varying combinations of membranous and proliferative changes. Granular deposits of immunoglobulins and complement components have been described along glomerular capillary walls and sometimes in mesangial regions. Gamble and Reardon [171] have reported that specific antitreponemal antibodies are found in eluates of renal biopsy specimens, and treponemal antigens may have been shown within glomerular deposits by immunofluorescence [523]. The apparent beneficial response to penicillin in some of the reported cases provides additional evidence for a causative role of the treponema [570].

Hepatitis B Virus–Associated Glomerulonephritis

In view of the established role of viruses in several forms of experimentally induced or spontaneously occurring immune complex glomerulonephritis in animals, viral agents are considered likely causes of some cases of human glomerulonephritis. However, hepatitis B is the only virus that has been convincingly implicated. The hepatitis B virus has certain properties in common with the lymphocytic choriomeningitis virus, which has been shown to produce immune complex glomerulonephritis in animals. Both are relatively noncytopathic, and both can induce a chronic carrier state characterized by antigenemia.

Many cases of membranous or membranoproliferative glomerulonephritis have been described in patients with hepatitis B infection, especially in children with the chronic carrier state. Furthermore, hepatitis B antigens have been found in glomerular immune deposits in many cases. There is, however, disagreement about the identity and importance of various antigens. Part of the problem may stem from lack of specificity of the reagents used. Investigators in Poland [78] and Hungary [382] have reported that HB_sAg or, less commonly, HB_cAg [488] is detectable by immunofluorescence in an appreciable percentage of patients with membranous glomerulonephritis or membranoproliferative glomerulonephritis, type I. In contrast, Takekoshi et al. [511] reported on the finding of HB_eAg by immunofluorescence in the glomerular deposits in two children with membranous glomerulonephritis in Japan. Collins et al. [103] described a patient with AIDS who had chronic hepatitis B infection and glomerulonephritis with features of membranous and membranoproliferative glomerulonephritis. HB_sAg was found in mesangial deposits, whereas only HB_eAg was demonstrable in epimembranous deposits. The latter observation supports the suggestion of Ito et al. [237] that HB_eAg is of major importance in membranous nephritis associated with hepatitis B infections. In a study of six HB_sAg-seropositive children with membranous glomerulonephritis, Ito et al. [237] found HB_eAg in glomeruli in four cases and HB_sAg in only one. HB_cAg was not demonstrable. The authors presented reasons for believing that the antisera that had been used in an earlier study [488] to detect HB_cAg probably contained anti-HB_e antibodies. Lin [316] also has found HB_eAg in a high percentage of hepatitis B–associated membranous glomerulonephritis. In a few cases, virus-like particles have been detected in glomeruli, but in most cases, the deposits are granular and lack structure.

Reports describing hepatitis antigens in glomerular deposits in appreciable numbers of patients with glomerulonephritis have not appeared from regions where hepatitis B infections or carrier states are uncommon, such as North America or Great Britain. However, isolated, well-documented cases have been described [105,289]. It is possible that the frequent detection of hepatitis B antigens in glomerular lesions of Polish children (who have a high carrier rate) reflects secondary trapping of these antigens in deposits containing complexes of other specificities. However, it has been reported from France that 42 percent of 33 children with membranous glomerulonephritis had HB_sAg detectable in the serum but not in renal tissue [282]. If technical factors did not account for these negative findings, the report provides evidence against secondary trapping.

Recent preliminary findings indicate that α-interferon therapy may induce remission of liver *and* renal disease in patients with chronic hepatitis B infection, which provides further evidence for a causative role of the viral infection [318].

Thus it seems likely that glomerular lesions can result from accumulation of immune complexes containing hepatitis antigens; however, it is not known whether the deposits result from trapping of circulating complexes or from in situ formation. Although circulating complexes are frequently found in patients with hepatitis B infection [236], no clear-cut relationship has been established between their presence and the development of glomerulonephritis.

Systemic Lupus Erythematosus (SLE)

Systemic lupus erythematosus is a disease of unknown cause, which, like its murine counterparts, is characterized by immune complex deposits in numerous sites, especially in glomeruli. The underlying immunologic derangements in SLE that lead to autoantibody formation are diverse and incompletely understood (for a recent review, see ref. 283). The present discussion will focus on the pathogenesis of the renal lesions. Many of the unresolved issues are similar to those already discussed in connection with murine models of lupus nephritis.

Lupus nephritis is considered to be one of the most thoroughly documented forms of human immune complex nephritis [348]. Abundant glomerular immune deposits are found in nearly all cases, in patterns that may be predominantly mesangial, subendothelial, intramembranous, or epimembranous; in addition, combinations of these patterns are seen. There is a general correlation between the distribution of glomerular deposits and the histologic form of lupus nephritis [349]. Tubulointerstitial deposits are also frequently found in lupus nephritis, especially in severe forms.

Although multiple autoantibodies are seen in SLE, there is considerable evidence that antibodies against native (double-stranded) DNA are of major pathogenetic importance [147]. For one thing, there is a good correlation between high levels of serum anti-DNA antibodies and signs of activity of disease. Furthermore, anti-DNA antibodies were convincingly demonstrated by Koffler et al. [288] many years ago to be concentrated in glomeruli of patients with severe lupus nephritis, as shown by analysis of eluates of renal specimens. At that time, glomerular immune deposits were thought to result exclusively from deposition of circulating immune complexes. Subsequent studies revealed evidence of circulating complexes in a high percentage of patients with SLE, although, as noted earlier, some of the results are spurious. However, contradictory results have been obtained concerning the presence of DNA–anti-DNA complexes or of free DNA in the circulation [145,240]. It is now generally believed that DNA–anti-DNA complexes constitute at most a very small percentage of the circulating complexes found in SLE, and that free DNA is either an artifact resulting from cell lysis after collection of the blood specimen or the result of cell lysis in vivo that occurs in a variety of diseases [145].

In more recent years, attention has focused on the possibility that DNA–anti-DNA complexes form within glomeruli. DNA has been shown to have an affinity for the GBM [239], possibly because DNA combines with histones, which are positively charged molecules that aggregate spontaneously to form stable complexes [471].

Lately, another mechanism has been proposed to account for the formation of glomerular deposits, namely that anti-DNA antibodies combine with antigens other than DNA within glomeruli [145]. As noted earlier, there is evidence that anti-DNA antibodies, especially monoclonal antibodies, cross-react with phospholipids, cell-surface proteins, cytoskeletal proteins, and glycosaminoglycans. Sabbaga et al. [458] have recently reported that anti-DNA antibodies eluted from two specimens of lupus nephritis exhibited more cross-reactivity than serum antibodies. The eluted antibodies reacted with ss-DNA, multiple polynucleotides, SmRNP, and phospholipids. These observations provide indirect evidence for formation of deposits through cross-reacting anti-DNA antibodies. A crucial consideration is therefore whether DNA itself is present in the glomerular deposits. As Eilat has pointed out [145], the reported evidence for DNA in glomerular deposits is questionable, since it is based on immunofluorescence studies employing anti-DNA antibodies, which might themselves cross-react with other antigens. If DNA itself is the antigen in glomerular deposits, it is not clear whether it is of exogenous or endogenous origin.

To complicate matters further, it is possible that different mechanisms and different antigens account for immune deposits in different forms of lupus nephritis. Experimental studies favor the interpretation that circulating complexes may account for mesangial or subendothelial deposits and that in situ formation may account for epimembranous or intramenbranous deposits.

A few cases of lupus nephritis have been described with severe necrotizing glomerular lesions and only scanty immune deposits, which suggests that mechanisms other than immune complex accumulation may be important in some cases [196,476].

Glomerulonephritis in Essential Mixed Cryoglobulinemia

Patients with essential mixed cryoglobulinemia, especially type II, commonly develop a distinctive form of glomerulonephritis [106,120,368] characterized by diffuse glomerular hypercellularity, due mainly to an influx of monocytes, and by intraluminal or subendothelial deposits of immunoglobulins and complement. In addition, arteritis and tubulointerstitial deposits are sometimes seen. There is strong evidence that accumulation of circulating mixed cryoglobulins is responsible for the lesions. Type II cryoglobulins are composed of monoclonal anti-IgG antibodies, usually of the IgM class, combined with polyclonal IgG. Monoclonal IgM rheumatoid factors from patients with mixed cryoglobulinemia have been shown to express cross-reactive idiotypes [120], and apparently this is due to the use of an unmutated germline V_K gene [437].

The glomerular deposits in a given patient have been shown to have the same composition as cryoglobulins isolated from the circulation, including the possession of common idiotopes on the anti-IgG components [120] and identical cylindrical structures seen by electron microscopy. It has been postulated that local precipitation in glomeruli is favored because of high concentrations of cryoglobulins resulting from filtration. In any case, the findings in essential mixed cryoglobulinemia provide impressive evidence that subendothelial deposits can result from accumulation of circulating immune complexes (that the intraluminal deposits form in the circulation goes without saying). Curiously, mesangial deposits are unusual, although this is the pattern seen following intravenous injection of most types of preformed complexes in animals.

It is believed that type II essential mixed cryoglobulinemia is basically a lymphoproliferative condition leading to clonal production of anti-IgG antibodies. However, overt evidence of malignancy is rarely found.

IgA Nephritis

Pathogenic mechanisms in IgA nephritis are reviewed in Chapter 6. The available evidence strongly favors the conclusion that the glomerular deposits are immune complexes and that they are probably derived from circulating complexes. However, although a variety of dietary or microbial antigens may have been identified in circulating complexes, there is apparently no conclusive evidence about the identity of antigens in glomerular deposits. The hypothesis that multiple antigens may be involved, even in a given patient, is attractive.

Membranoproliferative Glomerulonephritis, Type I

Possible pathogenetic mechanisms in membranoproliferative glomerulonephritis type I (with subendothelial deposits) are reviewed in Chapter 7. The close resemblance of the glomerular abnormalities to those seen in association with bacterial endocarditis or infected ventriculoatrial shunts favors the interpretation that immune complexes formed in the circulation over prolonged periods are responsible. In addition, evidence of circulating complexes has been obtained in some patients. It is possible that chronic unidentified infectious diseases are responsible, and indeed, chronic hepatitis B infections may be associated with glomerular lesions similar to those of idiopathic membranoproliferative glomerulonephritis. It also may be that the basic problem is defective elimination of complexes, such as may form in small amounts from time to time in all people during infections. This suggestion is supported by the occurrence of membranoproliferative glomerulonephritis, type I in some patients with inherited complement deficiencies, as discussed later.

Idiopathic Membranous Glomerulonephritis

Causative factors and primary pathogenetic mechanisms in membranous glomerulonephritis are extensively reviewed in Chapter 8. There is indirect evidence favoring an autoimmune basis, in particular the association with HLA-DR3 and the association with a T cell receptor phenotype similar to that seen in known autoimmune diseases, type 1 diabetes, and Graves disease [128]. Although the conclusion that the glomerular lesions result from immune complexes is generally accepted, the identity of the antigen is unknown and need not be the same, even in cases considered to be idiopathic. Because of the close resemblance of the glomerular abnormalities to those of Heymann nephritis, it is considered likely that the deposits form in situ, probably as a result of autoantibodies against podocyte surface antigens. However, as summarized in Chapter 8, attempts to implicate renal antigens similar to nephritogenic antigens of Heymann nephritis have been almost entirely unsuccessful. Nevertheless, preliminary observations obtained by Niles et al. [405] suggest that the search for antibodies against autologous renal antigens should be continued. They found that eluates from a specimen of membranous glomerulonephritis reacted with a human renal glycoprotein that may be homologous to rat gp330. Of interest, the specimen was obtained from a patient who died of a cerebral vascular accident, apparently early in the course of her renal disease. It is possible that only early deposits contain high concentrations of the relevant antibodies.

HOST FACTORS PREDISPOSING TO IMMUNE COMPLEX GLOMERULONEPHRITIS

Identification of relevant antigens, although an important goal, is only one step toward the understanding of immune complex glomerulonephritis. Clearly, the nature of the host response to the antigen is of crucial importance. Thus only a minority of individuals exposed to agents believed to induce immune complex glomerulonephritis develop disease.

For the most part, host factors that predispose to immune complex glomerulonephritis are unknown. It is not even certain to what extent susceptibility is under genetic control, although genetic influences have been clearly implicated in some diseases. The importance of genetic susceptibility in membranous glomerulonephritis was mentioned earlier. If membranous glomerulonephritis is mediated by autoantibodies against glomerular antigens, it may be that susceptibility is determined in part at least by class II MHC products, as has been shown in certain experimental models discussed earlier.

There is also evidence that genetic factors play a role in IgA nephritis, although the data are difficult to interpret, as discussed in Chapter 6. The evidence suggests that there are multiple immunoregulatory defects in patients with IgA nephritis, but how they may relate to the development of the renal disease is not known. Genetic factors are known to be important in SLE, where an association with HLA-DR2 and HLA-DR3 has been shown [441]. However, genetic factors do not account entirely for the disease; although there is a high concordance of SLE in monozygotic twins, it is closer to 60 than to 100 percent.

Deficiencies of Erythrocyte CR1

Many patients with SLE have decreased numbers of CR1 detectable on erythrocytes [140,235,373, 374]. Apparently, both genetic and acquired factors contribute to the reduction [450,565]. Reduced erythrocyte CR1 levels may aggravate the pathogenic importance of circulating complexes by interfering with their clearance.

It also has been suggested that the failure of IgA-containing complexes to bind to erythrocyte CR1 (because they do not activate the classical pathway) may be a factor in their deposition in glomeruli in IgA nephritis [469].

Reduction in Glomerular CR1

The role of glomerular CR1 in health and disease is at present totally obscure. The early suggestion that the receptors might serve to trap circulating complexes became untenable when it was learned that the receptors are restricted to podocytes. There have been, however, some interesting observations on reductions in levels of podocyte CR1 in various forms of glomerular disease. Many patients with lupus nephritis show reduced levels or absence of podocyte CR1. Minota et al. [373] reported that there is a close correlation between the reduction of CR1 on erythrocytes and on glomerular podocytes in patients with SLE, even among those without glomerular immune deposits. Although this probably reflects a genetic reduction in CR1 in SLE, several studies have shown that podocyte CR1 levels may be reduced in forms of glomerulonephritis other than lupus nephritis, with or without evidence of immune complex deposits [413,429].

Association of Genetic Complement Deficiencies with Human Immune Complex Diseases

The association of several immune complex diseases with deficiencies of complement components, especially C2, C1, or C4, strongly suggests that the complement system, and in particular the classical pathway, normally protects against these diseases [5,187,296]. It has been proposed that the association is due to an effect of a linked immune-response gene, because the genes that encode for C2 and C4 are in the region of the MHC. However, this would not account for the occurrence of immune complex diseases with C1 or C3 deficiencies [434], since these components are not encoded for in the MHC region. It has been proposed that complement deficiencies predispose to chronic microbial infections and that this accounts for the development of immune complex disorders. However, in my opinion, *the most plausible explanation for the association between complement deficiencies and immune complex diseases is that the lack of complement-mediated inhibition of immune precipitation favors the formation of insoluble deposits.* Nevertheless, it remains to be explained why so many of the patients have lupus-like syndromes in which autoantibodies against nuclear antigens play a dominant role. It is possible that complement deficiencies involve derangements in immune regulation in addition to defects in the handling of immune complexes [66].

Saturation of the Mononuclear Phagocyte System

As discussed earlier, there is experimental evidence that the capacity of mononuclear phagocyte system to clear circulating immune complexes can be saturated, which can lead to increased glomerular deposition of complexes. It has been suggested that dysfunction of the mononuclear phagocyte system may contribute to the development or intensification of human "immune complex diseases" (a description that is sometimes used to refer to SLE, immune complex glomerulonephritis, and certain forms of vasculitis thought to result from immune complexes). Frank et al. [164] and Roccatello et al. [446] have reported that patients with lupus nephritis and some other forms of immune complex nephritis clear antibody-coated erythrocytes more slowly than controls. However, reduced clearance was not found by Solomon and colleagues [489] in most patients with glomerulonephritis. In any case, the behavior of complexes composed of particulate antigens, as used in these studies, is quite different from that of complexes containing soluble antigens thought to be responsible for most immune complex deposits. At present, there is only suggestive evidence that impaired clearance of immune complexes by the mononuclear phagocyte system is important in the development of immune complex glomerulonephritis in man.

Anti-GBM Nephritis

Anti-GBM nephritis and related anti-basement-membrane disorders are reviewed in Chapter 10. Here only a few points and recent developments will be highlighted.

Anti-GBM nephritis is one of the most thoroughly documented autoimmune diseases in man. Autoantibodies against GBM components have been demonstrated in the serum and in eluates of kidney obtained from patients with anti-GBM nephritis. A faithful model has been described in sheep [493] in which the GBM antigen is the same as that involved in the human disease [81]. Transfer of human anti-GBM antibodies to nonhuman primates results in glomerular fixation of human IgG and glomerular lesions [309].

The most important recent progress in research on anti-GBM nephritis has been the characterization of the Goodpasture antigen by Wieslander and associates (for recent review, see Hudson [229]). In brief, the evidence indicates that the major antigen recognized by human anti-GBM antibodies (the Goodpasture antigen) is in a noncollagenous (NC1) domain of type IV collagen and more specifically on the newly discovered α_3 chain. The anti-GBM antibodies found in the serum and in the kidneys were shown to have the same specificity [463]; these findings support the potential therapeutic value of removal of circulating anti-GBM antibodies.

Pusey et al. [433] have reported evidence that indicates that human anti-GBM antibodies react with a very limited number of determinants. Thus a monoclonal antibody against the Goodpasture antigen was shown to block much of the binding of circulating human anti-GBM antibodies. In addition to antibodies against the Goodpasture antigen, some patients with anti-GBM nephritis have low titers of antibodies against laminin, the 7 S domain of type IV collagen and entactin [464]. The pathogenetic significance of these antibodies is unknown; they are occasionally found in other renal diseases or even in normal subjects. Newly developed assays, which employ purified antigens with ELISAs or Western blot analysis using collagenase GBM digests, permit the detection of antibodies specifically directed against the Goodpasture antigen [464]. In contrast, immunochemical assays using collagenase GBM digests detect other specificities and are therefore of less value in the diagnosis of anti-GBM nephritis [564].

The factors that initiate the formation of anti-GBM autoantibodies are unknown. Evidence that susceptibility to anti-GBM nephritis is under genetic control includes its occurrence in some identical twins and an association with HLA-DR2 and HLA-B7, as reviewed in Chapter 10. The evidence that exposure to hydrocarbons or viral infections is responsible is suggestive at best. It has been postulated that the stimulus for autoantibody formation is provided by the Goodpasture antigen itself, following release from a sequestered site. In support of this, it has been shown that the Goodpasture antigen is buried within the NC1 domain [229]. Exposure requires dissociation of the NC1 hexamer into its subunits. The sequestered-antigen hypothesis might account for the development of anti-GBM antibodies in some patients with other forms of glomerulonephritis that are associated with damage to the basement membrane [244,277,407]. However, it seems that factors other than release of antigen must be involved in the initiation of autoantibody formation in many cases of anti-GBM nephritis.

Further evidence that renal antigens may trigger the anti-GBM response has been provided by a patient with anti-GBM nephritis who received a renal transplant from an identical twin 22 months after bilateral nephrectomy [9]. The disease in the recipient appeared to have become inactive; anti-GBM antibodies were not detectable during an 18-month period prior to transplantation. Following transplantation, the patient again developed anti-GBM antibodies. The findings suggest that the reintroduction of renal tissue (which was not allogeneic) stimulated the reappearance of anti-GBM antibodies [9]. However, it is not clear that autologous renal basement-membrane antigens provided the original stimulus.

Role of T Cells in Human Glomerulonephritis

There is substantial, although largely indirect, evidence for a pathogenic role of T cells in certain human glomerular diseases [362]. As discussed earlier, the most conclusive evidence for T cell mediation of disease can be obtained through transfer studies, which obviously cannot be performed in man. The approaches that have been taken to obtain evidence of a role of T cells in human diseases include (1) demonstration of in vitro correlates of T cell reactions, for example, T cell proliferation or lymphokine production upon exposure of the patient's peripheral blood or tissue infiltrating lymphocytes to suspected pathogenic antigens; (2) analysis of phenotype of infiltrating cells in tissue sections by immunohistochemical techniques; and (3) studies in vitro of functional properties and antigenic specificities of cells recovered from lesions.

Using the first approach, Rocklin et al. [447] reported many years ago that peripheral blood lymphocytes obtained from patients with anti-GBM nephritis exhibit macrophage inhibitory factor (MIF) production upon exposure to basement membrane preparations. It would be desirable to repeat these observations using purified Goodpasture antigens and newer methods of assessing T cell responses in vitro. Even if peripheral blood T cells with specificity to the Goodpasture antigen were demonstrated, it would not prove that they directly mediated glomerular injury; they might function rather as helper cells for anti-GBM antibody production [132].

Several investigators have analyzed infiltrating mononuclear cells in various forms of glomerulonephritis using immunohistochemical techniques [22,92,154,225,329,362,377]. Mononuclear phagocytes (monocytes/macrophages) have been demonstrated in glomeruli in various forms of glomerulonephritis [92,154,378]. As discussed earlier, experimental studies have shown that their influx can be triggered by T cells. However, monocyte accumulation can result from other mechanisms, and in some diseases, notably in essential mixed cryoglobulinemia, the occurrence of mononuclear phagocytes appears to correlate with immunoglobulin deposits, which suggests that the cells accumulate by means of Fc receptors. However, in some cases, monocyte accumulation appears to be independent of immunoglobulin deposits and is associated with T cells.

A few reports have documented the presence of T cells in human glomerular diseases, especially in postinfectious glomerulonephritis or necrotizing and crescentic glomerulonephritis [22,57,92,387, 412,491,492]. The numbers have generally been small, and in most cases, $CD4^+$ T cells have predominated. Parra et al. [426] reported that early in poststreptococcal glomerulonephritis $CD4^+$ T cells predominated over $CD8^+$ cells, whereas later (>28 days) the reverse ratio was found. The finding of $CD4^+$ T cells, together with mononuclear phagocytes, offers evidence of a DTH mechanism.

Attempts to isolate and propagate T cells from human glomeruli and study their antigenic specificities and functions in vitro have apparently not been reported.

Glomerular Diseases with Obscure Immunologic Mechanisms

GLOMERULONEPHRITIS ASSOCIATED WITH ANTI-NEUTROPHIL CYTOPLASMIC ANTIBODIES (ANCA)

It has long been suspected that the conditions generally classified as necrotizing and/or crescentic glomerulonephritis, whether idiopathic or associated with Wegener's granulomatosis or some form of systemic vasculitis, are immunologically mediated. However, the immunologic mechanisms are obscure. In most cases, immunoglobulin deposits are scanty or absent, and there are no satisfactory experimental models. A role of T cells has been postulated, in large part because other mechanisms could not be documented, and also because T cells have been demonstrated in glomeruli in some cases [22,57,492].

The recent description of circulating autoantibodies against neutrophil (and monocyte) cytoplasmic antigens (ANCA) in patients with necrotizing and crescentic glomerulonephritis has heightened interest in immunologic mechanisms in necrotizing and crescentic glomerulonephritis. ANCA have been detected most often by indirect immunofluorescence using ethanol-fixed normal human neutrophils as substrates. Two staining patterns are observed. One is characterized by granular cytoplasmic staining (C-ANCA) [125,320, 326,535], which usually results from antibodies that react with a novel 29-kD serine protease (p29), which is probably proteinase 3 [191,327,406]. Nearly all patients diagnosed as having active Wegener's granulomatosis with systemic manifestations have C-ANCA [326,414,535] as well as some patients diagnosed as having idiopathic necrotizing and crescentic glomerulonephritis, which usually is associated with an ill-defined systemic illness often classified as microscopic polyarteritis nodosa [101,245].

The second type of ANCA produces nuclear or perinuclear staining (P-ANCA), which usually results from antibodies against myeloperoxidase (MPO) [101,151,245]. The P-ANCA pattern results from artifactual redistribution of MPO in ethanol-fixed neutrophils [151]. P-ANCA have been described in some patients with necrotizing and crescentic glomerulonephritis, either primary or associated with a disease often classified as microscopic polyarteritis nodosa, as well as in a very few patients with biopsy-proven Wegener's granulomatosis [11,172].

Niles et al. [407] recently conducted a study on the diagnostic usefulness of ANCA in 123 patients who presented with the clinical picture of rapidly progressive glomerulonephritis, using radioimmunoassays with purified p29 and MPO, the two best characterized antigens recognized by ANCA [407]. Twenty-six of 42 patients with necrotizing and crescentic glomerulonephritis with scanty or no immune deposits (so-called pauci-immune) had anti-MPO antibodies, and 14 had anti-p29 antibodies. No patient had both types of ANCA. ANCA were also found by RIA in 8 of 18 patients with anti-GBM nephritis (with documented antibodies to the Goodpasture antigen [464]). However, among 976 additional control specimens, including 225 from patients with other forms of renal disease, there were six apparently false positive tests for ANCA. If one excludes the patients with anti-GBM nephritis, the RIAs for ANCA had a 99.4 percent specificity for pauci-immune necrotizing and crescentic glomerulonephritis.

The finding of the combined presence of anti-GBM antibodies and ANCA in some patients confirms results obtained in two other studies [244,416]. Since both anti-GBM antibodies and ANCA have a very low prevalence, their coexistence cannot be coincidental. The cause of the phenomenon is unknown. It is possible that anti-GBM antibodies were produced secondary to release of GBM antigens. At present, it is not clear how patients with both ANCA and anti-GBM antibodies should be classified.

The study of Niles et al. [407] differs from several earlier investigations in that these authors studied patients in whom renal disease was a prominent part of their presentation, whereas others dealt with patients having a wider spectrum of clinical manifestations. Patients with Wegener's granulomatosis may present with localized necrotizing granulomatous lesions, generally in the respiratory tract, and are frequently negative for C-ANCA [414,535]. Some of these patients may continue to have localized lesions for years [155]. The vast majority of these become C-ANCA positive (and a very few P-ANCA positive) when they develop more diffuse lesions, including pulmonary capillaritis and/or necrotizing and crescentic glomerulonephritis [414]. Patients with characteristic necrotizing or granulomatous lesions, with or without systemic disease, are appropriately called *Wegener's granulomatosis,* and C-ANCA has been described as highly specific for patients with these features in several large series [414,535]. However, some patients, as in the study of Niles et al., as well as in other studies [101,245], have had C-ANCA with pulmonary capillaritis and/or necrotizing and crescentic glomerulonephritis without evidence of granulomatous lesions. Furthermore, other patients can have indistinguishable pulmonary capillaritis and/or necrotizing and crescentic glomerulonephritis in association with P-ANCA. In view of the specificity of the tests, it seems unlikely that patients with ANCA and necrotizing and crescentic glomerulonephritis, with or without classical features of Wegener's granulomatosis, are suffering from basically different glomerular diseases. The findings indicate, however, that different mechanisms may underly the glomerular and granulomatous lesions. From the point of view of terminology, *p29-ANCA– and MPO-ANCA–associated vasculitis, capillaritis, or glomerulonephritis* may be appropriate. The term *Wegener's granulomatosis* should probably be restricted to patients with typical necrotizing or granulomatous lesions, whether or not they have associated systemic manifestations or ANCA. The limitations of the term *microscopic polyarteritis nodosa* are fully discussed in Chapter 16.

Although ANCA are reliable markers of pauci-immune necrotizing and crescentic glomerulonephritis, it is not clear what their pathogenetic role is, if any. Titers of ANCA fall in most patients who undergo remission, but this does not happen invariably. It has been suggested that ANCA activate and release mediators from neutrophils, and there is in vitro evidence to support this [151,151*a*]. However, the glomerular lesions are distinctive and severe, and it seems that special, unrecognized pathogenetic mechanisms are involved. The role of T cells in the mediation of the glomerular lesions is totally unknown. It is not known what induces the production of ANCA.

Tubulointerstitial Nephritis: Immunologic Mechanisms

Evidence of immunologic mechanisms has been obtained in several human tubulointerstitial renal diseases [16,351,353,354,361] (see Table 3-3). It is convenient to consider antibody and cell-mediated mechanisms separately, although they often appear to operate simultaneously, as in some experimental models discussed earlier.

TUBULOINTERSTITIAL IMMUNE COMPLEXES

Evidence of tubulointerstitial immune complex deposits is provided by the detection of distinct granular deposits containing immunoglobulins and complement along the TBM or in the interstitium

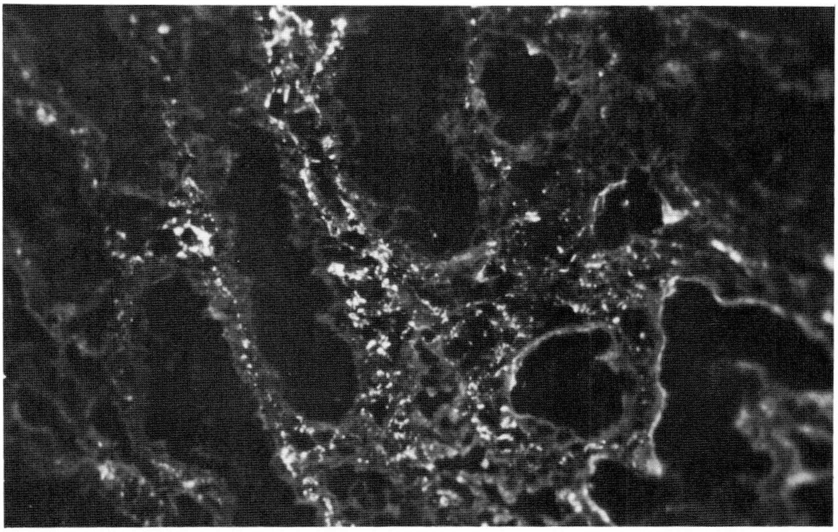

Fig. 3-13. *Frozen section of a renal biopsy specimen from a patient with idiopathic mixed cryoglobulinemia. Extensive granular tubulointerstitial deposits of IgM are seen.* ×400. *(Courtesy of Mr. A. B. Collins.)*

[16,73,276]. The condition in which prominent deposits are most often found is lupus nephritis; deposits are seen in about 50 percent of biopsies and are frequently associated with tubulointerstitial damage [73,307]. Antibodies reactive with thymidine, cytosine, or both have been shown to bind to the deposits in a few cases, providing evidence that the deposits may contain DNA [73]. In most cases of lupus nephritis, the severity of the tubulointerstitial damage parallels that of the glomerular disease. In a few patients, however, extensive tubulointerstitial deposits and severe tubulointerstitial damage have been seen with only minimal glomerular disease [115,148]. This indicates that the deposits do not result merely from saturation of normal removal mechanisms of circulating complexes. It is possible that Fc receptors present in the interstitium are involved in localization of the complexes [177].

Tubulointerstitial immunoglobulin-containing deposits have been described only infrequently in conditions other than lupus nephritis [351]. Extensive and conspicuous deposits have been described in a few patients with mixed cryoglobulinemia (Fig. 3-13), in Sjögren syndrome [566], in two patients with hypocomplementemic vasculitis, severe interstitial nephritis, mild mesangial glomerular lesions, and no conclusive evidence of systemic lupus erythematosus [109,411], and in a patient with atypical membranous nephritis with anti-brush border antibodies [136]. Less conspicuous deposits have been found in a few cases of renal allografts and with various forms of glomerulonephritis (membranous, membranoproliferative, crescentic, and shunt-associated) [276]. Small, irregular masses of IgG have been described in a few patients with chronic pyelonephritis and chronic interstitial nephritis [109].

Antigens in deposits have apparently been identified only in a few cases of lupus nephritis, as noted earlier, and in a patient with membranous nephritis (brush border antigens) [136]. In mixed cryoglobulinemia, the deposits presumably contain IgM–anti-IgG complexes, as evidenced by the presence of these reactants and the demonstration of anti-IgG activity through binding of fluoresceinated aggregated IgG [351].

ANTI-TBM NEPHRITIS

Anti-TBM antibodies have been thoroughly documented in human disease, but only in a relatively small number of cases [351]. The presence of anti-TBM antibodies is suggested by linear TBM staining for IgG and C3. (Staining for C3 alone in an interrupted linear pattern is not regarded as evidence for anti-TBM antibodies; this finding is often made in normal kidneys and is of uncertain significance.) Definitive evidence can be provided by the demonstration, by indirect immunofluorescence, of anti-TBM antibodies in the circulation or, when adequate tissue is available, in eluates of kidney.

Evidence of anti-TBM autoantibodies has been obtained in some patients with anti-GBM nephritis, in some renal allograft recipients, in a few patients with glomerulonephritis presumably mediated by immune complexes, in rare patients with lupus nephritis, in a small number of patients with drug-induced tubulointerstitial nephritis, and in a few patients with isolated tubulointerstitial disease [351].

More than half the patients with anti-GBM nephritis have associated anti-TBM antibodies, and Andres et al. [15] showed that the patients with anti-TBM antibodies have more severe tubulointerstitial damage than those without. IgG in eluates of renal tissue prepared from some patients with anti-GBM nephritis produce linear TBM staining along most of the cortical tubules, whereas other eluates react with only a few tubules, which suggests that antibodies in anti-GBM nephritis recognize more than one TBM antigen [563,564]. The target antigens have apparently not been characterized.

Serum antibodies from two patients with anti-TBM nephritis without anti-GBM antibodies (one idiopathic and one after renal transplantation) were shown to react with a proximal tubular basement membrane antigen termed *H3M-1*, which is a glycoprotein with an estimated weight of 48 to kD [97]. H3M-1 is analogous to the rabbit TBM antigen, designated *R3M-1*, which, as noted earlier, can induce experimental anti-TBM nephritis in guinea pigs.

Role of T Cells in Renal Diseases with Interstitial Mononuclear-Cell Infiltrates

In many renal diseases, prominent interstitial mononuclear-cell infiltrates are seen. Immunohistochemical studies with monoclonal antibodies performed in recent years have shown that T cells predominate in most cases. In addition to providing information about the phenotype of the infiltrating cells, immunohistochemical studies have revealed increased numbers of interstitial mononuclear cells even in conditions where their presence was not recognized in histologic preparations [119].

Interstitial T cell infiltrates are seen not only in diseases classified as interstitial (or tubulointerstitial) nephritis, but also in various forms of glomerulonephritis. The mechanisms leading to the accumulation of T cells in the interstitium are probably diverse and are mostly unknown. Current thinking about the nature and significance of the infiltrating cells is heavily influenced by immunohistochemical studies employing monoclonal antibodies.

I have already discussed the value and limitations of analysis of the phenotypes of mononuclear infiltrates in tissue sections [354]. The presence of large numbers of T cells with activation markers (Ia, transferrin receptors) in the renal interstitium probably indicates an ongoing T cell reaction initiated by an antigen native to or bound to the kidney. However, the presence of small lymphocytes, as is seen in many chronic renal diseases, including ischemic disorders, is of uncertain significance. It is not clear that the cells are functioning immunologically, since they lack activation markers.

In conditions characterized by activated T cells, T cell subset analysis can provide indirect evidence of the type of T cell reaction, as discussed earlier; a predominance of $CD4^+$ T cells, espe-

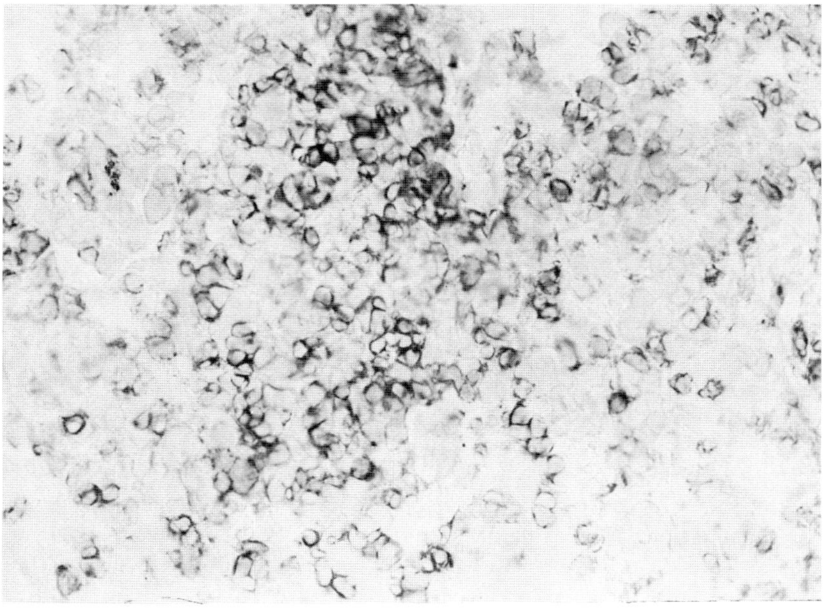

Fig. 3-14. *Frozen section of a renal biopsy specimen from a patient with anti-GBM nephritis. Numerous $CD4^+$ cells are seen in the interstitium.* ×313. *(Courtesy of Mr. A. B. Collins.)*

cially if accompanied by macrophages or granulomas, suggests a DTH reaction, and a predominance of $CD8^+$ T cells suggests a cytolytic reaction. However, for reasons already discussed, firm conclusions can rarely be drawn. Furthermore, immunohistochemical studies of cells infiltrating renal tissue have provided no information of diagnostic value [77].

T CELLS IN INTERSTITIAL INFILTRATES ASSOCIATED WITH GLOMERULONEPHRITIS

In most patients with anti-GBM nephritis, intense lymphocytic infiltrates are seen, some of which are concentrated around glomeruli. Interstitial infiltrates may be found in patients with or without TBM-bound IgG but appear to be more intense in the former group. In the few cases that have been studied by immunohistochemical techniques, numerous $CD4^+$ T cells have been found, many with activation markers (Ia, transferrin receptors) [57,491] (Fig. 3-14). In addition, numerous macrophages have been found. It is reasonable to assume that some of the infiltrating activated T cells are specifically sensitized to basement membrane antigens. However, direct evidence for this conclusion, as might be obtained by in vitro studies of T cells propagated from renal infiltrates, is lacking. Some of the infiltrating $CD4^+$ T cells may function as helper cells for antibody production (including anti-GBM antibodies), since some B cells and plasma cells are generally present in the infiltrates. Another likely role is induction of DTH reactions, an interpretation that is supported by the presence of numerous macrophages and occasional multinuclear cells.

Numerous interstitial T cells have been found in association with other forms of glomerulonephritis, including necrotizing and crescentic, and various forms of proliferative glomerulonephritis [57,67,225], lupus nephritis, mixed cryoglobulinemias, and others [77,119]. The mechanisms leading to interstitial infiltrates in these disorders are unknown; it may be that the antigens involved in the glomerular damage are also present in the interstitium. Evidence of this has been obtained in some cases of lupus nephritis and mixed cryoglobulinemias.

In most forms of glomerulonephritis, $CD4^+$ T cells predominate or are roughly equal to the number of $CD8^+$ cells in the interstitium [67]. However, there is considerable variation in the ratios, even within a given disease category.

In lupus nephritis, $CD8^+$ cells have been found to outnumber $CD4^+$ cells in half or more of the cases in some studies [8,117], whereas in another study [82], $CD4^+$ T cells predominated. Interstitial infiltrates are found in cases of lupus nephritis with or without tubulointerstitial immune deposits [8]. Alexopoulos et al. [8] observed expression of HLA-DR by tubular cells, which correlated with expression of DR in infiltrating interstitial cells. This group also found interstitial macrophages and cells with NK markers. NK cells were present in higher numbers in specimens with interstitial immune deposits than in those without; these authors interpreted this as indicative of antibody-dependent cell-mediated cytotoxicity. In one study, the degree of renal functional impairment at the time of biopsy correlated with the intensity of interstitial inflammation [8], but in another study, such a correlation was not found [117].

T CELLS IN INTERSTITIAL NEPHRITIS

Interstitial nephritis is commonly divided into acute and chronic forms (see Chap. 19). Acute interstitial nephritis, characterized by mononuclear cell infiltrates, was described many years ago in association with certain infections, such as scarlet fever or diphtheria, in the absence of bacteria in the kidneys. These forms are rarely seen today, and information on the phenotype of infiltrating cells is not available. The most common types of acute interstitial nephritis seen today are those associated with certain therapeutic drugs, with uveitis, or as idiopathic diseases [512].

Drug-Induced Acute Interstitial Nephritis: The Role of T Cells

It is well established that certain medications, notably beta-lactam antibiotics and nonsteroidal anti-inflammatory drugs, can induce acute tubulointerstitial nephritis. Furthermore, there is considerable evidence that the renal lesions result from immunologic mechanisms rather than toxic effects of the drug [361]. Thus only a small percentage of the patients who take the medication develop acute interstitial nephritis, and the reactions are not dose related. Furthermore, some patients with renal lesions, especially those associated with beta-lactam antibiotics, have systemic manifestations of hypersensitivity, including fever, rash, arthralgia, and eosinophils.

It seems likely that a hapten derivative of the drug becomes bound to certain sites in renal tissue, and that the reactivity is directed against a conjugate consisting of the hapten and the host component. Indeed, a drug hapten has been demonstrated in the TBM or interstitium by immunofluorescence in a few cases of methicillin-or penicillin-associated interstitial nephritis [361]. A model in which this type of mechanism operates has been described by Rennke et al. [442], as discussed earlier.

However, the immunologic mechanisms in drug-induced acute interstitial nephritis have not been completely elucidated. Apparently several mechanisms participate, and these appear to vary in importance from one case to another. In some patients, antibodies appear to be important, as evidenced by the presence of plasma cells and eosinophils. Moreover, anti-TBM antibodies have been described, but only in a few patients [361]. However, three considerations suggest that cell-mediated mechanisms are more important than antibody mechanisms: (1) T cells invariably predominate in the renal infiltrates (as discussed below), (2) granulomas are found in some cases, and (3) immunoglobulin accumulation is lacking in most specimens.

Immunohistochemical Studies of Infiltrating Cells in Drug-Induced Nephritis. Studies employing monoclonal antibodies have revealed that the majority of infiltrating mononuclear cells in drug-induced acute interstitial nephritis are T lymphocytes, with smaller percentages of mononuclear phagocytes and B cells [67,118]. Among the T cells, the percentage of $CD4^+$ and $CD8^+$ cells has varied in different patients and in various studies. In a few patients receiving beta-lactam antibiotics, $CD4^+$ cells have outnumbered $CD8^+$ cells [67,361]. However, in other cases, the ratio of $CD4^+$ to $CD8^+$ cells has been less than 1 [118]. In most patients with acute interstitial nephritis associated with nonsteroidal anti-inflammatory drugs, $CD8^+$ cells have predominated. However, D'Agati et al. [118] found no statistically significant differences in the ratio of $CD4^+$ to $CD8^+$ cells in patients receiving beta-lactam antibiotics or nonsteroidal anti-inflammatory drugs. Such differences as have been reported in individual cases are difficult to evaluate and may simply reflect the stage when the biopsies were performed. HLA-DR has been found on an appreciable number of T cells, indicating activation [232].

Expression of HLA-DR by tubule cells has been found in some cases of drug-induced acute interstitial nephritis [67]. As discussed earlier, this could play a role in the induction or, more probably, in intensification of the reaction.

Although the predominance of T cells favors a role for these cells, it is not clear whether delayed-type hypersensitivity or cytotoxic effects or both are involved. The finding of granulomas in some cases clearly points to delayed-type hypersensitivity. However, the high percentage of $CD8^+$ cells favors a cytotoxic reaction, which might be directed against parenchymal cells bearing drug derivatives.

Acute Tubulointerstitial Nephritis with Uveitis: The Role of T Cells

The features of this syndrome are described in Chapter 19. The evidence that the renal lesions are mediated by T cells consists of the finding of numerous infiltrating T cells in the absence of immunoglobulin deposits. $CD4^+$ T cells have been found to predominate in two cases studied [67]. The responsible antigen is unknown, but an autologous antigen is suspected. In this connection, autoimmune uveitis has been induced experimentally by immunization with ocular extracts in adjuvants [91]. Furthermore, reactivity of peripheral blood lymphocytes to a crude renal preparation was reported in two patients with uveitis and acute interstitial nephritis [275].

Secondary Pathogenetic Mechanisms in Human Renal Disease

Secondary pathogenetic mechanisms in human immunologic renal diseases are difficult to document or test directly. However, the presence in the kidneys of complement components, leukocytes, platelets, and coagulation factors in various human diseases supports pathogenic roles similar to those demonstrated in experimental models. In addition, there is reason to suspect the importance of cytokines, eicosanoids, oxygen species, and other mediators that are difficult to detect in man.

ROLE OF LEUKOCYTES

Neutrophils are present in various forms of glomerulonephritis and may contribute to injury, as in certain models. Mononuclear phagocytes (including activated macrophages) [92] have been shown to be prominent in acute glomerulonephritis [329,378], various forms of "proliferative" glomerulonephritis [225], essential mixed cryoglobulinema [377,378], and lupus nephritis [22]. Based on experimental studies, it seems probable that the monocytes contribute to glomerular damage, and some evidence for this is provided by an apparent correlation between the degree of monocyte infiltration and proteinuria [154]. Macrophages also have been demonstrated in human crescents [26], where they may contribute appreciably to the cell mass and generate procoagulant activity, as well as growth factors that may be essential for crescent formation.

ROLE OF THE COAGULATION SYSTEM AND PLATELETS

The finding of fibrin (or other fibrinogen derivatives) in early crescents is similar to that in experimental models, where defibrination, fibrinolysis by t-PA, or anticoagulation with dicumarol prevent crescent formation, as discussed earlier. Studies on the effects of anticoagulant therapy in human crescentic glomerulonephritis have been inconclusive [355]. However, in some of the studies, heparin has been used, and this has been found to be relatively ineffective in experimental models. Furthermore, to have any effect, therapy would have to be started very quickly, because of the rapidity with which most crescents undergo fibrosis. The apparent beneficial effects of plasmapheresis in some cases of crescentic glomerulonephritis could conceivably be *in part* due to lowering of fibrinogen levels.

Fibrinogen-reactive materials or fibrin thrombi also may be found in glomerular tufts in certain conditions, such as acute glomerulonephritis [364] and necrotizing and crescentic glomerulonephritis, where they may contribute to injury.

Platelets are observed in glomerular capillaries in various forms of glomerulonephritis. Moreover, increased intrarenal platelet consumption has been found to occur in some patients with glomerular disease, including those with severe lupus nephritis [95]. In addition, platelet antigens have been demonstrated in glomeruli by immunohistochemical techniques in patients with membranoproliferative glomerulonephritis and lupus nephritis [89,372]. As noted earlier, the localization of cationic platelet proteins in the GBM could increase permeability and promote the deposition of circulating immune complexes. Numerous other factors released from platelets might participate in injury, as discussed earlier.

ROLE OF THE COMPLEMENT SYSTEM

A pathogenic role of the complement system is supported by the finding of complement components in glomerular deposits, usually in association with immunoglobulins. Based on early experimental studies, most consideration has been given to the possibility that complement activation led to accumulation of leukocytes, which could result in glomerular damage. More recently, evidence has been obtained that C5b-9, whose effect is independent of leukocytes, may play a pathogenic role in certain human renal diseases [111]. Thus C5b-9 neoantigen accumulation has been demonstrated in human membranous glomerulonephritis, membranoproliferative glomerulonephritis [111,150], poststreptococcal glomerulonephritis [426], and lupus nephritis [218]. As in experimental models, the C5b-9 complex may produce damage that results in proteinura, although direct evidence of this is lacking.

The possible role of various complement components in acute glomerulonephritis and membranoproliferative glomerulonephritis has been reviewed in Chapters 5 and 7.

ROLE OF CYTOKINES AND EICOSANOIDS

Investigation of the role of cytokines and eicosanoids is in an early stage in experimental models and has barely begun in human diseases. Increased urinary excretion of IL-6 has been reported in patients with mesangial proliferative glomerulonephritis [228]. Indirect evidence of cytokine effects on glomeruli may be obtained by demonstration of endothelial cell activation [110]. With the development of new methods of detection and measurement of cytokines and eicosanoids, new information about their participation may be forthcoming.

GENERAL COMMENTS ABOUT MEDIATORS IN RENAL INJURY

The ultimate goal of investigating secondary mediators in renal disease is to find ways in which their injurious effects can be blocked therapeutically. For a number of reasons, many of which I have already discussed, this goal will be difficult to attain. For one thing, as learned from experimental studies, multiple, often overlapping pathways to injury exist, and if one is blocked, another is followed. In only a few models has a dominant mechanism been clearly documented. For example, fibrin accumulation in Bowman's space is essential for crescent formation, and activation of C5b-9 is required for proteinuria in Heymann nephritis. Another problem is that interference with mediators would have to be undertaken early to prevent irreparable damage in most renal diseases. The best hope for effective interaction would appear to be in rapidly progressive glomerular diseases, where the prevention of effect of mediators *combined* with measures that suppress the underlying immunologic mechanisms might be beneficial.

Control of nonimmunologic mechanisms of renal injury, such as hypertension, may offer more effective means of slowing the progression of various forms of chronic renal disease [422].

CONCLUDING REMARKS

In the third edition of this book, published in 1983, I concluded my chapter with a summary of the major changes in thinking about immunologic mechanisms in glomerular diseases that had occurred in the preceding decade (tubulointerstitial disease was not covered). Most of the advances came from experimental studies and included the following: the recognition that in situ formation is a mechanism of glomerular immune deposit formation, which had previously been assumed to result only from deposition of circulating immune complexes; the demonstration that T cell (DTH) mechanisms can produce glomerular disease; and the recognition of the importance of mononuclear phagocytes in the production of glomerular injury.

I also commented on how little progress had been made in the preceding decade in understanding human glomerular diseases, in particular in the following areas: in the identification of antigens involved in immune complex glomerulonephritis, in the documentation and measurement of anti-GBM antibodies, and in the elucidation of host factors that predispose to immunologic glomerular disease (although there was fragmentary information about the relationship of certain diseases with complement deficiencies and certain MHC associations).

What can be said of progress made in the past 8 years or so in understanding of immunologically mediated renal disease, including tubulointerstitial disease? Again, most progress has been made in studies of experimental models. The major advances, in my opinion, include the following: the further elucidation of the mechanisms of in situ formation of glomerular immune deposits, in particular the phenomenon of shedding of complexes from cell surfaces into adjacent basement membranes; identification of gp330 as the major pathogenic antigen of Heymann nephritis; the increasing recognition of the role of charge as a factor in localization of antigens or immune complexes in glomeruli; the recognition of the importance of the complement system in protection against immune complex diseases, through the erythrocyte CR1 mechanism for clearance of circulating immune complexes and through prevention or solubilization of immune precipitates; the role of the C5b-9 complex in glomerular injury; increasing knowledge of the importance and complexity of T cell mechanisms in glomerular, and especially tubulointerstitial, injury; recognition of the role of mesangial cells in the production of glomerular abnormalities; and expanding knowledge about mediators of injury, in particular, cytokines, oxygen metabolites, and eicosanoids.

With respect to understanding of immunologic mechanisms in human renal diseases, progress has continued to be slow. Among the major advances are the following: the identification of the antigen (the Goodpasture antigen) recognized by pathogenic anti-GBM antibodies, as a component of the α_3-chain type IV collagen in the NC1 region, which has led to the development of sensitive and specific assays for circulating anti-GBM antibodies; the recognition that anti-neutrophil cytoplasmic antibodies (ANCA) are sensitive and specific diagnostic markers for certain forms of necrotizing and crescentic glomerulonephritis; and the increasing recognition of the role of T cells in renal diseases, especially in tubulointerstitial diseases, largely as a result of analysis of infiltrating cells through the use of monoclonal antibodies and immunoperoxidase techniques.

Areas in which little or no progress has been made in human disease include the identification of antigens in immune complex glomerulonephritis; the identification of mediators of renal injury, and in particular the relevance of mediators demonstrated in experimental studies; the development of reliable assays for the detection and measurement of circulating pathogenic immune complexes; further understanding of the genetic basis for susceptibility to human diseases; and most important, in the development of safe, effective, and specific methods of treatment of immunologically mediated renal diseases.

In my opinion, the greatest hope for progress in the next decade is based on knowledge obtained in basic immunology, in particular in the elucidation of how the immune response is initiated and controlled. The ultimate hope for the prevention or treatment of immunologic diseases, including renal diseases, is to identify and eliminate specifically the immune response that leads to tissue injury. In view of the ignorance of pathogenic antigens in human renal diseases and the complexity of the immune response, this goal is still a long way off.

REFERENCES

1. Acha-Orbea, H., Mitchell, D. J., Timmermann, L., Wraith, D. C., Tausch, G. S., Waldor, M. K., Zamvil, S. S., McDevitt, H. O., and Steinman, L. Limited heterogeneity of T cell receptors from lymphocytes mediating autoimmune encephalomyelitis allows specific immune intervention. *Cell* 54:263, 1988.
2. Acha-Orbea, H., Steinman, L., and McDevitt, H. O. T-cell receptors in murine autoimmune diseases. *Annu. Rev. Immunol.* 7:371, 1989.
3. Ada, G. L., and Rose, N. R. The initiation and early development of autoimmune diseases. *Clin. Immunol. Immunopathol.* 41:3, 1988.
4. Adorini, L., and Nagy, Z. A. Peptide competition for antigen presentation. *Immunol. Today* 11:21, 1990.
5. Agnello, V. Complement deficiency states. *Medicine* (Baltimore) 57:1, 1978.
6. Agodoa, L. Y. C., Gauthier, V. J., and Mannik, M. Precipitating antigen-antibody systems are required for the formation of subepithelial electron-dense immune deposits in rat glomeruli. *J. Exp. Med.* 158:1259, 1988.
7. Albini, B., Penner, E., Stinson, M. W., Andres, G. A., and Milgrom, F. Identification of Antigens in Immune Complexes. In F. Milgrom, C. J. Abeyounis, and B. Albini (Eds.), *Antibodies: Protective, Destructive, and Regulatory Role. 9th International Convocation in Immunology, Amherst, N. Y.* Basel: Karger, 1985. P. 371.
8. Alexopoulos, E., Seron, D., Hartley, R. B., and Cameron, J. S. Lupus nephritis: Correlation of interstitial cells with glomerular function. *Kidney Int.* 37:100, 1990.
9. Almkuist, R. D., Buckalew, V. M., Hirszel, P., Maker, J. F., James, P. M., and Wilson, C. B. Recurrence of anti-glomerular basement membrane antibody-mediated glomerulonephritis in an isograft. *Clin. Immunol. Immunopathol.* 18:54, 1981.
10. Alousi, M. A., Post, R. A., and Heymann, W. Experimental autoimmune nephrosis in rats. Morphogenesis of the glomerular lesion: Immunohistochemical and electron microscopic studies. *Am. J. Pathol.* 54:47, 1969.
11. Andrassy, K., Koderisch, J., Erb, A., Waldherr, R., and Ritz, E. Detection and clinical implication of anti-neutrophil cytoplasm antibodies in Wegener's granulomatosis and rapidly progressive glomerulonephritis. *Clin. Nephrol.* 32:159, 1989.
12. Andres, G. A., Accinni, L., Hsu, K. C., Zabriskie, J. B., and Seegal, B. C. Electron microscopic studies of human glomerulonephritis with ferritin conjugated antibody: Localization of antigen-antibody complexes in glomerular structures of patients with acute glomerulonephritis. *J. Exp. Med.* 123:399, 1966.
13. Andres, G., Brentjens, J., Caldwell, P., Camussi, G., Kitazawa, K., Noble, B., and Matsuo, S. A New Look at the Mechanisms Responsible for In Situ Formation of Immune Deposits. In F. Milgrom, C. J. Abeyounis, and B. Albini (Eds.), *Antibodies: Protective, Destructive and Regulatory Role. 9th International Convocation on Immunology.* Karger: New York, 1985. P. 351.
14. Andres, G., Brentjens, J. R., Caldwell, P. R. B., Camussi, G., and Matsuo, S. Biology of disease: Formation of immune deposits and disease. *Lab. Invest.* 55:510, 1986.
15. Andres, G. A., Brentjens, J., Kohli, R., Anthone, R., Baliah, T., Montes, M., Mookerjee, B. K., Prezyna, A., Sepulveda, M., Venuto, R., and Elwood, C. Histology of human tubulointerstitial nephritis associated with antibodies to renal basement membranes. *Kidney Int.* 13:480, 1978.

16. Andres, G. A., and McCluskey, R. T. Tubular and interstitial renal disease due to immunologic mechanisms. *Kidney Int.* 7:271, 1975.
17. Andre-Schwartz, J., Datta, S. K., Shoenfeld, Y., Isenberg, D. A., Stollar, B. D., and Schwartz, R. S. Binding of cytoskeletal proteins by monoclonal anti-DNA lupus autoantibodies. *Clin. Immunol. Immunopathol.* 31:261, 1984.
18. Andrews, B. S., Eisenberg, R. A., Theofilopoulos, A. N., Izui, S., Wilson, C. B., McConahey, P. J., Murphy, E. D., Roths, J. B., and Dixon, F. J. Spontaneous murine lupus-like syndromes. *J. Exp. Med.* 148:1198, 1978.
19. Andrews, J., Hang, L., Theofilopoulos, A. N., and Dixon, F. J. Lack of relationship between serum gp70 levels and the severity of systemic lupus erythematosus in MRL/l mice. *J. Exp. Med.* 163:458, 1986.
20. Arisz, L., Noble, B., Milgrom, M., Brentjens, J. R., and Andres, G. A. Experimental chronic serum sickness in rats: A model of immune complex glomerulonephritis and systemic immune complex deposition. *Int. Arch. Allergy Appl. Immunol.* 60:80, 1979.
21. Arnaout, M. A., and Colten, H. R. Complement C3 receptors: Structure and function. *Molec. Immunol.* 21:1191, 1984.
22. Arrizabalaga, P., Mirapeix, E., Darnell, A., Torras, A., and Revert, L. Cellular immunity analysis using monoclonal antibodies in human glomerulonephritis. *Nephron* 53:41, 1989.
23. Assmann, K. J. M., Ronco, P., Tangelder, M. M., Lange, W. P. H., Verroust, P., and Koene, R. A. P. Comparison of antigenic targets involved in antibody-mediated membranous glomerulonephritis in the mouse and rat. *Am. J. Pathol.* 121:112, 1985.
24. Assmann, K. J. M., Ronco, P., Tangelder, M. M., Lange, W. P. H., Verroust, P., and Koene, R. A. P. Involvement of an antigen distinct from the Heymann antigen in membranous glomerulonephritis in the mouse. *Lab Invest.* 60:138, 1989.
25. Assmann, K. J. M., Tangelder, M. M., Lange, W. P. J., Tadema, T. M., and Koene, R. A. P. Membranous glomerulonephritis in the mouse. *Kidney Int.* 24:303, 1983.
26. Atkins, R. C., and Holdsworth, S. R. Cellular Mechanisms of Immune Glomerular Injury. In C. B. Wilson, B. M. Brenner, and J. H. Stein (Eds.), *Immunopathology of Renal Disease.* New York: Churchill Livingstone, 1988. P. 111.
27. Baker, P. J., Ochi, R. F., Schulze, M., Johnson, R. J., Campbell, C., and Couser, W. G. Depletion of C6 prevents development of proteinuria in experimental membranous nephropathy in rats. *Am. J. Pathol.* 135:185, 1989.
28. Balkwill, F. R., and Burke, F. The cytokine network. *Immunol. Today* 10:299, 1989.
29. Bannister, K. M., Ulich, T. R., and Wilson, C. B. Induction, characterization, and cell transfer of autoimmune tubulointerstitial nephritis in the Lewis rat. *Kidney Int.* 32:642, 1987.
30. Bannister, K. M., and Wilson, C. B. Transfer of tubulointerstitial nephritis in the Brown Norway rat with anti-tubular basement membrane antibody: Quantitation and kinetics of binding and effect of decomplementation. *J. Immunol.* 135:3911, 1985.
31. Barabas, A. Z., and Lannigan, R. Induction of an autologous immune complex glomerulonephritis in the rat by intravenous injection of heterologous anti-rat kidney tubular antibody: I. Production of chronic progressive immune-complex glomerulonephritis. *Br. J. Exp. Pathol.* 55:47, 1974.
32. Barba, L. M., Caldwell, P. R. B., Downie, G. H., Camussi, G., Brentjens, J. R., and Andres, G. Lung injury mediated by antibodies to endothelium: I. In the rabbit a repeated interaction of heterologous anti–angiotensin-converting enzyme antibodies with alveolar endothelium results in resistance to immune injury through antigenic modulation. *J. Exp. Med.* 158:2141, 1983.
33. Barnes, J. L., Camussi, G., Tetta, C., and Venkatachalam, M. A. Glomerular localization of platelet cationic proteins after immune complex–induced platelet activation. *Lab. Invest.* 63:755,1990.
34. Barnes, J. L., and Hevey, K. A. Glomerular mesangial cell migration in response to platelet-derived growth factor. *Lab. Invest.* 62:379, 1990.
35. Barnes, J. L., Levine, S. P., and Venkatachalam, M. A. Binding of platelet factor four (PF4) to glomerular polyanion. *Kidney Int.* 25:759, 1984.
36. Barnes, J. L., and Venkatachalam, M. A. The role of platelets and polycationic mediators in glomerular vascular injury. *Semin. Nephrol.* 5:57, 1985.
37. Bar-Shavit, R., Kahn, A., Fenton, J. W., and Wilner, G. D. Chemotactic response of monocytes to thrombin. *J. Cell Biol.* 96:282, 1983.
38. Bartolotti, S. R. Quantitative elution studies in experimental immune complex and nephrotoxic nephritis. *Clin. Exp. Immunol.* 29:334, 1977.
39. Bartolotti, S. R., and Peters, D. K. Delayed removal of renal-bound antigen in decomplemented rabbits with acute serum sickness. *Clin. Exp. Immunol.* 32:199, 1978.
40. Bayer, A. S., Theofilopoulos, A. N., Tillman, D. B., Dixon, F. J., and Guze, L. B. Use of circulating immune complex levels in the serodifferentiation of endocarditic and nonendocarditic septicemias. *Am. J. Med.* 66:58, 1979.
41. Beaufils, M., Gibert, C., Morel-Maroger, L.,

Sraer, J. D., Kanfer, A., Meyrier, A., Kourilsky, O., Vachon, F., and Richet, G. Glomerulonephritis in severe bacterial infections with and without endocarditis. *Adv. Nephrol.* 7:217, 1977.
42. Beaufils, M., Morel-Maroger, L., Sraer, J.-D., Kanfer, A., Kourilsky, O., and Richet, G. Acute renal failure of glomerular origin during visceral abscesses. *N. Engl. J. Med.* 295:185, 1976.
43. Becker, C. G., and Murphy, G. E. The experimental induction of glomerulonephritis like that in man by infection with group A streptococci. *J. Exp. Med.* 127:1, 1967.
44. Bellon, B., Belair, M. F., Kuhn, J., Druet, P., and Bariety, J. Trapping of circulating proteins in immune deposits of Heymann nephritis. *Lab. Invest.* 46:306, 1982.
45. Benacerraf, B. A hypothesis to relate the specificity of T lymphocytes and the activity of I region-specific Ir genes in macrophages and B lymphocytes. *J. Immunol.* 120:1809, 1978.
46. Benacerraf, B. Role of MHC gene products in immune regulation. *Science* 212:1229, 1981.
47. Benacerraf, B., McCluskey, R. T., and Patras, D. Localization of colloidal substances in vascular endothelium. A mechanism of tissue damage: I. Factors causing the pathologic deposition of colloidal carbon. *Am. J. Pathol.* 35:75, 1959.
48. Benacerraf, B., Sebestyen, M., and Cooper, N. S. The clearance of antigen-antibody complexes from the blood by the reticuloendothelial system. *J. Immunol.* 82:131, 1959.
49. Bene, M-C., Derennes, V., Faure, G., Thomas, J. L., Duheille, J., and Leclere, J. Graves' disease: In situ localization of lymphoid T cell subpopulations. *Clin. Exp. Immunol.* 52:311, 1983.
50. Bhan, A. K., Collins, A. B., Schneeberger, E. E., and McCluskey, R. T. A cell-mediated reaction against glomerular-bound immune complexes. *J. Exp. Med.* 150:1410, 1979.
51. Bhan, A. K., Schneeberger, E. E., Baird, L. G., Collins, A. B., Kamata, K., Bradford, D., Erikson, M. E., and McCluskey, R. T. Studies with monoclonal antibodies against brush border antigens in Heymann nephritis. *Lab. Invest.* 53:421, 1985.
52. Bhan, A. K., Schneeberger, E. E., Collins, A. B., and McCluskey, R. T. Evidence for a pathogenic role of a cell-mediated immune mechanism in experimental glomerulonephritis. *J. Exp. Med.* 148: 246, 1978.
53. Bhan, A. K., Schneeberger, E. E., Collins, A. B., and McCluskey, R. T. Systemic cell-mediated reactions in vivo: Effect of the interaction of circulating antigen with sensitized lymphocytes on glomeruli and pulmonary alveoli. *Am. J. Pathol.* 116:77, 1984.
54. Bjorkman, P. J., Saper, M. A., Samraoui, B., Bennett, W. S., Strominger, J. L., and Wiley, D. C. Structure of the human class I histocompatibility antigen, HLA-A2. *Nature* 329:506, 1987.
55. Bolton, W. K., Benton, F. R., and Sturgill, B. C. Autoimmune glomerulotubular-nephropathy in mice. *Clin. Exp. Immunol.* 33:463, 1978.
56. Bolton, W. K., Chandra, M., Tyson, T. M., Kirkpatrick, P. R., Sadovnic, M. J., and Sturgill, B. C. Transfer of experimental glomerulonephritis in chickens by mononuclear cells. *Kidney Int.* 34:598, 1988.
57. Bolton, W. K., Innes, D. J., Jr., Sturgill, B. C., and Kaiser, D. L. T-cells and macrophages in rapidly progressive glomerulonephritis: Clinicopathologic correlations. *Kidney Int.* 32:869, 1987.
58. Bolton, W. K., Tucker, F. L., and Sturgill, B. C. New avian model of experimental glomerulonephritis consistent with mediation by cellular immunity. Nonhumorally mediated glomerulonephritis in chickens. *J. Clin. Invest.* 73:1263, 1984.
59. Bona, C. A. V genes encoding autoantibodies: Molecular and phenotypic characteristics. *Annu. Rev. Immunol.* 6:327, 1988.
60. Border, W. A., Okuda, S., Languino, L. R., and Ruoslahti, E. Transforming growth factor β regulates production of proteoglycans by mesangial cells. *Kidney Int.* 37:689, 1990.
61. Borel, Y., Lewis, R. M., Andre-Schwartz, J., Stollar, B. D., and Diener, E. Treatment of lupus nephritis in adult (NZB+NZW) F_1 mice by cortisone-facilitated tolerance to nucleic acid antigens. *J. Clin. Invest.* 61:276, 1978.
62. Boros, P., Chen, J., Bona, C., and Unkeless, J. C. Autoimmune mice make anti-Fcγ receptor antibodies. *J. Exp. Med.* 171:1581, 1990.
63. Borrero, J., Todd, M. E., Becker, C. G., and Becker, E. L. Masugi nephritis: The renal lesion and the coagulation processes. *Clin. Nephrol.* 1: 86, 1973.
64. Boswell, J. M., Yui, M. A., Burt, D. W., and Kelley, V. E. Increased tumor necrosis factor and IL-1 β gene expression in the kidneys of mice with lupus nephritis. *J. Immunol.* 141:3050, 1988.
65. Bottazzo, G. F., Pujol-Borrell, R., Hanafusa, T., and Feldmann, M. Role of aberrant HLA-DR expression and antigen presentation in induction of endocrine autoimmunity. *Lancet* 2:1115, 1983.
66. Bottger, E. C., Hoffmann, T., Hadding, U., and Bitter-Suermann, D. Influence of genetically inherited complement deficiencies on humoral immune response in guinea pigs. *J. Immunol.* 135: 4100, 1985.
67. Boucher, A., Droz, D., Adafer, E., and Noel, L.-H. Characterization of mononuclear cell subsets in renal cellular interstitial infiltrates. *Kidney Int.* 29:1043, 1986.

68. Boyce, N. W., and Holdsworth, S. R. Macrophage–Fc-receptor affinity: Role in cellular mediation of antibody initiated glomerulonephritis. *Kidney Int.* 36:537, 1989.
69. Boyce, N. W., Tipping, P. G., and Holdsworth, S. R. Glomerular macrophages produce reactive oxygen species in experimental glomerulonephritis. *Kidney Int.* 35:778, 1989.
70. Boyns, A. R., and Hardwicke, J. The relationship between circulating soluble antigen-antibody complexes and the production of chronic glomerulonephritis in the rabbit. *Immunology* 14:367, 1968.
71. Brentjens, J. R., and Andres, G. Interaction of antibodies with renal cell surface antigens. *Kidney Int.* 35:954, 1989.
72. Brentjens, J. R., O'Donnell, D. W., Pawlowski, I. B., and Andres, G. A. Extraglomerular lesions associated with deposition of circulating antigen-antibody complexes in kidneys of rabbits with chronic serum sickness. *Clin. Immunol. Immunopathol.* 3:112, 1974.
73. Brentjens, J. R., Sepulveda, M., Baliah, T., Bentzel, C., Erlanger, B. F., Elwood, C., Montes, M., Hus, K. C., and Andres, G. A. Interstitial immune complex nephritis in patients with systemic lupus erythematosus. *Kidney Int.* 7:342, 1975.
74. Brinkman, K., Termaat, R. M., deJong, J., van den Brink, H. G., Berden, J. H. M., and Smeenk, R. J. T. Cross-reactive binding patterns of monoclonal antibodies to DNA are often caused by DNA/anti-DNA immune complexes. *Res. Immunol.* 140:595, 1989.
75. Bruijn, J. A., van Elven, E. H., Hogendoorn, P. C. W., Corver, W. E., Hoedemaeker, P. J., and Fleuren, G. J. Animal model of human diseases: Murine chronic graft-versus-host disease as a model for lupus nephritis. *Am. J. Pathol.* 130:639, 1988.
76. Bruijn, J. A., van Leer, E. H. G., Baelde, H. J. J., Corver, W. E., Hogendoorn, P. C. W., and Fleuren, G. J. Characterization and in vivo transfer of nephritogenic autoantibodies directed against dipeptidyl peptidase IV and laminin in experimental lupus nephritis. *Lab. Invest.* 63:350, 1990.
77. Brunati, C., Brando, B., Confalonieri, R., Belli, L. S., Lavagni, M. G., and Minetti, L. Immunophenotyping of mononuclear cell infiltrates associated with renal disease. *Clin. Nephrol.* 26:15, 1986.
78. Brzosko, W. J., Krawczynski, K., Nazarewicz, T., Morzychor, M., and Nowosanki, A. Glomerulonephritis associated with hepatitis B surface antigen immune complexes in children. *Lancet* 2: 477, 1974.
79. Burnet, F. M. *The Clonal Selection Theory of Acquired Immunity.* New York: Cambridge University Press, 1959.
80. Buus, S., Sette, A., Colon, S. M., Miles, C., and Grey, H. M. The relation between major histocompatibility complex (MHC) restriction and the capacity of Ia to bind immunogenic peptides. *Science* 235:1353, 1987.
81. Bygren, P., Wieslander, J., and Heinegard, D. Glomerulonephritis induced in sheep by immunization with human glomerular basement membrane. *Kidney Int.* 31:25, 1987.
82. Caligaris-Cappio, F., Bergui, L., Tesio, L., Ziano, R., and Camussi, G. HLA-DR$^+$ T cells of the Leu 3 (helper) type infiltrate the kidneys of patients with systemic lupus erythematosus. *Clin. Exp. Immunol.* 59:185, 1980.
83. Cameron, J. S. Platelets in glomerular disease. *Annu. Rev. Med.* 35:175, 1984.
84. Cameron, J. S., and Clark, W. F. A role for insoluble antibody-antigen complexes in glomerulonephritis? *Clin. Nephrol.* 18:55, 1982.
85. Camussi, G., Brentjens, J. R., Noble, B., Kerjaschki, D., Malavasi, F., Roholt, O. A., Farquhar, M. G., and Andres, G. Antibody-induced redistribution of Heymann antigen on the surface of cultured glomerular visceral epithelial cells: Possible role in the pathogenesis of Heymann glomerulonephritis. *J. Immunol.* 135:2409, 1985.
86. Camussi, G., Kerjaschki, D., Gonda, M., Nevins, T., Rielle, J.-C., Brentjens, J., and Andres, G. Expression and modulation of surface antigens in cultured rat glomerular visceral epithelial cells. *J. Histochem. Cytochem.* 37:1675, 1989.
87. Camussi, G., Tetta, C., Bussolino, F., Turello, E., Brentjens, J., Baglioni, C., and Andres, G. The effect of leukocyte stimulation on rabbit immune complex glomerulonephritis. *Kidney Int.* 38:1047, 1990.
88. Camussi, G., Tetta, C., Deregibus, M. C., Bussolino, F., Segoloni, G., and Vercellone, A. Platelet-activating factor (PAF) in experimentally induced rabbit acute serum sickness: Role of basophil-derived PAF in immune complex deposition. *J. Immunol.* 128:86, 1982.
89. Camussi, G., Tetta, C., Mazzucco, G., Monga, G., Roffinello, C., Alberton, M., Dellabona, P., Malavasi, F., and Vercellone, A. Platelet cationic proteins are present in glomeruli of lupus nephritis patients. *Kidney Int.* 30:555, 1986.
90. Carson, D. A., Chen, P. P., Fox, R. I., Kipps, T. J., Jirik, F., Goldfien, R. D., Silverman, G., Radoux, V., and Fong, S. Rheumatoid factor and immune networks. *Annu. Rev. Immunol.* 5:109, 1987.
91. Caspi, R. R., Roberge, F. G., Chan, C.-C., Wiggert, B., Chader, G. J., Rozenszajn, L. A., Lando, Z., and Nussenblatt, R. B. A new model of

autoimmune disease: Experimental autoimmune uveoretinitis induced in mice with two different retinal antigens. *J. Immunol.* 140:1490, 1988.

92. Castiglione, A., Bucci, A., Fellin, G., d'Amico, G., and Atkins, R. C. The relationship of infiltrating renal leukocytes to disease activity in lupus and cryoglobulinaemic glomerulonephritis. *Nephron* 50:14, 1988.
93. Caulfield, J. P., and Farquhar, M. G. Distribution of anionic sites in glomerular basement membranes: Their possible role in filtration and attachment. *Proc. Natl. Acad. Sci. USA* 73:1646, 1976.
94. Chatelet, F., Brianti, E., Ronco, P., Roland, J., and Verroust, P. Ultrastructural localization by monoclonal antibodies of brush border antigens expressed by glomeruli. *Am. J. Pathol.* 122:512, 1986.
95. Clark, W. F., Lewis, M. L., Cameron, J. S., and Parsons, V. Intrarenal platelet consumption in the diffuse proliferative nephritis of systemic lupus erythematosus. *Clin. Sci. Mol. Med.* 49:247, 1975.
96. Clayman, M. D., Martinez-Hernandez, A., Michaud, L., Alper, R., Mann, R., Kefalides, N. A., and Neilson, E. G. Isolation and characterization of the nephritogenic antigen-producing antitubular basement membrane disease. *J. Exp. Med.* 161:290, 1985.
97. Clayman, M. D., Michaud, L., Brentjens, J., Andres, G. A., Kefalides, N. A., and Neilson, E. G. Isolation of the target antigen of human anti-tubular basement membrane antibody-associated interstitial nephritis. *J. Clin. Invest.* 77:1143, 1986.
98. Cochrane, C. G. Mechanisms involved in the deposition of immune complexes in tissues. *J. Exp. Med.* 134:75S, 1971.
99. Cochrane, C. G., and Aikin, B. S. Polymorphonuclear leukocytes in immunologic reations: The destruction of vascular basement membrane in vivo and in vitro. *J. Exp. Med.* 124:733, 1966.
100. Cochrane, C. G., Unanue, E. R., and Dixon, F. J. A role of polymorphonuclear leukocytes and complement in nephrotoxic nephritis. *J. Exp. Med.* 122:99, 1965.
101. Cohen Tervaert, J. W., Goldschmeding, R., Elema, J. D., van der Giessen, M., Huitema, M. G., van der Hem, G. K., The, T. H., von dem Borne, A. E. G. Kr., and Kallenberg, C. G. M. Autoantibodies against myeloid lysosomal enzymes in crescentic glomerulonephritis. *Kidney Int.* 37:799, 1990.
102. Cole, E. H., Glynn, M. F. X., Laskin, C. A., Sweet, J., Mason, N., and Levy, G. A. Ancrod improves survival in murine systemic lupus erythematosus. *Kidney Int.* 37:29, 1990.
103. Collins, A. B., Bhan, A. K., Dienstag, J. C., Colvin, R. B., Haupert, G. T., Jr., Mushahwar, I. K., and McCluskey, R. T. Hepatitis B immune complex glomerulonephritis: Simultaneous glomerular deposition of hepatitis B surface and e antigens. *Clin. Immunol. Immunopathol.* 26:137, 1983.
104. Colvin, R. B. Wound Healing Processes in Hemostasis and Thrombosis. In M. A. Gimbrone (Ed.), *Contemporary Issues in Hemostasis and Thrombosis,* Vol. 2: *Vascular Endothelium in Hemostasis and Thrombosis.* New York: Churchill-Livingstone, 1986. P. 220.
105. Combes, B., Seastry, P., Shorey, J. Eigenbrodt, E. H., Barrera, A., Hull, A. K., and Carter, N. W. Glomerulonephritis with deposition of Australia antigen-antibody complexes in glomerular basement membrane. *Lancet* 2:234, 1971.
106. Cordonnier, D. J., Renversez, J. C., Vialtel, P., and Dechelette, E. The kidney in mixed cryoglobulinemias. *Springer Semin. Immunopathol.* 9:395, 1987.
107. Cosio, F. G., Bakaletz, A. P., and Mahan, J. D. Role of precipitating and nonprecipitating antibodies in glomerular immune complex formation. *Kidney Int.* 37:1429, 1990.
108. Cosio, F. G., Hebert, L. A., Birmingham, D. J., Dorval, B. L., Bakaletz, A. P., Kujala, G. A., Edberg, J. C., and Taylor, R. P. Clearance of human antibody/DNA immune complexes and free DNA from the circulation of the nonhuman primate. *Clin. Immunol. Immunopathol.* 42:1, 1987.
109. Cotran, R. S., and Galvanek, E. Immunopathology of human tubulointerstitial diseases: Localization of immunoglobulins, complement and Tamm-Horsfall protein. *Contrib. Nephrol.* 16:126, 1979.
110. Cotran, R. S., and Pober, J. S. Effects of cytokines on vascular endothelium: Their role in vascular and immune injury. *Kidney Int.* 35:969, 1989.
111. Couser, W. G., and Abrass, C. K. Pathogenesis of membranous nephropathy. *Annu. Rev. Med.* 39:517, 1988.
112. Couser, W. G., Baker, P. J., and Adler, S. Complement and the direct mediation of immune glomerular injury: A new perspective. *Kidney Int.* 28:879, 1985.
113. Couser, W. G., Steinmuller, D. R., Stilmant, M. M., Salant, D. J., and Lowenstein, L. M. Experimental glomerulonephritis in the isolated perfused rat kidney. *J. Clin. Invest.* 62:1275, 1978.
114. Couser, W. G., Stilmant, M. M., and Jermanovich, N. B. Complement-independent nephrotoxic nephritis in the guinea pig. *Kidney Int.* 11:170, 1977.
115. Cunningham, E., Provost, T., Brentjens, J. R., and Venuto, R. Acute renal failure secondary to

interstitial lupus nephritis associated with changes in immunological abnormalities (Abstract). *Kidney Int.* 12:464, 1977.
116. Cybulsky, A. V., Quigg, R. J., Badalementi, J., and Salant, D. J. Anti-Fx1A induces association of Heymann nephritis antigens with microfilaments of cultured glomerular visceral epithelial cells. *Am. J. Pathol.* 129:373, 1987.
117. D'Agati, V. D., Appel, G. B., Estes, D., Knowles, D. M., II, and Pirani, C. L. Monoclonal antibody identification of infiltrating mononuclear leukocytes in lupus nephritis. *Kidney Int.* 30:573, 1986.
118. D'Agati, V. D., Theise, N. D., Pirani, C. L., Knowles, D. M., and Appel, G. B. Interstitial nephritis related to nonsteroidal anti-inflammatory agents and beta-lactam antibiotics: A comparative study of the interstitial infiltrates using monoclonal antibodies. *Mod. Pathol.* 2:390, 1989.
119. D'Amico, G. Role of interstitial infiltration of leukocytes in glomerular diseases. *Nephrol. Dial. Transplant.* 3:596, 1988.
120. D'Amico, G., Colasanti, G., Ferrario, F., and Sinico, R. A. Renal involvement in essential mixed cryoglobulinemia. *Kidney Int.* 35:1004, 1989.
121. Damle, N. K., and Engleman, E. G. Antigen-specific suppressor T-lymphocytes in man. *Clin. Immunol. Immunopathol.* 53:S17, 1989.
122. Dang, H., and Harbeck, R. J. A comparison of anti-DNA antibodies from serum and kidney eluates of NZB × NZW F_1 mice. *J. Clin. Lab. Immunol.* 9:139, 1982.
123. Dang, H., and Harbeck, R. J. The in vivo and in vitro glomerular deposition of isolated anti-double-stranded-DNA antibodies in NZB/W mice. *Clin. Immunol. Immunopathol.* 30:265, 1984.
124. Datta, S. K. Short analytical review: A search for the underlying mechanisms of systemic autoimmune disease in the NZB × SWR model. *Clin. Immunol. Immunopathol.* 51:141, 1989.
125. Davies, D. J., Moran, J. E., Niall, J. F., and Ryan, G. B. Segmental necrotising glomerulonephritis with antineutrophil antibody: Possible arbovirus aetiology? *Br. Med. J.* 285:606, 1982.
126. Davis, M. M., and Bjorkman, P. J. T-cell antigen receptor genes and T-cell recognition. *Nature* 334:395, 1988.
127. De Heer, E., Daha, M. R., Bhakdi, S., Bazin, H., and Van Es, L. A. Possible involvement of terminal complement complex in active Heymann nephritis. *Kidney Int.* 22:388, 1985.
128. Demaine, A. G., Vaughan, R. W., Taube, D. H., and Welsh, K. I. Association of membranous nephropathy with T-cell receptor constant beta chain and immunoglobulin heavy chain switch region polymorphisms. *Immunogenetics* 27:19, 1988.
129. Devey, M. E., Bleasdale, K., Collins, M., and Steward, M. W. Experimental antigen-antibody complex disease in mice. *Int. Arch. Allergy Appl. Immunol.* 68:47, 1982.
130. Devey, M., and Steward, M. W. The induction of chronic antigen-antibody complex disease in selectively bred mice producing either high or low affinity antibody to protein antigens. *Immunology* 41:303, 1980.
131. di Giovine, F. S., and Duff, G. W. Interleukin 1: The first interleukin. *Immunol. Today* 11:13, 1990.
132. Dixon, F. J. What are sensitized cells doing in glomerulonephritis? *N. Engl. J. Med.* 283:536, 1970.
133. Dixon, F. J., Feldman, J. D., and Vazquez, J. J. Experimental glomerulonephritis: The pathogenesis of a laboratory model resembling the spectrum of human glomerulonephritis. *J. Exp. Med.* 113: 899, 1961.
134. Dixon, F. J., Oldstone, M. B. A., and Tonetti, G. Pathogenesis of immune complex glomerulonephritis of New Zealand mice. *J. Exp. Med.* 134: 65S, 1971.
135. Dixon, F. J., Vazquez, J. J., Weigle, W. O., and Cochrane, C. G. Pathogenesis of serum sickness. *AMA Arch. Pathol.* 65:18, 1958.
136. Douglas, M. F. S., Rabideau, D. P., Schwartz, M. M., and Lewis, E. J. Evidence of autologous immune-complex nephritis. *N. Engl. J. Med.* 305:1326, 1981.
137. Doxsey, S., Kerjaschki, D., and Farquhar, M. G. A large membrane glycoprotein (gp330) is a resident of coated pits of several absorbtive epithelia. *J. Cell Biol.* 97:778a, 1983.
138. Easley, J. R., and Halliwell, W. H. Relationship of proteinuria to glomerular basement membrane deposits in serum-sickness glomerulonephritis in rabbits. *Vet. Pathol.* 14:482, 1977.
139. Ebling, F., and Hahn, B. H. Restricted subpopulations of DNA antibodies in kidneys of mice with systemic lupus: Comparison of antibodies in serum and renal eluates. *Arthritis Rheum.* 23:392, 1980.
140. Edberg, J. C., Wright, E., and Taylor, R. P. Quantitative analyses of the binding of soluble complement-fixing antibody/dsDNA immune complexes to CR1 on human red blood cells. *J. Immunol.* 139:3739, 1987.
141. Edberg, J. C., Tosic, L., and Taylor, R. P. Immune adherence and the processing of soluble complement-fixing antibody/DNA immune complexes in mice. *Clin. Immunol. Immunopathol.* 51:118, 1989.
142. Eddy, A. A. Interstitial nephritis induced by

protein-overload proteinuria. *Am. J. Pathol.* 135: 719, 1989.

143. Edgington, T. S., Glassock, R. J., and Dixon, F. J. Autologous immune complex pathogenesis of experimental allergic glomerulonephritis. *Science* 155:1432, 1967.

144. Edgington, T. S., Glassock, R. J., and Dixon, F. J. Autologous immune complex nephritis induced with renal tubular antigen: I. Identification and isolation of the pathogenic antigen. *J. Exp. Med.* 127:555, 1968.

145. Eilat, D. Cross-reactions of anti-DNA antibodies and the central dogma of lupus nephritis. *Immunol. Today* 6:123, 1985.

146. Emlen, W., and Burdick, G. Clearance and organ localization of small DNA–anti-DNA immune complexes in mice. *J. Immunol.* 140:1816, 1988.

147. Emlen, W., Pisetsky, D. S., and Taylor, R. P. Antibodies to DNA: A perspective. *Arthritis Rheum.* 29:1417, 1986.

148. Epstein, F., and McCluskey, R. T. Case records of the Massachusetts General Hospital. *N. Engl. J. Med.* 294:100, 1976.

149. Faaber, P., Rijke, T. P. M., van de Putte, L. B. A., Capel, P. J. A., and Berden, J. H. M. Cross-reactivity of human and murine anti-DNA antibodies with heparan sulfate. *J. Clin. Invest.* 77: 1824, 1986.

150. Falk, R. J., Dalmasso, A. P., Kim, Y., Tsai, C. H., Scheinman, J. I., Gewurz, H., and Michael, A. F. Neoantigen of the polymerized ninth component of complement: Characterization of a monoclonal antibody and immunohistochemical localization in renal disease. *J. Clin. Invest.* 72: 560, 1983.

151. Falk, R. J., and Jennette, J. C. Anti-neutrophil cytoplasmic autoantibodies with specificity for myeloperoxidase in patients with systemic vasculitis and idiopathic necrotizing and crescentic glomerulonephritis. *N. Engl. J. Med.* 318:1651, 1988.

151a. Falk, R. J., Terrell, R. S., Charles, L. A., and Jennette, J. C. Anti-neutrophil cytoplasmic autoantibodies induce neutrophils to degranulate and produce oxygen radicals in vivo. *Proc. Natl. Acad. Sci. USA* 87:4115, 1990.

152. Feenstra, K., Lee, R. V. D., Greben, H. A., Arends, A., and Hoedemaeker, P. J. Experimental glomerulonephritis in the rat induced by antibodies directed against tubular antigens: I. The natural history: A histologic and immunohistologic study at the light microscopic and ultrastructural level. *Lab. Invest.* 32:235, 1975.

153. Feldman, J. D., Mardiney, M. R., and Shuler, S. E. Immunology and morphology of acute poststreptococcal glomerulonephritis. *Lab. Invest.* 15:283, 1966.

154. Ferrario, F., Castiglione, A., Colasanti, G., Di Belgioioso, G. B., Bertoli, S., and D'Amico, G. The detection of monocytes in human glomerulonephritis. *Kidney Int.* 28:513, 1985.

155. Fienberg, R. The protracted superficial phenomenon in pathergic (Wegener's) granulomatosis. *Hum. Pathol.* 12:458, 1981.

156. Finbloom, D. S., Magilavy, D. B., Harford, J. B., Rifai, A., and Plotz, P. H. Influence of antigen on immune complex behavior in mice. *J. Clin. Invest.* 68:214, 1981.

157. Fink, P. J., Shimonkevitz, R. P., and Bevan, M. J. Veto cells. *Annu. Rev. Immunol.* 6:115, 1988.

158. Fish, A. J., Michael, A. F., Vernier, R. L., and Good, R. A. Acute serum sickness nephritis in the rabbit (an immune deposit disease). *Am. J. Pathol.* 49:997, 1966.

159. Fleuren, G. J., Grond, J., and Hoedemaeker, P. J. The pathogenic role of free circulating antibody in autologous immune complex glomerulonephritis. *Clin. Exp. Immunol.* 41:205, 1980.

160. Fleuren, G., Grond, J., and Hoedemaeker, P. J. In situ formation of subepithelial glomerular immune complexes in passive serum sickness. *Kidney Int.* 17:631, 1980.

161. Ford, P. M., and Kosatka, I. The effect of in situ formation of antigen-antibody complexes in the glomerulus on subsequent glomerular localization of passively administered immune complexes. *Immunology* 39:337, 1980.

162. Ford, P. M., and Kosatka, I. The effect of human IgM rheumatoid factor on renal glomerular immune complex deposition in passive serum sickness in the mouse. *Immunology* 46:761, 1982.

163. Fox, B. S. Interaction of major histocompatibility complex molecules with immunogenic peptides. *Curr. Opin. Immunol.* 1:103, 1988.

164. Frank, M. M., Hamburger, M. I., Lawley, T. J., Kimberly, R. P., and Plotz, P. H. Defective reticuloendothelial system Fc-receptor function in systemic lupus erythematosus. *N. Engl. J. Med.* 300:518, 1979.

165. Friedman, J., Hoyer, J. R., and Seiler, M. W. Formation and clearance of tubulointerstitial immune complexes in kidneys of rats immunized with heterologous antisera to Tamm-Horsfall protein. *Kidney Int.* 21:575, 1982.

166. Fujinami, R. S., and Oldstone, M. B. A. Amino acid homology between the encephalitogenic site of myelin basic protein and virus: Mechanism for autoimmunity. *Science* 230:1043, 1985.

167. Fukatsu, A., Brentjens, J. R., Killen, P. D., Kleinman, H. K., Martin, G. R., and Andres,

G. A. Studies on the formation of glomerular immune deposits in Brown Norway rats injected with mercuric chloride. *Clin. Immunol. Immunopathol.* 45:35, 1987.
168. Gabbiani, G., Badonnel, M. C., and Vassalli, P. Experimental focal glomerular lesions elicited by insoluble immune complexes: Ultrastructural and immunofluorescent studies. *Lab. Invest.* 32:33, 1975.
169. Gallo, G. R., Caulin-Glaser, T., Emancipator, S. N., and Lamm, M. E. Nephritogenicity and differential distribution of glomerular immune complexes related to immunogen charge. *Lab. Invest.* 48:353, 1983.
170. Gallo, G. R., Caulin-Glaser, T., and Lamm, M. E. Charge of circulating immune complexes as a factor in glomerular basement membrane localization in mice. *J. Clin. Invest.* 67:1305, 1981.
171. Gamble, C. N., and Reardon, J. B. Immunopathogenesis of syphilitic glomerulonephritis: Elution of antitreponemal antibody from glomerular immune complex deposits. *N. Engl. J. Med.* 292:449, 1975.
172. Gans, R. O. B., Goldschmeding, R., Donker, A. J. M., Hoorntje, S. J., Kuizinga, M. C., Cohen Tervaert, J. W., Kallenberg, C. G. M., and von dem Borne, A. E. G. Kr. Neutrophil cytoplasmic autoantibodies and Wegener's granulomatosis. *Lancet* 1:269, 1989.
173. Gaulton, G. N., Bangs, J., Maddock, S., Springer, T., Eardley, D. D., and Strom, T. B. Characterization of a monoclonal rat anti-mouse interleukin 2 (IL-2) receptor antibody and its use in the biochemical characterization of the murine IL-2 receptor. *Clin. Immunol. Immunopathol.* 36:18, 1985.
174. Gauthier, V. J., and Mannik, M. Only the initial binding of cationic immune complexes to glomerular anionic sites is mediated by charge-charge interactions. *J. Immunol.* 136:3266, 1986.
175. Gauthier, V. J., Mannik, M., and Striker, G. E. Effect of cationized antibodies in preformed immune complexes on deposition and persistence in renal glomeruli. *J. Exp. Med.* 156:766, 1982.
176. Gauthier, V. J., Striker, G. E., and Mannik, M. Glomerular localization of preformed immune complexes prepared with anionic antibodies or with cationic antigens. *Lab. Invest.* 50:636, 1984.
177. Gelfand, M. C., Frank, M. M., Green, I., and Shin, M. L. Binding sites for immune complexes containing IgG in the renal interstitium. *Clin. Immunol. Immunopathol.* 13:19, 1979.
178. Geppert, T. D., and Lipsky, P. E. Antigen presentation at the inflammatory site. *Crit. Rev. Immunol.* 9:313, 1989.
179. Germuth, F. G., Jr. Comparative histologic and immunologic study in rabbits of induced hypersensitivity of serum sickness type. *J. Exp. Med.* 97:257, 1953.
180. Germuth, F. G., and Rodriguez, E. *Immunopathology of the Renal Glomerulus.* Boston: Little, Brown, 1973.
181. Germuth, F. G., Rodriguez, E., Lorelle, C. A., Trump, E. I., Melano, L., and Wise, O. Passive immune complex glomerulonephritis in mice: Models for various lesions found in human disease. II. Low-avidity complexes and diffuse proliferative glomerulonephritis with subepithelial deposits. *Lab. Invest.* 41:366, 1979.
182. Germuth, F. G., Jr., Senterfit, L. B., and Dreesman, G. R. Immune complex disease: V. The nature of the circulating complexes associated with glomerular alterations in the chronic BSA-rabbit system. *Johns Hopkins Med. J.* 130:344, 1972.
183. Germuth, F. G., Jr., Senterfit, L. B., and Pollack, A. D. Immune complex disease: I. Experimental acute and chronic glomerulonephritis. *Johns Hopkins Med. J.* 120:225, 1967.
184. Germuth, F. G., Valdes, A. J., Taylor, J. J., Wise, O., and Rodriguez, E. Fatal immune complex glomerulonephritis without deposits. *Johns Hopkins Med. J.* 136:189, 1975.
185. Giroux, L., Verroust, P., Morel-Maroger, L., Delarue, F., Delauche, M., and Sraer, J. D. Glomerular fibrinolytic activity during nephrotoxic nephritis. *Lab. Invest.* 40:415, 1979.
186. Gitlin, D., Latta, H., Batchelor, W. H., and Janeway, C. A. Experimental hypersensitivity in the rabbit: Disappearance rates of native and labeled heterologous proteins from the serum after intravenous injection. *J. Immunol.* 66:451, 1951.
187. Glass, D., Raum, D., Gibson, D., Stillman, J. S., and Schur, P. H. Inherited deficiency of the second component of complement: Rheumatic disease associations. *J. Clin. Invest.* 58:853, 1976.
188. Glassock, R. J., Edgington, T. S., Watson, J. I., and Dixon, F. J. Autologous immune complex nephritis induced with renal tubular antigen: II. The pathogenetic mechanism. *J. Exp. Med.* 127:573, 1968.
189. Golbus, S. M., and Wilson, C. B. Experimental glomerulonephritis induced by in situ formation of immune complexes in glomerular capillary wall. *Kidney Int.* 16:148, 1979.
190. Goldman, M., Rose, L. M., Hochmann, A., and Lambert, P. H. Deposition of idiotype–anti-idiotype immune complexes in renal glomeruli after polyclonal B cell activation. *J. Exp. Med.* 155:1385, 1982.
191. Goldschmeding, R., Ten Bokkel Huinink, D., Faber, N., Tetteroo, P. A. T., Vroom, T. M., Hack, C. E., and von dem Borne, A. E. G. Kr. Iden-

tification of the ANCA-antigen as a novel myeloid lysosomal serine protease. *APMIS* 97(S):46, 1989.

192. Goodwin, J. S., and Cuppens, J. Regulation of the immune response by prostaglandins. *J. Clin. Immunol.* 3:295, 1983.
193. Gregersen, P. K. Biology of disease. HLA class II polymorphism: Implications for genetic susceptibility to autoimmune disease. *Lab. Invest.* 61:5, 1989.
194. Gregersen, P. K., Silver, J., and Winchester, R. J. The shared epitope hypothesis: An approach to understanding the molecular genetics of susceptibility to rheumatoid arthritis. *Arthritis Rheum.* 30:1205, 1987.
195. Grey, H. M., Sette, A., and Lamont, A. Biologic significance and therapeutic implications of antigen/MHC interactions. *Clin. Immunol. Immunopathol.* 53:S47, 1989.
196. Grishman, E., and Churg, J. Focal segmental lupus nephritis. *Clin. Nephrol.* 17:5, 1982.
197. Groggel, G. C., and Terreros, D. A. Role of the terminal complement pathway in accelerated autologous anti-glomerular basement membrane nephritis. *Am. J. Pathol.* 136:533, 1990.
198. Grupe, W. E., and Kaplan, M. H. A proximal tubular antigen in the pathogenesis of autoimmune nephrosis. *Fed. Proc.* 26:573, 1967.
199. Grupe, W. E., and Kaplan, M. H. Demonstration of an antibody to proximal tubular antigen in the pathogenesis of experimental autoimmune nephrosis in rats. *J. Lab. Clin. Med.* 74:400, 1969.
200. Guillet, J.-G., Lai, M.-Z, Briner, T. J., Buus, S., Sette, A., Grey, H. M., Smith, J. A., and Gefter, M. L. Immunological self, nonself discrimination. *Science* 235:865, 1987.
201. Gutmann, E., Niles, J. L., McCluskey, R. T., and Brown, D. Loss of antigens associated with the apical endocytotic pathway in proximal tubules from rats with Heymann nephritis. *Am J. Pathol.* 138:1243, 1991.
202. Haakenstad, A. O., and Mannik, M. Saturation of the reticuloendothelial system with soluble immune complexes. *J. Immunol.* 112:1939, 1974.
203. Haakenstad, A. O., and Mannik, M. The Biology of Immune Complexes. In N. Talal (Ed.), *Autoimmunity: Genetic, Immunologic, Virologic, and Clinical Aspects.* New York: Academic Press, 1977. P. 278.
204. Haakenstad, A. O., Striker, G. E., and Mannik, M. The glomerular deposition of soluble immune complexes prepared with reduced and alkylated antibodies and with intact antibodies in mice. *Lab. Invest.* 35:293, 1976.
205. Haakenstad, A. O., Striker, G. E., and Mannik, M. Removal of glomerular immune deposits by excess antigen in chronic mouse model of immune complex disease. *Lab. Invest.* 48:323, 1983.
206. Hall, C. L., Colvin, R. B., Carey, K., and McCluskey, R. T. Passive transfer of autoimmune disease with isologous IgG_1 and IgG_2 antibodies to the tubular basement membrane in strain XIII guinea pigs. *J. Exp. Med.* 146:1246, 1977.
207. Hall, C. L., Colvin, R. B., and McCluskey, R. T. Human Immune Complex Diseases. In S. Cohen, P. A. Ward, and R. T. McCluskey (Eds.), *Mechanisms of Immunopathology.* New York: Wiley, 1979. P. 203.
208. Haqqi, T. M., and David, C. S. T-cell receptor V_β genes repertoire in mice: Possible role in resistance and susceptibility to type II collagen-induced arthritis. *J. Autoimmun.* 3:113, 1990.
209. Haverty, T. P., Watanabe, M., Neilson, E. G., and Kelly, C. J. Protective modulation of class II MHC gene expression in tubular epithelium by target antigen-specific antibodies: Cell-surface-directed down-regulation of transcription can influence susceptibility to murine tubulointerstitial nephritis. *J. Immunol.* 143:1133, 1989.
210. Hawkins, D. Basement membrane material excreted during acute immunologic renal injury. *Fed. Proc.* 26:744, 1967.
211. Hawn, C. V. Z., and Janeway, C. A. Histological and serological sequences in experimental hypersensitivity. *J. Exp. Med.* 85:571, 1947.
212. Heber-Katz, E. Short analytical review. The autoimmune T-cell receptor: Epitopes, idiotopes, and malatopes. *Clin. Immunol. Immunopathol.* 55:1, 1990.
213. Hebert, L. A., and Cosio, F. G. The erythrocyte–immune complex–glomerulonephritis connection in man. *Kidney Int.* 31:877, 1987.
214. Heidelberger, M. Quantitative chemical studies on complement or alexin. *J. Exp. Med.* 73:681, 1941.
215. Henson, P. M. Mechanisms of exocytosis in phagocytic inflammatory cells. *Am. J. Pathol.* 101: 494, 1980.
216. Henson, P. M., and Cochrane, C. G. Acute immune complex disease in rabbits: The role of complement and of a leukocyte-dependent release of vasoactive amines from platelets. *J. Exp. Med.* 133:554, 1971.
217. Heymann, W., Hackel, D. B., Harwood, S., Wilson, S. G. F., and Hunter, J. L. P. Production of nephrotic syndrome in rats by Freund's adjuvants and rat kidney suspensions. *Proc. Soc. Exp. Biol. Med.* 100:660, 1959.
218. Hinglais, N., Kazatchkine, M. D., Bhakdi, S., Appay, M.-D., Mandet, C., Grossetete, J., and Bariety, J. Immunohistochemical study of the C5b-9 complex of complement in human kidneys. *Kidney Int.* 30:399, 1986.
219. Hogendoorn, P. C. W., Bruijn, J. A., Broek, L.

J. C. M., De Heer, E., Foidart, J. M., Hoedemaeker, P. J., and Fleuren, G. J. Antibodies to purified renal tubular epithelial antigens contain activity against laminin, fibronectin, and type IV collagen. *Lab. Invest.* 58:278, 1988.

220. Holdsworth, S. R. Fc dependence of macrophage accumulation and subsequent injury in experimental glomerulonephritis. *J. Immunol.* 130: 735, 1983.

221. Holdsworth, S. R., Neale, T. J., and Wilson, C. B. The participation of macrophages and monocytes in experimental immune complex glomerulonephritis. *Clin. Immunol. Immunopathol.* 15: 510, 1980.

222. Holdsworth, S. R., Neale, T. J., and Wilson, C. B. Abrogation of immune glomerulonephritis (GN) in rabbits by anti-macrophage (M) serum. *Kidney Int.* 19:193, 1981.

223. Holdsworth, S. R., Thomson, N. M., Glasgow, E. F., Dowling, J. P., and Atkins, R. C. Tissue culture of isolated glomeruli in experimental crescentic glomerulonephritis. *J. Exp. Med.* 147:98, 1978.

224. Hong, K., Takata, Y., Sayama, K., Kozono, H., Takeda, J., Nakano, Y., Kinoshita, T., and Inoue, K. Inhibition of immune precipitation by complement. *J. Immunol.* 133:1464, 1984.

225. Hooke, D. H., Gee, D. C., and Atkins, R. C. Leukocyte analysis using monoclonal antibodies in human glomerulonephritis. *Kidney Int.* 31:964, 1987.

226. Hooper, D. C., Bayer, A. S., Karchmer, A. W., Theofilopoulos, A. N., and Swartz, M. N. Circulating immune complexes in prosthetic valve endocarditis. *Arch. Intern. Med.* 143:2081, 1983.

227. Hori, M. T., and Abrass, C. K. Isolation and characterization of circulating immune complexes from rats with experimental membranous nephropathy. *J. Immunol.* 144:3849, 1990.

228. Horii, Y., Muraguchi, A., Iwano, M., Matsuda, T., Hirayama, T., Yamada, H., Fujii, Y., Dohi, K., Ishikawa, H., Ohmoto, Y., Yoshizaki, K., Hirano, T., and Kishinoto, T. Involvement of IL-6 in mesangial proliferative glomerulonephritis. *J. Immunol.* 143:3949, 1989.

229. Hudson, B. G., Wieslander, J., Wisdom, B. J., Jr., and Noelken, M. E. Biology of disease. Goodpasture syndrome: Molecular architecture and function of basement membrane antigen. *Lab. Invest.* 61:256, 1989.

230. Hunsicker, L. G., Shearer, T. P., Plattner, S. B., and Weisenburger, D. The role of monocytes in serum sickness nephritis. *J. Exp. Med.* 150:413, 1979.

231. Hurd, E. R., Johnston, J. M., Okita, J. R., MacDonald, P. C., Ziff, M., and Gilliam, J. N. Prevention of glomerulonephritis and prolonged survival in New Zealand Black/New Zealand White F_1 hybrid mice fed an essential fatty acid-deficient diet. *J. Clin. Invest.* 67:476, 1981.

232. Husby, G., Tung, K. S., and Williams, R. C., Jr. Characterization of renal tissue lymphocytes in patients with interstitial nephritis. *Am. J. Med.* 70:31, 1981.

233. Hyman, L. R., Steinberg, A. D., Colvin, R. B., and Bernard, E. F. Immunopathogenesis of autoimmune tubulointerstitial nephritis: II. Role of an immune response gene linked to the major histocompatibility locus. *J. Immunol.* 117:1894, 1977.

234. Hyman, L. R., Colvin, R. B., and Steinberg, A. D. Immunopathogenesis of autoimmune tubulointerstitial nephritis: I. Demonstration of differential susceptibility in strain II and strain III guinea pigs. *J. Immunol.* 116:327, 1976.

235. Iida, K., Mornaghi, R., and Nussenzweig, V. Complement receptor (CR1) deficiency in erythrocytes from patients with systemic lupus erythematosus. *J. Exp. Med.* 155:1427, 1982.

236. Inman, R. D., McDougal, J. S., Redecha, P. B., Lockshin, M. D., Stevens, C. E., and Christian, C. L. Isolation and characterization of circulating immune complexes in patients with hepatitis B systemic vasculitis. *Clin. Immunol. Immunopathol.* 21:364, 1981.

237. Ito, H., Hattori, S., Matsuda, I., Amamiya, S., Hajikano, H., Yoshizawa, H., Miyakawa, Y., and Mayumi, M. Hepatitis B_e antigen-mediated membranous glomerulonephritis: Correlation of ultrastructural changes with HB_eAg in the serum and glomeruli. *Lab. Invest.* 44:214, 1981.

238. Izui, S., Kelley, V. E., McConahey, P. J., and Dixon, F. J. Selective suppression of retroviral gp70–anti-gp70 immune complex formation by prostaglandin E_1 in murine systemic lupus erythematosus. *J. Exp. Med.* 152:1645, 1980.

239. Izui, S., Lambert, P. H., and Miescher, P. A. In vitro demonstration of a particular affinity of glomerular basement membrane and collagen for DNA: A possible basis for a local formation of DNA–anti-DNA complexes in systemic lupus erythematosus. *J. Exp. Med.* 144:428, 1976.

240. Izui, S., Lambert, P. H., and Miescher, P. A. Failure to detect circulating DNA–anti-DNA complexes by four radioimmunological methods in patients with systemic lupus erythematosus. *Clin. Exp. Immunol.* 30:384, 1977.

241. Jacob, L., Lety, M.-A., Louvard, D., and Bach, J.-F. Binding of a monoclonal anti-DNA autoantibody to identical protein(s) present at the surface of several human cell types involved in lupus pathogenesis. *J. Clin. Invest.* 75:315, 1985.

242. Jacob, L., Tron, F., Bach, J. F., and Louvard, D. A. A monoclonal anti-DNA antibody also

binds to cell-surface protein(s). *Proc. Natl. Acad. Sci. USA* 81:3843, 1984.

243. Jayaraman, S., Martin, C. A., and Dorf, M. E. Enhancement of in vivo cell-mediated immune responses by three distinct cytokines. *J. Immunol.* 144:942, 1990.
244. Jayne, D. R. W., Marshall, P. D., Jones, S. J., and Lockwood, C. M. Autoantibodies to GBM and neutrophil cytoplasm in rapidly progressive glomerulonephritis. *Kidney Int.* 37:965, 1990.
245. Jennette, J. C., Wilkman, A. S., and Falk, R. J. Anti-neutrophil cytoplasmic autoantibody-associated glomerulonephritis and vasculitis. *Am. J. Pathol.* 135:921, 1989.
246. Jensen, P. E., Kapp, J. A., and Pierce, C. W. The role of suppressor T cells in the expression of immune response gene function. *J. Mol. Cell. Immunol.* 3:267, 1987.
247. Jeraj, K., Vernier, R. L., Sisson, S. P., and Michael, A. F. A new glomerular antigen in passive Heymann nephritis. *Br. J. Exp. Pathol.* 65:485, 1984.
248. Johnson, K. J., and Ward, P. A. Biology of disease: Newer concepts in the pathogenesis of immune complex–induced tissue injury. *Lab. Invest.* 47:218, 1982.
249. Johnson, R. J., Alpers, C. E., Pritzl, P., Schulze, M., Baker, P., Pruchno, C., and Couser, W. G. Platelets mediate neutrophil-dependent immune complex nephritis in the rat. *J. Clin. Invest.* 82: 1225, 1988.
250. Johnson, R. J., Alpers, C. E., Pruchno, C., Schulze, M., Baker, P. J., Pritzl, P., and Couser, W. G. Mechanisms and kinetics for platelet and neutrophil localization in immune complex nephritis. *Kidney Int.* 36:780, 1989.
251. Johnson, R. J., Garcia, R. L., Pritzl, P., and Alpers, C. E. Platelets mediate glomerular cell proliferation in immune complex nephritis induced by anti-mesangial cell antibodies in the rat. *Am. J. Pathol.* 136:369, 1990.
252. Johnson, R. J., Klebanoff, S. J., and Couser, W. G. Oxidants in Glomerular Injury. In C. B. Wilson, B. M. Brenner, and J. H. Stein (Eds.), *Contemporary Issues in Nephrology: Immunopathology of Renal Disease.* New York: Churchill-Livingstone, 1988, P. 87.
253. Johnson, R. J., Klebanoff, S. J., Ochi, R. F., Adler, S., Baker, P., Sparks, L., and Couser, W. G. Participation of the myeloperoxidase-H_2O_2-halide system in immune complex nephritis. *Kidney Int.* 33:342, 1987.
254. Jones, F. S., Pisetsky, D. S., and Kurlander, R. J. Defects in mononuclear phagocytic system (MPS) function in autoimmune MRL-lpr/lpr mice. *Clin. Immunol. Immunopathol.* 36:30, 1985.
255. Jordan, S. C., Buckingham, B., Sakai, R., and Olson, D. Studies of immune complex glomerulonephritis mediated by human thyroglobulin. *N. Engl. J. Med.* 304:1212, 1981.
256. Kagami, S., Kawakami, K., Okada, K., Kuroda, Y., Morioka, T., Shimizu, F., and Oite, T. Mechanism of formation of subepithelial electron-dense deposits in active in situ immune complex glomerulonephritis. *Am. J. Pathol.* 136:631, 1990.
257. Kamata, K., Baird, L. G., Erikson, M. E., Collins, A. B., and McCluskey, R. T. Characterization of antigens and antibody specificities involved in Heymann nephritis. *J. Immunol.* 135: 2400, 1985.
258. Kanalas, J. J., and Makker, S. P. A possible ligand of serum origin for the kidney autoantigen of Heymann nephritis. *J. Immunol.* 141:4152, 1988.
259. Kanwar, Y. S., Caulin-Glaser, T., Gallo, G. R., and Lamm, M. E. Interaction of immune complexes with glomerular heparan sulfate-proteoglycans. *Kidney Int.* 30:842, 1986.
260. Kanwar, Y. S., and Farquhar, M. G. Anionic sites in the glomerular basement membrane: In vivo and in vitro localization to the laminae rarae by cationic probes. *J. Cell Biol.* 81:137, 1976.
261. Kappler, J. W., Roehm, N., and Marrack, P. T-cell tolerance by clonal elimination in the thymus. *Cell* 49:273, 1987.
262. Kauffmann, R. H., Thompson, J., Valentijn, R. M. Daha, M. R., and Van Es, L. A. The clinical implications and the pathogenetic significance of circulating immune complexes in infective endocarditis. *Am. J. Med.* 71:17, 1981.
263. Kelley, J. Cytokines of the lung. *Am. Rev. Respir. Dis.* 141:765, 1990.
264. Kelley, V. E., Winkelstein, A., and Izui, S. Effects of prostaglandin E on immune complex nephritis in NZB/W mice. *Lab. Invest.* 41:531, 1979.
265. Kelley, V. E., Winkelstein, A., Izui, S., and Dixon, F. J. Prostaglandin E_1 inhibits T-cell proliferation and renal disease in MRL/l mice. *Clin. Immunol. Immunopathol.* 21:190, 1981.
266. Kelly, C. J., Zurier, R. B., Krakauer, K. A., Blanchard, N., and Neilson, E. G. Prostaglandin E_1 inhibits effector T-cell induction and tissue damage in experimental murine interstitial nephritis. *J. Clin. Invest.* 79:782, 1987.
267. Kennedy, T. L., Merrow, M., Phillips, S. M., Norman, M., and Neilson, E. G. Macrophage chemotaxis in anti-tubular basement membrane induced interstitial nephritis in guinea pigs. *Clin. Immunol. Immunopathol.* 36:243, 1985.
268. Kerjaschki, D., and Farquhar, M. G. The pathogenic antigen of Heymann nephritis is a membrane glycoprotein of the renal proximal tubule brush border. *Proc. Natl. Acad. Sci. USA* 79:5557, 1982.
269. Kerjaschki, D., and Farquhar, M. G. Immuno-

cytochemical localization of the Heymann nephritis antigen (gp330) in glomerular epithelial cells of normal Lewis rats. *J. Exp. Med.* 157:667, 1983.

270. Kerjaschki, D., and Farquhar, M. G. Participation of the Antigen of Heymann Nephritis—gp330—in the Formation of Immune Deposits. In F. Milgrom, C. J. Abeyounis, and B. Albini (Eds.), *Antibodies: Protective, Destructive, and Regulatory Role. 9th International Convocation on Immunology, Amherst, N. Y.* Basel: Karger, 1985. P. 340.
271. Kerjaschki, D., Horvat, R., Binder, S., Susani, M., Dekan, G., Ojha, P. P., Hillemanns, P., Ulrich, W., and Donini, U. Identification of a 400-kD protein in the brush borders of human kidney tubules that is similar to gp330, the nephritogenic antigen of rat Heymann nephritis. *Am. J. Pathol.* 129:183, 1987.
272. Kerjaschki, D., Miettinen, A., and Farquhar, M. G. Initial events in the formation of immune deposits in passive Heymann nephritis. *J. Exp. Med.* 166:109, 1987.
273. Kerjaschki, D., Noronha-Blob, L., Sacktor, B., and Farquhar, M. G. Microdomains of distinctive glycoprotein composition in the kidney proximal tubule brush border. *J. Cell Biol.* 98:1505, 1984.
274. Kerr, M. A. Detection and characterization of antibodies. *Curr. Opin. Immunol.* 1:948, 1989.
275. Kikkawa, Y., Sakura, M., Mano, T., Hirabayashi, K., and Kitagawa, T. Interstitial nephritis with concomitant uveitis. Report of two cases. *Contrib. Nephrol.* 4:1, 1975.
276. Klassen, J., Andres, G. A., Brennan, J. C., and McCluskey, R. T. An immunologic renal tubular lesion in man. *Clin. Immunol. Immunopathol.* 1:69, 1972.
277. Klassen, J., Elwood, C., Grossberg, A. L., Milgrom, F., Montes, M., Sepulveda, M., and Andres, G. A. Evolution of membranous nephropathy into anti-glomerular-basement-membrane glomerulonephritis. *N. Engl. J. Med.* 290: 1340, 1974.
278. Klassen, J., McCluskey, R. T., and Milgrom, F. Nonglomerular renal disease produced in rabbits by immunization with homologous kidney. *Am. J. Pathol.* 63:333, 1971.
279. Klassen, J., and Milgrom, F. Autoimmune concomitants of renal allografts. *Transplant. Proc.* 1:605, 1969.
280. Klassen, J., Milgrom, F. M., and McCluskey, R. T. Studies of the antigens involved in an immunologic renal tubular lesion in rabbits. *Am. J. Pathol.* 88:135, 1977.
281. Klassen, J., Sugisaki, T., Milgrom, F., and McCluskey, R. T. Studies on multiple renal lesions in Heymann nephritis. *Lab. Invest.* 25:577, 1971.
282. Kleinknecht, C., Levy, M., Peix, A., Broyer, M., and Courtecuisse, V. Membranous glomerulonephritis and hepatitis B surface antigen in children. *J. Pediatr.* 95:946, 1979.
283. Klinman, D. M. Recent advances in systemic lupus erythematosus. *Curr. Opin. Immunol.* 1:740, 1989.
284. Klinman, D. M. Regulation of B-cell activation in autoimmune mice. *Clin. Immunol. Immunopathol.* 53:S25, 1989.
285. Klinman, D. M., Eisenberg, R. A., and Steinberg, A. D. Development of the autoimmune B-cell repertoire in MRL-lpr/lpr mice. *J. Immunol.* 144:506, 1990.
286. Klinman, D. M., and Steinberg, A. D. Systemic autoimmune disease arises from polyclonal B-cell activation. *J. Exp. Med.* 165:1755, 1987.
287. Kniker, W. T., and Cochrane, C. G. The localization of circulating immune complexes in experimental serum sickness: The role of vasoactive amines and hydrodynamic forces. *J. Exp. Med.* 127:119, 1968.
288. Koffler, D., Agnello, V., Thoburn, R., and Kunkel, H. G. Systemic lupus erythematosus: Prototype of immune complex nephritis in man. *J. Exp. Med.* 134:169s, 1971.
289. Kohler, P. F., Cronin, R. E., Hammond, W. S., Olin, D., and Carr, R. I. Chronic membranous glomerulonephritis caused by hepatitis B antigen-antibody immune complexes. *Ann. Intern. Med.* 81:448, 1974.
290. Kondo, Y., Shigematsu, H., and Kobayashi, Y. Cellular aspects of rabbit Masugi nephritis. *Lab. Invest.* 27:620, 1972.
291. Koyama, A., Niwa, Y., Shigematsu, H., Taniguichi, M., and Tada, T. Studies on passive serum sickness: II. Factors determining the localization of antigen-antibody complexes in the murine renal glomerulus. *Lab. Invest.* 38:253, 1978.
292. Kraus, W., Ohyama, K., Snyder, D. S., and Beachey, E. H. Autoimmune sequence of streptococcal M protein shared with the intermediate filament protein, vimentin. *J. Exp. Med.* 169:481, 1989.
293. Krensky, A. M., Clayberger, C., Reiss, C. S., Strominger, J. L., and Burakoff, S. J. Specificity of $OKT4^+$ cytotoxic T-lymphocyte clones. *J. Immunol.* 129:2001, 1982.
294. Krieger, A., Thoenes, G. H., and Gunther, E. Genetic control of autoimmune tubulointerstitial nephritis in rats. *Clin. Immunol. Immunopathol.* 21:301, 1981.
295. Kurnick, J. T., and McCluskey, R. T. Perspectives on Cell-Mediated Immunity in Vivo. In S. Cohen (Ed.), *Lymphokines and the Immune Response.* Boca Raton, Fla.: CRC Press, 1990. P. 1.

295a. Kurnick, J. T., McCluskey, R. T., Bhan, A. K., Wright, K. A., Wilkinson, R., and Rubin, R. H. *Escherichia coli*-specific T lymphocytes in experimental pyelonephritis. *J. Immunol.* 141:3220, 1988.

296. Lachmann, P. J. Heberden oration 1986. Complement—Friend or foe? *Br. J. Rheumatol.* 26:409, 1987.

297. Lafer, E. M., Rauch, J., Andrzejewski, C., Jr., Mudd, D., Furie, B., Furie, B., Schwartz, R. S., and Stollar, B. D. Polyspecific monoclonal lupus autoantibodies reactive with both polynucleotides and phospholipids. *J. Exp. Med.* 153:897, 1981.

298. Lambert, P. H., and Dixon, F. J. Pathogenesis of the glomerulonephritis of NZB/W mice. *J. Exp. Med.* 127:507, 1968.

299. Lambert, P. H., Goldman, M., Renversez, J. C., Montagnino, G., and Tarantino, A. Pathological Consequences of Idiotype–Anti-Idiotype Interactions. In F. Milgrom, C. J. Abeyounis, and B. Albini (Eds.), *Antibodies: Protective, Destructive and Regulatory Role. 9th International Convocation on Immunology, Amherst, N. Y.* Basel: Karger, 1985. P. 356.

300. Lange, K., Wachstein, M., and McPherson, S. E. Immunologic mechanism of transmission of experimental glomerulonephritis in parabiotic rats. *Proc. Soc. Exp. Biol. Med.* 106:13, 1961.

301. Leber, P. D., and McCluskey, R. T. Immune Complex Diseases. In B. W. Zweifach, L. Grant, and R. T. McCluskey (Eds.), *The Inflammatory Process*, 2nd Ed. New York: Academic Press, 1974. P. 401.

302. Lefkowith, J. B. A., Morrison, A. R., and Schreiner, G. F. Murine glomerular leukotriene B_4 synthesis: Manipulation by (n-6) fatty acid deprivation and cellular origin. *J. Clin. Invest.* 82:1655, 1988.

303. Lefkowith, J. B. A., and Schreiner, G. F. Essential fatty acid deficiency depletes rat glomeruli of resident macrophages and inhibits angiotensin II–induced eicosanoid synthesis. *J. Clin. Invest.* 80: 947, 1987.

304. Lehman, D. H., Marquardt, H., Wilson, C. B., and Dixon, F. J. Specificity of autoantibodies to tubular and glomerular basement membranes induced in guinea pigs. *J. Immunol.* 112:241, 1974.

305. Lehman, D. H., and Wilson, C. B. Role of sensitized cells in anti-tubular basement membrane interstitial nephritis. *Int. Arch. Allergy Appl. Immunol.* 51:168, 1976.

306. Lehman, D. H., Wilson, C. B., and Dixon, F. J. Interstitial nephritis in rats immunized with heterologous tubular basement membrane. *Kidney Int.* 5:187, 1974.

307. Lehman, D. H., Wilson, C. B., and Dixon, F. J. Extraglomerular immunoglobulin deposits in human nephritis. *Am. J. Med.* 58:765, 1975.

308. Lerner, R. A., and Dixon, F. J. Transfer of ovine experimental allergic glomerulonephritis (EAG) with serum. *J. Exp. Med.* 124:431, 1966.

309. Lerner, R. A., Glassock, R. J., and Dixon, F. J. The role of anti-glomerular basement membrane antibody in the pathogenesis of human glomerulonephritis. *J. Exp. Med.* 126:989, 1967.

310. Levy, R. L., and Hong, R. The immune nature of subacute bacterial endocarditis (SBE) nephritis. *Am. J. Med.* 54:645, 1973.

311. Lew, A. M., Staines, N. A., and Steward, M. W. Glomerulonephritis induced by preformed immune complexes containing monoclonal antibodies of defined affinity and isotype. *Clin. Exp. Immunol.* 57:413, 1984.

312. Lew, A. M., Tovey, D. G., and Steward, M. W. Localization of covalent immune complexes on the epithelial side of the glomerular basement membrane in mice. *Int. Arch. Allergy Appl. Immunol.* 75:242, 1984.

313. Lewis, R. M., Armstrong, M. Y. K., Andre-Schwartz, J., Muftuoglu, A., Beldotti, L., and Schwartz, R. S. Chronic allogeneic disease: I. Development of glomerulonephritis. *J. Exp. Med.* 128:653, 1968.

314. Lianos, E. A. Eicosanoids and the modulation of glomerular immune injury. *Kidney Int.* 35:985, 1989.

315. Lianos, E. A., Andres, G. A., and Dunn, M. J. Glomerular prostaglandin and thomboxane synthesis in rat nephrotoxic serum nephritis. *J. Clin. Invest.* 72:1439, 1983.

316. Lin, C.-Y. Hepatitis B virus–associated membraneous nephropathy: Clinical features, immunological profiles and outcome. *Nephron* 55:37, 1990.

317. Lindberg, L. H., Vosti, K. L., and Raffel, S. Experimental streptococcal glomerulonephritis in rats. *J. Immunol.* 98:1231, 1967.

318. Lisker-Melman, M., Webb, D., Di Bisceglie, A. M., Kassianides, C., Martin, P., Rustgi, V., Waggoner, J. G., Park, Y., and Hoofnagle, J. H. Glomerulonephritis caused by chronic hepatitis B virus infection: Treatment with recombinant human alpha-interferon. *Ann. Intern. Med.* 111:479, 1989.

319. Livingstone, A. M., and Fathman, C. G. The structure of T-cell epitopes. *Annu. Rev. Immunol.* 5:477, 1987.

320. Lockwood, C. M., Bakes, D., Jones, S., Whitaker, K. B., Moss, D. W., and Savage, C. O. S. Association of alkaline phosphatase with an autoantigen recognized by circulating anti-neutrophil antibodies in systemic vasculitis. *Lancet* 1:716, 1987.

321. Lockwood, C. M., Bowman, C., Bakes, D., Pressey, A., and Dash, A. Autoimmunity and glomerulonephritis. *Adv. Nephrol.* 16:291, 1987.
322. Lohse, A. W. Autoreactive T cells. *Curr. Opin. Immunol.* 1:718, 1989.
323. Long, E. O. Processing requirements for presentation of antigens to T-lymphocytes. *Curr. Opin. Immunol.* 1:98, 1988.
324. Lovett, D. H., Resch, K., and Gemsa, D. Interleukin I and the glomerular mesangium: II. Monokine stimulation of mesangial cell prostanoid secretion. *Am. J. Pathol.* 129:543, 1987.
325. Lovett, D. H., Ryan, J. L., and Sterzel, R. B. A thymocyte-activating factor derived from glomerular mesangial cells. *J. Immunol.* 130:1796, 1983.
326. Ludemann, J., and Gross, W. L. Autoantibodies against cytoplasmic structures of neutrophil granulocytes in Wegener's granulomatosis. *Clin. Exp. Immunol.* 69:350, 1987.
327. Ludemann, J., Utecht, B., and Gross, W. L. Anti-neutrophil cytoplasm antibodies in Wegener's granulomatosis recognize an elastinolytic enzyme. *J. Exp. Med.* 171:357, 1990.
328. Madaio, M. P., Carlson, J., Cataldo, J., Ucci, A., Migliorini, P., and Pankewycz, O. Murine monoclonal anti-DNA antibodies bind directly to glomerular antigens and form immune deposits. *J. Immunol.* 138:2883, 1987.
329. Magil, A. B., Wadsworth, L. D., and Loewen, M. Monocytes and human renal glomerular disease: A quantitative evaluation. *Lab. Invest.* 44:27, 1981.
330. Makino, H., Lelongt, B., and Kanwar, Y. S. Nephritogenicity of proteoglycans: II. A model of immune complex nephritis. *Kidney Int.* 34:195, 1988.
331. Makker, S. P., and Kanalas, J. J. Renal antigens in mercuric chloride–induced, anti-GBM autoantibody glomerular disease. *Kidney Int.* 37:64, 1990.
332. Malissen, B. Autoimmunity: A T-cell receptor perspective. *J. Autoimmun.* 3:109, 1990.
333. Mampaso, F. M., and Wilson, C. B. Characterization of inflammatory cells in autoimmune tubulointerstitial nephritis in rats. *Kidney Int.* 23: 448, 1983.
334. Mann, R., and Neilson, E. G. The induction of antigen-specific suppressor cells diminishes disease expression in mice with interstitial nephritis. *Ann. N.Y. Acad. Sci.* 475:338, 1986.
335. Mann, R., Zakheim, B., Clayman, M., McCafferty, E., Michaud, L., and Neilson, E. G. Murine interstitial nephritis: IV. Long-term cultured L3T4^{+} T cell lines transfer delayed expression of disease as I-A-restricted inducers of the effector T cell repertoire. *J. Immunol.* 135:286, 1985.
336. Mannik, M. Pathophysiology of circulating immune complexes. *Arthritis Rheum.* 25:783, 1982.
337. Mannik, M., Agodoa, L. Y. C., and David, K. A. Rearrangement of immune complexes in glomeruli leads to persistence and development of electron-dense deposits. *J. Exp. Med.* 157:1516, 1983.
338. Mannik, M., and Arend, W. P. Fate of preformed immune complexes in rabbits and rhesus monkeys. *J. Exp. Med.* 134:19S, 1971.
339. Mannik, M., and Gauthier, V. J. Glomerular Deposition of Circulating Immune Complexes. In F. Milgrom, C. J. Abeyounis, and B. Albini (Eds.), *Antibodies: Protective, Destructive and Regulatory Role. 9th International Convocation on Immunology, Amherst, N. Y.* Basel: Karger, 1985. P. 363.
340. Mannik, M., Gauthier, V. J., Stapleton, S. A., and Agodoa, L. Y. C. Immune complexes with cationic antibodies deposit in glomeruli more effectively than cationic antibodies alone. *J. Immunol.* 38:4209, 1987.
341. Mannik, M., Haakenstad, A. O., and Arend, W. P. The Fate and Detection of Circulating Immune Complexes. In E. L. Brent and J. Holborrow (Eds.), *Progress in Immunology,* Vol. 5. New York: North-Holland, 1974. P. 91.
342. Mannik, M., and Jimenez, R. A. H. The Mononuclear Phagocyte System in Immune Complex Diseases. In F. Milgrom and B. Albini (Eds.), *Immunopathology. 6th International Convocation on Immunology, Niagara Falls, N. Y.* Basel: Karger, 1979. P. 212.
343. Mannik, M., and Striker, G. E. Removal of glomerular deposits of immune complexes in mice by administration of excess antigen. *Lab. Invest.* 42:483, 1980.
344. Matsuo, S., Caldwell, P. R. B., Brentjens, J. R., and Andres, G. In vivo interaction of antibodies with cell surface antigens: A mechanism responsible for in situ formation of immune deposits in the zona pellucida of rabbit oocytes. *J. Clin. Invest.* 75:1369, 1985.
345. Matsuo, S., Fukatsu, A., Taub, M. L., Caldwell, P. R. B., Brentjens, J. R., and Andres, G. Glomerulonephritis induced in the rabbit by antiendothelial antibodies. *J. Clin. Invest.* 79:1798, 1987.
346. Mauer, S. M., Sutherland, D. E. R., Howard, R. J., Fish, A. J., Najarian, J. S., and Michael, A. T. The glomerular mesangium: III. Acute immune mesangial injury: A new model of glomerulonephritis. *J. Exp. Med.* 137:533, 1973.
347. McCluskey, R. T. An Evaluation of Current Knowledge of Glomerular Diseases. In C. H. Coggins and N. B. Cummings (Eds.), *Prevention of Kidney and Urinary Tract Diseases. Fogarty Inter-*

national Center Series on Preventive Medicine, Vol. 5. Washington: DHEW Publication No. (NIH) 78-855, 1978. P. 49.

348. McCluskey, R. T. Evidence for an immune complex disorder in systemic lupus erythematosus (SLE). *Am. J. Kidney Dis.* 11:119, 1982.
349. McCluskey, R. T. The value of the renal biopsy in lupus nephritis. *Arthritis Rheum.* 25:867, 1982.
350. McCluskey, R. T. Modification of glomerular immune complex deposits (Editorial). *Lab. Invest.* 48:241, 1983.
351. McCluskey, R. T. Immunologically Mediated Tubulointerstitial Nephritis. In B. M. Brenner, J. H. Stein and R. S. Cotran (Eds.), *Contemporary Issues in Nephrology,* Vol. 10. New York: Churchill-Livingstone, 1983. P. 121.
352. McCluskey, R. T. Immunologic Mechanisms in Glomerular Diseases. In R. H. Heptinstall (Ed.), *Pathology of the Kidney,* 3rd Ed. Boston: Little, Brown, 1983. P. 301.
353. McCluskey, R. T. Immunopathogenetic mechanisms in renal disease. *Am. J. Kidney Dis.* 10:172, 1987.
354. McCluskey, R. T. Renal Diseases. In R. B. Colvin, A. K. Bhan, and R. T. McCluskey (Eds.), *Diagnostic Immunopathology.* New York: Raven Press, 1988. P. 41.
355. McCluskey, R. T., and Andres, G. A. Does t-PA have a role in the treatment of crescentic glomerulonephritis? (Editorial). *Lab. Invest.* 62:1, 1990.
356. McCluskey, R. T., and Benacerraf, B. Localization of colloidal substances in vascular endothelium. A mechanism of tissue damage: II. Experimental serum sickness with acute glomerulonephritis induced passively in mice by antigen-antibody complexes in antigen excess. *Am. J. Pathol.* 35:275, 1959.
357. McCluskey, R. T., Benacerraf, B., and McCluskey, J. W. Studies on the specificity of the cellular infiltrate in delayed hypersensitivity reactions. *J. Immunol.* 90:466, 1963.
358. McCluskey, R. T., Benacerraf, B., and Miller, F. Passive acute glomerulonephritis induced by antigen-antibody complexes solubilized in hapten excess. *Proc. Soc. Exp. Biol. Med.* 111:764, 1962.
359. McCluskey, R. T., Benacerraf, B., Potter, J. L., and Miller, F. The pathologic effects of intravenously administered soluble antigen-antibody complexes: I. Passive serum sickness in mice. *J. Exp. Med.* 111:181, 1960.
360. McCluskey, R. T., and Bhan, A. K. Cell-Mediated Reactions in Vivo. In I. Green, S. Cohen, and R. T. McCluskey (Eds.), *Mechanisms of Tumor Immunity.* New York: Wiley, 1977. P. 1.
361. McCluskey, R. T., and Bhan, A. K. Immunological Mechanisms in Drug-Induced Acute Interstitial Nephritis (AIN). In G. Porter (Ed.), *Nephrotoxic Mechanisms of Drugs and Environmental Toxins.* New York: Plenum Press, 1982. P. 393.
362. McCluskey, R. T., and Bhan, A. K. Cell-mediated immunity in renal disease. *Hum. Pathol.* 17:146, 1986.
363. McCluskey, R. T., Bhan, A. K., and Colvin, R. B. Experimental and Human Anti-Tubular Basement Membrane Nephritis. In N. Cummings, A. Michael, and C. Wilson (Eds.), *Immune Mechanisms in Renal Disease.* New York: Plenum Press, 1982. P. 279.
364. McCluskey, R. T., Vassalli, P., Gallo, G., and Baldwin, D. S. An immunofluorescent study of pathogenic mechanisms in glomerular diseases. *N. Engl. J. Med.* 274:695, 1966.
365. McCormick, N. N., Day, J., Morris, C. J., and Hill, A. G. S. The potentiating effect of rheumatoid arthritis serum in the immediate phase of nephrotoxic serum nephritis. *Clin. Exp. Immunol.* 4:19, 1969.
366. McLeish, K. R., Gohara, A. F., and Gunning, W. T. Suppression of antibody synthesis of prostaglandin E as a mechanism for preventing murine immune complex glomerulonephritis. *Lab. Invest.* 47:147, 1982.
367. Mellors, R. C., Ortega, L. G., and Holman, H. R. Role of gamma globulins in pathogenesis of renal lesions in systemic lupus erythematosus and chronic membranous glomerulonephritis, with an observation on the lupus erythematosus cell reaction. *J. Exp. Med.* 106:191, 1957.
368. Meltzer, M., Franklin, E. C., Elias, K., McCluskey, R. T., and Cooper, N. Cryoglobulinemia—a clinical and laboratory study: II cryoglobulins with rheumatoid factor activity. *Am. J. Med.* 40:837, 1966.
369. Meuer, S. C., Hussey, R. E., Hodgdon, J. C., Hercend, T., Schlossman, S. F., and Reinherz, E. L. Surface structures involved in target recognition by human cytotoxic T-lymphocytes. *Science* 218:471, 1982.
370. Michael, A. F., Drummond, K. N., Good, R. A., and Vernier, R. L. Acute poststreptococcal glomerulonephritis: Immune deposit disease. *J. Clin. Invest.* 45:237, 1966.
371. Miller, G. W., and Nussenzweig, V. A new complement function: Solubilization of antigen-antibody aggregates. *Proc. Natl. Acad. Sci. USA* 72:418, 1975.
372. Miller, K., Dresner, I. G., and Michael, A. F. Localization of platelet antigens in human kidney disease. *Kidney Int.* 18:472, 1980.
373. Minota, S., Terai, C., Nojima, Y., Takano, K., Yamada, A., Miyakawa, Y., and Takaku, F. Cor-

relative expression of C3b receptors in the glomerulus and on erythrocytes. *Clin. Immunol. Immunopathol.* 38:85, 1986.
374. Miyakawa, Y., Yamada, A., Kosaka, K., Tsuda, F., Kosugi, E., and Mayumi, M. Defective immune-adherence (C3b) receptor on erythrocytes from patients with systemic lupus erythematosus. *Lancet* 2:493, 1981.
375. Mohammed, I., Ansell, B. M., Holborow, E. J., and Bryceson, A. D. M. Circulating immune complexes in subacute infective endocarditis and poststreptococcal glomerulonephritis. *J. Clin. Pathol.* 30:308, 1977.
376. Moller, N. P. H. Fc-mediated immune precipitation: I. A new role of the Fc-portion of IgG. *Immunology* 38:631, 1979.
377. Monga, G., Mazzucco, G., Barbiano di Belgiojoso, G., and Busnack, G. The presence and possible role of monocyte infiltration in human chronic proliferative glomerulonephritis: Light microscopic immunofluorescence and histochemical correlations. *Am. J. Pathol.* 94:271, 1979.
378. Monga, G., Mazzucco, G., Barbiano di Belgiojoso, G., and Busnack, G. Monocyte infiltration and glomerular hypercellularity in human acute and persistent glomerulonephritis: Light and electron microscopic, immunofluorescence and histochemical investigation on 28 cases. *Lab. Invest.* 44:381, 1981.
379. Morrison, W. I., and Wright, N. B. Viruses associated with renal disease of man and animals. *Prog. Med. Virol.* 23:22, 1977.
380. Most, J., and Wick, G. Class II antigens in Hashimoto thyroiditis: II. Expression of HLA-DR on infiltrating mononuclear cells in peripolesis. *Clin. Immunol. Immunopathol.* 41:175, 1986.
381. Moulder, K., and Steward, M. W. Capillary-localized low-affinity antibody-antigen complexes act as a focus for the deposition of high-affinity complexes. *Clin. Exp. Immunol.* 77:275, 1989.
382. Nagy, J., Bajtai, G., Brasch, H., Sule, T., Ambrus, M., Diak, G., and Hamori, A. The role of hepatitis surface antigen in the pathogenesis of glomerulopathies. *Clin. Nephrol.* 12:109, 1979.
383. Naish, P., Penn, G. B., Evans, D. J., and Peters, D. K. The effect of defibrination on nephrotoxic serum nephritis in rabbits. *Clin. Sci.* 42:643, 1972.
384. Naish, P. F., Thomson, N. M., Simpson, I. J., and Peters, D. K. The role of polymorphonuclear leucocytes in the autologous phase of nephrotoxic nephritis. *Clin. Exp. Immunol.* 22:102, 1975.
385. Nathan, C. F. Secretory products of macrophages. *J. Clin. Invest.* 79:319, 1987.
386. Natori, Y., Hayakawa, I., and Shibata, S. Role of dipeptidyl peptidase IV (gp108) in passive Heymann nephritis. *Am. J. Pathol.* 134:405, 1989.
387. Neale, T. J., Carson, S. D., Tipping, P. G., and Holdsworth, S. R. Participation of cell-mediated immunity in deposition of fibrin in glomerulonephritis. *Lancet* 2:421, 1988.
388. Neale, T. J., and Wilson, C. B. Glomerular antigens in Heymann's nephritis: Reactivity of eluted and circulating antibody. *J. Immunol.* 128:323, 1982.
389. Neild, G. H., Ivory, K., Hiramatsu, M., and Williams, D. G. Cyclosporin A inhibits acute serum sickness nephritis in rabbits. *Clin. Exp. Immunol.* 52:586, 1983.
390. Neilson, E. G. Pathogenesis and therapy of interstitial nephritis. *Kidney Int.* 35:1257, 1989.
391. Neilson, E. G., Clayman, M. D., Haverty, T., Kelly, C. J., and Mann, R. Experimental strategies for the study of cellular immunity in renal disease. *Kidney Int.* 30:264, 1986.
392. Neilson, E. G., Gasser, D. L., McCafferty, E., Zakheim, B., and Phillips, S. M. Polymorphism of genes involved in anti-tubular basement membrane disease in rats. *Immunogenetics* 17:55, 1983.
393. Neilson, E. G., Jimenez, S. A., and Phillips, S. M. Cell-mediated immunity in interstitial nephritis: III. T-lymphocyte–mediated fibroblast proliferation and collagen synthesis: An immune mechanism for renal fibrogenesis. *J. Immunol.* 125:1708, 1980.
394. Neilson, E. G., Kelly, C. J., Clayman, M. D., Hines, W. H., Haverty, T., Sun, M. J., and Blanchard, N. Murine interstitial nephritis: VII. Suppression of renal injury after treatment with soluble suppressor factor TsF_1. *J. Immunol.* 139:1518, 1987.
395. Neilson, E. G., and Phillips, S. M. Cell-mediated immunity in interstitial nephritis: I. T-lymphocyte systems in nephritic guinea pigs: The natural history and diversity of the immune response. *J. Immunol.* 123:2373, 1979.
396. Neilson, E. G., and Phillips, S. M. Cell-mediated immunity in interstitial nephritis: II. T-lymphocyte effector mechanisms in nephritic guinea pigs: Analysis of the renotropic migration and cytotoxic response. *J. Immunol.* 123:2381, 1979.
397. Neilson, E. G., and Phillips, S. M. Cell-mediated immunity in interstitial nephritis: IV. Anti-tubular basement membrane antibodies can function in antibody-dependent cellular cytotoxicity reactions: Observations on a nephritogenic effector mechanism acting as an informational bridge between the humoral and cellular immune response. *J. Immunol.* 126:1990, 1981.
398. Neilson, E. G., and Phillips, S. M. Suppression

of interstitial nephritis by auto-anti-idiotypic immunity. *J. Exp. Med.* 155:179, 1982.
399. Neilson, E. G., Phillips, S. M., and Jimenez, S. Lymphokine modulation of fibroblast proliferation. *J. Immunol.* 128:1484, 1982.
400. Neilson, E. G., and Zakheim, B. T-cell regulation, anti-idiotypic immunity, and the nephritogenic immune response. *Kidney Int.* 24:289, 1983.
401. Nelson, R. A. Jr. The immune adherence phenomenon: An immunologically specific reaction between microorganisms and erythrocytes leading to enhanced phagocytes. *Science* 118:733, 1953.
402. Nepom, G. T. Determinants of genetic susceptibility in HLA-associated autoimmune disease. *Clin. Immunol. Immunopathol.* 53:S53, 1989.
403. Neugarten, J., and Baldwin, D. S. Glomerulonephritis in bacterial endocarditis. *Am. J. Med.* 77:297, 1984.
404. Neugarten, J., Gallo, G. R., and Baldwin, D. S. Glomerulonephritis in bacterial endocarditis. *Am. J. Kidney Dis.* 111:371, 1984.
405. Niles, J. L., Collins, B., Baird, L., Erikson, M., Bradford, D., Pan, G., Hsiung, C. K., Schneeberger, E., Bhan, A., and McCluskey, R. Antibodies reactive with a renal glycoprotein and with deposits in membranous nephritis (Abstract). *Kidney Int.* 31:338, 1987.
406. Niles, J. L., McCluskey, R. T., Ahmad, M. F., and Arnaout, M. A. Wegener's granulomatosis is a novel serine proteinase. *Blood* 74:1888, 1989.
407. Niles, J. L., Pan, G. L., Collins, A. B., Shannon, T., Skates, S., Fienberg, R., Arnaout, M. A., and McCluskey, R. T. Value of antigen-specific radioimmunoassays for measuring anti-neutrophil cytoplasmic antibodies (ANCA) in the differential diagnosis of rapidly progressive glomerulonephritis. *JASN (in press).*
408. Nishi, T., Bhan, A. K., Collins, A. B., and McCluskey, R. T. Effect of circulating immune complexes on Fc and C3 receptors of Kupffer cells in vivo. *Lab. Invest.* 44:442, 1981.
409. Noble, B., Ren, K., Taverne, J., and DiPirro, J. Mononuclear cells in glomeruli and cytokines in urine reflect the severity of experimental proliferative immune complex glomerulonephritis. *Clin. Exp. Immunol.* 80:281, 1990.
410. Noble, B., Steward, M. W., Vladutiu, A., and Brentjens, J. R. Relationship of the quality and quantity of circulating anti-BSA antibodies to the severity of glomerulonephritis in rats with chronic serum sickness. *Clin. Exp. Immunol.* 67:277, 1987.
411. Nojima, Y., Terai, C., Takano, K., Takehara, K., Yamada, A., and Takudu, F. Tubulointerstitial immune complex nephritis in a patient with cutaneous vasculitis. *Clin. Nephrol.* 25:48, 1986.
412. Nolasco, F. E. B., Cameron, J. S., Hartley, B., Coelho, A., Hildreth, G., and Reuben, R. Intraglomerular T cells and monocytes in nephritis: Study with monoclonal antibodies. *Kidney Int.* 31:1160, 1987.
413. Nolasco, F. E. B., Cameron, J. S., Hartley, B., Coelho, R. A., Hildreth, G., and Reuben, R. Abnormal podocyte CR1 expression in glomerular diseases: Association with glomerular cell proliferation and monocyte infiltration. *Nephrol. Dial. Transplant.* 2:304, 1987.
414. Nolle, B., Specks, U., Ludemann, J., Rohrbach, M. S., DeRemee, R. A., and Gross, W. L. Anticytoplasmic autoantibodies: Their immunodiagnostic value in Wegener granulomatosis. *Ann. Intern. Med.* 111:28, 1989.
415. Norris, D. A., Clark, R. A. F., Surgard, L. M., Huff, J. C., Weston, W. L., and Howell, S. E. Fibronectin fragment(s) are chemotactic for human peripheral blood monocytes. *J. Immunol.* 129:1612, 1982.
416. O'Donoghue, D. J., Short, C. D., Brenchley, P. E. C., Lawler, W., and Ballardie, F. W. Sequential development of systemic vasculitis with anti-neutrophil cytoplasmic antibodies complicating anti-glomerular basement membrane disease. *Clin. Nephrol.* 32:251, 1989.
417. Okumura, K., Kondo, Y., and Tada, T. Studies on passive serum sickness: I. The glomerular fine structure of serum sickness nephritis induced by preformed antigen antibody complexes in the mouse. *Lab. Invest.* 24:383, 1971.
418. Oldstone, M. B. A. Virus-Induced Immune Complex Formation and Disease: Definition, Regulation, Importance. In A. L. Notkins and M. B. A. Oldstone (Eds.), *Concepts in Viral Pathogenesis.* New York: Springer-Verlag, 1984. P. 201.
419. Oldstone, M. B. A. Molecular mimicry and autoimmune disease. *Cell* 50:819, 1987.
420. Oldstone, M. B. A., and Dixon, F. J. Immune complex disease in chronic viral infections. *J. Exp. Med.* 134:32S, 1971.
421. Oliveira, D. B. G., and Peters, D. K. Autoimmunity and the kidney. *Kidney Int.* 35:923, 1989.
422. Olson, J. L., and Heptinstall, R. H. Biology of disease: Nonimmunologic mechanisms of glomerular injury. *Lab. Invest.* 59:564, 1988.
423. Pankewycz, O. G., Migliorini, P., and Madaio, M. P. Polyreactive autoantibodies are nephritogenic in murine lupus nephritis. *J. Immunol.* 139:3287, 1987.
424. Parfrey, N. A., and Prud'homme, G. J. Patterns of MHC antigenic modulation in cyclosporine-induced autoimmunity. *Am. J. Pathol.* 136:479, 1990.
425. Paronetto, F. Cell-mediated immunity in liver disease. *Hum. Pathol.* 17:168, 1986.
426. Parra, G., Platt, J. L., Falk, R. J., Rodriguez-Iturbe, B., and Michael, A. F. Cell populations

and membrane attack complex in glomeruli of patients with poststreptococcal glomerulonephritis: Identification using monoclonal antibodies by indirect immunofluorescence. *Clin. Immunol. Immunopathol.* 33:324, 1984.
427. Pascal, R. R., Koss, M. N., and Kassel, R. L. Glomerulonephritis associated with immune complex deposits and viral particles in spontaneous murine leukemia. *Lab. Invest.* 29:159, 1973.
428. Penner, E., Albini, B., Glurich, I., Andres, G. A., and Milgrom, F. Dissociation of immune complexes in tissue sections by excess of antigen. *Int. Arch. Allergy Appl. Immunol.* 67:245, 1982.
429. Pettersson, E. E., Bhan, A. K., Schneeberger, E. E., Collins, A. B., Colvin, R. B., and McCluskey, R. T. Glomerular C3 receptors in human renal disease. *Kidney Int.* 13:245, 1978.
430. Pettersson, E. E., and Colvin, R. B. Cold-insoluble globulin (fibronectin, LETS protein) in normal and diseased human glomeruli: Papain-sensitive attachment to normal glomeruli and deposition in crescents. *Clin. Immunol. Immunopathol.* 11:425, 1978.
431. Pincus, T., Haberkern, R., and Christian, C. L. Experimental chronic glomerulitis. *J. Exp. Med.* 127:819, 1968.
432. Piquet, P. F., Grau, G. E., and Vassalli, P. Subcutaneous perfusion of tumor necrosis factor induces local proliferation of fibroblasts, capillaries, and epidermal cells, or massive tissue necrosis. *Am. J. Pathol.* 136:103, 1990.
433. Pusey, C. D., Dash, A., Kershaw, M. J., Morgan, A., Reilly, A., Rees, A. J., and Lockwood, C. M. A single autoantigen in Goodpasture's syndrome identified by a monoclonal antibody to human glomerular basement membrane. *Lab. Invest.* 56:23, 1987.
434. Pussell, B. A., Nayef, M., Bourke, E., Morris, S., and Peters, D. K. Complement deficiency and nephritis: A report of a family. *Lancet* 1:675, 1980.
435. Queluz, T. H., Pawlowski, I., Brunda, M. J., Brentjens, J. R., Vladutiu, A. O., and Andres, G. Pathogenesis of an experimental model of Goodpasture's hemorrhagic pneumonitis. *J. Clin. Invest.* 85:1507, 1990.
436. Radeke, H. H., Meier, B., Topley, N., Floge, J., Habermehl, G. G., and Resch, K. Interleukin 1-α and tumor necrosis factor α induce oxygen radical production in mesangial cells. *Kidney Int.* 37:767, 1990.
437. Radoux, V., Chen, P. P., Sorge, J. A., and Carson, D. A. A conserved human germline V_K gene directly encodes rheumatoid factor light chains. *J. Exp. Med.* 164:2119, 1986.
438. Rahman, M. A., Stork, J. E., and Dunn, M. J. The roles of eicosanoids in experimental glomerulonephritis. *Kidney Int.* 32:S40, 1987.
439. Ralfkiaer, E., and Lange-Wantzin, G. In situ immunological characterization of the infiltrating cells in positive patch tests. *Br. J. Dermatol.* 111:13, 1984.
439a. Ramsdell, F., and Fowlkes, B. J. Clonal deletion versus clonal anergy: The role of the thymus in inducing self tolerance. *Science* 248:1342, 1990.
440. Raychowdhury, R., Niles, J. L., McCluskey, R. T., and Smith, J. A. Autoimmune target in Heymann nephritis is a glycoprotein with homology to the LDL receptor. *Science* 244:1163, 1989.
441. Reinertsen, J. L., Klippel, J. H., Johnson, A. H., Steinberg, A. B., Decker, J. L., and Mann, D. L. B-lymphocyte alloantigens associated with systemic lupus erythematosus. *N. Engl. J. Med.* 299:515, 1978.
442. Rennke, H. G., Klein, P. S., and Mendrick, D. L. Cell-mediated immunity (CMI) in hapten-induced interstitial nephritis and glomerular crescent formation in the rat. *Kidney Int.* 37:428, 1990.
443. Robertson, J. L., Hill, G. S., and Rowlands, D. T., Jr. Tubulointerstitial nephritis and glomerulonephritis in Brown Norway rats immunized with heterologous glomerular basement membrane. *Am. J. Pathol.* 88:53, 1977.
444. Robinson, D. R., Prickett, J. D., Makoul, G. T., Steinberg, A. D., and Colvin, R. B. Dietary fish oil reduces progression of established renal disease in (NZB × NZW) F_1 mice and delays renal disease in BXSB and MRL/l strains. *Arthritis Rheum.* 29:539, 1986.
445. Robinson, D. R., Tateno, S., Knoell, C., Olesiak, W., Xu, L., Hirai, A., Guo, M., and Colvin, R. B. Dietary marine lipids suppress murine autoimmune disease. *J. Int. Med.* 225:211, 1989.
446. Roccatello, D., Martina, G., Coppo, R., Piccoli, G., Sena, L. M., and Cordonnier, D. Clinical significance of an impaired mononuclear phagocyte system immune clearance in human nephritis. *Nephron* 51:428, 1989.
447. Rocklin, R. E., Lewis, E. J., and David, J. R. In vitro evidence for cellular hypersensitivity to glomerular-basement-membrane antigens in human glomerulonephritis. *N. Engl. J. Med.* 283:497, 1970.
448. Ronco, P., Verroust, P., and Morel-Maroger, L. Viruses and glomerulonephritis. *Nephron* 31:97, 1982.
449. Rose, N. R. Pathogenic mechanisms in autoimmune diseases. *Clin. Immunol. Immunopathol.* 53:S7, 1989.
450. Ross, G. D., Yount, W. J., Walport, M. J., Winfield, J. B., Parker, C. J., Fuller, C. R., Taylor, R. P., Myones, B. L., and Lachmann, P. J. Dis-

ease-associated loss of erythrocyte complement receptors (CR1, C3b receptors) in patients with systemic lupus erythematosus and other diseases involving autoantibodies and/or complement activation. *J. Immunol.* 135:2005, 1985.

451. Rudofsky, U. Spontaneous and induced autoantibodies to renal and non renal basement membranes in mice. *Clin. Immunol. Immunopathol.* 15:200, 1980.
452. Rudofsky, U., Dilwith, R. L., and Tung, K. S. K. Susceptibility differences of inbred mice to induction of autoimmune renal tubulointerstitial lesions. *Lab. Invest.* 43:463, 1980.
453. Rudofsky, U. H., McMaster, P. R. B., Ma, W. S., Steblay, R. W., and Pollara, B. Experimental autoimmune renal cortical tubulointerstitial disease in guinea pigs lacking the fourth component of complement (C4). *J. Immunol.* 112:1387, 1974.
454. Rudofsky, U. H., and Pollara, B. Studies on the pathogenesis of autoimmune renal tubulointerstitial disease in guinea pigs: I. Inhibition of tissue injury in leukocyte-depleted passive transfer recipients. *Clin. Immunol. Immunopathol.* 4:425, 1975.
455. Rudofsky, U., and Steblay, R. W. Studies on autoimmune nephritis in sheep: II. Passive transfer of nephritis in sheep by plasma. *Fed. Proc.* 25:659, 1966.
456. Rudofsky, U. H., Steblay, R. W., and Pollara, B. Inhibition of experimental autoimmune renal tubulointerstitial disease in guinea pigs by depletion of complement with cobra venom factor. *Clin. Immunol. Immunopathol.* 3:396, 1975.
457. Rydel, J. J., Schwartz, M. M., and Singh, A. K. Sequential localization of antibody to multiple regions of the glomerular capillary wall in passive Heymann nephritis. *Lab. Invest.* 60:492, 1989.
458. Sabbaga, J., Pankewycz, O. G., Lufft, V., Schwartz, R. S., and Madaio, M. P. Cross-reactivity distinguishes serum and nephritogenic anti-DNA antibodies in human lupus from their natural counterparts in normal serum. *J. Autoimmun.* 3:215, 1990.
459. Salant, D. J., Adler, S., Darby, C., Capparell, N. J., Groggel, G. C., Feintzeig, I. D., Rennke, H. G., and Dittmer, J. E. Influence of antigen distribution on the mediation of immunological glomerular injury. *Kidney Int.* 27:938, 1985.
460. Salant, D. J., Belok, S., Madaio, M. P., and Couser, W. G. A new role for complement in experimental membranous nephropathy in rats. *J. Clin. Invest.* 66:1339, 1980.
461. Salant, D. J., Quigg, R. I., and Cybulsky, A. V. Heymann nephritis: Mechanisms of renal injury. *Kidney Int.* 35:976, 1989.
462. Sano, M. Participation of monocytes in glomerulonephritis in acute serum sickness of rabbits. *Acta Pathol. Jpn.* 26:423, 1976.
463. Saxena, R., Bygren, P., Butkowski, R., and Wieslander, J. Specificity of kidney-bound antibodies in Goodpasture's syndrome. *Clin. Exp. Immunol.* 78:31, 1989.
464. Saxena, R., Isaksson, B., Bygren, P., and Wieslander, J. A rapid assay for circulating anti-glomerular basement membrane antibodies in Goodpasture's syndrome. *J. Immunol. Meth.* 118:73, 1989.
465. Schifferli, J. A., Bartolotti, S. R., and Peters, D. K. Inhibition of immune precipitation by complement. *Clin. Exp. Immunol.* 42:387, 1980.
466. Schifferli, J. A., Ng, Y. C., and Peters, D. K. The role of complement and its receptor in the elimination of immune complexes. *N. Engl. J. Med.* 315:488, 1986.
467. Schifferli, J. A., and Peters, D. K. Complement, the immune-complex lattice, and the pathophysiology of complement-deficiency syndromes. *Lancet* 2:957, 1983.
468. Schifferli, J. A., Steiger, G., Hauptmann, G., Spaeth, P. J., and Sjoholm, A. G. Formation of soluble immune complexes by complement in sera of patients with various hypocomplementemic states: Difference between inhibition of immune precipitation and solubilization. *J. Clin. Invest.* 76:2127, 1985.
469. Schifferli, J. A., and Taylor, R. P. Physiological and pathological aspects of circulating immune complexes. *Kidney Int.* 35:993, 1989.
470. Schifferli, J. A., Woo, P., and Peters, D. K. Complement-mediated inhibition of immune precipitation: I. Role of the classical and alternative pathways. *Clin. Exp. Immunol.* 47:555, 1982.
471. Schmiedeke, T. M. J., Stockl, F. W., Weber, R., Sugisaki, Y., Batsford, S. R., and Vogt, A. Histones have high affinity for the glomerular basement membrane. *J. Exp. Med.* 169:1879, 1989.
472. Schneeberger, E. E., Leber, P. D., Karnovsky, M. J., and McCluskey, R. T. Altered functional properties of the renal glomerulus in autologous immune complex nephritis. An ultrastructural tracer study. *J. Exp. Med.* 139:1283, 1974.
473. Schreiner, G. F., Cotran, R. S., Pardo, V., and Unanue, E. R. A mononuclear cell component in experimental immunological glomerulonephritis. *J. Exp. Med.* 147:369, 1978.
474. Schreiner, G. F., Kiely, J.-M., Cotran, R. S., and Unanue, E. R. Characterization of resident glomerular cells in the rat expressing Ia determinants and manifesting genetically restricted interaction with lymphocytes. *J. Clin. Invest.* 68:920, 1981.
475. Schreiner, G. F., Rovin, B., and Lefkowith, J. B. The antiinflammatory effects of essential fatty acid

deficiency in experimental glomerulonephritis. *J. Immunol.* 143:3192, 1989.
476. Schwartz, M. M., Roberts, J. L., and Lewis, E. J. Necrotizing glomerulitis of systemic lupus erythematosus. *Hum. Pathol.* 14:158, 1983.
477. Schwartz, R. S. Immunologic and genetic aspects of systemic lupus erythematosus. *Kidney Int.* 19:474, 1981.
478. Schwartz, R. S. Editorial overview. *Curr. Opin. Immunol.* 1:695, 1989.
479. Seegal, B. C. The value of immunofluorescent antibody technique in the study of experimental nephritis: Possible application for the interpretation of the pathogenesis of certain forms of human nephropathy (Italian). *Rass. Fisiopatol. Clin. Ter.* 31:1063, 1959.
480. Shah, S. V. Role of reactive oxygen metabolites in experimental glomerular disease. *Kidney Int.* 35:1093, 1989.
481. Shigematsu, H., Niwa, Y., Takijawa, J., and Akikusa, B. Arthus-type nephritis: I. Characterization of glomerular lesions induced by insoluble and poorly soluble immune complexes. *Lab. Invest.* 40:492, 1979.
482. Shimonkevitz, R., Kappler, J., Marrack, P., and Grey, H. Antigen recognition by H2-restricted T cells: I. Cell-free antigen processing. *J. Exp. Med.* 158:303, 1983.
483. Shoenfeld, Y., and Mozes, E. Pathogenic idiotypes of autoantibodies in autoimmunity: Lessons from new experimental models of SLE. *FASEB J.* 4:2646, 1990.
484. Silva, F. G., Hoyer, J. R., and Pirani, C. L. Sequential studies of glomerular crescent formation in rats with antiglomerular basement membrane–induced glomerulonephritis and the role of coagulation factors. *Lab. Invest.* 51:404, 1984.
485. Simpson, I. J., Thomson, N. M., and Peters, D. K. Mediator Systems in Experimental Allergic Glomerular Injury. In *Proceedings of the Sixth International Congress of Nephrology.* Basel: Karger, 1976. P. 431.
486. Sindrey, M., Barratt, J., Hewitt, J., and Naish, P. Infective endocarditis–associated glomerulonephritis in rabbits: Evidence of a pathogenetic role for antiglobulins. *Clin. Exp. Immunol.* 45:253, 1981.
487. Sindrey, M., and Naish, P. The mediation of the localization of polymorphonuclear leucocytes in glomeruli during the autologous phase of nephrotoxic nephritis. *Clin. Exp. Immunol.* 35:350, 1979.
488. Slusarczyk, J., Michalak, T., Nazarewicz-de Mezer, T., Krawczynski, K., and Nowostawski. A. Membranous glomerulopathy associated with hepatitis B core antigen immune complexes in children. *Am. J. Pathol.* 98:29, 1980.
489. Solomon, L. R., Rawlinson, V. I., Howarth, S., and Mallick, N. P. Reticuloendothelial function in glomerulonephritis. *Nephron* 37:54, 1984.
490. Stachura, I., Jayakumar, S., and Bourke, E. T- and B-lymphocyte subsets in fenoprofen nephropathy. *Am. J. Med.* 75:9, 1983.
491. Stachura, I., Si, L., Madan, E., and Whiteside, T. Mononuclear cell subsets in human renal disease enumeration in tissue sections with monoclonal antibodies. *Clin. Immunol. Immunopathol.* 30:362, 1984.
492. Stachura, I., Si, L., and Whiteside, T. L. Mononuclear-cell subsets in human idiopathic crescentic glomerulonephritis (ICGN): Analysis in tissue sections with monoclonal antibodies. *J. Clin. Immunol.* 4:202, 1984.
493. Steblay, R. W. Glomerulonephritis induced in sheep by injections of heterologous glomerular basement membrane and Freund's complete adjuvant. *J. Exp. Med.* 116:253, 1962.
494. Steblay, R. W. Anti-tubular-basement-membrane-antibody tubulointerstitial nephritis. *Am. J. Pathol.* 97:649, 1979.
495. Steblay, R. W., and Rudofsky, U. Further evidence for autoantibodies as mediators of experimental autoimmune nephritis in sheep. *J. Lab. Clin. Med.* 68:1021, 1966.
496. Steblay, R. W., and Rudofsky, U. Renal tubular disease and autoantibodies against tubular basement membrane induced in guinea pigs. *J. Immunol.* 107:589, 1971.
497. Stenglein, B., Thoenes, G. H., and Gunther, E. Genetically controlled autologous immune complex glomerulonephritis in rats. *J. Immunol.* 115:895, 1975.
498. Steward, M. W. Chronic immune complex disease in mice: The role of antibody affinity. *Clin. Exp. Immunol.* 38:414, 1979.
499. Steward, M. W., Collins, M. J., Stanley, C., and Devey, M. E. Chronic antigen-antibody-complex glomerulonephritis in mice. *Br. J. Exp. Pathol.* 62:614, 1981.
500. Stow, J. L., Sawada, H., and Farquhar, M. G. Basement membrane heparan sulfate proteoglycans are concentrated in the laminae rarae and in podocytes of the rat renal glomerulus. *Proc. Natl. Acad. Sci. USA* 82:3296, 1985.
501. Strife, C. F., McDonald, B. M., Ruley, E. J., McAdams, A. J., and West, C. D. Shunt nephritis: The nature of the serum cryoglobulins and their relation to the complement profile. *J. Pediatr.* 88:403, 1976.
502. Striker, G. E., Mannik, M., and Tung, M. Y. The role of marrow-derived monocytes and mesangial cells in removal of immune complexes from renal glomeruli. *J. Exp. Med.* 149:127, 1979.

503. Strom, T. B., and Kelley, V. E. Toward more selective therapies to block undesired immune responses. *Kidney Int.* 35:1026, 1989.
504. Sugisaki, T., Klassen, J., Milgrom, F., Andres, G. A., and McCluskey, R. T. Immunopathologic study of an autoimmune tubular and interstitial renal disease in Brown Norway rats. *Lab. Invest.* 28:658, 1973.
505. Sugisaki, T., Yoshida, T., McCluskey, R. T., Andres, G. A., and Klassen, J. Autoimmune cell-mediated tubulointerstitial nephritis induced in Lewis rats by renal antigens. *Clin. Immunol. Immunopathol.* 15:33, 1980.
506. Sy, M.-S., and Benacerraf, B. Suppressor T cells, immunoglobulin and Igh restriction. *Immunol. Rev.* 101:133, 1988.
507. Takahashi, M., Czop, J., Ferreira, A., and Nussenzweig, V. Mechanism of solubilization of immune aggregates by complement: Implication for immunopathology. *Transplant. Rev.* 32:121, 1976.
508. Takahashi, M., Tack, B. F., and Nussenzweig, V. Requirements for the solubilization of immune aggregates by complement: Assembly of a factor B-dependent C3-convertase on the immune complexes. *J. Exp. Med.* 145:86, 1977.
509. Takahashi, M., and Takahashi, S. Complement-dependent solubilization of immune complexes. *Clin. Immunol. Allergy* 1:261, 1981.
510. Takahashi, M., Takahashi, S., and Hirose, S. Solubilization of antigen-antibody complexes: A new function of complement as a regulator of immune reactions. *Prog. Allergy* 27:134, 1980.
511. Takekoshi, Y., Tanaka, M., Miyakawa, Y., Yoshizawa, H., Takahashi, K., and Mayumi, M. Free "small" and IgG-associated "large" hepatitis B_e antigen in the serum and glomerular capillary walls of two patients with membranous glomerulonephritis. *N. Engl. J. Med.* 300:814, 1979.
512. Ten, R. M., Torres, V. E., Milliner, D. S., Schwab, T. R., Holley, K. E., and Gleich, G. J. Subspecialty clinics: Nephrology. Acute interstitial nephritis: Immunologic and clinical aspects. *Mayo Clin. Proc.* 63:921, 1988.
513. Thaiss, F., Batsford, S., Mihatsch, M. J., Heitz, P. U., Bitter-Suermann, D., and Vogt, A. Mediator systems in a passive model of in situ immune complex glomerulonephritis: Role for complement, polymorphonuclear granulocytes and monocytes. *Lab. Invest.* 54:624, 1986.
514. Theofilopoulos, A. N., and Dixon, F. J. Immune complexes in human diseases. *Am. J. Pathol.* 100:531, 1980.
515. Theofilopoulos, A. N., and Dixon, F. J. Murine models of systemic lupus erythematosus. *Adv. Immunol.* 37:269, 1985.
516. Theofilopoulos, A. N., Kofler, R., Singer, P. A., and Dixon, F. J. Molecular genetics of murine lupus models. *Adv. Immunol.* 46:61, 1989.
517. Thompson, N. M., Ian, J. M., Simpson, I. J., and Peters, D. K. Defibrination with ancrod in nephrotoxic nephritis in rabbits. *Kidney Int.* 10:343, 1976.
518. Thompson, N. M., Simpson, I. J., Evans, D. J., and Peters, D. K. Defibrination with ancrod in experimental chronic immune complex nephritis. *Clin. Exp. Immunol.* 20:527, 1975.
519. Tipping, P. G., and Holdsworth, S. R. The participation of macrophages, glomerular procoagulant activity, and factor VII in glomerular fibrin deposition: Studies in anti-GBM antibody induced glomerulonephritis in rabbits. *Am. J. Pathol.* 124:10, 1986.
520. Tipping, P. G., Neale, T. J., and Holdsworth, S. R. T lymphocyte participation in antibody-induced experimental glomerulonephritis. *Kidney Int.* 27:530, 1985.
521. Todd, J. A., Acha-Orbea, H., Bell, J. I., Chao, N., Fronek, Z., Jacob, C. O., McDermott, M., Sinha, A. A., Timmerman, L., Steinman, L., and McDevitt, H. O. A molecular basis for MHC class II–associated autoimmunity. *Science* 240:1003, 1988.
522. Tomer, Y., and Shoenfeld, Y. The significance of T suppressor cells in the development of autoimmunity. *J. Autoimmun.* 2:739, 1989.
523. Tourville, D. R., Byrd, L. H., Kim, D. V., Zajd, D., Lee, I., Reichman, L. B., and Baskin, S. Treponemal antigen in immunopathogenesis of syphilitic glomerulonephritis. *Am. J. Pathol.* 82:479, 1976.
524. Treser, G., Semar, M., McVicas, M., Franklin, M., Ty, A., Sagel, I., and Lange, K. Antigenic streptococcal components in acute glomerulonephritis. *Science* 163:676, 1969.
525. Tucker, F. L., Sturgill, B. C., and Bolton, W. K. Ultrastructural studies of experimental autoimmune glomerulonephritis in normal and bursectomized chickens. *Lab. Invest.* 53:563, 1985.
526. Ueda, S., Wakashin, M., Wakashin, Y., Mori, T., Yoshida, H., Mori, Y., Iesato, K., Ogawa, M., Azemoto, R., Kato, I., and Okuda, K. Suppressor system in murine interstitial nephritis: Analysis of tubular basement membrane (TBM)–specific suppressor T cells and their soluble factor in C57BL/6 mice using a syngeneic system. *Clin. Immunol. Immunopathol.* 45:78, 1987.
527. Ulich, T. R., Bannister, K. M., and Wilson, C. B. Tubulointerstitial nephritis induced in the Brown Norway rat with chaotropically solubilized bovine tubular basement membrane: The model and the humoral and cellular responses. *Clin. Immunol. Immunopathol.* 36:187, 1985.
528. Ulich, T. R., Bannister, K. M., and Wilson, C. B. Inhibition of neutrophilic infiltrate of ex-

perimental tubulointerstitial nephritis in the Brown Norway rat by decomplementation. *Clin. Immunol. Immunopathol.* 42:288, 1987.
529. Ulich, T. R., and Ni, R.-X. Inhibition of experimental autoimmune tubulointerstitial nephritis in Brown Norway rats by (15S)-15-methyl prostaglandin E_1: Analysis of the effect of prostaglandin E_1 on the induction of the humoral immune response and the elucitation of humorally mediated inflammation. *Am. J. Pathol.* 124:286, 1986.
530. Unanue, E. R., and Dixon, F. J. Experimental glomerulonephritis: IV. Participation of complement in nephrotoxic nephritis. *J. Exp. Med.* 119:965, 1964.
531. Unanue, E. R., and Dixon, F. J. Experimental glomerulonephritis: VI. The autologous phase of nephrotoxic serum nephritis. *J. Exp. Med.* 121: 715, 1965.
532. Unanue, E. R., and Dixon, F. J. Experimental glomerulonephritis: Immunological events and pathogenetic mechanisms. *Adv. Immunol.* 6:1, 1967.
533. Uwatoko, S., Aotsuka, S., Okawa, M., Egusa, Y., Yokohari, R., Aizawa, C., and Suzuki, K. C1q solid-phase radioimmunoassay: Evidence for the detection of antibody directed against the collagen-like region of C1q in sera from patients with systemic lupus erythematosus. *Clin. Exp. Immunol.* 69:98, 1987.
534. Van Damme, B. J. C., Fleuren, G. J., Bakker, W. W., Vernier, R. L., and Hoedemaeker, P. J. Experimental glomerulonephritis in the rat induced by antibodies directed against tubular antigens: V. Fixed glomerular antigens in the pathogenesis of heterologous immune complex glomerulonephritis. *Lab. Invest.* 38:502, 1978.
535. van der Woude, F. J., Rasmussen, N., Lobatto, S., Wiik, A., Permin, H., Van Es, L. A., van der Giessen, M., van der Hem, G. K., and The, T. H. Autoantibodies against neutrophils and monocytes: Tool for diagnosis and marker of disease activity in Wegener's granulomatosis. *Lancet* 1:806, 1985.
536. Van Zwieten, M. J., Bhan, A. K., McCluskey, R. T., and Collins, A. B. Studies on the pathogenesis of experimental anti-tubular basement membrane nephritis in guinea pig. *Am. J. Pathol.* 83:531, 1976.
537. Van Zwieten, M. J., Leber, P. D., Bhan, A. K., and McCluskey, R. T. Experimental cell-mediated interstitial nephritis induced with exogenous antigens. *J. Immunol.* 118:589, 1977.
538. Vassalli, P., and McCluskey, R. T. The coagulation process in rabbit Masugi nephritis. *Am. J. Pathol.* 45:653, 1964.
539. Vassalli, P., and McCluskey, R. T. The pathogenic role of fibrin deposition in immunologically induced glomerulonephritis. *Ann. N.Y. Acad. Sci.* 116:1052, 1964.
540. Vassalli, P., Simon, G., and Rouiller, C. Electron microscopic study of glomerular lesions resulting from intravascular fibrin formation. *Am. J. Pathol.* 43:579, 1963.
541. Vissers, M. C. M., Fantone, J. C., Wiggins, R., and Kunkel, S. L. Glomerular basement membrane–containing immune complexes stimulate tumor necrosis factor and interleukin-1 production by human monocytes. *Am. J. Pathol.* 134:1, 1989.
542. Vissers, M. C. M., Wiggins, R., and Fantone, J. C. Comparative ability of human monocytes and neutrophils to degrade glomerular basement membrane in vitro. *Lab. Invest.* 60:831, 1989.
543. Vissers, M. C. M., Winterbourn, C. C., and Hunt, J. S. Degradation of glomerular basement membrane by human neutrophils in vitro. *Biochim. Biophys. Acta* 804:154, 1984.
544. Vogt, A. New aspects of the pathogenesis of immune complex glomerulonephritis: Formation of subepithelial deposits. *Clin. Nephrol.* 21:15, 1984.
545. Vogt, A., Rohrbach, R., Shimizu, F., Takamiya, H., and Batsford, S. Interaction of cationized antigen with rat glomerular basement membrane: In situ immune complex formation. *Kidney Int.* 22:27, 1982.
546. Voorby, H. A. M., Kabel, P. J., De Haan, M., Jeucken, P. H. M., Van Der Gaag, R. D., De Baets, M. H., and Drexhage, H. A. Dendritic cells and class II MHC expression on thyrocytes during the autoimmune thyroid disease of the BB rat. *Clin. Immunol. Immunopathol.* 55:9, 1990.
547. Vosti, K. L., Lindberg, L. H., Kosek, J. C., and Raffel, S. Experimental streptococcal glomerulonephritis: Longitudinal study of a laboratory model resembling human acute poststreptococcal glomerulonephritis. *J. Infect. Dis.* 122:249, 1970.
548. Vyas, G. N., Roberts, I., Peterson, D. L., and Holland, P. V. Nonspecific test reactions for antibodies to hepatitis B surface antigen in chronic HB_sAg carriers. *J. Lab. Clin. Med.* 89:428, 1977.
549. Walport, M. J., and Lachmann, P. J. Erythrocyte complement receptor type 1, immune complexes, and the rheumatic diseases. *Arthritis Rheum.* 31:153, 1988.
550. Warren, J. S., Kunkel, S. L., Johnson, K. J., and Ward, P. A. In vitro activation of rat neutrophils and alveolar macrophages with IgA and IgG immune complexes. *Am. J. Pathol.* 129:578, 1987.
551. Warren, J. S., Ward, P. A., Johnson, K. J., and Ginsburg, I. Modulation of acute immune complex–mediated tissue injury by the presence of polyionic substances. *Am. J. Pathol.* 128:67, 1987.
552. Warren, J. S., Ward, P. A., and Johnson, K. J.

Tumor necrosis factor: A plurifunctional mediator of acute inflammation. *Mod. Pathol.* 1:242, 1988.

553. Waxman, F. J., Hebert, L. A., Cornacoff, J. B., VanAman, M. E., Smead, W. L., Kraut, E. H., Birmingham, D. J., and Taguiam, J. M. Complement depletion accelerates the clearance of immune complexes from the circulation of primates. *J. Clin. Invest.* 74:1329, 1984.
554. Waxman, F. J., Hebert, L. A., Cosio, F. G., Smead, W. L., VanAman, M. E., Taguiam, J. M., and Birmingham, D. J. Differential binding of immunoglobulin A and immunoglobulin G_1 immune complexes to primate erythrocytes in vivo: Immunoglobulin A immune complexes bind less well to erythrocytes and are preferentially deposited in glomeruli. *J. Clin. Invest.* 77:82, 1986.
555. Weber, K., Hawruk, E., and DeBari, V. A. Interaction of anti-DNA antibodies with synthetic polyanionic antigens. *J. Autoimmun.* 2:851, 1989.
556. Weiss, S. J. Mechanisms of disease: Tissue destruction by neutrophils. *N. Engl. J. Med.* 320: 365, 1989.
557. Werber, H. I., Emancipator, S. N., Tykocinski, M. L., and Sedor, J. R. The interleukin 1 gene is expressed by rat glomerular mesangial cells and is augmented in immune complex glomerulonephritis. *J. Immunol.* 138:3207, 1987.
558. Werdelin, O., and McCluskey, R. T. The nature of the specificity of mononuclear cells in experimental autoimmune inflammation and mechanisms leading to their accumulation. *J. Exp. Med.* 133:1242, 1971.
559. West, C. D. Immunology in Pediatric Renal Disease—Recent Advances. In K. Murakami et al. (Eds.), *Recent Advances in Pediatric Nephrology.* New York: Elsevier, Science Publishers, 1987. P. 29.
560. Wiggins, R. C. Hageman factor in experimental nephrotoxic nephritis in the rabbit. *Lab. Invest.* 53:335, 1985.
561. Wiggins, R. C., and Cochrane, C. G. Immune-complex–mediated biologic effects. *N. Engl. J. Med.* 304:518, 1981.
562. Wilson, C. B. Nephritogenic antibody mechanisms involving antigens within the glomerulus. *Immunol. Rev.* 55:257, 1981.
563. Wilson, C. B. Study of the immunopathogenesis of tubulointerstitial nephritis using model systems. *Kidney Int.* 35:938, 1989.
564. Wilson, C. B., and Dixon, F. J. The Renal Response to Immunological Injury. In B. M. Brenner and F. C. Rector (Eds.), *The Kidney,* 2nd Ed. Philadelphia: Saunders, 1981. P. 1237.
565. Wilson, J. G., Wong, W. W., Schur, P. H., and Fearon, D. T. Mode of inheritance of decreased C3b receptors in erythrocytes of patients with systemic lupus erythematosus. *N. Engl. J. Med.* 307:981, 1982.
566. Winer, R. L., Cohen, A. H., Sawhney, A. S., and Gorman, J. T. Sjögren's syndrome with immune complex tubulointerstitial renal disease. *Clin. Immunol. Immunopathol.* 8:494, 1977.
567. Wright, N. G., Morrison, W. I., Thompson, H., and Cornwell, H. J. C. Mesangial localization of immune complexes in experimental canine adenovirus glomerulonephritis. *Br. J. Exp. Pathol.* 55:458, 1974.
568. Wuthrich, R. P., Yui, M. A., Mazoujian, G., Nabavi, N., Glimcher, L. H., and Kelley, V. E. Enhanced MHC class II expression in renal proximal tubules precedes loss of renal function in MRL/lpr mice with lupus nephritis. *Am. J. Pathol.* 134:45, 1989.
569. Young, J. D. E., Damiano, A., DiNome, M. A., Leong, L. G., and Cohn, Z. A. Disassociation of membrane binding and lytic activities of the lymphocyte pore-forming protein (perforin). *J. Exp. Med.* 165:1371, 1987.
570. Yuceoglu, A. M., Sagel, I., Treser, G., Wasserman, E., and Lange, K. The glomerulopathy of congenital syphilis. A curable immune-deposit disease. *JAMA* 229:1085, 1974.
571. Zakheim, B., McCafferty, E., Phillips, S. M., Clayman, M., and Neilson, E. G. Murine interstitial nephritis: II. The adoptive transfer of disease with immune T-lymphocytes produces a phenotypically complex interstitial lesion. *J. Immunol.* 133:234, 1984.
572. Zaller, D. M., Osman, G., Kanagawa, O., and Hood, L. Prevention and treatment of murine experimental allergic encephalomyelitis with T cell receptor V_β-specific antibodies. *J. Exp. Med.* 171:1943, 1990.
573. Zinkernagel, R. M., Haenseler, E., Leist, T., Cerny, A., Hengartner, H., and Althage, A. T cell–mediated hepatitis in mice infected with lymphocytic choriomeningitis virus. *J. Exp. Med.* 164: 1075, 1986.
574. Zinkernagel, R. M., Leist, T., Hengartner, H., and Althage, A. Susceptibility to lymphocytic choriomeningitis virus isolates correlates directly with early and high cytotoxic T cell activity, as well as with foot pad swelling reaction, and all three are regulated by H-2D. *J. Exp. Med.* 162:2125, 1985.
575. Zoja, C., Corna, D., Macconi, D., Zilio, P., Bertani, T., and Remuzzi, G. Tissue plasminogen activator therapy of rabbit nephrotoxic nephritis. *Lab. Invest.* 62:34, 1990.
576. Zurier, R. B., Damjanov, I., Miller, P., and Biewer, B. Prostaglandin E_1 treatment prevents progression of nephritis in murine lupus erythematosus. *J. Clin. Lab. Immunol.* 1:95, 1978.

Robert H. Heptinstall

4
Classification of Glomerulonephritis; Focal, and Mesangial Proliferative Forms of Glomerulonephritis; Recurrent Hematuria

SCOPE OF CHAPTER

This chapter gives a brief account of the classification of glomerulonephritis and describes the way in which it is presented in the next several chapters. It will also provide an introduction to focal, and mesangial proliferative forms of glomerulonephritis, which share many common features and can be different manifestations of such conditions as systemic lupus erythematosus, Schönlein-Henoch syndrome, and IgA nephritis. Also included is an account of the clinical syndrome of recurrent hematuria with descriptions of the various conditions that can cause it.

CLASSIFICATION OF GLOMERULONEPHRITIS

Historical Aspects

There have been numerous attempts to classify glomerulonephritis over the years, and notable among them are those of Volhard and Fahr [125], Addis [3], Ellis [33], and Longcope [78,79]. All were devised before the renal biopsy was introduced, and all were dependent on autopsy material for the pathologic aspects when clinicopathologic correlations were made. Although this meant that the renal lesions were often at an advanced stage, this was not always the case, for many patients with severe forms of disease died quickly and others died from nonrenal causes. Particularly from the writings of Fahr [34,125], a considerable body of information on the pathology of glomerulonephritis was built up, and some of his descriptions stand unrivaled even today. Those seeking further information on these earlier classifications are directed to the first and second editions of this book, where more detailed accounts were given.

Present-Day Views

The percutaneous renal biopsy was introduced as a relatively safe, routine procedure by Iversen and Brun [63] in 1951, although for the sake of historical accuracy it should be pointed out that Alwall [4] had previously used a similar technique on several patients. The effect on our understanding of renal disease was remarkable, for not only could tissue now be obtained at an early stage of the disease in question, but sequential biopsies allowed a study of its progress. Furthermore, an opportunity was provided to see the pathology of conditions about which we had either no knowledge or only scanty information. An example of this is the entity of recurrent hematuria, study of which eventually led to confirmation of the concept of focal glomerulonephritis and later, when immunofluorescence techniques were introduced, to the discovery of IgA nephritis. The availability of fresh tissue allowed electron microscopic studies to be carried out so that over the years the combined use of light, electron, and immunohistologic microscopy on renal biopsies, coupled with appropriate experimental models, led to our present concepts and classification of renal disease.

Apart from various individual efforts to define and classify renal disease—for our purpose at this point, glomerulonephritis—there have been two major attempts to do so by committee. The first of these dealt mainly with definitions [61] and was less concerned with classification. The second, sponsored by the World Health Organization (WHO), was involved in the production of a histopathologic classification of glomerular disease [24], the major recommendations of which will be presented next.

The main division was twofold: (1) primary glomerulonephritis and (2) those forms of glomerulonephritis which accompany systemic diseases. The term *diffuse* was used to indicate that all glomeruli were affected, and the term *focal* was used to denote that only a certain number were involved.

PRIMARY GLOMERULONEPHRITIS

1. Focal and segmental glomerulonephritis
2. Diffuse glomerulonephritis
   a. Membranous glomerulonephritis
   b. Proliferative glomerulonephritis
      (i) Mesangial proliferative glomerulonephritis
      (ii) Endocapillary proliferative glomerulonephritis
      (iii) Mesangiocapillary glomerulonephritis (or membranoproliferative glomerulonephritis types I and III)

(iv) Dense deposit glomerulonephritis (membranoproliferative glomerulonephritis type II)
(v) Crescentic glomerulonephritis
c. Sclerosing glomerulonephritis.

GLOMERULONEPHRITIS OF SYSTEMIC DISEASES

This division included such conditions as systemic lupus erythematous (SLE), Schönlein-Henoch syndrome, Goodpasture's syndrome (anti-GBM antibody disease would have been more accurate), systemic infections, parasitic infections, and IgA nephritis. Other categories embraced the forms of glomerulonephritis accompanying polyarteritis nodosa, Wegener's syndrome, and Alport's syndrome. It is not clear to me why IgA nephritis was included as a manifestation of systemic disease; perhaps its overlap with Schönlein-Henoch syndrome prompted the WHO committee to regard it as such.

Nomenclature and Classification Used in Ensuing Chapters

The format to be used in the following chapters differs only slightly from that of the WHO classification, but certain adjustments have been made. For example, rather than having a chapter specifically designated endocapillary proliferative glomerulonephritis, we have chosen to include it in one headed "Acute Postinfectious Glomerulonephritis and Glomerulonephritis Complicating Persistent Bacterial Infection" (Chap. 5). The reason for this is to allow the inclusion of other glomerular manifestations of infections such as bacterial endocarditis and thereby avoid excessive fragmentation.

We also have chosen to use the old term *membranoproliferative glomerulonephritis* rather than *mesangiocapillary glomerulonephritis* and to depart from the WHO terminology by using the more appropriate term *anti-glomerular basement membrane antibody disease*—which accommodates certain cases without pulmonary hemorrhage—rather than the contentious eponym *Goodpasture's syndrome.*

IgA nephritis is treated in a separate chapter (Chap. 6) because it is such a common form of glomerulonephritis that takes on several histologic appearances. It is coupled with Schönlein-Henoch syndrome and hepatobiliary disease because of certain common features, chief of which is mesangial deposition of IgA.

Finally, we find ourselves bedfellows (figuratively speaking) with the WHO committee in perpetuating the term *proliferative,* appreciating full well that the hypercellularity in various forms of glomerulonephritis is not solely a hyperplasia of resident cells, but also an infiltration by those of exogenous origin.

The following list summarizes the categories of glomerulonephritis to be discussed and their locations in the book.

1. Focal glomerulonephritis	This chapter
2. Mesangial proliferative glomerulonephritis	This chapter
3. Acute postinfectious glomerulonephritis and glomerulonephritis complicating persistent bacterial infection	Chapter 5
4. IgA nephritides (including Schönlein-Henoch syndrome)	Chapter 6
5. Membranoproliferative glomerulonephritis types I and III and dense deposit disease.	Chapter 7
6. Membranous glomerulonephritis	Chapter 8
7. Crescentic glomerulonephritis	Chapter 9
8. Anti-GBM antibody disease	Chapter 10
9. Chronic glomerulonephritis	Chapter 11

FOCAL GLOMERULONEPHRITIS AND MESANGIAL PROLIFERATIVE GLOMERULONEPHRITIS

Definitions

FOCAL GLOMERULONEPHRITIS

By definition, focal glomerulonephritis is a form of glomerulonephritis in which by light microscopy only a certain number of the glomeruli are affected, the others being normal. A further feature is the way in which the affected glomeruli show changes in only part of the tuft; the term *segmental* is applied to this. The more precise designation, therefore, is focal and segmental glomerulonephritis. It is important to appreciate that many forms of focal glomerulonephritis display the presence of immunoglobulins and complement with a widespread distribution in the mesangium, and this is so even in those glomeruli which appear normal by light microscopy. Electron-dense deposits are usually present in a similar distribution. As a consequence, the definition of focal glomerulonephritis should be qualified by including "by light microscopy."

MESANGIAL PROLIFERATIVE GLOMERULONEPHRITIS

Mesangial proliferative glomerulonephritis is defined by the WHO committee [24] as "an essentially uniform increase in mesangial cells (with clusters of four or more per mesangial area) in all or nearly all glomeruli. Cell proliferation may be accompanied by an increase in the mesangial matrix." The committee goes on to point out that the capillary lumens are patent; this was done in order to separate it from what they call "endocapillary proliferative glomerulonephritis" (the type found typically in poststreptococcal glomerulonephritis), in which there is swelling of endothelial cells, infiltration by inflammatory cells, and mesangial proliferation. The capillary walls are not thickened, and neutrophil infiltration is not present. Immunofluorescence techniques demonstrate mesangial immunoglobulins in some forms but not in others, and the same is true of mesangial electron-dense deposits.

The term *mesangial proliferative glomerulonephritis* is contentious in implying that the increased numbers of cells represent replication of cells (most of which are of a modified smooth-muscle type) normally resident in the mesangium. Since bone marrow–derived monocytes are now recognized to contribute to the cellular increase in many forms of glomerulonephritis, some authors have contested use of the word *proliferative* [25]. They considered alternative names for mesangial proliferative glomerulonephritis and felt that *mesangiopathic glomerulonephritis* might be more appropriate. More will be said about the term *mesangiopathic* later in this account.

A further problem arises when mesangial hypercellularity is found in patients with either focal and segmental glomerular sclerosis and hyalinosis or what would otherwise be called *minimal-change disease* (Fig. 4-1). While it is often labeled *mesangial proliferative glomerulonephritis*, some contest this on the ground that it implies a distinct form of glomerulonephritis and use the term *diffuse mesangial proliferation* [50]. Others choose to call it *diffuse mesangial hypercellularity* [108,115]. Since this issue is more appropriately considered in Chapter 12, no more will be said at this stage except to record that I have chosen to list such cases under *mesangial proliferative glomerulonephritis*.

Evolution of the Concept of Focal Glomerulonephritis

In their 1914 monograph, Volhard and Fahr [125] separated focal nephritis from the diffuse variety and subdivided it into three main forms: (1) focal glomerulonephritis, with acute and chronic forms, (2) interstitial nephritis, and (3) embolic focal nephritis.

The acute form of focal glomerulonephritis began with the appearance of hematuria *at the height* of an infective condition such as tonsillitis or scarlatina. There was *no* rise in blood pressure, edema only exceptionally, and nitrogen retention only when oliguria occurred as part of a very severe infection. The urine contained very small amounts of albumin, but red and white blood cells and hyalin and granular casts were present in the sediment. The various features distinguishing it from classic poststreptococcal glomerulonephritis will be appreciated. In general, the prognosis was excellent, with disappearance of the hematuria after a few days; however, hematuria could persist for much longer periods and was assessed in terms of years in some patients. An important feature was the way in which attacks of infection could cause a recurrence of hematuria. These authors also described the way in which a chronic stage could develop with persistent hematuria and proteinuria.

In the ensuing years, similar views were expressed by Baehr [7], Ellis [33], and Fishberg [36]. The occurrence of hematuria at the height of an infection, the recurrent nature of the hematuria, the absence of hypertension and edema, the gen-

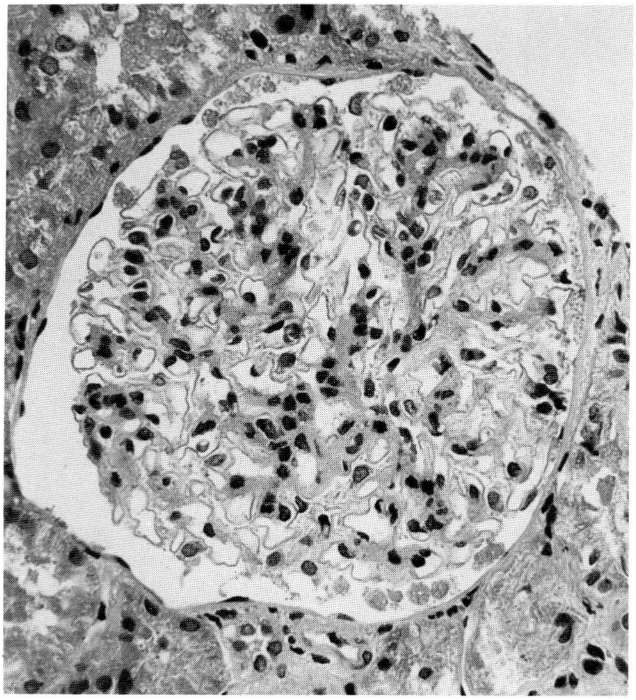

FIG. 4-1. *Glomerulus from patient with nephrotic syndrome. Pathologic features are restricted to mild increase in mesangial cellularity. H&E; ×320.*

erally good prognosis, and the existence of persistent forms were features that were repeatedly stressed. With great prescience, Baehr [7] imagined that the histologic changes would resemble those found in subacute bacterial endocarditis, a picture that he [6] and Löhlein [77] had described as showing focal and segmental glomerular lesions.

Apart from autopsy reports describing focal and segmental endothelial cell proliferation in patients with a variety of fatal infective conditions [36], the lesion in subacute bacterial endocarditis was the only recognized histologic picture of focal glomerulonephritis.

The introduction of the percutaneous renal biopsy in 1951 permitted examination of tissue at an early stage of evolution or from conditions that were not usually fatal. Thus by 1961 focal glomerulonephritis was clearly established as a pathologic entity [8,53,54,103]. It was found in systemic diseases such as SLE and Schönlein-Henoch syndrome, and in apparently primary glomerular disease with the clinical settings of recurrent hematuria, nephrotic syndrome, and chance proteinuria. Since that time, other systemic diseases have been added, and various primary forms of glomerular disease have been identified.

The application of immunofluorescence techniques to renal biopsies led to the interesting discovery in 1965 [15] that in children with recurrent hematuria and focal segmental glomerulonephritis, human globulin was present in those glomeruli showing no change by light microscopy and was distributed in a diffuse way in those showing segmental lesions by light microscopy. This was followed by the demonstration of Berger and Hinglais [11] that diffuse mesangial staining for immunoglobulins—predominantly IgA—was present in certain cases of focal glomerulonephritis. This

TABLE 4-1. *Immunofluorescence in focal glomerular lesions*

Disease	IgA	IgG	IgM	C3	Fibrinogen
Systemic lupus erythematosus (focal form)	Neg.	+ +[a] Diffuse, mesangial, and parietal[b]	Neg.	+ Diffuse, mesangial, and parietal	Neg. or very limited amounts focally
Schönlein-Henoch syndrome	+ + Diffuse, mesangial, and parietal	+ + Diffuse, mesangial, and parietal	Neg.	+ + Diffuse, mesangial, and parietal	+ + + Diffuse, mesangial, and parietal
Polyarteritis nodosa	Neg.	Neg.	Neg.	Neg.	+ + Focal in glomeruli and some vessels
Anti-GBM antibody disease	Neg.	+ + + Linear parietal and diffuse	Neg.	± Linear parietal and diffuse	Neg.
IgA nephritis	+ + + Diffuse and mesangial	+ Diffuse and mesangial	Neg.	+ Diffuse and mesangial	+ Diffuse when present
Focal segmental glomerular sclerosis and hyalinosis	Neg.	Neg.	+ Focal and segmental	+ Focal and segmental	Neg.

[a]+ to + + + = staining intensity; Neg. = no staining.
[b]Parietal refers to deposits along capillary walls.
Source: Modified from Morel-Maroger et al., *Am. J. Med.* 53:170, 1972, by permission of Dr. L. Morel-Maroger and the Editor of the *American Journal of Medicine*.

not only confirmed the earlier observation of a widespread distribution of immunoglobulins—now shown to be mesangial in position—in focal glomerulonephritis, but in addition identified a new entity referred to as *IgA nephritis.* As will be described in Chapter 6, this is a common condition [31], and in certain parts of the world, it is the most frequently encountered form of glomerulonephritis. With greater experience of immunofluorescence techniques, it became appreciated [91] that focal glomerulonephritis accompanying certain systemic diseases also displayed diffuse distribution of immunoglobulins and C3 (Table 4-1). As was the case with primary glomerulonephritis, positive immunofluorescence was present in a diffuse pattern not only in the glomeruli displaying segmental lesions by light microscopy, but also in those without lesions. The various proteins were situated predominantly in the mesangium but were sometimes also seen in relation to the glomerular capillary walls in SLE and Schönlein-Henoch syndrome. In anti-GBM antibody disease with focal segmental lesions, all glomeruli showed a linear distribution of IgG along the capillary walls, with or without C3 in a similar distribution. Inspection of Table 4-1 reveals that not all forms of focal glomerulonephritis have this diffuse positive fluorescence, and polyarteritis nodosa is an example of this. The same is true of primary focal segmental necrotizing glomerulonephritis.

Common Features of Focal Glomerulonephritis and Mesangial Proliferative Glomerulonephritis

Mesangial proliferative glomerulonephritis occurs either as a primary glomerulonephritis or as part of various systemic diseases. IgA nephritis is one of the best recognized primary forms of mesangial proliferative glomerulonephritis, and as was described earlier, it may also be manifest as focal glomerulonephritis. In both histologic types there is a diffuse mesangial deposition of immunoglobulins and C3, with IgA being the dominant immunoglobulin. Electron-dense deposits are present in the mesangium. Without going into details, it should be noted that other forms of mesangial proliferative glomerulonephritis of primary type show a diffuse mesangial distribution of immunoglobulins, with IgG predominating in some and IgM in others.

One of the common expressions of SLE is a diffuse mesangial hypercellularity that is accompanied by widespread deposition of immunoglobulins and C3 in the mesangium and by the presence of mesangial electron-dense deposits. Again, the similarity to focal glomerulonephritis is apparent because this is a common variant of lupus nephritis. Schönlein-Henoch syndrome, too, may be manifest as either focal or mesangial proliferative glomerulonephritis, with diffuse mesangial immunofluorescence patterns in both.

It is apparent that there are great similarities and overlap between certain types of focal and mesangial proliferative glomerulonephritis that are highly suggestive of a common pathogenesis.

Pathogenesis of Focal Glomerulonephritis and Mesangial Proliferative Glomerulonephritis

The studies of Germuth and Rodriguez [42,43] showed that under certain circumstances, the rabbit treated with foreign protein may exhibit a localization of immune complexes in the mesangium rather than in the capillary loops. The histologic picture seen with deposition in the loops was one of a widespread proliferative glomerulonephritis, whereas with deposition confined to the mesangium the proliferative changes were localized to the mesangium and were sometimes very mild. It was found that there were several factors involved in determining the site of deposition of complexes. One of these was the *size* of the complex formed, and good evidence for this was brought forward in experiments on the rabbit injected with bovine serum albumin. It was shown that whereas complexes of relatively small size localized in the glomerular capillary loops and produced a widespread proliferative picture, larger complexes (over 1 million daltons) lodged in the mesangium causing a less severe hypercellular reaction.

The importance of *complex size* was further shown in two studies in which rabbits were immunized with porcine thyroglobulin, which is of larger molecular size than bovine serum albumin [44,74]. It was felt that this would preclude the formation of small complexes capable of penetrating the capillary walls, and would facilitate the formation of intermediate-sized complexes over a wider range of antigen-antibody ratios with resultant sustained exposure of the glomeruli to these intermediate-sized complexes. Although the dosage schedule differed in these two experiments, in both it was found that repeated intravenous injections of thyroglobulin caused increased cellularity in the mesangium; electron-dense deposits were present and were confined to the mesangium and immediately adjacent subendothelial space. Rabbit immunoglobulins, C3, and porcine thyroglobulins also were found in the mesangium. Similar results were obtained when mice were immunized with ferritin, which also has a large molecular size [117].

Size is not the only factor that facilitates the mesangial localization of immune complexes. Changes in *permeability* of the capillary wall were considered to play an important role in experiments that allowed small complexes to deposit in the mesangium rather than penetrate and localize in the capillary wall [45]. This was found in studies in which cortisone was administered to rabbits with circulating small-sized complexes; in these animals, complexes were confined to the mesangial areas instead of penetrating and becoming deposited in the glomerular capillary walls [45]. It was believed that the cortisone interfered with the permeability of the basement membrane.

Hemodynamic factors are also clearly important in determining the site of deposition of complexes because glomeruli appear to be "protected" by narrowing of the renal artery in diffuse proliferative glomerulonephritis in man [98] and in experimental immune-complex disease [41] in the rabbit. Presumably a decreased perfusion pressure prevents the penetration of complexes into the glomerular capillary basement membranes in the same way as postulated in the cortisone experiments. Experiments on rats with streptozotocin-induced diabetes mellitus also have shown the importance of hemodynamic factors in the deposition of immunoglobulins in the mesangium and on the production of mesangial matrix [86]. In diabetic rats with 2 kidney, 1 clip hypertension, mesangial IgG, IgM, C3, and matrix were increased in the kidney subjected to high blood pressure and decreased in the kidney with the clip on its renal artery compared with normal rat kidneys. Infusion of angiotensin II has a comparable effect on the deposition of ferritin in the mesangium [116].

The idea of the importance of *class of immunoglobulin* in causing a mesangial proliferative lesion was tested by Border and Cohen [18], who immunized rabbits with either heat-denatured DNA or ultraviolet-irradiated DNA. Since the former of these antigens gives rise to an IgM antibody response and the second to IgG antibody, it was possible to compare the ability of the two antibodies to mediate a histologic reaction. It was found that both antigens produced diffuse mesangial hypercellularity, deposition of either IgG or IgM accompanied by C3, and the appearance of electron-dense deposits in the mesangium. Although the immunoglobulin class did not influence the development of the lesions, the experiment did show that DNA could produce a diffuse mesangial hypercellularity.

While the models described have been mainly concerned with circulating immune complexes, studies have been performed to examine the effects of circulating antibody on fixed antigens. Mauer et al. [87] injected aggregated human IgG intravenously into rabbits, and 10 hours later, at which time the aggregates were shown to be localized within the mesangium, removed one kidney and transplanted it into a normal rabbit. Injection of antibody to aggregated human IgG into the transplanted rabbit resulted in a prompt fall in serum complement with a reaction in the mesangium consisting of cellular proliferation and an increase in mesangial matrix. The resultant picture was one of a diffuse or localized mesangial proliferation with localized areas of glomerular sclerosis. The significance of these studies is that antigen present in the mesangium is accessible to, and capable of reacting with, circulating antibody to produce a form of glomerular injury. In this way, glomerulonephritis could develop without need of circulating complexes.

In summary, immune complexes in the mesangium have been shown to be associated with mesangial proliferation. Some are carried there in soluble form, but local formation has been demonstrated. In the case of circulating complexes, various factors determine their mesangial localization; these include size, hemodynamic conditions, and possibly changes in capillary wall permeability. *Electrostatic charge* is another possible factor, and cationic antigens have been shown not only to localize in the mesangium in greater amounts, but also to persist longer than their neutral counterparts [27]. The subject of immune complexes in the mesangium is well discussed by Couser et al. [30].

Factors responsible for mesangial cell proliferation have been explored outside the framework of immune-complex formation. For example, in a discussion of this matter, Kurokawa et al. [71] described the effect on mesangial cell growth in vitro of various growth-promoting peptides. Cell growth was shown to be stimulated by insulin, insulin-like growth factor I, and epidermal growth factor. The role of macrophages (now known to be common participants in many forms of glomerulonephritis) in causing stimulation of mesangial cell growth has been studied on several occasions. In one of these studies, interleukin I (a product of macrophages), in conjunction with platelet factors, was shown to enhance mesangial cell proliferation in vitro [80]. In another study, macrophage supernatatants stimulated the proliferation of mesangial cells; this was related in part to enhancement of endogenous mesangial cell PGE products [81]. The stimulating effect of macrophage products was prevented by pretreatment of mesangial cells with indomethacin, and exogenous PGE_2 was found to stimulate mesangial cell proliferation. While macrophages may play a role in causing mesangial cell proliferation in certain forms of glomerulonephritis, their apparent absence in the milder cases of mesangial proliferative glomerulonephritis suggests that other mechanisms for mesangial cell increase are at work.

All the work quoted so far relates to the production of a picture comparable with mesangial proliferative glomerulonephritis, but Germuth and Rodriguez [42,43] extended the concept of mesangial immune injury to focal glomerulonephritis. They used the term *mesangiopathic glomerulonephritis* for the situation in which there is primary deposition of immune complexes in the mesangium that provokes a proliferation of mesangial cells and matrix. Using their observations on the rabbit subjected to daily injections of moderate amounts of bovine serum albumin (12.5 mg), they proposed that as long as the immune deposits are confined to the mesangium, damage to the capillary loops will be prevented. If, however, the complexes are laid down so rapidly that their mass exceeds the capacity of the mesangium to accommodate them, some will in addition accumulate in the capillary wall and produce a local (segmental) proliferative or necrotizing lesion. They used the term *focal mesangiopathic glomerulonephritis* for this occurrence. As mentioned earlier, it is now clear that the immunofluorescence pattern in many—indeed most—forms of focal glomerulonephritis in man is diffuse throughout the mesangial regions; these include SLE, Schönlein-Henoch syndrome, bacterial endocarditis, and IgA nephritis. Further, these conditions may in certain patients be manifest as mesangial proliferative glomerulonephritis. The similarity to the experimental observations of Germuth and Rodriguez is apparent; that is, there is a basic lesion of mesangial involvement, which in some patients may be the sole lesion, but which in others has the localized or segmental proliferative component superadded. Mesangial proliferation is often inapparent by light microscopy—although immunoglobulins and complement are demonstrable—and the segmental lesion superimposed on this constitutes what all would recognize as focal and segmental glomerulonephritis. When a segmental proliferative or segmental necrotizing lesion is present in a kidney with clearly recognizable increased numbers of cells in the mesangium, the diagnosis of focal and segmental glomerulonephritis is difficult to sustain because, by definition, the glomeruli without the segmental lesions should be normal by light microscopy. Such cases are probably best referred to as *mesangial proliferative glomerulonephritis with segmental accentuation,* but doubtless many of them have been and still are labeled as focal and segmental glomerulonephritis. Fig. 4-2, from a patient with SLE, is an example of this. Only an occasional glomerulus showed the localized or segmental areas of cellular increase as demonstrated in this picture, the others showing no apparent change or mild increase in mesangial hypercellularity, as seen in the main part of this glomerulus. I originally diagnosed this case as focal glomerulonephritis.

While many cases of focal glomerulonephritis in man can be explained in this way, there are others that cannot. It will be noted in the next section that certain patients may show a focal and segmental glomerulonephritis in the absence of immunoglobulins and complement and that in others a patchy, nondescript immunohistologic pattern is identified. Severe injury to mesangial cells by Habu snake venom [21] or anti-thymocyte antiserum (mesangial cells have a thymocyte-like antigen on their surfaces) [62,130] leads to lesions of focal mesangial proliferative glomerulonephritis. Although heterologous IgG and rat C3 were found at an early stage in the mesangium of rats treated with anti-thymocyte antiserum, they disappeared rapidly and were not apparent by the time the cellular proliferation occurred. Whether selective mesangial cell necrosis can be a forerunner of these cases of focal glomerulonephritis without immune deposits in man is speculative.

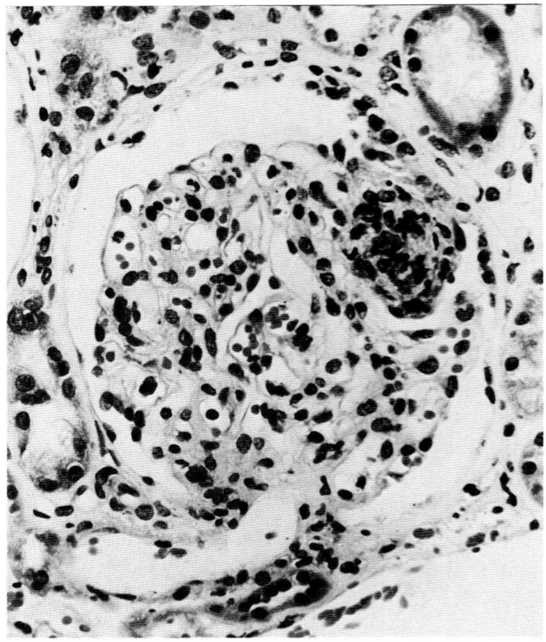

FIG. 4-2. *Glomerulus from 44-year-old woman with SLE to show localized (segmental) area of cellular increase and mild increase in mesangial cellularity in remaining lobules. Other glomeruli were normal or showed mild diffuse mesangial hypercellularity. Only a small number showed the segmental accentuation seen here. H&E; ×320.*

FOCAL GLOMERULONEPHRITIS

Focal glomerulonephritis may occur as part of various systemic diseases or as a primary form of glomerulonephritis. Table 4-2 gives a listing of these and the places in the book where they are discussed. Those conditions not described elsewhere are considered here.

Different Types

BEHÇET'S SYNDROME

Focal glomerulonephritis has been described in the occasional patient with this syndrome [39,67]. I have seen only one example, and this was in consultation with Dr. R. Singh.

PRIMARY FOCAL PROLIFERATIVE GLOMERULONEPHRITIS WITH MESANGIAL C3 ALONE OR COMBINED WITH IGG OR IGM

Although IgA nephritis—in which IgA is the predominant mesangial immunoglobulin—has emerged as a definite entity, certain patients are encountered in whom a focal form of glomerulonephritis is attended either by mesangial deposits of C3 alone [97], IgG and C3 together [43,92], or

Table 4-2. *Focal glomerulonephritis*

Accompanying systemic diseases:	
1. Systemic lupus erythematosus	Chapter 13
2. Infective endocarditis	Chapter 5
3. Schönlein-Henoch syndrome	Chapter 6
4. Anti-GBM antibody disease	Chapter 10
5. Polyarteritis and Wegener's syndrome	Chapter 16
6. Relapsing polychondritis	Chapter 16
7. Behçet's syndrome	This chapter
Primary forms of glomerulonephritis:	
1. IgA nephritis	Chapter 6
2. Focal proliferative glomerulonephritis with mesangial C3 alone or combined with IgG or IgM	This chapter
3. Focal proliferative glomerulonephritis with no immune deposits	This chapter
4. Focal segmental necrotizing glomerulonephritis	This chapter and Chapter 9

a combination of IgM and C3 [92,123] in the absence of IgA. The histologic picture is invariably of a focal proliferative type. These various patterns in which IgA is lacking are rare in focal glomerulonephritis, although, as will be seen later, IgM either by itself or in combination with C3 or other immunoglobulins occurs sufficiently often in patients with mesangial proliferative glomerulonephritis to warrant the name *IgM nephritis.*

PRIMARY FOCAL PROLIFERATIVE GLOMERULONEPHRITIS WITHOUT DEMONSTRABLE IMMUNOGLOBULINS

In several accounts of primary focal glomerulonephritis, appreciable numbers of cases have been recorded in which no immunoglobulins could be demonstrated in the glomeruli [70,92,123,129]. In three series with a histologic diagnosis of focal and segmental proliferative glomerulonephritis, no immunoglobulins were demonstrable in 10 of 21 cases [70], 10 of 26 [92], and 5 of 10 [129]. The pathogenesis of the segmental hypercellularity is not apparent in this group.

FOCAL SEGMENTAL NECROTIZING GLOMERULONEPHRITIS

This form may be found as part of a generalized vasculitis (polyarteritis or Wegener's syndrome), as the renal lesion of anti-GBM antibody disease, or as primary glomerulonephritis. The first two are discussed in Chapters 16 and 10, respectively, and no further mention will be made of them here.

Since necrotizing glomerulonephritis of all types is commonly accompanied by crescent formation, its primary form is traditionally described under primary or idiopathic crescentic glomerulonephritis, as it is in this book (Chap. 9). As a result, its identity is often submerged, as was pointed out in a recent review [38]. This brief section is included here mainly to establish that it is a definite entity.

Focal necrotizing glomerulonephritis is characterized by segmental areas of necrosis of the glomerular tuft in only a certain number of glomeruli (Fig. 4-3). It is therefore a focal segmental form of glomerulonephritis. In some instances only a few glomeruli are involved, but in others considerable numbers may be damaged. The areas of necrosis are sometimes accompanied by a reaction on the part of endocapillary cells, but this is usually overshadowed by the formation of crescents, which consist of proliferating epithelial cells from Bowman's capsule and infiltrating mononuclear cells (Figs. 4-4 and 4-5). Variable numbers of glomeruli show partial or total sclerosis. Although fibrin-fibrinogen can be demonstrated in the damaged parts of the glomerular tuft and in the crescents, immunoglobulins are either absent or scanty with no recognized pattern [38, 128,129a]. For this reason, the resultant picture is included under group 3 primary crescentic glomerulonephritis (see Chap. 9).

The overall spectrum of focal necrotizing glomerulonephritis has been discussed several times over the past few years [38,100,128,129a], and in all of these reports the primary form accounted for a substantial proportion of cases. The prognosis in the primary form is generally regarded as poor, and in one series, 78 percent of patients developed chronic renal failure [128]. In other series, the outlook was not so bleak; in one of them describing eight patients with this diagnosis, only two were on dialysis at follow-up, one had a very high

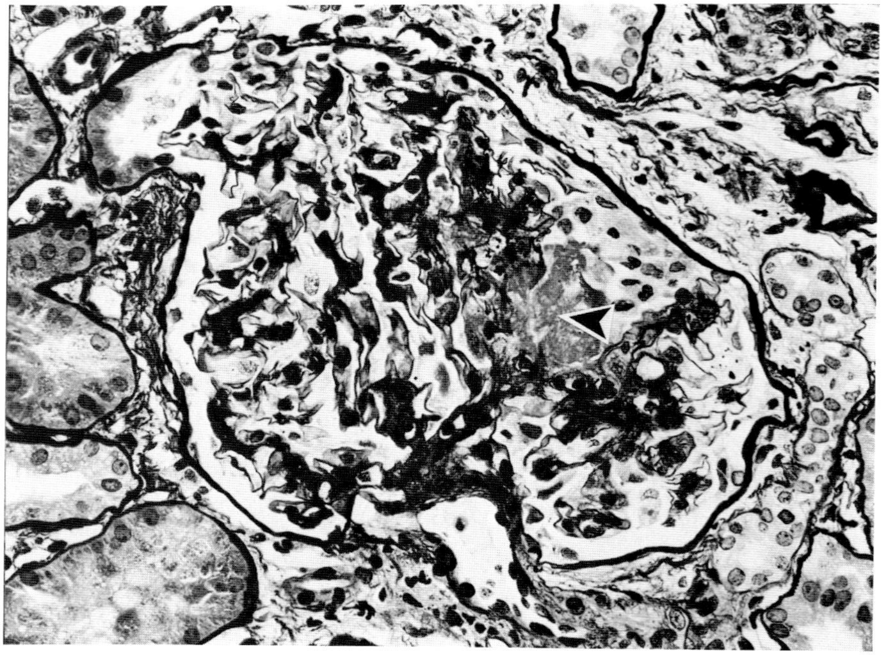

FIG. 4-3. *Glomerulus from biopsy with focal necrotizing glomerulonephritis of primary type. Arrowhead shows fibrin in capsular space in relation to disruption of capillary walls. Early crescent formation can be seen adjacent to lesion. Periodic acid–silver methenamine;* ×325.

serum creatinine level, another had a modest elevation, and four had normal levels [38]. Even better was the prognosis in the Mayo Clinic series [129a] of 170 patients with focal segmental glomerulonephritis (108 of the primary form and 62 as a feature of vasculitis); 61 percent were alive after 5 years. Overall, 22 patients developed end-stage renal failure. There was no significant difference in prognosis between the group with primary glomerulonephritis and those with vasculitis. The difference in outlook from one series to another is probably a reflection of the range of severity of glomerular involvement that exists in this condition.

Clinical Features of Focal Glomerulonephritis

The clinical features are varied, even when conditions such as SLE, Schönlein-Henoch syndrome, polyarteritis, and anti-GBM antibody disease are excluded. No further reference will be made here to the clinical features of these syndromes, for they are adequately treated in their respective chapters. This short account deals mainly with the primary proliferative form; further details of IgA nephritis are provided in Chapter 6, and of the primary necrotizing form in Chapter 9.

Hematuria is the main clinical manifestation, and it may be gross and readily noticed by the patient. In other instances it is only detected when the urinary sediment is examined. Microscopic hematuria tends to be persistent and may be found in the periods between recurrent attacks of gross hematuria; one of the features of the gross form is that it tends to be recurrent. The syndrome of recurrent hematuria will be described in detail in the section entitled Recurrent Hematuria.

Proteinuria is more variable; it may be absent,

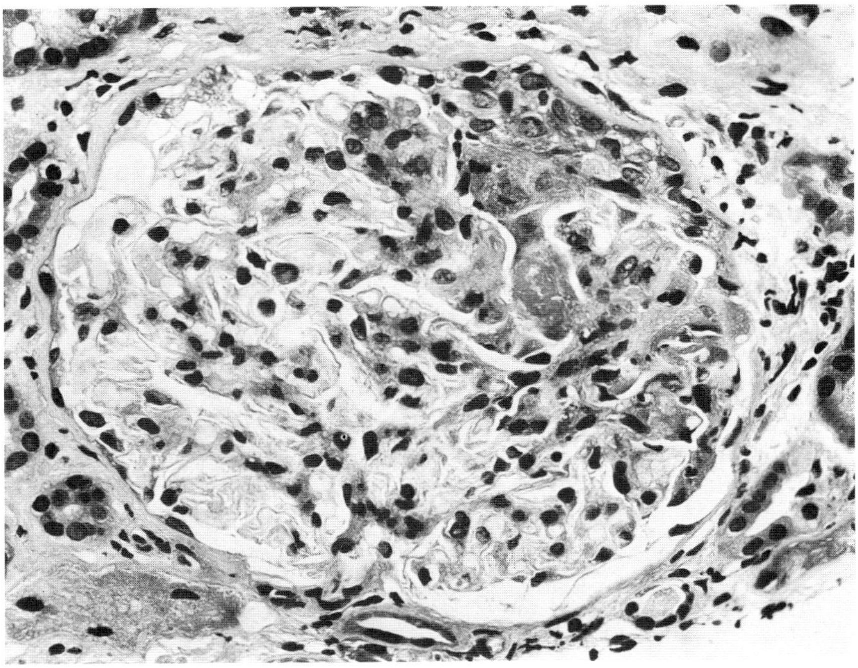

Fig. 4-4. *Glomerulus from same biopsy as Fig. 4-3 to show segmental lesion with localized cellular proliferation that appears to be in both the tuft and in relation to Bowman's capsule. The main part of the glomerulus appears normal. H&E; ×500.*

slight, moderate, or heavy. It is commonly absent in those with hematuria, giving rise to the old term *isolated hematuria,* and only rarely is it sufficiently great to give rise to the nephrotic syndrome. It is highly likely that cases of the nephrotic syndrome formerly claimed to be caused by focal glomerulonephritis were in fact examples of focal segmental glomerular sclerosis and hyalinosis, which is described in Chapter 12.

The outlook has generally been regarded as favorable, but increasingly it is becoming appreciated that renal failure and hypertension occur not infrequently in IgA nephritis, which is the most common form of primary focal glomerulonephritis. The prognosis clearly depends on the type of primary focal glomerulonephritis being considered, and the necrotizing form has a more ominous outlook than those with focal proliferative changes.

Pathologic Features of Focal Glomerulonephritis

It is important to realize that focal glomerulonephritis is a pathologic diagnosis, and although it may occur as part of a number of systemic diseases or as a primary glomerular disease, the histologic picture by light microscopy is remarkably similar in all of them. The following account concerns the primary forms, and descriptions of those attending systemic diseases are given in the appropriate places.

The single most important feature is the way in which, by light microscopy, only a certain number of glomeruli are affected, with the rest showing no abnormality (Fig. 4-6). The numbers affected vary from case to case, and as few as one in five or six may be affected in a biopsy specimen. Within an affected glomerulus, the change is often confined

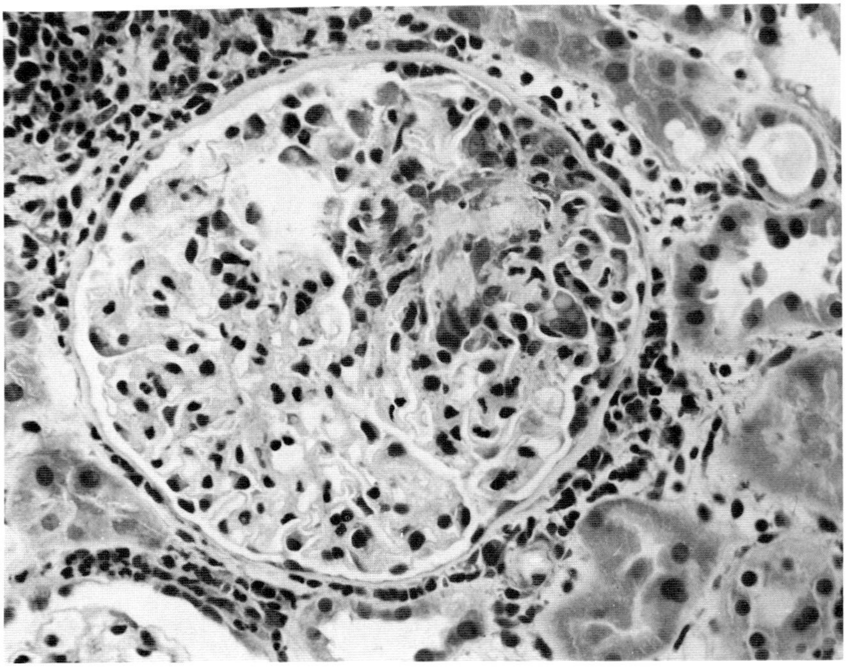

FIG. 4-5. *The glomerulus shows a segmental lesion with features similar to those in Fig. 4-4. This is from a biopsy showing focal segmental necrotizing glomerulonephritis in a patient with polyarteritis nodosa. H&E; ×340.*

to one or two lobules; this localized type of change is very characteristic and is usually referred to as *segmental.* The lesion is therefore focal and segmental. In many cases, the segmental lesion consists of increased numbers of cells, most of them probably being mesangial cells (Fig. 4-7). *Focal segmental proliferative glomerulonephritis* is the term applied to this group. In contrast is the focal segmental necrotizing type, which was described earlier. In this form, necrotizing changes are found instead of a cellular increase (Figs. 4-3 and 4-8), although there may be some proliferation of endocapillary cells, presumably as a reaction to injury. Crescent formation often accompanies those cases with necrotizing lesions, and when appreciable numbers of glomeruli are so affected, the appellation *crescentic glomerulonephritis* is used.

Segmental areas of solidification are often seen, and these may show adherence to Bowman's capsule (Fig. 4-9). These solidified areas are usually present in the longer-standing cases, and there is reason for considering them to be previously damaged areas. In our original study [54] we found that whereas an initial biopsy would sometimes show a predominance of the proliferative or necrotizing type of lesion, the reverse was true in repeat biopsies, with the solidified type of lesion being the most common. The solidified areas may be indistinguishable from the changes in focal segmental glomerular sclerosis, and this is a considerable source of confusion [129]. The capsular space may contain red blood cells.

Tubules in many cases show no striking changes, but in others there are localized areas of atrophy that become more extensive when glomerular changes are more profound. Blood vessels show no remarkable change in most cases, but arteriolar thickening and intimal increase in small arteries

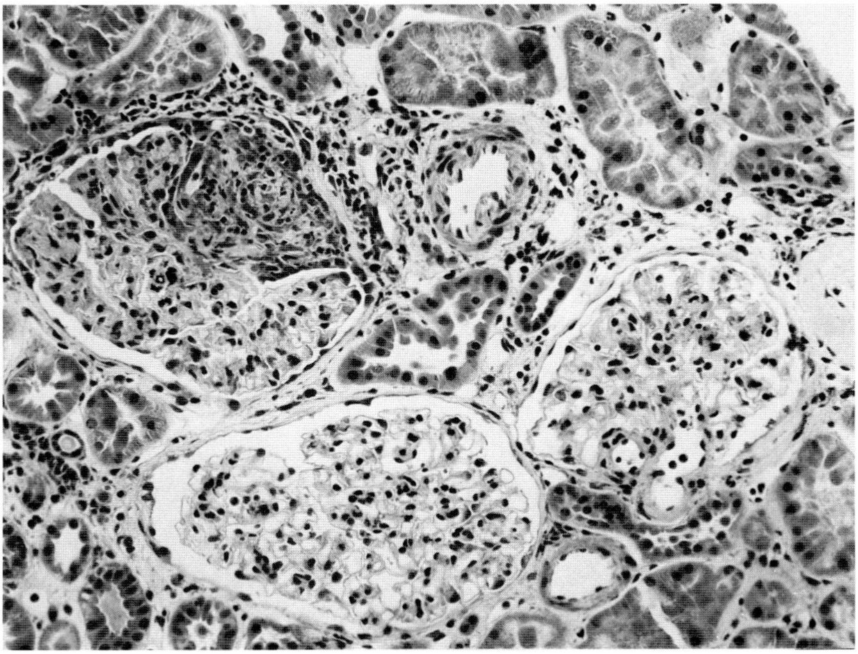

FIG. 4-6. *Three glomeruli from a biopsy of focal necrotizing glomerulonephritis. The two lower glomeruli appear normal, but the other shows a segmental area of cellular increase in continuity with Bowman's capsule. H&E; ×185.*

can be seen in some. The interstitial tissue shows no abnormality in mild cases, but lymphocytes and plasma cells may be present in those with more extensive damage. In this situation, there is also increased fibrosis.

IMMUNOFLUORESCENCE FINDINGS

As described earlier, one of the most interesting points to have emerged in the evolution of our concepts of focal glomerulonephritis is the demonstration of immunoglobulins and complement in the mesangial regions of all glomeruli in biopsies judged by light microscopy to have focal glomerulonephritis. This is so in SLE, Schönlein-Henoch syndrome, infective endocarditis, and several of the forms of primary glomerulonephritis, of which IgA nephritis is the best recognized and most common. In anti-GBM antibody disease there is a universal linear fluorescence for IgG and C3 along glomerular capillary walls, even though the histologic manifestation may be of a focal and segmental type. These findings are summarized in Table 4-1.

Confining ourselves to primary forms, IgA nephritis is characterized by the diffuse mesangial deposition of IgA in various combinations with C3, IgG, and, to a lesser extent, IgM in all glomeruli. In some cases there may be extension of the deposits for short distances along the adjacent capillary loops. A more extensive discussion of the various immunohistologic features of IgA nephritis is provided in Chapter 6.

More rarely, primary focal segmental proliferative glomerulonephritis shows a mesangial distribution of IgG and C3 [43,92] or of IgM and C3 [92,123] without IgA. In others there may be a

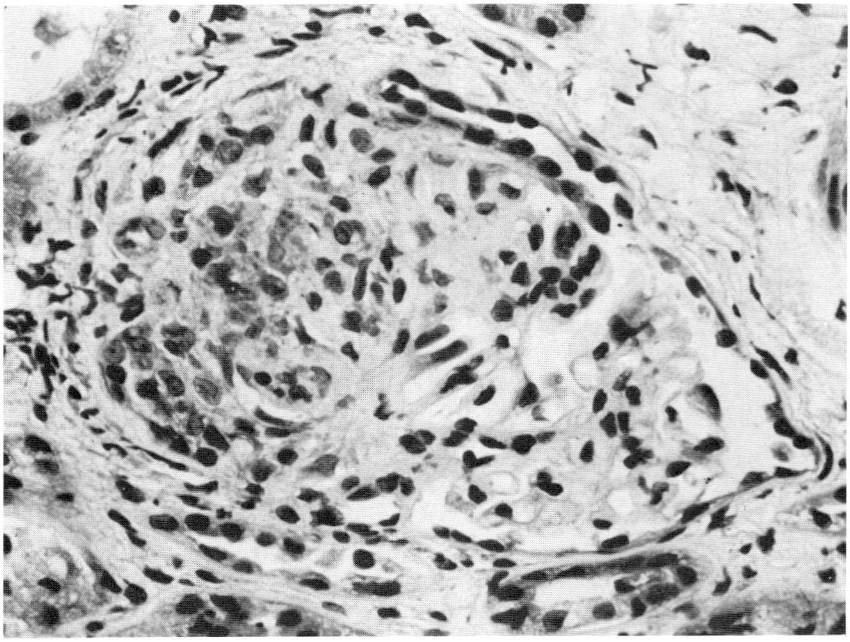

FIG. 4-7. *Glomerulus to show the localized lesion usually encountered in focal glomerulonephritis. The portion of the tuft to the left shows increased cellularity with some breaking up of nuclei, whereas the right side is spared. The majority of glomeruli in this case were normal. H&E; ×450.*

focal and local deposition of immunoglobulins [91].

An appreciable number of cases of focal segmental proliferative glomerulonephritis completely lack deposition of immunoglobulins and C3 [70,92,123,129]. The same absence of immunoglobulins or their presence in small amounts with no regular pattern of distribution is seen in focal segmental necrotizing glomerulonephritis [38, 128,129a].

ELECTRON MICROSCOPIC FINDINGS

In those cases in which there is widespread distribution of immune deposits, electron-dense deposits are commonly seen in a predominantly mesangial distribution. In general they are absent from those cases with the necrotizing forms.

MESANGIAL PROLIFERATIVE GLOMERULONEPHRITIS

Mesangial proliferative glomerulonephritis was defined and the various problems relating to its name and identity were briefly discussed earlier in the section entitled Focal Glomerulonephritis and Mesangial Proliferative Glomerulonephritis. As pointed out, I intend to be liberal in interpreting its content, fully aware of the pitfalls attending this approach. Like focal glomerulonephritis, it is found either as a manifestation of certain systemic diseases or as primary glomerulonephritis in its own right. Primary mesangial proliferative glomerulonephritis is a far from homogeneous entity, and a tentative breakdown is given in Table 4-3. This table also lists the various systemic diseases and gives the location in the book of those conditions not discussed below.

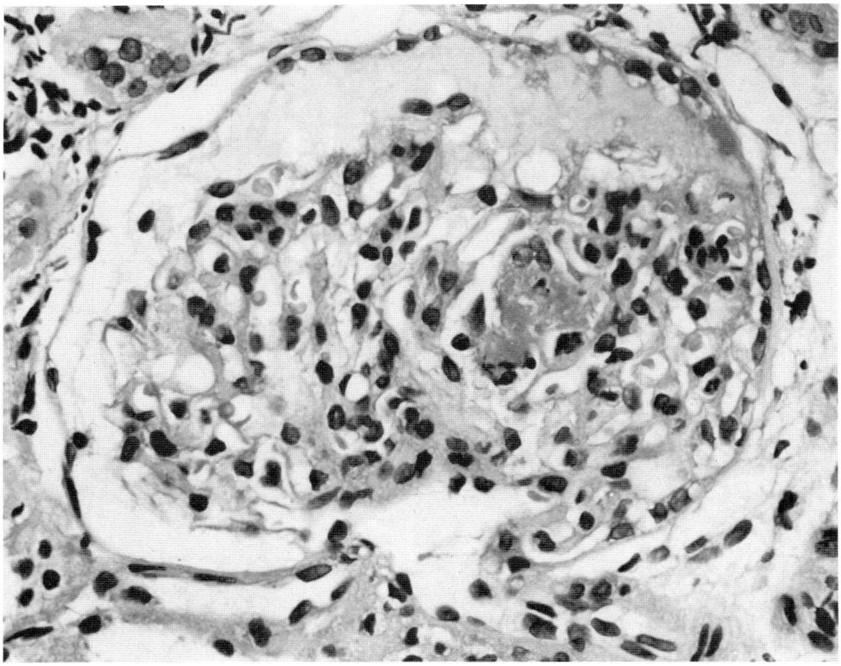

Fig. 4-8. *Glomerulus from patient with syndrome of recurrent hematuria. There is a localized or segmental area of necrosis to right of center. H&E; ×450. (From Heptinstall, R. H. In P. Kincaid-Smith, T. H. Mathew, and E. L. Becker (Eds.),* Glomerulonephritis: Morphology, Natural History and Treatment. *New York: Wiley, 1973. Used by permission.)*

Different Types

RETINITIS PIGMENTOSA

Two patients with retinitis pigmentosa were described who showed a mesangial proliferative glomerulonephritis on renal biopsy [66]. One had IgA deposition in the mesangium, making the diagnosis of IgA nephritis highly likely. No immunohistologic studies were carried out in the other, although electron microscopy was performed. The results were not stated, but the comment that the diagnosis of mesangial proliferative glomerulonephritis was supported by electron microscopy would suggest the presence of mesangial deposits. The authors felt that the relation of the glomerulonephritis to the retinitis pigmentosa was more than a chance association. If this is so, it is remarkable that more cases have not been uncovered.

RESOLVING POSTINFECTIOUS GLOMERULONEPHRITIS

Postinfectious glomerulonephritis, typically the poststreptococcal type, resolves in such a way that the excessive numbers of cells in the mesangium are the last to disappear. The resultant picture is that of mesangial proliferative glomerulonephritis (Fig. 4-10). This may be accompanied by IgG and C3 in a mesangial pattern as well as by mesangial electron-dense deposits [25]. Resolving postinfectious glomerulonephritis is therefore in every way a mesangial proliferative glomerulonephritis.

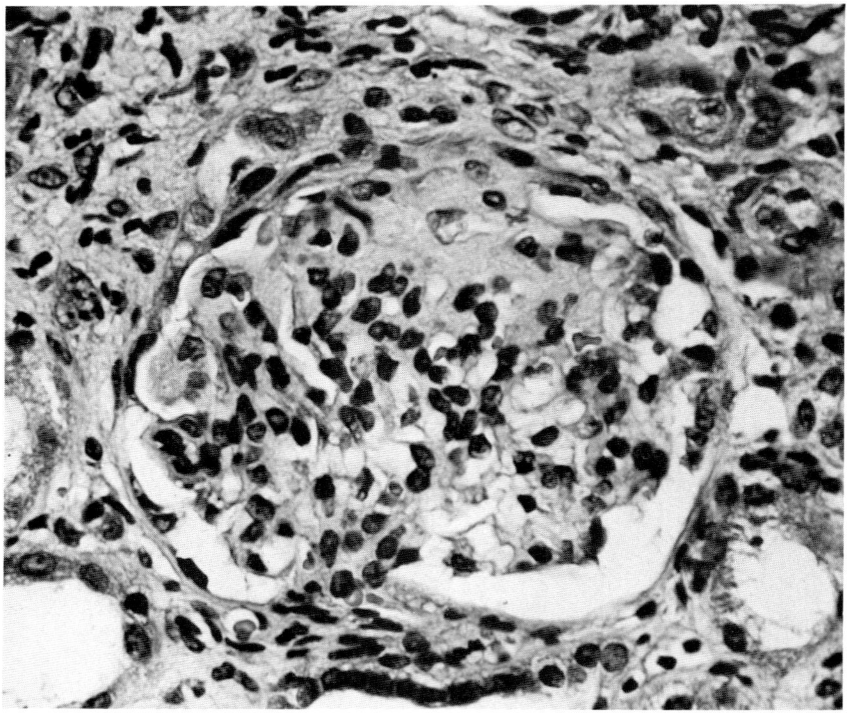

FIG. 4-9. *Glomerulus showing older solidified area at periphery of glomerulus (top), with adherence to Bowman's capsule, from a case of focal glomerulonephritis. H&E; ×500.*

IGM NEPHRITIS (IGM NEPHROPATHY)

What is referred to as *IgM nephritis* or *IgM nephropathy* was described almost simultaneously by Cohen et al. [26] and Bhasin et al. [13], although van de Putte et al. [123] had earlier called attention to the frequent presence of mesangial IgM in patients with recurrent or persistent hematuria. Despite the fact that certain of the latter authors' cases also had IgA present, some at least showed only IgM coupled with C3 and C1q. The patients of Cohen et al. and Bhasin et al. were mainly children and young adults with the nephrotic syndrome, sometimes complicated by hematuria. There was an increase in mesangial cellularity—usually mild to moderate—and the changes affected all glomeruli, each of which was involved to a more or less equal degree (Fig. 4-11). IgM, with or without C3, was present in the mesangium, usually in a

TABLE 4-3. *Mesangial proliferative glomerulonephritis*

Accompanying systemic diseases:	
1. Systemic lupus erythematosus	Chapter 13
2. Infective endocarditis	Chapter 5
3. Schönlein-Henoch syndrome	Chapter 6
4. Mixed connective tissue disease	Chapter 13
5. Retinitis pigmentosa	This section
Primary forms of glomerulonephritis:	
1. Resolving postinfectious glomerulonephritis	Chapter 5 and this section
2. IgA nephritis	Chapter 6
3. IgM nephritis	Chapter 12 and this section
4. With C3 alone or with C3 and IgG	This section
5. With no immunoglobulins or C3	This section

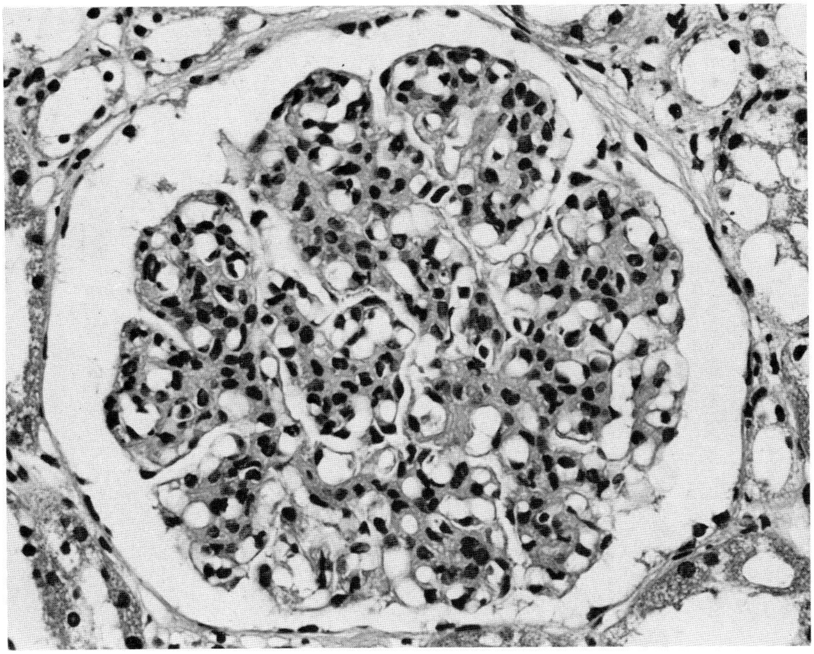

FIG. 4-10. *Glomerulus from a 23-year-old woman with resolving acute glomerulonephritis but with persistent hypercellularity in the mesangium. The capillaries are widely patent. H&E;* ×*350.*

diffuse pattern, and sometimes along capillary walls. Electron-dense deposits were recorded in the mesangium in some but not all cases; they were present in 2 of 11 cases in one series [26] and in 4 of 11 in the other [13]. Whether it is a distinct clinicopathologic entity has aroused considerable controversy, but for purposes of convenience, I have chosen to regard it as a form of mesangial proliferative glomerulonephritis.

Most of the cases described have been associated with the nephrotic syndrome or with persistent proteinuria [17,22,52,57,69,73,75,90,115, 118,124,127]. In many of these cases there is only a mild increase in the number of cells in the mesangium, and rather than use mesangial proliferative glomerulonephritis, some authors have opted for such noncommittal terms as *diffuse mesangial proliferation* [127] or *diffuse mesangial hypercellularity* [115].

IgM nephropathy also may be associated with recurrent attacks of gross hematuria or with persistent microscopic hematuria [52,56,58,69,90,99, 123,124]. In these cases, proteinuria is either absent or only mild. It is becoming increasingly apparent that IgM nephropathy makes a significant contribution to the considerable group of patients with recurrent hematuria. It is somewhat paradoxical that the same histologic and immunohistologic picture can on the one hand be associated with proteinuria of such severity as to cause the nephrotic syndrome, yet on the other be found along with hematuria and no proteinuria.

The immunohistologic picture in the various papers quoted earlier and in two others dealing purely with the immunohistology of mesangial proliferative glomerulonephritis [40,73] is one of mesangial IgM alone; IgM and C3 (Fig. 4-12); IgM, IgG, and C3; or IgM, IgA, and C3. IgM is

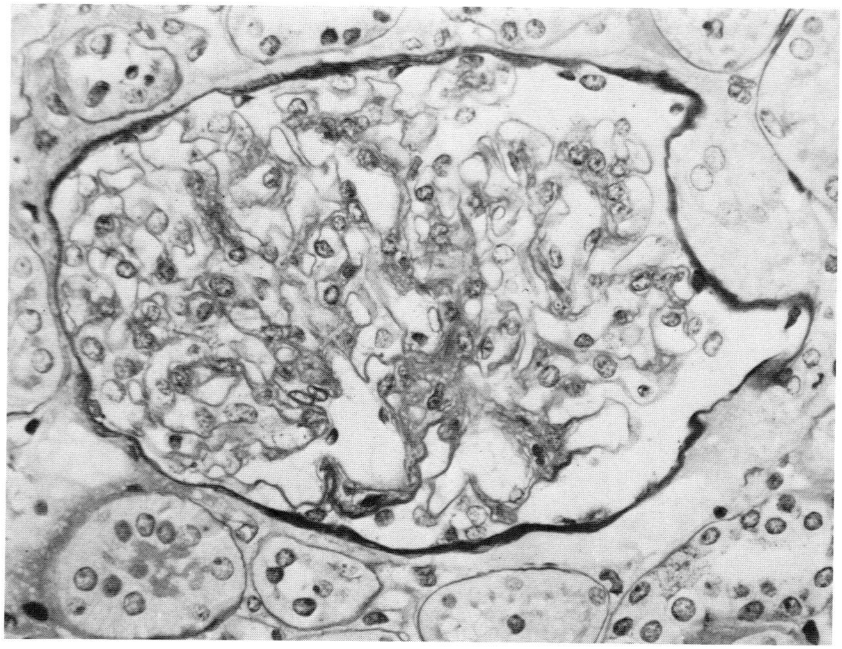

FIG. 4-11. *Glomerulus showing modest increase in cells in mesangium. From patient with nephrotic syndrome accompanied by IgM and C3 deposits in mesangium. PAS; ×400. (Prepared from slide supplied by Dr. Arthur Cohen.)*

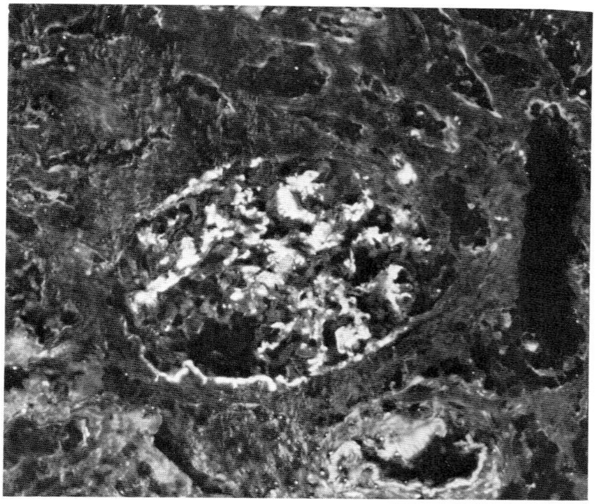

FIG. 4-12. *Immunofluorescence micrograph to show mesangial deposition of IgM from the same case as in Fig. 4-11. (Courtesy of Dr. Wayne Border.)*

predominant whenever several immunoglobulins are present. Electron-dense deposits in the mesangium are sometimes reported but appear to be absent in many patients. In this respect, the picture is unlike that of IgA nephritis, in which electron-dense deposits are almost invariably present.

The paper by Hughson et al. [58] on Zuni Indians (Pueblo Indians living in the village of Zuni) is of great interest. Despite the very high prevalence of IgA nephritis and Schönlein-Henoch syndrome among Pueblo Indians [113], it was found that among 14 Zuni Indians with mesangial hypercellularity and asymptomatic microscopic hematuria, 3 had mesangial IgM by itself and 4 had IgM with only segmental IgA. The others had predominant IgA, yet IgM was present in all. There is considerable inbreeding in this population, and many of the relatives had hematuria. Several of the patients also had thin basement membrane disease (described later), which in many instances is a hereditary condition attended clinically by hematuria. The significance of the large numbers of patients with IgM among the Zuni Indians is not clear.

MESANGIAL PROLIFERATIVE GLOMERULONEPHRITIS WITH MESANGIAL C3 ALONE OR WITH C3 AND IgG

A diffuse granular deposition of C3 in the mesangium without immunoglobulins has been recorded in association with mesangial proliferative glomerulonephritis [73] and in what was described as mesangial cellular proliferation and an increase in mesangial matrix [49]. A comparable pattern was referred to on page 270 under Focal Glomerulonephritis [97]. In all patients there was either gross or microscopic hematuria and a good prognosis, despite the fact that microscopic hematuria commonly persisted.

In other cases of mesangial proliferative glomerulonephritis, a combination of IgG and C3 without other immunoglobulins may be seen in a mesangial pattern [40,43,48,70]. There have been no claims that this represents a unique clinicopathologic entity, and it is recorded here merely to show that it is a distinct immunohistologic pattern. An example will be illustrated later (Fig. 4-13) in the section headed Pathologic Features.

MESANGIAL PROLIFERATIVE GLOMERULONEPHRITIS WITH ABSENCE OF IMMUNOGLOBULINS AND COMPLEMENT

As was the case with focal glomerulonephritis, a completely negative immunohistologic picture is also commonly found in mesangial proliferative glomerulonephritis or diffuse mesangial hypercellularity [16,93,110,115,127]. In the enormous series of Bohle et al. [16], 204 of 603 patients (34 percent) with mesangial proliferative glomerulonephritis had negative immunohistologic findings when all grades of the condition were considered. The proportion of biopsies with negative findings was higher in those with minimal proliferative changes, but even in those with moderate and severe mesangial hypercellularity, 24 of 154 patients (16 percent) were negative. The clinical features were varied; some were predominantly proteinuric, but others had hematuria as the main feature. The mean age for the whole group was 31 years. Sinniah [110] studied biopsies in 39 patients with mesangial proliferative glomerulonephritis (262 patients with IgA nephritis were considered separately), and of these, no fewer than 33 (85 percent) had negative immunofluorescence findings. The clinical presentations were variable and included recurrent microscopic and gross hematuria, proteinuria and nephrotic syndrome, microscopic hematuria as part of "postacute" glomerulonephritis, and chronic renal failure. All nine patients in another study had recurrent hematuria [95]. On biopsy they were shown to have either slight proliferative glomerulonephritis or normal biopsies by light microscopy, but no complement or immunoglobulins by immunofluorescence were reported in the mesangium.

In three series consisting of children with the nephrotic syndrome in which the glomeruli showed diffuse mesangial hypercellularity, negative immunohistologic findings were recorded in 55 percent [127], 64 percent [115], and 100 percent [93] of cases.

These various findings would suggest that appre-

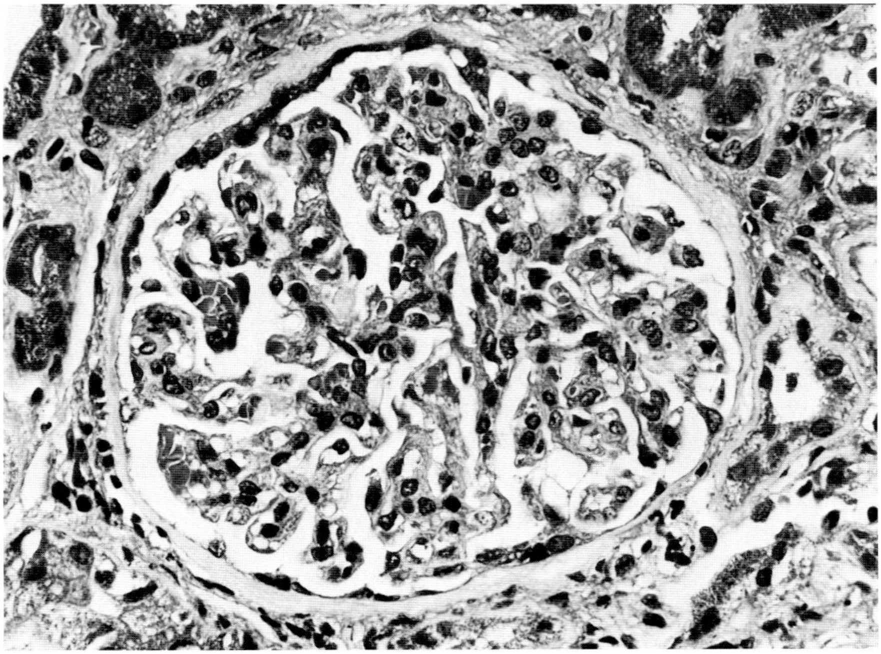

FIG. 4-13. *Glomerulus with mesangial hypercellularity from 36-year-old woman with nephrotic syndrome. Immunofluorescence microscopy of this biopsy revealed mesangial IgG and C3. Trichrome stain;* ×450.

ciable numbers of cases of what are variously labeled mesangial proliferative glomerulonephritis or diffuse mesangial hypercellularity lack an immunologic pathogenesis of the types commonly encountered in glomerulonephritis. The reason for the cellular increase is not apparent. It should be noted that clinical pictures represented by severe proteinuria on the one hand and isolated hematuria on the other can occur with this pathologic picture.

Clinical Features

Because the term is so all-embracing, many different clinical features are encountered; these are described in the appropriate chapters in the case of those accompanying systemic diseases, IgA nephritis, and IgM nephropathy.

The rest show various degrees of proteinuria, often severe enough to cause a nephrotic syndrome, and are frequently accompanied by microhematuria. Other cases present with recurrent attacks of gross hematuria or have microscopic hematuria found on routine examination. Those with hematuria may have no proteinuria—so-called isolated hematuria—but others may pass appreciable amounts of protein in the urine.

Pathologic Features

The basic change is one of an increase in mesangial cellularity (Fig. 4-13), and this may be accompanied by an increase in mesangial matrix and a widening of the mesangial areas (Fig. 4-14). According to the WHO committee [24], there should be four or more cells per mesangial area, and all or

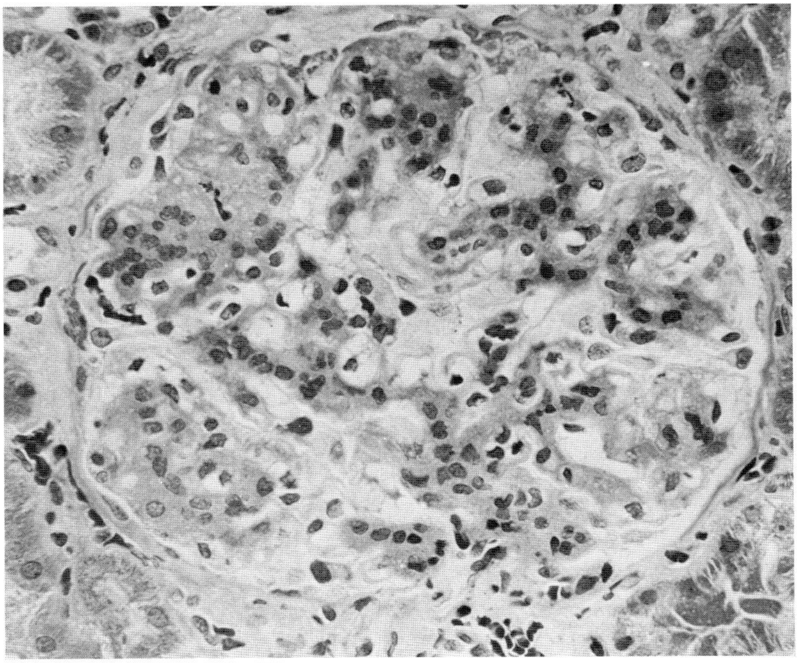

Fig. 4-14. *Glomerulus from patient with mesangial proliferative variant of IgA nephritis. There is increased cellularity and mild increase in mesangial matrix. Trichrome stain;* ×390. *(Courtesy of Dr. T. Ideura.)*

nearly all (over 80 percent) of the glomeruli should be involved. The increased cellularity within a given glomerulus is more or less uniform. There is a wide range of glomerular hypercellularity from one case to another, but most show only minor increases (see Fig. 4-1), as was clear from the large series of Bohle et al. [16]. In this group of 603 patients, the mesangial hypercellularity was graded from minimal to severe with two intermediate grades. Three-fourths fell into the two minor grades, and in only 3 percent was it regarded as severe. There are no significant changes in the glomerular capillary walls. Although crescents may be present in IgA nephritis and were seen in large numbers in one of our cases of IgM nephropathy (nephritis), they are not a significant feature of the other primary glomerular forms. Tubular and interstitial changes are absent or trivial.

IMMUNOFLUORESCENCE AND ELECTRON MICROSCOPIC FINDINGS

As was mentioned earlier, many different patterns of immunoglobulins, complement, and fibrin-fibrinogen are encountered; they will not be repeated. Figure 4-15 reveals the predominantly mesangial location of IgA in a case of IgA nephritis. Electron microscopy reveals electron-dense mesangial deposits in IgA nephritis, but even though they may be seen in other forms, they are inconstant.

RECURRENT HEMATURIA

At various points in this chapter we have made reference to patients who had recurrent attacks of gross hematuria or who had persistent microscopic hematuria. These patients are usually either children or young adults, with in most instances a predominance of males. The attacks are often precipitated by upper respiratory tract infections, and hematuria occurs at the height of the infection or a day or so later. The relatively long latent interval seen with poststreptococcal glomerulonephritis is lacking. Other factors such as exercise, inoculation with vaccines, and surgical or dental procedures also may precipitate attacks. Microscopic hematuria often persists between the attacks of overt hematuria, and in many patients, persistent microscopic hematuria may occur without gross attacks. Proteinuria is absent or minor in most patients.

It has become abundantly clear that no single disease accounts for this clinical picture, and the gradual recognition of the various entities responsible is reminiscent of the way in which the nephrotic syndrome was broken down into its various constituent parts. The renal biopsy was responsible for identifying focal glomerulonephritis as an important cause [54,103], and Joekes et al. [64] demonstrated that diffuse glomerular proliferative changes could occur just as often, thus providing evidence for the role of mesangial proliferative glomerulonephritis.

These findings were confirmed on many occasions [15,23,35,46,47,72,89,102,104,109,122], and with the introduction of immunofluorescence techniques, the entity of IgA nephritis was established [10,11] and appreciated to be a potent cause of recurrent or persistent hematuria [31,70,89, 111,123].

It also was realized that genetic influences were at work in a certain group of patients with recurrent or persistent hematuria [5,84,88,102]. These patients were found to have an excellent prognosis in contrast to those with Alport's syndrome, with its sinister outlook. With the application of electron microscopic techniques to renal biopsies, the concept of thin basement membrane disease was conceived in this group, to which such names as *benign familial hematuria* [84] and *benign recurrent hematuria* [5] had been applied.

These and other pioneering efforts have brought us to recognize a sizable list of causes of recurrent or persistent hematuria, and those which are primary renal diseases—as opposed to renal manifestations of systemic disease—are given in Table 4-4.

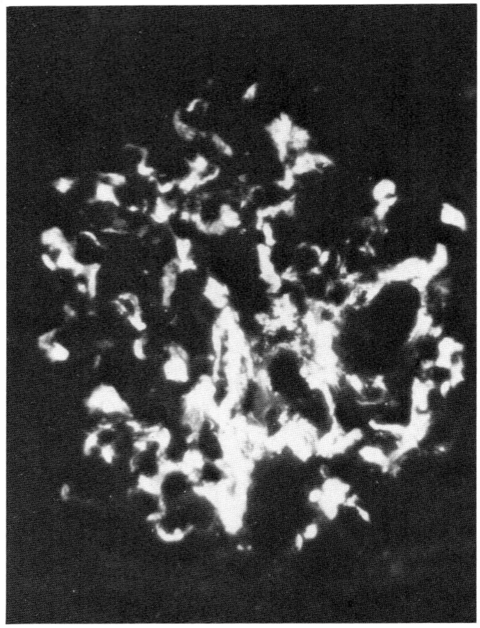

FIG. 4-15. *Immunofluorescence of glomerulus with widespread mesangial distribution of IgA. (Prepared from transparency supplied by Dr. L. Morel-Maroger.)*

Mesangial C3 Deposition

Under both focal, and mesangial proliferative glomerulonephritis it was recorded that hematuria may occur in patients whose biopsies show diffuse mesangial C3 deposition [49,97]. In some of these authors' cases, the glomeruli with mesangial C3 were normal by light microscopy or showed only trivial changes. Further, it was found that of the 43 biopsies subjected to electron microscopy in the two studies combined, only 1 showed glomerular basement membrane thinning. This is important because, as we shall see, basement membrane thinning is a common accompaniment and a likely cause of hematuria. In contrast is the experience

TABLE 4-4. *Primary renal causes of recurrent or persistent hematuria*

1. IgA nephritis	Chapter 6
2. IgM nephritis	This chapter (pp. 278–281)
3. Focal glomerulonephritis	This chapter (pp. 270–276)
4. Mesangial proliferative glomerulonephritis	This chapter (pp. 276–283)
5. Mesangial C3 deposition	This section
6. Thin basement membrane disease, including benign familial hematuria	This section
7. Alport's syndrome (hereditary nephritis)	Chapter 30
8. Loin pain–hematuria syndrome	This section
9. Kidneys apparently normal by light, immunohistologic, and electron microscopy	This section
10. Forniceal hemorrhage	This section

of Tiebosch et al. [119], who observed eight patients with a clinical picture of either recurrent gross hematuria or persistent microhematuria, whose biopsies had normal-appearing glomeruli by light microscopy but with diffuse mesangial C3 demonstrable by immunohistologic techniques. Despite the normal appearance by light microscopy, seven of the biopsies revealed thin glomerular capillary basement membranes by electron microscopy, thus providing an explanation for the leakage of blood into the urine. While the mechanism for hematuria in cases with diffuse deposition of C3 is not clear, it certainly can occur in the absence of thin glomerular basement membranes [49,97]. It is, however, important to exclude this condition when a given case is being investigated.

Thin Basement Membrane Disease

GENERAL FEATURES

Recurrent hematuria or permanent microhematuria in children has long been known to occur in a familial form [5,84,88]. The use of such terms as *benign recurrent hematuria* [5] and *benign familial hematuria* [84] symbolizes the good prognosis Stigmata of Alport's syndrome with its usual grim outlook are lacking in these cases. Renal biopsies revealed that the glomeruli were normal or showed only insignificant abnormalities by light microscopy, and when immunofluorescence techniques were employed [84], the results were negative. A further family with persistent microscopic hematuria was described by Rogers et al. [102], in which 8 of 34 members in four generations were affected. The important observation made in this study was that despite the lack of significant glomerular abnormalities by light or immunofluorescence microscopy, there was thinning of the glomerular capillary basement membrane by electron microscopy. As with one of the other series quoted [88] and a more recent report [85], the mode of inheritance was regarded as autosomal dominant. The presence of thin glomerular capillary basement membranes in patients with benign familial hematuria was rapidly confirmed by Hill et al. [55], who described it in four patients (children and adults). They also pointed out that in contrast to several other conditions in which irregular attenuation of the capillary wall could occur, the thinning was extreme and involved long stretches of capillary loops in the benign familial form. Further confirmation has been provided on numerous occasions in both children [28,120,121,126,131–133] and adults [1,28,29,32,119,133]. From these various writings it is clear that basement membrane thinning is a very common accompaniment of benign familial forms of hematuria. For convenience, these studies will be discussed under the headings of Children and Adults.

Children

The condition is common among children with asymptomatic hematuria, and this was clearly shown in a group of 76 pediatric patients (3 to 19 years old) with isolated hematuria persisting for more than 6 months [121]. Of the 43 patients with abnormal renal biopsies, 17 had thin glomerular capillary basement membranes as the sole abnormality. To put this into perspective, it should be noted that this was twice the number with IgA nephritis (8). A family history was established in five of the patients, but as in all series dealing with thin basement membranes, this figure is likely to be conservative. Because it has such a good prognosis, affected members of a pedigree cannot be identified simply by obtaining a history of renal disease or death from renal failure, as in Alport's syndrome. Instead, proof of hematuria in individual relatives is necessary, and this is a big undertaking. Tina et al. [120] addressed this matter in 19 children (aged 1 to 14 years) with asymptomatic hematuria. Ten children from nine families were considered to have benign familial hematuria by virtue of a history of hematuria in their siblings, parents, or grandparents; the other nine were from families without hematuria and were designated as having idiopathic recurrent hematuria. Apart from rare obsolescent glomeruli in a minority of biopsies in both groups and weakly staining mesangial deposits of IgM and C3 in one case from the second group, there were no glomerular abnormalities either by light or electron microscopy. Ultrastructural measurements of the width of the glomerular capillary basement membranes revealed the mean thickness to be significantly less in the familial group, and this was even more convincing when measurements of the lamina densa were used. The study is of importance for several reasons. First, it establishes an identifiable lesion in benign familial hematuria; second, it demonstrates that certain forms of recurrent or persistent hematuria need have no identifiable lesion; and third, it calls into question the existence of thin basement membranes in children lacking a family history.

In addition to the paper quoted earlier [121], a Japanese study [131] also claimed to have seen thin basement membranes with hematuria in a nonfamilial group of patients. In an electron microscopic study of renal biopsies from 218 children, thin glomerular capillary basement membranes were found in 23. Three of these were from patients with Alport's syndrome—which, as is discussed in Chapter 31, may show this change—and 20 were from children with persistent microscopic hematuria in the absence of proteinuria. Hematuria was found in family members of 10 of the children, putting these children in the category of benign familial hematuria with thin basement membranes, but the other 10 were alleged to have no family involvement. It is not clear how diligent the authors were in searching for familial involvement.

It is also apparent that not all patients with benign familial hematuria exhibit thinning of basement membranes. In the Japanese study just quoted [131], 21 of 31 patients with this condition had no thinning. Also, in a series of five children from the United Kingdom [132], thinning was absent in two, and in a single family (two children and two adults) from Germany with persistent microscopic hematuria and no progression of the disease [126], renal biopsy disclosed no attenuation of the basement membranes.

Adults

One of the early studies on the ultrastructure of benign familial hematuria in adults was published only in abstract form [29], but one of the authors (Dr. M. M. Schwartz) has kindly provided me with further details. Twelve of 58 patients being evaluated for asymptomatic hematuria without significant proteinuria were found to have family members with hematuria. Seven of the 12 were biopsied, and all had thin glomerular capillary basement membranes; 6 were adults and the seventh was a 14-year-old boy. The study is important not only for providing further evidence for thin glomerular basement membranes in benign familial hematuria, but also for demonstrating that it is a significant cause of hematuria in an adult population.

Later studies in adults have shown a significant familial component in recurrent or persistent hematuria [1,28,133] and have confirmed the presence of thin basement membranes in this group. Strong family histories of hematuria in patients with thin basement membranes were obtained in 8 of 12 [28], 5 of 7 [133], and 4 of 8 biopsies [1] in the absence of Alport's syndrome. As was the case in children, an appreciable number of adult cases with thin basement membranes have been reported in the apparent absence of familial involvement. A Dutch study [119] consisting of 80 patients—26 with recurrent macroscopic hematuria and 54 with persistent microscopic hematuria—specifically excluded patients with hereditary forms of renal disease. Biopsy revealed that 27 had

IgA nephritis, 11 had various abnormalities such as membranoproliferative glomerulonephritis, and the remaining 42 were normal by light microscopy. Ultrastructural measurements of glomerular basement membranes were made in these last 42; thin glomerular basement membranes were noted in 18, and the width was normal in 24. Thus, of the total group of 80, thin glomerular basement membrane disease accounted for 23 percent compared with IgA nephritis, which was responsible for 34 percent. When the analysis was restricted to the 54 patients with persistent microscopic hematuria, thin basement membrane disease and IgA nephritis occurred equally; there were 17 cases (31 percent) of each. The group with recurrent macroscopic hematuria (26 patients) contained only 1 example of thin basement membrane disease (4 percent) compared with 10 of IgA nephritis (38 percent).

The adult patients described by Dische et al. [32] differ somewhat from those in most other series. Whereas the patients in most series have hematuria alone or small amounts of protein in the urine, their series contained 8 of 14 patients with moderate to heavy proteinuria, 1 of them passing 9 g in 24 hours. Hypertension and renal failure were also present in several patients. Despite this, thin basement membranes were encountered in all 14 patients. The findings in this series indicate that the condition is not a uniform entity.

CLINICAL FINDINGS

Both sexes are evenly involved in thin basement membrane disease, and as noted earlier, it may occur in children and adults. It is seldom reported after the age of 50 years, and mean ages of 35 [32], 35 [119], and 40 years [1] were recorded in three series. Many cases are familial but lack extrarenal manifestations such as are found in Alport's syndrome. Nonfamilial cases have been described, but as discussed earlier, rigorous attempts to test family members are not always evident.

Hematuria is usually microscopic and persistent, although in some cases it is macroscopic and recurrent with persistence of red cells in the urine between the attacks. Recurrent attacks of gross hematuria have been noted to decrease with increasing age [133]. Red cell casts are common [29]. Proteinuria is either absent or slight in most cases, although in several series a small number of patients have significant amounts [1,28,119]; as noted earlier, one series had moderate to heavy proteinuria in over half the patients [32]. Blood pressure and serum creatinine levels are almost invariably normal and tend to remain so, although in one series hypertension and renal failure were recorded [32]. The overall prognosis is excellent [1,29,131,132], although microscopic hematuria commonly persists [119,131,133].

PATHOLOGIC FINDINGS

Light Microscopy

In most accounts, the glomeruli are normal, except for occasional ones showing total sclerosis as part of an aging phenomenon. Clearly, this is greater in adult biopsies. Slight increases in mesangial matrix or mesangial cells have been described [28,131] but are probably of little moment. Small foci of tubular atrophy may be found [55,120,131], and hemosiderin has been noted in the cytoplasm of tubular epithelium; this is clearly related to the hematuria [55]. The only series in which significant glomerular sclerosis and tubular atrophy have been described is the one referred to earlier in which severe proteinuria, hypertension, and renal failure were noted clinically [32].

Immunofluorescence Microscopy

In general, the glomerular staining is negative for all immunoglobulins, complement, and fibrinogen. Occasional biopsies have shown patchy mesangial deposition of IgM [28]; IgG, IgM, IgA, and C3 [131]; or C3 [55,132]. These are probably of little consequence, but the finding of diffuse granular mesangial deposition of C3 without immunoglobulins in 7 of 18 adult cases of thin basement membrane disease [119] should be noted.

Electron Microscopy

Extensive and severe thinning of the glomerular basement membrane is a universal finding (Fig. 4-16). It is to be distinguished from the localized areas of thinning found in a variety of conditions, such as diffuse types of glomerulonephritis and fo-

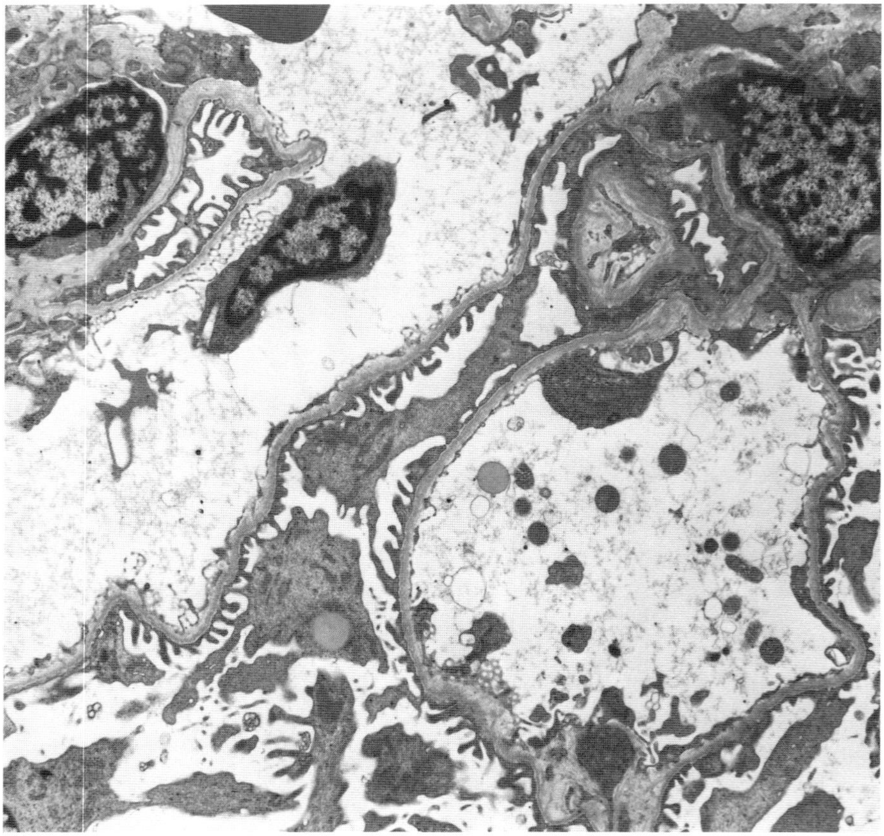

FIG. 4-16. *Electron micrograph from 18-year-old man with thin basement membrane disease. There is widespread thinning of the GBM, and multiple measurements revealed a mean width of 176 nm with a range of 146 to 220 nm.* ×5100. *(Prepared by Dr. Jean Olson.)*

cal segmental glomerulosclerosis [55]. The characteristic lamellar or basket-weave thickening seen in Alport's syndrome is completely lacking, and the nearest approach to this is the occasional report of splitting of the basement membrane, which may occur over short lengths of capillary walls [32,55,133]. It should be recorded that thinning of the basement membrane may occur in Alport's syndrome and may be extensive. More will be said of this in Chapter 30. Other ultrastructural changes described in thin basement membrane disease are localized stretches of foot-process effacement [1,32,131,132], in some cases accompanied by foot-process loss, leaving small bare areas on the epithelial side of the basement membrane.

Many morphometric studies have now been carried out to more accurately identify and document thinning of the basement membrane. The width of the basement membrane is judged as the distance between the outer aspect of an endothelial cell and the inner aspect of a visceral epithelial cell, and measurements are made on peripheral parts of the capillary loops. Some observers also measure the width of the lamina densa and consider this more meaningful [120,121]. Numbers of measurements made and the numbers of glomeruli studied vary from one observer to another. In various representative childhood series, basement membrane widths have been 225 to 241 [132], 211 to 267 [131], and 207.1 ± 11.89 nm [120]. When control values were quoted, they were 303 ± 16.9 nm (children with idiopathic recurrent hematuria) [120] and over 300 nm (minimal-change nephrotic syndrome) [131]. In adults, measurements in thin glomerular basement membrane disease were 153 to 213 [1], 191 ± 28 [119], 206 to 301 [32], and 235 to 327 nm [28]. When control widths were provided, they were 350 ± 43 nm (normal renal tissue) [119], 356 to 464 nm (IgA nephritis) [32], and 356 to 432 nm (nonhematuric biopsies) [28]. In an extended discussion of morphometric aspects, Tiebosch et al. [119] considered that 264 nm is an appropriate cutoff point in judging thinness in adults when a limited amount of tissue (one glomerulus) is available for study.

SUMMARY

Benign familial hematuria has been shown in certain cases to be accompanied by thin glomerular basement membranes, although this is not a universal finding [126,131,132]. It occurs equally in both sexes and may be encountered in children and adults. Although microscopic hematuria is persistent, there is very little evidence of progression to renal failure or the development of hypertension. It is differentiated from Alport's syndrome by a lack of extrarenal manifestations such as neurosensory deafness, absence of the characteristic lamellar (basket-weave) thickening of glomerular basement membranes, and failure to progress to chronic renal failure. In the few cases in which tests were performed to demonstrate the so-called Goodpasture antigen in basement membranes (it is lacking in many cases of Alport's syndrome), the results indicated it was present in benign familial hematuria [68,105,124a]. Further studies are necessary to define benign familial hematuria and its relation to Alport's syndrome, because cases have been identified in which family members have hearing loss [85], and because glomerular basement membrane thinning may be the predominant change in some patients with Alport's syndrome [51].

Thin glomerular basement membrane disease also has been described in patients with no apparent evidence of familial hematuria. While the prognosis is generally excellent, one series [32] revealed progressive decline in renal function, hypertension, and heavy proteinuria, suggesting that it is not a homogeneous entity.

Loin Pain–Hematuria Syndrome

Little et al. [76] described a syndrome in three young women in whom attacks of severe loin pain occurred over many years, accompanied by gross hematuria and fever. The pain was felt on one or both sides, and although pyelograms and cystoscopy revealed no abnormalities, renal arteriograms showed focal disorganization of peripheral renal arteries with relatively avascular areas of renal parenchyma. The patients were demanding, exaggerated their symptoms, and had been seen by a variety of specialists. Renal biopsy showed interstitial fibrosis, varying degrees of glomerular capsular fibrosis, and intimal thickening of small blood vessels. There was no abnormality of renal function.

Subsequent reports have confirmed most of the features originally described and have added others [2,9,12,14,19,20,37,59,106]. It appears that patients may have pain and gross hematuria, pain and microscopic hematuria, or loin pain only; hypertension is not a feature [2]. Females predominate, but the idea that the condition is restricted to women is no longer valid [2,14,106]. In the largest series to date [2], there were 48 women and 3 men; their ages ranged from 16 to 50 years.

In order to elucidate the syndrome, renal angiography and histologic study of kidney tissue have been performed. Angiography has revealed focal or widespread tortuosity, beading, stenosis, or occlusion of interlobar, arcuate, and interlobular arteries [2,19], but other studies have shown no organic vascular changes [12,14,59,107]. Spasm of intrarenal arteries has been reported [12].

Renal tissue has been obtained by renal biopsy or nephrectomy. Renal biopsies have shown glomeruli that were normal [9,112] or had mild mesangial hypercellularity [20,59,107]. The only report of positive immunofluorescence in glomeruli was one describing a finely granular pattern of C3 along capillary walls, small amounts of fibrin-fibrinogen, and IgA on occasional capillary walls in a minority of cases; IgA was absent from the mesangium in all biopsies [94]. Intimal thickening of small blood vessels has been recorded [2,107], and an almost constant feature has been the presence of C3 in arterioles [2,9,59,94,106,112]. When three nephrectomy specimens were examined, "atherosclerotic" changes were reported in large arteries down to arcuate size [37]. Interlobular arteries showed occlusive lesions, and the cortex contained areas of infarction or tubular loss and interstitial fibrosis. These vascular lesions presumably correspond to those seen in renal angiographic studies. In another nephrectomy specimen [14], intimal hyalin plaques and medial hypertrophy were reported in some of the arcuate arteries. In addition, this kidney showed what was described as segmental glomerulonephritis in a few glomeruli and interstitial nephritis.

Never having seen material from a case of loin pain–hematuria syndrome, I am in a poor position to comment on these findings. When arteriographic and histologic features are considered together, the significant changes appear to be those in the arteries and could well represent the result of intravascular thrombosis. Some of the patients have been on oral contraceptive agents [2,37], and in one report [2] several patients lost both their pain and hematuria when these agents were discontinued. The idea of platelet activation and fibrin formation has received support [65,107], and factor XII deficiency has been reported [112]. The frequent demonstration of C3 in arterioles should not evoke too much enthusiasm, since it is a common finding in many other conditions. The significance of an exaggerated type 3 hypersensitivity response to a variety of agents—particularly tuberculin [9]—is not apparent.

A follow-up of 43 patients for periods of 2 to 17 years (mean 5.3 years) revealed the following [2]: In 16 the symptoms abated spontaneously (mean time of 3.5 years); in 5 the pain and hematuria cleared when oral contraceptives were discontinued; in 2 there was relief following pregnancy; 1 became symptom-free after hysterectomy and bilateral oophorectomy; 2 obtained relief by taking sulfinpyrazone; but the remainder (almost half) still had problems.

The pain may be so debilitating that renal autotransplantation has been undertaken with the object of interrupting nerve fibers. This or the simple cutting of the renal nerves has been successful in some instances [14,106,107], although not in others [59]. In two cases the hematuria persisted despite relief of pain [106].

A group of patients that differs somewhat from those just described was recorded by MacDonald et al. [82]. It consisted of 36 males and 18 females who gave a history of a continuous ache in the region of both kidneys. Thirty-eight of them had gross hematuria, and 44 of the total group had an underlying focal and segmental glomerulonephritis on renal biopsy. Of the biopsies from these 44 patients, 15 were studied with immunofluorescence techniques and 7 were considered to be suffering from IgA nephritis. It also was noted that the vascular lesions seen on biopsy were out of proportion to the ages of the patients or to the levels of blood pressure. These patients differ from those mentioned earlier; first, the sex predominance is male rather than female; second, the quality of the pain is aching rather than severe; and third, the renal biopsy findings are mainly of focal and segmental glomerulonephritis, whereas this was not described in any for the previous series. Common to both is the severity of the vascular changes. Severe loin pain and hematuria have been recorded in isolated instances in both IgA and IgM nephritis [96], but its rarity in IgA nephritis is stressed in another paper [89].

In summary, loin pain–hematuria syndrome is a condition found mainly in women—often taking oral contraceptives—in whom severe bilateral or unilateral loin pain occurs with or without hematuria. There is often a psychogenic component, and the condition may be difficult to treat. The finding of narrowed intrarenal arteries by angiography or histology, coupled with some coagulation defects, has prompted the idea of intravascular thrombus formation. The evidence for this is incomplete, but if true, it might be asked why there are so few of the stigmata of thrombotic microangiopathy. The pain and the cause of the hematuria are largely unexplained.

Hematuria with Kidneys Apparently Normal by Light, Immunohistologic, and Electron Microscopy

In three series of *children* with recurrent gross hematuria or persistent microscopic hematuria [120, 121,133], a substantial number showed no abnormalities in the glomeruli when biopsies were examined by light, immunohistologic, and electron microscopy. The numbers falling into this category were 5 of 19 [120], 33 of 76 [121], and 8 of 19 [133]. In a series of 80 *adults* with hematuria, there were 24 with completely negative glomerular findings [119]. Thirteen had macroscopic and 11 had microscopic hematuria.

The reasons for the hematuria were not determined, but such causes as stone formation were excluded. Proteinuria was absent or slight in the great majority of cases, and the prognosis was excellent.

Hematuria from Forniceal Hemorrhage

An interesting but largely ignored cause of gross hematuria is that of forniceal hemorrhage. In this condition, the bleeding is unilateral and often of sufficient intensity to warrant removal of the kidney. When the excised kidney is examined, a direct communication between the lumen of the calyx and the veins of the renal sinus is revealed, and it is considered that the copious hematuria is caused by rupture of a vein [83,101]. Physical strain has sometimes preceded the episode of hematuria, but this is not invariable; the mechanism is not apparent. The papers on this topic were written before the present-day awareness of vesicoureteral reflux, and it is entirely likely that this could be the means by which the rupture occurs.

I have seen three cases that may provide the link between reflux and profuse hemorrhage, although certain important pieces of information are lacking [60,114]. These were all cases of gross unilateral hematuria in young people, in whom nephrectomy was performed to control the hemorrhage. In them, communications between renal tubules and intrarenal veins were present, with urine being found in the veins using Tamm-Horsfall protein as a marker and detecting it by fluorescent-antibody techniques. Considerable quantities of blood were found in the renal tubules, and mucosal hemorrhage was present in the pelvis and calyces. Although micturating cystograms were not performed, the tubulovenous communications are suggestive that reflux had taken place. It is tempting in retrospect to suggest that vesicoureteral reflux had caused communications between the calyx and renal veins with extensive bleeding into the pelvicalyceal system; the forces exerted by vesicoureteral reflux would thus cause blood to be propelled up the ducts of Bellini into the tubular system. As will be seen in Chapter 21, certain types of renal papillae permit calicotubular reflux, so the suggested sequence of events is entirely feasible.

Forniceal bleeding is mentioned because certain cases of hematuria cannot be explained by loss of blood across the glomeruli or by tumor or stone. Careful examination of the excised kidney—when the opportunity presents—is therefore essential to determine whether forniceal hemorrhage is present or not.

REFERENCES

1. Abe, S., Amagasaki, Y., Iyori, S., Konishi, K., Kato, E., Sakaguchi, H., and Shimoyama, K. Thin basement membrane syndrome in adults. *J. Clin. Pathol.* 40:318, 1987.
2. Aber, G. M., and Higgins, P. M. The natural history and management of the loin pain/haematuria syndrome. *Br. J. Urol.* 54:613, 1982.
3. Addis, T. *Glomerular Nephritis: Diagnosis and Treatment.* New York: Macmillan, 1949.
4. Alwall, N. Aspiration biopsy of the kidney: Including a report of a case of amyloidosis diagnosed through aspiration biopsy of the kidney in 1944 and investigated as an autopsy in 1950. *Acta Med. Scand.* 143:430, 1950.
5. Ayoub, E. M., and Vernier, R. L. Benign recurrent hematuria. *Am. J. Dis. Child.* 109:217, 1965.
6. Baehr, G. The significance of the embolic glo-

merular lesions of subacute streptococcus endocarditis. *Arch. Intern. Med.* 27:262, 1921.
7. Baehr, G. A benign and curable form of hemorrhagic nephritis. *JAMA* 86:1001, 1926.
8. Bates, R. C., Jennings, R. B., and Earle, D. P. Acute nephritis unrelated to group A hemolytic streptococcus infection: Report of 10 cases. *Am. J. Med.* 23:510, 1957.
9. Bell, G. M., Williams, P., and Thomson, D. Is the loin pain and haematuria syndrome a renal manifestation of hypersensitivity? *Lancet* 1:340, 1984.
10. Berger, J. IgA glomerular deposits in renal disease. *Transplant Proc.* 1:939, 1969.
11. Berger, J., and Hinglais, N. Les dépôts intercapillaires d'IgA-IgG. *J. Urol. Nephrol. (Paris)* 74:694, 1968.
12. Bergroth, V., Konttinen, Y. T., Nordström, D., and Laasonen, L. Loin pain and haematuria syndrome: Possible association with intrarenal arterial spasms. *Br. Med. J.* 294:1057, 1987.
13. Bhasin, H. K., Abuelo, J. G., Nayak, R., and Esparza, A. R. Mesangial proliferative glomerulonephritis. *Lab. Invest.* 39:21, 1978.
14. Bloom, P. B., Viner, E. D., Mazala, M., Jannetta, P. J., Stieber, A. C., and Simmons, R. L. Treatment of loin pain hematuria syndrome by renal autotransplantation. *Am. J. Med.* 87:228, 1989.
15. Bodian, M., Black, J. A., Kobayashi, N., Lake, B. D., and Shuler, S. E. Recurrent haematuria in childhood. *Q. J. Med.* 34:359, 1965.
16. Bohle, A., Gärtner, H.-V., Laberke, H.-G., and Krück, F. *Die Niere: Struktur und Funktion.* Stuttgart: Schattauer Verlag, 1984.
17. Border, W. A. Distinguishing minimal-change disease from mesangial disorders. *Kidney Int.* 34:419, 1988.
18. Border, W. A., and Cohen, A. H. Role of immunoglobulin class in mediation of experimental mesangial glomerulonephritis. *Clin. Immunol. Immunopathol.* 27:187, 1983.
19. Burden, R. P., Booth, L. J., Ockenden, B. G., Boyd, W. N., Higgins, P. M., and Aber, G. M. Intrarenal vascular changes in adult patients with recurrent haematuria and loin pain: A clinical, histological and angiographic study. *Q. J. Med.* 44:433, 1975.
20. Burden, R. P., Dathan, J. R., Etherington, M. D., Guyer, P. B., and MacIver, A. G. The loin-pain/haematuria syndrome. *Lancet* 1:897, 1979.
21. Cattell, V., and Bradfield, J. W. B. Focal mesangial proliferative glomerulonephritis in the rat caused by Habu snake venom: A morphologic study. *Am. J. Pathol.* 87:511, 1977.
22. Cavallo, T., and Johnson, M. P. Immunopathologic study of minimal change glomerular disease with mesangial IgM deposits. *Nephron* 27:281, 1981.
23. Chen, B. T. M., Ooi, B. S., Tan, K. K., and Khoo, O. T. Causes of recurrent haematuria. *Q. J. Med.* 41:141, 1972.
24. Churg, J., and Sobin, L. H. *Renal Disease: Classification and Atlas of Glomerular Diseases.* Tokyo: Igaku-Shoin, 1982.
25. Cohen, A. H., and Border, W. A. Mesangial proliferative glomerulonephritis. *Semin. Nephrol.* 2:228, 1982.
26. Cohen, A. H., Border, W. A., and Glassock, R. J. Nephrotic syndrome with glomerular mesangial IgM deposits. *Lab. Invest.* 38:610, 1978.
27. Cohen, S., Vernier, R. L., and Michael, A. F. The effect of charge on the renal distribution of ferritin. *Am. J. Pathol.* 110:170, 1983.
28. Coleman, M., Haynes, W. D. G., Dimopoulos, P., Barratt, L. J., and Jarvis, L. R. Glomerular basement membrane abnormalities associated with apparently idiopathic hematuria: Ultrastructural morphometric analysis. *Hum. Pathol.* 17:1022, 1986.
29. Cotton, J. R., Schwartz, M. M., Antonovych, T. T., and Hunsicker, L. G. Benign familial hematuria (BFH): Frequency and studies in 12 families (Abstract). *Kidney Int.* 8:408, 1975.
30. Couser, W. G., Adler, S., Baker, P. J., Johnson, R. J., and Perkinson, D. A. Mechanisms of Immune Complex Formation and Deposition in Glomeruli. In R. R. Robinson (Ed.), *Nephrology: Proceedings of the IXth International Congress of Nephrology.* New York: Springer-Verlag, 1984. P. 508.
31. D'Amico, G. The commonest glomerulonephritis in the World: IgA nephropathy. *Q. J. Med.* 64:709, 1987.
32. Dische, F. E., Weston, M. J., and Parsons, V. Abnormally thin glomerular basement membranes associated with hematuria, proteinuria or renal failure in adults. *Am. J. Nephrol.* 5:103, 1985.
33. Ellis, A. Natural history of Bright's disease: Clinical, histological and experimental observations. *Lancet* 1:1, 1942.
34. Fahr, T. Pathologische Anatomie des Morbus Brightii. In F. Henke, and O. Lubarsch (Eds.), *Handbuch der Speziellen Pathologischen Anatomie und Histologie,* Vol. 6, Part 1. Berlin: Springer, 1925. P. 156.
35. Ferris, T. F., Gorden, P., Kashgarian, M., and Epstein, F. H. Recurrent hematuria and focal nephritis. *N. Engl. J. Med.* 276:770, 1967.
36. Fishberg, A. M. *Hypertension and Nephritis,* 4th Ed. Philadelphia: Lea & Febiger, 1939.
37. Fletcher, P., Al-Khader, A. A., Parsons, V., and

Aber, G. M. The pathology of intrarenal vascular lesions associated with the loin-pain–haematuria syndrome. *Nephron* 24:150, 1979.
38. Furlong, T. J., Ibels, L. S., and Eckstein, R. P. The clinical spectrum of necrotizing glomerulonephritis. *Medicine* 66:192, 1987.
39. Gamble, C. N., Wiesner, K. B., Shapiro, R. F., and Boyer, W. J. The immune complex pathogenesis of glomerulonephritis and pulmonary vasculitis in Behçet's disease. *Am. J. Med.* 66:1031, 1979.
40. Gärtner, H. V., Wehner, H., and Bohle, A. The immunohistological findings in various forms of glomerulonephritis: A comparative investigation based on 335 renal biopsies. Part I: Endocapillary glomerulonephritis, mesangioproliferative glomerulonephritis, mesangioproliferative glomerulonephritis with focal crescents, minimal proliferating intercapillary glomerulonephritis (without nephrotic syndrome). *Pathol. Res. Pract.* 162:178, 1978.
41. Germuth, F. G., Jr., Kelemen, W. A., and Pollack, A. D. Immune complex disease: II. The role of circulatory dynamics and glomerular filtration in the development of experimental glomerulonephritis. *Johns Hopkins Med. J.* 120:252, 1967.
42. Germuth, F. G., Jr., and Rodriguez, E. *Immunopathology of the Renal Glomerulus: Immune Complex Deposit and Antibasement Membrane Disease.* Boston: Little, Brown, 1973.
43. Germuth, F. G., Jr., and Rodriguez, E. Focal mesangiopathic glomerulonephritis: Prevalence and pathogenesis. *Kidney Int.* 7:216, 1975.
44. Germuth, F. G., Jr., Rodriguez, E., Siddiqui, S. Y., Lorelle, C. A., McGee, S., Milano, L. L., and Wise O'L. Immune complex disease: VII. Experimental mesangiopathic glomerulonephritis produced by chronic immunization with thyroglobulin. *Lab. Invest.* 38:404, 1978.
45. Germuth, F. G., Jr., Valdes, A. J., Senterfit, L. B., and Pollack, A. D. A unique influence of cortisone on the transit of specific macromolecules across vascular walls in immune complex disease. *Johns Hopkins Med. J.* 122:137, 1968.
46. Gervais, M., and Drummond, K. N. L'hématurie récidivante chez l'enfant. *Union Med. Can.* 77: 406, 1970.
47. Glasgow, E. F., Moncrieff, M. W., and White, R. H. R. Symptomless haematuria in childhood. *Br. Med. J.* 2:687, 1970.
48. Glassock, R. J. Natural history and treatment of primary proliferative glomerulonephritis: A review. *Kidney Int.* 28(Suppl.17):S-136, 1985.
49. Grekas, D., Morley, A. R., Wilkinson, R., and Kerr, D. N. S. Isolated C3 deposition in patients without systemic disease. *Clin. Nephrol.* 21:270, 1984.
50. Habib, R., and Churg, J. Minimal Change Disease, Mesangial Proliferative Glomerulonephritis and Focal Sclerosis: Individual Entities or a Spectrum of Disease? In R. R. Robinson (Ed.) *Nephrology: Proceedings of the IXth International Congress of Nephrology.* New York: Springer-Verlag, 1984. P. 634.
51. Habib, R., Gubler, M.-C., Hinglais, N., Noël, L.-H., Droz, D., Levy, M., Mahieu, P., Foidart, J.-M., Perrin, D., Bois, E., and Grünfeld, J.-P. Alport's syndrome: Experience at Hôpital Necker. *Kidney Int.* 21(Suppl. 11):S-20, 1982.
52. Helin, H., Mustonen, J., Pasternack, A., and Antonen, J. IgM-associated glomerulonephritis. *Nephron* 31:11, 1982.
53. Heptinstall, R. H., and Joekes, A. M. Focal glomerulonephritis: A study based on renal biopsies. *Q. J. Med.* 28:329, 1959.
54. Heptinstall, R. H., and Joekes, A. M. Focal Glomerulonephritis. In G. E. W. Wolstenholme and M. P. Cameron (Eds.), *Ciba Foundation Symposium on Renal Biopsy.* Boston: Little, Brown, 1961. P. 194.
55. Hill, G. S., Jenis, E. H., and Goodloe, S., Jr. The nonspecificity of the ultrastructural alterations in hereditary nephritis: With additional observations on benign familial hematuria. *Lab Invest.* 31:516, 1974.
56. Hirszel, P., Yamase, H. T., Carney, W. R., Galen, M. A., Graeber, C. W., Johnson, K. J., Kennedy, T. L., Lapkin, R. A., McLean, R. H., Rosenworcel, E., and Rowett, D. A. Mesangial proliferative glomerulonephritis with IgM deposits: Clinicopathologic analysis and evidence for morphologic transitions. *Nephron* 38:100, 1984.
57. Hsu, H.-C., Chen, W.-Y., Lin, G.-J., Chen, L., Kao, S.-L., Huang, C.-C., and Lin, C.-Y. Clinical and immunopathologic study of mesangial IgM nephropathy: Report of 41 cases. *Histopathology* 8:435, 1984.
58. Hughson, M. D., Megill, D. M., Smith, S. M., Tung, K. S. K., Miller, G., and Hoy, W. E. Mesangiopathic glomerulonephritis in Zuni (New Mexico) Indians. *Arch. Pathol. Lab. Med.* 113: 148, 1989.
59. Hutchison, S. M. W., Doig, A., and Jenkins, A. McL. Recurrence of loin pain/haematuria syndrome after renal autotransplantation. *Lancet* 1:1501, 1987.
60. Iliff, W. J., and Galdabini, J. J. Massive intratubular hemorrhage with herniations into renal veins requiring nephrectomy. *J. Urol.* 108:44, 1972.
61. International Committee for Nomenclature and

Nosology of Renal Disease. *A Handbook of Kidney Nomenclature and Nosology: Criteria for Diagnosis Including Laboratory Procedures.* Boston: Little, Brown, 1975.

62. Ishizaki, M., Masuda, Y., Fukuda, Y., Sugisaki, Y., Yamanaka, N., and Masugi, Y. Experimental mesangioproliferative glomerulonephritis in rats induced by intravenous administration of antithymocyte serum. *Acta Pathol. Jpn.* 36:1191, 1986.
63. Iversen, P., and Brun, C. Aspiration biopsy of the kidney. *Am. J. Med.* 11:324, 1951.
64. Joekes, A. M., Pugh, R. C. B., and Pryor, J. S. Recurrent haematuria. *Br. J. Urol.* 34:463, 1962.
65. Jones, K., Naish, P. F., and Aber, G. M. Oestrogen-associated disease of the renal microcirculation. *Clin. Sci. Mol. Med.* 52:33, 1977.
66. Kalra, P. A., and Turney, J. H. Mesangioproliferative glomerulonephritis associated with retinitis pigmentosa. *Br. J. Ophthalmol.* 72:210, 1988.
67. Kansu, E., Deglin, S., Cantor, R. I., Burke, J. F., Jr., Cho, S. Y., and Cathart, R. T. The expanding spectrum of Behçet syndrome: A case with renal involvement. *JAMA* 237:1855, 1977.
68. Kashtan, C., Fish, A. J., Kleppel, M., Yoshioka, K., and Michael, A. F. Nephritogenic antigen determinants in epidermal and renal basement membranes of kindreds with Alport-type familial nephritis. *J. Clin. Invest.* 78:1035, 1986.
69. Kopolovic, J., Shvil, Y., Pomeranz, A., Ron, N., Rubinger, D., and Oren, R. IgM nephropathy: Morphological study related to clinical findings. *Am. J. Nephrol.* 7:275, 1987.
70. Kupor, L. R., Mullins, J. D., and McPhaul, J. J., Jr. Immunopathologic findings in idiopathic renal hematuria. *Arch. Intern. Med.* 135:1204, 1975.
71. Kurokawa, K., Okuda, T., Matsunaga, H., Chang, H., and Yamashita, N. Calcium-Activated Chloride Conductance in Mesangial Cells: Its Regulation by Vasoactive Peptides and Growth Promoting Factors. In A. M. Davison (Ed.), *Nephrology: Proceedings of the Xth International Congress of Nephrology.* London: Baillière Tindall, 1988. P. 541.
72. Labovitz, E. D., Steinmuller, S. R., Henderson, L. W., McCurdy, D. K., and Goldberg, M. "Benign" hematuria with focal glomerulitis in adults. *Ann. Intern. Med.* 77:723, 1972.
73. Larsen, S. Immune deposits in generalized mesangioproliferative glomerulonephritis: Fluorescent microscopy findings correlated to symptoms, clinical course and immunosuppressive therapy. *Acta Pathol. Microbiol. Scand.* [A] 86:543, 1978.
74. Lawler, W. Experimental mesangial proliferative glomerulopathy. *J. Pathol.* 133:107, 1981.
75. Lawler, W., Williams, G., Tarpey, P., and Mallick, N. P. IgM associated primary diffuse mesangial proliferative glomerulonephritis. *J. Clin. Pathol.* 33:1029, 1980.
76. Little, P. J., Sloper, J. S., and de Wardener, H. E. A syndrome of loin pain and haematuria associated with disease of peripheral renal arteries. *Q. J. Med.* 36:253, 1967.
77. Löhlein, M. Ueber hämorrhagische Nierenaffektionen bei chronischer ulzeröser Endokarditis (Embolische nichteiterige Herdnephritis). *Med. Klin.* 10:375, 1910.
78. Longcope, W. T. Studies of the variations in the antistreptolysin titer of the blood serum from patients with hemorrhagic nephritis: II. Observations on patients suffering from streptococcal infections, rheumatic fever and acute and chronic hemorrhagic nephritis. *J. Clin. Invest.* 15:277, 1936.
79. Longcope, W. T. Some observations on the course and outcome of hemorrhagic nephritis. *Trans. Am. Clin. Climatol. Assoc.* 53:153, 1937.
80. Lovett, D. H., Ryan, J. L., and Sterzel, R. B. Stimulation of rat mesangial cell proliferation by macrophage interleukin 1. *J. Immunol.* 131:2830, 1983.
81. MacCarthy, E. P., Hsu, A., Ooi, Y. M., and Ooi, B.S. Modulation of mouse mesangial cell proliferation by macrophage products. *Immunology* 56: 695, 1985.
82. MacDonald, I., Fairley, K. F., Hobbs, J. B., and Kincaid-Smith, P. Loin pain as a presenting symptom in idiopathic glomerulonephritis. *Clin. Nephrol.* 3:129, 1975.
83. MacMahon, H. E., and Latorraca, R. Essential renal hematuria. *J. Urol.* 71:667, 1959.
84. Marks, M. I., and Drummond, K. N. Benign familial hematuria. *Pediatrics* 44:590, 1969.
85. Matsui, A., Tomiyama, S., Baba, S., and Matsuda, T. Medical and genetic study of benign familial hematuria associated with sensorineural hearing loss (Abstract). *Pediatr. Nephrol.* 1:C40, 1987.
86. Mauer, S. M., Steffes, M. W., Azar, S., Sandberg, S. K., and Brown, D. M. The effects of Goldblatt hypertension on development of the glomerular lesions of diabetes mellitus in the rat. *Diabetes* 27:738, 1978.
87. Mauer, S. M., Sutherland, D. E. R., Howard, R. J., Fish, A. J., Najarian, J. S., and Michael, A. F. The glomerular mesangium: III. Acute immune mesangial injury: A new model of glomerulonephritis. *J. Exp. Med.* 137:553, 1973.
88. McConville, J. M., West, C. D., and McAdams, A. J. Familial and nonfamilial benign hematuria. *J. Pediatr.* 69:207, 1966.
89. Michael, J., Jones, N. F., Davies, D. R., and

Tighe, J. R. Recurrent haematuria: Role of renal biopsy and investigative morbidity. *Br. Med. J.* 1: 686, 1976.
90. Migone, L., Olivetti, G., Allegri, L., and Dall'Aglio, P. Mesangioproliferative glomerulonephritis. *Clin. Nephrol.* 13:219, 1980.
91. Morel-Maroger, L., Leathem, A., and Richet, G. Glomerular abnormalities in nonsystemic diseases: Relationship between findings by light microscopy and immunofluorescence in 433 renal biopsy specimens. *Am. J. Med.* 53:170, 1972.
92. Morel-Maroger, L., and Verroust, P. J. Clinicopathological Correlations in Glomerular Diseases. In N. F. Jones (Ed.), *Recent Advances in Renal Disease.* Edinburgh: Churchill-Livingstone, 1975. P. 48.
93. Murphy, W. M., Jukkola, A. F., and Roy, S., III. Nephrotic syndrome with mesangial-cell proliferation in children: A distinct entity? *Am. J. Clin. Pathol.* 72:42, 1979.
94. Naish, P. F., Aber, G. M., and Boyd, W. N. C3 deposition in renal arterioles in the loin pain and haematuria syndrome. *Br. Med. J.* 3:746, 1975.
95. Nomoto, Y., Sakai, H., Arimori, S., Iwagaki, H., Osamura, R. Y., Hata, J., and Tamaoki, N. Immunopathologic and histologic studies on benign recurrent hematuria: Clinicopathologic similarities with IgA nephropathy. *Am. J. Pathol.* 94:51, 1979.
96. Nortman, D. F., Rever, B. L., Stanley, T. M., and Kurokawa, K. The loin pain–hematuria syndrome in two cases of IgA and IgM nephropathy. *Arch. Intern. Med.* 141:1782, 1981.
97. Orfila, C., Pieraggi, M.-T., and Suc, J.-M. Mesangial isolated C3 deposition in patients with recurrent or persistent hematuria. *Lab. Invest.* 43:1, 1980.
98. Palmer, J. M., Eversole, S. L., and Stamey, T. A. Unilateral glomerulonephritis: Virtual absence of nephritis in a kidney with partial occlusion of the main renal artery. *Am. J. Med.* 40:816, 1966.
99. Pardo, V., Berian, M. G., Levi, D. F., and Strauss, J. Benign primary hematuria: Clinicopathologic study of 65 patients. *Am. J. Med.* 67:817, 1979.
100. Parfrey, P. S., Hutchinson, T. A., Jothy, S., Cramer, B. C., Martin, J., Hanley, J. A., and Seely, J. F. The spectrum of diseases associated with necrotizing glomerulonephritis and its prognosis. *Am. J. Kidney Dis.* 6:387, 1985.
101. Pytel, A. Renal fornical hemorrhages: Their pathogenesis and treatment. *J. Urol.* 83:783, 1960.
102. Rogers, P. W., Kurtzman, N. A., Bunn, S. M., Jr., and White, M. G. Familial benign essential hematuria. *Arch. Intern. Med.* 131:257, 1973.
103. Ross, J. H. Recurrent focal nephritis. *Q. J. Med.* 29:391, 1960.
104. Roy, L. P., Fish, A. J., Vernier, R. L., and Michael, A. F. Recurrent macroscopic hematuria, focal nephritis, and mesangial deposition of immunoglobulin and complement. *J. Pediatr.* 82:767, 1973.
105. Savage, C. O. S., Pusey, C. D., Kershaw, M. J., Cashman, S. J., Harrison, P., Hartley, B., Turner, D. R., Cameron, J. S., Evans, D. J., and Lockwood, C. M. The Goodpasture antigen in Alport's syndrome: Studies with a monoclonal antibody. *Kidney Int.* 30:107, 1986.
106. Sheil, A. G. R., Ibels, L. S., Thomas, M. A. B., and Graham, J. C. Renal autotransplantation for severe loin-pain/haematuria syndrome. *Lancet* 2:1216, 1985.
107. Siegler, R. L., Brewer, E. D., and Hammond, E. Platelet activation and prostacyclin supporting capacity in the loin pain hematuria syndrome. *Am. J. Kidney Dis.* 12:156, 1988.
108. Silva, F. G. Overview of pediatric nephropathology. *Kidney Int.* 33:1016, 1988.
109. Singer, D. B., Hill, L. L., Rosenberg, H. S., Marshall, J., and Swenson, R. Recurrent hematuria in childhood. *N. Engl. J. Med.* 279:7, 1968.
110. Sinniah, R. Renal disease in Singapore with particular reference to glomerulonephritis in adults. *Singapore Med. J.* 21:583, 1980.
111. Sinniah, R., Pwee, H. S., and Lim, C. H. Glomerular lesions in asymptomatic microscopic hematuria discovered on routine medical examination. *Clin. Nephrol.* 5:216, 1976.
112. Smellie, S. W., Lambert, M., Lavenne, E., and van Cangh, P. J. Factor XII deficiency associated with loin pain/haematuria syndrome. *Lancet* 2:1330, 1987.
113. Smith, S. M., and Tung, K. S. K. Incidence of IgA-related nephritides in American Indians in New Mexico. *Hum. Pathol.* 16:181, 1985.
114. Solez, K., and Heptinstall, R. H. Intrarenal urinary extravasation with formation of venous polyps containing Tamm-Horsfall protein. *J. Urol.* 119:180, 1978.
115. Southwest Pediatric Nephrology Study Group. Childhood nephrotic syndrome associated with diffuse mesangial hypercellularity: A report of the Southwest Pediatric Nephrology Study Group. *Kidney Int.* 23:87, 1983.
116. Stein, H. D., Feddergreen, W., Kashgarian, M., and Sterzel, R. B. Role of angiotensin II–induced renal functional changes in mesangial deposition of exogenous ferritin in rats. *Lab. Invest.* 49:270, 1983.
117. Stilmant, M. M., Couser, W. G., and Cotran, R. S. Experimental glomerulonephritis in the

mouse associated with mesangial deposition of autologous ferritin immune complexes. *Lab. Invest.* 32:746, 1975.
118. Tejani, A., and Nicastri, A. D. Mesangial IgM nephropathy. *Nephron* 35:1, 1983.
119. Tiebosch, T. M. G., Frederik, P. M., van Breda Vriesman, P. J. C., Mooy, J. M. V., van Rie, H., van de Wiel, T. W. M., Wolters, J., and Zeppenfeldt, E. Thin-basement-membrane nephropathy in adults with persistent hematuria. *N. Engl. J. Med.* 320:14, 1989.
120. Tina, L., Jenis, E., Jose, P., Medani, C., Papadopoulou, Z., and Calcagno, P. The glomerular basement membrane in benign familial hematuria. *Clin. Nephrol.* 17:1, 1982.
121. Trachtman, H., Weiss, R. A., Bennett, B., and Greifer, I. Isolated hematuria in children: Indications for a renal biopsy. *Kidney Int.* 25:94, 1984.
122. Travis, L. B., Daeschner, C. W., Dodge, W. F., Hopps, H. C., and Rosenberg, H. S. "Idiopathic" hematuria. *J. Pediatr.* 60:24, 1962.
123. Van de Putte, L. B. A., Brutel de la Riviere, G., and van Breda Vriesman, P. J. C. Recurrent or persistent hematuria: Sign of mesangial immune-complex deposition. *N. Engl. J. Med.* 290:1165, 1974.
124. Vangelista, A., Frasca, G., Biagini, G., and Bonomini, V. Long-term study of mesangial proliferative glomerulonephritis with IgM deposits. *Proc. EDTA* 18:503, 1981.
124a. Venkataseshan, V. S., Jovanovic, G., Kim, D. U., Andres, G. A., and Churg, J. Anti-GBM antibody staining in thin basement membrane (TBM) disease and Alport's syndrome (AS) (Abstract). *Kidney Int.* 37:252, 1990.
125. Volhard, F., and Fahr, T. *Die Brightsche Nierenkrankheit.* Berlin: Springer, 1914.
126. Waldherr, R. Familial glomerular disease. *Contrib. Nephrol.* 33:104, 1982.
127. Waldherr, R., Gubler, M. C., Levy, M., Broyer, M., and Habib, R. The significance of pure diffuse mesangial proliferation in idiopathic nephrotic syndrome. *Clin. Nephrol.* 10:171, 1978.
128. Weiss, M. A., and Crissman, J. D. Segmental necrotizing glomerulonephritis: Diagnostic, prognostic, and therapeutic significance. *Am. J. Kidney Dis.* 6:199, 1985.
129. Whitworth, J. A., Turner, D. R., Leibowitz, S., and Cameron, J. S. Focal segmental sclerosis or scarred focal proliferative glomerulonephritis? *Clin Nephrol.* 9:229, 1978.
129a. Wilkowski, M. J., Velosa, J. A., Holley, K. E., Offord, K. P., Chu, C.-P., Torres, V. E., McCarthy, J. T., Donadio, J. V., Jr., and Wagoner, R. D. Risk factors in idiopathic renal vasculitis and glomerulonephritis. *Kidney Int.* 36:1133, 1989.
130. Yamamoto, T., and Wilson, C. B. Quantitative and qualitative studies of antibody-induced mesangial cell damage in the rat. *Kidney Int.* 32:514, 1987.
131. Yoshikawa, N., Hashimoto, H., Katayama, Y., Yamada, Y., and Matsuo, T. The thin glomerular basement membrane in children with haematuria. *J. Pathol.* 142:253, 1984.
132. Yoshikawa, N., White, R. H. R., and Cameron, A. H. Familial hematuria: Clinicopathological correlations. *Clin. Nephrol.* 17:172, 1982.
133. Yum, M., and Bergstein, J. M. Basement membrane nephropathy: A new classification for Alport's syndrome and asymptomatic hematuria based on ultrastructural findings. *Hum. Pathol.* 14:996, 1983.

Fred G. Silva

5

Acute Postinfectious Glomerulonephritis and Glomerulonephritis Complicating Persistent Bacterial Infection

This chapter deals first with acute postinfectious glomerulonephritis, which is the type of glomerulonephritis that *follows* infections. Since acute poststreptococcal glomerulonephritis is the most common and best understood form, it serves as the prototype and will be described in detail. The less commonly encountered forms of postinfectious glomerulonephritis will be discussed only briefly.

The rest of the chapter deals with the forms of glomerulonephritis that *accompany* such persistent bacterial infections as infective endocarditis, deep-seated abscesses, and infected ventriculoatrial shunts inserted for the relief of hydrocephalus.

ACUTE POSTSTREPTOCOCCAL GLOMERULONEPHRITIS

Background

Acute glomerulonephritis has long been known to follow certain acute infections. Although Hippocrates over two millennia ago described the occurrence of back pain and gross hematuria leading to oliguria or anuria [189], it was Wells [491] who noted bloody urine in patients with scarlet fever and postscarlatinal anasarca. Bright, too [62], noted the association with scarlatina, and described the finding of blood in the urine and swelling of the face in what were probably attacks of acute poststreptococcal glomerulonephritis. He further observed that with or without treatment the patient's urine lost its "red particles" and that the swelling subsided, although in some instances he recorded that the patient returned at a later time with what we would now regard as chronic renal failure. With the introduction of microscopic examination of the kidney over the ensuing decades, it became appreciated that changes occurred in the glomeruli, and Langhans [253,254] described a category of Bright's disease with glomerular inflammation. Schick [412] commented on the similarity of the latent period in serum sickness to that of acute glomerulonephritis.

The first major clinicopathologic treatise on renal disease appeared in 1914 with the publication of Volhard (the clinician) and Fahr's (the pathologist) work *Die Brightsche Nierenkrankheit* [476]; they classified Bright's disease into a variety of different categories, including inflammatory diseases of the glomerulus. Longcope [281,282] recognized two general forms of glomerulonephritis, the first of which was associated with preceding bacterial infections and had a quick recovery and a good prognosis (acute glomerulonephritis). Ellis [121] distinguished two types of glomerulonephritis. Type 1 nephritis, usually seen in young patients, was characterized by an abrupt onset, constitutional symptoms, gross hematuria following infection, and a high recovery rate; this corresponded to the first type described by Longcope [281–283]. Fahr [124] described those cases of glomerulonephritis with no crescent formation as "intracapillary glomerulonephritis," and this association with infection is now clear.

Scarlet fever was noted to be associated with acute glomerulonephritis in the late 1800s and early 1900s, and it soon became apparent that there was a common association with a previous infection of group A streptococcus [176,179,346]. Varying attack rates of acute glomerulonephritis were noted in patients with scarlet fever, ranging from 3 [70] to 18 percent [480] of patients. Caiger [70] found a greater attack rate of nephritis in children under 15 years of age as compared with adults. These varying rates were probably largely dependent on the strain of streptococcus causing the infection, and it is now well recognized that only a relatively limited number of certain types of the organism are capable of inducing acute postinfectious glomerulonephritis. Ophüls [344] as early as 1917 had suggested that only certain strains of streptococci appeared to have a nephritogenic capacity.

Most cases of acute glomerulonephritis seen today are caused by the streptococcus, without the clinical signs and symptoms of scarlet fever [117]. In colder northern climates, most cases of acute glomerulonephritis follow upper respiratory tract infections, such as pharyngitis or tonsillitis [371,372], but cases also can follow skin infections, especially in warmer climates [102,358]. Most cases of acute poststreptococcal glomerulonephritis are caused by group A streptococci, which are also responsible for rheumatic fever. There are many differences, however, between the epidemiology of acute glomerulonephritis and that of rheumatic fever [37,421]. For example, the constant attack rate of 3 percent found in patients with rheumatic fever following group A streptococcal infections has not been found in patients with acute glomerulonephritis [370,373]. A likely explanation for the different patterns is that only certain strains of group A streptococci lead to acute glomerulonephritis [370,373,384–390,421, 448]. Types 12, 4, and 1 are more likely to cause acute glomerulonephritis after throat infections than other types [373,448,492,502]. Type 12 is especially common as a strain leading to acute glomerulonephritis. However, even with the same type of streptococcal organism, there are differences in the attack rate. Siegel et al. [426] showed that only 1 of 58 patients with well-documented type 12 streptococcal infection developed acute glomerulonephritis; this was a convincing demonstration that not all strains of type 12 are nephritogenic. The attack rate (variably defined and detected) with certain nephritogenic strains ranges from 1 to 33 percent of patients [376]. Type 4 also occurs frequently [372], as does type 1 [164]. It has been suggested that differences in the host, such as the antibody status (or T cell status), could lead to this variability. It is also possible that of all children infected with the various strains of streptococci, less than 2 percent develop clinically obvious acute glomerulonephritis.

Acute glomerulonephritis resulting from skin infections is not uncommon, especially in the warmer climates [10,99–102,149,227,238,358,362, 363,371,387,467,483]. Streptococcal infections of the throat are more common in the winter and early spring, whereas streptococcal pyoderma or impetigo tends to occur in temperate climates in the late summer and early fall [483]. The same seasonal pattern is found for acute glomerulonephritis when this occurs. When skin infections lead to acute glomerulonephritis, certain serotypes of streptococci are isolated more commonly than others; streptococcal M types 49, 42, 2, 57, and 60 seem to be common, and types 49, 42 and 2 are particularly potent [483]. The nephritogenic strains from the throat and skin show, in general, comparable attack rates of glomerulonephritis [483]. However, it also has been noted that type 49 infections occurring in the skin have much different attack rates of acute glomerulonephritis (24 percent) than does type 49 occurring in the throat (5 percent) [11]. Frequently, the same bacteria can be demonstrated in the throat and the skin; in these instances, the skin infection precedes that in the throat [11]. The concomitant occurrence of acute poststreptococcal glomerulonephritis and acute rheumatic fever has been noted [33,75, 244,399]. Acute glomerulonephritis related to infection has been associated with ear piercing [4], traumatic blister (new "thongs") [339], and lobar pneumonia due to streptococci [407] and was recorded in an allografted kidney from a renal transplant patient with a mycotic aneurysm of his coronary artery [332].

Many of the important observations on the epidemiology of acute postinfectious glomerulonephritis were made on the Red Lake Indian Reservation in Minnesota, where outbreaks of acute glomerulonephritis occurred in 1953 and again in 1966 [11]. A study of the second epidemic (both caused by type 49) showed that all cases occurred in children too young to have been infected in the first epidemic [10]. The lack of type-specific immunity was responsible for this fact. Recent studies from the Red Lake Reservation suggested that hereditary polymorphic light eruption may be a causative factor in streptococcal pyoderma in the Native Americans [146]. Epidemic outbreaks tend to occur in closed communities [380,384,448,517] or in highly populated areas in which poor hygiene, malnutrition, anemia, and parasites are common [358,384,387]. Some epidemics in certain communities tend to recur and are separated by 5 to 7 years [358,384]. The reason(s) for this recurrence is unclear

The number of patients with poststreptococcal glomerulonephritis has diminished significantly in the United States and Europe in the last two to three decades. However, postinfectious glomerulonephritis continues to have a high incidence in other parts of the world, such as Africa [342], the Caribbean [358], and South America [384].

General Properties of Streptococci, Antibody Formation, and Complement Changes

STREPTOCOCCUS PYOGENES

Streptococcus pyogenes (group A streptococcus, GAS) produces many virulence-enhancing extracellular products and toxins, including erythrogenic toxin, DNase, hyaluronidase, streptokinase, NADase, proteinases, and the hemolysins-streptolysin-O (oxygen labile) and streptolysin-S (oxygen stable). GAS is the etiologic agent of a number of suppurative infections, including pharyngitis, cellulitis, scarlet fever, erysipelas, pyoderma, puerperal sepsis, and impetigo. GAS infection can be diagnosed/monitored with many laboratory procedures that detect the organism, its antigens, or antibodies to it.

Conventional methods for the identification of viable organisms include finding beta-hemolytic colonies on 5% sheep blood agar with a subsequent presumptive identification based on sensitivity to bacitracin on streptococcal selective agar or hydrolysis of L-pyrrolidonyl-beta-naphthylamide. Presumptive identification usually takes from 18 to 48 hours and is inexpensive. Other common serologic procedures are latex agglutination, coagglutination, and immunofluorescent antibody staining [123]. An infrequently used reference method is the Lancefield precipitin test, in which cell-wall antigens must be extracted by heating or chemical treatment prior to testing [18]. Throat cultures are the most reliable method for finding GAS, but they have a long turnaround time.

Rapid methods for the detection of organism antigen directly from throat swabs include latex agglutination, coagglutination, and enzyme immunoassay [96,329]. These methods require extraction of the carbohydrate antigen from the throat swab with enzyme or acid reagents. More than 30 commercial detection kits are available. These kits are inexpensive, and it takes 5 to 20 minutes to perform the test. Many of these tests claim to have excellent specificity, sensitivity, and predictive positive and negative values based on scientific studies. However, it is difficult to compare and validate the above-mentioned parameters among different kits because of differences in the following variables: testing laboratories and their experimental design, prevalence of streptococcal infection in the test group, experience of the laboratorian, and proper identification of endpoints and minimum colony-forming units per milliliter for detection (i.e., sensitivity). These rapid methods are considered helpful if results are positive, but negative results do not necessarily mean the specimen-collection site was free of *S. pyogenes*. In addition, cultures with less than 10 colonies (with false-negative rapid test results) yielded positive serologic test results (i.e., fourfold or greater rise in antibody titers). Therefore, small numbers of GAS can be meaningful.

There is much information on the biologic characteristics of the streptococcal organism as well as the strains that lead to acute glomerulonephritis. Poststreptococcal glomerulonephritis is almost always due to strains of the serogroup A; however, several well-documented outbreaks have been due to group C organisms in patients with septic arthritis, pneumonia, and septicemia [21,113] and to group G (skin infections) streptococci [378]. Rammelkamp et al. [372] have shown that nephritogenic strains (especially M types 12, 4, 25, and 49) are more susceptible than other non-nephritogenic strains to lysis with bacteriophages. Despite the strong association of certain types of streptococcal organisms with glomerulonephritis (M types 1, 2, 4, 12, 18, 25, 49, 55, 57, and 60 have all been reported), as mentioned before, not all strains of the same type are nephritogenic. As described earlier, the attack rate varies considerably even among those strains which have a strong propensity for leading to poststreptococcal glomerulonephritis. Khandke et al. [235] have noted differences in the structural features of the streptococcal M proteins from nephritogenic and rheumatogenic subtypes. Others [175] have studied the presence or absence of lysogeny of group A streptococci with regard to their nephritogenicity; these investigators did not find a direct correlation between lysogeny and acute glomerulonephritis. Nontypable group A streptococci also have been cultured from patients with acute glomerulonephritis; these presumably represent unclassified nephritogenic strains [384]. It is likely that multiple factors (of the bacteria and the host) contribute to the differences in the attack rates for different strains of streptococcal organisms.

Lange et al. [248] have described an antigen that is present in all nephritogenic strains of streptococci tested. This antigen is immunologically identical in all and is unlike any known extracellular product of streptococci. Others [472] describe that the extracellular products of strains of streptococci isolated from patients with acute poststreptococcal glomerulonephritis possess a protein that is unique for these strains; this protein is not produced by streptococci recovered from patients lacking renal involvement [472]. These "nephritogenic" proteins will be discussed later.

ANTIBODY FORMATION

Both intracellular and extracellular antigenic components of the streptococcus stimulate the production of antibodies in the infected patient. Antibodies against the various streptococcal products, although probably not all are involved with the conferring of immunity, are of great help in clinical medicine because their presence provides evidence for a preceding streptococcal infection [219,269,494]. These antibodies include antistreptolysin-O (ASO), antistreptokinase (ASK), antihyaluronidase (AH), antideoxyribonuclease-B (anti-DNase-B), anti-diphosphopyridine nucleotidase (anti-DPNase), and anti-nicotinamide adenine dinucleotidase (anti-NADase). The "streptozyme" antibody test was introduced as a latex agglutination method in a kit intended to simultaneously measure antibodies to five streptococcal extracellular antigens (exoenzymes), including streptolysin, streptokinase, hyaluronidase, DNase, and NADase. It should be noted, however, that approximately 20 percent of healthy children have elevated streptozyme titers. Also, some investigators believe that the reliability of the "streptozyme" is not as good as the conventional methods for the single-antibody determinations [126]. At this time, it appears that the current technology for a home test kit for antistreptococcal antibodies is inaccurate because of the low levels of specificity and sensitivity. Most physicians seeing patients who had used a home test kit would probably retest irrespective of what the reaction.

Two of the most useful antibody determinations in the evaluation of patients with recent streptococcal infections are the ASO and the anti-DNase-B [126]. The ASO is the best known and the one most frequently ordered [126]. For example, in one study [36], the ASO titer was above 160 units in 92 percent of patients with acute glomerulonephritis; ASK and AH titers were raised in less than 50 percent. The ASO titer is usually greater than 250 Todd units, with most patients having a threefold or greater rise. A rising titer provides the best proof of a streptococcal infection. The ASO titer begins to rise within a few days of the infection and reaches a peak level after several weeks; as a rule, it then declines [281]. Normal levels were noted in 75 percent of subjects within 1 to 2 years after the infection [284]. However, the ASO titer does not increase in all patients with streptococcal infections; thus the absence of a high titer does not exclude a streptococcal infection. This is especially noted in patients with skin infections (pyoderma). Conversely, the ASO titer can rise modestly in patients with nonstreptococcal disease, and up to one-third of patients with other forms of nonstreptococcal glomerulonephritis may have mild elevations of ASO. Because the ASK or AH titer may be elevated when the ASO titer does not rise (as in skin infections), some have suggested that a combination of all three tests is of advantage in diagnosing acute poststreptococcal glomerulonephritis. False-positive results are caused by betalipoprotein in liver disease, some other bacteria, and oxidation of streptolysin-O. False-negative results can occur after antibiotic treatment of the patient.

AH and anti-DNase-B titers are commonly raised in patients with skin infections [43,101, 362], more so than ASO, as indicated above. Anti-DNase-B testing is more sensitive than AH and is the test of choice in the investigation of skin infections. Anti-DNase-B titer remains elevated longer than the ASO titer.

There is no direct correlation between the height of the antibody titer to these bacterial products and the occurrence and severity of acute glomerulonephritis [284,448]. Some investigators, however, have suggested that there is a significantly greater immune response in patients with acute glomerulonephritis and skin infections than in patients with comparable clinical and bacteriologic evidence of streptococcal skin infection and no evidence of acute glomerulonephritis [101, 227]. Dodge et al. [107] showed that the highest titers of ASO on admission were distinctly higher in those children whose lesions healed than in those whose lesions did not heal. Analogy was drawn by these authors to the work of Dixon et al. [103], who showed in experimental studies that rabbits that were the best antibody producers did not develop chronic renal lesions when subjected to multiple infections of small amounts of foreign protein. It is unusual for patients to develop a second attack of poststreptococcal glomerulonephritis; this is probably due to the relatively limited number of nephritogenic strains of streptococci and to the acquisition of type-specific protective immunity to the serotype of streptococcus that elicited the initial attack. It is likely that other factors may explain the relative resistance to another nephritic attack, such as the presence of antibodies to the specific nephritogenic factor(s); cross-reacting neutralizing antibodies may be directed at one potential factor but cross-react with another [192]. When second attacks do occur [396], they are similar clinically and morphologically to the initial attack. A more frequent phenomenon is the propensity for streptococcal infections to precipitate exacerbations of chronic glomerulonephritis [421]; these exacerbations often occur after a latent period of only 1 to 4 days. This feature of immunity and lack of a second bout of acute glomerulonephritis is shared by all streptococci with nephritogenic potential [384].

Penicillin interferes with both the production of type-specific antibody and ASO when significant dosages are given [426]. It may also affect the renal response, and in a series of patients followed with respiratory tract infection at a community care center, it was noted that patients with group A streptococcal acute glomerulonephritis had been treated with antibiotics significantly later than patients without signs of acute glomerulonephritis [201]. Experimental evidence in a rabbit model of poststreptococcal glomerulonephritis utilizing viable group A streptococci suggested that penicillin therapy within the first 3 days of infection prevented the acute nephritic process [34].

COMPLEMENT CHANGES

Serum complement is decreased during the acute episode in almost all patients with acute postinfectious glomerulonephritis [32,267,432] and is considered evidence in favor of the diagnosis and of an antigen-antibody reaction [133]. Serum complement levels return to normal within 6 weeks of the acute onset of the nephritis [236]. In patients in whom the serum complement level is normal, serial determinations will often show a further elevation during the recovery stage. There is activation of both the classical and the alternative pathways of the complement cascade; Levy et al. [265] suggested that although both pathways are implicated in the early stages of the disease, continued C3 depression is probably through the alternative pathway.

Clinical Features

Acute postinfectious glomerulonephritis most commonly affects children and young adults, although no age group is exempt from this disorder. Although the peak incidence is in the first decade of life, more than half the patients described by Sapir et al. [403] and a third of the patients in another study [299] were over the age of 40 years. Occurrence in older patients has been noted [1,116, 308,320]. Males seem to be affected more commonly than females [179,384], the ratio often being 2 : 1 [20]; this ratio is in marked contrast to patients with rheumatic fever, which affects both sexes equally [421]. The distribution of acute postinfectious (especially poststreptococcal) glomerulonephritis is worldwide. In North America it affects groups equally in the northern and southern parts, also in contrast to rheumatic fever. Acute poststreptococcal glomerulonephritis mav occur in either sporadic or epidemic form; children are the group most commonly affected in the epidemic forms.

For diagnosis of an "acute postinfectious glomerulonephritis," clear evidence that infection preceded the glomerulonephritis is required. A preceding infective episode (such as pharyngitis, tonsillitis, mastoiditis, peritonsillar abscess, or otitis media) is the *sine qua non* for diagnosis of an acute poststreptococcal glomerulonephritis [282]. Airborne droplets are responsible for the spread of streptococcal pharyngitis [335,336]. Skin infection also may lead to nephritis [102,227,282,358, 387]; this is most often associated with epidemics. The offending organism is virtually always a group A streptococcus; types 12, 4, 1, and 49 appear to be the most common nephritogenic types. However, the same glomerular pattern has been described with a number of different organisms, including bacteria (e.g., pneumococcus, etc.), fungi, and even viruses.

There is a delay or latent (or gap) period between the streptococcal infection and the onset of signs and symptoms of acute glomerulonephritis; this is often 1 to 4 weeks (average 10 to 11 days) before the onset of the acute nephritic syndrome. In general, the latent period is 1 to 2 weeks after a throat infection but 3 to 6 weeks after a skin infection.

The onset of clinical symptoms is typically abrupt. At the onset of the clinical symptomatology, the urine becomes dark, smoky, or "coke" or coffee colored [3]. Puffiness of the face or eyelids as a manifestation of edema is sudden and common; in some cases there also may be edema of the legs and sacrum. The periorbital edema is characterized by prominence on awakening in the morning and a tendency to subside or decrease if the patient is up and about in the morning. The edema, as well as other features of the circulatory congestion, such as dyspnea, cardiomegaly, and increased venous pressure, is thought to be the result of a defect in the renal excretion of sodium and water [160,230,418], although heart failure is also a factor both in children and older patients [67,178,308]. The severity of edema in poststreptococcal glomerulonephritis is often disproportionate to the degree of renal impairment. Compromise of the intraglomerular blood flow (due to the glomerular hypercellularity resulting in progressive encroachment on the cross-sectional area of the glomerular capillaries), in part, leads to a prerenal condition that is manifested by a low fractional excretion of sodium, low urinary sodium concentrations, and concentrated urine [161, 162]. This salt and water retention often results in a dilutional anemia, hypertension, and edema [161]. Experimental models of acute glomerulonephritis have demonstrated appropriate depression of proximal tubular reabsorption of sodium and water, which suggests that there may be inappropriate sodium retention at a distal site [162]. In patients with impaired cardiac function, this sodium retention may lead to pulmonary edema.

In patients with severe proliferative glomerulonephritis, progression of the lesion may result in oliguria or even anuria. Oliguria may be either short-lived or persist and possibly be indicative of a severe form of glomerular disease (i.e., crescentic glomerular form). Oliguria tends to be transient, with diuresis usually occurring within 1 to 2 weeks. Anuria is less common. During the onset of oliguria/anuria, the proteinuria may actually diminish because of a decrease in the glomerular filtration rate [270]. With resolution of the glomerular process, increasing proteinuria may parallel increasing glomerular filtration rate or even precede it.

Hypertension commonly occurs (half or more of patients) [236], especially in the more severe cases; it is usually transient, with a rapid return to normal levels of blood pressure. Plasma renin activity is usually low. Although generally thought to be the result of sodium and water retention, studies by Parra et al. [349] suggested that inhibition of the angiotensin-converting enzyme by captopril could be an effective short-term treatment of low-renin hypertension in this disease. However, hypertension may persist, and where this occurs, it indicates either progression to a more chronic stage (the likelihood of this happening is discussed later) or the possibility that the disorder is not "classic" acute postinfectious glomerulonephritis. Hypertensive encephalopathy is noted in no more than 5 to 10 percent of patients. The cause of the hypertension is uncertain, but it has been attributed to sodium/fluid retention with volume expansion or increased vascular tonus from neurogenic or humoral influences [160,418]. Successful pregnancy can occur in patients with acute poststreptococcal glomerulonephritis [145,431].

Subclinical forms of acute poststreptococcal glomerulonephritis are more frequent than symptomatic disease [10,107,108,201,386,398,423]. In a prospective study of 248 children with group A streptococcal infections, Sagel et al. [398] measured serum complement levels and ASO titers and performed urinalysis. They found that subclinical disease was almost 20 times more common than overt acute glomerulonephritis. Over a 6-week period, 54 children showed either transient depression of serum complement (19 children), mild urinary abnormalities (proteinuria, hematuria, or leukocyturia; 15 children), or both (20 children). All patients were asymptomatic, except for one who was edematous; hypertension was present in half the patients. Renal biopsy was performed in 20 patients in whom depressed complement and urinary abnormalities were present, and a proliferative glomerular change, ranging from mild to severe, was noted; a granular immunofluorescence pattern was noted in 15 of the 20 biopsies. This indicates that morphologic glomerular involvement following a streptococcal infection is not an uncommon event, and the pronounced glomerular lesions can occur with few obvious clinical changes in the urine and without the usual clinical signs and symptoms of glomerulonephritis. Derrick et al. [98] have also shown that serum complement levels can be low in patients without clinical manifestations in acute glomerulonephritis, and hypocomplementemia has been noted in siblings of children and adolescents with acute glomerulonephritis caused by streptococcal skin infections. Some of these siblings developed hematuria. These authors [98] felt that this indicated a subclinical attack, since the serum complement level was depressed and the epidemiologic data on the serotypes of the streptococcal organisms cultured from the skin were akin to previous studies of clinically obvious acute poststreptococcal glomerulonephritis.

Laboratory Findings

Elevations in BUN and serum creatinine levels reflect the disease in the glomerular filtration rate, and they are often noted during the acute stages; like the hypertension, however, the BUN and serum creatinine elevations are usually only transient and quickly subside. Failure of normalization of these values suggests that one may not be dealing with a true case of acute postinfectious glomerulonephritis. BUN and serum creatinine levels may remain elevated in those patients who develop the crescentic form of postinfectious glomerulonephritis [91,395]. The decreased glomerular filtration rate is not totally dependent on compromise of the glomerular capillaries by the hypercellular process but also may be due to other factors, because changes in the permeability characteristics of the glomerular capillary basement membrane (i.e., reduced K_f) and increased glomerular hydraulic pressures are known to occur in experimental acute proliferative glomerulonephritis [45,209]. The filtering capacity of the glomerular filtration barrier is known as the *glomerular filtration coefficient* K_f; K_f is the product of the hydraulic conductivity of the glomerular basement membrane (L_p) and the total surface area of the glomerular filter (A or S_f). Early in the course of the disease there is an increase in the glomerular plasma flow that partially compensates for the decrease in K_f and helps to maintain the glomerular filtration rate. Later on (or in more severe disease) the glomerular plasma flow decreases and the glomerular filtration rate falls.

Proteinuria may be mild or so severe as to cause hypoalbuminemia and severe edema. Proteinuria is less than 5 g/24 hours in most cases [182]. The nephrotic syndrome has been described in approximately 5 to 10 percent of patients [236,503]; in one series [20] it was noted in 20 percent. The proteinuria usually disappears within 6 months, and it cleared in all but 4 of the 23 patients with clinical healing in the studies of Jennings and Earle [212]. Proteinuria may persist for longer periods, but complete clinical recovery has been noted after it has been maintained for as long as 15 [207] and 26 months [212]. McCluskey and Baldwin [299] described a well-documented patient with disappearance of proteinuria after 6 years. However, others [406] have described a patient in which the proteinuria disappeared, only to be followed by the onset of chronic renal failure at a later date.

The urine of patients with acute poststreptococcal glomerulonephritis has a high specific gravity, and the brown/smoky color is caused by hemolysis of erythrocytes that have penetrated the glomerular basement membrane and have passed into the tubular system; both are particularly common in patients in whom the urine volume is reduced.

The urinary sediment shows red blood cells and red blood cell casts; granular casts and sometimes leukocyte casts are noted. Microscopic hematuria often persists longer than proteinuria and may be present in patients in whom the disease has otherwise completely disappeared clinically [212]. Hematuria may persist for as long as 18 months, and in a few patients, it persists for much longer periods, even up to 5 years. The presence of red blood cell casts is of great importance because they indicate that the bleeding is of glomerular origin. Such casts are best discovered in first early morning urine specimens studied by the physician shortly after voiding. Distorted red blood cells, sometimes termed *dysmorphic,* are also thought to be indicative of glomerular disease by some investigators [42,127,468].

A clinical picture has been noted in which the urine shows only a few erythrocytes or trace amounts of proteinuria despite other classic signs and symptoms of acute glomerulonephritis (e.g., edema, hypertension, decreased serum complement) [203]; recovery is generally the rule.

It is an old observation that red blood cells (microhematuria) and proteinuria (albuminuria) may be found in the urine during the latent period between initial infection and the clinical onset of the acute glomerulonephritic process [455]. Albuminuria and red cells were present during the first week after infection in a group of patients with scarlet fever; this was termed *early albuminuria,* in contrast to *late albuminuria,* which developed between the ninth and forty-eighth days. Others have noted this too [142,448]. It therefore appears that some changes are taking place quite early in the course of the disease; the exact nature of this glomerular involvement is unclear, but it could represent a "planting of the antigen" or a toxic effect of bacterial products on the glomeruli. The albuminuria and microhematuria found in the interval between infection and nephritis can be detected in up to half the patients with streptococcal upper respiratory tract infections and are thought by some to be more likely to occur in patients who subsequently develop acute glomerulonephritis [335,336]. Renal biopsies have been taken shortly after the onset of infection [142], and mild focal hypercellularity of the glomeruli has been noted. It is of historical interest that one of the 19th-century students of the kidney believed that this early proteinuria is only of importance when it "joins hands" with the later proteinuria [455].

The serum albumin level is sometimes low because of the loss of albumin in the urine in those patients with severe proteinuria. The serum cholesterol level may be elevated in some children [186].

As noted before, antibodies to various streptococcal products can be found in patients with acute glomerulonephritis; these are used diagnostically to establish the presence of a preceding streptococcal infection. Comparisons of acute and subsiding titers are of great importance clinically. A rise in titer of two or more dilution increments between the acute and the convalescent serum is usually considered significant regardless of the magnitude of the titer. The upper limit of the normal range varies with the season, geographic area, and age of the patient; thus each laboratory should establish its own limits of normality. Patients who are treated with antibiotics early in the course of the infectious episode, or elderly patients, may not exhibit a significant rise in antibody titers; thus the diagnosis may be difficult in the absence of positive cultures.

Anemia is commonly noted in the early stages, and this is thought to be primarily a dilutional phenomenon as a consequence of the expanded extracellular fluid, although cases of hemolytic anemia [307] and thrombocytopenia have been reported [97,288,307,382].

Glomerular filtration rate is reduced in the acute stage, whereas the effective renal plasma flow is normal or reduced; therefore, the filtration fraction is generally reduced [61,118]. Tubular function may be altered, as assessed by Tm_{pah} and Tm glucose, but this is usually less than the reduction in the glomerular filtration rate.

Pathogenesis

The relationship between streptococcal infection and acute glomerulonephritis is well established, and much has been learned about the exact mechanism by which the infection leads to the characteristic glomerular changes. It has been known for a long time that the blood and urine are sterile in patients with acute glomerulonephritis [283], and the kidney parenchyma is also sterile [31]. The renal changes in acute glomerulonephritis were noted to be unlike those in patients with streptococcal septicemia, in which the major change is interstitial nephritis and abscess formation. However, some studies have shown that streptococcal septicemia can lead to a proliferative glomerulonephritis, a finding that is especially common in patients with acute bacterial endocarditis. Although streptococcal toxins could conceivably play a role in acute glomerulonephritis, this is unlikely because the renal injury would be expected to occur at the height of the infection (whereas it occurs during the subsidence of the infection). Also, an acute proliferative glomerulonephritis is not the type of morphologic change usually noted in patients with a variety of circulating toxins; additionally, it would be anticipated that the renal changes would be proportional to the severity of the infection, which is not the case.

IMMUNE-MEDIATED DISEASE AND EXPERIMENTAL STUDIES

It is now well accepted that acute poststreptococcal and other forms of postinfectious glomerulonephritis are secondary to an immunologic phenomenon. There is much to support an immune complex mechanism [105,155]. Schick et al. [412] noted the latent interval between the clinical infection and the onset of acute glomerulonephritis and likened it to the course of events in acute serum sickness and other allergic states. The latent interval after infection has been well documented [165,295,504] and usually ranges between 7 and 21 days (average about 10 to 11 days) [504].

The immune reactions occurring in the glomeruli could theoretically be brought about in several ways. A streptococcal antigen could be directly planted in the glomerulus, or alternatively, a cross-reacting or altered antigen could act as an immunogen and incite an immunologic response [192]. Deposited immune complexes could consist of either streptococcal antigen-antibody complexes or autologous antigen-antibody complexes. All these possibilities have been considered and studied in this form of glomerulonephritis.

Much of the support for an immune complex pathogenesis comes from the analogy with acute "one-shot" serum sickness in the rabbit. When human acute postinfectious glomerulonephritis is compared with acute serum sickness, there are obvious similarities. Von Pirquet [478] in 1911 felt that the similarities between postinfectious glomerulonephritis and the acute serum sickness syndrome supported his concept of allergy. Longcope [280] showed that parenteral administration of foreign protein in experimental animals could induce a glomerulonephritis, and other aspects of this are covered in Chapter 3. As noted in that chapter, there is a latent interval between the injection of foreign protein and development of the acute glomerulonephritis that is quite reminiscent of the latent interval between streptococcal infection and the clinical onset of human renal disease. By immunofluorescence techniques, it is possible to demonstrate antigen, antibody, and complement in the glomeruli. This correlates with the formation of a variety of circulating immune complexes. Ultrastructural studies in both human beings and experimental animals also show similar glomerular subepithelial electron-dense "immune-type" deposits [104,136,154,156,300]. Low levels of serum complement are found in both instances. Like the human counterpart, experimental acute serum sickness is a self-limited disease that generally resolves over a period of weeks. Some investigators have suggested that the macrophage is the predominant mediator of glomerular injury in acute serum sickness in rabbits [457–459]. However, the lack of an exact animal model for postinfectious glomerulonephritis in the past has made it difficult to clarify certain issues in the pathogenesis of this disease [384].

Many attempts have been made to induce an animal model of acute poststreptococcal glomerulonephritis by the injection of intact streptococci [28,120,314,365], crude culture supernatants [192], or specific components of the streptococci [192, 213]. Although some of these experimental manipulations produced histologic lesions somewhat similar to the disease pattern in man, most involved the periodic administration of the putative factors thought to be involved; this, of course, does not precisely mimic the gradual release of streptococcal products that probably occurs at the site of infection seen in the clinical situation in man [192]. Also, many of the experimental studies were performed at a time when electron and immunofluorescence microscopy and other biochemical determinations were not available, making it difficult to carry out an adequate comparison [192].

Holm et al. [192] developed an animal model that permitted the establishment of a focal infection (using subcutaneous tissue cages) and continuous monitoring of the infection and the release of streptococcal factors. This simulates acute poststreptococcal glomerulonephritis clinically, histologically, and immunologically. Rabbits infected with streptococci containing the *nephritis strain-associated protein (NSAP)* exhibited glomerular deposits that contained NSAP by the end of the first week (in the absence of antibody to NSAP); the glomeruli 3 weeks later showed a pattern similar to human acute poststreptococcal glomerulonephritis. Animals infected with streptococci that were NSAP-negative did not develop glomerulonephritis. The ability of NSAP to bind to glomerular structures suggested to these authors that it has unique nephrotoxic properties. In a later study [193–195] these same authors demonstrated that infusion of purified NSAP over an 8-day period (by means of osmotic pump) led to a similar glomerulonephritic process. No renal changes were noted after exposure to streptokinase C. This suggested to these investigators that the nephritogenic capacity of NSAP is distinct from that of streptokinase C despite the similarity between these molecules. These authors [193–194] identified NSAP in the glomeruli (in both the infection model and the infusion model) using a monoclonal antibody to NSAP, but they were unable to demonstrate NSAP in the kidneys of rabbits given streptokinase C or infected with streptococci not having NSAP. These studies await confirmation.

Holm [192] theorized that the NSAP molecule has unique domains responsible for its binding to a specific receptor in the kidney. He suggested that the ability of NSAP to convert plasminogen to plasmin (possibly in situ) might be related to many of the pathologic events taking place in acute poststreptococcal glomerulonephritis [192]. The plasmin formed by the interaction between NSAP and plasminogen splits the C3 molecule and activates the alternative pathway of complement activation, thereby initiating the inflammatory glomerular response. C3b deposits have been noted in man before immunoglobulins are detected, and plasma fibrinolytic hyperreactivity has been demonstrated in children with poststreptococcal glomerulonephritis (coinciding with a decrease in the plasminogen levels) [289].

SEARCH FOR THE ANTIGEN

The identity of the nephritogenic fractions of the bacteria is controversial. Rodriguez-Iturbe [384] has suggested two major possibilities: (1) that the nephritogenic antigen is a specific component of some streptococci or (2) that the streptococcal infection itself triggers an autoantigenic reactivity in the host. However, as noted later, it has been very difficult to demonstrate streptococcal antigen either within the presumed immune complexes in the glomeruli or in the circulating immune complexes [128,301]; Seegal et al. [419], Michael et al. [310], and Andres et al. [9] have all demonstrated streptococcal antigens by a variety of techniques.

Treser et al. [464] described how IgG fractions from the serum of patients with acute postinfectious glomerulonephritis caused staining of the glomerular capillaries and mesangium of patients with early acute glomerulonephritis. This staining was abolished if the serum fraction was previously absorbed with frozen and thawed nephritogenic beta-hemolytic streptococcal organisms. The plasma membrane appeared to be the fraction responsible. This staining activity was not abolished by absorption with other bacteria, and the antisera against streptococcal plasma membranes had similar staining properties to those of the sera of the patients with acute postinfectious glomerulonephritis. The conclusion drawn was that the streptococcal plasma membrane constituents were present in the glomeruli of patients with acute poststreptococcal glomerulonephritis [511]. These same workers

[511] were able to show antigenic sites in the mesangial matrix and on the glomerular subendothelial region using immunoferritin ultrastructural techniques [511]. Studies by Lange et al. [247,248] and others [9,119,163,174,177,231,232,245,264] have suggested that free antigen may be found in situ in the glomeruli and is available for the deposition of circulating antibodies. Cationic antigens, which are able to penetrate the fixed glomerular polyanionic charge barrier of the capillary wall, could be likely candidates for triggering an in situ immune complex reaction [22,341].

Traditionally, streptococcal M-protein has been thought to be the relevant antigenic bacterial fraction [479]. M-protein fractions can complex with fibrinogen and localize in the glomerulus [225, 228], and glomerulonephritis can be induced with injection of M-protein–M-protein/fibrinogen complexes [205]. M-protein may be antigenically cross-reactive with the GBM [297]. However, Treser et al. [464,465] have suggested that the nephritogenic fraction is different from the M-protein. Serum from patients convalescing from poststreptococcal glomerulonephritis, when labeled, could identify free antigenic sites in renal biopsy specimens showing poststreptococcal glomerulonephritis; because this serum had these antibodies independent of the M type of the original infection, it suggested that a non-M antigen was present in the glomerulus.

Several streptococcal fractions have been studied in search of the trigger for glomerulonephritis. One streptococcal fraction has been extensively studied by workers at the New York Medical College [247–251,422,464,511,512]. Endostreptosin was obtained after disruption of nephritogenic streptococci, and it had the ability to preabsorb the specific antibody of convalescent sera. This antigen is demonstrable in the glomerulus only during the initial phase of acute glomerulonephritis and reacts with antibodies present in the convalescent sera of acute glomerulonephritic patients. In the late phases of the disease, the antigen can no longer be detected, presumably because all the previously noted antigenic sites have been covered by the specific antibody [247]. Endostreptosin's molecular weight is between 40,000 and 50,000 [213] and is most likely derived from the streptococcal cytoplasm. Seligson et al. [422] have suggested that acute elevations of endostreptosin titers are generally diagnostic for acute poststreptococcal glomerulonephritis. Although low levels of antibody titers have been found in as many as 70 percent of normal individuals, significantly higher titers of antibodies are found in patients with poststreptococcal glomerulonephritis [422]. The majority of patients with acute rheumatic fever do not have these high levels of antibody titer. Thus Lange et al. [249] believe that elevated levels of antibody to endostreptosin are diagnostic for postinfectious glomerulonephritis and correlate well with the course of the pathologic disease process. This factor is similar to the preabsorbing antigen described by Yoshizawa et al. [511,512] and to that of Holm et al. [196]. Lange et al. [247] have suggested that endostreptosin may act as a planted antigen for an in situ immune-complex reaction along the glomerular capillary wall.

Villarreal et al. [472], in Zabriskie's laboratory, identified an extracellular protein unique to nephritogenic strains from cultures of the type 12 organisms. This fraction [called *nephritis strain-associated protein (NSAP)*] was noted in 56 percent of renal biopsies showing poststreptococcal glomerulonephritis; this fraction was not found in biopsies from patients with other forms of nonstreptococcal glomerulonephritis or rheumatic fever. The vast majority of patients with glomerulonephritis had serum antibodies to the fraction [340]. This NSAP has a subunit of 46 kD. The molecule has recently been isolated and purified [213]; it has antigenic, biochemical, and structural similarities to streptokinase from group C streptococcal organisms as well as being a plasminogen activator.

Vogt et al. [475] isolated and identified a number of different cationic proteins from nephritogenic streptococci. Cationic moieties are known to have affinity for the GBM. Antibodies raised againt these cationic proteins enabled Vogt et al. to demonstrate the existence of these protein antigens (a shared antigenic cross-reactivity) in almost half the renal biopsies studied showing acute poststreptococcal glomerulonephritis. Serum antibodies to these cationic antigens were noted in the poststreptococcal patients studied. The cationic antigens were not identified in renal biopsies showing immune complex (but nonstreptococcal) glomerulonephritis. The authors suggested that this antigen possibly initiated acute glomerulonephritis by means of in situ immune complex formation.

CIRCULATING IMMUNE COMPLEXES AND CRYOGLOBULINS

Ninety percent of patients with acute postinfectious glomerulonephritis have elevated serum levels of IgG and IgM. A number of techniques have been utilized to detect circulating immune complexes [55,140,144,274,309,512]. Border [55] summarized some of the literature and found that 58 percent of patients with acute glomerulonephritis had evidence of circulating immune complexes, compared with 4 percent of normal controls. Circulating immune complexes (as measured by C1q-binding activity) are found in the serum of two-thirds of patients in the first week of the disease. After 4 weeks of the disease, they are noted in about 20 percent of patients [316, 343,385]. It has been suggested that circulating immune complexes correlate with the severity of the renal disease and with the demonstration of renal immune deposits [22]. However, Rodriguez-Iturbe et al. [385] and others [140,309] did not note a correlation between this assay and the intensity of the clinical manifestations. Lin [274] noted that patients with poststreptococcal glomerulonephritis had significantly elevated levels of circulating immune complexes during the acute phases; 6 months later, the levels were only slightly elevated, and by 9 months after the initial attack, no circulating immune complexes were detectable. Patients who had persistent hematuria and proteinuria, however, continued to have detectable immune complexes during this time. It has been suggested that the acute arthritis and skin rash sometimes noted in patients with acute poststreptococcal glomerulonephritis are due to circulating immune complexes [277].

Cryoglobulins are frequently found in patients with acute poststreptococcal glomerulonephritis [2,304,305]. In fact, Rodriguez-Iturbe [384] noted cryoglobulins in two-thirds of patients in the first 2 weeks of the disease. Most of these studies have noted that the cryoglobulins contain combinations of IgG, C3, and/or IgM. IgA is less commonly found in the precipitates. Streptococcal antigens are not generally found in the cryoprecipitates [305]. McIntosh and coworkers [304] suggested that the detection of serum cryoglobulins was a better indicator of clinical and morphologic renal disease than was measurement of serum complement.

Serum from patients with acute postinfectious glomerulonephritis contains components of mesangial matrix and glomerular basement membranes [9,232,248,310,419,464,511], and nephritogenic antigens have been observed in circulating immune complexes in patients with acute poststreptococcal glomerulonephritis (but not in patients with acute rheumatic fever) [144]. Yoshimoto et al. [510] noted high levels of antibodies to streptococcal cell membrane antigens. Kefalides et al. [232] recorded that the sera from patients with postinfectious glomerulonephritis contained antibodies against all the major macromolecular components of the GBM (i.e., type IV collagen, laminin). Because circulating immune complexes of various types have been observed in patients with streptococcal infections alone (without glomerulonephritis), it is possible that these complexes represent a systemic inflammatory response in the patients rather than the cause of glomerular damage [512]. A similar suggestion with regard to lymphocyte-cell subpopulations and their binding to group A streptococcal membranes was noted by Williams [500]. Cryoglobulinemic glomerulonephritis is described in Chapter 24.

COMPLEMENT AND COMPLEMENT RECEPTORS

Early in the 1900s, Hedinger [180] demonstrated low serum complement levels in two patients with acute nephritis with uremia. Since that time, many workers have shown either a virtual absence or low levels of complement [72,98,134,250,252, 270,485]. Serum complement levels are almost always low in the acute stages of acute poststreptococcal glomerulonephritis. Rodriguez-Iturbe [384] noted depressed levels in 93 percent of patients. Lange et al. [248] suggest that in the acute stage of the clinical disease thought to be postinfectious glomerulonephritis, the absence of a low complement level indicates that the patient does not have postinfectious glomerulonephritis. Wasserman et al. [485] found low serum complement levels in 445 of 446 patients. Serum complement levels soon rise to normal levels after several weeks and almost always returns to normal within 6 weeks. In over half the patients of Fischel and Gajdusek [134], normal serum complement levels had been attained within 3 weeks of the acute clinical onset of disease. All 32 patients studied by Cameron et al. [72] had regained normal serum complement levels within 4 months, and all but 2 within 2 months.

It has been suggested that the persistence of low serum complement levels is associated with a poor prognosis [252]; however, renal biopsy must be performed in these patients to exclude a non-postinfectious glomerulonephritis, such as membranoproliferative glomerulonephritis. Most authors have not found a correlation between the level of serum complement and the degree of proteinuria [134], confirming the fact that complement was not decreased because of loss of complement in the urine. As noted before, the low serum complement level is evidence in favor of an antigen-antibody reaction. Because the serum complement level rises soon after the acute phase of the disease, it is generally not thought that there is a generalized disorder in the synthesis of complement [134]. However, one study [7] did show that children with postinfectious glomerulonephritis had reduced synthesis of C3 relative to normal subjects. Serum complement levels are depressed even in patients with subclinical glomerulonephritis [98,398].

The serum complement studies performed have measured either total hemolytic complement or fractions of the complement cascade, such as C3. Many studies have shown that although serum levels of C3 are depressed, the early components of the complement cascade, such as C1q, C2, or C4, have been normal or only slightly depressed [72,267,432,498]. These studies suggest that the alternative pathway of complement activation is operating, a suggestion strengthened by immunofluorescence studies showing the deposition of properdin in the glomeruli [304,311,322,493]. Other studies showing C3 deposition but no apparent IgG [2,135,311,470,507] also suggest that the alternative pathway often operates in acute postinfectious glomerulonephritis.

Other investigators propose that C3 activation can occur by both the classical and alternative pathways in acute glomerulonephritis [498,507]. It has been suggested that the classical pathway is involved primarily during the early stages of the process, but less so later [266].

Gelfand et al. [152] first demonstrated receptors for complement on the glomerular visceral epithelial cells. There is a loss of these complement receptors in patients with acute glomerulonephritis [152,321]. Whether this is pathogenetically important or just a secondary epiphenomenon is unclear at the present time, but there is not much evidence to suggest that the receptors are important in human disease.

OTHER MECHANISMS OF RENAL INJURY

In addition to the classic concept that streptococcal organisms produce a protein fraction that is immunogenic and causes an antibody response, there is also a suggestion that the streptococcal organism may trigger an autologous immune complex disease by inducing antigenic modification of a normal component of the streptococcal organism. McIntosh et al. [303] and others [12,325,388,390] have suggested that acute postinfectious glomerulonephritis is in part or totally an autologous immune complex disease in which autologous IgG is modified by a number of streptococcal enzymes or products of the bacterial organism released during infection (e.g., neuraminidase). In this way, IgG becomes autoimmunogenic and stimulates the production of antibodies against itself [303,325, 340]. Subsequent formation of endogenous antibody to the altered IgG could result in the formation of antigen-antibody complexes that act as the immune complexes responsible for the glomerular injury. Depletion of the sialic acid by neuraminidase was considered to be probable even in the rendering of the IgG autoimmunogenic. Mosquera and Rodriguez-Iturbe [325] reported that nephritogenic streptococci were frequently neuraminidase producers. Others have described similar findings [388], although not all agree [360]. Circulating anti-immunoglobulins have been detected in half the patients [384], and glomerular fixed antiglobulins were detected in most renal biopsy specimens from patients with poststreptococcal glomerulonephritis [303–305]. IgG eluted from the kidney shows anti-IgG reactivity [385]. Rheumatoid factor also has been noted in patients with acute poststreptococcal glomerulonephritis [452]. Vilches and Williams [471] found persistent anti-DNA antibodies and DNA–anti-DNA complexes in two patients with poststreptococcal glomerulonephritis. Fillit et al. [130] noted that sera from patients with poststreptococcal glomerulonephritis contained antibodies to glomerular heparan sulfate proteoglycan, and Kemeny et al. [233] demonstrated intact linear GBM staining with monoclonal antibodies to heparan sulfate proteoglycan, in contrast to other forms of glomerulonephritis, in which the staining was lost.

Cell-mediated mechanisms have traditionally not been considered an important factor in the initiation of the acute glomerular injury. Increasingly, however, they have been studied and are now thought to play an ancillary role in the progression of acute glomerulonephritis to a chronic stage [39,40,48,50–52,132,256,379,383,515]. They also may be important in those patients with severe acute postinfectious glomerulonephritis who have few immune deposits [132]. Zabriskie et al. [515] have suggested that proteins from nephritogenic streptococci may deposit in the glomerulus and release a glycopeptidase capable of altering the composition of the GBM and exposing new antigens. Progression might occur through antibodies on sensitized lymphocytes now directed against the "new" GBM antigens. The same workers demonstrated that lymphocytes from patients with nonresolving poststreptococcal glomerulonephritis showed significant inhibition of cell migration and increased DNA synthesis in the presence of group A streptococcal antigens; lymphocytes from patients with unrelated renal diseases showed lesser degrees of reactivity [379,515]. The same workers [93] have also recorded similar findings in cases of chronic proliferative glomerulonephritis. However, demonstration of the renal morphologic changes in these papers was not forthcoming.

Altered lymphocyte transformation using streptococcal protoplast-membrane antigens in 12 patients known to have had acute poststreptococcal glomerulonephritis with persistent renal disease has been noted by Bhat et al. [41]. A depressed immune response was noted in these patients compared with normal subjects. The authors concluded that the depressed cellular immune response could be responsible for the chronicity by facilitating the persistence of a humoral immune mechanism. Reid et al. [379] also suggested that the percentage of T lymphocytes (especially T gamma, the T cells bearing Fc receptors for IgG) is reduced, although others found evidence of neither enhanced lymphocyte response to nonspecific mitogens [239] nor leukocyte migration inhibition [168]. Patients with a well-documented history of postinfectious glomerulonephritis and end-stage renal disease respond to altered basement membrane antigens, whereas patients with end-stage renal disease secondary to other renal conditions do not [131]. None of these patients respond to native GBM antigens [131]. Prutis et al. [366] studied the activity of helix-destabilizing protein (indispensable in basic genetic processes such as DNA replication, genetic recombination, and transcription) in lymphocytes and found it in especially high levels in patients with acute glomerulonephritis, in whom it correlated with the activity of the glomerulonephritic process. In a study by Rodriguez-Iturbe et al. [390], using a skin window technique, evidence was found of activation of the patient's lymphocytes by normal human IgG. Reactive oxygen species produced by glomerular macrophages have been shown to contribute to GBM injury in a rabbit model of diffuse proliferative glomerulonephritis [58], but macrophages also can contribute to the glomerular handling of circulating immune complexes [57].

FIBRIN/FIBRINOLYSIS

Various studies on coagulation have been performed in patients with acute glomerulonephritis [6,223]. One study showed that during the acute phase, there was evidence of fibrin formation—as judged by an increase in plasma high-molecular-weight fibrinogen complexes—and the development of either hypo- or hyperfibrinogenemia, gross depression of coagulation factor XIII, and decreased levels of α_2-macroglobulin. When recovery occurred, these abnormalities waned. Fibrinolysis was found to increase, as determined by an elevation of fibrin degradation (split) products in the urine [6]. This last change also has been noted by others [84,95]. In most series, the degradation products in the urine decreased as recovery occurred.

Patients with persistent clinical activity and progressive disease have large daily fluctuations in urinary fibrin split products [84]. This cyclical activity was thought to represent either fluctuating inflammatory activity or periodic attempts by the fibrinolytic pathways to degrade the glomerular fibrin. There is no correlation between the levels of serum C3 and serum fibrinogen degradation products [361]. Platelets may play a role in various forms of glomerulonephritis [181], and glomerular platelet antigens have been noted in a variety of human glomerular diseases [312]. Ultrastructural demonstration of platelets in acute poststreptococcal glomerulonephritis in man is unusual; however, platelets are thought to be evanescent and may be missed by electron microscopic studies, especially if the biopsy is late in the course of the disease.

GENETIC PREDISPOSITION

Acute poststreptococcal glomerulonephritis occurs in siblings of patients with this disease [107]. Dodge et al. [107,108] reported that 20 percent of index cases had siblings with subclinical or clinical acute glomerulonephritis. Rodriguez-Iturbe et al. [386] noted an attack rate for siblings in affected families in nonepidemic conditions of 38.5 percent. This is even higher than the attack rate in epidemic conditions; thus a familial susceptibility to the disease was suggested [386,423]. Lange et al. [249] also found a high rate of asymptomatic glomerulonephritis (detected by urinalysis, hypocomplementemia, or elevated antibody titers to streptococcal antigens) in the family members of patients with symptomatic poststreptococcal glomerulonephritis (22 percent). It is conceivable, of course, that these findings could be explained on the basis of shared environments and shared infections. Layrisse et al. [257] suggested that HLA-DRw4 was more common in patients with acute poststreptococcal glomerulonephritis, but at present, no firm conclusions can be reached about the association between certain HLA antigens and the development of acute poststreptococcal glomerulonephritis [125,259,375,377,417].

Pathologic Changes

As with most of the glomerulonephritides, our early knowledge of the pathology of acute glomerulonephritis was derived mostly from autopsy material. With the advent of renal biopsy, it became possible to compare the morphologic pattern of the glomerular involvement in the living patient with that seen in patients dying with glomerulonephritis. Renal biopsy studies have shown that the morphologic picture described from autopsy material is virtually identical with that found on renal biopsy. This is probably because death in patients with acute glomerulonephritis was attributable to congestive heart disease, not to the renal injury. Recently, fewer biopsies showing acute glomerulonephritis have been available, since the clinician (especially the pediatric nephrologist) is nowadays less likely to biopsy a patient with "classic" or "typical" signs and symptoms of acute postinfectious glomerulonephritis. Indications for considering renal biopsy in children with acute nephritic syndrome include (1) persistent gross hematuria beyond 1 month or persistent hypocomplementemia beyond 6 weeks, (2) progressive deterioration of glomerular filtration rate, (3) hypertension persisting beyond 2 months, (4) extrarenal manifestations of systemic disease, (5) family history of renal disease, (6) age less than 2 years, or (7) onset of nephritis within 48 hours of pharyngitis [190,331] (Table 5-1). The indications for renal biopsy in adults are not so clear but are probably more liberal because of the less common occurrence of poststreptococcal glomerulonephritis in the adult. A number of glomerular diseases may present in a manner clinically indistinguishable from acute poststreptococcal glomerulonephritis; they include membranoproliferative glomerulonephritis (various types), Schönlein-Henoch syndrome, polyarteritis, and crescentic glomerulone-

Table 5-1. *Atypical features that suggest a need for renal biopsy*

I. Absence of evidence for immune complex disease
  A. No rise in antistreptococcal antibodies
  B. Normal serum complement level
II. Atypical early features
  A. No latent period
  B. Anuria
  C. No improvement or continued decrease in GFR at 2 weeks
  D. Persistence of hypertension beyond 2 weeks
  E. Nephrotic syndrome
III. Atypical features during presumed recovery
  A. Failure of normalization of GFR by 4 weeks
  B. Depression of serum complement level beyond 6 weeks
  C. Persistence of proteinuria beyond 6–8 months
  D. Persistence of hematuria beyond 18 months

Source: Modified with permission from Dr. Martin Nash, Renal Biopsy in Medical Diseases of the Kidney. Postgraduate Course, Department of Pathology, Columbia-Presbyterian Medical Center, New York, 1989.

phritis (of different forms). The most frequent example of another disease process masquerading as acute postinfectious glomerulonephritis in a child is one of the types of membranoproliferative glomerulonephritis.

GROSS APPEARANCE

The kidneys are symmetrically enlarged, generally 25 to 50 percent larger than normal. They are pallid in appearance, and the cut surfaces bulge because of interstitial edema. The main thickening is noted in the cortex. The glomeruli may stand out as gray, translucent dots. Although Wilks [497] in 1853 described "large white kidneys" in some patients with Bright's disease preceded by scarlatina, it is more likely that he was dealing with the various pathologic conditions that give rise to the nephrotic syndrome.

MICROSCOPIC FINDINGS

Glomeruli

Hypercellularity and Other Common Findings. The glomeruli are all affected (diffuse involvement) and usually to an approximately equal degree (global involvement) (Figs. 5-1 through 5-3). The glomerular tufts are larger than normal and contain an increase in the number of cells. Many cell types can be identified, including native endocapillary cells (endothelial and mesangial cells from the tuft itself) and migrant inflammatory cells, including polymorphonuclear leukocytes and monocytes (Figs. 5-4 and 5-5). The extent to which endocapillary cells contribute to the hypercellularity is debated and will be discussed later. Polymorphonuclear leukocytes are the most easily identified cells and may be present in large numbers—hence the term *exudative glomerulonephritis.* In other cases they are inconspicuous. It has been suggested by Jennings and Earle [212] that polymorphonuclear leukocytes may be more frequently found in biopsies performed shortly after the clinical onset of the disease. Occasionally, other inflammatory cells such as eosinophils [135,270] and lymphocytes can be noted, but this is unusual. Eosinophils are sometimes present in large numbers in cases from the tropics [182]. Necroses in the glomerular tuft are unusual (Fig. 5-6).

The individual lobules of the glomeruli are wider than normal and sometimes assume a clubbed appearance. The glomerular capillary lumina are often reduced by the hypercellularity so that erythrocytes may be difficult to see. The stalk region of the mesangium may be quite hypercellular [212]. The glomerular capillary walls are generally not thickened, although there occasionally may be some mild thickening noted by light microscopy. The combination of expansion of the lobules, hypercellularity of the tuft, and some localized thickening of the glomerular capillary walls may produce a picture almost identical to that of a membranoproliferative glomerulonephritis. Ultrastructural and immunofluorescence studies and clinical findings at the time of biopsy and follow-up will generally allow easy separation of these two morphologically and clinically distinct entities.

In some patients it is possible, especially with the oil-immersion lens, to detect tiny nodules on the epithelial side of the glomerular capillary wall. These can be identified either as fuchsinophilic dots with the trichrome stain (Masson or Mallory) on thin (3-μm) sections, or in 0.5-μm plastic-embedded sections stained with toluidine blue (Fig. 5-7). These minute structures correspond to

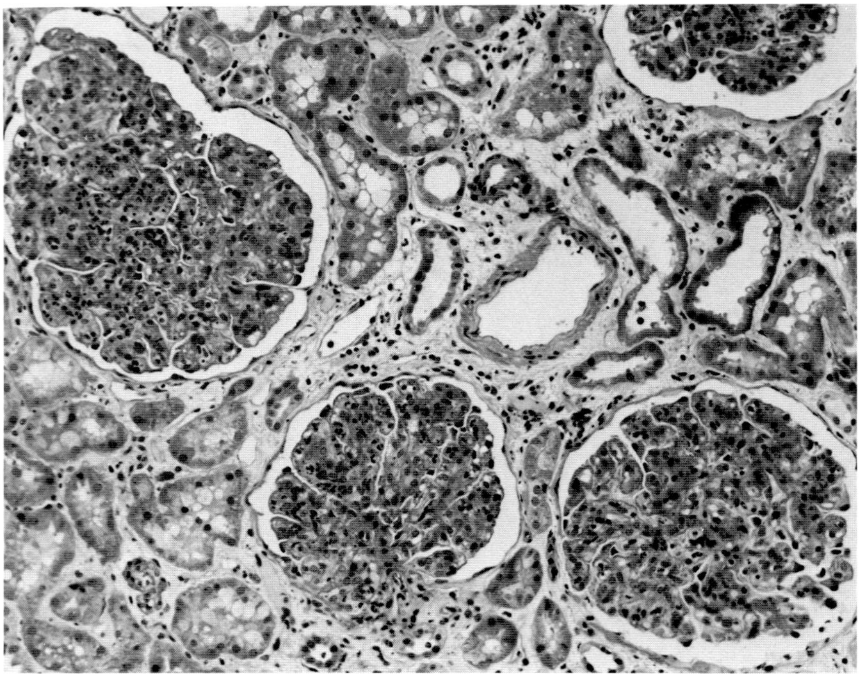

FIG. 5-1. *Three glomeruli showing diffuse intracapillary hypercellularity with closure of all the glomerular capillaries. The glomeruli are all increased in size and cellularity. H&E;* $\times$ *160.*

the subepithelial deposits ("humps") noted by electron microscopy. It is important to study all renal biopsies with the oil-immersion lens and the trichrome stain because these small deposits may be overlooked on casual examination with the high-dry objective alone. Although the glomerulonephritis is diffuse (involving all or almost all glomeruli equally), there may be lesser focal and segmental change in some glomeruli (Fig. 5-8).

In some patients there may be crescent formation [124*a*, 157,315,393,427] and/or early adhesions (synechiae) (Fig. 5-9). In a few patients the crescent formation is so prominent that the term *crescentic glomerulonephritis* may be used. Bowman's space also may contain erythrocytes; this is evidence in a percutaneous renal biopsy that the hematuria is caused by glomerular bleeding. Polymorphonuclear leukocytes also may be noted in Bowman's space.

CELL TYPES. There is still considerable controversy over the type of cell leading to the glomerular hypercellularity. The old term *proliferative glomerulonephritis* would indicate that the increased cellularity is restricted to native glomerular cells, either endocapillary cells (endothelial and/or mesangial) or extracapillary cells (parietal cells). However, recent evidence has suggested that much of the glomerular hypercellularity (as well as the crescent formation in Bowman's space) is secondary to infiltrating monocytic cells from the peripheral circulation. Langhans [253,254] initially suggested that the major cause of the cellular increase in the glomerular tuft was a proliferation of endothelial cells. This concept was responsible for the designation *intracapillary glomerulonephritis* and has been championed by a number of authors [30, 31,114,212,302]. McGregor [302] supported the idea of proliferation of endothelial cells, but did

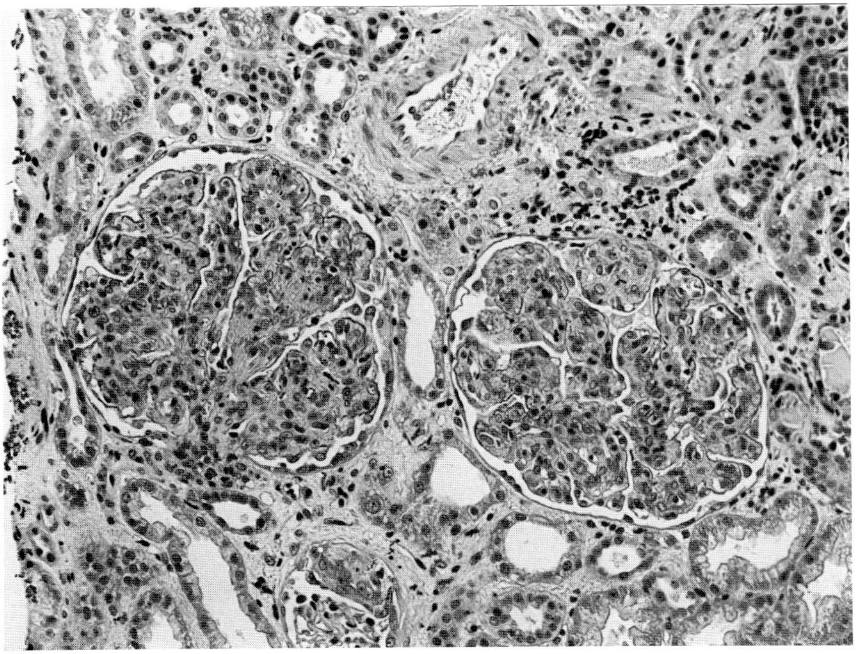

FIG. 5-2. *Two glomeruli with severe intracapillary hypercellularity and closure of the glomerular capillaries. Because of the increased cellularity within each lobule, there is an accentuation of the lobularity. H&E; ×200. (Courtesy of Dr. Edith Hawkins.)*

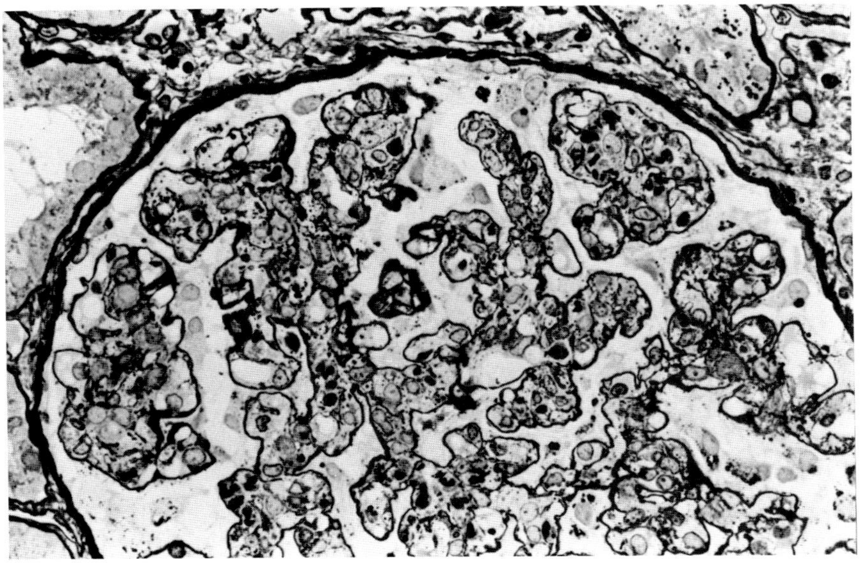

FIG. 5-3. *Silver impregnation of a glomerulus from a patient with acute poststreptococcal glomerulonephritis. Note that all the hypercellularity is confined within the glomerular capillaries (intracapillary hypercellularity). There is only a slight increase in silver-positive mesangial matrix fibrils. Jones silver methenamine; ×400.*

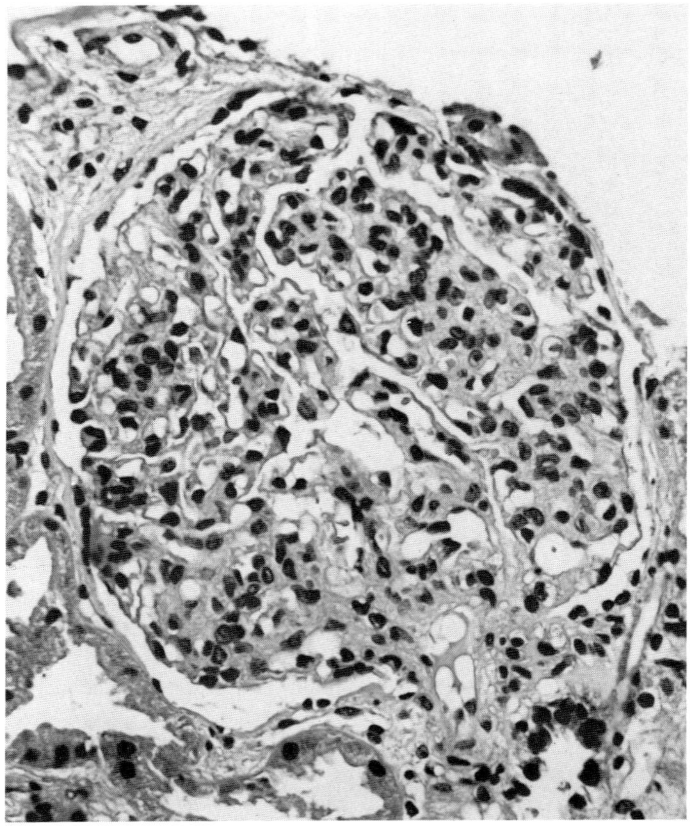

FIG. 5-4. *Renal biopsy from a 24-year-old woman with acute poststreptococcal glomerulonephritis. The glomerulus shows a broadening of the lobules, increase in cellularity with moderate numbers of neutrophils, and reduction of the capillary lumens. Complete clinical recovery took place in a period of weeks. H&E; ×400.*

not deny a role for monocytes in acute glomerulonephritis. Jennings and Earle [212] favored the notion that hypercellularity was due to native intraglomerular cells because of the presence of mitotic figures in "cells inside and attached to the glomerular capillary basement membrane (by definition, endothelial cells). . . ." These authors also used electron microscopy to strengthen their view, and described cells—in what they considered the resolving phases of the disease process—in which inclusions of electron-dense material resembling glomerular basement membrane were seen; they stated that such inclusions were not seen in mononuclear inflammatory cells [212]. This argument, however, did not resolve the question over which endocapillary cells (mesangial and/or endothelial) were participating in the proliferation. The newly described Ia-bearing mesangial cell [415,416] also could conceivably play a role in hypercellularity, but few studies in man have been forthcoming.

Jones [214–217] suggested that polymorphonuclear leukocytes appeared at an early stage in the mesangial regions, followed by mononuclear cells,

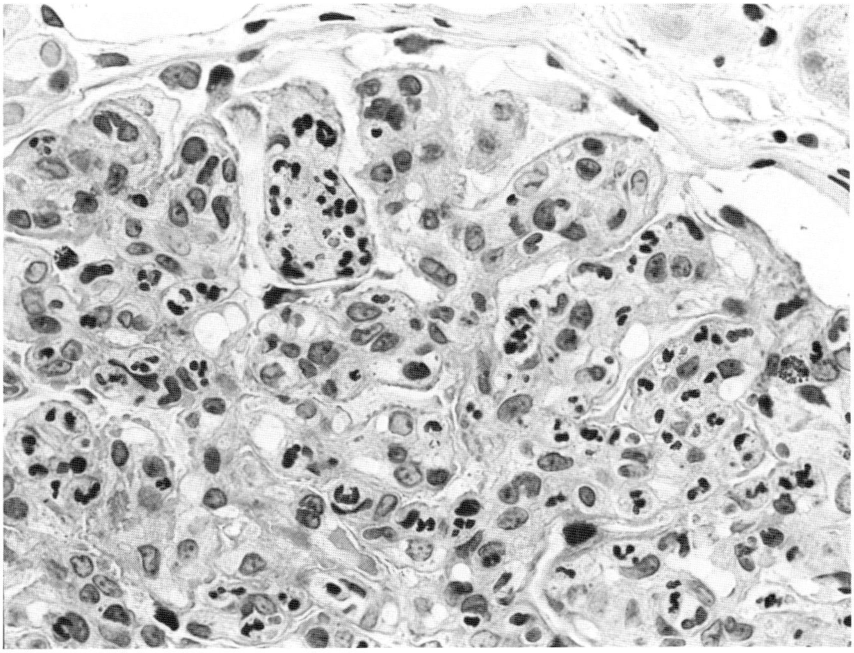

Fig. 5-5. *Acute diffuse intracapillary glomerulonephritis with considerable infiltration of the glomerulus by neutrophils. This "exudative" change is not uncommon in acute postinfectious glomerulonephritis. H&E; ×650. (Courtesy of Drs. William Murphy and Lillian Gaber.)*

which later were dominant. The contribution by endothelial cells to the hypercellularity was considered negligible. Using similar techniques to those of Jones (i.e., thin sectioning), Grishman and Churg [169] agreed that the major changes were in the mesangium; they described proliferation of mesangial cells but did not commit themselves as to the nature of the cells. Many other investigators have mentioned the great difficulty in distinguishing between endothelial and mesangial cells; for some time even the actual existence of the mesangial cell distinct from a deep endothelial cell was debated [107,270].

Experimental studies also have contributed to the concept that mononuclear phagocytes appear in the glomerular tuft in various forms of experimentally induced glomerulonephritis [59,60,76, 77,191,206,256,290,291,415,416,451]. Although most of these studies utilized models of Masugi nephritis and Habu snake venom, some did use the acute serum sickness models in the rabbit [191, 206]. Monocytes were demonstrated in this last model of acute glomerulonephritis by Hunsicker et al. [206] and by Holdsworth et al. [191] using electron microscopy and staining for nonspecific esterase. Thus it appears that bone marrow–derived mononuclear cells play a significant part of the hypercellularity noted in the glomeruli of certain experimental diseases. In human studies using staining for nonspecific esterase and electron microscopy, it has been recorded that monocytes are identified in less than half the biopsies of acute glomerulonephritis examined, especially in the early stages of the disease [317,318]. Specimens with mesangial hypercellularity but less exudative change had fewer esterase-positive cells. There

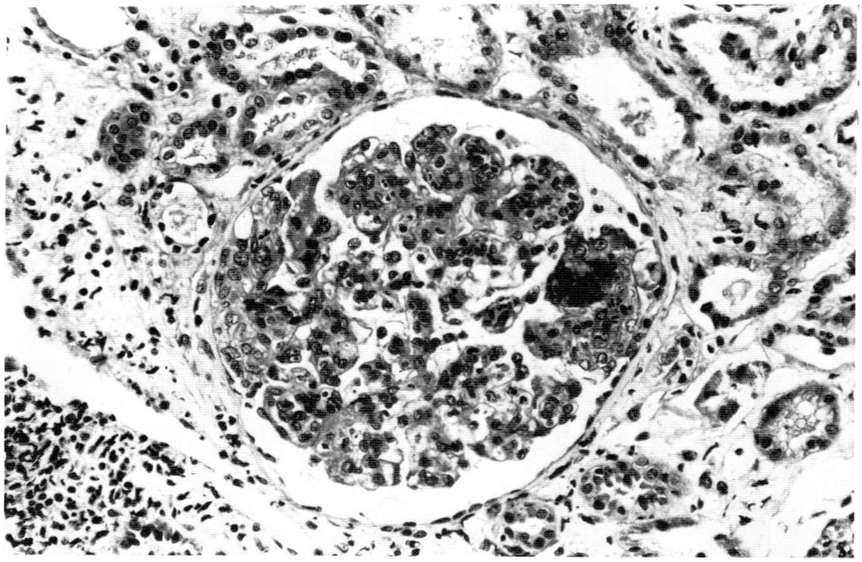

FIG. 5-6. *A glomerulus from a patient with classic acute poststreptococcal glomerulonephritis. Note the focal intracapillary region of necrosis at approximately 3 o'clock. This is an unusual feature in acute postinfectious glomerulonephritis. H&E; ×400. (Courtesy of Drs. William Murphy and Lillian Gaber.)*

was a good correlation between the degree of monocytic infiltration, polymorph involvement, and hypercellularity. It was concluded that early glomerular hypercellularity was due to an influx of blood borne cells but at a later stage was caused mainly by proliferation of intrinsic glomerular cells [292,293]. Magil et al. [292,293] demonstrated glomerular intraluminal monocytes that correlated positively with the presence of deposits. They also described dissection of the glomerular endothelium from the capillary wall adjacent to deposits by the monocytes. Studies utilizing α_1-antitrypsin as a marker of monocytes revealed similar findings [255]. Ferrario et al. [129] showed that the degree of proteinuria correlated well with the degree of glomerular mononuclear-cell infiltration. It should be noted that the greatest degree of glomerular mononuclear infiltration appears to be found in essential cryoglobulinemia.

However, ultrastructural studies in experimental immune complex glomerulonephritis do show proliferation of endogenous glomerular cells of endothelial and mesangial type [76,77,112]. Several investigators have suggested that infiltrating mononuclear cells and their soluble factors (mediators) can be responsible for increasing the growth and proliferation of endothelial and mesangial cells [89,112]. On the other hand, mesangial cells may regulate the physiology of the infiltrating mononuclear cells and modify the local immune response [287]. Sano [402] and Striker et al. [451] have shown that much of the glomerular tuft hypercellularity in experimental serum sickness models is due to infiltrating macrophages of bone marrow origin.

The controversy over the nature of the cells contributing to glomerular tuft hypercellularity is somewhat reminiscent of the one concerning the type of cell comprising the glomerular crescent. The exact cell type involved may relate to timing, with macrophages appearing early and native cellular proliferation occurring later. Schiffer and Mi-

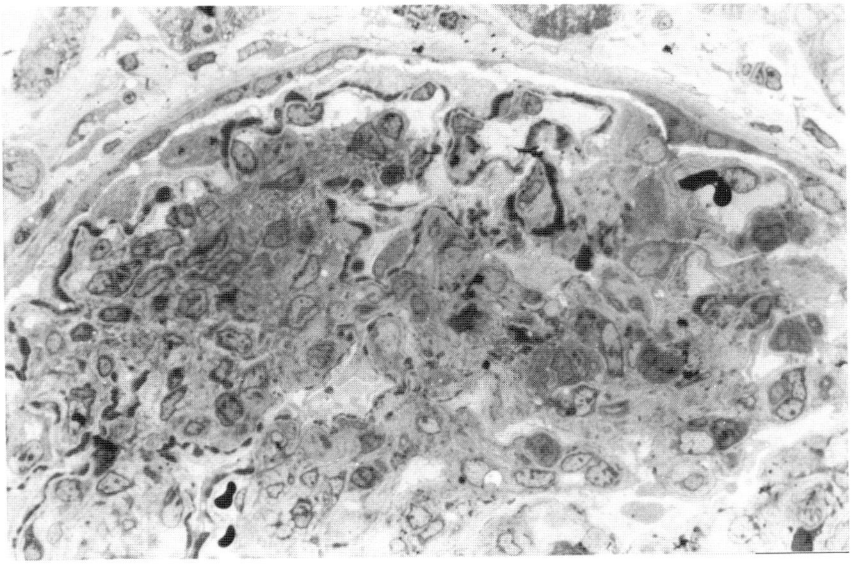

Fig. 5-7. *High magnification of a plastic section from a renal biopsy with acute postinfectious (poststreptococcal) glomerulonephritis. Note the osmiophilic (dense) deposits along the glomerular capillary walls (best noted from 10 to 1 o'clock) at the periphery of the glomerular capillaries. Although this patient had "classic" poststreptococcal glomerulonephritis, the glomerular subepithelial deposits were quite large, numerous, and confluent. Toluidine blue stain of Epon-embedded section; ×600. (Courtesy of Dr. Edith Hawkins.)*

chael [413], utilizing Y bodies as markers for male cells in renal transplants between males and females, noted that in grafts that developed glomerular mesangial hyperplasia (presumably as a recurrence of the original disease in the host), it was not possible to identify bone marrow–derived mononuclear cells despite the demonstration of Y-body–positive extrarenal cells in crescents and the interstitial infiltration. This suggested that the hypercellularity represented endogenous mesangial proliferation. Of course, the situation studied is somewhat different from "naturally occurring" acute glomerulonephritis [182].

There is little information at this time regarding the immunophenotyping of inflammatory cells in acute diffuse proliferative glomerulonephritis [64,198]. Cameron et al. [73] observed the presence of T cells and macrophages in proliferative glomerulonephritis without crescents. There was a direct correlation between the numbers of T lymphocytes and of macrophages. Parra et al. [348] studied the cell populations in glomeruli of patients with acute poststreptococcal glomerulonephritis using monoclonal antibodies and indirect immunofluorescence. They found infiltration of the glomeruli by monocytes, granulocytes, and lymphoid cells; T cells were noted adjacent to Bowman's capsule. $CD4^+$ (helper/inducer) lymphocytes were noted in the glomeruli early in the course of the disease, whereas $CD8^+$ (cytotoxic/suppressor) cells were noted later. The role of the monocyte in crescent formation is described in Chapter 9.

Polymorphonuclear leukocytes can be found, although large numbers of these cells do not indicate a poor outcome. The leukotactic properties of complement have been demonstrated; Lewy et al. [270] noted a case with predominant polymorpho-

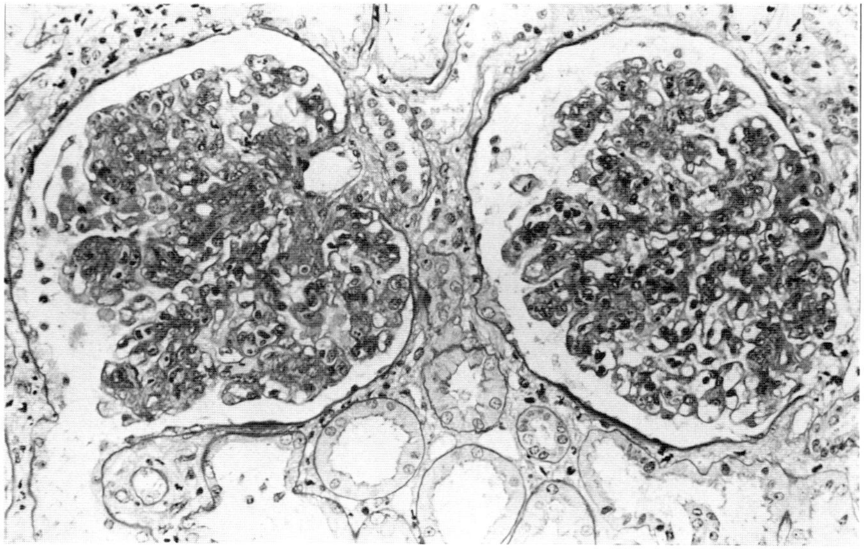

A

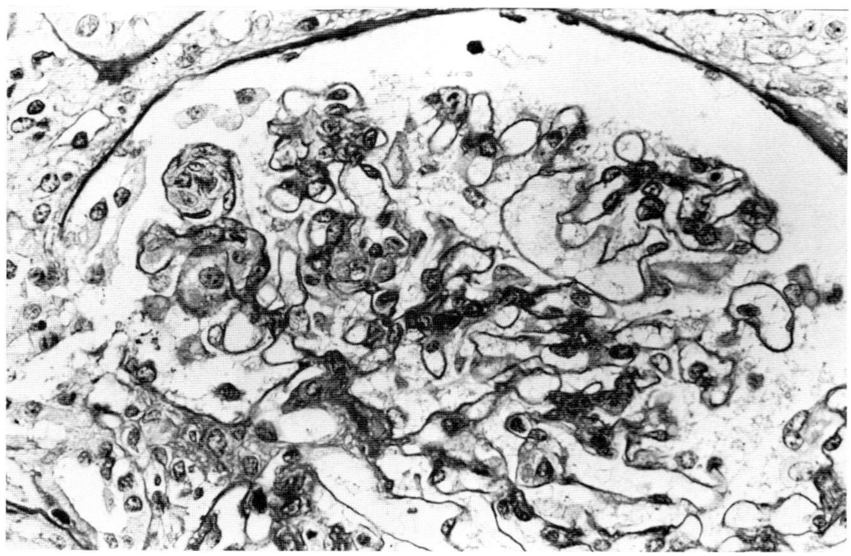

B

FIG. 5-8. *Renal biopsy from a patient with acute poststreptococcal glomerulonephritis. (A) Most of the glomeruli showed global severe intracapillary hypercellularity (acute diffuse intracapillary glomerulonephritis). H&E; ×250. (B) An occasional glomerulus showed only mild and/or segmental intracapillary hypercellularity (upper left). Note that most of the glomerular capillaries are patent. Jones silver methenamine; ×400. (Courtesy of Dr. Marc Stegman.)*

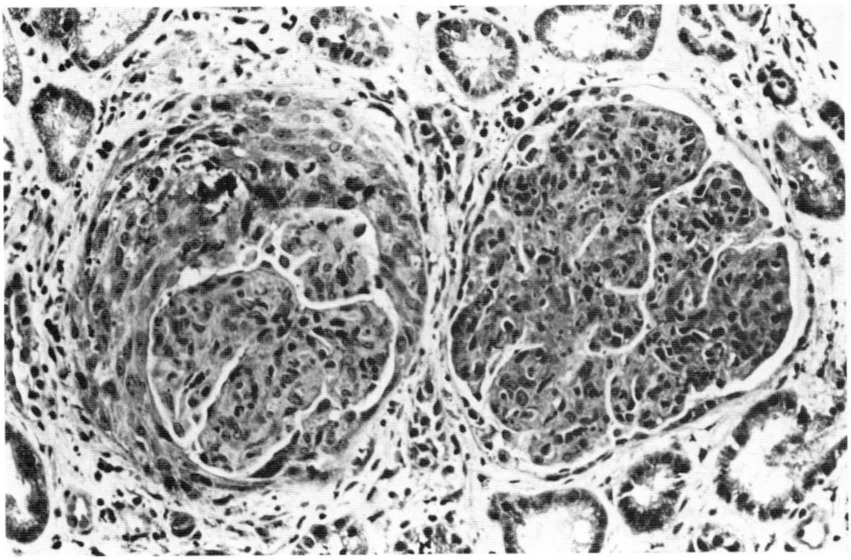

Fig. 5-9. *Two glomeruli, one of which shows a crescent. Note that both show a global increase in cellularity. H&E; ×250. (Courtesy of Drs. Srinivasan Rajaraman and Tito Cavallo.)*

nuclear leukocytic reaction in which there were large numbers of glomerular subepithelial humps; these authors commented that in other cases the greatest numbers of polymorphonuclear leukocytes were found when there were large numbers of humps.

Other Mesangial Changes. Other mesangial abnormalities have been noted. MacCallum [286] was particularly impressed by changes occurring in the mesangium, a structure he termed the *intercapillary space.* He considered that there was an exudation into this space and suggested that this exudate could be organized during the transition to chronic glomerulonephritis. He spoke of an intercapillary rather than an intracapillary glomerulonephritis, a distinction that was quite controversial at the time. The concept of involvement of the mesangium was further extended by Jones [214–217], who in a study of serial sections and with the use of thin sections focused his attention on changes occurring in this structure. Initially, there was edema and enlargement; in glomerulonephritis with scarring there was an increase in the fibers of the mesangial regions. McGregor [302] noted mesangial fibrils or fibers between proliferating endothelial cells and leukocytes in a high proportion of cases. In those cases which progressed rather than resolved, the fibers increased in number and size, finally forming a hyalin mass. Bell [31] suggested that these fibers could be formed by a splitting of the inner part of the glomerular capillary wall; he described how they progressed to form a hyalin mass in the center of the lobule in cases of latent chronic glomerulonephritis. All these observed findings were similar and the confusion lay only in the individual author's concept of the structure of the glomerulus. McGregor [302] and Bell [30,31] believed that there was no intercapillary space (mesangium), and what they referred to as "intracapillary fibers" were in all likelihood in the intercapillary space or mesangium. These fibers in the mesangial region gradually increase in cases failing to resolve, and although the exact evolution is controversial, they apparently give rise to centrilobular hyalin nodules. By ultrastructural study, these lesions consist of basement membrane–like material or mesangial matrix. McCluskey and Baldwin [299] suggested that lesser degrees of change might resolve.

Several probes have shown increases in some naturally occurring substances in the glomeruli in postinfectious glomerulonephritis. Actomyosin has been shown to be mildly increased in the mesangial regions [409], but the significance of this finding is unclear. Likewise, fibronectin has been demonstrated in a similar site [408,490]. This protein is present in the normal mesangium and is significantly increased in a variety of conditions associated with mesangial increase [276,356]. Mosquera and Rodriguez-Iturbe [326] demonstrated glomerular binding sites for fluoresceinated peanut agglutination (PNA) lectin in renal biopsies showing acute poststreptococcal glomerulonephritis. PNA has specificity for galactosyl radicals that are exposed after sialic acid removal, as one would see with neuraminidase. These findings suggested to the authors that sialic acid–depleted material was present in glomeruli early in the course of the glomerulonephritic process.

Renal biopsies in patients with minimal urinary changes have been performed (usually in prospective studies) and show differing results. Some find no obvious abnormalities except for a "proximalization" of the parietal epithelium of Bowman's capsule [207]. Increased cellularity of the glomeruli also has been noted, as have changes indistinguishable from characteristic acute diffuse proliferative poststreptococcal glomerulonephritis [5, 35,87,115,166,203,222,224].

RESOLVING GLOMERULONEPHRITIS. In renal biopsies taken several weeks after the clinical onset of disease or in those patients in whom repeated biopsies are performed, there is a diffuse cellular increase in the mesangial regions of the glomeruli; the glomerular capillaries are now patent and the capillary walls appear thin and delicate [393,469] (Figs. 5-10 and 5-11). It appears that some degree of resolution of the hypercellular process has taken place, and the number of polymorphonuclear leukocytes is decreased [212]. Mesangial hypercellularity appears to persist for many months in patients who eventually undergo complete resolution of their glomerular lesion [182,393]. An old term for this morphologic picture is *chronic latent glomerulonephritis*. However, caution needs to be exercised for two reasons. First, an unusually thick paraffin section may give the false appearance of diffuse mesangial hypercellularity or, more likely, cause one to interpret it as diffuse proliferative glomerulonephritis. Second, a great many cases termed *chronic latent glomerulonephritis* are not resolving/resolved acute postinfectious glomerulonephritis, in my opinion, but rather a nonspecific histologic pattern associated with a variety of renal injuries unrelated to previous infections [85,86, 87,364].

It has been considered that patients with well-documented poststreptococcal glomerulonephritis who show a mesangial proliferative picture on a subsequent biopsy appear to have a worse renal prognosis than those with typical resolving streptococcal glomerulonephritis. Patients with isolated C3 mesangial deposits in association with a mesangial proliferative glomerulonephritis may actually have a poststreptococcal glomerulonephritis, but there is little proof of this in most patients. It is likely that several entities may show this pattern, since the kidney responds in a limited fashion to many different injurious stimuli. Complete morphologic resolution often occurs following acute poststreptococcal glomerulonephritis [392,469].

Tubules

The tubular changes are not as pronounced as those involving the glomeruli [182]. When proteinuria is present, there may be hyalin droplets (protein reabsorption droplets—phagolysosomes) in the proximal convoluted tubular epithelium. Erythrocytes may be seen in the lumen of the tubules, and they are sometimes mixed with eosinophilic cast-like material. Polymorphonuclear leukocytes also can be present in the lumen, especially in the first portions of the proximal tubules; this finding is most commonly seen in patients with severe exudation or infiltration of polymorphonuclear leukocytes in the glomeruli. In a few patients, polymorphonuclear leukocytes can be seen between the tubular basement membrane and the overlying tubular epithelial cells (Fig. 5-

12). Hutt et al. [207] described "advanced focal degeneration" of the tubules, more commonly noted in the distal tubules than in the proximal tubules. This consisted of dilatation of the distal convoluted tubules with degeneration of the epithelium and sometimes breaks in the tubular basement membranes. There was interstitial inflammation, as well as some flattening of the epithelium and focal dilatation of the proximal tubules. These authors suggested that the lesions were not due to ischemia but instead were secondary to a process similar to the one responsible for the glomerular lesion. Watt et al. [486] described a fine vacuolization of the proximal tubular epithelial cells; with serial renal biopsies, these changes resolved, the dilatation being the slowest to recover. There was no apparent relationship between the morphologic tubular changes and Tm_{PAH}.

In the most florid cases of acute glomerulonephritis with extensive crescent formation, there may be tubular atrophy and loss, as well as tubulitis (inflammatory cells between the tubular basement membranes and the tubular epithelium, or within the tubular epithelium). Morel-Maroger et al. [322] described a severe example of acute postinfectious glomerulonephritis with tubular damage that was accompanied by anti-tubular basement membrane antibodies. Immunofluorescence demonstrated a linear pattern with anti-IgG along most of the tubular basement membranes; C3 was demonstrated only focally. There was a pronounced inflammatory-cell infiltrate in the interstitium.

Interstitium

The degree of interstitial involvement is variable. In fact, one of the first demonstrations of interstitial nephritis in any renal disease was by Councilman [90] in 1897 in association with scarlatina. The interstitial areas may show edema with separation of the tubules from one another. Scattered foci of inflammatory cells, made up of mixtures of polymorphonuclear leukocytes, mononuclear cells, and lymphocytes, are sometimes present. There may occasionally be a severe interstitial mononuclear-cell infiltration [428]. Scattered regions of interstitial fibrosis also may occur. Usually, however, the interstitial changes are not remarkable or severe. As noted earlier, interstitial changes may be found in relation to tubular changes [207,243]. Bohle et al. [47], using morphometric methods on tissue sections, showed that the level of serum creatinine correlated with the increase in interstitial volume. They explained this on the basis of a reduction of renal blood flow, and hence glomerular filtration rate, brought about by compression of the postglomerular vasculature.

Blood Vessels

The arteries and arterioles generally do not show many changes. In older patients, preexisting vascular abnormalities, such as arterial and arteriolar sclerosis, may be seen, and according to Gallo et al. [150], these may accentuate and lead to increased renal parenchymal injury. Arteritis has been described [46], but obviously in such cases polyarteritis must be excluded. I have seen one case typical of acute postinfectious glomerulonephritis with a necrotizing arteritis. There are other accounts of arteritis [139,211] as well, but these are rare. Heptinstall [182] noted it twice in well-documented cases of poststreptococcal glomerulonephritis, one of these being in the crescentic form of the disease. Fibrinoid necrosis of the arterioles may occur and is usually associated with severe hypertension.

ELECTRON MICROSCOPIC FINDINGS

There are many reports of the ultrastructural findings in acute glomerulonephritis [107,128,135,184, 212,237,240, 270, 310, 436, 438, 453, 454, 460]. Many of the findings merely confirm what has long been noted at the light microscopic level, that is, increased numbers of endocapillary and infiltrative inflammatory cells in the glomerular tuft. There is swelling of glomerular cells (both endothelial and mesangial) with closure of the capillary lumens by the increased numbers of cells and/or swelling of the native glomerular cells. The glomerular basement membranes generally appear normal in contour, thickness, and texture, although patchy thickening may occasionally be noted. There may be widening of the lamina rara interna by subendothelial electron-lucent "fluff" or fibrillar/finely granular electron-dense material.

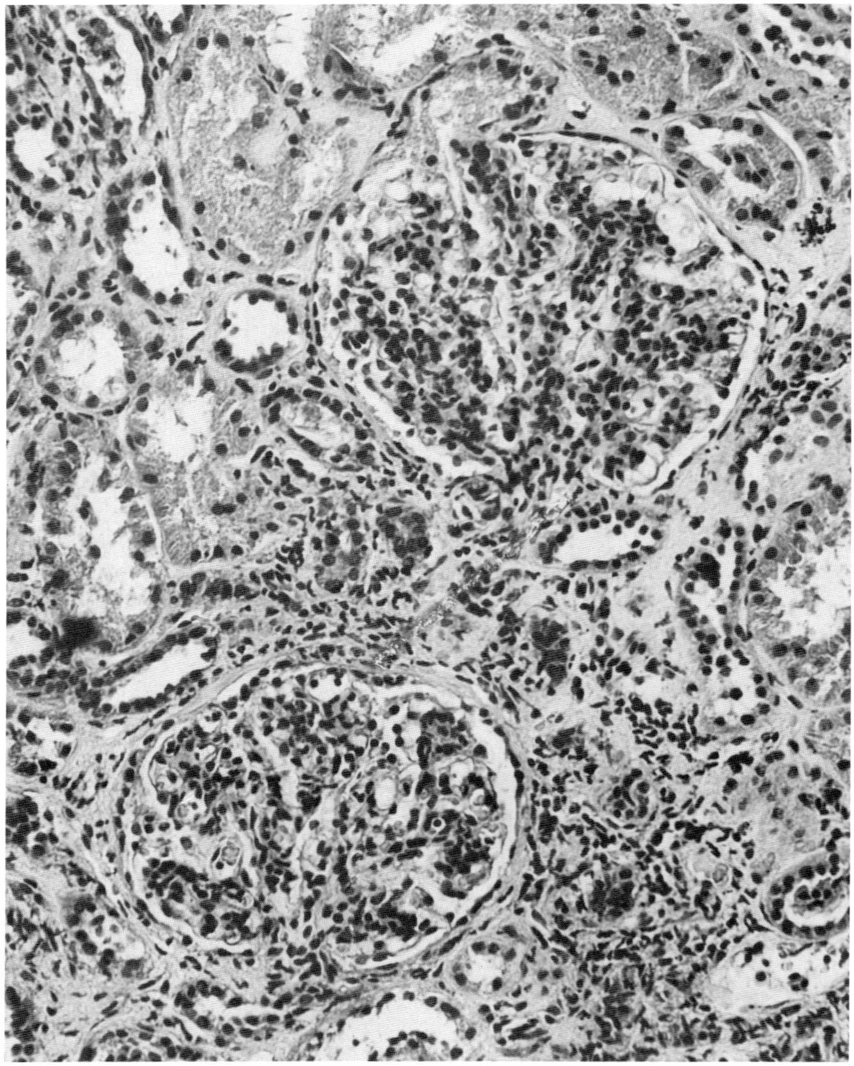

A

FIG. 5-10. *(A) Two glomeruli from a 42-year-old man with acute glomerulonephritis. Considerable cellular increase has occurred and appears to be mainly centrilobular. (B) Second biopsy from same patient taken after 6 months. Considerable resolution has taken place, with a decrease in cells and development of patency of the capillary lumens. Hypercellularity persists in the mesangium, however. H&E; (A) ×250; (B) ×500.*

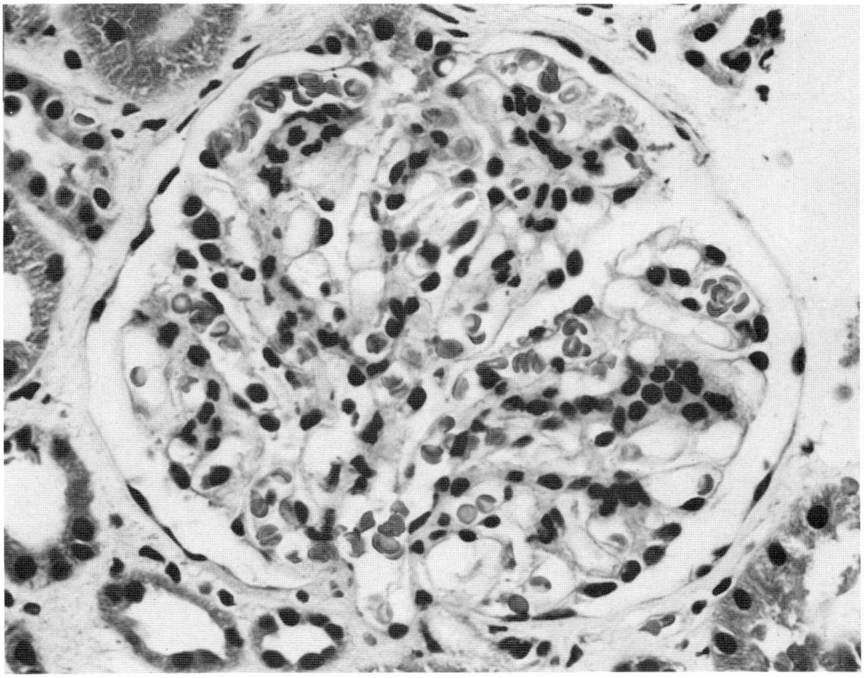

B

Fig. 5-10. (continued)

The outer layer of the glomerular basement membrane may show "scalloping" or irregularity of the lamina rara externa and lamina densa. The GBM may contain lucent areas; these may represent resolving deposits, which will be described and discussed later. Often the glomerular endothelium is disrupted and denuded, with polymorphonuclear leukocytes directly adjacent to the denuded glomerular basement membranes.

The most consistent classic diagnostic change is the presence of glomerular subepithelial electron-dense "immune type" deposits, often referred to as "humps" (Figs. 5-13 and 5-14). They are especially abundant in the first few weeks of acute postinfectious glomerulonephritis, and they decrease in number after this time. They are usually less than 1 μm wide and long, but they sometimes measure up to 3 μm wide and 6 μm long [283]. In the study of Lewy et al. [270], two patients had quite elongated cigar-shaped glomerular subepithelial humps; these patients also had the nephrotic syndrome. The subepithelial humps are sometimes separated from the lamina densa by a zone of translucence that is continuous with the lamina rara externa; on other occasions they merge with the underlying lamina densa. The deposits often bulge or project toward the cytoplasm of the overlying glomerular visceral epithelial cell, which often shows effacement of foot processes just above the deposit. There is frequent condensation of the microfilaments (possibly myofilaments) at the base of the effaced glomerular visceral epithelial cell adjacent to the hump. The electron density of the deposits is variable, and the granularity may range from fine to coarse [82] (Figs. 5-15 and 5-16). Although there is no direct correlation between the fine ultrastructural appearance of the deposit and the clinical or nonultrastructural morphologic find-

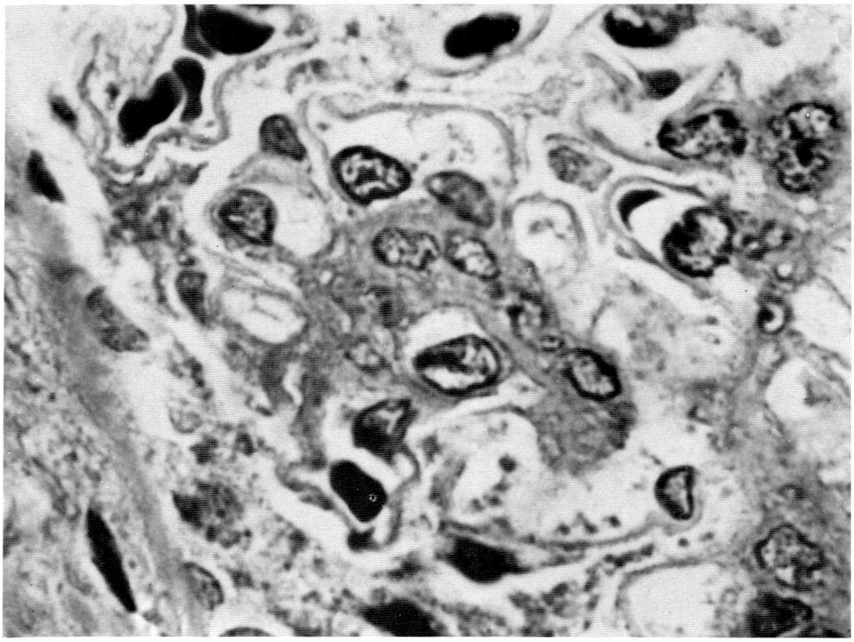

FIG. 5-11. *Resolving glomerulonephritis showing cells still remaining in the mesangium. Urine had become normal before the biopsy was taken. Heidenhain's connective-tissue stain on a 2-μm section; ×2370. (From Earle, D. P., and Jennings, R. B. In G. E. W. Wolstenholme and M. P. Cameron (Eds.), Ciba Foundation Symposium on Renal Biopsy: Clinical and Pathological Significance. Edinburgh: Churchill Livingstone, 1962.)*

ings, Tornroth et al. [460] have suggested that electron-lucent regions in the deposit may represent regions of resolution.

The deposits are usually plentiful, discrete, and most commonly found on that part of the GBM overlying the mesangial regions [182]. At times the subepithelial deposits may be confluent along short stretches of the basement membranes. Similar discrete electron-dense "immune type" deposits may be seen in the lamina densa, the subendothelial regions [135,240,270,393,436,438,460] (Fig. 5-17), and even occasionally along Bowman's capsule [270]. Glomerular subendothelial deposits are noted in those patients with inconspicuous changes in the urine; they tend to appear early in the course of the disease and generally disappear by 6 weeks after the acute episode. Although the glomerular subepithelial hump is the most characteristic lesion by electron microscopy, similar deposits are seen in a variety of other glomerular disorders, such as membranous glomerulonephritis, membranoproliferative glomerulonephritis (types I, II, and III), systemic lupus erythematosus (SLE), and Schönlein-Henoch syndrome.

The mesangial regions contain large numbers of cells whose identity is often elusive. In addition to native mesangial cells, there appear to be varying quantities of infiltrating inflammatory cells from the peripheral circulation. Polymorphonuclear leukocytes are the easiest cells to identify in the glomerular mesangial regions and may be extensive in the exudative form of glomerulonephritis. There may be a mild increase in the amount of mesangial-matrix–basement membrane–like material, probably corresponding to the fibers seen by several au-

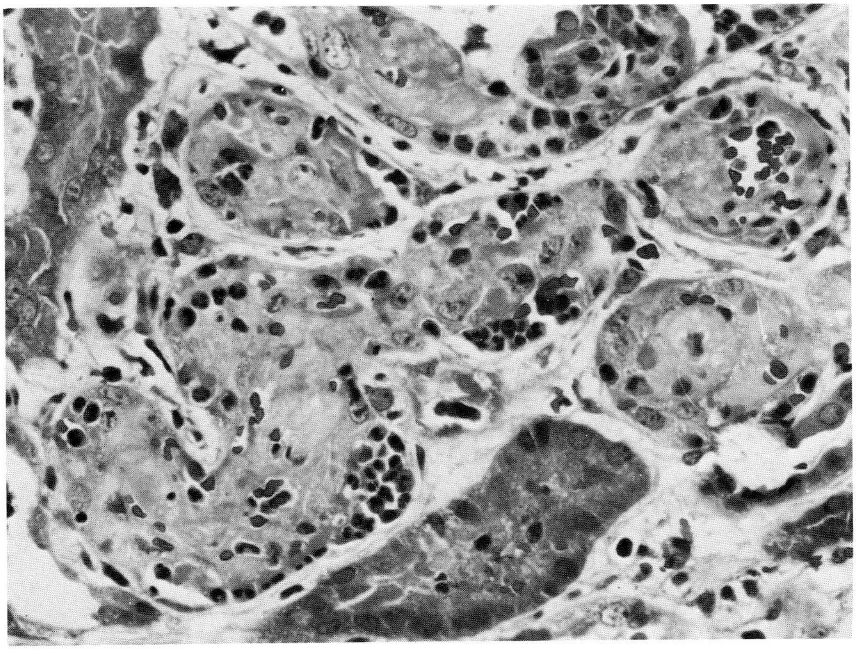

FIG. 5-12. *Proximal convoluted tubules with neutrophils situated between tubular basement membranes and tubular epithelium. This biopsy showed postinfectious glomerulonephritis, crescents, and adhesions. The patient made a complete recovery. H&E; ×400.*

thors noted earlier by light microscopy [217,302]. Irregular fibrillar amorphous masses may be seen in the mesangial regions [128]. Discrete, electron-dense, "immune type" deposits also may be seen in the mesangial regions in some cases of classic post-infectious glomerulonephritis [393,436,438]. Bowman's space may contain debris, fibrin, large epithelial cells, crescents, erythrocytes, and polymorphonuclear leukocytes.

During the recovery phase (based on serially biopsied patients), the glomerular subepithelial humps tend to disappear quite rapidly (usually within 6 weeks of the clinical onset of disease) [184]. Sometimes they persist for longer periods of time [240], but the clinical course in such cases is not clear. The fate of the glomerular subepithelial deposits has been studied by Tornroth [460], who has shown that the electron density (osmiophilia) of the deposits decreases with time so that translucent or electron-lucent regions are formed. Empty spaces can be seen that presumably collapse and are replaced by the overlying glomerular visceral epithelium. The deposits may disappear by simple dissolution and/or by removal by epithelial vesicles. Glomerular intramembranous electron-lucent regions were seen in later biopsies (after 1 month), and in some cases these regions protruded toward the epithelium and were covered on that side by a thick layer of basement membrane–like material. Other deposits were found deeper in the lamina densa, giving it a somewhat mottled appearance [460]. Kobayashi et al. [240] showed that the deposits became buried in the GBM and also acquired a fine granularity with an electron density less than that of the original humps. Glomerular subendothelial deposits that were present early disappeared with time [240,460]. The GBM became irregular in thickness and contour. In-

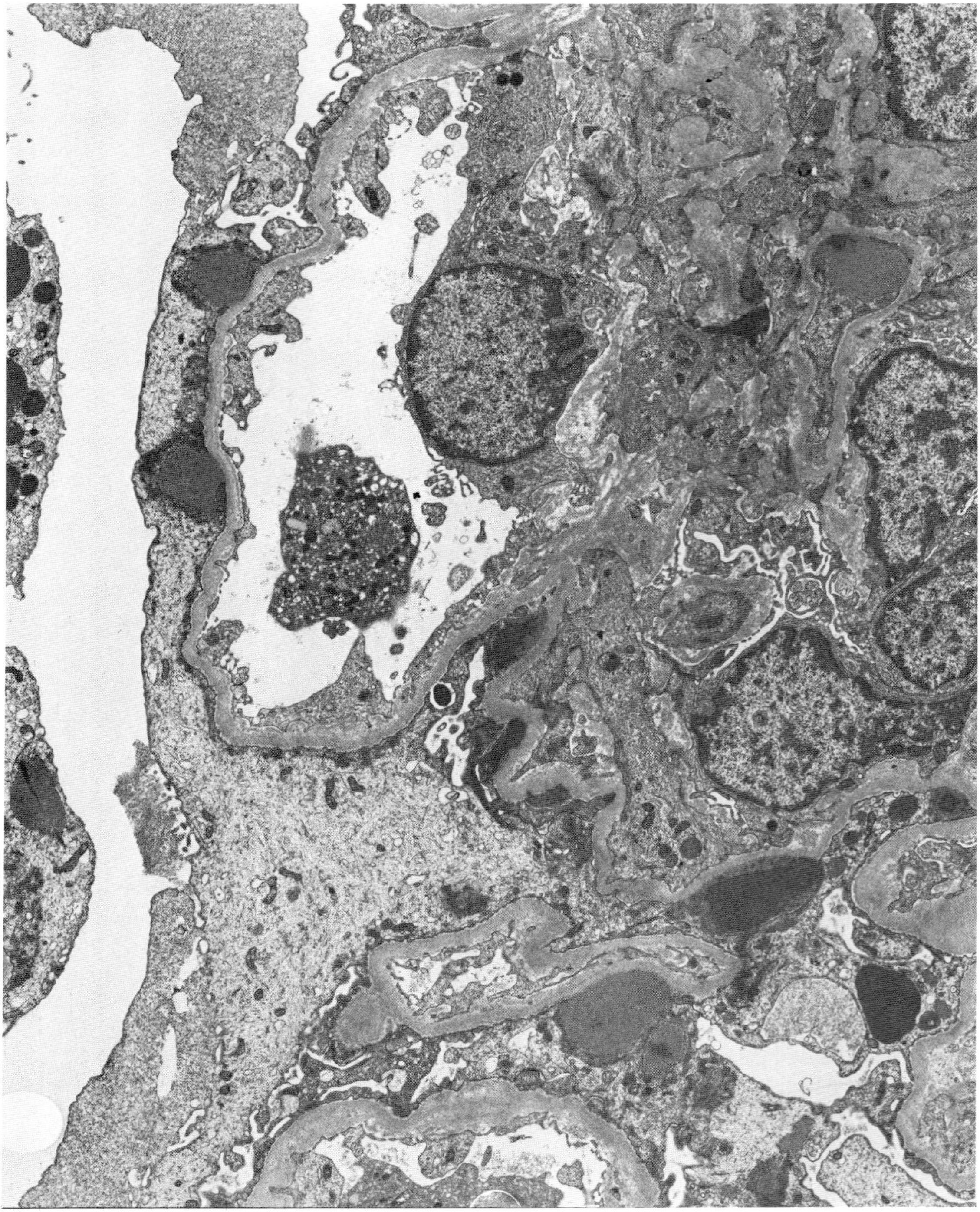

creased cellularity may persist in the mesangial regions for many months, even in those patients in whom the clinical picture and urinary sediment have returned to normal. In patients who have persistent proteinuria, increased mesangial matrix is often found. It appears that more subepithelial humps are noted in those patients with a severe, protracted clinical picture than in those with immediate clinical recovery [240]. Size of the deposits does not seem to correlate with clinical course or outcome [182].

Ultrastructural studies in prospective series of patients with minimal urinary findings have shown either a lack of electron-dense deposits [115] or glomerular subepithelial [203,222,224] or subendothelial deposits [203,224]; in one case the deposits were confined to the glomerular subendothelial zone [166]. As Heptinstall has indicated [182], the position of electron-dense deposits is of interest in this group of patients. While glomerular subendothelial deposits may be seen in the classic form of acute poststreptococcal glomerulonephritis, they are not so plentiful nor so consistent as glomerular subepithelial deposits. In the patients referred to earlier, however, the glomerular subendothelial deposits were conspicuous, and in one patient, they were the only deposits noted [166]. The pathogenetic mechanism(s) responsible for this are uncertain, but much discussion has ensued [182].

In another series, the ultrastructural findings in patients with subclinical glomerulonephritis were studied [398]. The only biopsies in which glomerular subepithelial deposits were noted were from cases that were severe by light microscopy. Combined glomerular intramembranous and mesangial deposits were seen in one of these two patients with severe light microscopic changes; the other patient with these deposits had only mild disease by light microscopy. Isolated glomerular intramembranous deposits were seen in two additional cases, both of which were mild in their light microscopic appearance. No deposits were identified in the remaining seven cases studied by electron microscopy.

Focal disruptions or gaps of the GBM have been identified [53,298,447], and rarely, mononuclear cells and erythrocytes can be seen migrating through these gaps [298]. Usually, however, the gaps are filled by glomerular endocapillary and visceral epithelial cells. Scanning electron microscopic studies following the selective removal of glomerular visceral epithelial cells by a sequence of lytic and solubilization procedures by Bonsib et al. [53] are of interest. The changes seen in acute postinfectious glomerulonephritis are illustrated in Figure 5-18. There are several distinct crater-like GBM formations (Fig. 5-18*B*); these are empty, reflecting the solubilization of the subepithelial immune complexes. The craters are uniform in size and shape. Every glomerulus studied contained at least several craters, which were located in various sites within the glomerular tuft. The case from which Figure 5-18C was prepared was unique by virtue of the presence of subepithelial humps several years following the acute nephritic episode and the large size of GBM craters.

IMMUNOFLUORESCENCE FINDINGS

Immunofluorescence studies have been performed by a large number of investigators [2,128,135,301,304, 310,311,323,324,419,435–439,463,470,507]. Classically, in biopsies taken early in the clinical course (first 2 or 3 weeks) of the illness, small, finely granular deposits are noted along the glomerular capillary walls following treatment with anti-IgG and often anti-C3 fluoresceinated antisera (Figs. 5-19 and 5-20). The pattern is granular ("lumpy bumpy"), although it may not be as coarse as noted in patients with idiopathic membranous glomerulonephritis. These deposits may assume a linear pattern in some areas owing to the confluence of deposits. It is highly likely that the granular deposits correspond to the glomerular

Fig. 5-13. *Segment of a glomerulus from a patient with acute poststreptococcal glomerulonephritis. This electron micrograph shows a number of discrete electron-dense osmiophilic deposits in the subepithelial portions of the glomerular capillary walls. Some of the glomerular capillaries are narrowed or compressed, but one is patent. Uranyl acetate and lead citrate;* $\times 6930$. *(Courtesy of Drs. William Murphy and Lillian Gaber.)*

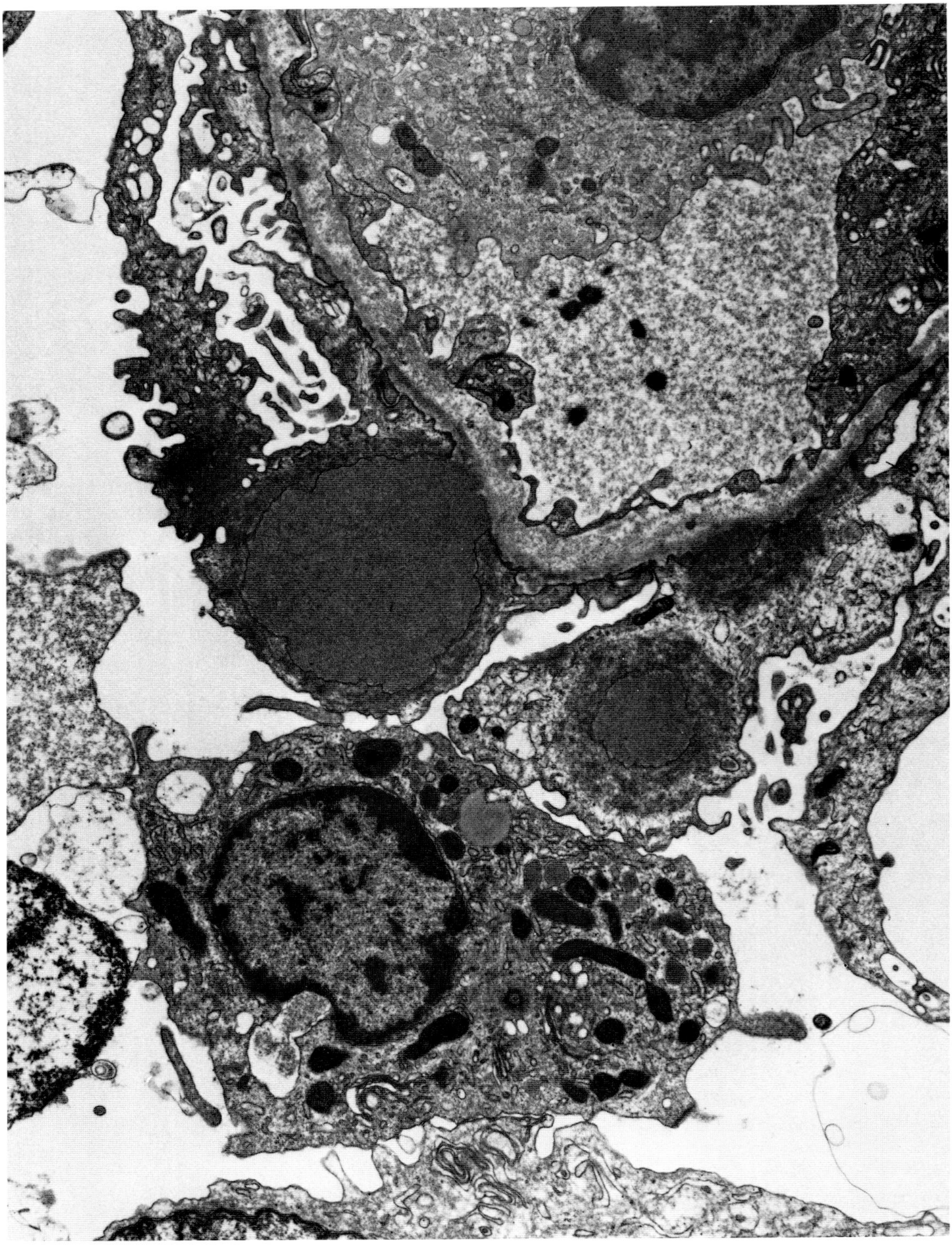

subepithelial deposits noted by electron microscopy, although not all authors are sure of this [68].

Recently, Sorger et al. [435–439] have described additional immunofluorescence patterns different from the classic picture. They noted three different patterns, called (1) the "garland" pattern, (Fig. 5-21), (2) the "starry sky" pattern (Fig. 5-22), and (3) the mesangial pattern (Fig. 5-23). The *garland pattern* is manifest by a discrete, more densely packed, and sometimes confluent heavy disposition of IgG and C3, probably corresponding to the numerous humps noted on the subepithelial side of the glomèrular capillary wall [437,438]; this pattern is most often seen in patients with acute glomerulonephritis in whom severe proteinuria (often with the nephrotic syndrome) is present (see Fig. 5-21). Other glomerular deposits are rare. In younger patients, both the clinical and morphologic findings usually regress after a month-long course; in older patients, both the clinical (proteinuria) and morphologic findings persist even after months. The *starry sky pattern* has a more irregular, finely granular pattern with the deposits (IgG, IgM, C3, IgA) being smaller and often situated on the GBM overlying the mesangial regions; this pattern was most commonly seen in early cases (see Fig. 5-22). Only a few large, typical humps were noted. This picture may turn into the *mesangial pattern,* characterized by a granular deposition of IgG and C3 (usually with predominance of C3). It seems to be most closely related to a resolving pattern (see Fig. 5-23). The deposits are generally noted in the stalk region of the glomerulus and are accompanied by mesangial hypercellularity. There is no evidence so far that different etiologic factors are responsible for these three subtypes [439]; the individual immune response of the host is likely to play a role in their genesis.

A diffuse granular pattern for IgG and usually C3 is also noted in patients with subclinical glomerulonephritis [2,310,323,324,470,507] and in those with minimal urinary changes [203].

Some authors have described more intense and more constant staining with anti-C3 than with anti-IgG [2,310,323,324,470,507]; some of these same authors have described the presence of C3 without any demonstrable IgG. Others have noted the combination of granular and patchy, interrupted linear staining along the glomerular capillary wall and in the mesangial regions [20,128, 135,310]. At times, there seems to be an exclusively patchy, interrupted linear pattern for C3 along GBMs close to the mesangium, as well as in the mesangium, with no staining for IgG [135, 310]. This interrupted linear pattern has been found most commonly either in patients in whom the initial renal biopsy was performed at a later stage than usual or in repeat biopsies [135,310]. C3 without the presence of IgG has been recorded in the mesangial areas with no capillary wall deposits [438]; this pattern also tends to be seen in patients who are biopsied later than usual (i.e., several weeks after the clinical onset of disease). Fish et al. [135] have advanced a variety of explanations as to why C3 is present in the absence of IgG. They suggested that there may have been covering of IgG by C3 that prevented its detection. Another explanation could be that C3 reaches detectable levels for the immunofluorescence technique while IgG remains below the threshold level. It was considered that the interrupted linear deposits of C3 in the absence of IgG could be the result of a direct toxic effect of the organism (i.e., streptococcus) on the glomerulus and that only a certain percentage of patients (especially those destined to develop severe acute nephritis) proceed to nodular deposits. Finally, these authors [135] raised the possibility that variations in streptococci causing skin infection—most patients reported had skin infections—are responsible, although it is well documented that C3 but not IgG can be found in patients with throat infections. A few patients with documented acute

Fig. 5-14. *Glomerular capillary wall from a patient with acute poststreptococcal glomerulonephritis. There is a large, discrete, electron-dense (osmiophilic) "immune type" deposit in the glomerular subepithelial region of the capillary wall. This hump, or deposit, is large and abuts on the glomerular capillary wall. There is effacement or fusion of the glomerular visceral epithelial cell over the deposit. Uranyl acetate and lead citrate;* × *10,125. (Courtesy of Drs. Tito Cavallo and Srinivasan Rajaraman.)*

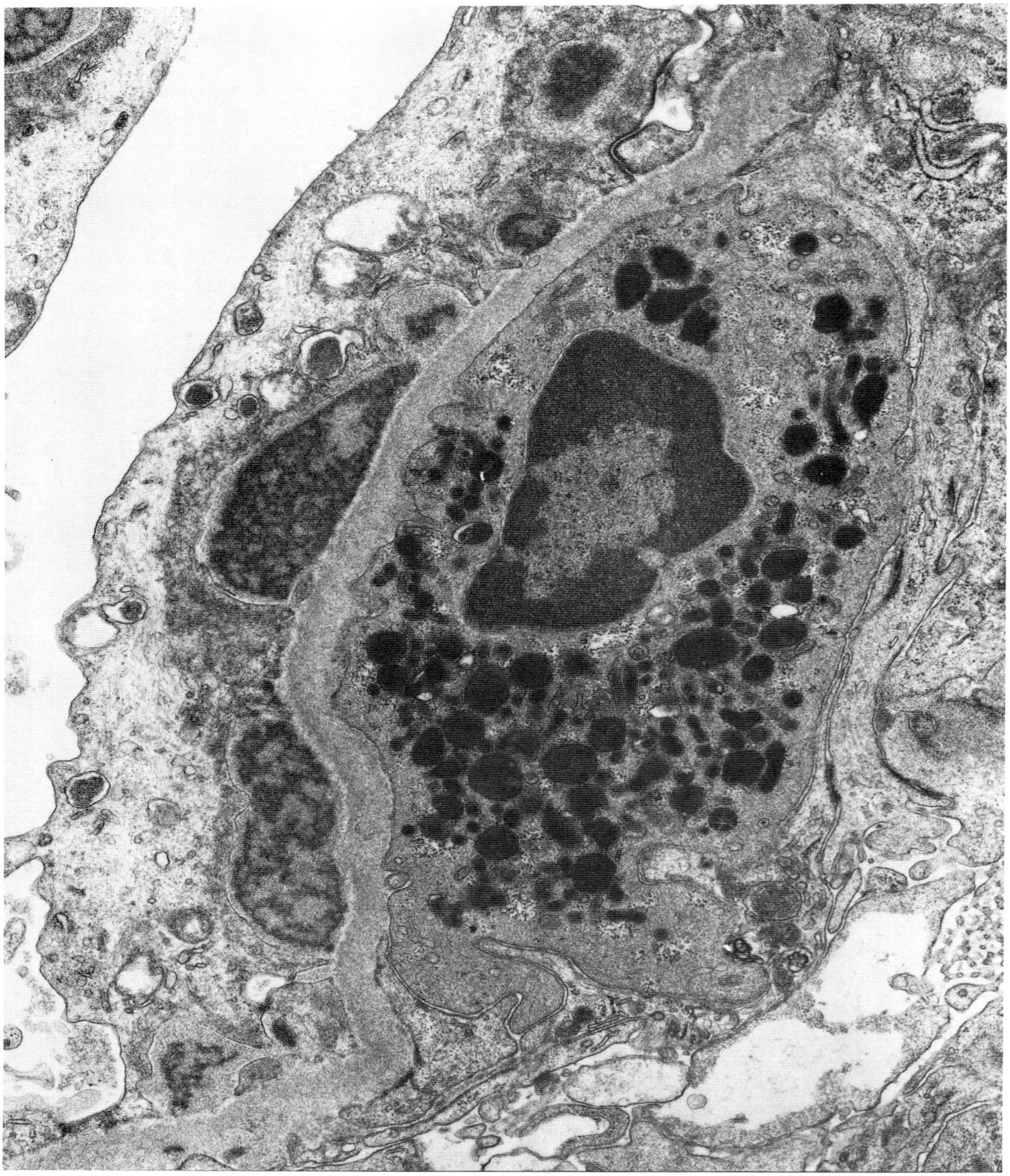

poststreptococcal glomerulonephritis have linear glomerular capillary wall deposits of IgG by immunofluorescence in the absence of anti-GBM antibodies as studied by radioimmunoassay. Thus acute glomerulonephritis represents yet another glomerular disease that may show nonspecific linear staining.

IgM is frequently present and was recorded in over 50 percent of cases in one series [304]. Other authors [135,310,323,324] have not found IgM. IgA is usually absent [2,135,323,324] but has occasionally been noted [304,470,507]. IgE has seldom been sought; in one series of 10 patients it was present in five biopsies [507], but in another study of three patients it was absent in all [311]. Fibrin/fibrinogen-related antigen also can be detected in the mesangial regions (as well as in Bowman's space in the crescentic form) [128,135, 301,323,324].

Westberg et al. [493] noted properdin in the glomeruli in eight cases of postinfectious glomerulonephritis. In three of these patients the pattern was granular along the glomerular capillary walls, whereas in five it was noted in the mesangium together with C3. Various other authors [323, 324,470] have also found properdin in several biopsies. Early components of complement, such as C1q and C4, are generally lacking [311,323, 324,507]. These various observations support the role of the alternative pathway of complement activation in postinfectious glomerulonephritis [507].

Parra et al. [348] studied the membrane attack complex in glomeruli of patients with acute poststreptococcal glomerulonephritis using monoclonal antibodies and indirect immunofluorescence. Membrane attack complex was noted along the GBM early, and within the mesangial regions later in the course of the disease (a distribution similar to the deposition of C3 and C5). Rarely, immunoglobulins and complement components may be detected in renal arterioles, especially in those patients with necrotizing arteritis. Immunohistochemical studies by Kamitsuji et al. [223] localized intraglomerular deposits of fibrin and cross-linked fibrin in the proliferative glomerulonephritides.

As noted earlier, attempts to identify and localize the streptococcal antigen have usually failed [128,301]. However, studies by Seegal [419] demonstrated streptococcal antigen in over half the cases studied. Michael et al. [310] found evidence of a type 1 group A streptococcus in the glomeruli in 2 of 10 patients' biopsies. Andres et al. [9], using ferritin-conjugated antibodies to type 12 streptococcal products, showed labeled antibody in the GBM, mesangium, and arterioles. No staining was noted in the glomerular subepithelial deposits. The discrepancy between the results of various studies suggests that either the wrong antibody or the wrong antigen is being studied or that the antigen is being lost or masked in the glomeruli in these studies [247,248,251]. I have the intuitive feeling that antigen is present in the glomeruli and that identification awaits development of the correct technology.

Deposits of immunoglobulins and especially complement may be detected in the glomeruli for months to years after apparent clinical resolution. The intensity of the immunofluorescence staining usually correlates with the severity of the glomerular lesion, although a severe diffuse glomerulonephritis may be seen with unimpressive or negligible deposits.

FIG. 5-15. *Electron micrograph of a segment of the glomerular capillary wall showing large, discrete, subepithelial electron-dense deposits. Note the heterogeneous or variegated appearance of these humps (i.e., varying degrees of osmiophilia or electron density). There is loss of the glomerular endothelium, and a polymorphonuclear leukocyte abuts the naked or denuded GBM. Polymorphonuclear leukocytes are often noted near these glomerular subepithelial deposits. Uranyl acetate and lead citrate;* × *14,400.*

Clinicopathologic Correlations

Many studies have been performed to correlate the various clinical and pathologic aspects [207, 212,270,350]. There is no correlation between the presence of hematuria and/or proteinuria and the severity of the glomerular lesion. This is not surprising because proven histologic glomerulonephritis has been noted in patients with minimal or absent hematuria and proteinuria [5,43,87,115, 166,203,222,224], and it is known that consider-

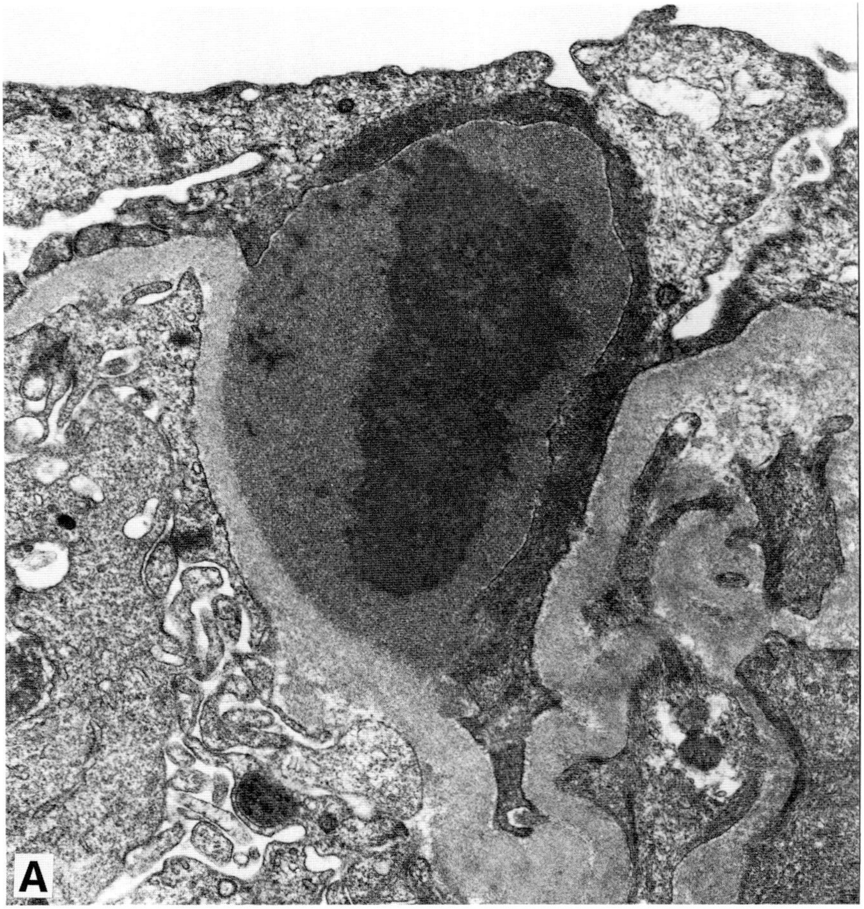

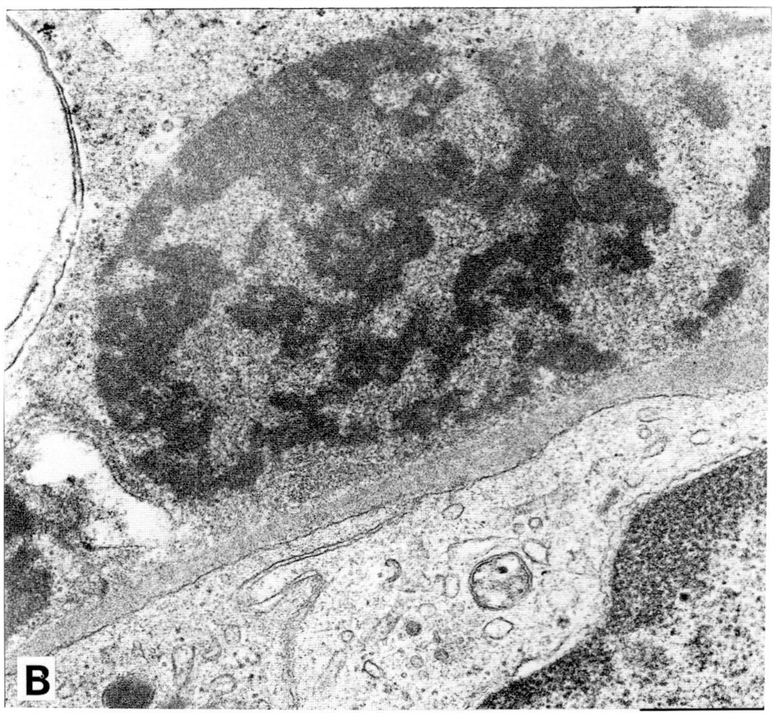

FIG. 5-16. *(A) Electron micrograph of a segment of the glomerular capillary wall from a patient with typical acute poststreptococcal glomerulonephritis. Note that the electron density (i.e., osmiophilia) of the glomerular subepithelial deposit is not homogeneous. (B) Similar variegated appearance of deposit. These regions of greater electron lucency suggest to some investigators that the deposit is being "washed out" or in the process of dissolution. Uranyl acetate and lead citrate; (A) ×20,100; (B) ×23,450. (Courtesy of Drs. William Murphy and Lillian Gaber and Drs. Conrad L. Pirani and Vivette D'Agati.)*

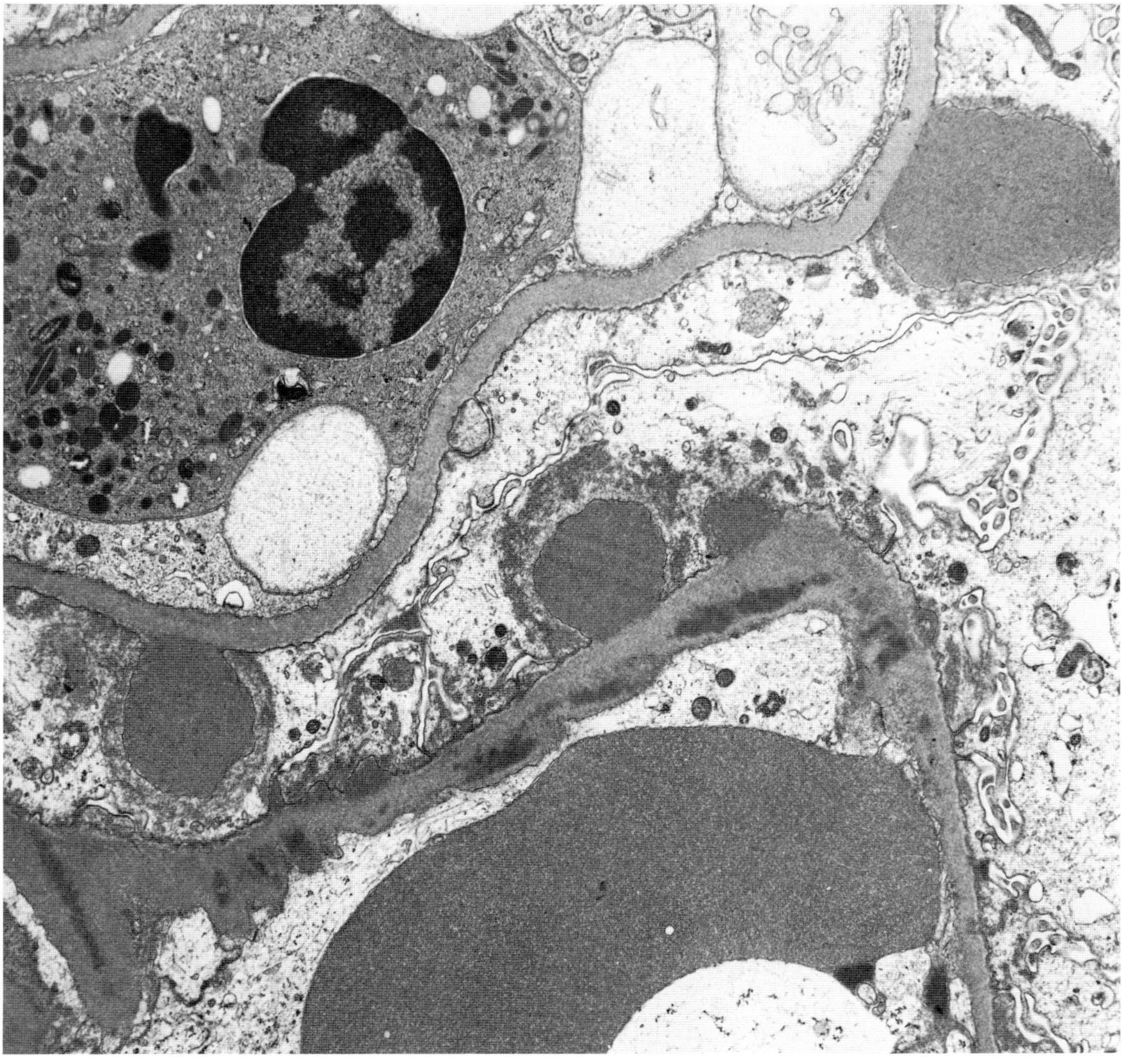

Fig. 5-17. *Electron micrograph of a segment of glomerular capillary wall from a patient with acute poststreptococcal glomerulonephritis. Glomerular subendothelial deposits can be occasionally found in these patients, although the predominant deposit is usually the typical subepithelial deposit. Uranyl acetate and lead citrate;* × 6090. *(Courtesy of Drs. Conrad L. Pirani and Vivette D'Agati.)*

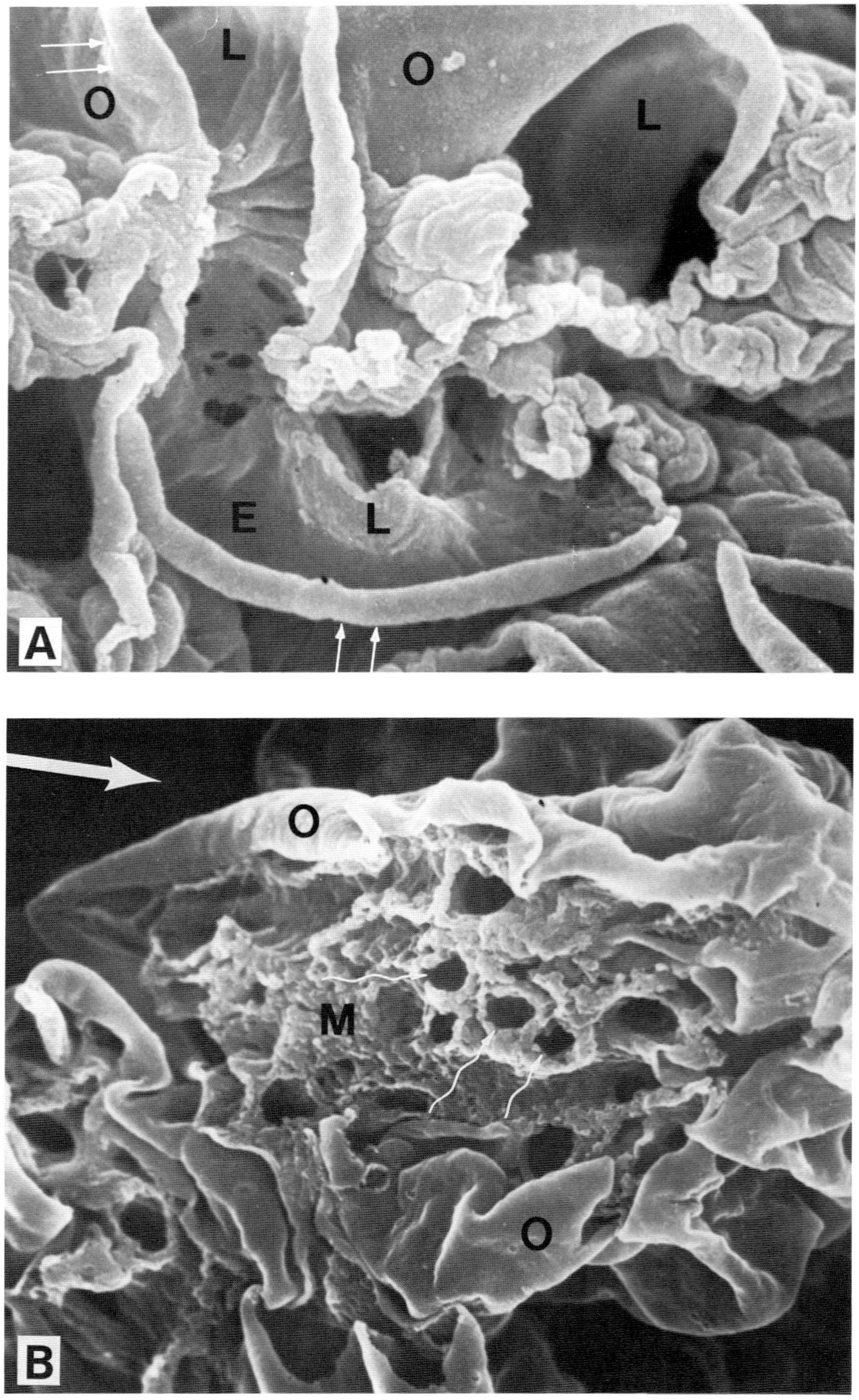
O
L
O
L
E
L
A
O
M
O
B

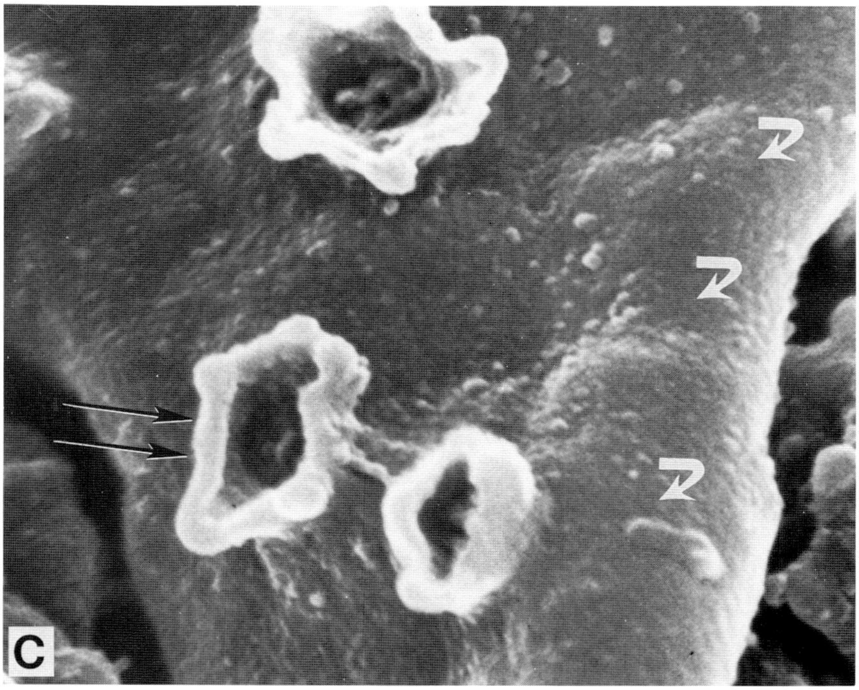

Fig. 5-18. *Scanning electron micrographs using technique of Bonsib et al. [53], in which the cellular elements have been removed by enzymatic digestion leaving behind only basement membrane, mesangial matrix, and other basement-membrane–like substances. (A) Segment of normal glomerulus for orientation showing open capillary lumen (L) and endothelial (E) aspect of GBM (thin arrows). Subepithelial outer (O) surface of GBM is also identified. (B) Segment of glomerulus from patient with acute proliferation as manifested by alterations in mesangial matrix (M) with holes (wavy white arrows) representing former site of either proliferating cells or deposits. Orientation is provided by outer (O) aspect of GBM and urinary space (thick white arrow). (C) Segment of glomerulus from patient with later changes seen in acute poststreptococcal glomerulonephritis showing subepithelial aspect of GBM (curved arrow) with reaction (dark arrows) to site of deposit. (A) ×6375; (B) ×2550; (C) ×13,125. (Courtesy of Dr. Steven M. Bonsib.)*

able hematuria can occur with no changes or only trivial changes in the glomeruli in the condition of recurrent hematuria [182]. Some authors, however, have suggested that red blood cell and protein excretion increases with increasing numbers of glomerular endocapillary cells until a point is reached at which there is a 75 percent occlusion of the glomerular capillary lumens; beyond this point there is diminishing excretion of red blood cells and protein because of decrease in the GFR [270]. Another study [396] showed that the quantitative 12-hour urinary protein excretion correlated directly with the severity of the light microscopic changes in the initial biopsy. No such correlation was noted for hematuria, azotemia, edema, or severity of hypertension.

Hutt et al. [207] did not find any correlation between edema and the glomerular changes. Al-

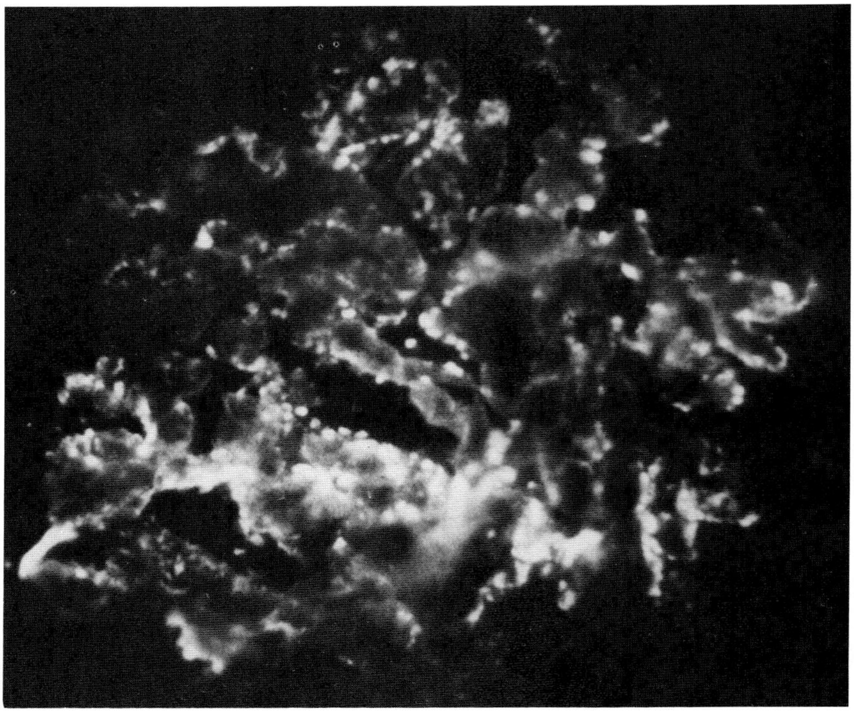

FIG. 5-19. *Immunofluorescence with IgG in a patient with acute poststreptococcal glomerulonephritis to show fine granular pattern along capillary walls. (Courtesy of Dr. Gloria Gallo.)*

though Jennings and Earle [212] found some correlation between the light microscopic appearances of the glomeruli and the various clinical parameters, certain exceptions were noted; there was a greater tendency for patients with the more severe glomerular changes to develop hypertension, although this was not absolute. These patients also tended to have high BUN values [212]. However, 7 of 11 patients of Hutt et al. [207] with renal biopsy–documented acute glomerulonephritis had blood urea concentrations below 40 mg/100 ml.

The GFR (determined by a variety of means) is often low, and the correlation with glomerular hypercellularity is good. Hutt et al. [207] felt that creatinine clearances gave a better indication of the structural abnormalities than blood urea concentrations. Parrish et al. [350] showed that the ratio of glomerular to tubular functions (GFR/Tm_{PAH}) gave a good indication of the progress of the renal disease, since the renal histology improved in those patients whose ratio rose during the course of the disease but remained unchanged in those whose ratio was low. Hutt et al. [207] also described severe impairment of renal concentrating ability in patients with tubular lesions. They also noted that the erythrocyte sedimentation rate correlated well with the structural changes—in fact, better than any other constant identified.

The most extensive clinicopathologic correlations to date have been the studies of Lewy et al. [270]. They found that glomerular tuft hypercellularity showed a significant inverse correlation with creatinine clearance and a good relationship

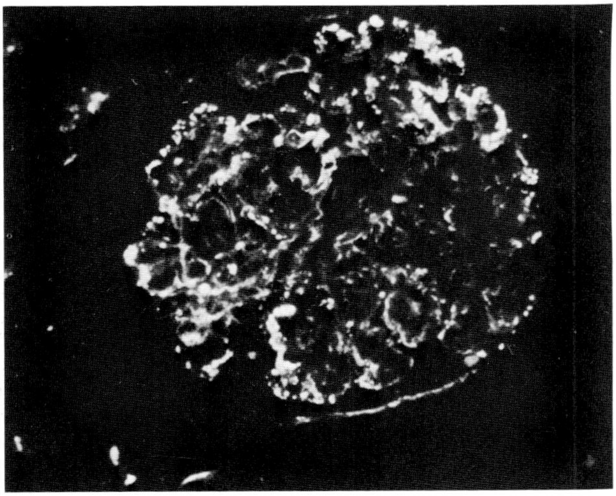

Fig. 5-20. *Fluorescence micrograph to show granular pattern for C3 along glomerular capillary walls in a patient with acute poststreptococcal glomerulonephritis. (Courtesy of Dr. George Bannayan.)*

with BUN. Glomerular tuft hypercellularity did not correlate with the ASO titer, presence of oliguria, or hypertension; it also showed no significant correlation with serum complement levels. However, the greatest degree of glomerular hypercellularity was associated with the lowest levels of serum complement. There was no correlation between the number of glomerular humps (by electron microscopy) and the level of serum complement. Total morphologic tubular damage related directly to the creatinine clearance and BUN. This is not surprising, since there may be a good correlation between the glomerular and tubular damage.

Haen et al. [173] showed with morphometric studies that there is a direct correlation between the serum creatinine level and the degree of interstitial volume. It was noted that even with severe glomerular changes, the serum creatinine level was not usually increased unless the interstitial volume was increased by 15 percent. Bohle et al. [47] and Hooke and Atkins [197] have also demonstrated a close relationship between the severity of interstitial inflammation and the GFR in a number of glomerulonephritides. The number of glomerular humps (by electron microscopy) was associated with a more severe and protracted clinical picture [240]. There was no apparent difference in the glomerular lesion nor in the clinical course when patients with and without hypocomplementemia were compared. Some authors state that up to 10 to 20 percent of patients may have normal serum complement levels [267]; others disagree [247,250,252]. There is no doubt that large numbers of crescents are associated with oliguria and rises in the BUN and serum creatinine levels.

Several investigators have suggested that initial and/or persistent nephrotic syndrome is a harbinger of a poor renal prognosis [430,474]. As noted before, there may be difficulty in distinguishing between exacerbations of nonstreptococcal chronic glomerulonephritis and true de novo attacks of acute poststreptococcal glomerulonephritis [242]. An added problem is the lack of demonstration of a streptococcal etiology in the cases studied [228]. Renal biopsy [387] of patients with decreased creatinine clearance, microscopic hematuria, and proteinuria usually show moderate to advanced

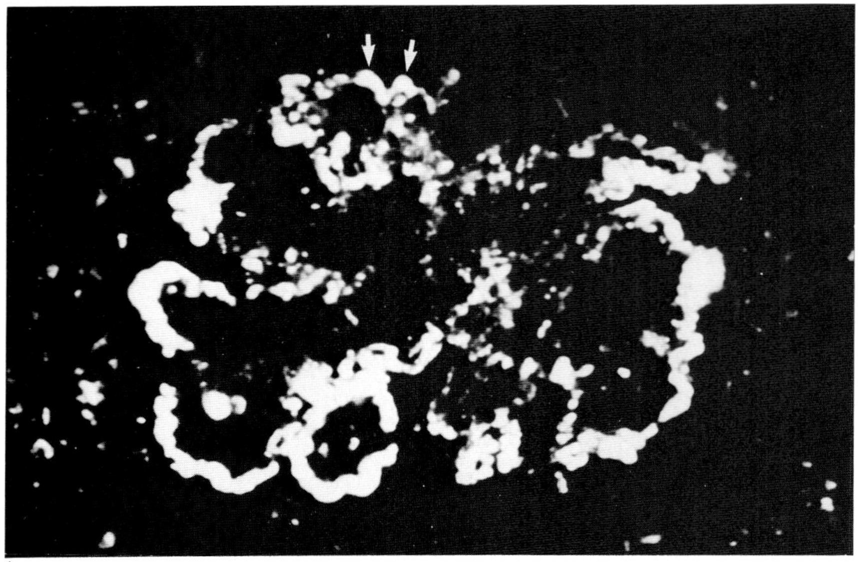

A

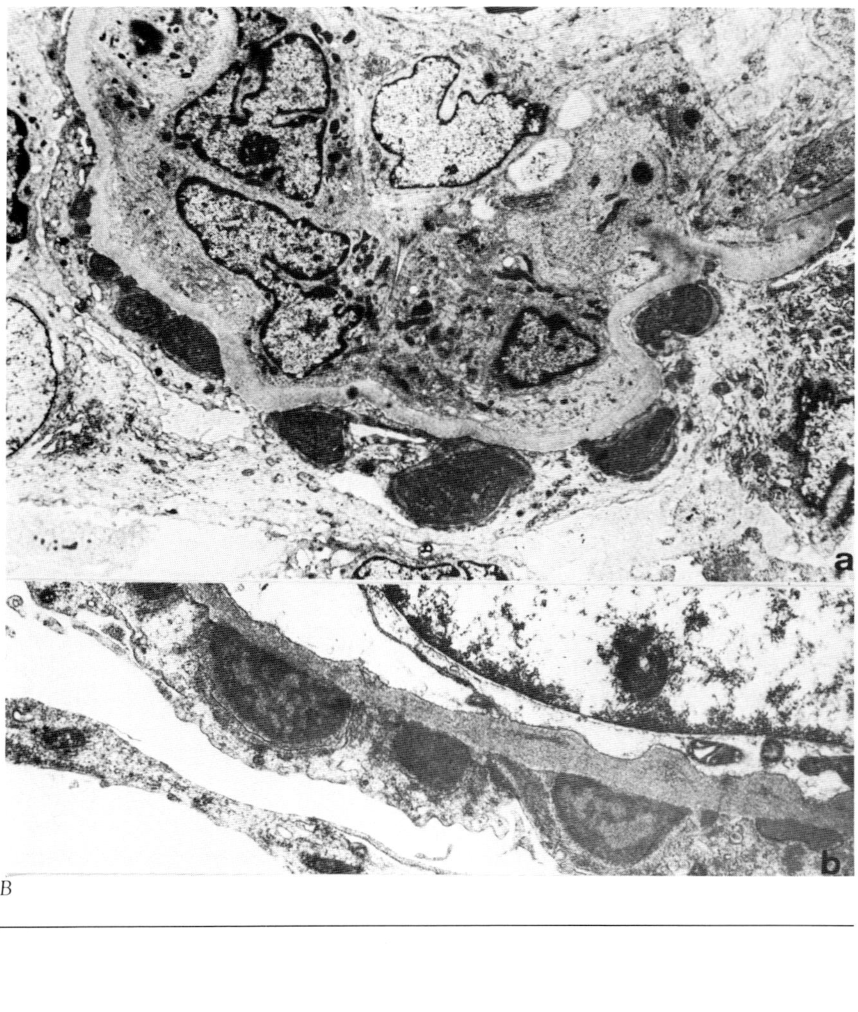

B

glomerular sclerosis, mesangial hypercellularity, and intense immunofluorescent staining for IgG and C3. However, patients without clinical or laboratory findings of disease can have moderate segmental mesangial sclerosis and positive glomerular immunofluorescence with IgG and C3 [387].

Patients older than 60 years of age tend to have a worse renal prognosis than do younger adults, according to some investigators [270,401,403]. One of three of the reported older individuals has evidence of persistent renal disease with mild impairment of renal function [270,401,403].

When adult patients with oliguria/anuria and crescent formation are considered, the prognosis is especially poor. As many as 50 percent of them progress to end-stage renal failure [81,430]. The 50 percent progression to end-stage renal disease is noted even in patients with crescentic glomerulonephritis (of the poststreptococcal type) without acute oliguria/anuria in one series [49]. The prognosis in adult patients with oliguria/anuria may be related to the availability and use of dialysis and other medical support.

Correlation of Light, Electron, and Immunofluorescence Microscopy

There is usually concordance or harmony between the light and the electron microscopic findings. The number of glomerular subepithelial deposits is directly correlated with the degree of polymorphonuclear leukocytic infiltrates in the glomeruli; however, humps can be seen in sections without polymorphs [270]. Those patients with the greatest glomerular tuft hypercellularity generally have the most numerous humps. There is an inconstant relationship between the presence of humps and damage to the glomerular endothelium, at least as manifested by ultrastructural studies.

There is generally thought to be a good correlation between the light microscopic appearance of diffuse glomerular hypercellularity and the characteristic diffuse granular staining along the glomerular capillary walls for IgG and C3 [135,463]. In certain cases, however, lesions thought by light microscopy to be well developed may not have glomerular staining for IgG and may show only an interrupted linear staining with C3 [135]. In biopsies in which light microscopy shows complete resolution of the hypercellularity, there is a loss of staining with IgG and C3 [135,310]. Biopsies in which the glomerular lesions persist with only mesangial hypercellularity show mainly C3 (and some IgG) in the mesangial areas [463]. In others in which mesangial prominence was present many months after the initial biopsy, there was only complement in the mesangium with a patchy, linear pattern along the glomerular capillaries for gamma globulin and IgG [128]. Michael et al. [310] noted only focal IgG and C3 in renal biopsies performed 10 years after the initial episode; by light microscopy, these patients showed only a focal and segmental mesangial hypercellularity.

There is usually granular immunofluorescent staining along the glomerular capillary walls corresponding to the humps noted in ultrastructural studies from the same biopsy. This, however, is not always the case, and some believe that the number and location of the immunofluorescent granules best match the various sizes of the glomerular subendothelial deposits [68,128]. It was felt that the humps noted on electron microscopic studies were too few to account for all the fluorescent granules. It also was believed that the irregular masses of amorphous and fibrillar mesangial material matched the gamma globulin and complement noted there by immunofluorescence studies. However, these electron microscopic findings also could be due to fibrin(ogen) because there was

Fig. 5-21. *(A) Immunofluorescence showing a garland pattern. Garland-like outline of the glomerular loops is due to large subepithelial deposits on the outer side of the GBM (arrows). The mesangial regions appear largely empty. IgG; ×450. (B) Accompanying electron micrographs showing a part of a glomerulus from a patient with a garland pattern. In (a), there is hypercellularity, and numerous subepithelial deposits of varying density are present. ×5700. In (b), taken at a higher magnification, there are spotted deposits of different sizes. ×9000. From a 37-year-old man with a 2-week history of poststreptococcal glomerulonephritis. (From Sorger, K. Postinfectious Glomerulonephritis. Stuttgart: Gustav Fischer Verlag, 1986; used by permission.)*

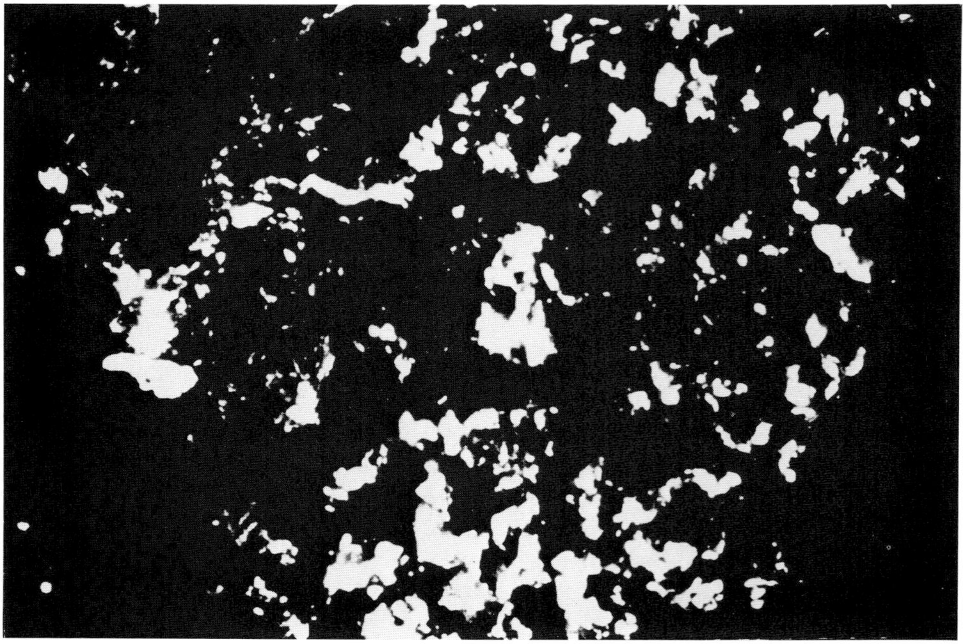

A

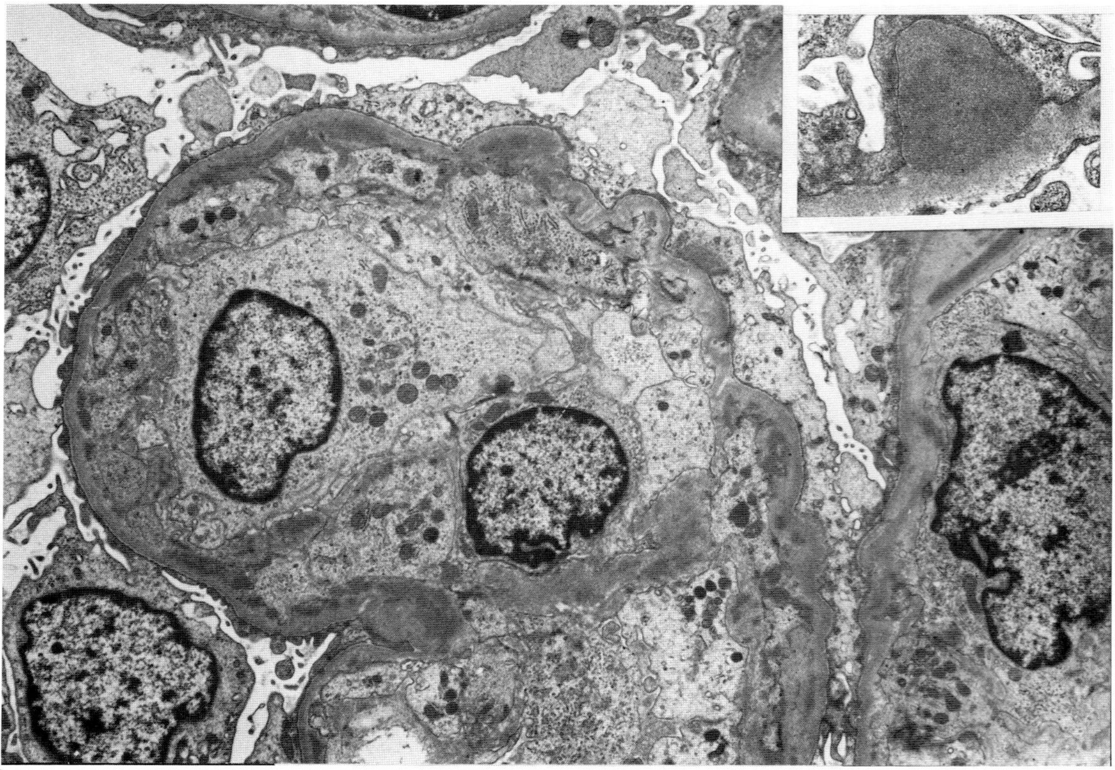

B

positive immunofluorescence for fibrin at this site. Fish et al. [135] also noted granular immunofluorescent staining in a patient with only glomerular subendothelial deposits by electron microscopy but stated that in general in their cases the distribution of immunofluorescent granules seemed to correlate with the humps. They also described an interrupted linear immunofluorescence for C3 without IgG staining in a patient with classic humps. Negative immunofluorescence was noted in one of their patients with well-developed glomerular subendothelial deposits. In the studies of Sagel et al. [398], a granular immunofluorescence pattern was noted for IgG and C3 along the glomerular capillary walls despite the absence of electron microscopic deposits (this was a case of subclinical glomerulonephritis).

As noted earlier, Sorger et al. [438] have provided the most detailed of the immunofluorescence studies. They described three patterns: (1) "starry sky," (2) "garland," and (3) mesangial patterns. In the starry sky type, there is a fine granular deposition of IgG and C3 along the glomerular capillary walls and mesangium. The garland pattern consists of densely packed, sometimes confluent or continuous deposits of IgG and C3 along the glomerular capillary walls. The mesangial pattern consists of the presence of C3 in the mesangial regions. When these three patterns were compared with the ultrastructural findings, the starry sky pattern corresponded in general to the glomerular subendothelial deposits, the garland pattern to the classic glomerular subepithelial deposits that tended to be elongated or confluent, and the mesangial pattern to electron-dense deposits in the mesangium and in a subepithelial pattern on the GBM overlying the mesangium (see Figs. 5-21, 5-22, and 5-23).

In summary, the correlations are good, although there are some anomalies. Chief among these is the sometime lack of concordance between the immunofluorescence and electron microscopic studies.

FIG. 5-22. *(A) Immunofluorescence showing a starry sky pattern. There is diffuse and irregularly distributed fine and coarse granular deposits in the glomerular capillary walls and in the glomerular mesangial regions.* C3; ×704. *(B) The accompanying electron micrograph shows a segment of a glomerular capillary loop from a patient with a starry sky pattern. The lumen of the glomerular capillary is totally occupied by a monocyte and by endothelial cells with prominent nuclei and swollen cell bodies. Numerous subendothelial deposits are present.* ×5280. (Inset) *A pointed, arch-like glomerular subepithelial deposit with sparse areas of higher electron density.* ×17,600. *From a 56-year-old man with a 3-week history of poststreptococcal glomerulonephritis.* (From Sorger, K. *Postinfectious Glomerulonephritis.* Stuttgart: Gustav Fischer Verlag, 1986; used by permission.)

Correlation of Morphologic Changes with Clinical Outcome

The most controversial facet of acute glomerulonephritis is its long-term outlook. This is a question on which there are strong opinions and often incomplete data. The difficulty in demonstrating with certainty that the glomerulonephritis in the individual patient is related to streptococcal infection has made it difficult to interpret follow-up studies on progression to a chronic stage. Information on the correlation of morphologic changes with clinical outcome was scanty before the days of the renal biopsy, although it was known that certain patients pursued a rather hectic course with death due to renal failure within a few months [279,476]. Most of these are poststreptococcal cases in which crescent formation is abundant; it was suggested that the presence of a large number of crescents was usually a sinister sign. However, it is quite common to have an acute postinfectious glomerulonephritis with a few crescents, and complete recovery is generally the rule [270]. Clinical recovery has been noted in half the patients with less than 40 percent crescents [270], as well as in certain patients with a greater percentage of crescents [440].

Crescentic glomerulonephritis as a severe manifestation of the postinfectious episode has been noted by many [8,63,81,91,122,124*a*,157,268,278,299,315,393,395,427,430,440,506]. The significance of crescentic glomerulonephritis in children with acute poststreptococcal glomerulonephritis has remained controversial [8,91,395,442]. In a comprehensive review of the natural history

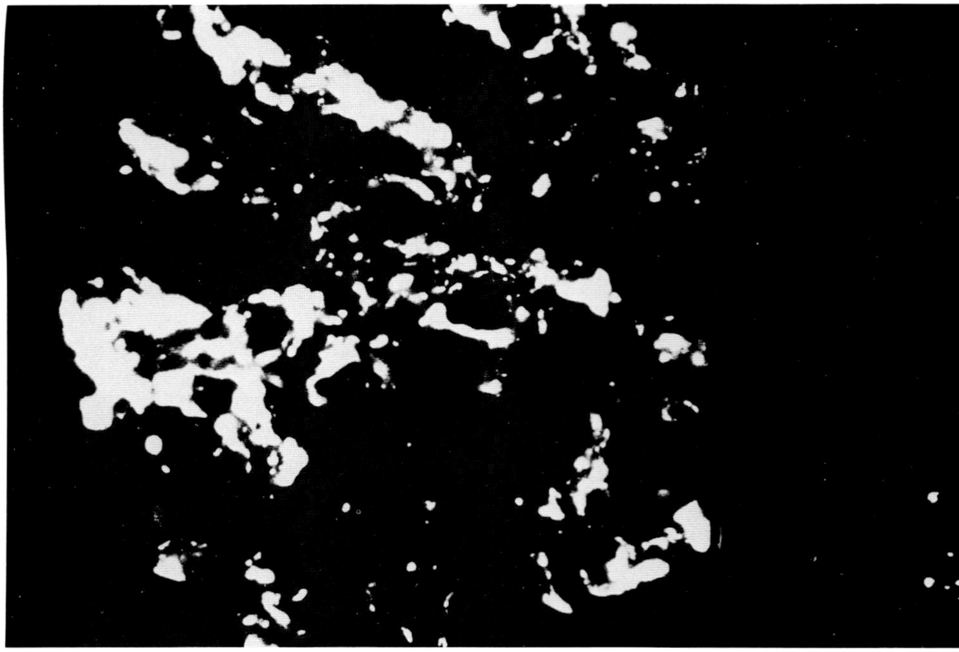

A

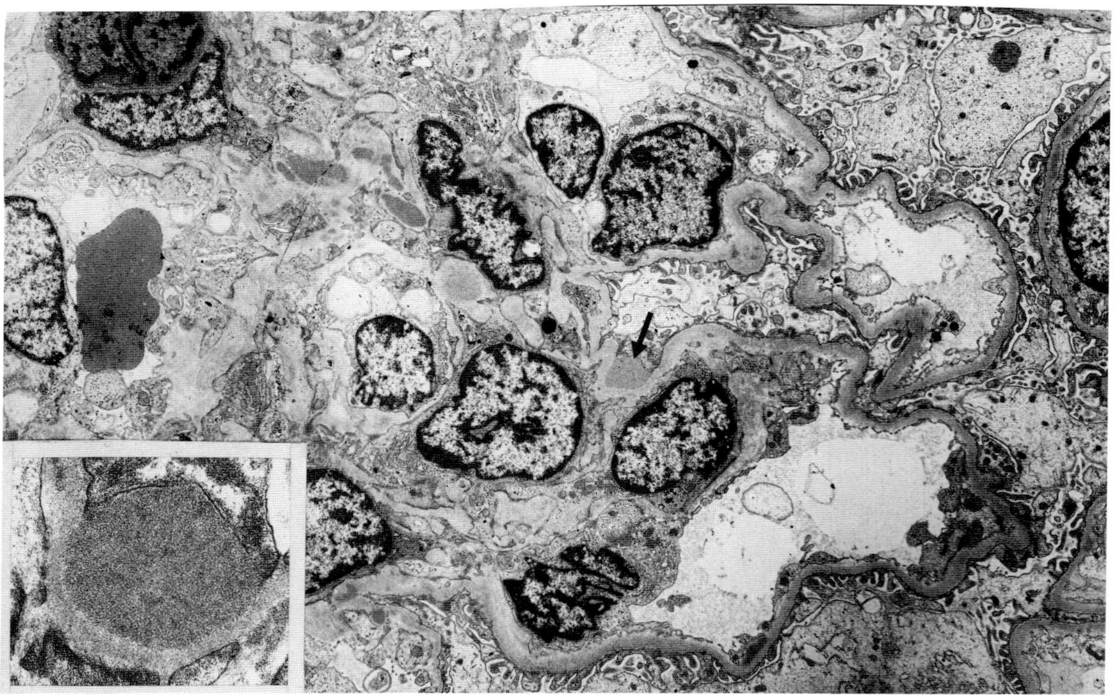

B

of glomerulonephritis, Cameron [71] described the actuarial survival of patients with severe crescentic glomerulonephritis based on the experiences of himself and Drs. Habib, Kincaid-Smith, and Morel-Maroger. He concluded that the prognosis of such patients (with all forms of nephritis) is "almost entirely dependent on the large numbers of crescents and that the prognosis normally associated with the underlying glomerular disease is no longer operative, because the prognosis of the crescent formation is so bad". He also furthered the argument that the apparently good prognosis in patients who had acute poststreptococcal glomerulonephritis with extensive crescents has been misrepresented because most of the patients in this group have had relatively minor degrees of crescent formation. In the investigation of the Southwest Pediatric Nephrology Study Group (SPNSG) [440], six patients with poststreptococcal glomerulonephritis and crescent formation in 51, 60, 87, 90, 92, and 100 percent of their glomeruli were identified. The crescents were generally cellular rather than fibrocellular or fibrous, and there was a low percentage of large crescents with little evidence of chronic histologic changes such as global glomerular sclerosis and interstitial fibrosis. It is likely, in the absence of constant or progressive injury to the glomerulus, that these cellular crescents will resolve without major sequelae [122]. Indeed, all five patients with adequate follow-up in the SPNSG series had normal GFRs at the latest evaluation, irrespective of whether treatment was given. The SPNSG concluded from the data in these patients that well-documented acute poststreptococcal glomerulonephritis with crescents in children is a self-limited disorder with an excellent clinical outcome. The study of Roy et al. [395] would further suggest that this outcome is unaffected by therapeutic intervention and that such patients should receive only supportive measures to control the consequences of their renal insufficiency and hypertension until a spontaneous remission occurs. However, Cunningham et al. [91] noted that 7 of 13 children with acute poststreptococcal glomerulonephritis and crescentic glomerulonephritis progressed to chronic renal failure; in some of their patients, anticoagulant and antiplatelet therapy appeared to improve survival. Thus the renal prognosis in this set of patients is still somewhat controversial. (See also Chapter 9.)

Jennings and Earle [212] have suggested that the severely exudative form with a large number of polymorphonuclear leukocytes is the forerunner of the most severe form; however, the mere presence of polymorphonuclear leukocytes in the glomerular tuft does not portend a poor prognosis. Polymorphonuclear leukocytes are often present in the glomeruli of patients who recover completely [107]. One group of investigators has noted a correlation between the number of glomerular subepithelial humps by electron microscopy and prolonged oliguria [240].

For some time, a number of authors have attempted to utilize other morphologic markers as prognostic indicators. Some suggest that the overall degree of glomerular tuft hypercellularity is related to either the degree of persistent proteinuria [188,212] or to outcome [406], but other authors have noted that there does not seem to be a good correlation between excessive glomerular hypercellularity and outcome [270,403]. Lesser degrees of hypercellularity also have been noted to be associated with "irreversible" renal changes [406]. There are so many exceptions to the suggested correlations that a rule of thumb probably does not exist. It is likely that several of these morphologic features taken together may be of greater prognostic value than any single finding, but this type of

←

Fig. 5-23. *(A) Immunofluorescence showing a mesangial pattern. Granular deposits are found in the mesangial regions while the glomerular capillary wall remains largely negative. C3;* $\times 704$. *(B) The accompanying electron micrograph shows the corresponding ultrastructural appearance. A portion of the glomerulus shows marked proliferation of mesangial cells but free and open glomerular capillary lumens. Mesangial deposits are located in the mesangial matrix, and individual subepithelial deposits are present in the region of the mesangial waist (arrow). Less frequently, glomerular subendothelial deposits are situated along the loop.* $\times 5280$. *(Inset) A glomerular subepithelial deposit with almost homogeneous, comparatively pale density.* $\times 17{,}600$. *This is from an 18-year-old man with a 5-week duration of the illness. (From Sorger, K. Postinfectious Glomerulonephritis. Stuttgart: Gustav Fischer Verlag, 1986; used by permission.)*

study has not been performed. Some investigators have demonstrated that glomerular necroses, adhesions, glomerular capillary thromboses, and crescent formation and interstitial nephritis were more commonly found in those patients whose disease progressed [81,182].

A study by Lien et al. [273] addressed the issue of obsolescent glomeruli in 57 patients (mostly adult) with acute poststreptococcal glomerulonephritis followed for 1 to 4 years. Twenty-six percent of these patients had combinations of hypertension, microscopic hematuria, proteinuria, and elevations in the serum creatinine level. Nine percent died. Renal biopsies in 33 patients during the follow-up period showed significant glomerular obsolescence in only 3 patients. These authors also raised the important point that one must exclude an underlying clinically covert glomerular disease that is brought to clinical attention because of a superimposed acute postinfectious glomerulonephritis.

Vascular changes such as arteriolar sclerosis and arterial sclerosis have been suggested to be a harbinger of a poor prognosis [19,150]. A direct correlation was noted between the presence of thickening of the vessel wall with narrowing of the lumen and the percentage of globally sclerotic glomeruli. Hypertension tended to develop in those patients with global glomerular sclerosis and morphologic evidence of vascular disease.

Ultrastructural changes such as large and confluent glomerular subepithelial electron-dense deposits have been thought to be indicators of a poor prognosis [188]. These "atypical" humps were invariably associated with renal failure following the initial attack, according to this report.

Persistence of immunoglobulins and complement, primarily in the glomerular mesangial regions, has been considered to be evidence of continuing immunologic involvement and injury [251,464]. Those patients who progress into a chronic stage show this finding. However, some authors have noted the final loss of immunoglobulins and complement as long as 5 years after the initial acute attack; therefore, the persistence of these immunoreactants beyond the acute stage of the disease cannot be universally regarded as an infallible sign of a poor prognosis.

Linear immunofluorescence for IgG was noted in certain patients who developed chronic renal failure [251,406]; anti-GBM antibodies were searched for but not identified [406]. The long-term study of Baldwin et al. [20] showed similar linear immunofluorescence in repeat renal biopsies with a significant number of globally sclerotic glomeruli; renal failure had not yet developed in these patients. It is unclear whether these changes will portend a poor prognosis.

Clinical Outcome

Despite much information gathered from long-term observations of patients surviving epidemics throughout the world over the last several decades [501], there is nothing as controversial in acute postinfectious glomerulonephritis as the eventual or final renal outcome. Some possible outcomes include (1) complete recovery, (2) death during the acute attack from either renal or cardiac failure or hypertensive encephalopathy, or (3) death from the infection itself. Those patients dying of uremia usually do so after a period of several months (and most of them show a crescentic form of glomerulonephritis). A *fourth* clinical possibility is that the patient continues to have various combinations of proteinuria, hematuria, hypertension, and renal insufficiency (persistently elevated BUN and serum creatinine levels). When these occur, it is difficult to know whether the findings represent a slow resolution of the original acute glomerulonephritis with potential for recovery, whether the kidney has suffered irreversible damage leading to progressive renal disease, or whether limited permanent injury has occurred with no further adverse progression. *Lastly,* the patient could develop chronic renal failure after variable and longer periods of time. The percentage of patients ending up with a chronic nephropathy is difficult to assess because of the differing criteria utilized to judge "chronicity."

Because it is often difficult to know with certainty whether the acute nephritis represents a new disease or an exacerbation of a preexisting disease, it is not always possible to be certain that the renal disease studied was indeed an acute post-streptococcal glomerulonephritis in a patient with previously normal kidneys. There are now many reported instances of an occult preexisting renal condition being brought to clinical attention because of a superimposed unrelated second disease. An example of this is acute glomerulonephritis being superimposed on diabetic nephropathy [38,78]. Transition of acute proliferative glomerulonephritis to membranous glomerulonephritis also has been reported [229,381].

The outcome of patients with acute postinfectious glomerulonephritis is shown in Table 5-2, but many important points need to be made before considering its contents. In many of the series quoted, renal biopsies were not performed; thus histologic proof of the acute glomerulonephritis is lacking. The criteria used for making the diagnosis of acute postinfectious glomerulonephritis were clinical and variable. Length of follow-up varies between series but is often short. The outcome indicators used are also different; some authors used the presence of mild proteinuria and microscopic hematuria, whereas others relied on BUN and serum creatinine levels and the presence of hypertension. As Heptinstall stated in the third edition of this book [182], "It is a human failing to include as many cases in a series as possible, yet the task of assessing prognosis from published series would be made much easier if a smaller number of cases, all with a minimum follow-up period of, say, 5 or 10 years, were described."

Short-term follow-up data can give an erroneous impression, because the disease resolves more slowly in some patients than in others, with the net result that the number of patients in the latent stage is exaggerated. Studies with short-term follow-up provide fewer opportunities for some patients with asymptomatic proteinuria to progress to the chronic stage with hypertension and raised levels of BUN and serum creatinine, or for other patients to recover completely.

It is important to remember that selection or entry bias plays a major role in the interpretation of these series. Patients studied in the hospital represent a highly selected population, and it is likely that the majority of mild cases—clinically thought to be postinfectious glomerulonephritis—may not be hospitalized or biopsied. Hospitalized patients are likely to have the most severe clinical course. Renal biopsy is usually reserved for those whose clinical picture is one *not* of a classic or typical acute postinfectious glomerulonephritis [190,331].

Despite these reservations, most investigators believe that the prognosis in children is good in both the epidemic and sporadic cases. Mortality in children in the acute stage is generally low, although some workers have noted higher death rates than others [148]. These high mortality rates are usually the result of either severe infection, cardiac failure, or hypertensive encephalopathy, not the nephritic process itself.

A review of 13 series confined to childhood (see Table 5-2) notes that up to 45 percent of children are found to have latent or chronic disease, usually defined as asymptomatic or intermittent proteinuria. As mentioned before, it is likely that short follow-up periods and highly selective admission policies contribute to this high figure. The morphologic findings in one of these large series, that of Travis et al. [461], have been described 3 years or more after the acute attack. Of the 54 children whose diagnosis of acute postinfectious glomerulonephritis was confirmed by biopsy, 1 died from a crescentic form of glomerulonephritis, 4 failed to show histologic healing, 3 had latent glomerulonephritis, and 1 had chronic glomerulonephritis. The authors thought that the 3 patients with latent glomerulonephritis were capable of spontaneous resolution of their glomerular process. If that were true and the patient with the crescentic form of acute glomerulonephritis was excluded, then the probability of recovery from the acute attack of postinfectious glomerulonephritis would be 98 percent. If resolution of the three with latent glomerulonephritis were not to take place, the probability of recovery would be 92 percent.

In a prospective study of children followed for 4 to 12 years after the onset of acute glomerulonephritis with sequential renal biopsies, healing occurred in 20 percent at 2 years, 46 percent at 4 years, 77 percent at 6 years, 94 percent at 10 years, and 97 percent at 12 years [396]. Although there was a very high rate of healing, this can be considerably delayed. There was less than perfect correlation between the morphologic findings and the results of the Addis counts of hematuria; for example, 6 patients (17 percent) had abnormal

TABLE 5-2. *Outcome of acute glomerulonephritis: adults, adults and children, and children only*

Author	Follow-up period (years)	Population studied	No. of patients	Died in acute stage (%)	Chronic or latent stage (%)	Not traced (%)	Recovery (%)
Richter [381*a*]	1–19	Adult	100	5 (5)[c]	15	13	62
Rudebeck [397]	Over 4	Adult[a]	318[b]	5 (2)[d]	9 (16)[i]	15	53
Jennings and Earle [212]	Short	Adult	36	3	36[j]	0	61
Kushner et al. [243]	Up to 4	Adult[a]	29	0	24	0	76
Longcope [282]	1/2–12	Adult and child	116	6 (4)[d]	9 (32)[g]	0	49
Hayman and Martin [179]	1/2–8	Adult and child	77	9	33[h]	0	67[h]
Ellis [121]	Years	Adult and child	173	4 (4)[d]	10	0	82
Murphy and Peters [327]	2–10	Adult and child	205	13[e]	36	17[k]	34
Ramberg [368*a*]	—	Adult and child	175	6	25	7	62
Addis [3]	Years	Adult and child	118	7[f]	20	0	73
Baldwin et al. [19,20]	2–18	Adult and child	168	5.4 (3.6)[d]	See text	—	—
Rodriguez-Iturbe et al. [387]	5–6	Adult and child[r]	120	1.3	13[s]	0	87
Nissenson et al. [336]	7–12	Adult and child[r]	722	0	See text	—	—
Garcia et al. [151]	11–12	Adult and child	71	0	21[v]	0	79
Chugh et al. [81]	2–10	Adult and child	146	14[m]	31[x]	27	28
Potter et al. [360]	12–17	Adult and child[r]	534	0[y]	3.5	0	96.5
Guild [171]	1–12	Child	34	0	18	0	82[n]
Gachet [148]	Over 1	Child	114[l]	7	9[l]	0	91[l]
Davis and Faber [94]	Over 2	Child	102	6	13[m]	0	81
Burke and Ross [68]	2	Child	90	3	3	0	94
Akerrén and Lindgren [4*a*]	—	Child	57	0	0	0	100
McCrory et al. [301*a*]	2	Child	35	0	3	0	97
Perlman et al. [354]	10	Child	62	1.6	0	0	98.4

Dodge et al. [107]	2	Child	20	0	45[o]	0	55
Lewy et al. [270]	5	Child	21	0[p]	24[q]	0	76
Schacht et al. [405]	2	Child	54	0[u]	38	0	62
	5	Child	31	0[u]	45	0	55
Travis et al. [461][t]	>3	Child	54	2	8	0	92[h]
Roy et al. [396][t]	4–12	Child	35	0	3	0	97
Drachman [110]	1/2–2	Child	155	0	0	0	100
	11–12	Child	80	0	0	75	100

[a]Over 10 years of age.
[b]Seen within 3 months of onset.
[c]Died from etiologic disease or incidental cause.
[d]Died in rapidly progressive phase.
[e]Died in acute stage or later.
[f]Died from unrelated disease; time not given.
[g]"Quiescent" cases (latent).
[h]Percentage of those who survived acute attack.
[i]Uncertain.
[j]Some followed for less than 1 year.
[k]All had recovered on discharge.
[l]Those who survived the acute phase.
[m]Includes 5 percent who died from chronic nephritis.
[n]Includes three with orthostatic proteinuria.
[o]Of nine patients, two had persistent and seven had intermittent proteinuria.
[p]Three deaths in initial 46 patients.
[q]Includes one death from chronic renal failure at 5 years.
[r]Mainly children.
[s]Nine percent in children, 37 percent in adults.
[t]By histologic outcome.
[u]Two had crescentic glomerulonephritis and became uremic.
[v]One patient with chronic renal failure.
[w]Died of uremia within 2 years.
[x]Half developed renal failure.
[y]Only one patient died in renal failure 6 to 10 years after the initial illness.

Addis counts at a time when histologic healing and resolution had occurred.

The patients with epidemic forms of poststreptococcal glomerulonephritis have almost uniformly shown excellent outcomes, and only a few have persisting renal abnormalities as determined by clinical and laboratory examinations (hematuria/proteinuria) [110,153,236,335,336,354,357, 359,360,387]. This is exemplified by long term follow-up of an epidemic in Trinidad of 760 patients, 87 percent of whom were below the age of 15 years. The excellent results at 2–6 years [359] were surpassed in the 7–12 year study by Nissenson et al. [336] in which of the 722 patients followed, persistent urinary abnormalities were present in only 0.8 percent, hypertension in 2.3 percent and serum creatinine levels over 1.2 mg/100 ml in as few as 3 patients. In the 12–17 year follow-up of 534 patients undertaken by Potter et al. [360] only 3.5 percent had urinary abnormalities, 3.7 percent were hypertensive, and no patient had a serum creatinine level greater than 1.25 mg/100ml. These figures did not differ from expected values in surveys of the normal population.

In an 11- to 12-year follow-up of an epidemic in children by Drachman et al. [110], no persistent urinary or serologic abnormalities (BUN, creatinine) were noted. Drukker et al. [111] studied the renal sodium handling (i.e., the natriuretic response to IV saline loading) in 11 patients (both children and adults) several years after acute poststreptococcal glomerulonephritis and found no evidence of exaggerated natriuresis.

Some series [81,405,474] suggest that children do not do as well as generally believed and that there is a high proportion with clinical or laboratory abnormalities at follow-up. It is also considered that patients who had poststreptococcal glomerulonephritis in childhood have an increased propensity or susceptibility to chronic glomerulonephritis as an adult [108,159,212,406]. In a series of 83 children who were followed for periods of up to 17 years (with renal biopsy being performed in 36 of them), proteinuria, hypertension, and decreased GFR were noted in 38 percent of the 54 children followed for at least 2 years, in 45 percent of 31 patients followed for 5 years or more, and in 47 percent of 17 patients followed for over 10 years [405]. Two of the patients, who were uremic from onset, showed progression from a diffuse proliferative glomerulonephritis with crescents to proliferative and sclerosing chronic glomerulonephritis. A study of 35 patients by Rodriguez-Iturbe [384] indicated that patients followed for up to 13 years after an episode of poststreptococcal glomerulonephritis had a diminished renal reserve capacity as determined by a decreased GFR after a challenge by acute oral protein load.

Thus these studies indicate that although uremia is rare, there is evidence of depressed renal function in some children. This dictates the need for continued follow-up. The following features have an adverse effect on clinical outcome: underlying renal disease, persisting proteinuria with or without the nephrotic syndrome, decreased renal function, oliguria/anuria, extensive crescent formation, atypical humps on electron microscopy, and the garland pattern on immunofluorescence. The prognosis for children with these features is worse than for those without them [81,91,188, 437,438,474]. Children with the crescentic form of postinfectious glomerulonephritis may or may not have a poor renal prognosis [8,91,440].

The prognosis in adults is even more controversial, and many authors consider that it is not as favorable as in children [20,260,261,273]. The proportion of complete recoveries ranges from 53 to 76 percent in a number of series (see Table 5-2), and death in the acute stage has been recorded in up to 9 percent of adults [179]. It should be noted that several of the series quoted in Table 5-2 that indicated a high mortality in the acute stage were compiled many years ago (circa 1940 and 1950). In those series containing only adults, the figures of "chronicity" range up to 36 percent [283,397]. The percentages might vary in part because of different durations of follow-up and uncertainty as to whether to include patients whose sole abnormality was hematuria and/or proteinuria [212].

The studies of Baldwin and colleagues [19,20, 406] are of great importance in determining prognosis in a predominantly adult population. In one of their series [20] of 89 adults and 37 children, 9 patients died within the first 6 months, 6 of them having the crescentic form of acute glomerulonephritis. Two others died in renal failure (one at 2 years, the other at 6 years); both showed extensive glomerular sclerosis at that time. Proteinuria was noted in half the patients followed from 5 to 7 years, and hypertension was seen in one-fourth to one-half. Repeat renal biopsies showed subsidence of the glomerular hypercellularity and an increase in the degree of glomerular sclerosis. The severity of glomerular sclerosis correlated with reductions in the GFR. Baldwin et al. [19] in a later study noted that 56 percent of renal biopsies obtained 3 years or more after the onset of the acute attack showed segmental to global glomerular sclerosis of 10 percent or more of glomeruli (an abnormally high percentage for patients under the age of 40 years [226]). Of the 95 patients followed for more than 2 years in this study, 46 percent had proteinuria, 42 percent had hypertension, and 38 percent had reduced GFRs. Some patients died in chronic renal failure [406]; this suggested that although improvement in renal function can occur after acute onset of the initial illness, chronic renal failure might nevertheless develop several years later. All the deaths were in adult patients.

In Baldwin's largest study, involving 168 patients who were followed for periods up to 18 years [19], the author noted proteinuria and/or hypertension in 50 percent (clinical uremia occurred in 6). Thus Baldwin and coworkers maintain that an appreciable number of patients developed irreversible sclerotic glomerular changes. The mechanism of such progression is unclear, although ischemia or enhancement by vascular disease was proposed. These results, however, have been widely challenged. It has been suggested that there is an inordinately high proportion of adult patients in the studies and that the patients are somewhat "atypical" for acute poststreptococcal glomerulonephritis. Also, the patient population had a much higher frequency of nephrotic syndrome and was clinically different from typical acute postinfectious glomerulonephritis. Indeed, reports from other investigators [151,273,320,462] fail to support the findings of Baldwin et al. and suggest that progression to chronicity is a rare event.

In summary, acute postinfectious (mostly poststreptococcal) glomerulonephritis has an excellent prognosis in children, although the outcome with the crescentic form is less clear, especially in epidemics. Complete clinical recovery usually takes place in children. It is difficult to determine whether patients with skin infections have a different prognosis from patients with throat infections, although the prognosis in either type of infection appears good in the epidemic variety [396]. Death may occur in the acute stage from infections, heart disease, or kidney failure; 7 percent appears to be one of the highest figures noted [148,270]. The outcome in adults is more controversial. Recovery appears to occur in most adults, although probably not to the same extent as in children. In most series, at least two-thirds of adults recover. Approximately 5 percent of adults die from the same causes as noted earlier in children, although death from renal failure appears to be more common. Up to 5 percent of adult patients die with a crescentic form of glomerulonephritis, and varying proportions of patients enter the latent or chronic stages. This number varies because of the different lengths of follow-up, the different criteria used to assess chronicity, and the fact that the patients in the various series are not strictly comparable [384,384*a*]. After review of all the studies with significant follow-up, Rodriguez-Iturbe [384,384*a*] suggested that regardless of the frequency of renal functional abnormalities and histologic changes, uremia is quite rare after a decade of follow-up. In his review of the combined series, terminal end-stage kidney disease developed in only about 1 percent of all patients.

ACUTE POSTINFECTIOUS GLOMERULONEPHRITIS OF NONSTREPTOCOCCAL ETIOLOGIES

Group A streptococcal organisms are not the only organisms with the ability to lead to an acute diffuse proliferative glomerulonephritis [147,158, 367,410,516]. A variety of bacterial, viral, and

Table 5-3. *Glomerulonephritis with other infections*

I. Bacterial	
A.	Shunt nephritis [13,24,29,44,74,141, 170,174,177,185,231,330,337,345,411, 414,449,450,481,488,499,508,509]
B.	Endocarditis [14–17,26,80,88,119,167, 172,210,245,262,316,333,334,351, 352,441,444]
C.	Pneumococcal pneumonia and infection [187,208,221,304,407,420]
D.	Syphilis [482]
E.	Salmonellosis [67,246]
F.	Brucellosis [477]
G.	Deep abscesses [25–27,92]
H.	Mycobacterial infection [466]
I.	Campylobacter enteritis [296]
J.	Staphylococcal infections [92,182,294,304,400,404,443]
K.	Yersinia infections [143]
L.	Q fever (*Coxiella burnetii*) [353]
M.	Legionnaire's disease [489]
N.	Mycoplasma infection [473,484]
II. Viral	
A.	Varicella [241,313,429]
B.	Coxsackie [433]
C.	Cytomegalovirus [79]
D.	Measles [109,275]
E.	Mumps [319]
F.	Epstein-Barr [424,487,505]
G.	Influenza [433,434]
H.	Hepatitis B [65]
I.	ECHO [204,433,434,513]
J.	Adenovirus [109,433,434,513]
K.	Vaccinia [183]
L.	Variola [183]
M.	Herpes [285,446]

fungal antigens are thought to give rise to acute glomerulonephritis (Table 5-3), and these antigens have been demonstrated in the glomeruli of the affected patients. Many of these patients present with an acute nephritic syndrome, but they do so with less frequency than with nephritogenic streptococci [218,516]. The glomerular diseases related to these nonstreptococcal antigens are generally associated with a broader spectrum of morphologic changes than noted earlier in typical acute poststreptococcal glomerulonephritis. There are also a number of patients with acute diffuse proliferative glomerulonephritis (appearing to be postinfectious) in whom no evidence of infection can be found. Some of these are still probably instances of poststreptococcal glomerulonephritis in which the relevant diagnostic laboratory studies were not performed. Occult suppurative infections (such as infective endocarditis) can result in a diffuse proliferative glomerulonephritis [27]; there are also likely instances in which the glomerular hypercellularity is confined to the mesangial regions and in which the typical humps and immunofluorescence findings are not identified. It should be commented on that the most common misdiagnosis I have noted in consultation (and even sometimes in the literature) is the erroneous interpretation of a pure mesangial hypercellularity (i.e., mesangial "glomerulitis") without closure of the glomerular capillary loops as a true acute diffuse proliferative glomerulonephritis. Another common reason for the inappropriate overuse of the diagnosis of acute proliferative glomerulonephritis is that the sections for light microscopy are too thick, which leads to an erroneous perception of hypercellularity.

Staphylococcal organisms (especially coagulase-positive staphylococci–*Staphylococcus aureus*) have on occasion led to a clinical and morphologic picture identical to that of poststreptococcal glomerulonephritis [92,294,400,443]. Most of these instances have been associated with infective endocarditis (see p. 364). However, some of these patients with staphylococcal glomerulonephritis have not had endocarditis [294,443]. McIntosh et al. [304] noted this in two patients with staphylococcal pneumonia, and Heptinstall [182] noted it in one patient with a staphylococcal septicemia without endocarditis. Acute diffuse proliferative glomerulonephritis also has been noted in patients with staphylococcal pneumonia and empyema [25,92,400], as well as arthritis and septicemia [294]. Sato et al. [404] noted the presence of an antistaphylolysin antibody in three patients with acute glomerulonephritis, and in two of these patients the staphylococcal antigen was demonstrated in the glomerular mesangium by immunofluorescence techniques. IgG, IgA, and C3 were noted in the mesangial and capillary walls of the glomeruli [443].

Coagulase-negative staphylococci (*Staphylococcus epidermidis*) have been implicated in acute postinfectious glomerulonephritis in patients with infected ventriculoatrial shunts used for the treatment of hydrocephalus. The morphologic picture found in these patients is most often of a membranoproliferative (mesangiocapillary) glomerulonephritis. This will be considered later under Glomerulonephritis with Infected Ventriculoatrial Shunts.

Pneumococcal infections may lead to acute proliferative glomerulonephritis [208,420], as well as to other morphologic patterns [187,208,221], such as a pure mesangial proliferative glomerulonephropathy. Hill et al. [187] described one patient who had antibodies against the pneumococcal capsular carbohydrate that gave positive fluorescence in the glomeruli when an indirect immunofluorescence study was performed. Heptinstall [182], McIntosh et al. [304], and Hyman et al. [208] each described patients with pneumococcal pneumonia and glomerular disease. Clinical signs are hematuria, proteinuria, edema, and renal insufficiency. Glomerular subepithelial humps are found, and C3 and pneumococcal antigens can be detected in the mesangial regions and along the glomerular capillaries by immunofluorescence techniques [187,221]. Properdin also has been noted in a similar distribution [208], and C3, C3 proactivator, and pneumococcal antigen are sometimes noted focally along the tubular basement membranes [221]. In view of these findings, it was suggested that the alternative pathway of complement activation had been stimulated by the pneumococcal polysaccharide. Complete recovery has been noted.

Meningococcal infections may lead to an acute proliferative glomerulonephritis [185,368]. Such patients may not have clinical evidence of glomerulonephritis but are biopsied because of laboratory evidence of circulating immune complexes. Immunofluorescence and electron microscopic studies reveal similar changes to those noted in typical poststreptococcal acute glomerulonephritis.

There are many other causes of acute postinfectious glomerulonephritis (see Table 5-3). Proliferative glomerulonephritis has been reported in patients with pneumonia due to *Klebsiella* and *Mycoplasma* [138,473,484]. This disease may be manifest by hematuria, proteinuria, or renal insufficiency, but it may be clinically occult [138, 473,484]. Klebsiella capsular polysaccharide antigens, immunoglobulins, and complement have been demonstrated in the glomerular capillaries and in the mesangial regions of a patient with focal proliferative glomerulonephritis and pneumonia caused by *Klebsiella* [138]. The eluate of the glomerular-bound IgG had antibody specific to *Klebsiella.* A similar demonstration of diffuse proliferative glomerulonephritis with mycoplasma antigen, immunoglobulin, and complement deposition along the glomerular capillary wall and mesangium was noted in a patient with pneumonia caused by *Mycoplasma* [473]. Disseminated *Mycobacterium gordonae* with glomerulonephritis also has been reported [466].

Deep-seated abscesses caused by a variety of organisms such as *Staphylococcus aureus* and *Pseudomonas aeruginosa* can lead to an acute glomerulonephritis [25–27] (see p. 354). The morphologic pattern ranges from an acute diffuse proliferative glomerulonephritis to a crescentic glomerulonephritis. *Salmonella typhi* has been noted to lead to a glomerulonephritis with glomerular deposition of immunoglobulins and complement [66,246], although the clinical evidence of glomerular disease was usually slight.

A variety of protozoan and viral organisms can produce glomerulonephritis, although the glomerular changes by light microscopy are not as marked as those in classic acute postinfectious glomerulonephritis (see Table 5-3). Renal disease caused by parasitic infections is covered in Chapter 28.

Viruses have been incriminated in the causation of acute (immune complex–mediated) glomerulonephritis [202,391,433,434,445] (see Table 5-3). Smith et al. [433] studied prospectively 240 previously healthy military personnel with nonstreptococcal upper respiratory tract infections for asymptomatic glomerulonephritis. Nine patients were found to have red blood cell casts in the urine and a focal or diffuse mesangial hypercellularity (with mesangial deposits of C3) on renal biopsy. Five of these nine patients had serologic evidence of viral infection with adenovirus or influenza A or B, and four of nine had hypocomplementemia. Repeat renal biopsies showed histologic improvement and/or loss of immunofluorescent staining.

GLOMERULONEPHRITIS ASSOCIATED WITH DEEP-SEATED VISCERAL ABSCESSES

Whitworth et al. [495] and Beaufils et al. [25–27] first described the association of glomerulonephritis and visceral suppuration in the absence of an infective endocarditis.

Clinical Features

The temporal association between the deep-seated infection and the glomerulonephritic "immune type" lesions suggests an etiologic relationship between these two conditions. Serum cryoglobulins and circulating immune complexes are often present [25–27] and usually disappear when the infection is cured. Hypocomplementemia is not generally a feature unless infective endocarditis is also present [25–27]; the data suggest activation of the alternative pathway of complement activation.

Deep suppurative infection can be caused either by gram-positive or gram-negative organisms; as noted before, bacterial endocarditis also can be present. Bacteremia may not be documented in all patients. The majority of the cases are due to intrathoracic abscesses, but wound infections, subphrenic abscess, appendiceal abscess, septic abortion, cutaneous abscess, mediastinitis, acute osteomyelitis, and infection of valvular and vascular Dacron prostheses have all been reported [25,54,88,92]. Lung abscesses were most commonly noted in those patients with the crescentic form of the disease [495]. The duration of the deep-seated abscess ranges from a few weeks to a few years [25–27]. The morphology correlates somewhat with the duration of the preceding infection. Those patients with infection of less than 2 months' duration had only mesangial hypercellularity, whereas patients with more than 2 months of infection had either an acute diffuse glomerulonephritis with crescents or a crescentic glomerulonephritis [25–27].

The patients are febrile and generally quite ill. Microhematuria is present in all patients, and gross hematuria is noted in approximately half of them. Proteinuria is usually present and may be marked. Hypertension is noted in about one-fourth of patients, and oliguria is present in almost half. Rapid progression of renal insufficiency can occur [25–27,495]. Some three-fourths of patients will require dialysis. Extrarenal manifestation include purpura, arthralgia, and cutaneous necrosis.

Pathologic Changes

A number of morphologic patterns have been noted [26], including crescentic glomerulonephritis [495], membranoproliferative glomerulonephritis with or without crescents [25–27,495], acute diffuse proliferative glomerulonephritis [92] with or without crescents [25–27], and mild mesangial hypercellularity [443]. Immunofluorescence staining is positive in the glomeruli in a granular pattern for immunoglobulins and complement. Electron microscopy most commonly demonstrates glomerular mesangial deposits; glomerular subepithelial deposits have been noted in one patient with *S. aureus* and acute diffuse proliferative glomerulonephritis [92].

Prognosis and Outcome

When there is complete eradication of the deep-seated infection (usually through surgical means), renal function generally recovers and cryoglobulinemia disappears [25–27,495]. Repeat renal biopsies show morphologic evidence of healing with only mild residual mesangial hypercellularity, capillary wall thickening, and some globally sclerotic glomeruli [25–27,495]. If infection cannot be controlled (noted in about one of three reported patients), the glomerulonephritis persists (as demonstrated on repeat biopsies), and patients succumb to renal failure [25–27,495]. Incomplete therapy (delayed or suboptimal) results in moderate to severe renal insufficiency that may require dialysis. Persistent microhematuria or proteinuria may be found in those who otherwise appear to have recovered normal renal function [25–27,495].

GLOMERULONEPHRITIS ASSOCIATED WITH INFECTIVE ENDOCARDITIS

Infection of the heart valves historically has been divided into *subacute bacterial endocarditis,* in which a previously damaged heart valve is susceptible to bacterial organisms of low virulence, and *acute bacterial endocarditis,* in which a previously normal heart valve is infected by a virulent bacterial organism. Infection of a rheumatic heart by organisms of the streptococcus viridans group is an example of the former, whereas *S. aureus* infection (in an intravenous drug abuser) is an example of the latter. The natural history of glomerulonephritis secondary to infective endocarditis has been dramatically influenced and changed by the advent of antibiotic therapy and the changing epidemiologic patterns. Although some authors have discontinued use of those two subdivisions (subacute and acute), I intend to retain them in this chapter for historical reasons.

Glomerulonephritis in Subacute Bacterial Endocarditis

Renal complications of subacute bacterial endocarditis include glomerulonephritis, renal infarction, abscesses, and therapy-related or therapy-induced interstitial nephritis. I will only consider glomerulonephritis here.

Embolic nonsuppurative focal nephritis was the name given by Löhlein at the turn of the century [279] to the renal lesions noted in seven patients with subacute bacterial endocarditis. Three of the patients were infected by organisms of the streptococcus viridans group. Baehr [14] and Bell [31] described glomerulonephritis at autopsy in patients with subacute and acute endocarditis. The lesion in subacute endocarditis was characterized by a number of glomeruli showing segmental or local necrosis, often with segmental hypercellularity and/or sclerosis. Polymorphonuclear leukocytes and nuclear fragments also were present. Thus different stages of the segmental lesions appeared to be represented. The majority of the glomeruli were histologically normal. The term *focal embolic nephritis* implied that the renal disease was secondary to embolization of infectious material; although most investigators do not now accept this pathogenetic mechanism, a few authors have described embolization of infectious material to glomeruli [456,518]. Because it is now apparent that the mechanism is virtually always an immunologic one, the term *focal and segmental proliferative, necrotizing, and/or sclerosing glomerulonephritis* is championed. The most common organisms leading to this pattern are those of the streptococcus viridans group and coagulase-negative staphylococci, including *S. epidermidis,* although *Actinobacillus actinomycetemcomitans, Streptococcus mitis, Hemophilus influenzae, Neisseria gonorrheae,* enterococci, and *Chlamydia psittaci* have all been reported.

The true incidence of glomerulonephritis associated with subacute bacterial endocarditis is difficult to determine; most reports do not emanate from prospective and consecutive examinations of clinical and morphologic material from unselected patients but instead come from retrospective postmortem or renal biopsy studies from selected patients, usually those with the most severe disease. Some series are derived from clinical observations without the benefit of histologic examination of renal tissues. Patients with clinical evidence of renal disease, that is, active urinary sediment such as hematuria, may have renal infarction rather than glomerulonephritis. Other published studies suffer from incomplete clinical data even to confirm the diagnosis of infective endocarditis and lack information on such essentials as blood cultures. Data collected from postmortem examinations have the drawback that they tend to overestimate the incidence and severity of endocarditis-related glomerulonephritis. Antibiotic therapy leads to resolution of milder forms of endocarditis-associated glomerulonephritis so that the preexisting glomerulonephritis may be modified or not even evident at the time of morphologic examination.

CLINICAL FEATURES

Renal involvement may occasionally be the presenting manifestation of subacute bacterial endocarditis; this happens when the diagnosis of endocarditis is not considered or when blood cultures are negative. The clinical findings of renal involvement may be mild and are usually overshadowed by the cardiac features and the effects of the systemic infection. Macroscopic hematuria may be present, but the microscopic form is more commonly noted. Hematuria may persist or resolve, only to appear again on several different occasions. It has been suggested that macroscopic hematuria is caused by renal infarctions rather than by the glomerular lesions [182]. Proteinuria (mild) and renal casts may be detected in the urine; nephrotic syndrome is unusual. Hypertension is also unusual. Depression in serum complement is frequent but not always present, nor is it specific for renal involvement even when present [23,56, 69,172,234,351]. Prior to the era of antibiotic therapy, hypocomplementemia was noted in 90 percent of patients with diffuse glomerulonephritis and 60 percent of patients with focal glomerulonephritis in subacute bacterial endocarditis. Most patients appear to have activation of the classical complement pathway [338].

When the BUN and serum creatinine levels are elevated, the renal pattern is more likely to be the diffuse form of glomerulonephritis [14,15,137] rather than the focal form. However, some authors have noted patients dying from renal failure in whom the renal pattern has been that of a focal glomerulonephritis [30,31,56,172,262,263,306, 441], but in most of these studies it appears that most of the glomeruli were involved and damaged. It is likely that these cases were examples of the diffuse form in which there was segmental accentuation of the glomerular lesion rather than a truly focal form [182]. Focal glomerulonephritis may occur in the absence of any clinical renal involvement [323]. Uremia was present in about 5 to 10 percent of patients with endocarditis in the preantibiotic era [167]. Following the introduction of antibiotics, this figure fell to 3 to 4 percent [167]. No uremic deaths were found in penicillin-treated patients with fatal subacute bacterial endocarditis in the series of Spain and King [441]. Eight patients with diffuse glomerulonephritis and one patient with focal glomerulonephritis developed uremia in the 52 untreated patients in the same series.

PATHOLOGIC CHANGES

Gross Appearance

The kidneys are either normal in size or enlarged. The largest kidneys are in those patients who have a concomitant widespread or diffuse glomerulonephritis. There are petechial hemorrhages in the subcapsular region of the kidney (hence the description "flea-bitten") [200]; two-thirds of the 30 patients studied by Barajas and Heptinstall had this appearance [182]. Either fresh or healed renal infarcts were identified in 57 percent of the cases; they were either single or multiple and were of a size suggesting obstruction of arcuate or large interlobular arteries.

Microscopic Findings

The infarcts noted grossly show a variety of ages; they are sterile and are not different from any other type of sterile infarct (see Chap. 18). Nothing more will be said about them at this point.

GLOMERULI. A number of different light microscopic glomerular patterns are noted. Focal and segmental glomerulonephritis is often present [14,31,56,263,279,323,441]. This type of lesion was noted in from 50 to 84 percent of patients studied [14,182,221,263,441]. Bell [31] found focal segmental lesions occurring with diffuse proliferation in over half his patients; focal glomerulonephritis alone also was noted in 18 percent. When focal and segmental glomerulonephritis occurs, only a portion of the total number of glomeruli seen are affected by light microscopy. This is in keeping with the World Health Organization (WHO) definition [83]. The focal and segmental glomerular changes are evenly distributed throughout the kidney, although the percentage of glomeruli with lesions varies widely. Baehr noted that 2 to 75 percent of the glomeruli were involved in his patients [14]. In over 70 percent of patients, the segmental glomerular lesions involved from 10 to 40 percent of the glomeruli [14–17]. In the series of Barajas and Heptinstall [182], of 15 patients with focal and segmental glomerulonephritis, 6 had 15 percent or more of the glomeruli involved, 7 had 5 to 14 percent, and 2 had 4 percent or less. Villarreal and Sokoloff [472*a*] described patients who had over 95 percent of their glomeruli affected as seen by light microscopy. These authors noted the difficulty in distinguishing widespread glomerulonephritis due to endocarditis from chronic glomerulonephritis when the lesions showed "advanced healing."

There are two histologic types of lesion. The first, called the *acute,* or *fresh, lesion,* consists of fibrinoid necrosis and/or intracapillary thrombosis confined to one or two glomerular lobules (Fig. 5-24). Polymorphonuclear leukocytes and nuclear debris may be present. There is usually segmental hypercellularity in the affected segment, but it is not always present. Adhesions or synechiae to Bowman's capsule may occur with adjacent crescent formation. Erythrocytes may be found in Bowman's space or in the renal tubular lumens. A few authors have demonstrated organisms in some of the involved segments [518], but this is very unusual. It is important to remember that even in the focal and segmental form of glomerulonephritis (by light microscopy) there are widespread de-

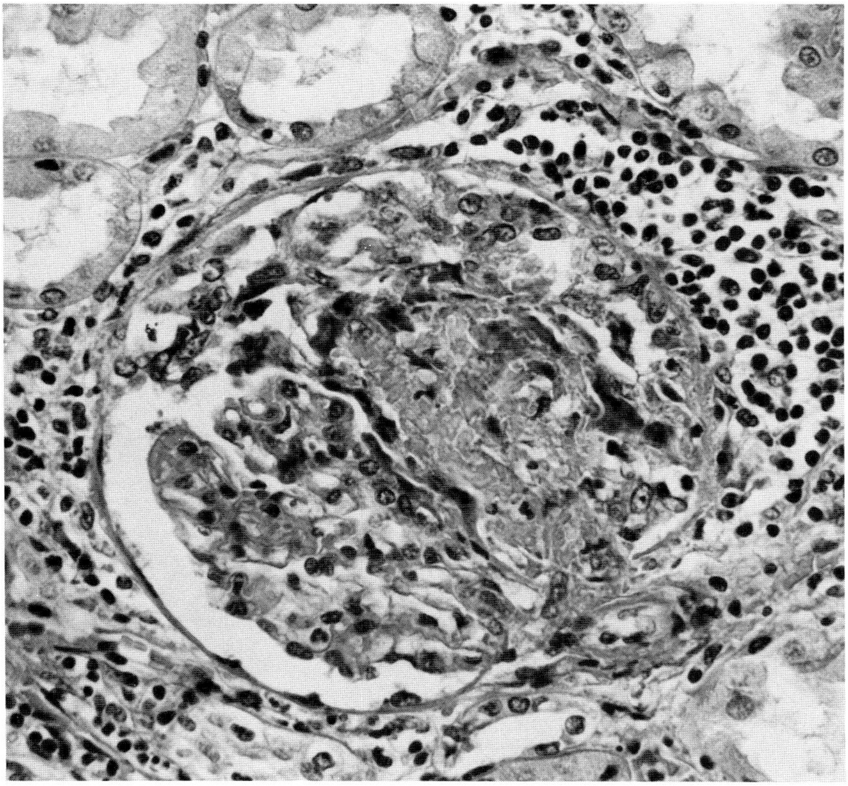

FIG. 5-24. *Glomerulus from patient with endocarditis of 3 months' duration caused by organism of streptococcus viridans group. There is necrosis in the right-hand side of the glomerulus together with early crescent formation. Between 5 and 10 percent of the glomeruli showed either fresh or healed lesions. H&E; ×440.*

posits throughout all glomeruli when they are studied by electron microscopy and/or immunofluorescence.

The second lesion is a *healed, scarred,* or more appropriately termed *sclerotic lesion.* It is usually situated at the periphery of one or of several lobules (Figs. 5-25 and 5-26). There is usually an adhesion or synechia between the sclerotic region and Bowman's capsule. There may be an adjacent fibrocellular crescent. Layers of fibrotic capsular bands encircling the involved glomerular tufts may be noted, but this is not a specific change. Collagen is not often present in the glomerular sclerotic region. Organisms are not demonstrable in these lesions either. This advanced, or scarred, lesion is most common in those cases of longer duration and is the exclusive lesion found in Libman's healed, or bacteria-free, stage [271,272].

The active segmental lesions are indistinguishable at the light microscopic level from other forms of focal segmental proliferative or necrotizing glomerulonephritis. The focal segmental sclerotic change may be difficult to distinguish from idiopathic focal and segmental glomerular sclerosis [496].

An acute diffuse and global endocapillary proliferative glomerulonephritis also may be encountered [16,31,56,80,172,234,352]. Bell [31] described "glomerulitis" in which there was mild endocapillary (now known to be mesangial) hypercellularity with little increase in mesangial matrix and little or no narrowing of the glomerular capillary lumina. Few polymorphonuclear leukocytes were present. A more severe form of acute diffuse and global endocapillary hypercellularity narrows or occludes the glomerular capillaries and may be associated with an increase in mesangial matrix; by light microscopy it is quite indistin-

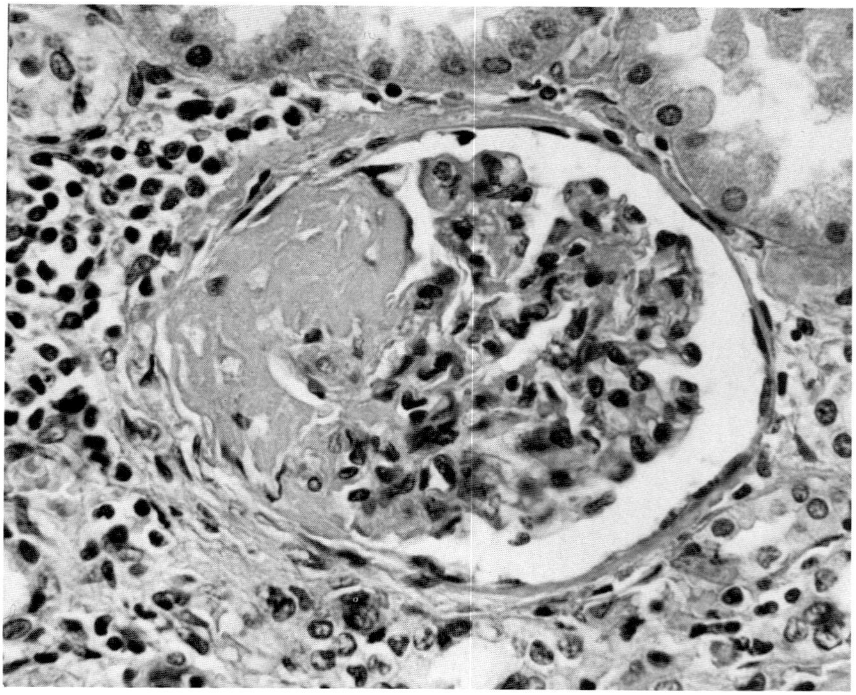

FIG. 5-25. *Old hyalin area at periphery of glomerulus merging with Bowman's capsule, from the same patient as in Fig. 5-24. H&E; ×235.*

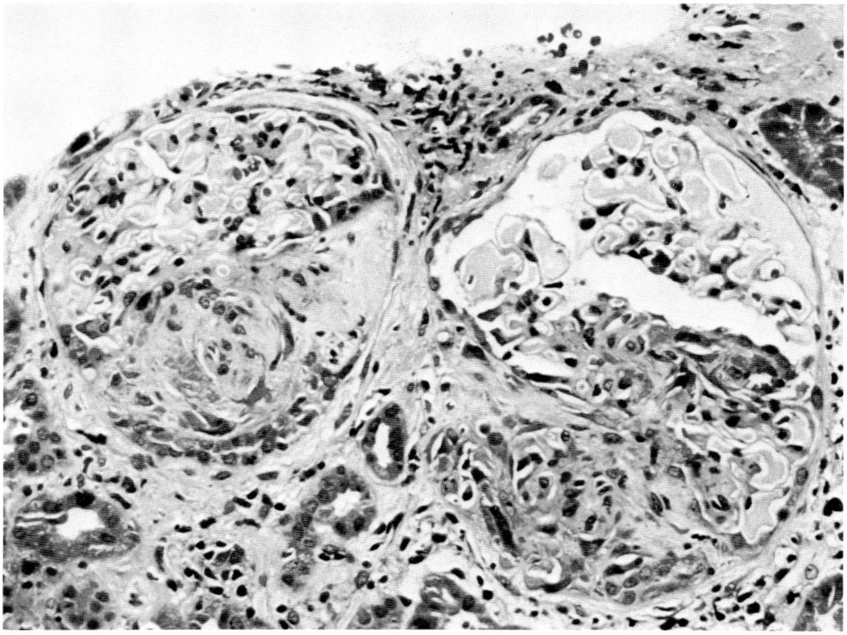

Fig. 5-26. *Two glomeruli from a biopsy on a 19-year-old man with subacute bacterial endocarditis. Both show segmental scarring. Most of the glomeruli in this biopsy showed no abnormalities. H&E; ×265. (Courtesy of Dr. George Bannayan.)*

guishable from typical postinfectious glomerulonephritis. The diffuse proliferative glomerulonephritic form shows increased cellularity of all glomeruli (or almost all glomeruli) with global involvement of the entire tuft. The term *proliferative* is utilized, and although many of the cells are likely to be endogenous endocapillary cells, migrant monocytes and/or polymorphonuclear leukocytes probably also contribute to the hypercellularity. There may be segmental necrosis, thrombosis, or sclerosis superimposed on the generalized hypercellularity [172,234]. Crescents also may be present but are generally not so numerous as to warrant the designation of *crescentic glomerulonephritis* [172,323].

Baehr and Lande [16] have noted the greater frequency of generalized changes in the so-called bacteria-free stage, and most of the patients studied by Gutman et al. [172] with repeated negative blood cultures showed widespread glomerular involvement. However, the diffuse glomerulonephritic form can occur in patients with positive blood cultures, and not all patients with negative cultures have the diffuse type of lesion. Bell [31] noted diffuse proliferation in 65 percent of his patients. The exact frequency of this pattern is difficult to determine because most series are small and the large series are based on autopsy findings. Most studies were performed many years ago when the value of thin sections was not well appreciated, and many of the sections demonstrated in the papers were quite thick, thereby exaggerating the cellularity of the glomerular tufts [182]. Barajas and Heptinstall [182] noted diffuse changes in 17 percent of patients, but Christian [80] described them in 80 percent. A marked focal segmental proliferation (hypercellularity with closure of the capillaries) may coexist with a mild diffuse global hypercellularity [31,172,333,334]. At times, the segmental lesions may be so numerous as to be virtually diffuse and global. Baehr [14–17] noted diffuse global and focal segmental hypercellularity in a third of his patients. It is at times difficult to know from the older literature whether the authors were describing pure mesangial hypercellularity without glomerular capillary lumen narrowing or closure, or a more severe mesangial hypercellularity with loss of the capillary lumens. It is obvious that thicker histologic sections create a hypercellular histologic appearance.

A further glomerular pattern noted is a membranoproliferative (mesangiocapillary) glomerulonephritis [26,109,444]. Most of the older studies are not detailed, and it is not possible to determine the precise characteristics of the lesion. The finding of membranoproliferative glomerulonephritis is not surprising considering that it is one of the most commonly encountered lesions in patients with shunt nephritis. Recovery can apparently take place in these patients [26].

INTERSTITIUM. There is interstitial inflammation regardless of the type of glomerular pattern, and it can be present even in treated patients with quiescent disease [323].

TUBULES. There may be tubular atrophy commensurate with the degree of glomerular damage. Tubular casts are frequent. Ultrastructural studies of tubular basement membranes may reveal discrete electron-dense deposits, but their nature is not understood at the present time.

ARTERIES. Arterial intimal thickening may be present [323]. It may be noted in quite young individuals, and the cause is uncertain.

Immunofluorescence Findings

Immunofluorescence studies in both the focal and segmental and in the diffuse forms of glomerulonephritis show widespread glomerular distribution of immunoglobulins and/or complement, even in the normal-appearing glomeruli. The glomerular staining is located in the mesangial regions and along the glomerular capillary walls. Morel-Maroger et al. [323*a*] described a series of patients, most treated with antibiotics, and demonstrated diffuse granular immunofluorescence along the glomerular capillaries for C3 and, in some patients, for IgG, IgM, and IgA in the mesangial regions. Other investigators have shown a granular pattern for immunoglobulins and C3 along the glomerular capillary walls [56,263] and in the mes-

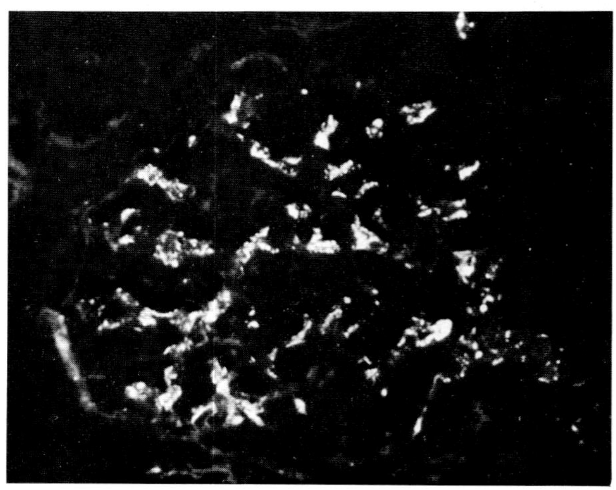

FIG. 5-27. *Immunofluorescence to demonstrate C3 in a glomerulus from same biopsy as in Fig. 5-26. There is a predominantly granular mesangial distribution of C3. IgG and IgM were present with a similar distribution. (Courtesy of Dr. George Bannayan.)*

angial regions [56]. Heptinstall [182] cites a case shown to him by George Bannayan in which the majority of glomeruli were normal by light microscopy but others showed segmental sclerosis. There was mesangial IgG, IgM, and C3 with less intense granular staining along the glomerular capillary walls (Fig. 5-27). Rarely, a linear pattern has been described, but it is not indicative of anti-GBM antibody formation. Immunofluorescence studies in the diffuse glomerulonephritic form, as noted, show diffuse granular deposition of immunoglobulins along the glomerular capillary walls and in the mesangial regions [172,234]. Diffuse coarse granular deposits of C3 along the glomerular capillary walls with large subendothelial deposits of IgG and IgM have been described [323*a*], but some authors have failed to demonstrate immunoglobulins or C3 [56]. Perez et al. [352] described granular deposition of IgM and C3 in the glomeruli, in addition to bacterial antigen demonstrated by the corresponding antiserum.

Electron Microscopic Findings

Ultrastructural studies show discrete electron-dense deposits on the endothelial side of the GBM, especially in the regions near the mesangial areas (Fig. 5-28). Boulton-Jones et al. [56] and others [172] have shown glomerular subendothelial and mesangial deposits.

PATHOGENESIS

Löhlein [279] was the first to describe the renal changes in this condition when he reported seven patients with endocarditis in some of whom organisms of the streptococcus viridans group were cul-

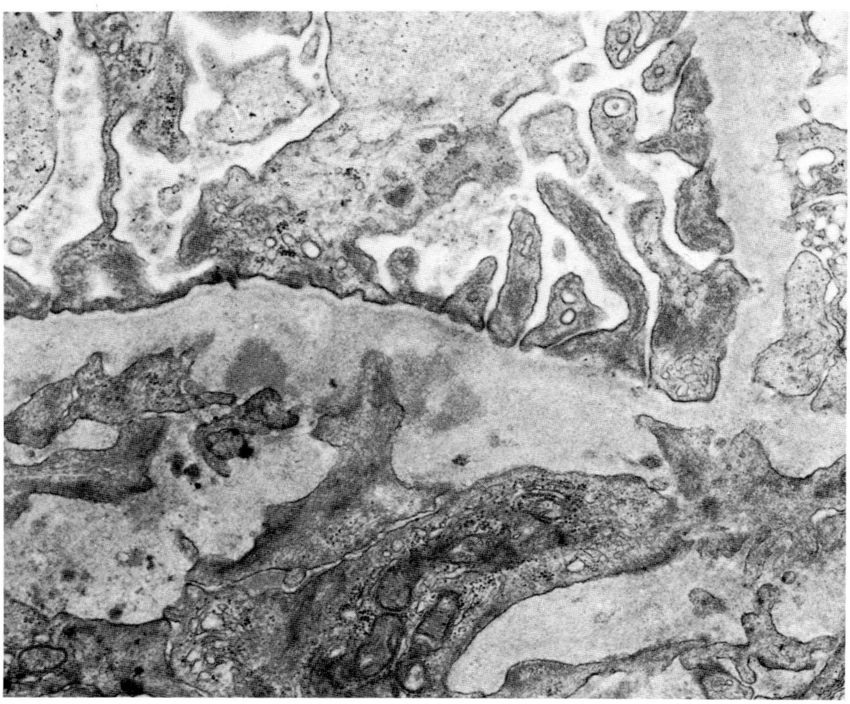

Fig. 5-28. *Electron micrograph from the same biopsy as shown in Fig. 5-26. It shows dense deposits in a subendothelial position where the capillary wall is reflected over the mesangium.* ×15,000. *(Courtesy of Dr. George Bannayan.)*

tured during life. He observed streptococci in an embolus that was impacted in an artery and had led to infarction; this suggested to him that the glomerulonephritis was caused by bacterial emboli. This idea was further supported by Baehr [14], who noted bacterial emboli in glomeruli in 5 of 25 patients. The segmentally scarred (sclerotic) lesion was thought to represent a later lesion resulting from healing of the necrotic lesion. Bell [30] considered that the acute glomerular lesion was a hyalin intracapillary thrombus, which in the larger but not the smaller lesions led to necrosis of the glomerular capillaries. He suggested that the first step was the lodgement of minute infected emboli or small clusters of bacterial organisms in the glomerular capillaries, with release of toxic substances by the bacteria leading to thrombosis and necrosis. He stated that in rare instances bacteria could be demonstrated in the glomeruli. Thörig et al. [456] recently came to the same conclusion after induction of bacterial endocarditis by intravenous injection of live streptococci into rabbits with a nonbacterial thrombotic endocarditis. Their view differs from other investigators in that they thought that the necrotic foci disintegrate and disappear and that the sclerotic lesion develops independently.

Longcope [280] suggested that the glomerulonephritic lesion was of allergic type; this idea was supported by others [220] who believed that the lesion differed only in degree from those in classic diffuse glomerulonephritis. Bell [31] did note in 1932 that "the fact that a certain duration of the infection is necessary suggests that immune bodies may play a role in the formation of the glomerular lesions." It is now apparent that both the focal and segmental glomerulonephritis and the acute diffuse glomerulonephritis are manifestations of an immunologic reaction, and that circulating immune complexes play the major role in the pathogenesis of the glomerular injury. Bacterial cultures from kidneys with this type of pattern show no growth. It is now recognized that focal glomerulonephritis can be seen in diseases in which there are no sources of emboli, such as systemic lupus erythematosus and polyarteritis nodosa. Patients with known true septic emboli do not generally have this type of glomerular response.

Williams and Kunkel [499] demonstrated depression in the level of serum complement in patients with subacute infective endocarditis. Subsequently, patients with focal or diffuse glomerulonephritis due to infective endocarditis also were noted to have hypocomplementemia [26,172, 234,352]. The degree of complement depression is directly correlated with the severity of renal involvement [338]. Persistent hypocomplementemia is associated with a failure to control the infection and prevent continuing renal insufficiency [333, 334], whereas normalization of the serum complement occurs with successful antibiotic therapy and the return of renal function [338].

Circulating immune complexes have been demonstrated in patients with infective endocarditis [23,69,316,499]. High levels of circulating immune complexes have been noted in patients with less virulent bacteria, right-sided cardiac involvement, and hypocomplementemia; many of these patients also had extracardiac manifestations of endocarditis [23,69]. Circulating immune complexes are persistent or rise when it is not possible to control the infection [69,199]; successful antibiotic therapy leads to falling levels of circulating immune complexes [23]. Rheumatoid factor also may be present [351,499], and the titer falls quickly after successful antibiotic therapy [499]. However, rheumatoid factor may not necessarily be indicative of renal involvement in patients with infective endocarditis [351].

Mixed cryoglobulinemia has been identified in the serum of most patients with infective endocarditis [69]. The levels of cryoglobulinemia (like the level of circulating immune complexes) fall with control of the infection [69]. However, the level of serum cryoglobulin is not directly correlated with the presence or absence of renal involvement [69]. Further study of the type(s) of cryoglobulin is required.

While some of the studies quoted were not accompanied by renal biopsies, others have been, and immunofluorescence and electron microscopic studies show evidence of an immune complex–mediated glomerulonephritis [26,56,172,234,263, 323,352]. Some studies have shown that the eluate from a kidney with focal glomerulonephritis due to infective endocarditis reacted specifically with bacteria cultured from the patient's blood [210,263]. Immunofluorescence studies have demonstrated bacterial antigens in glomerular deposits in infective endocarditis due to streptococcal infection [352]. Focal glomerulonephritis occurring in patients with infections involving only the right side of the heart suggests that embolization is not a major mechanism in this disorder. It is uncertain, however, whether the glomerular deposits form locally, with the binding of circulating antibodies to planted (possibly bacterial) or native glomerular antigens, or result from the deposition of circulating immune complexes.

In summary, there is now much evidence in support of an immunologic mechanism of the immune complex type in all forms of glomerular disease occurring in patients with subacute infective endocarditis.

EFFECT OF TREATMENT ON THE RENAL LESION

Most studies indicate that there is a partial to total resolution of the renal disease after successful antibiotic therapy [167]; however, repeat biopsies are generally not performed.

Observations on the incidence of glomerulonephritis in the early years of antibiotic therapy are few and contradictory. Spain and King [441] studied 77 patients with subacute bacterial endocarditis: 52 were not treated, whereas 25 were given penicillin, with treatment starting on average within 1 to 2 months after the clinical onset of the disease. The frequency of focal glomerulonephritis was reduced by one-half. Diffuse glomerulonephritis was noted in a third of untreated patients, but no case of diffuse glomerulonephritis was noted in the treated patients. Great numbers of sclerotic or healed lesions were identified in the treated group. The efficacy of antibiotic treatment with regard to glomerular damage is therefore apparent and has been confirmed by others [271,272,323]. The generalized acute diffuse form of glomerulonephritis was found to completely disappear. However, this is not invariable, because Jones et al. [216] noted 4 patients with diffuse glomerulonephritis among 15 deaths in their group of 33 patients. Recent studies suggest an incidence of glomerulonephritis in 2 to 60 percent of patients [70,333,334,338 351].

Glomerulonephritis in Acute Infective Endocarditis

Antibiotic therapy and prophylaxis, the decrease in rheumatic fever, and the marked increase in intravenous drug abuse have all altered the picture of infective endocarditis [333,334]. The routes of infection, types of organisms, and clinical manifestation have all undergone major changes. While the frequency of infection with organisms of the streptococcus viridans group has decreased [441], *S. aureus* has become a major cause of bacterial endocarditis [333,334]. This organism carries a high likelihood of glomerulonephritis, especially in patients with intravenous drug abuse. *S. aureus* is the etiologic agent in over a third of the fatal cases and is responsible for over half the cases of all types of endocarditis-associated glomerulonephritis in recent series [69,333,334, 338,351]. Glomerulonephritis may develop in intravenous drug abusers with *S. aureus* infections following a clinical illness of only 1 week [338].

Irrespective of the infecting organism, focal and segmental glomerulonephritis is rare in patients with acute bacterial endocarditis when this is defined as infective endocarditis lasting less than 6 weeks. A recent study by Neugarten and colleagues [333,334] at a large metropolitan hospital from 1965 to 1979 showed glomerulonephritis in 22 percent of patients with infective (mostly acute bacterial) endocarditis. Glomerulonephritis was focal in 8 percent and diffuse in 14 percent of the patients.

In the preantibiotic era, focal "embolic" glomerulonephritis appeared to occur less frequently in acute than in subacute bacterial endocarditis [14–17,31,333,334]. Bell [31] noted an incidence of 7 percent of focal glomerulonephritis in patients with what he termed the *acute primary form* (i.e., those forms which seemed to begin as a bacteremia) and of 6 percent in patients with the *secondary acute form* (i.e., his term for those patients in whom bloodstream bacterial invasion occurs from a known focus such as acute endometritis or lobar pneumonia). The incidence of focal glomerulonephritis in the subacute form was 53 percent. Bell found diffuse proliferative or exudative glomerulonephritis in 29 and 33 percent of patients with primary and secondary acute forms, respectively. Patients with infections caused by organisms of the streptococcus viridans group of less than 6 weeks' duration did not have focal glomerulonephritis. The experiences of other workers are similar [182].

The combination of acute infective endocarditis and diffuse glomerulonephritis is usually the result of infection by coagulase-positive staphylococci (*S. aureus*). But largely as a result of drug addiction, other organisms are being seen more frequently. These include coagulase-negative staphylococci (*S. epidermidis*) and *Pseudomonas aeruginosa* [26]. A wide range of other bacterial and fungal organisms has been described in those patients.

COAGULASE-POSITIVE STAPHYLOCOCCI

Diffuse proliferative glomerulonephritis is well documented in patients with acute endocarditis caused by coagulase-positive staphylococci (*S. aureus*) [26,172,333,334,355,374,514]. The clinical picture may be dominated by the underlying infective process, but oliguria may herald the onset of renal involvement. There is often a nephritic process with red blood cells and casts in the urine. Gross hematuria may occur secondary to glomerulonephritis, renal infarction, or a drug-related interstitial nephritis. Proteinuria is also often noted, but the nephrotic syndrome is unusual [333,334]. Most of these patients were intravenous drug abusers with *S. aureus* infections. The BUN level is often elevated, and the serum complement level is reduced [26,172,514]. Hypertension is unusual and when found may have been present before the acute onset of infective endocarditis [444,514]. These laboratory findings may show considerable resolution or improvement (within days to weeks) after the institution of antibiotic therapy. Renal insufficiency may be relatively mild or may lead to the need for dialysis [333,334]. The degree of renal insufficiency does not correlate with the clinical duration of the infective endocarditis [333,334]. In most patients, the serum creatinine level reaches its peak at or just into the beginning of successful antibiotic therapy and soon decreases with the therapy. Patients who present with renal failure fare less well than those in whom it is absent [333,334]. It has been suggested recently by two groups [306,394] that addition of plasmapheresis and steroids aids in renal recovery, but additional studies are needed to confirm these findings.

Although a transient worsening of renal function may occur prior to recovery, [262], mild to moderate renal insufficiency almost always resolves with proper antibiotic therapy [172,262]. Even severe renal failure may resolve with antibiotic therapy, although this may take weeks or months to achieve [262,352].

Repeat biopsies have shown almost complete morphologic resolution in those patients with clinical recovery [26]; the only renal parenchymal changes noted were a persistence of mesangial sclerosis and the presence of globally sclerotic glomeruli [26].

Occasionally, persistent renal insufficiency may occur despite proper antibiotic therapy and dialysis [56,333,334]. Marked residual morphologic changes have been noted long after apparent cure [56]. Progressive renal failure and uremic deaths have been reported occasionally in the antibiotic era [56,333,334]; this is not common, and once infective endocarditis has been effectively treated, complete renal healing should occur. There may be persistent proteinuria or hematuria in some patients despite effective therapy [119,168,323, 333,334,444].

PATHOLOGIC CHANGES

Microscopic Findings

The light microscopic features of an acute diffuse proliferative glomerulonephritis are present (Fig. 5-29). There is proliferation of native endocapillary cells as well as infiltration by mononuclear and polymorphonuclear cells. Crescents are often identified. The light microscopic changes closely resemble those already described in patients with acute postinfectious (poststreptococcal) glomerulonephritis.

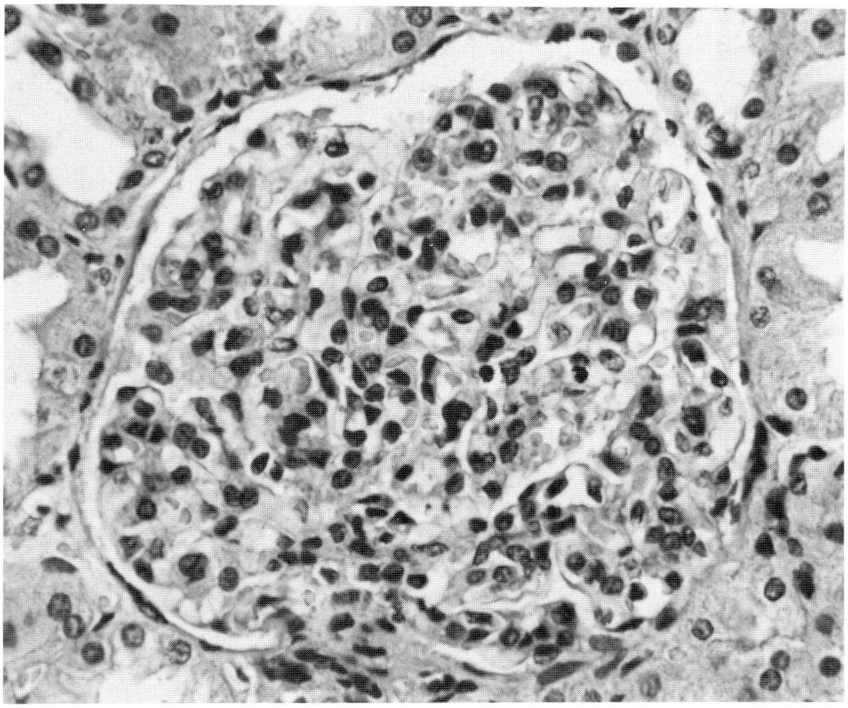

Fig. 5-29. *Diffuse proliferative lesion from a patient with an endocarditis caused by a coagulase-positive staphylococcus. All the glomeruli showed similar changes. H&E; ×430.*

Electron Microscopic Findings

Ultrastructural studies always show glomerular deposits, and discrete electron-dense glomerular subepithelial and intramembranous deposits are the most common [333,334,355,374,514] (Fig. 5-30). Glomerular subendothelial deposits also can be seen, and they sometimes occur in the mesangial regions [333,334], epecially in repeat biopsies studied months after the initial onset of the disease [172]. In some of these studies [172], glomerular subepithelial humps did not disappear on repeat biopsy, as they do in classic acute poststreptococcal glomerulonephritis; the persistence of these humps suggests either that immune complexes containing staphylococcal antigens disappear more slowly than those of streptococcal origin or that the source of the antigen has not been completely eliminated.

Immunofluorescence Findings

Immunofluorescence methods show granular deposits of IgG and C3 along the glomerular capillary walls and often in the mesangial regions [26,172,355,374,514]. Sometimes the mesangium is predominantly involved, with less conspicuous deposits along the capillary walls [172,514]. Immunofluorescence studies have demonstrated bacterial antigens in the glomerular deposits in patients with infective endocarditis due to *S. aureus* [355,514]; staphylococcal antigens also were demonstrated along tubular basement membranes in some patients [355].

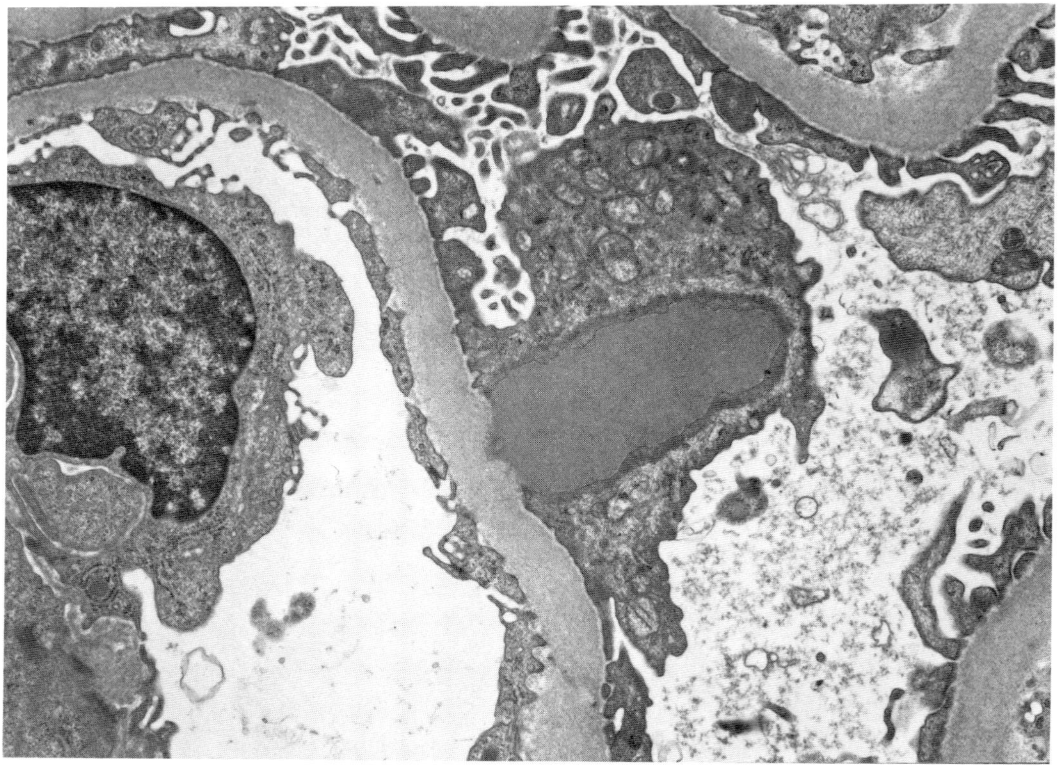

FIG. 5-30. *Electron micrograph showing hump on epithelial side of glomerular capillary basement membrane from a patient with coagulase-positive staphylococcal endocarditis. The hump is covered by a dense zone in the epithelial cytoplasm.* × *11,000. (Courtesy of Dr. G. Striker. From Gutman, R. A., et al.* Medicine *51: 1, 1972, Fig. 9. Copyright 1972 by The Williams & Wilkins Company, Baltimore. Used by permission.)*

PATHOGENESIS

The immunofluorescence and electron microscopic findings, along with the depression of serum C3, suggest an immune complex etiology and pathogenesis. The continued antigenemia (i.e., bacteremia) probably provides a propitious background for the development of these immune complexes.

Most of the cases of infective endocarditis now seen are secondary to drug addiction [172,374]. Narcotic addicts are particularly vulnerable to infective endocarditis [333,334]. Between 40 and 78 percent of intravenous drug abusers with acute endocarditis secondary to *S. aureus* have glomerulonephritis [70,333,334,338,351]. The reason for the high incidence in this group is not known but may be related to existing antibodies to staphylococcal antigens or to the nonimmune activation of the alternative complement pathway by staphylococcal cell-wall antigens.

Hypocomplementemia is noted in 70 percent of patients with acute bacterial endocarditis and diffuse glomerulonephritis. The frequency in patients with focal glomerulonephritis and acute endocarditis is not known. There appears to be a high frequency of activation of the alternative complement pathway in patients with *S. aureus* endocarditis and glomerulonephritis [338]. Several pieces of evidence suggest that there may be nonimmune activation of the alternative complement pathway by staphylococcal cell-wall antigens in acute endocarditis secondary to *S. aureus*. These are (1) an inability to demonstrate circulating immune complexes in some of these patients [333,334,338], (2) an absence of prolonged illness before evidence of glomerulonephritis, and (3) deposition of complement without accompanying immunoglobulins in immunofluorescence studies [231]. Other organisms have been associated with endocarditis, such as the gonococcus [119] and *Coxiella burnetii* [353].

GLOMERULONEPHRITIS WITH INFECTED VENTRICULOATRIAL SHUNTS

Infection of ventriculoatrial shunts (inserted for the relief of hydrocephalus) may lead to glomerulonephritis [13,29,44,106,231, 330, 369, 414, 449, 450,509]. This was first described by Black and colleagues [44] in two children with the nephrotic syndrome and gross hematuria who had developed bacterial colonization of a ventricovascular shunt. Over 100 patients with shunt nephritis have now been described. The infecting organism is usually a coagulase-negative staphylococcus (*S. epidermidis*) that has been introduced either intraoperatively, probably from a skin source, or as a result of transient bacteremia to which the shunt is exposed. The exact way in which the shunt becomes infected is not clear [13,170]. Other reported organisms include *Listeria monocytogenes* [450], peptococcus [74], *Corynebacterium bovis, Bacillus subtilis,* micrococcus, diphtheroid species, and gram-positive anaerobic rods, such as *Propionibacterium acnes* [29,141,170]. Between 6 and 27 percent of ventriculoatrial shunts have evidence of bacterial colonization [29,74,174], and low-grade bacteremia may be present for years before the onset of clinical symptomatology [13]. Cultures of the blood and cerebrospinal fluid may be sterile, and bacterial identification may only be achieved upon removal of the shunt [13]. Clinically overt glomerulonephritis occurs in about 4 to 5 percent of infected patients [170]; the true incidence is not known and would require prospective urinalysis to identify patients with subclinical renal involvement [264]. The latent period between shunt placement and the onset of clinical symptomatology ranges from 1 month to 15 years (mean 4 years). Renal involvement is almost exclusively noted in patients with ventriculoatrial or ventriculojugular shunts; renal involvement in patients with ventriculoperitoneal shunts is quite rare but has been reported and is similar to that seen with ventriculoatrial shunts [106,337]. Ventriculoatrial shunts have been almost totally replaced by ventriculoperitoneal shunts as a form of therapy for hydrocephalus.

Clinical Features

The clinical features include anorexia, anemia, malaise, and fever (all probably the result of the bacteremia); fever is noted in over four-fifths of patients. Most of the patients are children, although adults have been reported (age ranges from 2 months to over 50 years). Patients usually present with signs and symptoms of bacteremia and sepsis, although the renal involvement may be the presenting manifestation [29]. Purpura, arthralgias, lymphadenopathy, hepatosplenomegaly, hypergammaglobulinemia (IgA, IgM, and IgG), and anemia are common. Less common is leukocytosis, leukopenia [106], thrombocytopenia [449, 508], elevation of the erythrocyte sedimentation rate [13], and hypertension. Renal findings include edema, hematuria (gross in half), and proteinuria [24,29,74,245,337,414,449,450,481,509]. The proteinuria may be pronounced, and the nephrotic syndrome has been described in about half the patients [44,449]. One patient even had 38 g of proteinuria per 24 hours [509]. Acute oliguric renal failure has been noted [74]. Apparent recovery occurs in most patients whose infected shunts are removed [13,29,106,449,509], although there may be persistent proteinuria [106]. Death may occur from complications following removal of the shunt [231] or from the original neurologic disease for which the shunt was inserted [449].

Pathogenesis

There is evidence that the renal disease is caused by immune-complex deposition. As noted before in other infectious diseases, there is frequently a depression of the serum complement level [29,106,231,450,509]. Decreases in serum C3 levels are noted in over 85 percent of patients. One-half of patients with acute glomerulonephritis have reduced levels of C4, indicative of activation of the classical complement pathway. Evidence of activation of the alternative pathway is noted in only a few patients [106,444,450,508]. Patients with shunt infections without glomerulonephritis do not have hypocomplementemia [264]. Serum levels of C3 and C4 generally normalize after effective therapy (i.e., antibiotic therapy and/or shunt removal) [13,508]. If therapy is inadequate and the glomerulonephritis persists, then the serum complement level remains depressed [508].

Cryoglobulinemia has been noted [74,450]. Cryoglobulins are able to activate the classical complement pathway in vitro [450]. Circulating immune complexes and rheumatoid factors are found in most patients [411]. Circulating immune complexes, serum cryoglobulins, and serial titers of antibody to bacterial antigen all abate with removal of the shunt, control of the infection, and remission of the glomerulonephritic process [24, 264]. IgG, IgM, and C3 are present in the cryoglobulins, and there was evidence in one study for the presence of both antibody to the bacterial organism and the bacterial antigen [450].

Pathologic Changes

MICROSCOPIC FINDINGS

Renal biopsies show a diffuse proliferative glomerulonephritis or a typical membranoproliferative glomerulonephritis type I [74,369,450]. Polymorphonuclear leukocytes are often present. There is often an increase in the amount of mesangial matrix [44,106,509], and one case was referred to as *lobular glomerulonephritis* [106]. There is almost always accentuation of the lobular pattern. Crescents may be present [106,369]. A membranoproliferative glomerulonephritic pattern is found in approximately one-half of patients, diffuse (nonlobular) proliferative glomerulonephritis in about one-third, and pure mesangial proliferative glomerulonephropathy in the remainder. Focal segmental proliferative glomerulonephritis and crescentic glomerulonephritis have been noted but less commonly [13].

IMMUNOFLUORESCENCE FINDINGS

Immunofluorescence techniques show a granular to coarse broken-linear pattern along the glomerular capillary walls and in the mesangial regions [13,44,74,106,231,369,450,509]. Peripheral glomerular capillary wall immunofluorescent deposits are noted in over four-fifths of patients, whereas mesangial deposits are noted in slightly more than one-half. IgG and IgM are common, and C3 and the early complement components (C1q and C4) are present. IgG is noted in about two-thirds of patients [13], but IgM is sometimes the predominant immunoglobulin [106,170,345]. It was found in 84 percent of patients in one study [13]. IgA, usually less intense than IgG or IgM, is noted in less than one-half of cases [13]. Bacterial antigens have been demonstrated [106,170,231,345]. IgM and C1q have been described in peritubular capillaries [106], and immune complexes have been described along the tubular basement membranes [264].

ELECTRON MICROSCOPIC FINDINGS

Ultrastructural studies demonstrate the presence of discrete electron-dense "immune type" deposits on the subendothelial portions of the glomerular capillary walls and in the mesangial regions [106,369,450,509]. Glomerular intramembranous and subepithelial deposits also have been described but are rare [13,74]. Increased mesangial matrix and circumferential mesangial-cell interposition with creation of a new inner basement-membrane–like material also can be identified. Repeat renal biopsy after successful treatment reveals complete disappearance of the deposits noted by electron microscopy and immunofluorescence techniques [481].

Outcome

Serial renal biopsies have been performed before and after removal of the shunt; complete resolution of the glomerulonephritic process has been noted [481]. The only residua may be mild mesangial hypercellularity [488] or focal global glomerular sclerosis [264,488]. In most patients, the immunofluorescent and electron microscopic deposits completely disappear [264,488,509]. However, patients who develop crescentic glomerulonephritis may not resolve despite adequate therapy [488]. Full clinical recovery is noted in about two-thirds of patients; persistence of renal disease is noted in the remaining third and is manifested by proteinuria, microhematuria, hypertension, or renal insufficiency. Rarely, complete clinical recovery can occur after several months of proteinuria or hematuria [444]. Delay in diagnosis may prevent complete recovery [330] and lead to irreversible renal insufficiency [414].

It has been reported that the glomerulonephritic process may develop as long as 5 years after the apparent colonization of a shunt and the presence of low-grade bacteremia [24,29,74,245,449]. In some of these reports, culture of the blood and of cerebrospinal fluid obtained from the shunt during life was sterile, and identification of a bacterial infection was possible only on removal of the shunt [13]; in other cases, the organism was erroneously regarded as a contaminant [29] or the infection was thought to be controlled by antibiotic therapy [449]. If the shunt is not treated properly and the bacteria persist, mild renal involvement may progress to severe renal impairment [369,488]. Repeat renal biopsies in these cases have shown an increase in glomerular tuft hypercellularity, crescent formation, sclerotic glomeruli, and in the numbers of glomerular electron-dense deposits [369]. As noted before, eradication of the bacteremia (usually by removal of the shunt) leads to a subsidence of the glomerulonephritic process [264]. Although removal of the shunt is almost always needed to permanently eliminate the infection [13,369], remission of bacteremia and kidney disease has been achieved by antibiotic therapy alone [170, 264,509].

In summary, infected ventriculoatrial shunts may lead to a membranoproliferative glomerulonephritic pattern. It is of considerable interest that complete clinical cure can occur in the shunt type following eradication of infection. In contrast, most patients with the idiopathic form of membranoproliferative glomerulonephritis type I progress inexorably toward end-stage renal disease. It is intriguing to speculate that if we knew the etiology leading to the classic idiopathic membranoproliferative glomerulonephritis type I, withdrawal of that etiologic factor could allow repair, reconstitution, and recovery of the glomeruli and renal function.

REFERENCES

1. Abrass, C. K. Glomerulonephritis in the elderly. *Am. J. Nephrol.* 5:409, 1985.
2. Adam, C., Morel-Maroger, L., and Richet, G. Cryoglobulins in glomerulonephritis not related to systemic disease. *Kidney Int.* 3:334, 1973.
3. Addis, T. *Glomerular Nephritis: Diagnosis and Treatment.* New York: Macmillan, 1949.
4. Ahmed-Jushuf, I. H., Selby, P. L., and Brownjohn, A. M. Acute poststreptococcal glomerulonephritis following ear piercing. *Postgrad. Med. J.* 60:73, 1984.

4*a*. Akerrén, Y., and Lindgren, M. Investigation concerning early rising in acute hemorrhagic nephritis. *Acta Med. Scand.* 151:419, 1955.

5. Albert, M. S., Leeming, J. M., and Scaglione, P. R. Acute glomerulonephritis without abnormality of the urine. *J. Pediatr.* 68:525, 1966.
6. Alkjaersig, N. K., Fletcher, A. P., Lewis, M. L., Cole, B. R., Ingelfinger, J. R., and Robson, A. M. Pathophysiological response of the blood coagulation system in acute glomerulonephritis. *Kidney Int.* 10:319, 1976.
7. Alper, C. A., and Rose, F. S. Studies of the in vivo behavior of human C'3 in normal subjects and patients. *J. Clin. Invest.* 46:2021, 1967.
8. Anand, S. K., Trygstad, C. W., and Sharma, H. M. Extracapillary proliferative glomerulonephritis in children. *Pediatrics* 56:434, 1975.
9. Andres, G. A., Accinni, L., Hsu, K. C., Zabriskie, J. B., and Seegal, B. C. Electron microscopic studies of human glomerulonephritis with ferritin-conjugated antibody. *J. Exp. Med.* 123: 399, 1966.
10. Anthony, B. F., Kaplan, E. L., Chapman, S. S., Quie, P. G., and Wannamaker, L. W. Epidemic

acute nephritis with reappearance of type-49 streptococcus. *Lancet* 2:787, 1967.
11. Anthony, B. F., Kaplan, E. L., Wannamaker, L. W., Briese, F. W., and Chapman, S. S. Attack rates of acute nephritis after type-49 streptococcal infection of the skin and of the respiratory tract. *J. Clin. Invest.* 48:1697, 1969.
12. Asami, T., Tanaka, A., Gunji, T., and Sakai, K. Elevated serum and urine sialic acid levels in renal diseases of childhood. *Clin. Nephrol.* 23:112, 1985.
13. Arze, R. S., Rashid, H., Morley, R., Ward, M. K., and Kerr, D. N. Shunt nephritis: Report of two cases and review of the literature. *Clin. Nephrol.* 19:48, 1983.
14. Baehr, G. Glomerular lesions of subacute bacterial endocarditis. *J. Exp. Med.* 15:330, 1912.
15. Baehr, G. Renal complications of endocarditis. *Trans. Assoc. Am. Physicians* 46:87, 1931.
16. Baehr, G., and Lande, H. Glomerulonephritis as a complication of subacute streptococcus endocarditis. *JAMA* 75:789, 1920.
17. Baehr, G., and Sacks, B. The occurrence of glomerulonephritis in association with verrucous endocarditis. *Proc. N.Y. Pathol. Soc.* 23:64, 1923.
18. Bailey, R., and Scott, E. Streptococci, Including Enterococci and Pneumococci, and Aerococcus. In S. M. Finegold and E. J. Baron (Eds.), *Bailey and Scott's Diagnostic Microbiology,* 7th Ed. St. Louis: Mosby, 1986. P. 366.
19. Baldwin, D. S. Poststreptococcal glomerulonephritis: A progressive disease? *Am. J. Med.* 62:1, 1977.
20. Baldwin, D. S., Gluck, M. C., Schacht, R. G., and Gallo, G. The long-term course of poststreptococcal glomerulonephritis. *Ann. Intern. Med.* 80:342, 1974.
21. Barnham, M., Ljunggren, A., and McIntyre, M. Human infection with streptococcus zooepidemicus (Lancefield group C): Three case reports. *Epidemiol. Infect.* 98:183, 1987.
22. Batsford, S. R., Takamiya, H., and Vogt, A. A model of in-situ immune complex glomerulonephritis in the rat employing cationized ferritin. *Clin. Nephrol.* 14:211, 1980.
23. Bayer, A. S., Theofilopoulos, A. N., Tillman, D. B., Dixon, F. J., and Guze, L.B. Use of circulating immune complex levels in the serodifferentiation of endocarditic and non-endocarditic septicemias. *Am. J. Med.* 66:58, 1979.
24. Bayston, R., and Swinden, J. The aetiology and prevention of shunt nephritis. *Z. Kinderchir.* 28: 377, 1979.
25. Beaufils, M. Glomerular disease complicating abdominal sepsis (Clinical Conference). *Kidney Int.* 19:609, 1981.
26. Beaufils, M., Gilbert, C., Morel-Maroger, L., Sraer, J. D., Kanfer, A., Meyrier, A., Kourilsky, O., Vachon, F., and Richet, G. Glomerulonephritis in Severe Bacterial Infections with and without Endocarditis. In J. Hamburger, J. Crosnier, J. P. Grünfeld, and M. H. Maxwell (Eds.), *Advances in Nephrology,* Vol. 7. Chicago: Year Book Medical, 1977. P. 217.
27. Beaufils, M., Morel-Maroger, L., and Sraer, J. D. Acute renal failure of glomerular origin during visceral abscesses. *N. Engl. J. Med.* 295:185, 1976.
28. Becker, C. G., and Murphy, G. E. The experimental induction of glomerulonephritis like that in man by infection with group A streptococci. *J. Exp. Med.* 127:1, 1968.
29. Beeler, B. A., Crowder, J. G., Smith, J. W., and White, A. *Propionibacterium acnes:* Pathogen in central nervous system shunt infection. Report of three cases including immune complex glomerulonephritis. *Am. J. Med.* 61:935, 1983.
30. Bell, E. T. *Renal Diseases,* 2nd Ed. Philadelphia: Lea & Febiger, 1950.
31. Bell, E. T. Glomerular lesions associated with endocarditis. *Am. J. Pathol.* 8:639, 1932.
32. Benatar, A., Beatty, D. W., and Human, D. G. Immunological abnormalities in children with acute rheumatic carditis and acute post-streptococcal glomerulonephritis. *Int. J. Cardiol.* 21:51, 1988.
33. Ben-Dov, I., Berry, E. M., and Kopolovic, J. Poststreptococcal nephritis and acute rheumatic fever in two adults. *Arch. Intern. Med.* 145:338, 1985.
34. Bergholm, A. M., and Holm, S. E. Effect of early penicillin treatment on the development of experimental poststreptococcal glomerulonephritis. *Acta Pathol. Microbiol. Immunol. Scand.* [C] 91:271, 1983.
35. Berman, L. B., and Vogelsang, P. Poststreptococcal glomerulonephritis without proteinuria. *N. Engl. J. Med.* 268:1275, 1963.
36. Bernstein, S. H., and Stillerman, M. A study of the association of group A streptococci with acute glomerulonephritis. *Ann. Intern. Med.* 52:1026, 1960.
37. Berrios, X., Quesney, F., Morales, A., Blazquez, J., Lagomarsino, E., and Bisno, A. L. Acute rheumatic fever and poststreptococcal glomerulonephritis in an open population: Comparative studies of epidemiology and bacteriology. *J. Lab. Clin. Med.* 108:535, 1986.
38. Bertani, T., Mecca, G., Sacchi, G., and Remuzzi, G. Superimposed nephritis: A separate entity among glomerular diseases? *Am. J. Kidney Dis.* 7:205, 1986.
39. Bhan, A. K., Collins, A. B., Schneeberger, E. E.,

and McCluskey, R. T. A cell-mediated reaction against glomerular bound immune complexes. *J. Exp. Med.* 150:1410, 1979.
40. Bhan, A., Schneeberger, E., Collins, A., and McCluskey, R. Evidence for a pathogenic role of a cell-mediated immune mechanism in experimental glomerulonephritis. *J. Exp. Med.* 148:246, 1978.
41. Bhat, J. G., Gombos, E. A., and Baldwin, D. S. Depressed cellular immune response to streptococcal antigens in poststreptococcal glomerulonephritis. *Clin. Immunol. Immunopathol.* 7:230, 1977.
42. Birch, D. F., Fairley, K. F., Whitworth, J. A., Forbes, I., Fairley, J. K., Cheshire, G. R., and Ryan, G. B. Urinary erythrocyte morphology in the diagnosis of glomerular hematuria. *Clin. Nephrol.* 20:78, 1983.
43. Bisno, A. L., Nelson, K. E., Waytz, P., and Brunt, J. Factors influencing serum antibody responses in streptococcal pyoderma. *J. Lab. Clin. Med.* 81:410, 1973.
44. Black, J. A., Challacombe, D. N., and Ockenden, B. G. Nephrotic syndrome associated with bacteremia after shunt operations for hydrocephalus. *Lancet* 2:291, 1965.
45. Blantz, R., Tucker, B. J., and Wilson, C. B. The acute effects of anti-glomerular basement membrane antibody on the process of glomerular infiltration in the rat: The influence of dose and complement depletion. *J. Clin. Invest.* 61:910, 1978.
46. Bodaghi, E., Kheradpir, K. M., and Maddah, M. Vasculitis in acute streptococcal glomerulonephritis. *Int. J. Pediatr. Nephrol.* 8:69, 1987.
47. Bohle, A., Bader, R., Grund, K. E., Mackensen, S., and Neunhoeffer, J. Serum creatinine concentration and renal interstitial volume: Analysis of correlations in endocapillary (acute) glomerulonephritis and in moderately severe mesangioproliferative glomerulonephritis. *Virchows Arch. [Pathol. Anat.]* 375:87, 1977.
48. Bolton, W. K. The role of cell-mediated immunity in the pathogenesis of glomerulonephritis. *Plasma Ther. Transfusion Technol.* 5:415, 1984.
49. Bolton, W. K. The Role of High Dose Steroids in Nephritis Syndromes: The Case for Aggressively Using Them. In R. G. Narins (Ed.), *Controversies in Nephrology and Hypertension.* New York: Churchill-Livingstone, 1984. P. 421.
50. Bolton, W. K., Innes, D. J., Sturgill, B. C., and Kaiser, D. L. T-cells and macrophages in rapidly progressive glomerulonephritis: Clinicopathologic correlations. *Kidney Int.* 32:869, 1987.
51. Bolton, W. K., Chandra, M., Tyson, T. M., Kirkpatrick, P. R., Sadovnic, M. J., and Sturgill, B. C. Transfer of experimental glomerulonephritis in chickens by mononuclear cells. *Kidney Int.* 34: 598, 1988.
52. Bolton, W. K., Tucker, F. L., and Sturgill, B. C. A new avian model of experimental glomerulonephritis consistent with mediation by cellular immunity. *J. Clin. Invest.* 73:1263, 1984.
53. Bonsib, S. M. Glomerular basement membrane discontinuities. *Am. J. Pathol.* 119:357, 1985.
54. Boonshaft, B., Maher, J. F., and Schreiner, G. E. Nephrotic syndrome associated with osteomyelitis without secondary amyloidosis. *Arch. Intern Med.* 125:322, 1970.
55. Border, W. A. Immune complex detection in glomerular diseases. *Nephron* 24:105, 1979.
56. Boulton-Jones, J. M., Sissons, J. G. P., Evans, D. J., and Peters, D. K. Renal lesions of subacute infective endocarditis. *Br. Med. J.* 2:11, 1974.
57. Boyce, N. W., and Holdsworth, S. R. Quantitation of the intrarenal uptake of immunoglobulin aggregates by macrophages in diffuse proliferative glomerulonephritis. *Clin. Exp. Immunol.* 64:638, 1986.
58. Boyce, N. W., Tipping, P. G., and Holdsworth, S. R. Glomerular macrophages produce reactive oxygen species in experimental glomerulonephritis. *Kidney Int.* 35:778, 1989.
59. Bradfield, J. W. B., and Cattell, V. The mesangial cell in glomerulonephritis: I. Mechanisms of hypercellularity in experimental immune complex glomerulonephritis. *Lab. Invest.* 36:481, 1977.
60. Bradfield, J. W. B., Cattell, V., and Smith, J. The mesangial cell in glomerulonephritis: II. Mesangial proliferation caused by Habu snake venom in the rat. *Lab. Invest.* 36:487, 1977.
61. Bradley, S. E., Bradley, G. P., Tyson, C. J., Curry, J. J., and Blake, W. D. Renal function in renal diseases. *Am. J. Med.* 9:766, 1950.
62. Bright, R. Cases and observations illustrative of renal disease accompanied with the secretion of albuminous urine. *Guys Hosp. Rep.* 1:338,1836.
63. Brun, C., Gormsen, H., Hilden, T., Iversen, P., and Raaschou, F. Kidney biopsy in acute glomerulonephritis. *Acta Med. Scand.* 160:155, 1958.
64. Brunati, C., Brando, R., Confalonieri, R., Belli, L. S., Lavangni, M. G., and Minetti, L. Immunophenotyping of mononuclear cell infiltrates associated with renal disease. *Clin. Nephrol.* 26: 15, 1986.
65. Brzosko, W. J., Krawczynski, K., Nazarewicz, T., Morzycka, M., and Nowoslawski, A. Glomerulonephritis associated with hepatitis-B surface antigen immune complexes in children. *Lancet* 2: 477, 1974.
66. Buka, I., and Coovadia, H. M. Typhoid glomerulonephritis. *Arch. Dis. Child.* 55:305, 1980.
67. Burke, F. G., and Ross, S. Acute glomerulone-

phritis: A review of ninety cases. *J. Pediatr.* 30:157, 1947.
68. Burkholder, P. M. Atlas of Human Glomerular Pathology. New York: Harper & Row, 1974.
69. Cabane, J., Godeau, P., Herreman, G., Acar, J., Diegon, M., and Bach, J. F. Fate of circulating immune complexes in infective endocarditis. *Am. J. Med.* 66:277, 1979.
70. Caiger, F. F. Scarlet Fever. In T. C. Allbutt (Ed.), *A System of Medicine,* Vol. 3. New York: Macmillan, 1898. P. 122.
71. Cameron, J. S. The Natural History of Glomerulonephritis. In P. Kincaid-Smith, A. J. F. D'Apice, and R. C. Atkins (Eds.), *Progress in Glomerulonephritis.* New York: Wiley, 1979. P. 1.
72. Cameron, J. S., Vick, R. M., Ogg, C. S., Seymour, W. M., Chantler, C., and Turner, D. R. Plasma C3 and C4 concentrations in management of glomerulonephritis. *Br. Med. J.* 3:668, 1973.
73. Cameron, J. S., Nolasco, F., and Hartley, B. Glomerular T-cells and macrophages in crescentic and non-crescentic proliferative glomerulonephritis (Abstract). *Kidney Int.* 29:267, 1986.
74. Caron, C., Luneau, C., Gervais, M. H., Plante, G. E., Sanchez, G., and Blain, G. La glomérulonéphrite de shunt: Manifestations cliniques et histopathologiques. *Can. Med. Assoc. J.* 120:557, 1979.
75. Castillejos, G., Padilla, L. Lerma, A., Gonzalez, S., and Reyes, P. A. Coincidence of acute rheumatic fever and acute post-streptococcal glomerulonephritis. *J. Rheumatol.* 12:587, 1985.
76. Cattell, V., and Arlidge, S. The origin of proliferating cells in the glomerulus and Bowman's capsule in nephrotoxic serum nephritis: Effects of unilateral renal irradiation. *Br. J. Exp. Pathol.* 62:669, 1981.
77. Cattell, V., and Jamieson, S. W. The origin of glomerular crescents in experimental nephrotoxic serum nephritis in the rabbit. *Lab. Invest.* 39:584, 1978.
78. Cavallo, T., Pinto, J. A., and Rajaraman, S. Immune complex disease complicating diabetic glomerulosclerosis. *Am. J. Nephrol.* 4:347, 1984.
79. Chan, C. N., Lai, F. M., Lai, K. N., and Pang, J. A. Relapse of idiopathic pulmonary haemorrhage and glomerulonephritis associated with cytomegalovirus (CMV) infection. *Postgrad. Med. J.* 64:52, 1988.
80. Christian, H. A. The kidneys in subacute *Streptococcus viridans* endocarditis. *J. Mt. Sinai Hosp. New York* 8:427, 1941–1942.
81. Chugh, K. S., Halhotra, H. S., Sakhuja, V., Bhusnurmath, S., Singhal, P. C., Unni, V. N., Singh, N., Pirzada, R., and Kapoor, M. M. Progression to end-stage renal disease in poststreptococcal glomerulonephritis (PSGN)—Chandigarh Study. *Int. J. Artif. Organs* 10:189, 1987.
82. Churg, J., and Grishman, E. Ultrastructure of immune deposits in renal glomeruli. *Ann. Intern. Med.* 76:479, 1972.
83. Churg, J., and Sobin, L. H. *Renal Diseases: Classification and Atlas of Glomerular Diseases.* Tokyo: Igaku-Shoin, 1982.
84. Clarkson, A. R., MacDonald, M. K., Petrie, J. J. B., Cash, J. D., and Robson, J. S. Serum and urinary fibrin/fibrinogen degradation in glomerulonephritis. *Br. Med. J.* 3:447, 1971.
85. Cohen, A. H., and Border, A. H. Mesangial proliferative glomerulonephritis. *Semin. Nephrol.* 2:228, 1982.
86. Cohen, A. H., Border, W. A., and Glassock, R. J. Nephrotic syndrome with glomerular mesangial IgM deposits. *Lab. Invest.* 38:610, 1978.
87. Cohen, J. A., and Levitt, M. F. Acute glomerulonephritis with few urinary abnormalities: Report of two cases proved by renal biopsy. *N. Engl. J. Med.* 268:749, 1963.
88. Coleman, M., Burnett, J., Barratt, L. J., and Dupont, P. Glomerulonephritis associated with chronic bacterial infection of a dacron arterial prosthesis. *Clin. Nephrol.* 20:315, 1983.
89. Cotran, R. S. The Role of Monocytes and Macrophages in Glomerulonephritis: Introduction. In W. Zurukzoglu, M. Papadimitriou, M. Pyrpasopoulos, M. Sion, and C. Zamboulis (Eds.), *Proceedings of the Eighth International Congress of Nephrology.* Basel: Karger, 1981. P. 853.
90. Councilman, W. T. An anatomical and bacteriological study of acute diffuse nephritis. *Am. J. Med. Sci.* 114:23, 1897.
91. Cunningham, R. J., Gilfoil, M., Cavallo, T., Brouhard, B. H., Travis, L. B., Berger, M., and Petrusick, T. Rapidly progressive glomerulonephritis in children: A report of thirteen cases and a review of the literature. *Pediatr. Res.* 14:128, 1980.
92. Danovitch, G. M., Nord, E. P., Barki, Y., and Krugliak, L. Staphylococcal lung abscess and acute glomerulonephritis. *Isr. J. Med. Sci.* 15:840, 1979.
93. Dardenne, M., Zabriskie, J., and Bach, J. F. Streptococcal sensitivity in chronic glomerulonephritis. *Lancet* 1:126, 1972.
94. Davis, J. H., and Faber, H. K. The prognosis in acute glomerulonephritis in children. *J. Pediatr.* 27:453, 1945.
95. Dawson, K. P., and Flack, M. Urinary fibrin degradation products in childhood acute nephritis. *N.Z. Med. J.* 86:332, 1977.
96. DeBates, M. J., Thompson, K., Case, M. S., and McNally, C. Speed limit: Comparing direct de-

tection kits for group A strep. *Lab. Management* 26:26, 1988.
97. de Chadarévian, J. P., Goodyer, P. R., and Kaplan, B. S. Acute glomerulonephritis and hemolytic uremic syndrome. *Can. Med. Assoc. J.* 123:391, 1980.
98. Derrick, C. W., Reeves, M. S., and Dillon, H. C., Jr. Complement in overt and asymptomatic nephritis after skin infection. *J. Clin. Invest.* 49:1178, 1970.
99. Dillon, H. C., Jr. Pyoderma and nephritis. *Annu. Rev. Med.* 18:207, 1967.
100. Dillon, H. C., Jr., Moody, M. D., Maxted, W. R., and Parker, M. T. The epidemiology of impetigo and acute glomerulonephritis: Results of serological typing of group A streptococci. *Am. J. Epidemiol.* 86:710, 1967.
101. Dillon, H. C., and Reeves, M. S. A. Streptococcal immune responses in nephritis after skin infection. *Am. J. Med.* 56:333, 1974.
102. Dillon, H. C., Reeves, M. S., and Maxted, W. R. Acute glomerulonephritis following skin infection due to streptococci of M-type 2. *Lancet* 1:543, 1968.
103. Dixon, F. J., Feldman, J. D., and Vazquez, J. J. Experimental glomerulonephritis: The pathogenesis of a laboratory model resembling the spectrum of human glomerulonephritis. *J. Exp. Med.* 113:899, 1961.
104. Dixon, F. J., Vazquez, J. J., Weigle, W. O., and Cochrane, C. G. Pathogenesis of serum sickness. *Arch. Pathol.* 65:18, 1958.
105. Dixon, F. J., and Wilson, C. B. Immunological Renal Injury Produced by Formation and Deposition of Immune Complexes. In C. B. Wilson, B. M. Brenner, and J. H. Stein (Eds.), *Immunological Mechanisms of Renal Disease.* New York: Churchill-Livingstone, 1979. P. 1.
106. Dobrin, R. S., Day, N. K., Quie, P. G., Moore, H. L., Vernier, R. L., Michael, A. F., and Fish, A. J. The role of complement, immunoglobulins, and bacterial antigen in coagulase-negative staphylococcal shunt nephritis. *Am. J. Med.* 59:660, 1975.
107. Dodge, W. F., Spargo, B. H., Bass, J. A., and Travis, L. B. The relationship between the clinical and pathologic features of poststreptococcal glomerulonephritis: A study of the early natural history. *Medicine* 47:227, 1968.
108. Dodge, W. F., Spargo, B. H., Travis, L. B., Srivastava, R., Carrajal, H., DeBeukelaer, M., Longley, M., and Menchaca, J. Poststreptococcal glomerulonephritis: A prospective study in children. *N. Engl. J. Med.* 286:273, 1972.
109. Dormont, J., and Delfarissy, J. F. Infectious Diseases. In J. Hamburger, J. Crosnier, and J. P. Grünfeld (Eds), *Nephrology.* New York: Wiley, 1979. P. 769.
110. Drachman, R., Aldajem, M., and Vardy, P. A. Natural history of an acute glomerulonephritis epidemic in children: An 11 to 12 year follow-up. *Isr. J. Med. Sci.* 18:603, 1982.
111. Drukker, A., Pomeranz, A., Reichenberg, J., Mor, J., and Stankiewicz, H. Natriuretic response to I.V. saline loading after acute poststreptococcal glomerulonephritis. *Isr. J. Med. Sci.* 22:779, 1986.
112. Dubois, C. H., Foidart, J. B., Hautier, M. B., Dechenne, C. A., Lemaire, M. J., and Mahieu, P. R. Proliferative glomerulonephritis in rats: Evidence that mononuclear phagocytes infiltrating the glomeruli stimulate the proliferation of endothelial and mesangial cells. *Eur. J. Clin. Invest.* 11:91, 1981.
113. Duca, E., Teodorovici, Gr., Radu, C., Vîţă, A., Talaşman-Niculescu, P., Bernescu, E., Feldi, C. and Roşca, V. A new nephritogenic streptococcus. *J. Hyg.* 67:691, 1969.
114. Dunn, J. S. The fundamental lesion in acute diffuse intracapillary glomerulonephritis. *J. Pathol. Bacteriol.* 51:169, 1940.
115. Dunn, M. J. Acute glomerulonephritis with normal results from urinanalyses. *JAMA* 201:933, 1967.
116. Earle, D. P. Glomerulonephritis in the Adult Population. In E. L. Becker (Ed.), *Cornell Seminars in Nephrology.* New York: Wiley, 1973. P. 73.
117. Earle, D. P. Poststreptococcal acute glomerulonephritis. *Hosp. Pract.* 20:84, 1985.
118. Earle, D. P., Farber, S. J., Alexander, J. D., and Pellegrino, E. D. Renal function and electrolyte metabolism in acute glomerulonephritis. *J. Clin. Invest.* 30:421, 1951.
119. Ebright, J. R., and Koworoski, R. Gonococcal endocarditis associated with immune complex glomerulonephritis. *Am. J. Med.* 68:793, 1980.
120. Ehrich, J. H., Foellmer, H. G., Klöpper, J. W., Barmeier, F. W., and Sterzel, R. B. Experimental postinfectious glomerulonephritis in rodents. *Contrib. Nephrol.* 19:95, 1980.
121. Ellis, A. Natural history of Bright's disease: Clinical, histological and experimental observations. *Lancet* 1:1, 1942.
122. Faarup, P., Norgaard, T., Elling, F., and Jensen, H. Structural changes in kidneys of patients with oliguric extracapillary glomerulonephritis during immunosuppressive therapy. *Acta Pathol. Microbiol. Immunol. Scand.* 86:409, 1978.
123. Facklam, R. R., and Carey, R. B. Streptococci and Aerococci. In E. H. Lennette, A. Balows, W. J. Hausler, and H. J. Shadomy (Eds.), *Manual of Clinical Microbiology.* Washington: American So-

ciety of Microbiology, 1985. P. 154.
124. Fahr, T. Pathologische Anatomie des Morbus Brightii. In F. Henke, and O. Lubarsch (Eds.), *Handbuch der Speziellen Pathologischen Anatomie und Histologie,* Vol. 6, Part 1. Berlin: Springer, 1925. P. 156.
124*a*. Fairley, C., Mathews, D. C., and Becker, G. J. Rapid development of diffuse crescents in post-streptococcal glomerulonephritis. *Clin. Nephrol.* 28:256, 1987.
125. Falk, J. A., Fleishman, J. L., and Zabriskie, J. B. A study of HLA-antigen phenotype in rheumatic fever and rheumatic heart disease patients. *Tissue Antigens* 3:173, 1973.
126. Farmer, S. G. Immunology of Bacterial Infections. In E. H. Lennette, A. Balows, W. J. Hausler, and H. J. Shadomy (Eds.), *Manual of Clinical Microbiology,* 4th Ed. Washington: American Society for Microbiology, 1985. P. 898.
127. Fassett, R. G., Horgan, B., Gove, D., and Mathew, T. H. Scanning electron microscopy of glomerular and non-glomerular red blood cells. *Clin. Nephrol.* 20:11, 1983.
128. Feldman, J. D., Mardiney, M. R., and Shuler, S. E. Immunology and morphology of acute poststreptococcal glomerulonephritis. *Lab. Invest.* 15:283, 1966.
129. Ferrario, F., Kourilsky, O., and Morel-Maroger, L. Acute endocapillary glomerulonephritis in adults: A histologic and clinical comparison between patients with and without initial acute renal failure. *Clin. Nephrol.* 19:17, 1983.
130. Fillit, H., Damle, S. P., Gregory, J. D., Volin, C., Poon-King, T., and Zabriskie, J. Sera from patients with poststreptococcal glomerulonephritis contain antibodies to glomerular heparan sulfate proteoglycan. *J. Exp. Med.* 161:277, 1985.
131. Fillit, H., Read, S. E., Sherman, R. L., Zabriskie, J. B., and van de Rijn, I. Cellular reactivity to altered glomerular basement membrane in glomerulonephritis. *N. Engl. J. Med.* 298:861, 1978.
132. Fillit, H., Villarreal, H., Jr., and Zabriskie, J. B. The Role of Streptococcal and Glomerular Basement Membrane Antigens in Glomerulonephritis. In N. B. Cummings (Ed.), *Symposium on Immune Mechanisms in Renal Diseases.* New York: Plenum Press, 1983. P. 399.
133. Fischel, E. E. Immune reactions in human glomerulonephritis. *J. Chronic Dis.* 5:34, 1957.
134. Fischel, E. E., and Gajdusek, D. C. Serum complement in acute glomerulonephritis and other renal diseases. *Am. J. Med.* 12:190, 1952.
135. Fish, A. J., Herdman, R. C., Michael, A. F., Pickering, R. J., and Good, R. A. Epidemic acute glomerulonephritis associated with type 49 streptococcal pyoderma: II. Correlative study of light, immunofluorescent and electron microscopic findings. *Am. J. Med.* 48:28, 1970.
136. Fish, A. J., Michael, A. F., Vernier, R. L., and Good, R. A. Acute serum sickness nephritis in the rabbit: An immune deposit disease. *Am. J. Pathol.* 49:997, 1966.
137. Fishberg, A. M. *Hypertension and Nephritis,* 4th Ed. Philadelphia: Lea & Febiger, 1939.
138. Forrest, J. W., John, F., Mills, L. R., Buxton, T. B., Moore, W. L., Hudson, J. B., and Ozawa, T. Immune complex glomerulonephritis associated with *Klebsiella pneumoniae* infection. *Clin. Nephrol.* 7:76, 1977.
139. Fordham, C. C., Epstein, F. H., Huffines, W. D., and Harrington, J. T. Polyarteritis and acute poststreptococcal glomerulonephritis. *Ann. Intern. Med.* 61:89, 1964.
140. Franco, S., Moalem, T., Becker, M., Sadan, N., and Klajman, A. Circulating immune complexes in children with acute poststreptococcal glomerulonephritis. *Isr. J. Med. Sci.* 16:357, 1980.
141. Frank, J. A., Jr., Friedman, H. S., Davidson, D. M., Falletta, J. M., and Kinney, T. R. *Propionibacterium* shunt nephritis in two adolescents with medulloblastoma. *Cancer* 52:330, 1983.
142. Freedman, P., Meister, H. P., Co, B. S., Markowitz, A. S., and Dubin, A. Subclinical renal response to streptococcal infection. *N. Engl. J. Med.* 275:795, 1966.
143. Friedberg, M., Denneberg, T., Brun, C., Larsen, J. H., and Larsen, S. Glomerulonephritis in infections with *Yersinia enterocolitica* O-serotype 3. *Acta Med. Scand.* 209:103, 1981.
144. Friedman, J., van de Rijn, I., Ohkuni, H., Fischetti, V., and Zabriskie, J. Immunological studies of post-streptococcal sequelae: Evidence for presence of streptococcal antigens in circulating immune complexes. *J. Clin. Invest.* 74:1027, 1984.
145. Fukuda, O., Ito, M., Nakayama, M., Matsui, K., Fujisaki, S., and Okamura, H. Acute glomerulonephritis during the third trimester of pregnancy. *Int. J. Gynaecol. Obstet.* 26:141, 1988.
146. Fusaro, R. M., and Johnson, J. A. Hereditary polymorphic light eruption in American Indians: Photoprotection and prevention of streptococcal pyoderma and glomerulonephritis. *JAMA* 244:1456, 1980.
147. Futrakul, P., Boonpucknavig, V., Boonpucknavig, S., Mitrakul, C., and Bhamarapravati, N. Acute glomerulonephritis complicating *Plasmodium falciparum* infection. *Clin. Pediatr.* 13:281, 1974.
148. Gachet, F. S. Course and prognosis of hemorrhagic nephritis in children. *Am. J. Dis. Child.* 61:1175, 1941.
149. Gallagher, B. A., and Miller, C. G. Acute glo-

merulonephritis in Jamaican children. *West Indian Med. J.* 16:17, 1967.
150. Gallo, G. R., Feiner, H. D., Steele, J. M., Jr., Schacht, R. G., Gluck, M. C., and Baldwin, D. S. Role of intrarenal vascular sclerosis in progression of poststreptococcal glomerulonephritis. *Clin. Nephrol.* 13:49, 1980.
151. Garcia, R., Rubio, L., and Rodriguez-Iturbe, B. Long-term prognosis of epidemic poststreptococcal glomerulonephritis in Maracaibo: Follow-up studies 11 to 12 years after the acute episode. *Clin. Nephrol.* 15:291, 1981.
152. Gelfand, M. C., Shin, M. L., Nagle, R. B., Green, I., and Frank, M. M. The glomerular complement receptor in immunologically mediated renal glomerular injury. *N. Engl. J. Med.* 295:10, 1976.
153. George, J. T. A., McDonald, J. C., Payne, D. J. H., and Slade, D. A. Nephritis in North Yorkshire. *Br. Med. J.* 2:1381, 1958.
154. Germuth, F. G., Jr. A comparative histologic and immunologic study in rabbits of induced hypersensitivity of the serum sickness type. *J. Exp. Med.* 97:257, 1953.
155. Germuth, F. G., Jr., Kelemen, W. A., and Pollack, A. D. Immune complex disease: II. The role of circulatory dynamics and glomerular filtration in the development of experimental glomerulonephritis. *Johns Hopkins Med. J.* 120:252, 1967.
156. Germuth, F. G., Jr., and Pollack, A. D. The production of lesions of "serum sickness" in normal animals by the passive transfer of antibody in the presence of antigen. *Bull. Johns Hopkins Hosp.* 102:245, 1958.
157. Gill, D. G., Turner, D. R., Chantler, C., and Cameron, J. The progression of acute proliferative post streptococcal glomerulonephritis to severe epithelial crescent formation. *Clin. Nephrol.* 8:449, 1977.
158. Ginsburg, B. E., Wasserman, J., Huldt, G., and Bergstrand, A. Case of glomerulonephritis associated with acute toxoplasmosis. *Br. Med. J.* 3: 664, 1974.
159. Glassock, R. J. Clinicopathologic spectrum and therapeutic strategies in rapidly progressive glomerulonephritis. *Proc. Dialysis Tranplant. Forum* 5:109, 1975.
160. Glassock, R. J. Clinical Aspects of Acute, Rapidly Progressive and Chronic Glomerulonephritis. In L. E. Earley and C. W. Gottschalk (Eds.), *Strauss and Welt's Diseases of the Kidney,* 3rd Ed. Boston: Little, Brown, 1979. P. 691.
161. Glassock, R. J. Pathophysiology of acute glomerulonephritis. *Hosp. Pract.* 23(2):163, 1988.
162. Godon, J. P. Sodium and water retention in experimental glomerulonephritis. *Kidney Int.* 2:271, 1972.
163. Golbus, S. M., and Wilson, C. B. Experimental glomerulonephritis induced by in situ formation of immune complexes in glomerular capillary wall. *Kidney Int.* 16:148, 1979.
164. Goldsmith, H. J., Cowan, M. A., and Gooder, E. Familial outbreak of acute glomerulonephritis due to Griffith type-1 streptococcus. *Lancet* 2:674, 1958.
165. Goodall, E. W. On the etiology and clinical aspects of scarlatinal nephritis. *Guys Hosp. Rep.* 46:91, 1889.
166. Goorno, W., Ashworth, C. T., and Carter, N. W. Acute glomerulonephritis with absence of abnormal urinary findings: Diagnosis by light and electron microscopy. *Ann. Intern. Med.* 66:345, 1967.
167. Gorlin, R., Favour, C. B., and Emery, F. J. Long-term follow-up study of penicillin-treated subacute bacterial endocarditis. *N. Engl. J. Med.* 242:995, 1950.
168. Gowrishankar, R., and Agarwal, S. C. Leucocyte migration inhibition with human heart valve glycoproteins and group A streptococcal ribonucleic acid proteins in rheumatic heart disease and post-streptococcal glomerulonephritis. *Clin. Exp. Immunol.* 39:519, 1980.
169. Grishman, E., and Churg, J. Acute glomerulonephritis: A histopathologic study by means of thin sections. *Am. J. Pathol.* 33:993, 1957.
170. Groeneveld, A. B. J., Nommensen, F. E., Mullink, H., Ooms, E. C. M., and Bode, W. A. Shunt nephritis associated with *Propionibacterium acnes* with demonstration of the antigen in the glomeruli. *Nephron* 32:365, 1982.
171. Guild, H. G. The prognosis of acute glomerular nephritis in childhood. *Bull. Johns Hopkins Hosp.* 48:193, 1931.
172. Gutman, R. A., Striker, G. E., Gilliland, B. C., and Cutler, R. E. The immune complex glomerulonephritis of bacterial endocarditis. *Medicine (Baltimore)* 51:1, 1972.
173. Haen, M., Mackensen-Haen, S., Klingebiel, T., Stark-Jakob, B., Christ, H., and Bohle, A. Creatinine clearance and renal interstitium in diffuse endocapillary proliferative glomerulonephritis. *Pathol. Res. Pract.* 179:462, 1985.
174. Halmagyi, G. M., and Horvath, J. S. Acute glomerulonephritis in an adult with infected ventriculoatrial shunt. *Med. J. Aust.* 1:136, 1979.
175. Halperin, S. A., Ferrieri, P., Gray, E. D., Kaplan, E. L., and Wannamaker, L. W. Antibody response to bacteriophage hyaluronidase in acute glomerulonephritis after group A streptococcal infection. *J. Infect. Dis.* 155:253, 1987.
176. Hansborg, H. Untersuchungen über die Prog-

nose der Scharlachnephritis. *Acta Med. Scand.* 61:570, 1924.
177. Harkiss, G. D., Brown, D. L., and Evans, D. B. Longitudinal study of circulating immune complexes in a patient with *Staphylococcus albus*–induced shunt nephritis. *Clin. Exp. Immunol.* 37: 228, 1979.
178. Hart, D. H., Scheinkestel, C., Whitworth, J. A., and Kincaid-Smith, P. Acute post-streptococcal glomerulonephritis without proteinuria. *J. R. Soc. Med.* 78:842, 1985.
179. Hayman, J. M., and Martin, J. W. Acute nephritis: Review of 77 cases. *Am. J. Med. Sci.* 200:505, 1940.
180. Hedinger, E. Klinische Beiträge zur Frage der Hämolyse. *Dtsch. Arch. Klin. Med.* 74:24, 1902.
181. Henson, P. M., and Cochrane, C. G. Acute immune complex disease in rabbits: The role of complement and of a leukocyte-dependent release of vasoactive amines from platelets. *J. Exp. Med.* 133:554, 1971.
182. Heptinstall, R. H. Pathology of the Kidney, 3rd Ed. Boston: Little, Brown, 1983.
183. Herbut, P. A. Diffuse glomerulonephritis following revaccination for smallpox. *Am. J. Pathol.* 300:1011, 1944.
184. Herdson, P. B., Jennings, R. B., and Earle, D. P. Glomerular fine structure in poststreptococcal acute glomerulonephritis. *Arch. Pathol.* 81:117, 1966.
185. Herrin, J. T., Colvin, R. B., and Dibonna, D. R. Acute diffuse proliferative glomerulonephritis following meningococcal infection: A new antigen-antibody cause of acute nephritis. *Pediatr. Res.* 6:419, 1972.
186. Heymann, W., and Wilson, S. G. F. Hyperlipemia in early stages of acute glomerular nephritis. *J. Clin. Invest.* 38:186, 1959.
187. Hill, L. L., Guerra, S., and Rosenberg, H. Acute glomerulonephritis (AGN) secondary to pneumococcal infection. *J. Pediatr.* 67:904, 1965.
188. Hinglais, N., Garcia-Torres, R., and Kleinknecht, D. Long-term prognosis in acute glomerulonephritis: The predictive value of early clinical and pathologic features observed in 65 patients. *Am. J. Med.* 56:52, 1974.
189. Hippocrates: Coan Prognosis. In J. Chadwick and W. N. Mann (Trans.), *The Medical Works of Hippocrates* Oxford: Blackwell & Thomas, 1950. P. 219.
190. Hogg, R. J. Diagnostic, prognostic, and therapeutic implications of the renal biopsy in children with renal disease. *Semin. Nephrol.* 5:240, 1985.
191. Holdsworth, S. R., Neale, T. J., and Wilson, C. B. The participation of macrophages and monocytes in experimental immune complex glomerulonephritis. *Clin. Immunol. Immunopathol.* 15:510, 1980.
192. Holm, S. E. The pathogenesis of acute poststreptococcal glomerulonephritis in new lights. Review article. *APMIS* 96:189, 1988.
193. Holm, S. E., Bergholm, A.-M., and Johnston, K. H. A Possible Role of NSAP in the Pathogenesis of the Initial Phase of Experimental APSGN. In *Abstracts of Xth Lancefield International Symposium of Streptococci and Streptococcal Disease.* Cologne: 1987. P. 41.
194. Holm, S. E., Bergholm, A.-M., and Johnston, K. H. Evidence of NSAP as the Initiating Factor of Streptococcal Glomerulonephritis: Biological Findings in Rabbits Exposed to Pure NSAP Using Osmotic Pumps. In *Abstracts of Xth Lancefield International Symposium of Streptococci and Streptococcal Diseases.* Cologne: 1987. P. 41.
195. Holm, S. E., Bergholm, A.-M., and Johnston, K. H. A streptococcal plasminogen activator in the focus of infection and in the kidneys during the initial phase of experimental streptococcal glomerulonephritis. *APMIS* 96:1097, 1988.
196. Holm, S. E., Johnsson, J., and Zettergren, L. Experimental streptococcal nephritis in rabbits. *Acta Pathol. Microbiol. Scand.* 69:417, 1967.
197. Hooke, D. H., and Atkins, R. C. Quantitation of the Interstital Leucocyte Infiltrate in Human Glomerulonephritis and Interstitial Nephritis and Its Functional Correlation. In *Abstracts of the 9th International Congress of Nephrology.* 1984. P. 283A.
198. Hooke, D. H., Hancock, W. W., Gee, D. C., Kraft, N., and Atkins, R. C. Monoclonal antibody analysis of glomerular hypercellularity in human glomerulonephritis. *Clin. Nephrol.* 22:163, 1984.
199. Hooper, D. C., Bayer, A. S., Karchmer, A. W., Theofilopoulos, A. N., and Swartz, M. N. Circulating immune complexes in prosthetic valve endocarditis. *Arch. Intern. Med.* 143:2081, 1983.
200. Horder, T. Infective endocarditis with an analysis of 150 cases and with special reference to the chronic form of the disease. *Q. J. Med.* 2:289, 1909.
201. Hovelius, B., Bygren, P., Christensen, P. M., and Mårdh, P. A. Respiratory tract infections at a community care centre: With emphasis on group A streptococci. *Scand. J. Infect. Dis. Suppl.* 39:59, 1983.
202. Howard, R. J., and Balfour, H. H. Virus infection and kidney disease. *Minn. Med.* 58:809, 1975.
203. Hoyer, J. R., Michael, A. F., Fish, A. J., and Good, R. A. Acute poststreptococcal glomerulonephritis presenting as hypertensive encepha-

lopathy with minimal urinary abnormalities. *Pediatrics* 39:412, 1967.
204. Huang, T. W., and Wiegenstein, L. M. Mesangiolytic glomerulonephritis in an infant with immune deficiency and echovirus infection. *Arch. Pathol. Lab. Med.* 101:125, 1977.
205. Humair, L., Kwaan, H. C., and Potter, E. V. The role of fibrinogen in renal disease: II. Effect of anticoagulants and urokinase on experimental lesions in mice. *J. Lab. Clin. Med.* 74:72, 1969.
206. Hunsicker, L. G., Shearer, T. P., Plattner, S. B., and Weisenburger, D. The role of monocytes in serum sickness nephritis. *J. Exp. Med.* 150:413, 1979.
207. Hutt, M. S. R., Pinniger, J. L., and de Wardener, H. E. The relationship between the clinical and the histological features of acute glomerular nephritis: Based on a study of renal biopsy material. *Q. J. Med.* 27:265, 1958.
208. Hyman, L. R., Jenis, E. H., Hill, G. S., Zimmerman, S. W., and Burkholder, P. M. Alternate C3 pathway activation in pneumococcal glomerulonephritis. *Am. J. Med.* 58:810, 1975.
209. Ichikawa, I., Hoyer, J. R., Seiler, M. W., and Brenner, B. M. Mechanism of glomerulotubular balance in the setting of heterogeneous glomerular injury: Preservation of a close functional linkage between individual nephrons and surrounding microvasculature. *J. Clin. Invest.* 69:185, 1982.
210. Iida, H., Mizumura, Y., Uraoka, T., Takata, M., Sugimoto, T., Miwa, A., and Yamagishi, T. Membranous glomerulonephritis associated with enterococcal endocarditis. *Nephron* 40:88, 1985.
211. Inglefinger, J. R., McCluskey, R. T., Schneeberger, E. E., and Grupe, W. E. Necrotizing arteritis in acute poststreptococcal glomerulonephritis: Report of a recovered case. *J. Pediatr.* 91:228, 1977.
212. Jennings, R. B., and Earle, D. P. Poststreptococcal glomerulonephritis: Histopathologic and clinical studies of the acute, subsiding acute and early chronic latent phases. *J. Clin. Invest.* 40:1525, 1961.
213. Johnston, K. H., and Zabriskie, J. B. Purification and partial characterization of the nephritis strain-associated protein from *Streptococcus pyogenes*. *J. Exp. Med.* 163:697, 1986.
214. Jones, D. Inflammation and repair of the glomerulus. *Am. J. Pathol.* 27:991, 1951.
215. Jones, D. B. Glomerulonephritis. *Am. J. Pathol.* 29:33, 1953.
216. Jones, D. B. The Kidney: Inflammatory and Vascular Disease of the Glomerulus. In R. C. Mellors (Ed.), *Analytical Pathology.* New York: McGraw-Hill, 1957. P. 161.
217. Jones, D. B. The nature of scar tissue in glomerulonephritis. *Am. J. Pathol.* 42:185, 1963.
218. Jones, J. M., and Davison, A. M. Persistent infection as a cause of renal disease in patients submitted to renal biopsy: A report from the Glomerulonephritis Registry of the United Kingdom MRC. *Q. J. Med.* 58:123, 1986.
219. Jordan, S. C., and Lemire, J. M. Acute glomerulonephritis: Diagnosis and treatment. *Pediatr. Clin. North Am.* 29:857, 1982.
220. Jungmann, P. Ueber chronische Streptokokkeninfektionen. *Dtsch. Med. Wochenschr.* 50:71, 1924.
221. Kaehny, W. D., Ozawa, T., Schwartz, M. T., Stanford, R. E., Kohler, P. F., and McIntosh, R. M. Acute nephritis and pulmonary alveolitis following pneumococcal pneumonia. *Arch. Intern. Med.* 138:806, 1978.
222. Kahn, L. Acute glomerulonephritis with minimal urinary findings. *Clin. Pediatr.* 5:449, 1966.
223. Kamitsuji, H., Sakamoto, S., Matsunaga, T., Taira, K., Kawahara, S., and Nakajima, M. Intraglomerular deposition of fibrin/fibrinogen-related antigen in children with various renal diseases. *Am. J. Pathol.* 133:61, 1988.
224. Kandall, S., Edelmann, C. M., Jr., and Bernstein, J. Acute poststreptococcal glomerulonephritis: A case with minimal urinary abnormalities. *Am. J. Dis. Child.* 118:426, 1969.
225. Kantor, F. S. Fibrinogen precipitation by streptococcal M protein: I. Identity of the reactants and stoichiometry of the reaction. *J. Exp. Med.* 121:849, 1965.
226. Kaplan, C., Pasternack, B., Shah, H., and Gallo, G. Age-related incidence of sclerotic glomeruli in human kidneys. *Am. J. Pathol.* 80:227, 1975.
227. Kaplan, E. L., Anthony, B. F., Chapman, S. S., and Wannamaker, L. W. Epidemic acute glomerulonephritis associated with type 49 streptococcal pyoderma. *Am. J. Med.* 48:9, 1970.
228. Kaplan, M. H. Localization of streptococcal antigens in tissue: I. Histologic distribution and persistence of M protein, types 1, 5, 12, and 19 in the tissues of the mouse. *J. Exp. Med.* 107:341, 1958.
229. Kapur, S., Salcedo, J., Chandra, R., and Antonovych, T. Evolution of membranous nephropathy from a proliferative and exudative glomerulonephritis: A report of three cases studied by serial biopsies. *Int. J. Pediatr. Nephrol.* 6:105, 1985.
230. Kassirer, J. P., and Schwartz, W. B. Acute glomerulonephritis. *N. Engl. J. Med.* 265:686, 736, 1961.
231. Kaufman, D. B., and McIntosh, R. The pathogenesis of the renal lesion in a patient with streptococcal disease, infected ventriculoatrial shunt,

cryoglobulinemia and nephritis. *Am. J. Med.* 50:262, 1971.

232. Kefalides, N. A., Pegg, M. T., Ohno, N., Poon-King, T., Zabriskie, J., and Fillit, H. Antibodies to basement membrane collagen and to laminin are present in sera from patients with poststreptococcal glomerulonephritis. *J. Exp. Med.* 163:588, 1986.
233. Kemeny, E., Fillit, H. M., Damle, S., Mahabir, R., Kefalides, N. A., Gregory, J. D., Antonovych, T., Sabnis, S., and Zabriskie, J. B. Monoclonal antibodies to heparan sulfate proteoglycan: Development and application to the study of normal tissue and pathologic human kidney biopsies. *Connect. Tissue Res.* 18:9, 1988.
234. Keslin, M. H., Messner, R. P., and Williams, R. C., Jr. Glomerulonephritis with subacute bacterial endocarditis: Immunofluorescent studies. *Arch. Intern. Med.* 132:578, 1973.
235. Khandke, K. M., Fairwell, T., and Manjula, B. N. Difference in the structural features of streptococcal M proteins from nephritogenic and rheumatogenic serotypes. *J. Exp. Med.* 166:151, 1987.
236. Khuffash, F. A., Sharda, D. C., and Majeed, H. A. Sporadic pharyngitis associated acute poststreptococcal nephritis. *Clin. Pediatr. (Phila.)* 25:181, 1986.
237. Kimmelstiel, P., Kim, O. J., and Beres, J. Studies on renal biopsy specimens with the aid of the electron microscope: II. Glomerulonephritis and glomerulonephrosis. *Am. J. Clin. Pathol.* 38:280, 1962.
238. Kleinman, H. Epidemic acute glomerulonephritis at Red Lake. *Minn. Med.* 37:479, 1954.
239. Klinger, M. Response of lymphocytes to nonspecific mitogens (PHA, ConA, PWM) in patients with glomerulonephritis. *Arch. Immunol. Ther. Exp. (Warsz.)* 28:225, 1980.
240. Kobayashi, O., Okawa, K. I., Kamiyama, T., and Wada, H. Electron microscopic alterations of the glomerular capillaries in children with poststreptococcal glomerulonephritis. *Acta Med. Biol.* 19:75, 1971.
241. Krebs, R. A., and Burvant, M. V. Nephrotic syndrome in association with varicella. *JAMA* 222:325, 1972.
242. Kurtzman, N. A. Does acute poststreptococcal glomerulonephritis lead to chronic renal disease? *N. Engl. J. Med.* 298:795, 1978.
243. Kushner, D. S., Armstrong, S. H., Dubin, A., Szanto, P. B., and Markowitz, A. Acute glomerulonephritis in the adult: Longitudinal, clinical, functional and morphologic studies of rates of healing and progression to chronicity. *Medicine (Baltimore)* 40:203, 1961.
244. Kwong, Y. L., Chan, K. W., and Chan, M. K. Acute post-streptococcal glomerulonephritis followed shortly by acute rheumatic fever. *Postgrad. Med. J.* 63:209, 1987.
245. Lam, C. N., McNeish, A. S., and Gibson, A. A. M. Nephrotic syndrome associated with complement deficiency and *Staphylococcus albus* bacteremia. *Scott. Med. J.* 14:86, 1969.
246. Lamberticci, J. R., Godoy, P., Neves, J., Bambirra, E. A., and Ferreira, M. D. Glomerulonephritis in *Salmonella–Schistosoma mansoni* association. *Am. J. Trop. Med. Hyg.* 38:97, 1988.
247. Lange, K. Evidence for the in situ origin of poststreptococcal GN: Glomerular localization of endostreptosin. *Clin. Nephrol.* 19:3, 1983.
248. Lange, K., Ahmed, U., Kleinberger, H., and Treser, G. A hitherto unknown streptococcal antigen and its probable relation to acute poststreptococcal glomerulonephritis. *Clin. Nephrol.* 5:207, 1976.
249. Lange, K., Azadegan, A. A., Seligson, G., Bovie, R. C., and Majeed, H. Asymptomatic poststreptococcal glomerulonephritis in relatives of patients with symptomatic glomerulonephritis. *Child. Nephrol. Urol.* 9:11, 1988–1989.
250. Lange, K., Graig, F., Oberman, J., Slobody, L., Ogur, G., and Lo Casto, F. Changes in serum complement during the course and treatment of glomerulonephritis. *Arch. Intern. Med.* 88:433, 1951.
251. Lange, K., and Treser, G. Acute poststreptococcal glomerulonephritis: Mechanism and sequelae—Attempts at a unifying concept. *Clin. Nephrol.* 1:55, 1973.
252. Lange, K., Wasserman, E., and Slobody, L. B. The significance of serum complement levels for the diagnosis and prognosis of acute and subacute glomerulonephritis and lupus erythematosus disseminatus. *Ann. Intern. Med.* 53:636, 1960.
253. Langhans, T. Über die Veränderung der Glomeruli bei der Nephritis nebst einigen Bemerkungen über die Entstehung der Fibrincylinder. *Virchows Arch.* [A] 76:85, 1879.
254. Langhans, T. Über die entzündlichen Veränderungen der Glomeruli und die acute Nephritis. *Virchows Arch.* 99:193, 1885.
255. Laohapand, T., Cattell, V., and Gabriel, J. R. T. Monocyte infiltration in human glomerulonephritis: Alpha-antitrypsin as a marker for mononuclear phagocytes in renal biopsies. *Clin. Nephrol.* 19:309, 1983.
256. Lavelle, K. J., Durland, B. D., and Yum, M. N. The effect of antimacrophage antiserum on immune complex glomerulonephritis. *J. Lab. Clin. Med.* 98:195, 1981.
257. Layrisse, Z., Rodriguez-Iturbe, B., Garcia-Ramirez, R., Rodriguez, A., and Tiwari, J. Family

studies of the HLA system in acute poststreptococcal glomerulonephritis. *Hum. Immunol.* 7:177, 1983.
258. Lee, H. W. Korean hemorrhagic fever. *Prog. Med. Virol.* 28:96, 1982.
259. Leirisalo, M., Laifinen, O., and Tiilikaien, A. HLA phenotypes in patients with rheumatic fever, rheumatic heart disease and *Yersinia* arthritis. *J. Rheumatol.* 4(Suppl. 3):78, 1977.
260. Lemieux, G., Cuvelier, A. A., and Lefebvre, R. The clinical spectrum of renal insufficiency during acute glomerulonephritis in the adult. *Can. Med. Assoc. J.* 96:1129, 1967.
261. Leonard, C. D., Nagle, R. B., Striker, G. E., Cutler, R. E., and Scribner, B. H. Acute glomerulonephritis with prolonged oliguria: An analysis of 29 cases. *Ann. Intern. Med.* 73:703, 1970.
262. Lerner, I. L., and Weinstein, L. Infective endocarditis in the antibiotic era. *N. Engl. J. Med.* 274:199, 259, 320, 1966.
263. Levy, R. L., and Hong, R. The immune nature of subacute bacterial endocarditis. *Am. J. Med.* 54:645, 1973.
264. Levy, M., Gubler, M. C., and Habib, R. Pathology and Immunopathology of the Shunt Nephritis in Children: Report of 10 cases (Abstract). In *Proceedings of the Eighth International Congress of Nephrology.* Athens: 1981. P. 290.
265. Levy, M., Sich, M., Pirotzky, E., and Habib, R. Complement activation in acute glomerulonephritis in children. *Int. J. Pediatr. Nephrol.* 6:17, 1985.
266. Lewis, E. J. Patterns of circulating complement in renal diseases. *Annu. Rev. Med.* 30:445, 1979.
267. Lewis, E. J., Carpenter, C. B., and Schur, P. H. Serum complement component levels in human glomerulonephritis. *Ann. Intern. Med.* 75:555, 1971.
268. Lewis, E. J., Cavallo, T., Harrington, J. T., and Cotran, R. S. An immunopathologic study of rapidly progressive glomerulonephritis in the adult. *Human Pathol.* 2:185, 1971.
269. Lewy, J. E. Acute poststreptococcal glomerulonephritis. *Pediatr. Clin. North Am.* 23:751, 1976.
270. Lewy, J. E., Salinas-Madrigal, L., Herdson, P. B., Pirani, C. L., and Metcoff, J. Clinicopathologic correlations in acute poststreptococcal glomerulonephritis: A correlation between renal functions, morphologic damage and clinical course of 46 children with acute poststreptococcal glomerulonephritis. *Medicine (Baltimore)* 50:453, 1971.
271. Libman, E. A study of the endocardial lesions of subacute bacterial endocarditis with particular reference to healing or healed lesions: With clinical notes. *Am. J. Med. Sci.* 144:313, 1912.
272. Libman, E. The clinical features of cases of subacute bacterial endocarditis that have spontaneously become bacteria free. *Am. J. Med. Sci.* 146:625, 1913.
273. Lien, J. W. K., Mathew, T. H., and Meadows, R. Acute post-streptococcal glomerulonephritis in adults: A long-term study. *Q. J. Med.* 48:99, 1979.
274. Lin, C. Y. Serial studies of circulating immune complexes in poststreptococcal glomerulonephritis. *Pediatrics* 70:725, 1982.
275. Lin, C. Y., and Hsu, H. C. Measles and acute glomerulonephritis. *Pediatrics* 71:398, 1983.
276. Linder, E., Miettinen, A., and Tornroth, T. Fibronectin as a marker for the glomerular mesangium in immunohistology of kidney biopsies. *Lab. Invest.* 42:70, 1980.
277. Llach, F. Acute post-streptococcal glomerulonephritis, arthritis, and purpura. *J. Okla. State Med. Assoc.* 73:84, 1980.
278. Lockwood, C. M., Pinching, A. J., Sweny, P., Rees, A. J., Russell, B., and Uff, J. Plasma exchange and immunosuppression in the treatment of fulminating immune-complex crescentic nephritis. *Lancet* 1:63, 1977.
279. Löehlein, M. Ueber hämorrhagische Nierenaffektionen bei chronischer ulzeröser Endokarditis (Embolische nichteiterige Herdnephritis). *Med. Klin.* 10:375, 1910.
280. Longcope, W. T. The production of experimental nephritis by repeated protein intoxication. *J. Exp. Med.* 18:678, 1913.
281. Longcope, W. T. Studies of the variations in the antistreptolysin titer of the blood serum from patients with hemorrhagic nephritis: II. Observations on patients suffering from streptococcal infections, rheumatic fever and acute and chronic hemorrhagic nephritis. *J. Clin. Invest.* 15:277, 1936.
282. Longcope, W. T. Some observations on the course and outcome of hemorrhagic nephritis. *Trans. Am. Clin. Climatol. Assoc.* 53:153, 1937.
283. Longcope, W. T., O'Brien, D. P., McGuire, J., Hansen, O. C., and Denny, E. R. Relationship of acute infections to glomerular nephritis. *J. Clin. Invest.* 5:7, 1928.
284. Lyttle, J. D., Seegal, D., Loeb, E. N., and Jost, E. L. The serum antistreptolysin titer in acute glomerulonephritis. *J. Clin. Invest.* 17:631, 1938.
285. Ma, K. W., Golbus, S. M., Kaufman, R., Staley, N., Londer, H., and Brown, D. C. Glomerulonephritis with Hodgkin's disease and herpes zoster. *Arch. Pathol. Lab. Med.* 102:527, 1978.
286. MacCallum, W. G. Glomerular changes in nephritis. *Bull. Johns Hopkins Hosp.* 55:416, 1934.
287. MacCarthy, E. P., Hsu, A., Ooi, Y. M., and Ooi, B. S. Evidence for a mouse mesangial cell–derived factor that stimulates lymphocyte proliferation. *J. Clin. Invest.* 76:426, 1985.

289. Maggiore, Q., Jovanovich, B., and Baldini, G. Plasma fibrinolytic hyperactivity in children with acute post streptococcal glomerulonephritis. *Nephron* 6:81, 1969.
290. Magil, A. B. Histogenesis of glomerular crescents: Immunohistochemical demonstration of cytokeratin in crescent cells. *Am. J. Pathol.* 120:222, 1985.
291. Magil, A. B., and Wadsworth, L. D. Monocyte involvement in glomerular crescents: A histochemical and ultrastructural study. *Lab. Invest.* 47:160, 1982.
292. Magil, A. B., Wadsworth, L. D., and Loewen, M. Monocytes and human renal glomerular disease: A quantitative evaluation. *Lab. Invest.* 44:27, 1981.
293. Magil, A. B., and Wadsworth, L. D. Monocytes in human glomerulonephritis: An electron microscopic study. *Lab. Invest.* 45:77, 1981.
294. Maher, E. R., Hamilton, D. V., Thiru, S., and Wheatley, T. Acute renal failure due to glomerulonephritis associated with staphylococcal infection. *Postgrad. Med. J.* 60:433, 1984.
295. Mahomed, F. A. The etiology of Bright's disease and the prealbuminuric stage. *Med. Chir. Trans. (2nd Series)* 39:197, 1874.
296. Maidment, C. G., Evans, D. B., Coulden, R. A., and Thiru, S. Campylobacter enteritis complicated by glomerulonephritis (Letter). *J. Infect.* 10:177, 1985.
297. Markowitz, A. S., and Lange, C. F. Streptococcal related glomerulonephritis: I. Isolation, immunocytochemistry and comparative chemistry of soluble fractions from type 12 nephritogenic streptococci and human glomeruli. *J. Immunol.* 92: 565, 1964.
298. Mazzucco, G., and Monga, G. Monocyte escape through a glomerular capillary basement membrane gap: An ultrastructural observation in a case of acute glomerulonephritis. *Nephron* 39:272, 1985.
299. McCluskey, R. T., and Baldwin, D. S. Natural history of acute glomerulonephritis. *Am. J. Med.* 35:213, 1963.
300. McCluskey, R. T., Benacerraf, B., Potter, J. L., and Miller, F. The pathologic effects of intravenously administered soluble antigen-antibody complexes: I. Passive serum sickness in mice. *J Exp. Med.* 111:181, 1960.
301. McCluskey, R. T., Vassalli, P., Gallo, G., and Baldwin, D. S. An immunofluorescent study of pathogenic mechanisms in glomerular diseases. *N. Engl. J. Med.* 274:695, 1966.
301*a*. McCrory, W. W., Fleisher, D. S., and Sohn, W. B. Effects of early ambulation on the course of nephritis in children. *Pediatrics* 24:395, 1959.
302. McGregor, L. The cytological changes occurring in the glomerulus of clinical glomerulonephritis. *Am. J. Pathol.* 5:559, 1929.
303. McIntosh, R. M., Garcia, R., Rubio, L., Rabideau, D., Allen, J. E., Carr, R. I., and Rodriguez-Iturbe, B. Evidence for an autologous immune complex pathogenic mechanism in acute poststreptococcal glomerulonephritis. *Kidney Int.* 14: 501, 1978.
304. McIntosh, R. M., Griswold, W. R., Chernack, W. B., Williams, G., Strauss, J., Kaufman, D. B., Koss, M. N., McIntosh, J. R., Cohen, R., and Weil, R. Cryoglobulins III: Further studies on the nature, incidence, clinical, diagnostic, prognostic, and immunopathologic significance of cryoproteins in renal disease. *Q. J. Med.* 44:285, 1975.
305. McIntosh, R. M., Kulvinskas, C., and Kaufman, D. B. Cryoglobulins II: The biological and chemical properties of cryoproteins in acute poststreptococcal glomerulonephritis. *Int. Arch. Allergy* 41:700, 1971.
306. McKenzie, P. F., Taylor, A. E., Woodroffe, A. J., Seymour, A. E., Chan, Y. L., and Clarkson, A. R. Plasmapheresis in glomerulonephritis. *Clin. Nephrol.* 12:97, 1979.
307. Medani, C. L., Pearl, P. L., and Hall-Craggs, M. Acute renal failure, hemolytic anemia and thrombocytopenia in poststreptococcal glomerulonephritis. *South. Med. J.* 80:370, 1987.
308. Melby, P. C., Musick, W. D., Luger, A. M., and Khanna, R. Poststreptococcal glomerulonephritis in the elderly: Report of a case and review of the literature. *Am. J. Nephrol.* 7:235, 1987.
309. Mezzano, S., Olavarria, F., Ardiles, L., and Lopez, M. I. Incidence of circulating immune complexes in patients with acute poststreptococcal glomerulonephritis and in patients with streptococcal impetigo. *Clin. Nephrol.* 26:61, 1986.
310. Michael, A. F., Drummond, K. N., Good, R. A., and Vernier, R. L. Acute poststreptococcal glomerulonephritis: Immune deposit disease. *J. Clin. Invest.* 45:237, 1966.
311. Michael, A. F., and McLean, R. H. Evidence for Activation of the Alternate Pathway in Glomerulonephritis. In J. Hamburger, J. Crosnier, and M. H. Maxwell (Eds.), *Advances in Nephrology*, Vol. 4. Chicago: Year Book Medical, 1974. P. 49.
312. Miller, K., Dresner, I. G., and Michael, A. F. Localization of platelet antigens in human kidney disease. *Kidney Int.* 8:472, 1980.
313. Minkowitz, S., Wenk, R., Friedman, E., Yuceoglu, A., and Berkovich, S. Acute glomerulonephritis associated with varicella infection. *Am. J. Med.* 44:489, 1968.
314. Miyamoto, Y., Kotake, I., Ochiai, S., and Kodama, T. Experimental nephritis produced in rabbits by inoculation of group A hemolytic strep-

tococci isolated from epidemic nephritis patients: A focal infection experiment in the paranasal sinuses. *Jpn. J. Microbiol.* 4:105, 1960.
315. Modai, D., Pik, A., Behar, M., Eidelman, A., Averbukh, Z., Weissgarten, J., Gabizon, D., and Rosenmann, E. Biopsy-proven evolution of poststreptococcal glomerulonephritis to rapidly progressive glomerulonephritis of a post-infectious type. *Clin. Nephrol.* 23:198, 1985.
316. Mohammed, I., Ansell, B. M., Holbrow, E. J., and Cryceson, A. D. M. Circulating immune complexes in subacute infective endocarditis and poststreptococcal glomerulonephritis. *J. Clin. Pathol.* 30:308, 1977.
317. Monga, G., Mazzucco, G., and Castello, R. Monocytes in human glomerulonephritides: Immunohistochemical and ultrastructural correlations. *Contrib. Nephrol.* 45:141, 1985.
318. Monga, G., Mazzucco, G., Barbiano di Belgiojoso, G., and Busnach, G. Monocyte infiltration and glomerular hypercellularity in human acute and persistent glomerulonephritis: Light and electron microscopic, immunofluorescence, and histochemical investigation on 28 cases. *Lab. Invest.* 44:381, 1981.
319. Monteiro, G. E., and Lillicrap, C. A. Case of mumps nephritis. *Br. Med. J.* 4:721, 1967.
320. Montoliu, J., Darnell, A., Torres, A., and Revert, L. Acute and rapidly progressive forms of glomerulonephritis in the elderly. *J. Am. Geriatr. Soc.* 29:108, 1981.
321. Moran, J., Colasanti, G., Amos, N., and Peters, D. K. C3b receptors in glomerular disease. *Clin. Exp. Immunol.* 28:212, 1977.
322. Morel-Maroger, L., Kourilsky, O., Mignon, F., and Richet, G. Anti-tubular basement membrane antibodies in rapidly progressive poststreptococcal glomerulonephritis: Report of a case. *Clin. Immunol. Immunopathol.* 2:185, 1974.
323. Morel-Maroger, L., Leathem, A., and Richet, G. Glomerular abnormalities in nonsystemic diseases: Relationship between findings by light microscopy and immunofluorescence in 433 renal biopsy specimens. *Am. J. Med.* 53:170, 1972.
323*a*. Morel-Maroger, L., Sraer, J. D., Herreman, G., and Godeau, P. Kidney in subacute endocarditis: Pathological and immunofluorescence findings. *Arch. Pathol.* 94:205, 1972.
324. Morel-Maroger, L. J., and Verroust, P. J. Clinicopathological Correlations in Glomerular Diseases. In N. F. Jones (Ed.), *Recent Advances in Renal Disease.* Edinburgh: Churchill-Livingstone, 1975. P. 48.
325. Mosquera, J. A., and Rodriguez-Iturbe, B. Extracellular neuraminidase production of streptococci with acute nephritis. *Clin. Nephrol.* 21:21, 1984.
326. Mosquera, J. A., and Rodriguez-Iturbe, B. Glomerular binding sites for peanut agglutinin in acute poststreptococcal glomerulonephritis. *Clin. Nephrol.* 26:227, 1986.
327. Murphy, F. D., and Peters, B. J. Treatment of acute nephritis: The immediate results and outcome ten years later in 89 cases. *JAMA* 118:183, 1942.
328. Myers, B. D., Okarma, T. B., Friedman, S., Bridges, C., Ross, J., Asseff, S., and Deen, W. M. Mechanisms of proteinuria in human glomerulonephritis. *J. Clin. Invest.* 70:732, 1982.
329. Nadler, H. Group A strep detection. *Diagn. Clin. Test.* 27:34, 1989.
330. Narchi, H., Taylor, R., Azmy, A. F., Murphy, A. V., and Beattie, T. J. Shunt nephritis. *J. Pediatr. Surg.* 23:839, 1988.
331. Nash, M. Clinical Aspects of Glomerulonephritis. In *Renal Biopsy in Medical Diseases of the Kidneys* (postgraduate course). New York: Columbia Presbyterian Medical Center, 1988. P. 69.
332. Nebeker, H. G., Hercz, G., Feld, G. K., Stanley, T. M., Coburn, J. W., and Kurokawa, K. Postinfectious glomerulonephritis in a renal allograft associated with a mycotic aneurysm of a coronary artery. *Am. J. Med.* 76:940, 1984.
333. Neugarten, J., and Baldwin, D. S. Glomerulonephritis in bacterial endocarditis. *Am. J. Med.* 77:297, 1984.
334. Neugarten, J., Gallo, G. R., and Baldwin, D. S. Glomerulonephritis in bacterial endocarditis. *Am. J. Kidney Dis.* 3:371, 1984.
335. Nissenson, A. R., Baraff, L. J., Fine, R. N., and Knutson, D. Poststreptococcal acute glomerulonephritis: Fact and controversy. *Ann. Intern. Med.* 91:76, 1979.
336. Nissenson, A. R., Mayon-White, R., Potter, E. V., Mayon-White, V., Abidh, S., Poon-King, T., and Earle, D. P. Continued absence of clinical renal disease 7 to 12 years after poststreptococcal acute glomerulonephritis in Trinidad. *Am. J. Med.* 67:255, 1979.
337. Noe, H. N., and Roy, S. Shunt nephritis. *J. Urol.* 125:731, 1981.
338. O'Connor, D. T., Weisman, M. H., and Fierer, J. Activation of the alternate complement pathway in *Staph. aureus* infective endocarditis and its relationship to thrombocytopenia, coagulation abnormalities and acute glomerulonephritis. *Clin. Exp. Immunol.* 34:179, 1978.
339. O'Donnell, D., and Markowitz, S. Acute postinfection glomerulonephritis caused by new "thongs": A case report. *S. Afr. Med. J.* 69:575, 1986.
340. Ohkuni, H., Friedman, J., van de Rijn, I., Fischetti, V. A., Poon-King, T., and Zabriskie, J. B. Immunological studies of poststreptococcal sequelae: Serological studies with an extracellular pro-

tein associated with nephritogenic streptococci. *Clin. Exp. Immunol.* 54:185, 1983.
341. Oite, T., Batsford, S. R., Mihatsch, M. J., Takamiya, H., and Vogt, A. Quantitative studies of in situ immune complex glomerulonephritis in the rat induced by planted cationized antigen. *J. Exp. Med.* 155:460, 1982.
342. Onyewotu, I. I., and Mee, J. Circulating immune complexes and complement levels in relation to the clinical presentation of Nigerian children with acute poststreptococcal glomerulonephritis. *J. Clin. Pathol.* 31:817, 1978.
343. Ooi, Y. M., Vallota, E. H., and West, C. D. Serum immune complexes in membranoproliferative and other glomerulonephritides. *Kidney Int.* 11:275, 1977.
344. Ophüls, W. The etiology and development of nephritis. *JAMA* 69:1223, 1917.
345. O'Regan, S., and Makker, S. P. Shunt nephritis: Demonstration of diphtheroid antigen in glomeruli. *Am. J. Med. Sci.* 278:161, 1979.
346. Osman, A. A., Close, H. G., and Carter, H. Studies in Bright's disease: VIII. Observations on the aetiology of scarlatinal nephritis. *Guys Hosp. Rep.* 83:360, 1933.
347. Osorio, A. M., Thun, M. J., Novak, R. F., Van Cura, E. J., and Avner, E. D. Silica and glomerulonephritis: Case report and review of the literature. *Am. J. Kidney Dis.* 9:224, 1987.
348. Parra, G., Platt, J. L., Falk, R. J., Rodriguez-Iturbe, B., and Michael, A. F. Cell population and membrane attack complex in glomeruli of patients with poststreptococcal glomerulonephritis: Identification using monoclonal antibodies by indirect immunofluorescence. *Clin. Immunol. Immunopathol.* 33:324, 1984.
349. Parra, G., Rodriguez-Iturbe, B., Colina-Chourio, J., and Garcia, R. Short-term treatment with captopril in hypertension due to acute glomerulonephritis. *Clin. Nephrol.* 29:58, 1988.
350. Parrish, A. E., Kramer, N. C., Hatch, F. E., Watt, M. F., and Howe, J. S. The relation between glomerular function and histology in acute glomerulonephritis. *J. Lab. Clin. Med.* 58:197, 1961.
351. Pelletier, L. L., Jr., and Petersdorf, R. G. Infective endocarditis: A review of 125 cases from the University of Washington Hospitals, 1962–1972. *Medicine (Baltimore)* 56:287, 1977.
352. Perez, G. O., Rothfield, N., and Williams, R. C., Jr. Immune complex nephritis in bacterial endocarditis. *Arch. Intern. Med.* 136:334, 1976.
353. Perez-Fontan, M., Huarte, E., Tellez, A., Rodriguez-Carmona, A., Picazo, M. L., and Martinez-Ara, J. Glomerular nephropathy associated with chronic Q-fever. *Am. J. Kidney Dis.* 11:298, 1988.
354. Perlman, L. V., Herdman, R. C., Kleinman, H., and Vernier, R. L. Poststreptococcal glomerulonephritis: A ten year follow-up of an epidemic. *JAMA* 194:63, 1965.
355. Pertschuk, L. P., Woda, B. A., Vuletin, J. C., Brigati, D. J., Soriano, C. B., and Nicastri, A. D. Glomerulonephritis due to *Staphylococcus aureus* antigen. *Am. J. Clin. Pathol.* 65:301, 1976.
356. Pettersson, E. E., and Colvin, R. B. Cold-insoluble globulin (fibronectin, LETS protein) in normal and diseased human glomeruli: Papain-sensitive attachment to normal glomeruli and deposition in crescents. *Clin. Immunol. Immunopathol.* 11:425, 1978.
357. Pleydell, M. J., and Hall-Turner, W. J. A. An outbreak of nephritis in Northamptonshire. *Br. Med. J.* 2:1382, 1958.
358. Poon-King, T., Mohammed, I., Cox, R., Potter, E. V., Simon, N. M., Siegel, A. C., and Earle, D. P. Recurrent epidemic nephritis in South Trinidad. *N. Engl. J. Med.* 277:728, 1967.
359. Potter, E. V., Abidh, S., Sharrett, A. R., Burt, E. G., Svartmen, M., Finklea, J. F., Poon-King, T., and Earle, D. P. Clinical healing two to six years after poststreptococcal glomerulonephritis in Trinidad. *N. Engl. J. Med.* 298:767, 1978.
360. Potter, E. V., Lipschultz, S. A., Abidh, S., Poon-King, T., and Earle, D. P. Twelve to seventeen year follow-up of patients with post-streptococcal acute glomerulonephritis in Trinidad. *N. Engl. J. Med.* 307:725, 1982.
361. Potter, E. V., O'Keefe, T. J., Svartman, M., Poon-King, T., and Earle, D. P. Relationship of serum B1C globulin to fibrinolysis in patients with poststreptococcal acute glomerulonephritis. *J. Lab. Clin. Med.* 82:776, 1973.
362. Potter, E. V., Seigel, A. C., Simon, N. M., McAninch, J., Earle, D. P., Poon-King, T., Mohammed, I., and Abidh, S. Streptococcal infections and epidemic acute glomerulonephritis in South Trinidad. *J. Pediatr.* 72:871, 1968.
363. Potter, E. V., Vincente, J. B., Mayon-White, R. T., Shaughnessy, M. A., Poon-King, T., and Earle, D. P. Skin infections and immunoglobulin A in serum, sweat, and saliva of patients recovered from poststreptococcal acute glomerulonephritis or acute rheumatic fever and their siblings. *Am. J. Epidemiol.* 115:951, 1982.
364. Pound, S. E., McDonald, M. K., and Thomson, D. Diffuse proliferative glomerulonephritis: How many types? *Histopathology* 11:227, 1987.
365. Prakash, K., Pillai, P. K., and Sharma, K. B. Experimental production of acute glomerulonephritis by various subtypes of beta-hemolytic streptococci. *Indian J. Med. Res.* 75:192, 1982.
366. Prutis, K. B., Robak, M., Kopec, W., and Szewczyk, Z. Activity of helix: Destabilizing protein in lymphocytes of patients with glomerulopathies

and with chronic renal insufficiency. *Clin. Nephrol.* 23:142, 1985.
367. Queiroz, F. P., Brito, E., Martinelli, R., and Rocha, H. Nephrotic syndrome in patients with Schistosoma mansoni infection. *Am. J. Trop. Med. Hyg.* 22:622, 1973.
368. Rainford, D. J., Woodrow, D. F., Sloper, J. C., de Wardener, H. E., and Griffiths, I. Post-meningococcal acute glomerular nephritis. *Clin. Nephrol.* 9:249, 1978.
368*a*. Ramberg, R. The prognosis for acute nephritis. *Acta Med. Scand.* 127:396, 1947.
369. Rames, L., Wise, B., Goodman, J. R., and Piel, C. F. Renal disease with staphylococcus albus bacteremia: A complication in ventriculoatrial shunts. *JAMA* 212:1671, 1970.
370. Rammelkamp, C. H. Glomerulonephritis. *Proc. Inst. Med. Chicago* 19:371, 1953.
371. Rammelkamp, C. H. Acute Hemorrhagic Glomerulonephritis. In M. McCarty (Ed.), *Streptococcal Infections.* New York: Columbia University Press, 1954.
372. Rammelkamp, C. H. Microbiologic aspects of glomerulonephritis. *J. Chronic Dis.* 5:28, 1957.
373. Rammelkamp, C. H., and Weaver, R. S. Acute glomerulonephritis: The significance of the variations in the incidence of the disease. *J. Clin. Invest.* 32:345, 1953.
374. Rao, T. K. S., Nicastri, A. D., and Friedman, E. A. Renal Consequences of Narcotic Abuse. In J. Hamburger, J. Crosnier, J. P. Grünfeld, and M. H. Maxwell (Eds.), *Advances in Nephrology,* Vol. 7. Chicago: Year Book Medical, 1977, P. 261.
375. Read, S. E., Poon-King, T., Reid, H. F. M., and Zabriskie, J. B. HLA and Group A Streptococcal Sequelae. In S. E. Read and J. B. Zabriskie (Eds.), *Streptococcal Diseases and the Immune Response.* New York: Academic Press, 1980. P. 347.
376. Reed, R. W. An epidemic of acute nephritis. *Can. Med. Assoc. J.* 68:488, 1953.
377. Rees, A. J. The HLA complex and susceptibility to glomerulonephritis. *Plasma Ther. Transfusion Technol.* 5:455, 1984.
378. Reid, H. F., Bassett, D. C., Poon-King, T., Zabriskie, J. B., and Read, S.E. Group G streptococci in healthy school children and in patients with glomerulonephritis in Trinidad. *J. Hyg. (Lond.)* 94:61, 1985.
379. Reid, H. F., Read, S. E., Zabriskie, J. B., Ramkissoon, R., and Poon-King, T. Suppression of cellular reactivity to group A streptococcal antigens in patients with acute poststreptococcal glomerulonephritis. *J. Infect. Dis.* 149:841, 1984.
380. Reinstein, C. R. Epidemic nephritis at Red Lake, Minnesota. *J. Pediatr.* 47:25, 1955.
381. Richet, G., Fillastre, J. P., Morel-Maroger, L., and Bariety, J. Change from diffuse proliferative to membranous glomerulonephritis: Serial biopsies in four cases. *Kidney Int.* 5:57, 1974.
381*a*. Richter, A. B. Prognosis in acute glomerular nephritis. *Ann. Intern. Med.* 9:1057, 1936.
382. Rizkallah, M. F., Ghandour, M. H., Sabbah, R., and Akhtar, M. Acute thrombocytopenic purpura and poststreptococcal acute glomerulonephritis in a child. *Clin. Pediatr. (Phila.)* 23:581, 1984.
383. Rocklin, R., Lewis, E., and David, J. In vitro evidence for cellular hypersensitivity to glomerular basement membrane antigens in human glomerulonephritis. *N. Engl. J. Med.* 283:497, 1970.
384. Rodriguez-Iturbe, B. Epidemic post-streptococcal glomerulonephritis. *Kidney Int.* 25:129, 1984.
384*a*. Rodriguez-Iturbe, B. Poststreptococcal glomerulonephritis. In R. R. Robinson (Ed.), *Nephrology.* New York: Springer-Verlag, 1984. P. 623.
385. Rodriguez-Iturbe, B., Carr, R. I., Garcia, R., Rabideau, D., Rubio, L., and McIntosh, R. M. Circulating immune complexes and serum immunoglobulins in acute poststreptococcal glomerulonephritis. *Clin. Nephrol.* 13:1, 1980.
386. Rodriguez-Iturbe, B., Castillo, L., Valbuena, R., and Cuenca, L. Attack rate of poststreptococcal nephritis in families: A prospective study. *Lancet* 1:401, 1981.
387. Rodriguez-Iturbe, B., Garcia, R., Rubio, L., Cuenca, L., Treser, G., and Lange, K. Epidemic glomerulonephritis in Maracaibo: Evidence for progression to chronicity. *Clin. Nephrol.* 5:197, 1976.
388. Rodriguez-Iturbe, B., Katujar, V. N., and Coello, J. Neuraminidase activity and free sialic acid levels in the serum of patients with acute poststreptococcal glomerulonephritis. *N. Engl. J. Med.* 304: 1506, 1981.
389. Rodriguez-Iturbe, B., Rabideau, D., Garcia, R., Rubio, L., and McIntosh, R. M. Characterization of the glomerular antibody in acute poststreptococcal glomerulonephritis. *Ann. Intern. Med.* 92:478, 1980.
390. Rodriguez-Iturbe, B., Silva-Beauperthny, Y., Piarra, G., Ubio, L., and Garcia, E. Skin immune response to normal human IgG in patients with rheumatoid arthritis and acute poststreptococcal glomerulonephritis. *Am. J. Clin. Pathol.* 76:270, 1981.
391. Ronco, P., Verroust, P., and Morel-Maroger, L. Viruses and glomerulonephritis. *Nephron* 31:91, 1982.
392. Rosenberg, H. G., Donoso, P. L., Vial, S. U., Carranza, C., and Romero, P. Clinical and morphological recovery between two episodes of acute glomerulonephritis: A light and electron microscopic study with immunofluorescence. *Clin. Nephrol.* 21:350, 1984.

393. Rosenberg, H. G., Vial, S. U., Pomeroy, J., Figueroa, S., Donoso, P. L., and Carranza, C. Acute glomerulonephritis in children: An evolutive morphologic and immunologic study of the glomerular inflammation. *Pathol. Res. Pract.* 180: 633, 1985.
394. Rovzar, M. A., Logan, J. L., Ogden, D. A., and Graham, A. R. Immunosuppressive therapy and plasmapheresis in rapidly progressive glomerulonephritis associated with bacterial endocarditis. *Am. J. Kidney Dis.* 7:428, 1986.
395. Roy, S., III, Murphy, W. M., and Arant, B. S., Jr. Poststreptococcal crescentic glomerulonephritis in children: Comparison of quintuple therapy versus supportive care. *J. Pediatr.* 98:403, 1981.
396. Roy, S., III, Pitcock, J. A., and Ettledorf, J. N. Prognosis of acute poststreptococcal glomerulonephritis in childhood: Prospective study and review of the literature. *Adv. Pediatr.* 23:35, 1976.
397. Rudebeck, J. Clinical and prognostic aspects of acute glomerulonephritis. *Acta Med. Scand. (Suppl.)* 173:1, 1946.
398. Sagel, I., Treser, G., Ty, A., Yoshizawa, N., Kleinberger, H., Yuceoglu, A. M., Wasserman, E., and Lange, K. Occurrence and nature of glomerular lesions after group A streptococci infections in children. *Ann. Intern. Med.* 79:492, 1973.
399. Said, R., Hussein, M., and Hassan, A. Simultaneous occurrence of acute poststreptococcal glomerulonephritis and acute rheumatic fever. *Am. J. Nephrol.* 6:14, 1986.
400. Salyer, W. R., and Salyer, D. C. Unilateral glomerulonephritis. *J. Pathol.* 113:247, 1974.
401. Samiy, A. H., Field, R. A., and Merrill, J. P. Acute glomerulonephritis in older patients: Report of seven cases over 60 years of age. *Ann. Intern. Med.* 54:603, 1961.
402. Sano, M. Participation of monocytes in glomerulonephritis in acute serum sickness of rabbit. *Acta Pathol. Jpn.* 26:423, 1976.
403. Sapir, D. G., Yardley, J. H., and Walker, W. G. Acute glomerulonephritis in older patients. *Johns Hopkins Med. J.* 123:145, 1968.
404. Sato, M., Nakazora, H., and Ofuji, T. The pathogenic role of *Staphylococcus aureus* in primary human glomerulonephritis. *Clin. Nephrol.* 11:190, 1979.
405. Schacht, R. G., Gallo, G. R., Gluck, M. C., Iqbal, M. S., and Baldwin, D. S. Irreversible disease following acute poststreptococcal glomerulonephritis in children. *J. Chronic Dis.* 32:515, 1979.
406. Schacht, R. G., Gluck, M. C., Gallo, G. R., and Baldwin, D. S. Progression to uremia after remission of acute poststreptococcal glomerulonephritis. *N. Engl. J. Med.* 295:977, 1976.
407. Schachter, J., Pomeranz, A., Berger, I., and Wolach, B. Acute glomerulonephritis secondary to lobar pneumonia. *Int. J. Pediatr. Nephrol.* 8:211, 1987.
408. Scheinman, J. I., Fish, A. J., Matas, A. J., and Michael, A. F. The immunohistopathology of glomerular antigens: II. The glomerular basement membrane, actomyosin, and fibroblast surface antigens in normal, diseased, and transplanted human kidneys. *Am. J. Pathol.* 90:71, 1978.
409. Scheinman, J. I., Fish, A. J., and Michael, A. F. The immunohistopathology of glomerular antigens: The glomerular basement membrane, collagen, and actomyosin antigens in normal and diseased kidneys. *J. Clin. Invest.* 54:1144, 1974.
410. Schena, F. P. Renal manifestations in bacterial infections. *Contrib. Nephrol.* 48:125, 1985.
411. Schena, F. P., Pertosa, G., Pastore, A., de Tommasi, A., Montagna, M. T., and Bonomo, L. Circulating immune complexes in infected ventriculoatrial and ventriculoperitoneal shunts. *J. Clin. Immunol.* 3:173, 1983.
412. Schick, B. Die Nachkrankheiten des Scharlach: Pathogenese der Nachkrankheiten. In T. Escherich and B. Shick (Eds.), *Scharlach.* Leipzig: Holder, 1912. P. 151.
413. Schiffer, M. S., and Michael, A. F. Renal cell turnover studied by Y chromosome (Y body) staining of the transplanted human kidney. *J. Lab. Clin. Med.* 92:841, 1978.
414. Schoeneman, M., Bennett, B., and Greifer, I. Shunt nephritis progressing to chronic renal failure. *Am. J. Kidney Dis.* 2:375, 1982.
415. Schreiner, G. F., Cotran, R. S., and Unanue, E. R. Modulation of Ia and leukocyte common antigen expression in rat glomeruli during the course of glomerulonephritis and aminonucleoside nephrosis. *Lab. Invest.* 51:524, 1984.
416. Schreiner, G. F., Kiely, J., Cotran, R. S., and Unanue, E. R. Characterization of resident glomerular cells in the rat expressing Ia determinants and manifesting genetically restricted interactions with lymphocytes. *J. Clin. Invest.* 68:920, 1981.
417. Schur, P. H., and Carpenter, C. B. Host and Genetic Factors Contributing to Immunologic Renal Disease. In C. B. Wilson, B. M. Brenner, and J. H. Stein (Eds.), *Contemporary Issues in Nephrology,* Vol. 3: *Immunologic Mechanisms of Renal Disease.* New York: Churchill-Livingstone, 1978. P. 144.
418. Schwartz, W. B., and Kassirer, J. P. Clinical Aspects of Acute Glomerulonephritis. In M. B. Strauss and L. G. Welt (Eds.), *Diseases of the Kidney,* 2nd Ed. Boston: Little, Brown, 1971. P. 419.
419. Seegal, B., Andres, G. A., Hsu, K. C., and Zabriskie, J. B. Studies on the pathogenesis of acute and progressive glomerulonephritis in man

by immunofluorescein and immunoferritin techniques. *Fed. Proc.* 24:100, 1965.
420. Seegal, D. Acute glomerulonephritis following pneumococcic lobar pneumonia: Analysis of seven cases. *Arch. Intern. Med.* 56:912, 1935.
421. Seegal, D., and Earle, D. P., Jr. A consideration of certain biological differences between glomerulonephritis and rheumatic fever. *Am. J. Med. Sci.* 201:528, 1941.
422. Seligson, G., Lange, K., Majeed, H. A., Deol, H. L., Cronin, W., and Boyle, R. Significance of endostreptosin antibody titers in poststreptococcal glomerulonephritis. *Clin. Nephrol.* 24:69, 1985.
423. Sharret, A. R., Poon-King, T., and Potter, E. V. Subclinical nephritis in South Trinidad. *Am. J. Epidemol.* 94:231, 1971.
424. Shashaty, G. G., and Atamer, M. A. Hemolytic uremic syndrome associated with infectious mononucleosis. *Am. J. Dis. Child.* 127:720, 1974.
425. Sheridan, R. J., Roy, S., and Stapleton, F. B. Reflux nephropathy complicated by acute poststreptococcal glomerulonephritis. *Int. J. Pediatr. Nephrol.* 4:119, 1983.
426. Siegel, A. C., Johnson, E. E., and Stollerman, G. H. Controlled studies of streptococcal pharyngitis in a pediatric population: I. Factors related to the attack rate of rheumatic fever. *N. Engl. J. Med.* 265:559, 1961.
427. Silva, F., and Verani, R. Crescentic glomerulonephritis: Relationship of the stage of crescent formation to gaps in Bowman's capsule (Abstract). *Kidney Int.* 25:226, 1984.
428. Silverstein, R. L., Eigenbrodt, E. H., and McPhaul, J. J., Jr. Interstitial nephritis caused by methicillin: Studies in a case complicating staphylococcal sepsis with acute glomerulonephritis. *Am. J. Clin. Pathol.* 76:316, 1981.
429. Singhal, P. C., Chugh, K. S., and Muthusethupathi, M. A. Rapidly progressive glomerulonephritis associated with varicella infection. *J. Pediatr.* 91:680, 1977.
430. Singhal, P. C., Malik, G. H., Narayan, G., Khan, A. S., Bhusnurmath, S., and Datta, B. N. Prognosis of poststreptococcal glomerulonephritis: Chandigarh study. *Ann. Acad. Med. Singapore* 11:36, 1982.
431. Singson, E., Fisher, K. F., and Lindheimer, M. D. Acute poststreptococcal glomerulonephritis in pregnancy: Case report with an 18-year follow-up. *Am. J. Obstet. Gynecol.* 137:857, 1980.
432. Sjoholm, A. G. Complement components and complement activation in acute poststreptococcal glomerulonephritis. *Int. Arch. Allergy Appl. Immunol.* 58:274, 1979.
433. Smith, M. C., Cooke, J. R., Zimmerman, D. M., Bird, J. J., Feaster, B. D., Morrison, R. E., and Reimann, B. E. F. Asymptomatic glomerulonephritis after nonstreptotoccal upper respiratory infections. *Ann. Intern. Med.* 91:697, 1979.
434. Smith, R. D., and Aquino, J. Viruses and the kidney. *Med. Clin. North Am.* 55:89, 1971.
435. Sorger, K. Postinfectious glomerulonephritis: Subtypes, clinicopathological correlations, and follow-up studies. *Veroff. Pathol.* 125:1, 1986.
436. Sorger, K., and Thoenes, W. Zum Dynamik der akuten Glomerulonephritis. In U. von Gessler and D. Seybold (Eds.), *Glomerulonephritis.* Stuttgart: Thieme, 1980. P. 105.
437. Sorger, K., Balun, J., Hübner, F. K., Köhler, H., Olbing, H., Schulz, W., Seybold, D., Thoenes, G. H., and Thoenes, W. The garland type of acute postinfectious glomerulonephritis: Morphological characteristics and follow-up studies. *Clin. Nephrol.* 20:17, 1983.
438. Sorger, K., Gessler, U., Hübner, F. K., Köhler, H., Schulz, W., Stühlinger, W., Thoenes, G. H., and Thoenes, W. Subtypes of acute postinfectious glomerulonephritis: Synopsis of clinical and pathological features. *Clin. Nephrol.* 17:114, 1982.
439. Sorger, K., Gessler, U., Hübner, F. K., Köhler, H., Olbing, H., Schulz, W., Thoenes, G. H., and Thoenes, W. Follow-up studies of three subtypes of acute postinfectious glomerulonephritis ascertained by renal biopsy. *Clin. Nephrol.* 27:111, 1987.
440. Southwest Pediatric Nephrology Study Group. A clinicopathologic study of crescentic glomerulonephritis in 50 children. *Kidney Int.* 27:450, 1985.
441. Spain, D. M., and King, D. W. The effect of penicillin on the renal lesion of subacute bacterial endocarditis. *Ann. Intern. Med.* 36:1086, 1952.
442. Spargo, B. H., Dodge, W. F., and Travis, L. B. The relationships between the clinical course and pathologic features of poststreptococcal glomerulonephritis. *Contrib. Nephrol.* 2:130, 1976.
443. Spector, D. A., Millan, J., Zauber, N., and Burton, J. Glomerulonephritis and *Staphylococcus aureus* infections. *Clin. Nephrol.* 14:256, 1980.
444. Spitzer, R. E., Stitzel, A. E., and Urmson, J. R. Is glomerulonephritis after bacterial sepsis always benign? (Letter). *Lancet* 1:871, 1978.
445. Steciwko, A. Viral infections, their influence on some parts of the immune system and glomerulonephritis development. *Int. Urol. Nephrol.* 19:433, 1987.
446. Streitman, K., Beregi, E., Hollós, I., and Túri, S. Herpes nephropathy. *Clin. Nephrol.* 7:106, 1977.
447. Stejskal, J., Pirani, C. L., Okada, M., Mandelanakis, N., and Pollak, V. E. Discontinuities (gaps) of the glomerular capillary wall and basement membrane in renal disease. *Lab. Invest.* 28:149, 1973.

448. Stetson, C. A., Rammelkamp, C. H., Krause, R. M., Kohen, R. J., and Perry, W. D. Epidemic acute nephritis: Studies on etiology, natural history and prevention. *Medicine (Baltimore)* 34:431, 1955.
449. Stickler, G. B., Shin, M. H., Burke, E. C., Holley, K. E., Miller, R. H., and Segar, W. E. Diffuse glomerulonephritis associated with infected ventriculoatrial shunt. *N. Engl. J. Med.* 279:1077, 1968.
450. Strife, C. F., McDonald, B. M., Ruley, E. J., McAdams, A. J., and West, C. D. Shunt nephritis: The nature of the serum cryoglobulins and their relation to the complement profile. *J. Pediatr.* 88:403, 1976.
451. Striker, G. E., Mannik, M., and Tung, M. Y. Role of marrow-derived monocytes and mesangial cells in removal of immune complexes from renal glomeruli. *J. Exp. Med.* 149:127, 1979.
452. Suga, T., Endoh, M., Miura, M., Tomino, Y., Nomoto, Y., and Sakai, H. Two cases of acute poststreptococcal glomerulonephritis superimposed on rheumatoid arthritis. *Tokai J. Exp. Clin. Med.* 9:291, 1984.
453. Takebayashi, Sh., Giese, W., Manitz, G., Mönninghoff, W., and Themann, H. Feinstrukturelle Aspekte der menschlichen Glomerulonephritis: I. Proliferative Glomerulonephritis bei Erwachsenen. *Virchows Arch. [Pathol. Anat.]* 353:141, 1971.
454. Takebayashi, Sh., Giese, W., Manitz, G., Bassewitz, D. B. v., and Themann, H. Feinstrukturelle Aspekte der menschlichen Glomerulonephritis: II. Proliferative Glomerulonephritis bei Kindern. *Virchows Arch. [Pathol. Anat.]* 353:157, 1971.
455. Thompson, R. S. Scarlatinal albuminuria and the prealbuminuric stage, studied by frequent testing. *Med. Chir. Trans. (London)* 51(2nd Series): 97, 1886.
456. Thörig, L., Daha, M. R., Eulderink, F., Kooy-Bauer, W. C., and Thompson, J. Experimental *Streptococcus sanguis* endocarditis: Immune complexes and renal involvement. *Clin. Exp. Immunol.* 40:469, 1980.
457. Tipping, P. G., and Holdsworth, S. R. Effect of cyclosporine A on antibody-induced experimental glomerulonephritis. *Nephron* 40:201, 1985.
458. Tipping, P. G., and Holdsworth, S. R. The mechanism of action of corticosteroids on glomerular injury in acute serum sickness in rabbits. *Clin. Exp. Immunol.* 59:555, 1985.
459. Tipping, P. G., Neale, T. J., and Holdsworth, S. R. T-lymphocyte participation in antibody-induced experimental glomerulonephritis. *Kidney Int.* 27: 520, 1985.
460. Tornroth, T. The fate of subepithelial deposits in acute poststreptococcal glomerulonephritis. *Lab. Invest.* 35:461, 1976.
461. Travis, L. B., Dodge, W. F., Beathard, G. A., Spargo, B. H., Lorentz, W. B., Carvajal, H. F., and Berger, M. Acute glomerulonephritis in children: A review of the natural history with emphasis on prognosis. *Clin. Nephrol.* 1:169, 1973.
463. Treser, G., Ehrenreich, T., Ores, R., Sagel, I., Wasserman, E., and Lange, K. Natural history of "apparently healed" acute poststreptococcal glomerulonephritis in children. *Pediatrics* 43:1005, 1969.
464. Treser, G., Semar, M., McVicar, M., Franklin, M., Ty, A., Sagel, I., and Lange, K. Antigenic streptococcal components in acute glomerulonephritis. *Science* 163:676, 1969.
465. Treser, G., Semar, M., Sagel, I., Ty, A., Sterzel, R. B., Schaerf, R., and Lange, K. Independence of the nephritogenicity of group A streptococci from their M types. *Clin. Exp. Immunol.* 9:57, 1971.
466. Turner, D. M., Ransey, P. G., Ojemann, G. A., and Ralph, D. D. Disseminated *Mycobacterium gordonae* infection associated with glomerulonephritis. *West. J. Med.* 142:391, 1985.
467. Updyke, E. L., Moore, M. S., and Conroy, E. Provisional new type of group A streptococci associated with nephritis. *Science* 121:171, 1955.
468. Van Iseghem, P., Hauglustaine, D., Bollens, W., and Michielsen, P. Urinary erythrocyte morphology in acute glomerulonephritis. *Br. Med. J.* 287:1183, 1983.
469. Velhote, V., Saldanha, L. B., Malheiro, P. S., Praxedes, J. N., Penna, D. O., Marcondes, M., and Sabbaga, E. Acute glomerulonephritis: Three episodes demonstrated by light and electron microscopic and immunofluorescent studies—a case report. *Clin. Nephrol.* 26:307, 1986.
470. Verroust, P. J., Wilson, C. B., Cooper, N. R., Edgington, T. S., and Dixon, F. J. Glomerular complement components in human glomerulonephritis. *J. Clin. Invest.* 53:77, 1974.
471. Vilches, A. R., and Williams, D. G. Persistent anti-DNA antibodies and DNA–anti-DNA complexes in poststreptococcal glomerulonephritis. *Clin. Nephrol.* 22:97, 1984.
472. Villarreal, H., Jr., Fischetti, V. A., Van de Rijn, I., and Zabriskie, J. B. The occurrence of a protein in the extracellular products of streptococci isolated from patients with acute glomerulonephritis. *J. Exp. Med.* 149:459, 1979.
472*a*. Villarreal, H., and Sokoloff, L. The occurrence of renal insufficiency in subacute bacterial endocarditis. *Am. J. Med. Sci.* 220:655, 1950.
473. Vitullo, B. B., Renal, S. O., de Chadarevian, J.

P., and Kaplan, B. S. *Mycoplasma* pneumonia associated with acute glomerulonephritis. *Nephron* 21:284, 1978.
474. Vogl, W., Renke, M., Mayer-Eichberger, D., Schmitt, H., and Bohle, A. Long-term prognosis for endocapillary glomerulonephritis of poststreptococcal type in children and adults. *Nephron* 44:58, 1986.
475. Vogt, A., Batsford, S., Rodriguez-Iturbe, B., and Garcia, R. Cationic antigens in poststreptococcal glomerulonephritis. *Clin. Nephrol.* 20:271, 1983.
476. Volhard, F., and Fahr, T. *Die Brightsche Nierenkrankheit.* Berlin: Springer, 1914.
477. Volpi, A., Doregatti, C., Tarelli, T., Brognoli, M., Giordant, F., Meroni, M., Orlandini, G., and Sessa, A. Acute glomerulonephritis in human brucellosis. *Pathologica* 77:519, 1985.
478. Von Pirquet, C. E. Allergy. *Arch. Intern. Med.* 7:383, 1911.
479. Vosti, K. L., Johnson, R. H., and Dillon, M. F. Further characterization of purified fractions of M-protein from a strain of group A, type 12 streptococcus. *J. Immunol.* 107:104, 1971.
480. Wahrer, C. F. An epidemic of hemorrhagic nephritis following scarlet fever. *JAMA* 51:1410, 1908.
481. Wakabayashi, Y., Kobayashi, Y., and Shigematsu, H. Shunt nephritis: Histological dynamics following removal of the shunt. *Nephron* 40:111, 1985.
482. Walker, P. D., Deeves, E. C., Sahba, G., Wallin, J. D., and O'Neil, W. M. Rapidly progressive glomerulonephritis in a patient with syphilis. *Am. J. Med.* 76:1106, 1984.
483. Wannamaker, L. W. Differences between streptococcal infections of the throat and of the skin. *N. Engl. J. Med.* 282:23, 78, 1970.
484. Waskowski, S. D., and Powers, B. Glomerulonephritis and mycoplasma infection (Letter). *Ann. Intern. Med.* 97:112, 1983.
485. Wasserman, E., Schwarz, F., Wachstein, M., and Lange, K. Diagnostic value of serum complement determination in hereditary nephritis. *J. Lab. Clin. Med.* 65:589, 1965.
486. Watt, M. F., Howe, J. S., and Parrish, A. E. Renal tubular changes in acute glomerulonephritis. *Arch. Intern. Med.* 103:690, 1959.
487. Wedderburn, N., Davies, D. R., Mitchell, G. H., Desgrenges, C., and de Thé, G. Glomerulonephritis in common marmosets infected with *Plasmodium brasilianum* and Epstein-Barr virus. *J. Infect. Dis.* 158:789, 1988.
488. Wegmann, W., and Leumann, E. P. Glomerulonephritis associated with infected ventriculoatrial shunt: Clinical and morphological findings. *Virchows Arch.* [*Pathol. Anat.*] 359:185, 1973.
489. Wegmüller, E., Weldmann, P., Hess, T., and Reubi, F. C. Rapidly progressive glomerulonephritis accompanying Legionnaires disease. *Arch. Intern. Med.* 145:1711, 1985.
490. Weiss, M. A., Ooi, B. S., Ooi, Y. M., Engvall, E., and Ruoslahti, E. Immunofluorescent localization of fibronectin in the human kidney. *Lab. Invest.* 41:340, 1979.
491. Wells, W. C. *Transactions of a Society for the Improvement of Medical and Chirurgical Knowledge,* Vol. 3. London: The Society for the Improvement of Medical and Chirurgical Knowledge, 1812. P. 3.
492. Wertheim, A. R., Lyttle, J. D., Loeb, E. N., Earle, D. P., Seegal, B. C., and Seegal, D. The association of type-specific hemolytic streptococci with acute glomerulonephritis at the Presbyterian and Babies Hospitals, New York, N.Y., in the years 1936–1942. *J. Clin. Invest.* 32:359, 1953.
493. Westberg, N. G., Naff, G. B., Boyer, J. T., and Michael, A. F. Glomerular deposition of properdin in acute and chronic glomerulonephritis with hypocomplementemia. *J. Clin. Invest.* 50:642, 1971.
494. Whitley, K., Keane, W. F., and Vernier, R. L. Acute glomerulonephritis: A clinical overview. *Med. Clin. North Am.* 68:259, 1984.
495. Whitworth, J. A., Morel-Maroger, L., Mignon, F., and Richet, G. The significance of extracapillary proliferation: Clinicopathological review of 60 patients. *Nephron* 16:1, 1976.
496. Whitworth, J. A., Turner, D. R., Leibowitz, S., and Cameron, J. S. Focal segmental sclerosis or scarred focal proliferative glomerulonephritis? *Clin. Nephrol.* 9:229, 1978.
497. Wilks, S. *Guy's Hospital Report* 9 (second series). London: Guy's Hospital, 1853. P. 232.
498. Williams, D. G., Peters, D. K., Fallows, J., Petrie, A., Kourilsky, O., Morel-Maroger, L., and Cameron, J. S. Studies of serum complement in the hypocomplementaemic nephritides. *Clin. Exp. Immunol.* 18:391, 1974.
499. Williams, R. C., Jr., and Kunkel, H. G. Rheumatoid factor, complement and conglutinin aberrations in patients with subacute bacterial endocarditis. *J. Clin. Invest.* 41:666, 1962.
500. Williams, R. C. Jr., van de Rijn, I., Reid, H., Poon-King, T., and Zabriskie, J. B. Lymphocyte cell subpopulations during acute post-streptococcal glomerulonephritis: Cell surface antigens and binding of streptococcal membrane antigens and C-reactive protein. *Clin. Exp. Immunol.* 46:397, 1981.
501. Williams, W. Poststreptococcal glomerulonephritis: How important is it as a cause of chronic

renal diseases. *Transplant. Proc.* 19(Suppl. 2):97, 1987.
502. Wilmers, M. J., Cunliffe, A. C., and Williams, R. E. O. Type-12 streptococci associated with haemorrhagic nephritis. *Lancet* 2:17, 1954.
503. Wilson, S. G. F., and Heymann, W. Acute glomerulonephritis with the nephrotic syndrome. *Pediatrics* 23:874, 1959.
504. Winkenwerder, W. L., McLeod, N., and Baker, M. Infection and hemorrhagic nephritis. *Arch. Intern. Med.* 56:297, 1935.
505. Woodroffe, A. J., Row, P. G., Meadows, R., and Lawrence, J. R. Nephritis in infectious mononucleosis: An autopsy report. *Am. J. Pathol.* 23:463, 1947.
506. Wu, M. J., Osanloo, E. O., Molnar, Z. V., Daugirdas, J. T., Gandhi, V. C., and Ing, T. S. Poststreptococcal crescentic glomerulonephritis in a patient with preexisting membranous glomerulonephropathy. *Nephron* 35:62, 1983.
507. Wyatt, R. J., McAdams, A. J., Forristal, J., Snyder, J., and West, C. D. Glomerular deposition of complement-control proteins in acute and chronic glomerulonephritis. *Kidney Int.* 16:505, 1979.
508. Wyatt, R. J., Walsh, J. W., and Holland, N. H. Shunt nephritis. *J. Neurosurg.* 55:99, 1981.
509. Yeh, B. P. Y., Young, H. F., Schatzki, P. F., and Bear, E. S. Immune complex disease associated with an infected ventriculojugular shunt: A curable form of glomerulonephritis. *South. Med. J.* 70:1141, 1977.
510. Yoshimoto, M., Hosoi, S., Fujisawa, S., Sudo, M., and Okuda, R. High levels of antibodies to streptococcal cell membrane antigens specifically bound to monoclonal antibodies in acute poststreptococcal glomerulonephritis. *J. Clin. Microbiol.* 25:680, 1987.
511. Yoshizawa, N., Treser, G., Sagel, I., Ty, A., Ahmed, U., and Lange, K. Demonstration of antigenic sites in glomeruli of patients with acute poststreptococcal glomerulonephritis by immunofluorescein and immunoferritin technics. *Am. J. Pathol.* 70:131, 1973.
512. Yoshizawa, N., Treser, G., McClung, J. A., Sagel, I., and Takahashi, K. Circulating immune complexes in patients with uncomplicated group A streptococcal pharyngitis and patients with acute poststreptococcal glomerulonephritis. *Am. J. Nephrol.* 3:23, 1983.
513. Yuceoglu, A. M., Berkovich, S., and Minkowitz, S. Acute glomerulonephritis associated with ECHO virus type 9 infection. *J. Pediatr.* 69:603, 1966.
514. Yum, M., Wheat, L. J., Maxwell, D., and Edwards, J. L. Immunofluorescent localization of *Staphylococcus aureus* antigen in the acute bacterial endocarditis nephritis. *Am. J. Clin. Pathol.* 70:832, 1978.
515. Zabriskie, J. B., Lewshenia, R., Möller, G., Wehle, B., and Falk, R. E. Lymphocytic responses to streptococcal antigens in glomerulonephritis patients. *Science* 168:1105, 1970.
516. Zarconi, J., and Smith, M. C. Glomerulonephritis: Bacterial, viral, and other infectious causes. *Postgrad. Med.* 84:239, 251, 1988.
517. Zimmerman, R., Cross, M., Miller, D. R., and Sciple, G. W. A streptococcal epidemic in an isolated civilian population with institution of mass prophylaxis. *J. Pediatr.* 69:40, 1966.
518. Zollinger, H. U., and Mihatsch, M. J. *Renal Pathology in Biopsy.* Berlin: Springer-Verlag, 1978. P. 282.

Steven N. Emancipator

6

Primary and Secondary Forms of IgA Nephritis, Schönlein-Henoch Syndrome

The recorded history of IgA nephritides began with the recognition of a population of patients who had predominantly IgA in glomerular immunoglobulin deposits. In 1968, Berger and Hinglais [50] described a group of patients with episodic macrohematuria, persistent microhematuria, and moderate proteinuria who were characterized pathologically by a focal glomerulonephritis with predominant IgA in glomeruli. The disease likely existed prior to this recognition. Acute and chronic focal glomerulonephritides were distinguished by Volhard and Fahr [636]. The acute form, characterized by hematuria at the zenith of an infection, was clinically manifest by hematuria, usually without azotemia, edema, or hypertension. Thus this disease was distinguished from poststreptococcal glomerulonephritis. Although most patients clinically resolved, hematuria persisted in a few, and episodes of infection often exacerbated new bouts of hematuria. The chronic form of focal glomerulonephritis displayed persistent hematuria and proteinuria. The contemporary student of renal medicine will readily recognize the similarity these early reports bear to the patients Berger reported in 1968 and 1969 [49,50].

Slow progress over the five decades between Volhard and Fahr's studies and Berger's reports saw the development of renal biopsy techniques. Several investigators confirmed earlier observations and developed the concept that focal glomerulonephritis, and particularly mesangiopathic lesions, were associated with hematuria [25,36,65,109,150, 175,206,235,270,271,485,517,522,523,627,633]. Many, but certainly not all, of the patients who were the subjects of these reports likely suffered from IgA nephritis.

Progress in our understanding of focal glomerulonephritis with predominantly IgA deposits subsequently burgeoned. The number of publications has grown exponentially (Fig. 6-1). By the end of 1989, little more than 20 years after the original proposition that IgA nephritis is an entity, more than 1300 titles cited in *Index Medicus* included *IgA* and *glomerulonephritis* or *IgA nephropathy* as key words. Initial publications were descriptive case series, pondering if the observations represented an entity. Subsequently, more analytical

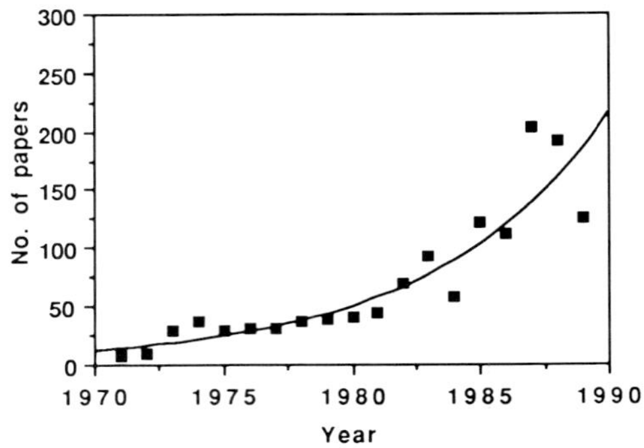

FIG. 6-1. *The number of publications indexed in Medline, plotted on the ordinate, is approximately an exponential function of time ($r^2 = 0.876$, $p < 0.01$), plotted on the abscissa. The data, obtained from an online search, consider all papers indexed under both glomerulonephritis and IgA until 1985 and thereafter include papers indexed under IgA nephropathy, a medical subject heading established in 1985.*

clinicopathologic studies that established correlations and prognostic indicators were published. Finally, during the current period, therapeutics and physiologic mechanisms form the focal point of most papers.

One consequence of the multidisciplinary approach toward mechanistic studies of IgA nephritides now underway has been the recognition that the syndrome originally described by Schönlein [548*a*] and expanded on decades later by Henoch [269] is an integral and conceptual part of the family of IgA nephritides, as are glomerular alterations secondary to a variety of clinical conditions, notably hepatobiliary disease [174,459]. Plainly, not all focal glomerulonephritis is IgA nephritis, and not all glomerular diseases associated with liver disorders are examples of secondary IgA nephritis. Focal segmental glomerulonephritis without predominant IgA immune deposits is discussed in Chapters 4, 5, and 13 in association with etiologically related conditions. This chapter considers, in turn, primary (idiopathic) IgA nephritis, secondary IgA nephritis, anaphylactoid purpura (Schönlein-Henoch syndrome), and glomerulonephritis associated with liver disease, including those forms which do not have predominantly IgA deposits. The reference list is intended to focus attention on the pathologic changes in IgA nephritides as they relate to the whole patient while still enabling the reader to unearth the full literature on the subject. As such, cognizant of the many recent extensive reviews and monographs in this field [97,127,128,132,177,180,304,663], only original papers or reviews that elucidate pathologic, clinicopathologic, or pathophysiologic concepts and more recent papers are cited. It is hoped that colleagues will not be slighted by omissions of those papers not oriented to pathology.

PRIMARY IgA NEPHRITIS

Glomerulonephritis characterized by the predominance of IgA among glomerular immunogloblin deposits, in the absence of systemic disease or other nonrenal disease, is considered primary, or idiopathic, IgA nephritis (IgAN). While initially regarded as a benign disease of questionable significance and relevance, IgAN is now considered the most prevalent form of glomerulonephritis worldwide and a major cause of end-stage kidney disease and chronic renal insufficiency [128,180].

The statistics presented in the sections entitled Clinical Features and Pathologic Changes represent a collation of data from many large series where sufficiently detailed databases were provided to allow codification of all variables considered [8, 22,49,98,122,135,139,147,159,204,291,317,318, 370,388,403,404,435,436,445,454,460,520,548, 555,571,576,589,619,638,664,670,677]. Unless otherwise indicated in the text, the specific estimates of frequency are means, weighted for the number of cases from each individual report, and are based on a total of 2287 cases of IgAN. Other series, which do not provide detail in all aspects, are cited in the context of their main thrust. The information provided in these papers agrees well with that which forms the basis for the general statistics on primary IgAN quoted.

Clinical Features

DEMOGRAPHICS

Patients with IgAN range in age from 4 to 80 years, but patients over 40 years of age account for less than 15 percent of all cases. The mean age overall is 28 years, and approximately 65 percent of patients are in the second and third decades of life. Worldwide, the male-to-female ratio is 2 : 1. Series of Asian patients show nearly equal involvement in males and females, while the male-to-female ratio in Europe and North America is 3.3 : 1. Series of IgAN patients have been reported from all over the world. Although the disease is observed in all races, there is a relative rarity in blacks, both in the United States and in Africa [222,301,362,403,549]. American Indians, on the other hand, have a higher incidence of IgAN than the world population at large [286, 572].

The frequency with which IgAN is diagnosed varies from 4 to 44 percent of all renal biopsies. The overall frequency shows decided geographic variation, with 5 to 10 percent being a typical estimate in North America, the United Kingdom, and northwestern Europe, through 20 to 35 percent in most European series and Australia, and from 25 to 45 percent in Asia [97,177]. Several authors have underscored the influence that policies on health screening and indications for renal biopsy bear on the frequency with which IgAN is diagnosed [128,180,198]. The impact of routine urine screening is best illustrated by the independent studies of Propper [493], Woo [659], and Feehally [198] and their respective colleagues. Patients with persistent microhematuria are routinely biopsied in Aberdeen, Scotland [493]; 37 percent of these individuals prove to have IgAN, and this diagnosis is established in 26 percent of all renal biopsies in that center. Another center within the United Kingdom with a more conservative biopsy policy recognizes IgAN in only 4 percent of its renal biopsies [571]. In Singapore, males actively screened by urinalysis at the time of examination for military service are biopsied if persistent abnormalities are detected [659]. Females are not subject to active urinalysis screening programs; the male-to-female ratio is more than 5 : 1 among asymptomatic IgAN patients but nearly equal among symptomatic patients. Using data obtained by questionnaire submitted by 90 percent of the nephrology centers in Britain, Feehally et al. [198] emphasized the important contribution that changing biopsy policy makes to the apparent increase in the incidence of IgAN in the United Kingdom. In Japan, the active screening of urine in people of both sexes and a policy of performing biopsies in all individuals with persistent urinary abnormalities account for the high apparent incidence of IgAN, the nearly equal male-to-female ratio, and the increased proportion of patients who have asymptomatic disease or mild signs (H. Sakai, personal communication).

If a disease can only be diagnosed by biopsy, as is the case for IgAN, biopsy policy can influence the spectrum of clinical manifestations of the disease as well as its apparent incidence (Fig. 6-2). In regions where there is no active urine screening program or where only patients with obvious signs of renal disease are biopsied, the apparent incidence of IgAN will correlate inversely with the frequency of severe signs among patients diagnosed as having the disease, because patients with mild changes are missed. The frequency of severe signs among IgAN patients also will be higher, since these patients are being positively selected. On the other hand, in places where there is active urinalysis screening and a policy of performing biopsies for mild signs such as persistent microhematuria or low-grade proteinuria, more patients will be biopsied and diagnosed. At the same time, however, severity of manifestations and frequency of diagnosis will no longer correlate, and the frequency of gross hematuria and heavy proteinuria among IgAN patients will be lower.

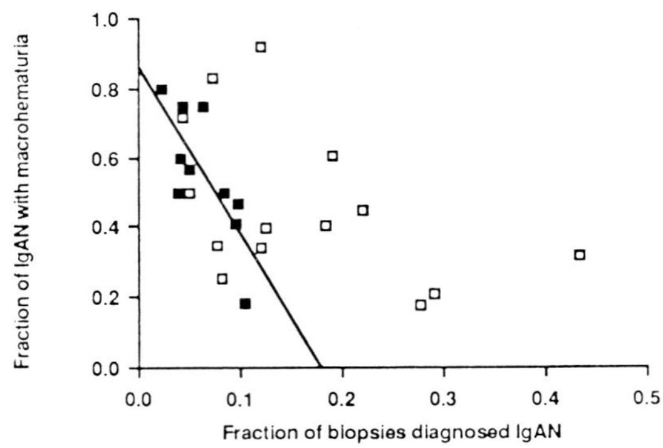

FIG. 6-2. *Scattergrams depict the frequency at which patients with IgAN manifest macrohematuria versus the frequency at which IgAN is diagnosed among all renal biopsies. Included are data from 25 series of cases for which complete information was available (see text). In studies from North America and the United Kingdom (closed squares), where biopsy policy is generally conservative, and where the frequency of diagnosis of IgAN is relatively low, the two frequencies are highly (inversely) correlated (solid line; $p < 0.01$). In contrast, in continental Europe, Australia, and Japan (open squares), where a more aggressive biopsy policy and more extensive urinalysis screening exist, there is no significant correlation. Since many patients with IgAN have only mild signs such as low-grade proteinuria and/or microhematuria, IgAN patients are underrepresented in geographic areas with a conservative biopsy policy; diagnosis depends on severe manifestations such as macrohematuria and/or proteinuria. In countries with a more aggressive biopsy policy, even patients with only mild disease are biopsied, diagnosed, and included in the data. This increases the prevalence of IgAN and at the same time removes the inverse correlation between macrohematuria (and also severe proteinuria, data not shown) and the rate of diagnosis of IgAN. (Reprinted from Emancipator, S. N., and Lamm, M. E.* Lab. Invest. 60: 168, 1989, *by permission of the U.S.–Canadian Academy of Pathology.)*

MANIFESTATIONS OF DISEASE

Hematuria is the most consistent element in the clinical expression of IgAN [342,361,425,471, 480,567,645,658]. Episodic macrohematuria and persistent microhematuria are present in approximately 54 and 78 percent of patients, respectively (Fig. 6-3A). The macrohematuria typically persists for a few days, but it may last for weeks. Ob-

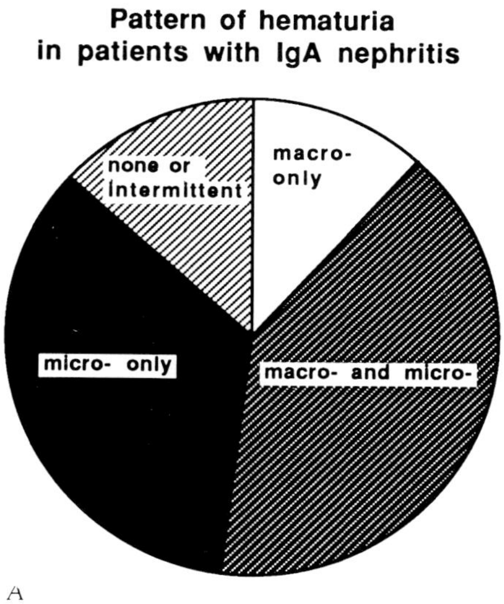

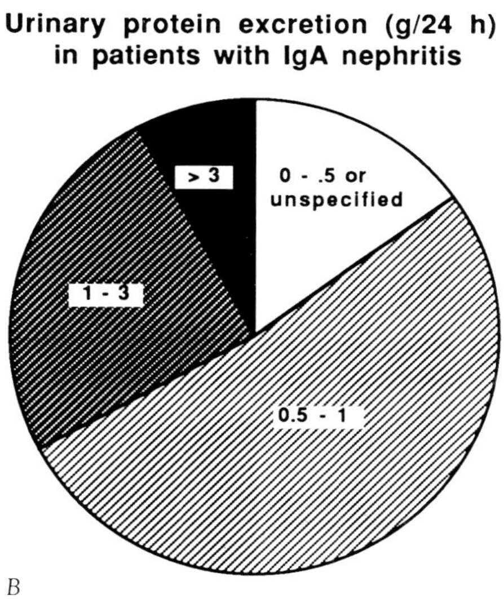

Fig. 6-3. *(A) The proportion of IgA nephritis patients with episodic macrohematuria, transient or persistent microhematuria, or macrohematuria superimposed on microhematuria. (B) The proportion of IgA nephritis patients with unspecified protein excretion or positive proteinuria less than 0.5 g daily, between 0.5 and 1 g daily, between 1 and 3 g daily, and more than 3 g daily. Note that few patients have no hematuria or no proteinuria. These data are based on a total of 2287 cases of IgA nephritis in children and adults reported worldwide (see text).*

viously, episodic macrohematuria and persistent microhematuria coexist in an appreciable number of individuals. In addition, intermittent microhematuria occurs in many IgAN patients, increasing the overall number of patients with some form of hematuria and the complexity of the various patterns of hematuria syndrome that can be encountered.

The incidence of macrohematuria in children is higher (80 percent) than in adults (45 percent) in the Western hemisphere, whereas in the Eastern hemisphere, the incidence of macrohematuria in children and adults tends to be similar (40 percent) [40,97,98,132,183,576,672]. In Japan, 60 percent is a maximal incidence of gross hematuria occurring at any time in children with IgAN [672]. The more conservative biopsy policy in the West selects for IgAN patients with more conspicuous clinical manifestations, which in children is likely to be hematuria rather than other signs of nephritis.

Proteinuria is also a frequent sign of IgAN, again encountered to some degree in nearly all patients; while the majority (52 percent) excrete less than 1 g per day, an appreciable number (33 percent) have greater proteinuria, including some 5 to 10 percent of all patients who present with heavy proteinuria or fully developed nephrotic syndrome (Fig. 6-3*B*). Hypertension, azotemia/acute renal failure, and chronic renal failure are observed in 15, 10, and 5 percent, respectively, of new patients, and each is the presenting sign or symptom in roughly 5 percent of all patients [487,585,593]. Heavy proteinuria and hypertension are correlated with increasing age at apparent onset, and children are less likely to have these features than adults [40,97,98,132,183]. Pain in the flank or abdomen also may be a presenting sign, but it is recognized in relatively few patients [477,646].

PREVALENT COMBINATIONS OF SIGNS AND SYMPTOMS

As already stated, hematuria is the presenting sign in more than 75 percent of all patients, is observed in more than 95 percent at some time during the clinical course, and is frequently accompanied by proteinuria, hypertension, and/or azotemia in variable combinations. However, recognition of characteristic syndromes is important from the perspective of diagnosis of the individual patient. Three major sign/symptom complexes have been recognized in IgAN (Fig. 6-4): (1) episodic macrohematuria with low-grade proteinuria and variable reduction in glomerular filtration rate (GFR), sometimes with concomitant or subsequent acute transient renal failure, (2) persistent or episodic microhematuria with variable proteinuria, and (3) chronic renal failure [60,100,133].

The first of these, accounting for approximately 60 percent of patients, is most frequent in young males. Exacerbation of gross hematuria is synpharyngitic (i.e., nephritis occurs at the height of pharyngitis) in 60 to 80 percent of patients. The association of hematuria, and perhaps renal insufficiency, with acute pharyngitis is superficially reminiscent of poststreptococcal glomerulonephritis. However, IgAN patients can be readily distinguished from those with poststreptococcal nephritis on clinical grounds, in that the interval between sore throat and nephritis is measured in days rather than weeks and the nephritis is recurrent, may frequently *precede* the sore throat, and is itself rarely streptococcal in etiology. Although not all patients have hematuric episodes accompanied by clinical pharyngitis, most have at least some of their episodes accompanied by "viral" illness. In this context, it is worth noting that acute gastroenteritis, bronchitis, and sinusitis are also associated with episodic macrohematuria in many patients and are conceptually related to, although not examples of, synpharyngitic nephritis. These patients with episodic macrohematuria also make up the majority of those with IgAN who have temporal association of "viral" illness with nephritis (50 percent overall but 80 percent or more among this group). These observations collectively suggest that the underlying mechanism of glomerular injury in this group is particularly related to immune responses to mucosal infections.

Despite accounts relating this syndrome to high-grade histologic lesions [46,47,576], patients with episodic bouts of gross hematuria have enjoyed the best long-term renal survival in several studies, as first proposed by D'Amico [128,130,

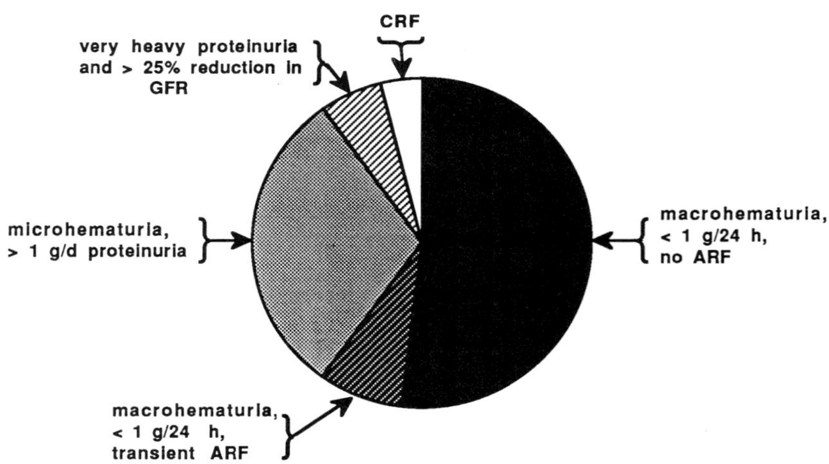

FIG. 6-4. *The proportion of IgA nephritis patients who present for medical attention with major sign/symptom complexes: episodic macrohematuria with 1 g or less daily protein excretion with or without acute renal failure (ARF); persistent or intermittent microhematuria with 1 g or more daily protein excretion, which is sometimes heavy and accompanied by reduction of GFR; and patients with chronic renal failure.*

131,157,291,330,555,571]. Several investigators have emphasized that episodes of acute renal failure associated with gross hematuria are typically transient [378,404,491,520], even though associated with more severe glomerular lesions, which include cellular crescents. Indeed, such nephritic episodes do not appear to have any long-term prognostic significance [378,491], and the glomerular lesions and tubular necrosis often observed in these patients generally resolve [324]. On the other hand, within the group of patients with macrohematuria, rapidly progressive renal failure with crescentic glomerulonephritis is also documented in IgAN [2,5,130,188,373,396,678]. Prospective clinical recognition of these patients can be difficult. IgAN with rapid progression to end-stage failure tends to occur in the younger patients, generally those less than 16 years of age. Acute renal failure is more frequent in the subset of patients with rapid progression. These patients are more frequently hypertensive and more severely azotemic upon presentation than those with IgAN without rapid progression to end-stage failure, but individual patients cannot be distinguished prospectively on clinical grounds.

The next most frequent group of patients (30 percent overall) presents with either persistent or intermittent microscopic hematuria; these patients, particularly in the United Kingdom and North America, where more severe clinical signs are required for biopsy to be indicated, are more likely to have moderate or heavy proteinuria (~1 g/24 h or more). They are also more likely to have persistent decreases in GFR, although the incidence of acute renal failure is much less than in the group with episodic gross hematuria. They also tend to be older (over 30 years of age), and the male-to-female ratio approaches parity. These patients account for the majority of cases of IgAN that progress to end-stage kidney disease.

Some patients in this group present with or develop the nephrotic syndrome [98,122,139,159, 571]. Although some investigators have argued that this subset of patients represents coexistence of two distinct processes, the number of such patients exceeds by far that predicted from the incidences of IgAN and minimal-change disease were these two diseases to coexist randomly in some individuals. Response of such patients to corticosteroid therapy, considered by some an indicator that primary nephrotic syndrome underlies the proteinuria, should not be construed as evidence that the IgA glomerular deposits in these patients are independent of the proteinuria; rather, the efficacy of steroids may indicate that the *mechanism* of proteinuria may be common to both pathophysiologic processes [14,32,318,345,370,373,564,576, 577,665]. Certainly, "collision" of IgAN and idiopathic nephrotic syndrome contributes to this pool of patients, although with current technology it is impossible to prove or disprove coexistence of these processes as independent. As discussed later (under Pathophysiology), mesangiopathic lesions can be associated with heavy proteinuria or nephrotic syndrome. Coincident IgAN and membranous nephropathy with nephrotic syndrome does occur, and the separate processes are indicated by the compartmentalization of IgG to the epimembranous deposits and IgA to the mesangium within the same glomeruli [300]. However, mesangiopathic lesions induced by immune deposits with predominantly IgA likely represent a distinct process, and therefore, IgAN must enter into the differential diagnosis of the nephrotic syndrome, although only a small proportion of nephrotic individuals will prove to have IgAN when biopsied.

The third group, namely patients with chronic renal failure, tend to be the oldest (over 50 years), the most likely to be hypertensive, and of course, those with the poorest prognosis.

Pathologic Changes

GROSS APPEARANCE

The kidneys of patients with IgAN are likely to appear grossly normal, but little information is available.

MICROSCOPIC FINDINGS

The morphologic expression of renal injury in IgAN is, like the clinical expression of the disease, wide ranging and variable. Yet much of this variability actually reflects different combinations of glomerular, tubular, vascular, and interstitial lesions. By presenting these in sequence, some of the diversity of the appearance of IgAN is obscured. It is important to be mindful that a spectrum of lesions in each part of the nephron can contribute to the overall appearance, as well as structural status, of the kidney afflicted with IgAN.

This potential for varying degrees of injury in the different regions of the kidney proves a stumbling block to classification of IgAN. Various classification schemes, effective for specific ad hoc purposes of the investigators devising them, do not consistently score glomerular, tubular, and vascular lesions, including presence and degree of crescents and sclerosis, as independent features. A short verbal description would ultimately prove best to allow for comparisons among series of patients. Table 6-1 provides a modified classification scheme that is essentially a shorthand notation of descriptive terms.

Glomeruli

All patterns of glomerular injury are observed in IgAN (Fig. 6-5), and IgAN is indeed a microcosm of glomerulonephritis in general, both clinically and pathologically [342,361,425,471,480,567, 645,658]. Mesangial proliferative and focal proliferative nephritides predominate, however, and IgAN is the first consideration when these patterns of glomerular disease are encountered in patients without systemic illness, particularly if the patient is hematuric.

By light microscopy, the most common appearance of the glomeruli is that of mesangiopathic glomerulonephritis (63 percent of all patients), defined as histologic changes confined to proliferation of cells and expansion of matrix within mesangial areas. The lesions in these patients are by no means homogeneous; in many, there is only matrix expansion (Fig. 6-6), whereas others show

TABLE 6-1. *Histopathologic classification of IgA nephritis**

Categories	
A	Normal or minimal glomerular lesions
B	Focal mesangial proliferation
C	Diffuse mesangial proliferation
D1	Focal and segmental endocapillary proliferation superimposed on mesangial proliferation
D2	Focal and segmental endocapillary proliferation alone
E	Diffuse endocapillary proliferation
F	Diffuse extracapillary proliferation (crescents in >70 percent), with or without endocapillary proliferation
G	Glomerular sclerosis (>70 percent glomeruli sclerotic)
H	Unclassifiable or combined lesions
Suffixes	
m, M	Mesangial matrix expansion is disproportionately prominent to a noticeable (m) or marked (M) degree
c, C	Mesangial hypercellularity is disproportionately prominent to a noticeable (c) or marked (C) extent
s, S	Sclerosis involving >10 percent and <30 percent of glomeruli (s) or ≥30 percent but ≤70 percent of glomeruli (S)†
k, K	Crescents involving >10 percent and <30 percent of glomeruli (k) or ≥30 percent but ≤70 percent of glomeruli (K)
a, A	Tubular atrophy and/or interstitial fibrosis, moderate (a) or severe (A) in degree
i, I	Interstitial nephritis, moderate (i) or severe (I) in degree
v, V	Arteriolar sclerosis, moderate (v) or severe (V) in degree

*The categories are based on the views of the writer and on the schemes developed by various authors. The scheme presented here is essentially a shorthand histologic description. For example, CmiV would denote a diffuse mesangial proliferative glomerulonephritis with a relative prominence of matrix, moderate focal lymphohistiocytic interstitial infiltrates, and marked vascular sclerosis.

†Sclerosis involving more than 70 percent of glomeruli makes a diagnosis of IgAN difficult, in that this extent of sclerosis would often restrict the patent glomeruli available to evaluate immunofluorescence, upon which a diagnosis of IgAN must reside, to too small a number. Category G should generally be reserved for repeat biopsies of patients with a diagnosis of IgAN already established who have progressed. If a sufficient number of patent glomeruli on which to make a diagnosis of IgAN does not exist but IgAN is considered the most probable diagnosis, the patient should be classified in group H.

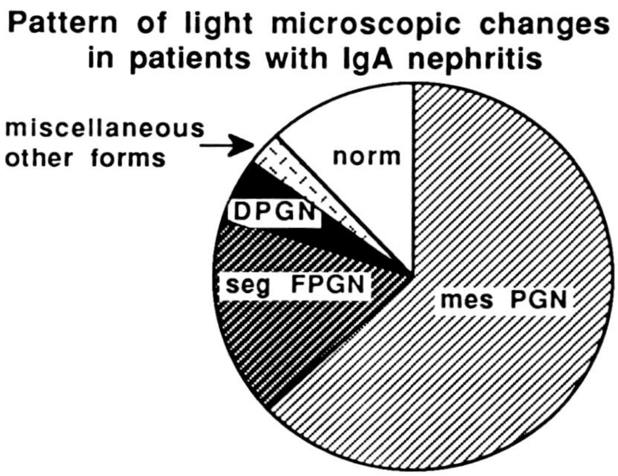

Fig. 6-5. *The distribution of the patterns of pathologic changes encountered in 2287 cases of IgA nephritis in selected series (see Figs. 6-3 and 6-4 and the text). Mesangial proliferative glomerulonephritis (mes PGN) is the major morphologic pattern of expression of glomerular injury, followed by approximately equal numbers of patients with somewhat more (focal and segmental proliferation, seg FPGN) or less (normal or near normal, norm) pronounced changes. Other patterns are a distinct minority.*

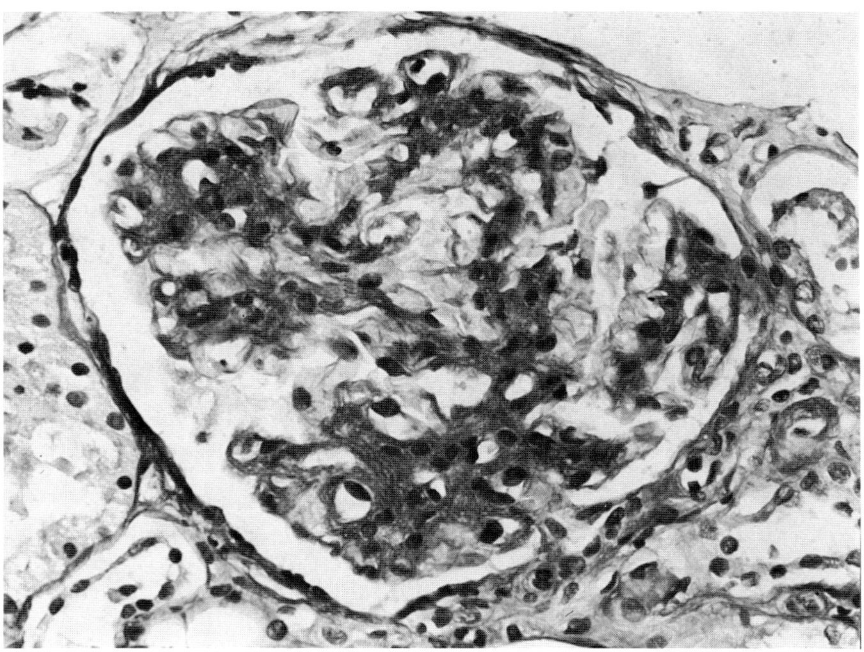

Fig. 6-6. *This glomerulus, from a patient with persistent microhematuria and approximately 1.5 g proteinuria daily, shows a moderate to marked expansion of mesangial matrix but only a mild to equivocal increase in mesangial cellularity. Capillaries are patent throughout. Note the lucencies within the matrix, which may represent immune deposits. PAS; ×400.*

nearly exclusive proliferation of cells (Fig. 6-7). Whether matrix changes, proliferation, or both are evident, there is additional variegation in that the severity of these histologic changes can vary from equivocal to florid (Fig. 6-8). Within an individual biopsy, the appearance of the glomeruli is usually fairly uniform, but the full range of variation can occasionally be encountered in a single biopsy core, with focal and segmental or diffuse mesangial lesions showing different severity and combinations of cellularity and matrix (Fig. 6-9). It is important to distinguish pure mesangiopathic focal or diffuse lesions from lesions that occlude capillaries in a focal-segmental or global distribution. Many authors reporting series of patients with IgAN have failed to make this distinction, making subsequent interpretation difficult.

The mesangial matrix expansion is often more conspicuous in PAS-stained sections than in silver-methenamine stains, perhaps owing to the fact that the deposits, while less argyrophilic than the extracellular matrix, do contain carbohydrate components stainable by PAS. In the usual case, the expansion of mesangial matrix is diffuse, global, and in keeping with the hypercellularity. However, segmental accentuation or diminution of matrix and expansion out of proportion to hypercellularity are frequent. Grading of the severity of mesangial lesions requires experience and is in part subjective. However, morphometric analysis

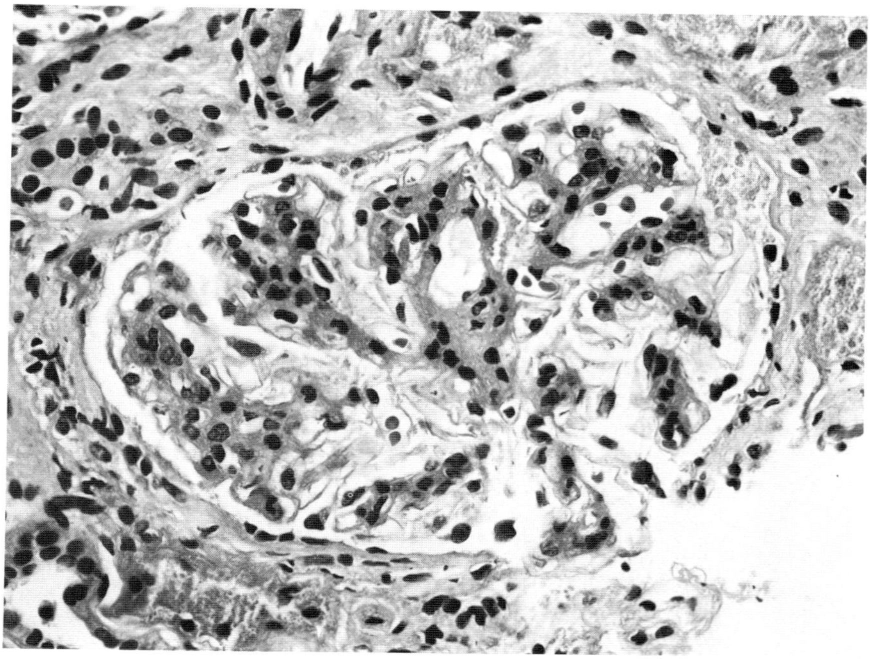

FIG. 6-7. *This glomerulus, from a patient with transient microhematuria and approximately 1.5 g proteinuria daily, shows a moderate to marked mesangial hypercellularity with a relatively modest increase in mesangial matrix. Capillary lumens are patent or equivocally compromised by the mesangial proliferative process. Although the proportion of cells to matrix differs markedly from that depicted in Fig. 6-6, both are examples of mesangial proliferative glomerulonephritis. H&E;* ×400.

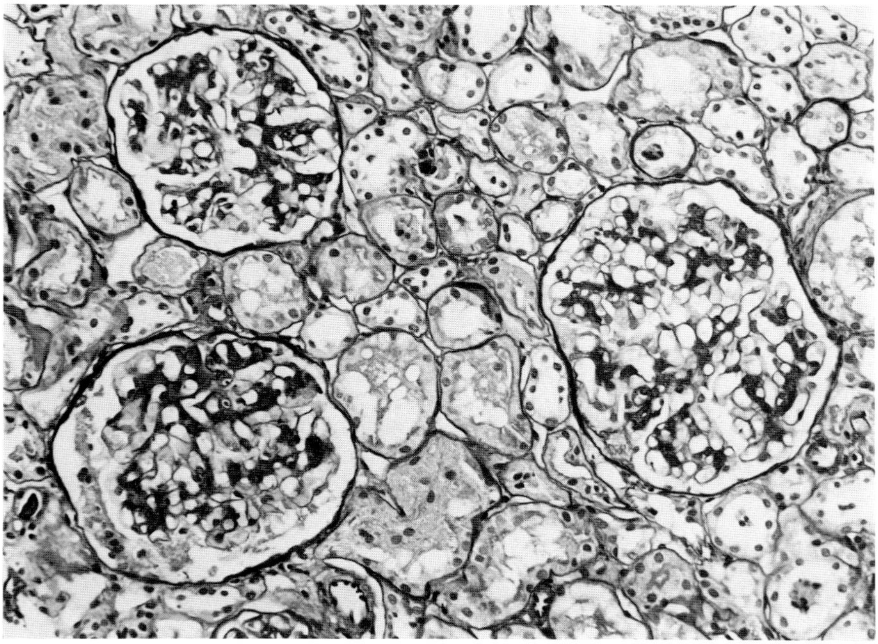

Fig. 6-8. *These three glomeruli, from a patient with episodic macrohematuria and approximately 1 g proteinuria daily, show variation in the severity of mesangial expansion from equivocal (right) to marked (lower left). Note the small crescent in the glomerulus in the lower left. PAS; ×200.*

verifies expanded mesangial volume in patients with IgAN, even when the glomeruli are judged to be minimally altered by an experienced renal pathologist [314,597,671]. In addition to immune deposits, the mesangium is expanded by increased extracellular matrix that is apparently normal in quality. By immunohistochemistry, collagen IV, fibronectin, and heparan sulfate appear dominant in mesangial proliferative glomerulonephritis, just as they are normally [583].

By all criteria, the increase in cellularity within the mesangium represents hyperplasia and hypertrophy of endogenous glomerular cells. Moreover, as discussed below, the ultrastructural appearance of these cells is similar to mesangial cells cultured in vitro from glomerular explants. Infiltration of the glomeruli by exogenous leukocytes does occur, but these cells represent a distinct minority of the intraglomerular cell population. Lymphocytes, monocyte/macrophages, and neutrophils are found at a frequency of only one cell of each lineage per glomerular cross section, on average, and are certainly neither a constant feature nor related to the overall grade of mesangial hypercellularity [326, 376,468].

Deposits are not conspicuous in this pattern of glomerulonephritis by routine light microscopy. However, Berger and others have reported small foci of mesangial lucency in silver-stained sections, and deposits are often evident in sections stained with trichrome. Segmental adhesions of glomerular tuft to parietal epithelium are present focally in many cases with mesangial proliferation, and hyperplasia of parietal epithelium is also en-

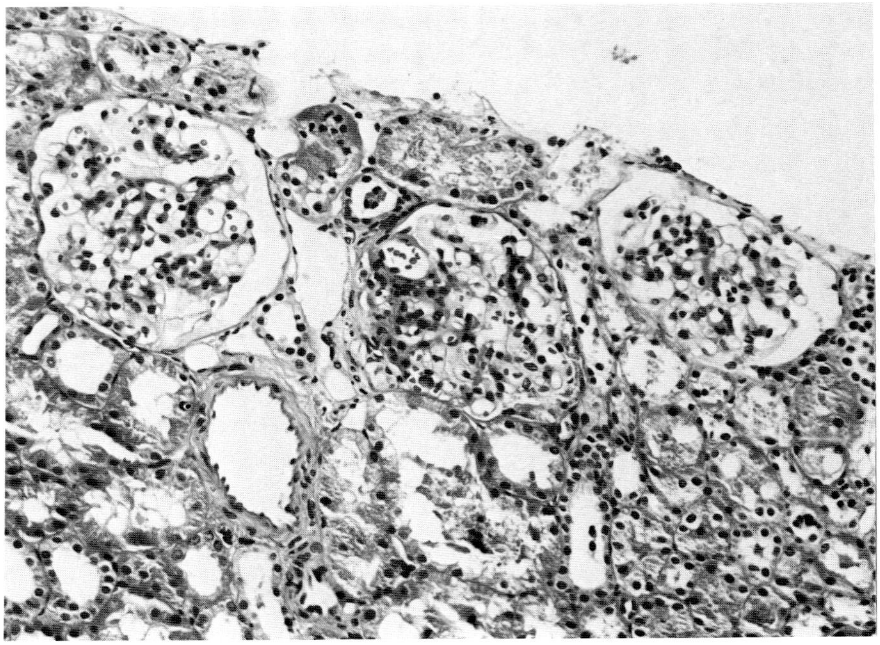

FIG. 6-9. *These three glomeruli, from a patient with intermittent microhematuria and 500 μg proteinuria daily, all show moderate mesangial hypercellularity but have different proportions of matrix expansion. This photograph emphasizes that even in the same biopsy core there is variability in the pattern of glomerular involvement. H&E; ×250.*

countered (Fig. 6-10). While the few prominent parietal cells usually seen in association with mesangiopathic IgAN do not merit the term *crescent,* this arbitrary distinction of degree is not embraced by all pathologists, and many refer to these foci of extracapillary proliferation as crescents. In any case, they are not so abundant, so large, or associated with segmental tuft necrosis or adhesions to prompt the pessimistic prognosis that widespread, large crescent formation does in higher-grade lesions.

Focal and segmental endocapillary proliferation is seen in approximately 17 percent of patients (see Fig. 6-10), and diffuse endocapillary proliferation is the predominant pattern in some 5 percent (Figs. 6-11 and 6-12). Both patterns are usually, but not necessarily, superimposed on mesangiopathic glomerulonephritis. The identity of the supernumerary cells in these cases, as in proliferative glomerulonephritis generally, is open to question. Leukocytes are more numerous in these forms of intracapillary proliferation than in glomeruli with pure mesangial lesions but are certainly less abundant than in typical postinfectious or connective-tissue disease–related proliferative glomerulonephritis. There are often segmental thickenings or irregularities of the capillary walls in glomeruli from patients with endocapillary lesions, even in lobules lacking endocapillary hypercellularity. Notwithstanding the typically focal-segmental distribution of endocapillary proliferation, immune deposits are diffuse and uniformly distributed throughout the mesangium. Capillary wall deposits can sometimes be recog-

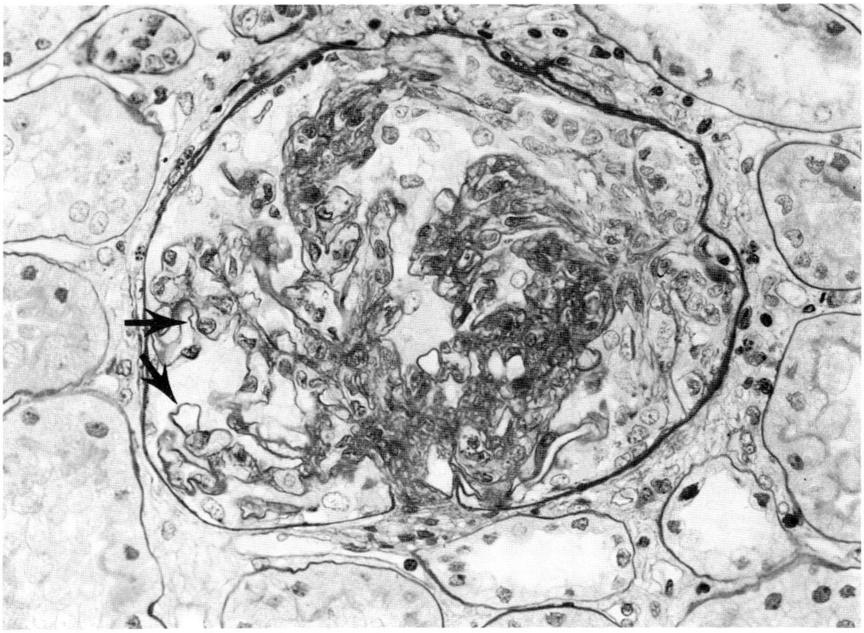

Fig. 6-10. *In this glomerulus there is segmental endocapillary proliferation and collapse of glomerular capillaries associated with adhesion of tuft to a partial crescent. Note the expansion of the vascular pole and the tortuosity of capillary walls (arrows) remote from the synechia. PAS;* ×400.

nized in sections stained with silver, PAS, or trichrome in subendothelial and, less frequently, subepithelial sites. The mesangial component of the proliferation is usually moderate to severe and typically more constant than in patients with pure mesangiopathic glomerulonephritis alone (discussed earlier). Segmental adhesions of tuft to parietal epithelium (synechiae) and focal parietal epithelial hyperplasia are more frequent in patients with these lesions than in patients with pure mesangiopathic disease.

Segmental tuft necrosis and/or focal crescent formation may accompany all patterns of proliferation. The proportion of cases with such lesions ranges from 20 percent in pure mesangial lesions to nearly 50 percent in cases with diffuse endocapillary proliferation [46,96,110,127,249,330,362]. Likewise, global glomerulosclerosis is encountered in some glomeruli in about 30 to 50 percent of biopsies [98,122,147,199,388,403,445,460,589, 677]. However, it is rare for tuft necrosis to be encountered diffusely, and cases in which glomerulosclerosis or crescent formation is encountered in more than 50 percent of glomeruli represent only 15 and 8 percent of patients, respectively.

As Abuelo et al. [5] noted, among others [130,188,373,396,678], some 5 to 8 percent of all IgAN patients progress rapidly to end-stage renal disease. The patients all have significant crescent formation and thus can be recognized by biopsy. Capillary wall deposits, especially large subepithelial deposits, are frequently associated with the crescents and synechiae.

Other patterns of glomerular injury have been

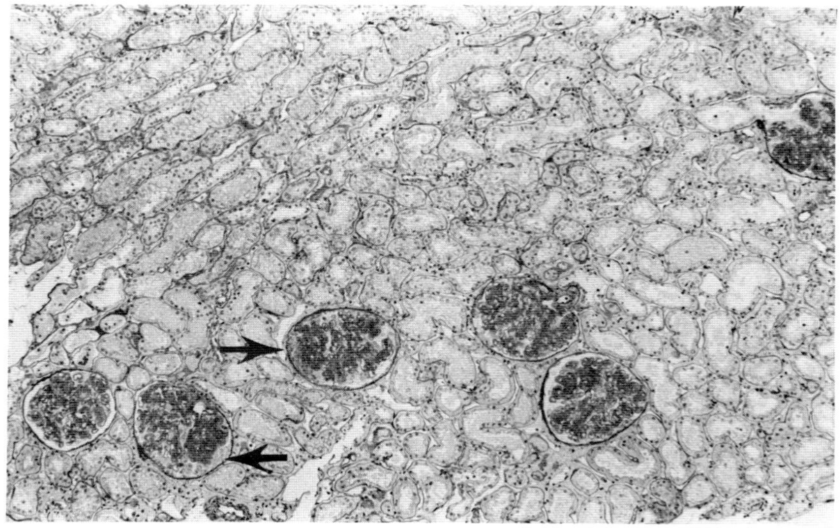

FIG. 6-11. *There is global endocapillary proliferation of all six glomeruli in this field, indeed representative of the entire open renal biopsy specimen. Note the lack of interstitial inflammatory infiltrate. The patient had recurrent episodic synpharyngitic macrohemturia. Note the small crescents in two glomeruli (arrows). PAS; ×35. (Photographed from material kindly provided by Dr. D. Sedmak.)*

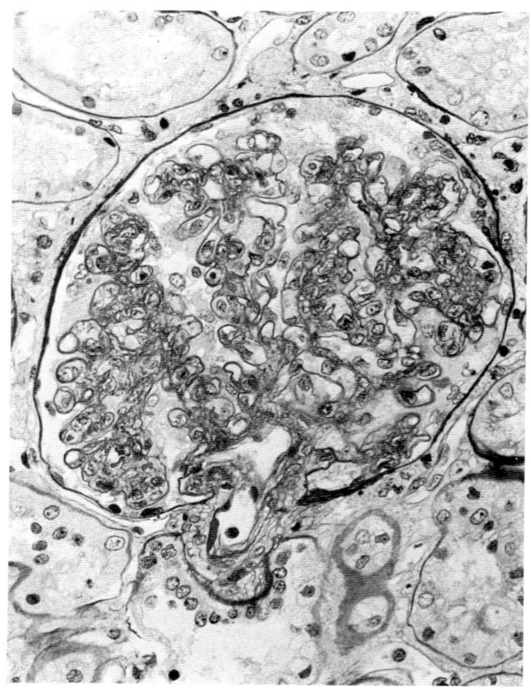

FIG. 6-12. *A higher magnification of a single glomerulus from Fig. 6-11 shows occlusion of most capillaries due to an increased cellularity and a mild expansion of matrix. In contrast to postinfectious glomerulonephritis, which this case otherwise resembles, there are few neutrophils or other leukocytes infiltrating the glomeruli in this patient. PAS; ×320. (Photographed from material kindly provided by Dr. D. Sedmak.)*

reported with low frequency (approximately 3 percent) or anecdotally in IgAN. Focal and segmental glomerular sclerosis with predominant IgA deposits and membranous, membranoproliferative (Fig. 6-13), and mixed glomerulonephritic lesions have all been described in addition to the necrotizing, crescentic, and sclerotic forms just mentioned. Finally, approximately 12 percent of all IgAN patients have normal or minimally altered glomeruli (Fig. 6-14).

Tubules

Perhaps the most frequent change observed in the tubules of IgAN is the presence of erythrocytes or erythrocyte casts. The presence of red cells in the tubules correlates well with clinical hematuria, but their absence does not imply that the patient is not hematuric. Several large series, collectively recording details on tubular and interstitial changes in 1311 biopsies of patients with IgAN, indicate that degenerative change (desquamation, loss of microvillous brush border, and vacuolization of tubular epithelium), generally focal, is frequently encountered (57 percent of patients), particularly in patients with acute renal failure or nephrotic syndrome [1,98,131,147,156,159,204,214,280,282, 315,318,325,330,378,388,403,418,443,448,450, 481,555,628,677]. Focal tubular atrophy, generally mild and confined to clusters of three to five tubules, is evident in 40 percent of patients (Fig. 6-15); it is typically associated with interstitial fibrosis (see below). Scattered casts are present in a few patients. Other, less detailed studies substantially corroborate these observations [122,130, 135,157,460,572].

Tubular lesions rarely involve loops of Henle or collecting ducts and are not confined to or associated with any particular pattern of glomerular involvement. Prognostic significance to date is restricted to atrophy, associated with fibrosis.

Morphometric analysis of tubular cross sections at sites apart from foci of atrophy can reveal pseudodilation of cortical tubules due to flattening of tubular cells and formation of small tubular casts

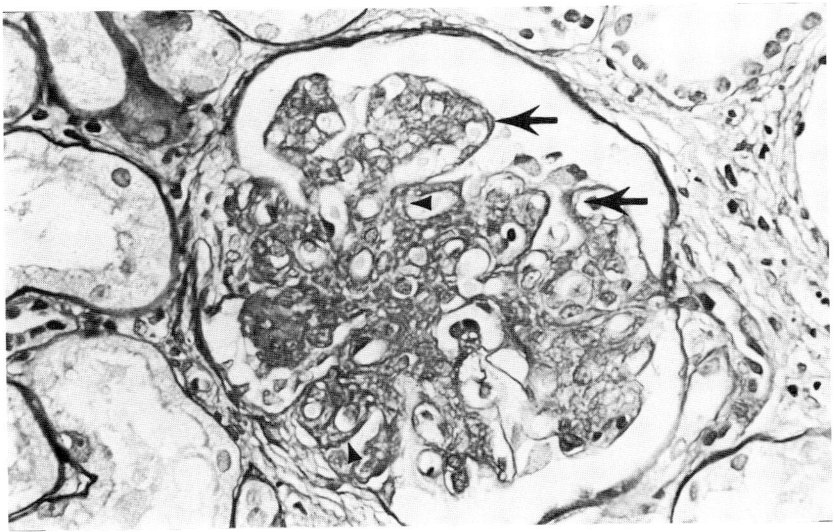

Fig. 6-13. *There is modest hypersegmentation of capillary tufts within this glomerulus. In addition, duplication or splitting of capillary walls (arrows) and mesangial interposition (arrowhead) are evident. This pattern, reminiscent of membranoproliferative glomerulonephritis, is encountered in only 1 to 2 percent of patients with IgA nephritis.* PAS; ×335.

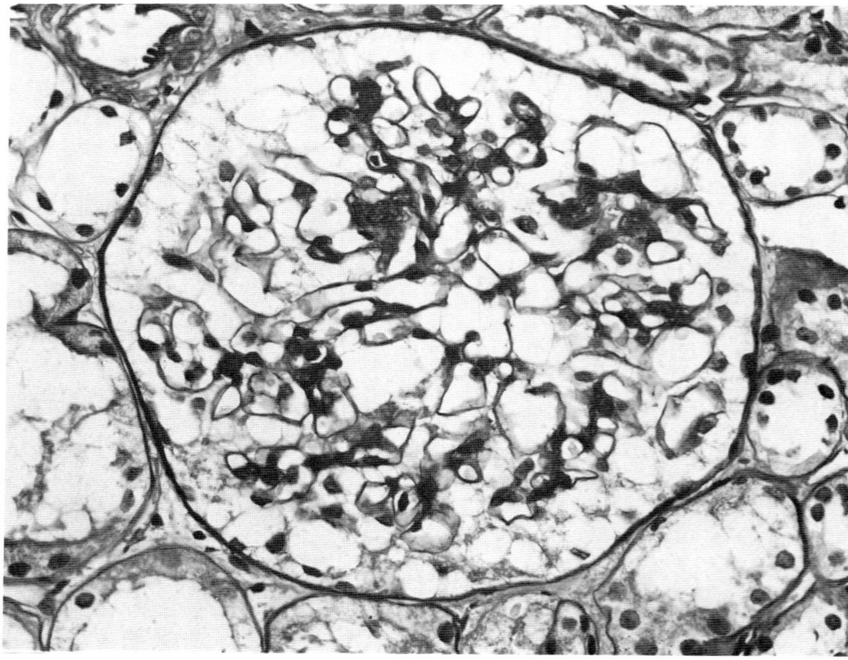

FIG. 6-14. *Normal glomeruli as seen by light microscopy are encountered in IgA nephritis. This glomerulus, representative of all those in the sample, is from a patient with episodic macrohematuria, daily urinary protein excretion of approximately 800 μg, and diffuse mesangial deposits of IgA, IgM, and C3 with electron-dense paramesangial deposits. PAS;* ×400.

with a frequency higher than expected [391]. These subtle changes may precede better developed foci of tubular atrophy and interstitial fibrosis and as such are potentially valuable prognostically.

Blood Vessels

Medial hypertrophy and/or hyalin arteriolosclerosis (Fig. 6-16) were present in arterioles and small arteries of 54 percent of IgAN patients, regardless of age, in one series [199]. Although other series report similar incidence figures for arteriosclerosis and arteriolosclerosis [98,101,127,128, 131,159,202,210,280,324,418,443,677], there is an impression, in at least some series, that vascular disease is less common in children [98,127]. Although many patients with arteriosclerotic lesions are hypertensive, many are normotensive, and there is no correlation between these two variables. Feiner et al. [199] have suggested that although systemic hypertension has an important role in the progression of renal disease, "a primary intrarenal vascular defect, independent of but enhanced by hypertension" underlies progressive renal damage in IgAN. Recently, these investigators have performed a morphometric analysis of vascular lesions. Morphometry is capable of making subtle vessel lesions more obvious and again showed a strong relationship between arteriolar hypertrophy and tendency for progression [223].

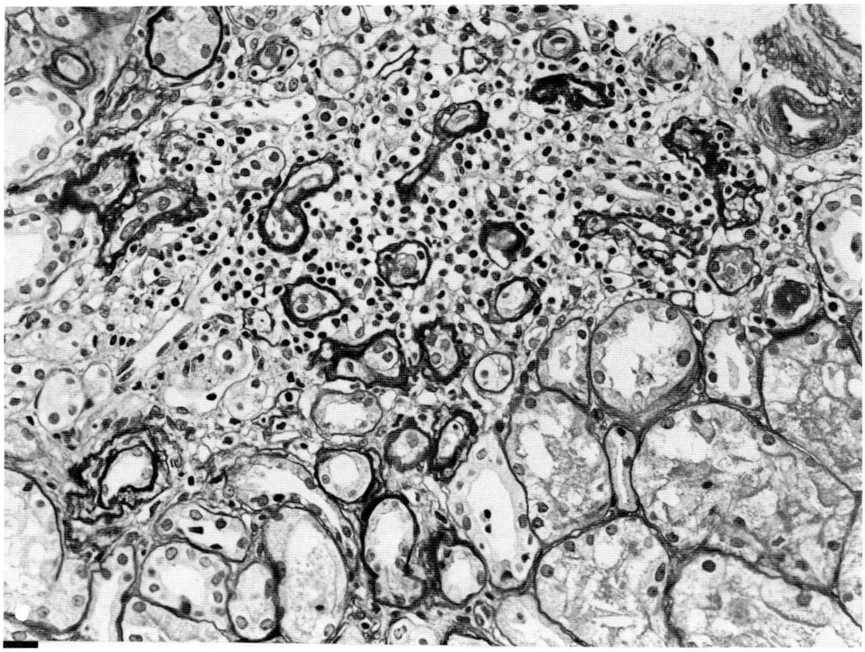

Fig. 6-15. *Focal tubular atrophy, evident by thickening of tubular basement membranes, reduction in tubular lumen area, and flattening of tubular epithelium, is often seen in IgA nephritis. The patchy process seen here is accompanied by a moderate lymphohistiocytic interstitial infiltrate and interstitial edema. PAS; ×250.*

Interstitium

In the studies that specifically discuss tubular and interstitial changes [9,450,460,481,527,555,628, 677], approximately 40 percent of IgAN patients have fibrosis within the cortical interstitium (Fig. 6-17). Generally focal, the fibrosis is mild in 15 percent of all patients, moderate in 15 percent, and severe in 7 percent. Only 3 to 5 percent of all patients have diffuse moderate or severe fibrosis. Focal tubular atrophy is typically present in relation to the fibrosis. There are patchy areas of sparse lymphohistiocytic infiltrate in as many as 20 percent of all patients (Fig. 6-18), nearly always associated with foci of fibrosis and tubular atrophy. Edema is generally inconspicuous in these individuals.

In perhaps 5 percent of IgAN patients there is a frank acute tubulointerstitial nephritis, with edema, irregular clusters of numerous lymphocytes and macrophages, and associated degenerative changes in tubules (Fig. 6-19). These foci tend to be accentuated around glomeruli, small arteries, and arterioles, and may be indistinguishable from primary interstitial nephritis.

IMMUNOHISTOCHEMICAL FINDINGS

Glomeruli

IgA is by definition the predominant immunoglobulin deposited in glomeruli in IgAN. However, IgA is the exclusive immunoglobulin in only 26 percent of cases (Fig. 6-20). IgG or IgM is codeposited in 37 and 13 percent of cases, respectively, and 25 percent of patients have deposits of all

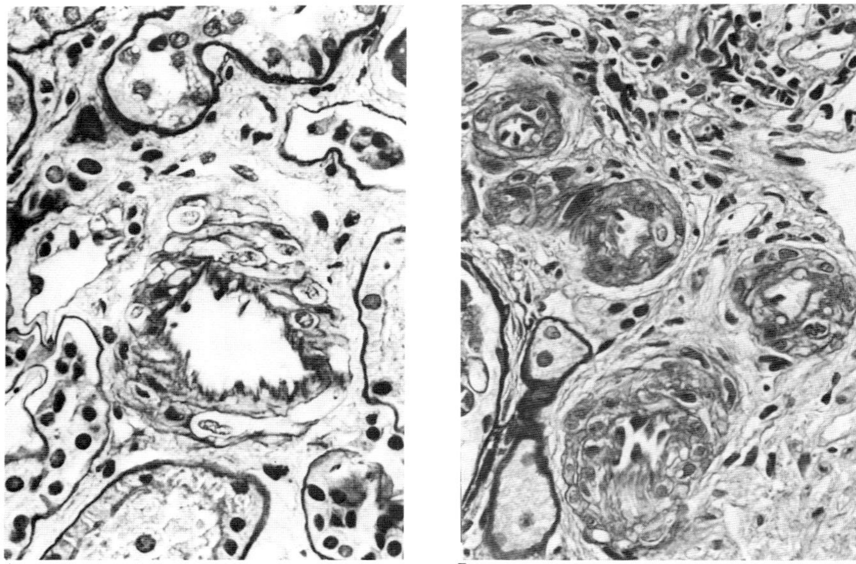

A B

FIG. 6-16. *Mild (A) to severe (B) arteriolosclerosis is encountered in approximately 54 percent of patients. Hyalin (not shown) is sometimes seen in association with the medial hypertrophy. (A) Silver methenamine; ×550; (B) PAS; ×400.*

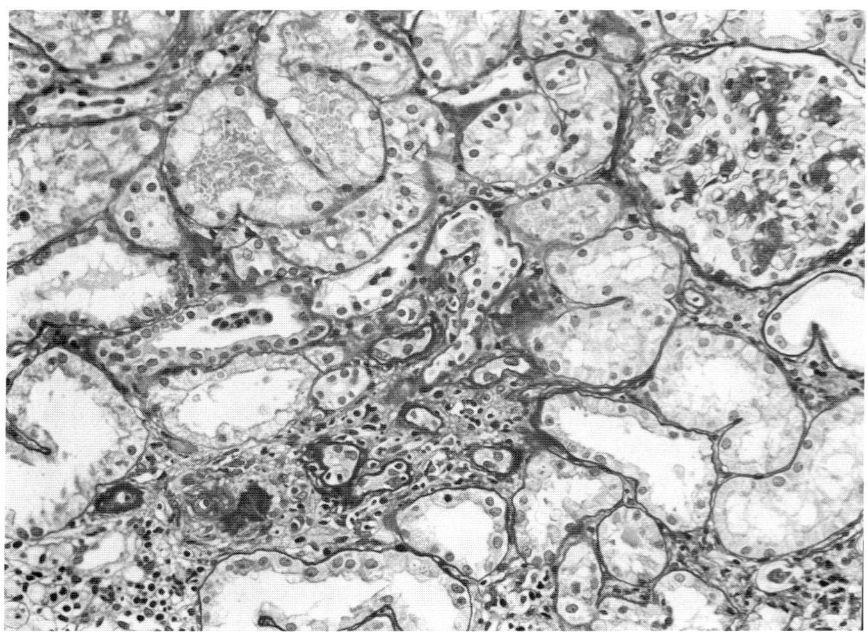

FIG. 6-17. *Interstitial fibrosis, almost always focal, is seen in up to 55 percent of patients with IgA nephritis. Note that the tubules within the scarred area are atrophic. The glomerulus shows moderate mesangial matrix expansion. PAS; ×200.*

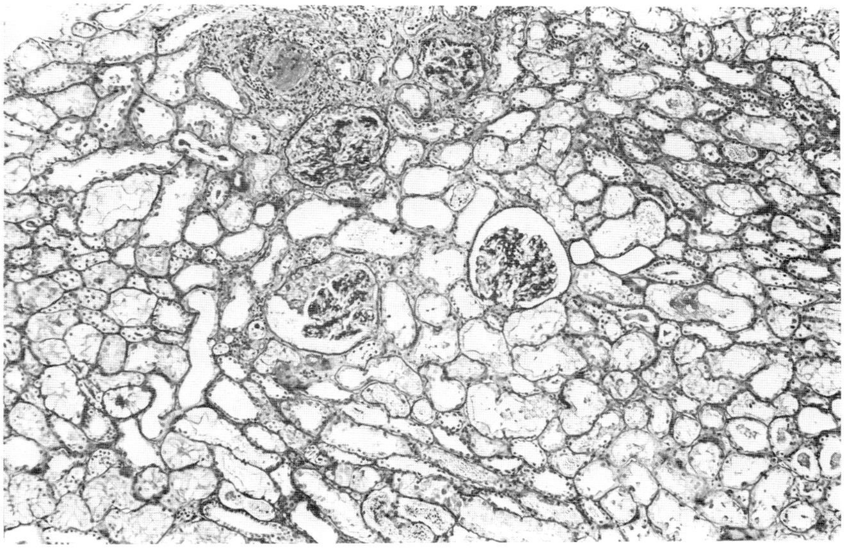

FIG. 6-18. *There is a focus of dense lymphohistiocytic interstitial infiltrate encompassing a sclerotic glomerulus in the upper left portion of this field. Note that the majority of the field is devoid of interstitial changes. Foci of interstitial nephritis are often seen in IgA nephritis.* PAS; ×80.

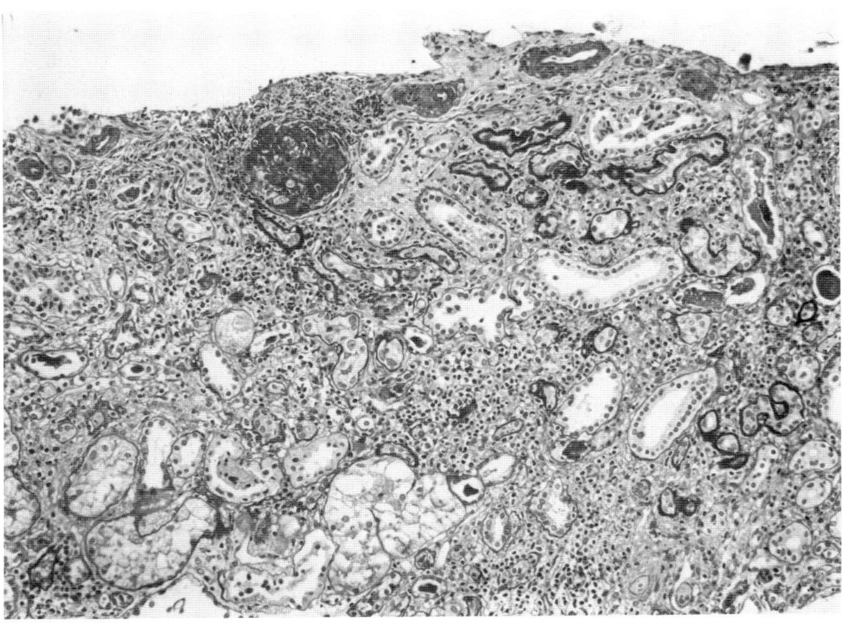

FIG. 6-19. *There is a diffuse lymphohistiocytic infiltrate associated with interstitial edema and focal tubular atrophy evident in this biopsy. A frank interstitial nephritis component is not frequent in IgA nephritis but is widely recognized in a small percentage of cases.* PAS; ×120.

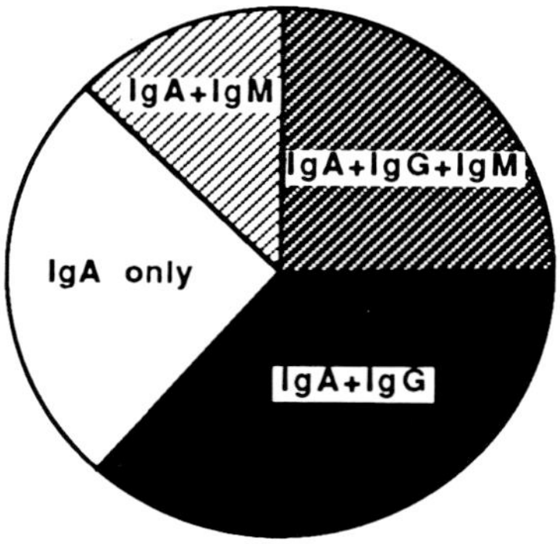

FIG. 6-20. *The proportion of patients with various codeposits of non-IgA immunoglobulin is presented. All patients, by definition, have glomerular IgA, and nearly all have C3 deposits. Note that most patients have IgG and/or IgM codeposits; few have deposits of classical pathway complement components (not shown, see text).*

three major immunoglubulin classes. Although capillary wall deposits of immune reactants are superimposed in some cases, diffuse mesangial deposits are the rule in all patients (Figs. 6-21 and 6-22). Mesangial deposits may be segmental in rare cases but are generally global. Rarely, linear capillary wall deposits are encountered [67,342].

Most evidence favors IgA-associated J-chain deposits with both kappa and lambda light chains, indicative of polyclonal oligomeric IgA [44,45,51, 344,350,382,383]. The ratio of light chain types within the immunoglobulin deposits remains controversial, however, as does the presence of J-chain and the degree of polymerization of the deposited IgA. It is now clear, despite initial confusion, that the IgA_1 subclass predominates by far over the IgA_2 subclass in glomerular immune deposits [43,107,383,439,494,525,605,625]. Glomerular deposits of secretory component are not a feature of IgAN.

Complement deposits indicate that activation occurs primarily along the alternative pathway. C3 is nearly always present (95 percent), yet the early components of the classical pathway (C1 and C4) are detected in only 12 percent of biopsies. This indirect evidence for the vast predominance of alternative pathway activation is corroborated by studies in a more limited number of patients; these demonstrate almost ubiquitous deposition of the alternative pathway components, properdin and factor B, in mesangial areas in IgAN patients [42, 98, 140, 157, 189, 191, 192, 278, 298, 317, 330, 403, 404, 418, 428, 502, 520, 576, 602, 607, 637, 677]. Hence, by immunohistology, IgAN can be recognized by the association of IgA and alternative pathway components of complement predominating over other immunoglobulin classes and the classical pathway components.

Recent unpublished observations by West and associates indicate that the C3 deposits in the glomeruli of IgAN patients are largely in the activated rather than the inactivated state (Fig. 6-23). Among various glomerulonephritides, only proliferative lupus nephritis and IgAN had significant percentages of the deposited C3 in the active form, emphasizng the capacity for alternative pathway activation in these diseases. This may be of pathogenetic significance. Receptors that bind C3b are present in glomeruli. Moreover, amplification of complement activation by means of the alternative pathway can occur in diseases such as IgAN and proliferative lupus nephritis, in which most C3 is in the active C3b form, but not in other diseases, where most deposited C3 is in the inactive iC3b form, since only C3b can serve in the amplification.

The membrane attack complex (MAC) of complement is very frequently detected in the glomerular immune deposits in IgAN; indeed, IgAN was the first disease in which glomerular deposits of MAC neoantigen were described [42,51,52,98, 157,189,298,317,403,576,604,607,613]. However, the inevitable codeposition of the regulatory S-protein casts some doubt as to the pathophysiologic significance of the MAC deposits, since factor S limits the biologic activity of MAC [298, 604,607,613]. Moreover, the near 100 percent frequency of MAC deposition does not support the concept that MAC can have prognostic or nosologic value.

Except in cases of necrotizing/crescentic glo-

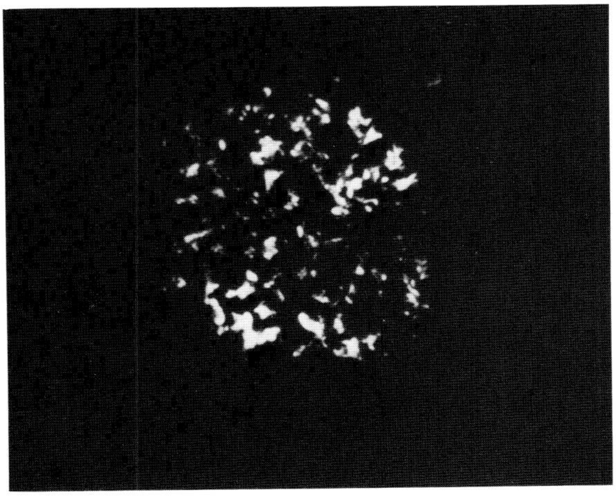

Fig. 6-21. *Glomerular deposits of IgA generally show a diffuse, global mesangial pattern, as seen here, even in glomeruli that appear normal by light microscopy. Deposits of C3 (not shown) parallel those of IgA, and less intense deposits of IgG and/or IgM are often seen in a similar pattern as well.* ×160.

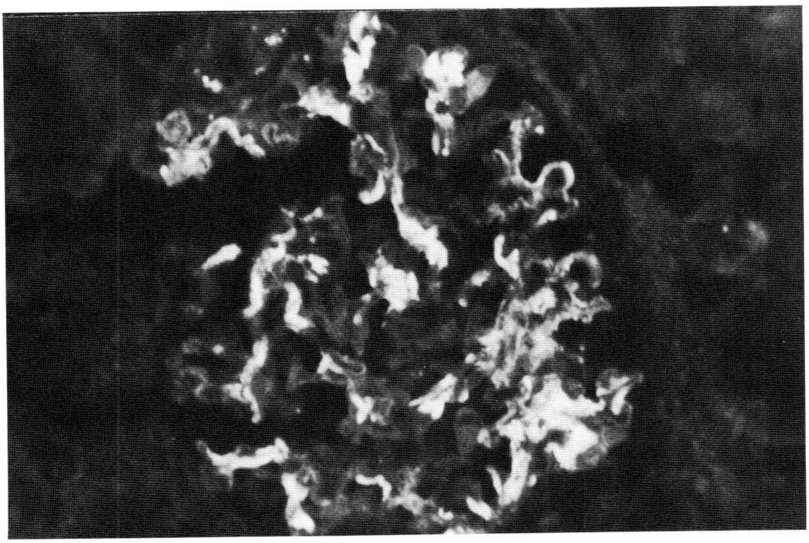

Fig. 6-22. *In addition to mesangial deposits, segmental capillary deposits are frequently seen, as shown here. These deposits are most commonly encountered in association with segmental (or diffuse) endocapillary proliferation.* ×400.

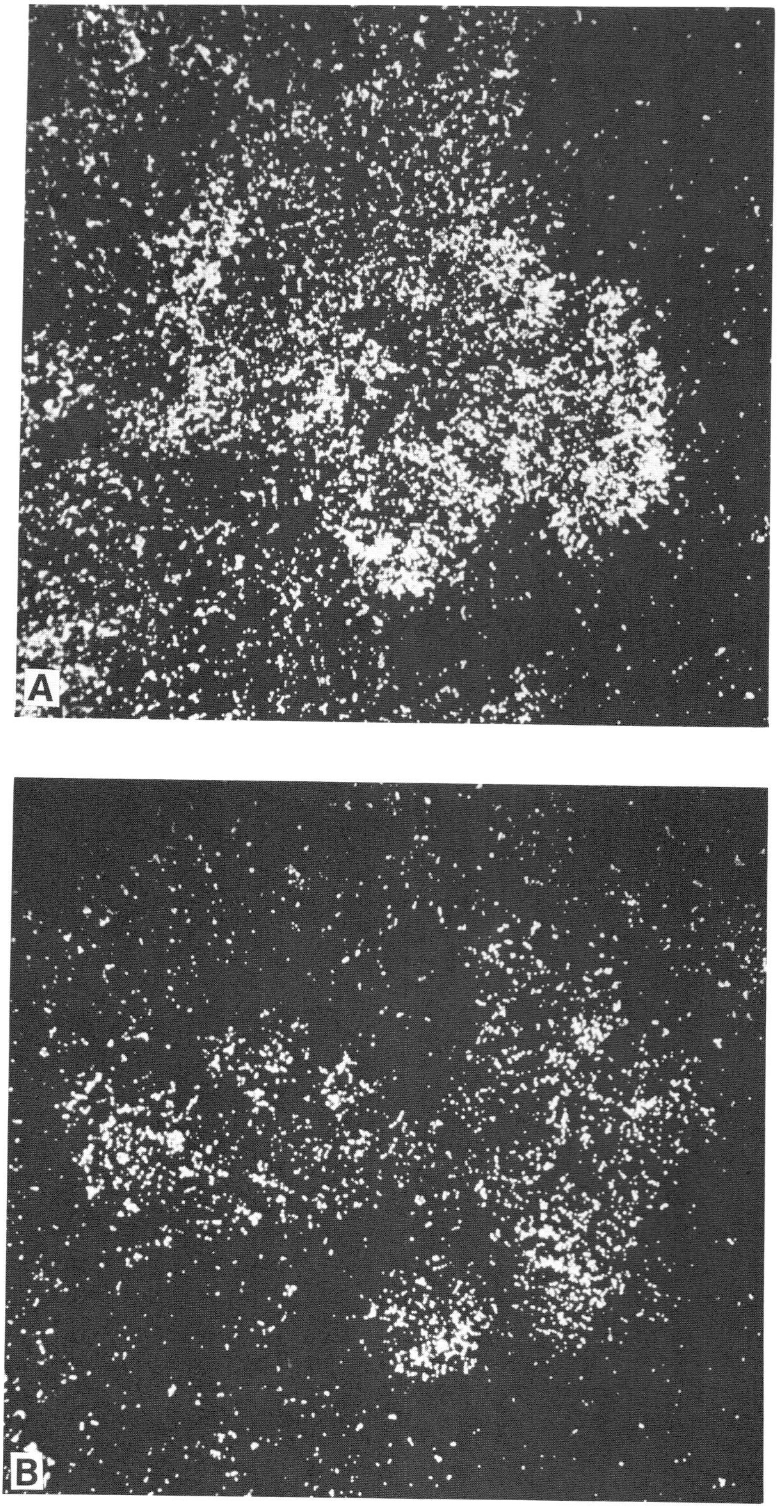

Fig. 6-23. *(A) Dark-field microscopic examination of an autoradiogram of a glomerulus with radioiodinated anti-C3c antiserum reveals large numbers of silver grains (white areas) in the photographic emulsion over the tissue section. (B) A serial section treated with trypsin prior to incubation with radiolabelled anti-C3c reveals persistence of approximately half the silver grains. Although both active C3b and inactive iC3b react with anti-C3c, C3b is resistant to digestion by trypsin, whereas the C3c component of iC3b is solubilized out of the tissue by trypsin proteolysis. Thus, in IgA nephritis, almost 50 percent of all C3 sites are in the active C3b form, capable of participating in the alternative (amplification) pathway of complement activation. In other proliferative and nonproliferative glomerulonephritides, except lupus nephritis, very little glomerular C3 is in the active C3b configuration.* ×340. *(Courtesy of Dr. C. D. West.)*

merulonephrits, significant capillary fibrin deposition is not frequent in cases of IgAN. Fibrin, of course, is deposited within glomerular crescents. When fibrin is encountered in capillaries, the histologic lesions are more likely to be severe [128,554]. Capillary wall fibrin deposition may therefore be of prognostic significance.

Extraglomerular Sites

Tubular and/or interstitial deposits of immunoglobulin or complement are distinctly unusual in biopsies of IgAN patients, even in the presence of foci of tubular atrophy and interstitial fibrosis [214]. Biopsies that have a florid interstitial nephritis component have scattered interstitial deposits of IgG, IgA, and sometimes C3, C1q, and/or IgM, usually in relation to tubular basement membranes or cortical capillaries; such biopsies are rare.

Occasionally (up to 20 percent of patients), there are deposits of IgA and/or C3 in the lamina media of cortical arterioles and/or the macula densa and glomerular vascular pole [8,98,131, 403,443]. This finding, rarely accompanied by deposits of IgA, may herald a progressive course [133,403,555].

Deposits of IgA, sometimes accompanied by C3, are also observed in superficial dermal capillaries in approximately 50 percent of patients with IgAN [22,98,354,496,599,604,616]. Infrequently, linear IgA at the dermal-epidermal junction—reminiscent of dermatitis herpetiformis—is present as well. Although these changes were initially considered valuable for recognition of IgAN, the low sensitivity (50 percent true positive rate) and nonspecificity (up to 20 percent of individuals without IgAN have similar deposits) combine to nullify the diagnostic value of such deposits.

ELECTRON MICROSCOPIC FINDINGS

Glomeruli

Ultrastructurally, electron-dense mesangial deposits are nearly always present. The distribution of electron-dense material correlates well with the routine immunohistologic procedures. Immunoglobulins and complement detected by immunoelectron microscopy in limited numbers of patients shows congruence with immunohistology at the light microscopic level [151,163,400,453,594].

By transmission electron microscopy, the deposits in many cases are at the periphery of the mesangium, at the interface of the capillary lumen with mesangium, and at the junction of the glomerular capillary wall and the mesangial matrix (paramesangium). These deposits are generally small (100–300 nm) and nearly always uniformly electron dense (Fig. 6-24). In the remaining cases, deposits are present not only within the paramesangium, but also deeper within the mesangial matrix (Fig. 6-25). The deposits in such patients are more variable in size (up to 1000 nm) and may show variation in density as well. Some investigators have proposed that deposits deeper in the mesangium denote more advanced cases [568]. In some cases, partially lucent deposits are present in the mesangium (Fig. 6-26).

Extramesangial deposits are segmental in nature (Figs. 6-27 and 6-28), and there is considerable variation in the frequency with which they are encountered (0 to 50 percent) [8,49,98,204,403, 404,454,553]. In 12 reports that emphasize ultrastructural study of glomerular capillaries, encompassing 414 biopsies, deposits within capillary walls were most frequently present in subendothelial sites (weighted mean, 19 percent of all patients) (see Fig. 6-27), with less frequent deposition in subepithelial (12 percent) and intramembranous (13 percent) sites [8,78,98,159, 262,362,403,457,532,576,677,678]. Clarkson et al. [98] characterized two patterns of epimembranous deposits that occurred with approximately equal frequency. In one pattern, large, widely spaced, electron-dense and, rarely, electron-lucent deposits were observed underlying visceral epithelium, reminiscent of the humps typical of postinfectious nephritis. Other patients had more numerous, small (<300 nm), electron-dense deposits at intervals along the lamina rara externa similar in character to, though more widely spaced than, those seen in membranous nephropathy.

Mesangial cells are frequently increased in size as well as in number and are enriched in organelles [370,404,568]. Microfilaments are usually conspicuous, in contrast to mesangial cells in patients with minimal change disease, and are frequently

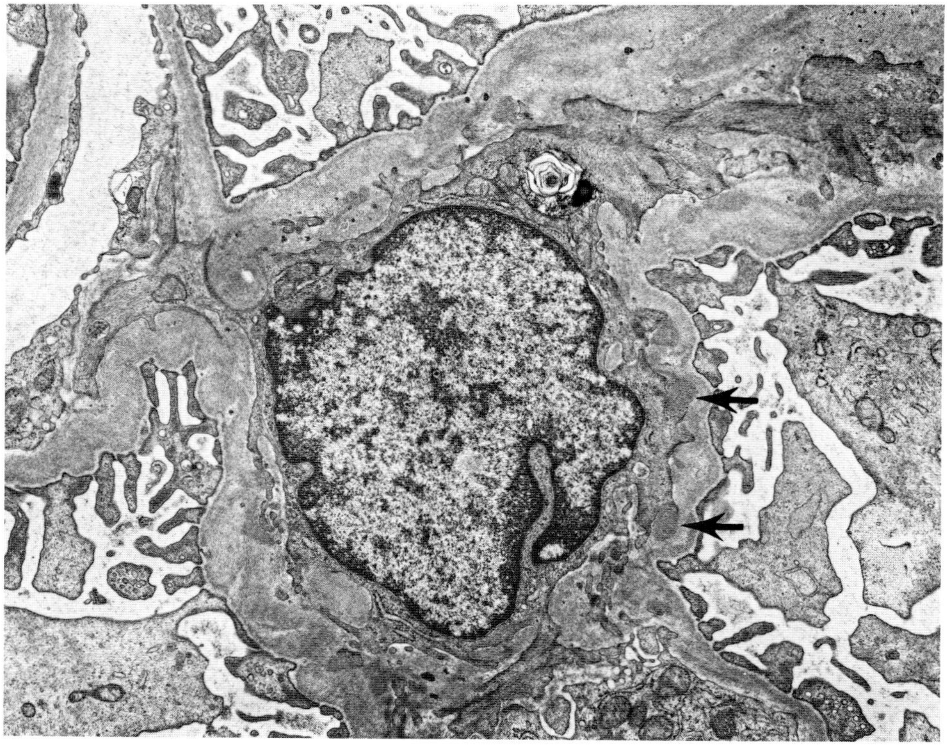

FIG. 6-24. *This representative electron micrograph shows small (100-nm) deposits (arrows) in the paramesangial area, where the capillary basement membrane joins and crosses over the mesangial matrix. Similar deposits are nearly ubiquitous in cases of IgA nephritis. Capillary walls are free of deposits.* × *10,200.*

organized into dense bodies (see Fig. 6-28). Mitochondria are typically more numerous, and occasionally, rough endoplasmic reticulum is conspicuous as well. Visceral epithelium may show broadening of podocytes and prominent endosomes when proteinuria is heavy; lysosomes are rarely evident. No changes in endothelium are recognized.

With respect to extracellular components of the glomerulus, the mesangial matrix is expanded and often appears fibrillar. In patients with more severe matrix expansion, long-spaced collagen is frequently recognized [78,262,473,532,553,568]. Polymerized fibrin is encountered rarely in capillary lumens and/or Bowman's space. The lamina densa of the GBMs may show thinning (12 percent) and/or splitting (11 percent), reminiscent of the changes seen in Alport's syndrome [98,204, 403,457,576] (Fig. 6-29). Some investigators also report thickening and/or etching of the basement membrane [98]. *Etching* refers to a segmental erosion of the outer portion of the lamina densa, to which it imparts a scalloped border (see Figs. 6-26 and 6-29). Gaps and interruptions in GBMs are also described [598]. These ultrastructural changes, some of which are very focal, have uncertain pathogenetic and prognostic significance. Their recognition and prevalence vary widely, even

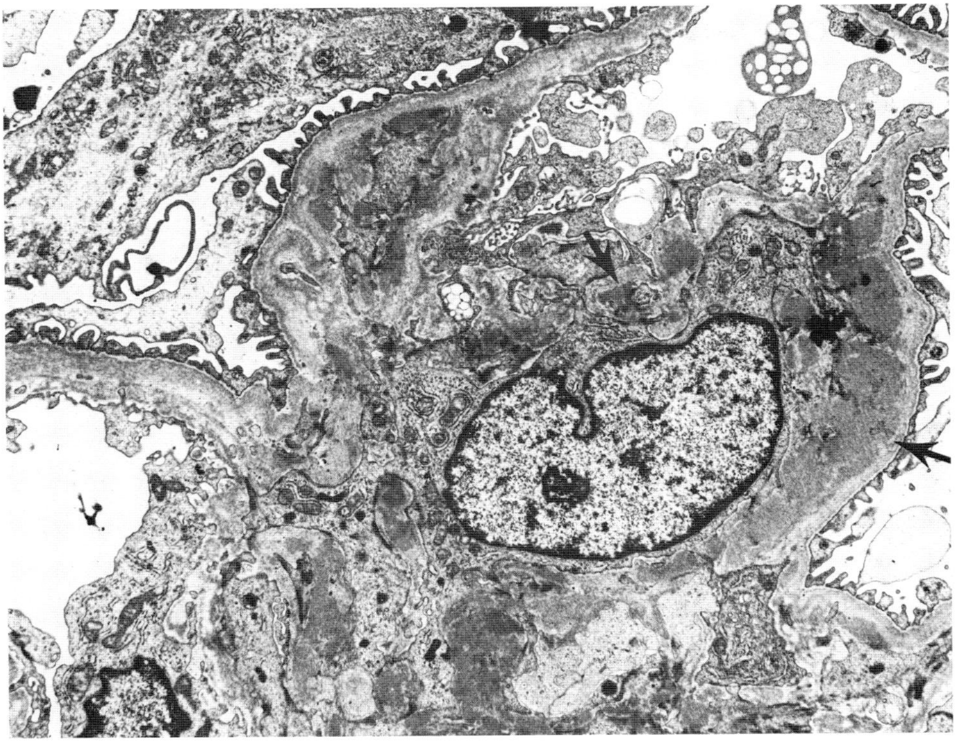

Fig. 6-25. *The deposits (arrows) in this electron micrograph are larger (up to 700 μm), more coalescent, and deeper within mesangial matrix than those in Fig. 6-24. Such deposits are typical of more advanced cases of IgA nephritis. Note the lamellation of capillary wall seen on the left and upper center (seen to better advantage in Fig. 6-29) and the increased organelle content within the cytoplasm of the mesangial cell (see also Fig. 6-28).* ×6300.

among series primarily directed to ultrastructural study of glomeruli. Further detailed study is required for appreciation of the significance and genesis of these lesions.

Extraglomerular Sites

In addition to the aforementioned glomerular changes, tubulointerstitial and vascular injury is also observed. These features are evident by light microscopy. Electron microscopy adds little, if any, insight. Rarely (0.7 percent), small, discrete, electron-dense deposits are present in arterioles.

Etiology and Pathogenesis

Knowledge of the etiology and pathogenesis of IgAN, like that of glomerulonephritis in general, is scant. The "facts," such as they are, represent attempts to correlate clinical observations and integrate such correlations with experimental data gleaned from animal models. This approach, although fraught with certain assumptions, offers at least a skeletal conception of the dynamic processes likely to be operative in IgAN. Progressively more refined and sophisticated schemata will emerge, it is hoped, from the current scaffolding.

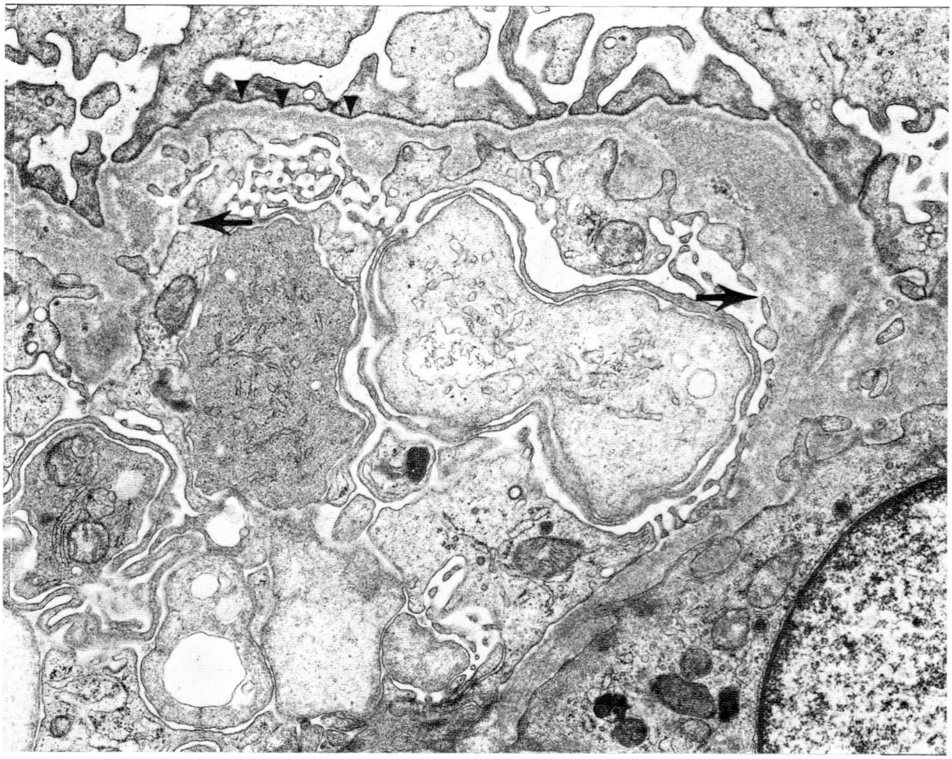

FIG. 6-26. *Partially resolving deposits with lucent as well as dense areas, such as the paramesangial and capillary deposits seen here (arrows), are often seen in IgA nephritis. Note also the scalloped appearance of the lamina rara externa (arrowheads), referred to as etching.* × 15,750.

An extensive review of how and why IgA immune deposits form, and of possible pathophysiologic mechanisms, was published recently [177]. In this section, experimental and clinical evidence are likewise interleaved to offer a current working hypothesis of the pathogenesis of IgAN. A schema of conceptually favored routes to glomerular injury is presented in Fig. 6-30.

SOURCE AND NATURE OF THE DEPOSITED IGA

On a mass basis, IgA content in human beings exceeds that of IgG, IgM, IgD, and IgE combined [416]. The IgA synthetic rate, approximately 2.7 mg/kg per hour, is highest because more plasma cells are committed to synthesis of IgA than to any other class of Ig. Although IgA-committed plasma cells are most abundant, serum IgA concentration is less than IgG concentration owing to the short (2–3 days) half-life of IgA [352,416,620].

Secretory mucosae contain the highest concentration of IgA-committed cells in the body and collectively account for most of the IgA produced systemically. However, the bone marrow and spleen also contain significant numbers of IgA-committed cells, although it appears that these cells are nevertheless regulated in part by T cells that reside in mucosae [352,416,620].

IgA exists as two distinct subclasses in man,

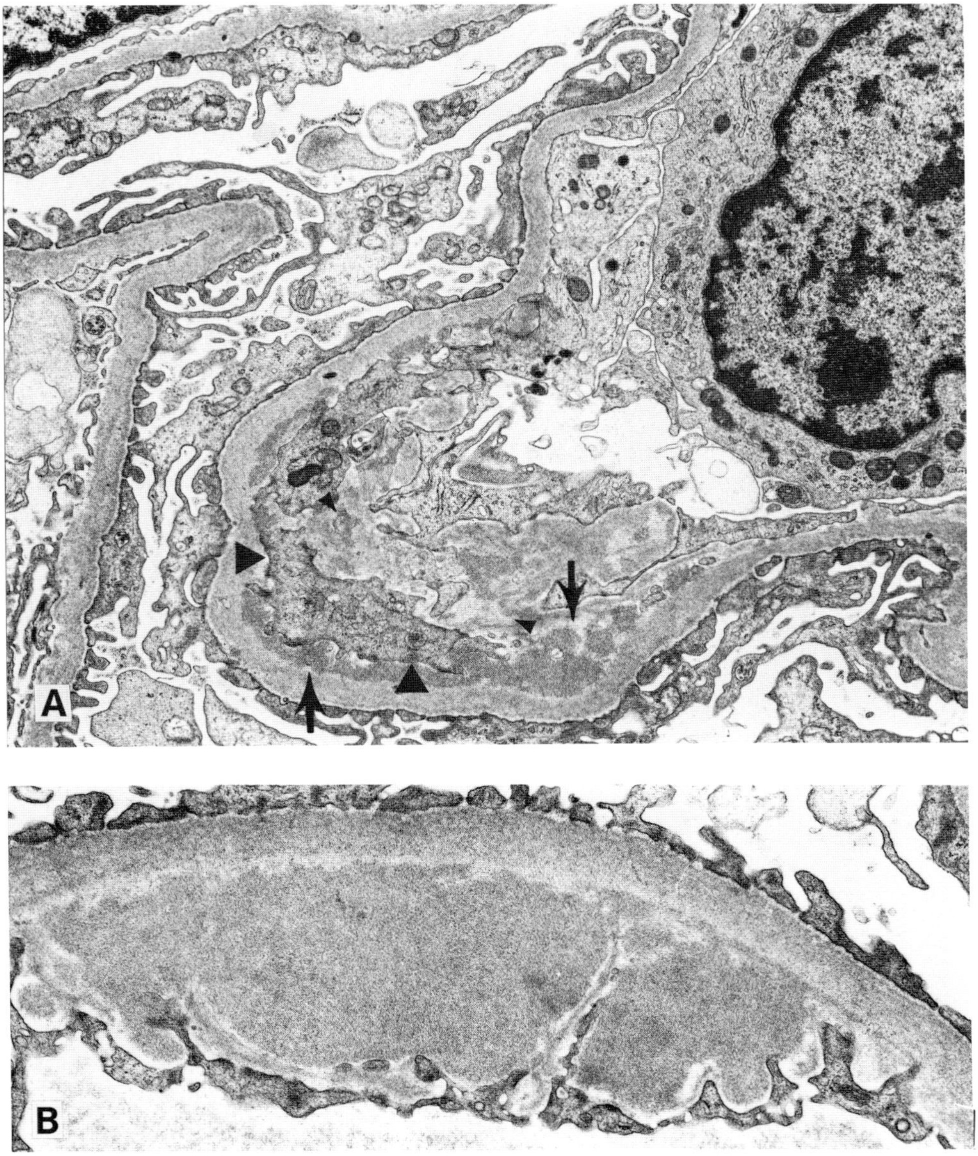

FIG. 6-27. *Capillary wall deposits, most often subendothelial, are seen in 10 to 20 percent of patients with IgA nephritis. (A) Advanced subendothelial deposits (arrows) are associated with new basement-membrane formation (small arrowheads) and cellular interposition (large arrowheads). Some etching is also evident in the lamina rara externa. (B) A very large subendothelial deposit is present with little reaction. Note the broadening of the epithelial podocytes. These deposits, reminiscent of membranoproliferative glomerulonephritis and lupus nephritis, contain IgA and C3 but little or no IgG, IgM, C1q, or C4 by immunoelectron microscopy, distinguishing the deposits of IgA nephritis from these other conditions. (A) ×9,675; (B) ×15,050.*

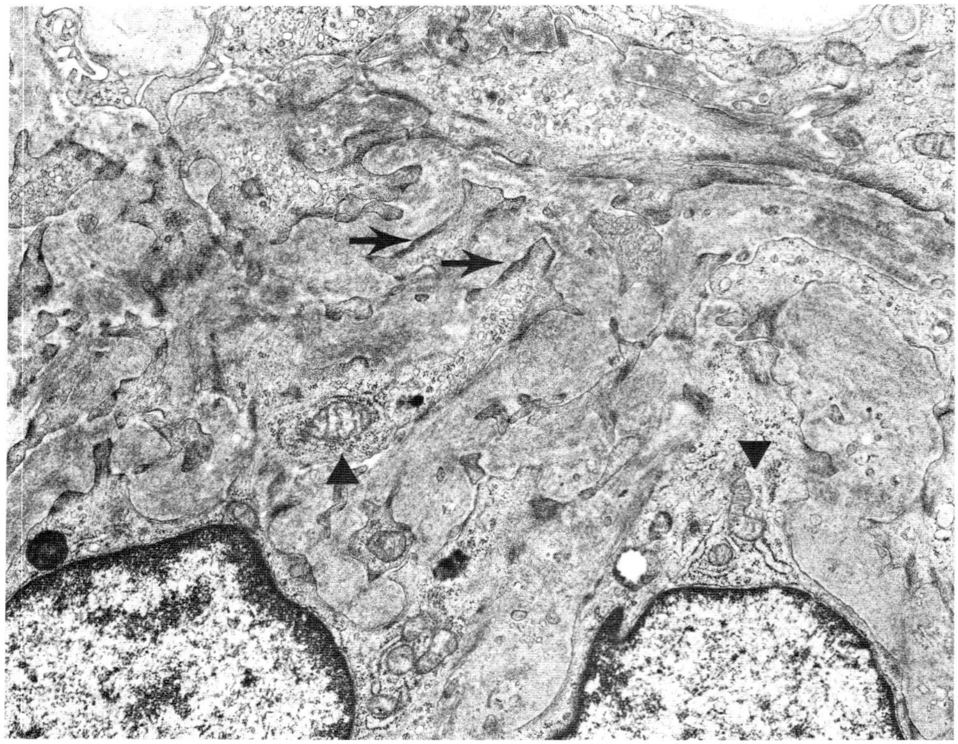

FIG. 6-28. *In this electron micrograph of a mesangial area of a patient with IgA nephritis, condensation of microfilaments onto the cytoplasmic membrane (dense bodies, arrows) and abundant mitochondria and rough endoplasmic reticulum (arrowheads) are evident in mesangial cell cytoplasm.* × *13,050.*

IgA_1 and IgA_2. Either subclass is synthesized by plasma cells as a 155 kD protein consisting of two immunoglobulin heavy alpha chains (55 kD each) and two light chains (22 kD each) or as dimers, trimers, tetramers, and pentamers of the basic four-chain immunoglobulin structure, with molecular weights that are integral multiples of 155 kD. Dimers and oligomers contain a joining chain (J-chain) and can be actively transported from the basolateral to the luminal surface of secretory epithelium by means of a specialized glycoprotein receptor (secretory component). During secretion, a portion of secretory component becomes covalently bound to IgA, and the presence of a secretory component in an IgA molecule therefore indicates that it has already traversed a secretory epithelium.

In human beings, serum IgA is predominantly monomeric, lacking J-chain, of the IgA_1 subclass, and is derived from plasmacytes within the marrow and spleen. Mucosa-associated plasmacytes produce predominantly dimeric and tetrameric IgA-containing J-chain [416,620,657]. Despite the presence of significant amounts of IgA_2, IgA_1 still predominates in the mucosae derived from the embryologic foregut, including the airways. Some investigators, citing the predominance of the IgA_1 subclass in glomerular deposits and questioning the presence of J-chain, propose that most of the IgA deposited in glomeruli arises from the bone

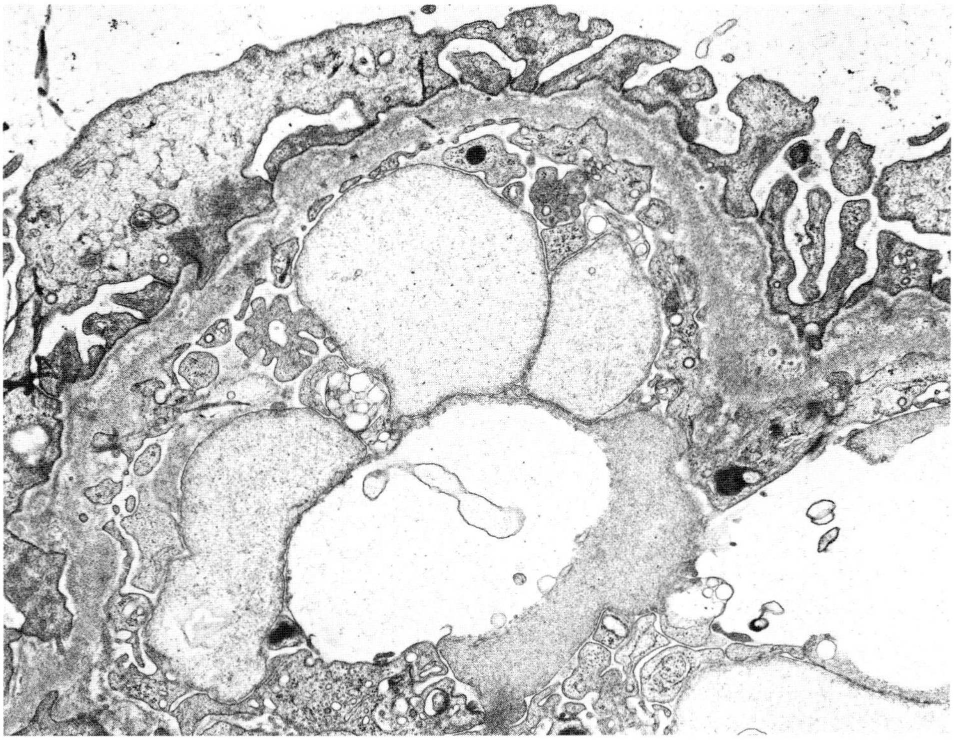

Fig. 6-29. *The capillary wall in this portion of the same glomerulus depicted in Fig. 6-28 is lamellated, with numerous intramembranous lucencies. There is also etching present in the lamina rara externa.* × *13,050.*

marrow and spleen [108,258,383,497,554,605, 626]. However, as pointed out by Rifai [506] and made obvious from the foregoing, a predominance of IgA_1 in glomerular deposits does not exclude a mucosal origin of the deposited IgA. Furthermore, it seems clear that at least a proportion of the IgA deposited in glomeruli in IgAN patients contains J-chain, and IgA eluted from glomeruli is predominantly oligomeric and associated with J-chain [13,44,111,149,154,173,331,383,386,429, 611,638]. The immunofluorescence studies demonstrating J-chain are not in universal agreement [366] and elution experiments are difficult to interpret because the acid elution procedure may have altered the glomerular deposits prior to their analysis. Nonetheless, all current evidence, taken together, implicates secretory mucosae as the primary source of IgA deposited in glomeruli in IgAN patients. This may be particularly relevant to the secondary forms of IgAN (see below), because most diseases that potentially underlie secondary IgAN involve mucosae.

Regarding the nature of the deposited IgA, deposits of immunoglobulin and complement in glomeruli are traditionally interpreted as evidence that the glomerular disease is caused by formation or deposition of antigen-antibody complexes within the glomeruli. In Chapter 3, McCluskey reviewed the experimental and clinical support for this view. Regarding IgAN, past controversy now seems resolved, and IgAN is perceived by virtually all investigators to be an immune complex depo-

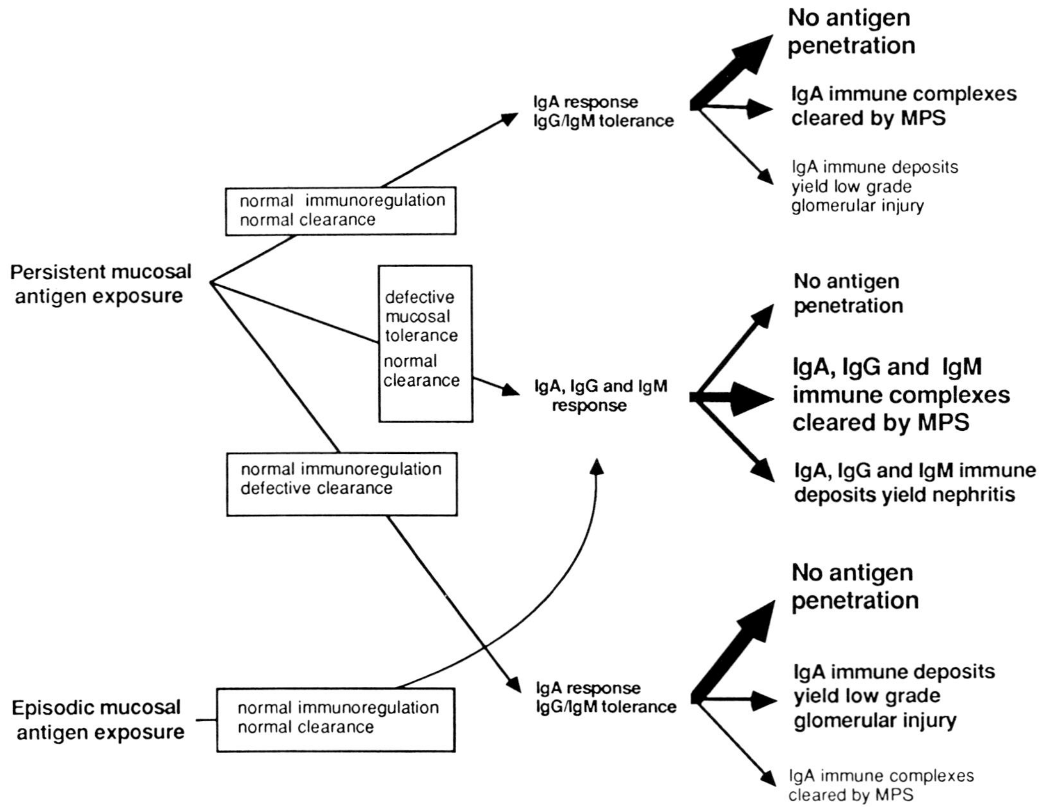

FIG. 6-30. *Schematic diagram of some of the ways in which a host can respond to mucosal antigenic stimulation. The heavy arrows and large type represent those pathways and outcomes considered most likely; the medium arrows and medium type, intermediate; and the small arrows and small type, least likely. Note that combined defects in immunoregulation and clearance (not shown) would synergize to elicit more severe nephritis. In situations with episodic antigen expsoure, either the same or different antigens could elicit individual bouts of nephritis; even in individuals with normal immunoregulation, the intrinsically weak "memory" of IgA responses and the interval usually required to establish mucosal tolerance with respect to IgG and IgM responses could promote nephritis. The responses in normal individuals with episodic antigen exposure could thus resemble the situation in which persistent antigen exposure occurs in individuals with defective mucosal tolerance. For simplicity, situations in which episodic antigen exposure occurs in hosts with abnormal immunoregulation or defective clearance are omitted. MPS, mononuclear phagocyte system. (Reprinted from Emancipator, S. N., and Lamm, M. E.* Lab. Invest. *60: 168, 1989, by permission of U.S.–Canadian Academy of Pathology.)*

sition disease in which most of the antibody is of the IgA class [97,127,128,132,177,180,304, 624,663]. Alternative hypotheses consider nonimmune aggregates of IgA, IgA with a structure that promotes glomerular binding, and situations in which IgA is the antigenic rather than the antibody component of rheumatoid factor–like immune complexes.

In favor of an immune complex pathogenesis, several investigators have demonstrated that many patients with IgAN have elevated levels of circulating IgA-containing macromolecular complexes thought to be immune [105,110–112,114,126, 256,258,273,321,339,366,385,444,536,545,580, 608,617,663]. While only 15 to 25 percent of single serum samples from IgAN patients are abnormal in terms of IgA-containing complexes, serial determinations improve the apparent sensitivity to roughly 50 percent. The frequency of an abnormal result for circulating IgA immune complex assays is higher among IgAN patients during clinical exacerbation than during periods of clinical quiescence, and the level of circulating immune complexes correlates well with the apparent severity of disease. Moreover, immune complexes of IgA antibody and specific antigen, if injected into mice, elicit hematuria; deposition of IgA, antigen, and complement in glomeruli; expansion of PAS-positive mesangial matrix by light microscopy; and electron-dense deposits in the mesangium [94, 179,180,294,509]. The extent of glomerular involvement is directly related to immune complex dose, and injection of nonimmune mixtures (controls) has no effect. Increased levels of IgA complexes in the circulation of patients with IgAN also may underlie changes in blood viscosity in these patients [551].

As already mentioned, Monteiro et al. [429, 430] were able to elute IgA from biopsy specimens. Physicochemically and immunochemically, this IgA was structurally normal, but the glycosylation pattern and amino acid sequence of the eluted material were not studied. Although the acid-elution method used would dissociate antigen-antibody complexes, it also might promote elution of material deposited on a nonimmune basis. On the other hand, these data render very unlikely the possibility that the deposited IgA represents covalent nonimmune aggregates, since the acid elution would not dissociate covalently bound macromolecules. After fractionation under acid conditions, the eluted IgA remained soluble at physiologic pH. This observation suggests that noncovalent autoaggregation per se is not a reason for deposition, as proposed earlier [53,135,149, 155,169,386,388,647]. Prior to fractionation, neutralization promoted reaggregation. In summary, IgA immune complexes can, when injected into animals, elicit the same pattern of glomerular injury observed in patients with IgAN, and clinical studies associate acid-soluble IgA-containing complexes with disease activity. If nonimmune aggregation underlies deposition of IgA complexes in patients, it is based on acid-labile, noncovalent binding, which includes at least one component other than IgA.

Recent data from Jackson [295] argue that an increased amount of IgA complexes in the circulation is not a sufficient factor per se to promote glomerular deposition of IgA. This investigator found increased, often very high, levels of circulating IgA complexes in patients with acquired immunodeficiency syndrome (AIDS), yet observed no renal deposits of IgA or complement. Indeed, although there is a nephropathy associated with AIDS, it is a focal and segmental glomerulosclerosis without immunoglobulin deposits (see Chap. 28). Clearly, factors in addition to the level of circulating IgA complexes must play a role in nephritogenesis.

Another possibility, proposed in general terms, is deposition of IgA within glomeruli for reasons related to IgA structure. Originally, this concept was predicated on some abnormality in the IgA molecule promoting binding to a glomerular component. However, several groups have recently reported that normal human IgA_1 binds to fibronectin, a major constituent of the extracellular mesangial matrix [417, A. Woodroffe and D. Schlondorff, independent personal communications]. Plasma and tissue forms of fibronectin exist, and IgA_1 apparently binds to both. Perhaps the level of IgA complexes and the amount of circulating fibronectin together determine whether deposition occurs. Among individuals with elevated circulating IgA complexes, those with high plasma fibronectin levels may deposit less IgA in the glomeruli, whereas among those with lower plasma fibronectin, more of the circulating IgA complexes would partition into mesangial areas. Parallel speculations related to other lectin-based nonimmune binding systems can be envisioned. For example, Amore et al. [11] have shown that gliadin binds both to mesangial cells in culture and to IgA. These bindings are inhibited by different saccharides, suggesting that two lectin domains allow gliadin to "bridge" IgA and mesangial cells. The role of gliadin as a bridge may be relevant to the apparent benefit of a gluten-free diet in patients with IgAN [113].

These concepts have no factual basis at present but warrant future investigation. Glycosylation patterns of IgA to date are established for only a few monoclonal IgA proteins derived from only a few individuals [416,620]. Conceivably, differences in glycation among individuals constitute a factor—in addition to increased circulating IgA complexes—that determines nephritis. Deposited IgA must be bound to another element noncovalently, as already discussed [429,430], and therefore, deposits cannot form simply on a lectin-based binding of IgA to the glomerulus unless the carbohydrate-binding protein naturally present in the glomerulus is also eluted under acid conditions. This does not appear to be the case with fibronectin or mesangial cell glycoproteins. Moreover, glomerular deposits of IgA itself appear innocuous (see below).

Interaction of carbohydrate side chains of IgA with a lectin-like glomerular component might attenuate the ability of IgA in an immune lattice to inhibit complement fixation by other components of the immune lattice. Although inhibition of complement fixation by IgA content in an immune lattice is documented [13,524,526], any effect of glycosyl-protein interaction on this inhibition is speculative currently. If this speculation is valid, the IgA component of an immune lattice may favor glomerular deposition (see Mononuclear Phagocyte Function below) and, when deposited, bind to lectin-like components to allow complement fixation within the glomerulus, leading to injury.

ANTIGENS

If the deposited IgA represents immune complexes bound to some glomerular component by means of immune specificity or not, the antigen component of the complex remains enigmatic. As already mentioned, one hypothesis considers that IgA itself can serve as the antigen component of an immune complex. Indeed, IgG and IgM antibodies specific for the constant region of the Fab fragment of IgA (i.e., antibodies that bind to the domain comprising the constant light chain sequence and the first constant region of IgA heavy chain) are described in normal individuals and observed at higher concentration in sera of some IgAN patients [126,296]. However, a more recent study by these investigators indicates that such autoantibodies have little or no pathogenetic significance [295].

Rheumatoid factors (IgG and/or IgM) specific for the Fc region of IgA might underlie complexes containing IgA as antigens, but this mechanism remains speculative at present. On the other hand, IgA antibodies specific for IgG are present in increased titers in IgAN patients [126,546, 563], but again, a more recent study suggests that the antibody titers are unrelated to disease propensity or severity [562]. Autoimmune IgA antibodies specific for endogenous components may promote formation of immune complexes rich in IgA and in a few cases are well documented [29,67,149, 388,668].

Many investigators have attempted to identify exogenous antigens as components of IgA immune complexes, both circulating in plasma and deposited in glomeruli. In a sense, the success encountered is the problem, because collectively these studies implicate a panoply of antigens centered principally on dietary constituents [82,113,212, 357,405,449,518,525,536,629,663,669] and components of infectious microorganisms, especially viruses [187,246,451,525,606,609,610,611]. Conflicting reports on the presence or absence of some particular agent abound, but nearly every group suggests a role for one or another antigen. The multitude of potentially culpable antigens could be due to the fact that disease is instigated by different antigens in different individuals. Indeed, multiple antigens, some infectious, others inert, may underlie nephritogenesis even in a single patient. Nevertheless, conclusions regarding an antigen's role in inciting causal immune complexes must be drawn with caution. To date, only serologic tests have implicated specific antigens. Hence controls must be critically designed to avoid errors borne of cross-reactions, possible even with panels of monoclonal antibodies [641].

MONONUCLEAR PHAGOCYTE FUNCTION AND CLEARANCE OF CIRCULATING IMMUNE COMPLEXES

Accumulation of immune complexes in glomeruli implies increased generation of complexes, impaired clearance, or both. There is substantial evidence in support of enhanced production of IgA immune complexes in IgAN patients, as already mentioned [57,105,110–112,114,126,258,292,366, 444,536,580,608,663]. The issue of clearance, however, is somewhat obscure, as pointed out in a recent editorial [181]. While several reports document defective clearance in IgAN patients, these studies used IgG-coated erythrocytes [358,463,514, 573]. A recently published study in human beings injected with model soluble IgA immune complexes revealed identical clearance rates in patients with IgAN and in controls [510]. On the other hand, heat-aggregated IgA was less rapidly cleared from the circulation of IgAN patients compared with controls [515]. These apparently antithetical results may be reconciled by recognition of the chemical differences between the IgA preparations. Which of the two chemical preparations, if either, is more relevant to physiologic IgA immune complexes remains an open issue. The significance of studies using IgG-coated particulates, however, is doubtful. IgG interacts with different receptor populations than IgA, is cleared from the circulation by different routes, and has a different potential for complement activation [181]. Moreover, addition of even relatively small amounts of IgA to an immune lattice containing predominantly IgG inhibits incorporation of complement into the lattice [524,526,612,643]. Hence, in terms of complement-mediated solubilization and complement receptor–mediated immune adherence and clearance, IgA immune complexes are closer to mixed IgG-IgA immune complexes than are IgG immune complexes. Once deposits localize within glomeruli, poorer complement fixation is beneficial. However, it is important to remember that poorer complement fixation impairs clearance and promotes glomerular deposition of immune complexes. In mice, blockade of the mononuclear phagocyte system is required to promote glomerular deposits in a chronic mucosal immunization model with one antigen (lactalbumin) [424,539] but not others (bovine gamma globulin, ferritin, gliadin) [178,182,232]. Indeterminate as the issue of clearance kinetics may be at present, emerging sophistication should clarify the role of clearance in nephritogenesis in the future. Uptake of IgA complexes by neutrophils and monocytes/macrophages has been recently emphasized and represents another area ripe for future clarification [333,513].

GENETICS AND IMMUNOREGULATION

There is significant evidence that risk for IgAN is in part heritable. Familial clustering [147,170, 306,316, 432, 528, 571, 601], racial sparing [222,301,362,403,549] or predilection [286,572], and association of major histocompatibility genetic loci (particularly HLA-Bw35, B12, and DR4) [56,72,170,195,276,306,313,316,332,365, 389,447,467,481,505] with risk or severity of disease are all documented in the literature. Genes encoding complement components 3 and 4 and the switch regions of immunoglobulin heavy chains also have been implicated [144,305,495,666,667]. The functional significance of these differences does not obviously relate to propensity for either increased formation or impaired clearance of IgA immune complexes. The data overall are difficult to interpret at present because of discrepant results and lack of clear causality. As reviewed in detail by Julian et al. [307], the only confirmed and uncontested data apply to the complement phenotypes. The data regarding HLA phenotypes are particularly controversial [16,62,92,98,122,146,

170,249,308,331,334,496,497,544,555]. When considered in the context of gene frequencies and nondisjunction through critical statistics, apparent relationships disappear.

As recently reviewed, several investigators implicate immunoregulatory dysfunction in IgAN patients, and these defects may be genetic in nature [116,136,177]. Peripheral blood B lymphocytes from IgAN patients may secrete abnormally high amounts of IgA, either spontaneously or after mitogen stimulation [81,116,165,168,169,211,256, 346,380,469,534,545,640]. Mitogen-stimulated T cells capable of suppressing IgA synthesis by B cells from non-IgAN glomerulonephritis patients do not suppress IgA synthesis by patients' B cells [7,81,165–169,186,205,256,531,533]. These data suggest a defect in patients' B cells. Approximately half of all IgAN patients have increased serum concentrations of IgA. Moreover, a higher proportion of B lymphocytes in the peripheral blood of IgAN patients bear surface IgA than in normal individuals, and compared with controls, enhanced specific IgA responses are measured in the sera of patients in response to a variety of antigens.

In addition, T cells and T cell culture supernatants from IgAN patients are less effective at suppressing mitogen-driven IgA secretion by normal or patient B cells than are control T cell preparations [7,81,93,116,165–169,256,531,533,661]. IgA-specific suppression by T cells from IgAN patients is inversely correlated with the concentration of IgA in their serum. Finally, T cells from IgAN patients promote IgA secretion in vitro more effectively than do T cells from controls [81,165–169,256,531,533]. Tonsillar lymphocytes, as a population of cells more similar to mucosal lymphocytes than blood lymphocytes, behave in essentially the same fashion as peripheral blood lymphocytes. Egido et al. [164] also observed increased production of polymeric IgA by tonsillar cells in IgAN patients during exacerbation when compared with patients in remission; this suggested alterations specifically in the mucosal immune system.

Abnormalities in IgG production are also recognized in IgAN patients [18,518,525,545]. Some subclasses of IgG are more abundant in patients' sera relative to controls, and reciprocal differences are observed in glomerular immune deposits. Schena et al. [545] report that IgG concentrations and IgG-containing immune complexes in serum increase significantly in IgAN patients during exacerbation relative to periods of remission, whereas IgA and complexes containing only IgA are at similar high levels in exacerbation and remission.

Collectively, these data suggest that there are differences in regulation of immune responses in patients with IgAN relative to normal individuals and to patients with glomerulonephritis without predominantly IgA deposits. Most recently, Gesualdo et al. [238] recognized that compared with those from age- and sex-matched normal individuals, peripheral blood lymphocytes from IgAN patients synthesize more interleukin 4 (IL-4), a polypeptide synthesized by T cells that dramatically influences B cell differentiation. Interestingly, serum concentrations of IL-4 in these patients were only 60 percent of the values of the controls. The disparity between in vitro secretion and serum levels is reminiscent of observations regarding production of specific IgA antibodies after oral challenge with polio vaccine [363,642]. In the case of IL-4, the data indicate increased catabolism and/or increased receptor-mediated uptake of IL-4 in IgAN patients with active disease. The results to date, intriguing though they may be, must be regarded as tentative. Patients with IgAN should be stratified according to immunoregulatory status, and correlation with clinical and pathologic criteria should be pursued.

Although it is very likely that some, perhaps many immunoregulatory defects occur in IgAN patients, the nature of these defects is obscure and may differ in the various IgAN patient subpopulations. One issue that must be considered is whether any immune defects are acquired or genetic. For example, exposure of chronically orally immunized mice to either cyclophosphamide or estradiol results in nephritis and altered immune responses compared with mice receiving an identical immunization protocol but given saline instead of drug [237]. These mice were given only two doses of the drugs, 6 weeks apart. It would therefore be very difficult to exclude acquired immune defects in patients due to random environmental exposure. Similar defects in immunoregulation occur on a genetic basis in selected strains of mice. The strain of mice is also an important factor in genesis of an IgA immune response and, therefore, in genesis of IgAN [232,293]. Therefore, a genetic basis may underlie IgAN in man as well. Abnormal function of T and B lymphocytes is documented in patients and their relatives (reviewed in ref. 177), further corroborating a genetic predisposition to IgAN.

Whether acquired or congenital, it is likely that defects in immunoregulation contribute to the genesis of IgAN in at least a number of patients. Indeed, consideration of clinical observations in the context of known immunologic concepts has led to the idea that the two major syndromes that herald onset of IgAN are related to two defects in immunoregulation. Specifically, episodic macrohematuria may result from hyperfunction of both suppressor (during antigen-free intervals) and helper (during antigen exposure) T cells, whereas the microhematuria/proteinuria form of IgAN is caused by defective mucosal tolerance. Although beyond the scope of this chapter, the data suggesting these principles are reviewed in detail elsewhere [177].

IgA DEPOSITION AS AN EPIPHENOMENON

Save for macrohematuria, the portents for long-term prognosis in IgAN are very similar to those in membranous nephropathy [71,652] and may be generic for glomerular disease in general. Histologically and clinically matched cases of mesangial proliferative glomerulonephritis, with and without dominant IgA, have similar long-term courses [286,474]. As already mentioned, only a minority (25 percent) of patients with IgAN have IgA as the only immunoglobulin deposited, whereas many asymptomatic patients have abundant mesangial IgA deposits without renal disease [3,4,52, 84,475,663]. In mice with IgAN induced by oral immunization or injection of immune complexes, codeposits of IgG and IgM are important elements, apparently because they promote glomerular C3 deposition, potent at nephritogenesis [182]. In another experimental system induced by injection of immune complexes, IgG/IgM codeposits are unimportant, but the antigen structure is critical for nephritogenesis [507]. Antigens capable of fixing complement themselves elicit injury when given with specific antibody, whereas structurally similar antigens that do not fix complement do not elicit injury. These observations collectively suggest that IgA per se is not noxious to the glomerulus and is not pathophysiologically important.

An alternative view holds that the IgA component of glomerular immune deposits in IgAN is a functionally important ingredient in immune deposition and pathogenesis [215]. Introduction of IgA, even as a small percentage of the total immunoglobulins, into an immune lattice profoundly affects the complement-activating potential of that lattice; it appears that IgA somehow *inhibits* IgG and/or IgM-mediated complement fixation [524,526,643]. Therefore, IgA-rich immune complexes are likely to have a complement-immunoglobulin ratio quite distinct from similar complexes lacking IgA. This could significantly influence the propensity for renal deposition of immune complexes from the circulation, since clearance mechanisms dependent on insertion of complement into the immune lattice would be impaired [172,181].

Another means by which IgA might serve a pathogenetic role is by virtue of its binding to fibronectin, an abundant constituent of the extracellular matrix of the glomerular mesangium, or to other, as yet unidentified elements within glomeruli [417, A. Woodroffe and D. Schlondorff, independent personal communications]. In this scenario, IgA immune complexes or perhaps IgA alone would preferentially accumulate in the mesangium by virtue of the binding of IgA to the acceptor component of the glomerulus. If IgG and/or IgM and C3 were associated with these immune complexes, they would likewise deposit to initiate nephritis. Some investigators have suggested that IgA immune complexes might deposit first, followed by accumulation of IgG and/or IgM with specificity either for an antigen component or for the IgA within the IgA immune complexes [94]. In either event, the affinity of IgA could serve as a means of "targeting" immune complexes to the mesangium. In addition, IgA immune complexes might interfere with cellular interactions with fibronectin or other components, altering mesangial function. The potential for interaction of glomerular IgA and acceptors in glomeruli as a factor in complement activation and in modulation of metabolic glomerular responses to immune deposits has been discussed already (at the end of the section entitled Source and Nature of the Deposited IgA).

Pathophysiology

IgAN is, as already noted, primarily a mesangiopathic disease. Therefore, when considering the pathophysiology of IgAN, it seems appropriate to focus on the mesangium. The normal physiology and biology of the glomerular mesangium and its potential contribution to glomerular pathophysiology have been reviewed on several occasions [66,414]. Immune complexes, the membrane attack complex of complement, and cytokines from inflammatory cells can all promote functional and morphologic changes in mesangial cells (reviewed in ref. 177). These include calcium mobilization and cell contraction, along with release of vasoactive prostaglandins, platelet-activating factor, proteolytic and endoglycosidase enzymes, reactive oxygen intermediates, and cytokines such as interleukin 1 and tumor necrosis factor. Mesangial cells synthesize platelet-derived growth factor, an autocrine mitogen, and may augment such synthesis after appropriate stimuli [559]. Proliferation of mesangial cells also may ensue upon insertion of the membrane attack complex into cell membranes. The precise interplay among these mechanisms and metabolites remains unclear, and the influence IgA exerts in their modulation is just now beginning to emerge. The basic elements of mesangial function and interaction with immune reactants likely underlie glomerular function in IgAN and other forms of glomerulonephritis equally. Moreover, it seems that IgA within the immune lattice promotes glomerular deposition (see IgA Deposition as an Epiphenomenon) and modulates glomerular responses to IgG, IgM, and complement.

The relationship between IgA and IgG and complement components of glomerular deposits may be at the level of amplification. Recently, Hernando et al. [274] reported that immune complexes prepared in vitro with only IgA antibody and similar immune complexes prepared with only IgG both elicited superoxide anion and tumor necrosis factor release from mesangial cells in culture. While either isotype elicited comparable responses, addition of fresh serum as a source of complement augmented the response to (complement-fixing) IgG-containing immune complexes but did not influence the response to IgA immune complexes. If these in vitro data can be extrapolated to in vivo conditions, they suggest several explanations. First, adding sufficient IgG (or perhaps IgM) to a predominantly IgA immune lattice would favor some complement fixation, albeit much less than would be the case were all the antibody of the IgG or IgM class. Complement fixation could then augment mesangial-cell responses, including contraction and production of eicosanoids and IL-1 as well as of superoxide and tumor necrosis factor. On the other hand, if the antigen itself could promote complement fixation [94], IgG or IgM codeposits would be unnecessary for the activation of complement. Moreover, if the antigen structure (such as a polymer) resulted in a high density of IgA antibody, the local concentration of IgA might be great enough to elicit maximal mesangial-cell responses, and augmentation by complement would be unnecessary.

While the cellular responses to immunoglobulin and complement are being elucidated in vitro, parallel work proceeds in vivo. Gesualdo et al. [236] have adapted the chronic oral immunization model of IgAN to rats in an effort to identify inflammatory mediators potentially important in nephritogenesis and to characterize glomerular hemodynamics. During an episode of microhematuria induced by systemic antigen challenge in mucosally immunized rats, glomerular thromboxane but not prostaglandin synthesis is increased. Deposits of predominantly IgA with admixtures of IgG, IgM, and C3 are present, with only mild expansion of mesangial matrix evident by light microscopy. These rats had a 20 percent decrement in both glomerular filtration rate and renal plasma flow but unchanged glomerular filtration fraction compared with controls. The investigators reasoned that glomerular synthesis of thromboxane unopposed by increments in vasodilator prostaglandins—a situation heretofore unrecognized in glomerulonephritis—might underlie hematuria and the hemodynamic changes. Indeed, treatment of similar rats with a thromboxane synthetase inhibitor, thromboxane receptor antagonist, or both eliminated hematuria and restored renal plasma flow to baseline levels. Glomerular filtration rate did not recover, suggesting a component of thromboxane-independent glomerular contraction no longer opposed by a thromboxane-induced efferent arteriolar constriction. Micropuncture study of single-nephron glomerular hemodynamics may shed added light on this issue.

Thromboxane synthesis in glomeruli may have other significant effects as well. Thromboxane analogues can stimulate in vitro synthesis of extracellular matrix by cultured cells [327]. Therefore, thromboxane may promote sclerosis in vivo. Preliminary extension of parallel studies to patients is underway, and data from therapeutic trials with diets rich in fish oil, deficient in essential fatty acids, or with antithromboxane drugs suggest that these mechanisms do, indeed, operate in man [39,48,153,261,489]. Angiotensin II also may play an important role, as inferred from studies in patients that suggest a therapeutic effect for antagonists of this mediator and an up-regulation of angiotensin II receptors in glomeruli of IgAN patients compared with controls [255,343,486].

In another model of IgAN induced in mice and characterized by pronounced increases of mesangial cells and/or matrix, Gesualdo et al. [236] detected parallel increases of messenger RNA encoding platelet-derived growth factor and interleukin 1, agents with known autocrine effects on mesangial-cell proliferation and synthesis of extracellular matrix. A role for platelet-derived growth factor is beginning to emerge in patients, since both the receptor for this polypeptide mediator [201] and the mediator itself (Fig. 6-31) are demonstrable in

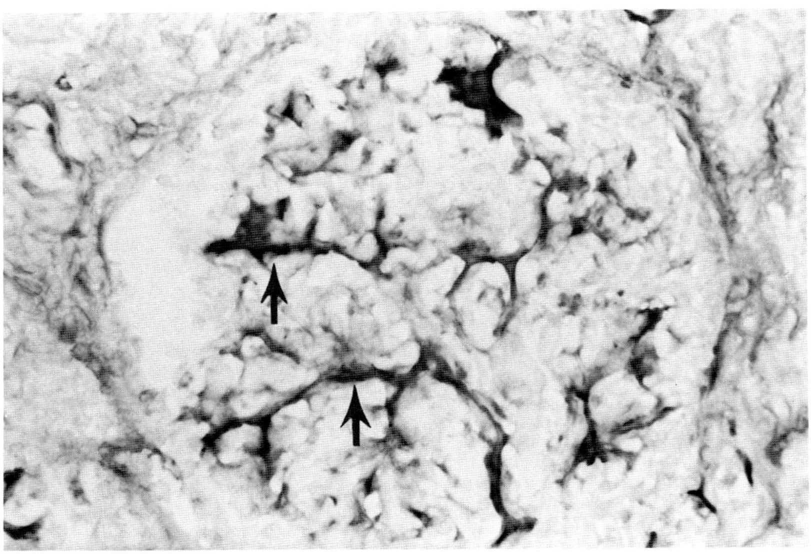

Fig. 6-31. *Insoluble grains of polymerized diaminobenzidine (arrows) lie within mesangial cells in this glomerulus, reacted sequentially with goat anti–platelet-derived growth factor (specific for the AB heterodimer) and a biotinyl rabbit anti-goat secondary antibody, detected with avidin peroxidase. Serial sections incubated with an irrelevant antibody as the primary serum or with the specific primary serum plus soluble recombinant platelet-derived growth factor revealed no staining in glomeruli (not shown).* ×450.

glomeruli of IgAN patients at levels that exceed (by immunoperoxidase staining) those observed in normal glomeruli. In addition to endogenous glomerular sources, intravascular or intraglomerular coagulation and platelet infiltration also may contribute to glomerular injury or progression [91, 621]. Quantitative assessments of these mediators and effects of antagonists on clinical status and course will be required before their role can be established.

Speculations based on these various data have obvious significance for our understanding of the pathophysiology of IgAN and its progression, with attendant ramifications for therapy. Interpretation of these data is still open to question. Nonetheless, these data provide a conceptual framework upon which we can gather clinical experience. The future will likely see substantial progress in this effort.

Clinical Outcome

Irrespective of the role IgA plays in promoting deposition and initiating pathophysiologic responses, immune deposits containing IgA can definitely be noxious to glomeruli. End-stage kidney disease requiring dialysis or transplantation therapy developed over a 20-year course in 20 to 50 percent of patients in several large long-term studies [46,58,60,70,96–99,106,110,111,115,117, 122,127–130,133,143,147,157,170,199,214,223, 227,280,283,291,308,318,325,330,340,342,347–349,351,356,359,362,371,373,378,385,406,425, 443,456,458,496,532,540,576,589,590,628,632, 635,638,639,658–660]. In most survival curves, it is noted that "renal death" ensued in approximately 1.5 percent of all patients annually for the first 5 years and in 1 percent of patients thereafter. These facts, taken together with the overall incidence of IgAN, suggest that IgAN accounts for 15 to 25 percent of all end-stage kidney disease. Chronic renal insufficiency is even more prevalent.

Clinical findings associated with increased likelihood of progression in many of the studies just cited and in more focused reports are older age at onset [135,370,460,570], lack of episodic macrohematuria [86,171,197,203,233,250,264], heavy proteinuria [242,263,458,555,571,659], hypertension [51,249,403,555,571,659], persistently decreased GFR or serum creatinine in excess of 1.4 mg/100 ml [370], and impaired ability to concentrate urine [446]. Pathologic features associated with a poor prognosis include severe glomerular histologic grade [46,96,280,362,570,589], including glomerular sclerosis, interstitial fibrosis, endocapillary proliferation, and/or numerous (>10 percent of glomeruli) circumferential crescents [2,249,330]; capillary immune deposits [227,288, 330,589]; presence of abundant codeposits of IgG or IgM; and hyalin arteriolosclerosis [98,127,199]. Capillary deposits of IgA and IgM and/or fibrin were particularly singled out as a premonitor of poor outcome in some studies [133,675] and were correlated with endocapillary proliferation and a more severe histologic grade [131].

Many of these clinical and pathologic features tend to be congruent. For example, proteinuria and severity of segmental endocapillary proliferation show coincidence, and both correlate with immune deposits in capillary walls [14,70]. Glomerular sclerosis, interstitial changes, and arteriolosclerosis are all very well correlated with each other. Crescents, deposits of non-IgA immunoglobulin classes, and capillary wall deposits of fibrin are all associated on the one hand with likelihood for a poor outcome and on the other hand with the occurrence of episodic macrohematuria, yet the occurrence of macrohematuria itself is a sign of a good prognosis. Hence the predictive value of these features might be predicated on intervening variables rather than on the features themselves, and each feature per se might lend an erroneous overall interpretation to the prognosis of an individual patient. Moreover, while many of these observations are associated with particular prognostic outcomes in the whole population of patients, all have relatively low predictive value when applied to an individual patient.

A more critical approach for assessing the predictive value of each clinical or pathologic feature that is associated with poor outcome on a population scale was taken by Clarkson and Woodroffe [100], D'Amico et al. [133], and by Beukhof et al. [59–61]. With multivariate analysis corrected for attrition from the population by development of chronic renal insufficiency, and with controls for intervening factors, only a few variables proved to be independent predictors of progression. Proteinuria exceeding 1 g daily, persistent defects in GFR, glomerular sclerosis, and vascular sclerosis were the only parameters that proved independent predictors of progression in the series mentioned and in other subsequent studies. Hence these variables are most likely to be useful in individual prognosis, in elucidation of mechanisms of progression, and in evaluation of the efficacy of therapeutic regimens. Interestingly, persistent heavy proteinuria is most frequently encountered in patients thought to have defective mucosal tolerance to environmental or commensal antigens [177]. Conversely, heavy proteinuria is least likely to be seen in acute episodic hematuria patients, who seldom progress to end-stage kidney.

The rate at which irreversible renal injury ensues is variable. As already mentioned, rapidly progressive renal failure, observed in roughly 5 percent of IgAN patients, is recognized clinically by inexorable deterioration in glomerular filtration and pathologically by circumferential crescents in more than 30 percent of glomeruli [5,99,130,188,373,396,678]. Among other patients with IgAN, slow and intermediate courses seem to be distinguishable on the basis of systemic hypertension and vascular sclerosis [60,128,133, 456]. Control of hypertension is an important component of management of IgAN, even though the salutary effects observed in populations with careful antihypertensive management may reflect a shift from a more to a less rapidly progressive course. More extensive long-term study of the role of hypertension and vascular sclerosis is required to determine if vascular changes per se lead to permanent renal damage or if they act synergistically with other factors to accelerate injury in hypertensive patients.

Renal Transplantation in IgAN

Some patients with end-stage kidney due to IgAN have, of course, been recipients of allografts. The indications for renal transplantation and the pathologic features and mechanisms encountered in grafted kidneys are discussed in Chapter 27. However, aspects of engraftment in IgAN relate specifically to this disease.

As first recognized by Berger, IgAN is among those diseases which recur in renal allografts [24,53,87,157,251,279,399,437]. Recurrence is observed in 20 to 25 percent of recipients and is generally confined to immunohistologic detection of IgA. Light microscopic or urinary changes occur only rarely in allografts, and graft function is typically unaffected. Hence IgAN underlying terminal renal failure is not a contraindication to transplantation therapy in otherwise eligible recipients with end-stage IgAN. Clinical recurrence in these patients with loss of the graft appears to be a very unusual problem. No data suggesting altered frequency or severity of rejection have been published, but some investigators propose that recurrence is more frequent in major histocompatibility antigen–identical transplants.

Transplantation of kidneys into recipients with end-stage IgAN has provided added insights that may be related to the special features of this disease. There is, as already mentioned, a genetic and perhaps familial basis for IgAN. Hence, if siblings of patients with end-stage IgAN are used as donors, it should be kept in mind that they are at higher risk for developing IgAN than the general population. A clinically healthy donor kidney may, at the time of grafting, show morphologic stigmata of IgAN, suggesting "latent" IgAN, which may evolve into clinically evident IgAN after grafting. While this may represent recurrence, it may as well indicate natural evolution of IgAN from an evanescent state [53]. Moreover, there are documented instances of allografts bearing IgA deposits at the time of transplantation into patients with terminal renal failure caused by diseases other than IgAN. In at least a few instances in which pre- and posttransplant biopsies were examined, the IgA deposits in such kidneys apparently dissipated after a variable period in the recipient [538,558]. In summary, study of IgA deposits in renal transplants serves to emphasize that mesangial IgA depostion is not itself sufficient to cause disease because IgA deposits can exist in clinically normal kidneys and resolve after grafting, and because the disease can recur in allografts.

SECONDARY IgA NEPHRITIS

Alcoholic cirrhosis, biliary ectasia, cholangitis, and cirrhosis associated with cystic fibrosis are all

TABLE 6-2. *Classification of diseases underlying secondary IgA nephritis, excluding hepatobiliary disease*

I. Mucosal diseases
  A. Chronic inflammation
    1. Hypersensitivity (Sjögren syndrome)
    2. Idiopathic (Crohn's disease, ulcerative colitis)
    3. Infectious (yersinosis, brucellosis)
  B. Neoplasia (Bronchogenic and colon carcinoma)
II. Hematologic diseases
  A. Lymphoproliferative disorders (lymphoma, cryoglobulinemia)
  B. Myeloproliferative states (polycythemia, thrombocytosis)
III. Systemic autoimmune/hypersensitivity diseases (ankylosing spondylitis, dermatitis herpetiformis)*

*Although systemic lupus erythematosus could fit into this category, the renal involvement in lupus rarely, if ever, fulfills the criteria of predominant IgA and C3 over IgG/IgM and C1q. I prefer to consider patients with lupus and glomerulonephritis with heavy IgA deposits within the context of lupus nephritis rather than secondary IgA nephritis.

conditions in which a high proportion of patients have mesangial deposits of IgA indistinguishable from those with primary IgAN. Renal involvement in these patients is discussed in a separate section at the end of the chapter. In addition, there are various other diseases that are associated with IgAN with a frequency significantly higher than that in the general population yet not so high as in hepatobiliary disease (Table 6-2).

Clinical Features

DEMOGRAPHICS

Diseases of secretory mucosae, including celiac disease [267,315,434], Crohn's disease [101,285], Sjögren's syndrome [218,313,426], and chronic infectious or inflammatory diseases of mucosae, especially lung [100,104,184,213,217,311,412,440, 470,482,483,676], and carcinomas of lung, colon, stomach, and breast [73,83,191,275,401,441,442, 565] make up the first category of illnesses associated with secondary IgAN. Although initially all associations were anecdotal, increasing experience shows that as many as 7 to 10 percent of patients with these diseases will have secondary IgAN, defined simply as mesangial deposits of IgA. This incidence exceeds that encountered in a large autopsy series (4 percent), which is considered a high estimate of IgA deposits in a normal population.

A second group of diseases includes lymphoproliferative diseases, such as mycosis fungoides [498], IgA gammopathies [155,158,194], non-Hodgkin's lymphomas [394], and cryoglobulinemia [394]. In these diseases, the incidence of secondary IgAN is perhaps 3 to 5 percent of all patients. Polycythemia and thrombocytic disorders, hematologic diseases that may be related in some way to the hematologic malignancies just mentioned, also have been associated with glomerular IgA deposits [289,394].

Finally, autoimmune and hypersensitivity diseases such as dermatitis herpetiformis [35,142, 148,220,266,267,434,479], ankylosing spondylitis [26,337,415,556] and related spondylarthropathies [76,299], scleritis, and sundry collagen-vascular diseases [394] are also seen in association with mesangial IgA deposits. Patients with IgAN secondary to autoimmune or hypersensitivity diseases are still a very small group of cases. The incidence of secondary IgAN is difficult to estimate, but it does appear higher than in the general population.

MANIFESTATIONS OF DISEASE

Most patients with secondary IgAN have been recognized at autopsy and were never observed to have had urinary or renal functional abnormalities during life. Asymptomatic microhematuria, with mild proteinuria (<0.5 g/24h) or without proteinuria, make up nearly all remaining patients. Episodic macrohematuria and/or renal insufficiency or proteinuria, common in primary IgAN, are rarely reported but do occur. Conceivably, the more clinically overt cases that are occasionally encountered represent coincidence of two independent processes, primary IgAN and the associated disease. On the other hand, the clinically latent examples may represent the true propensity of these diseases to generate IgA immune deposits with low nephritogenic potential.

Pathologic Changes

GROSS APPEARANCE

The kidneys of patients with secondary IgAN are likely to appear grossly normal, but no information is available.

MICROSCOPIC FINDINGS

Glomeruli

Glomeruli in secondary IgAN are often normal. Focal and segmental mesangial proliferation, usually mild, is seen in nearly all the remaining cases. Diffuse mesangial and focal and segmental endocapillary proliferation is infrequent, and diffuse endocapillary proliferation is not reported. Synechiae, necroses, and extracapillary proliferation are minor elements and are present only in rare cases.

Tubules

Tubules may show erythrocytes in the lumina in patients with hematuria. Otherwise, changes in tubules, blood vessels, and interstitium are inconspicuous in all but a few anecdotal cases. The relatively few cases with more than equivocal changes by light microscopy are from patients with clinically overt disease; these may represent coincidence of idiopathic IgAN and the disease purportedly underlying the renal disease.

IMMUNOHISTOCHEMICAL FINDINGS

Diffuse mesangial deposits of IgA are the rule in secondary IgAN, just as in the primary form. There is little information on the distribution of IgA subclasses or content of J-chain or secretory component, but it appears that secondary IgAN parallels primary IgAN. Codeposits of IgG and IgM, C1q, or C4 are much less frequent in secondary IgAN (~20 percent) compared with the primary disease. Interestingly, C3 deposits, although nearly ubiquitous in primary IgAN, are also relatively uncommon (25 to 35 percent of all patients) and tend to be segmental and of lower staining intensity. Membrane attack complex, properdin, and factor B are reported, but case series testing for these reactants are too few to allow generalization. Fibrin deposits, when reported, are sparse. Capillary wall deposits are rare and are associated with segmental endocapillary proliferation, and overt clinical signs of disease.

ELECTRON MICROSCOPIC FINDINGS

Ultrastructural studies of secondary IgAN are limited. Deposits are generally sparse, limited to the mesangium, and electron dense. Mesangial-cell hypertrophy and/or hyperplasia are infrequently observed, and matrix expansion is variable and mild, if present. Epithelial-cell changes and splitting, lamellation, or irregularities of basement membranes are only rarely encountered.

Etiology and Pathogenesis

It is tempting to speculate that disorders involving mucosae result in stimulation of mucosa-associated lymphoid tissue—the richest population of IgA-committed B cells—or that defects in immunoregulation due to hematopoietic neoplasms or underlying associated autoimmune diseases operate to promote vigorous IgA-rich immune responses. With respect to the mucosal diseases associated with IgAN, transforming growth factor (TGF-β), a product of injured epithelial cells [15], may play a role in increasing IgA production and altering mesangial-cell function [68,103,575]. Increased penetrability of mucosae by environmental antigens [137,449,541,669], overproduction of specific IgA antibodies, and impaired clearance may contribute alone or in concert to the genesis of secondary IgAN. However, as for the primary disease, the specific pathogenesis of the immune deposits is enigmatic. It is highly likely, though, that the pathophysiology of secondary IgAN is similar to the primary form.

As already intimated, it is possible that some instances of "secondary" IgAN are in fact an independent coincidence of two unrelated disease processes, IgAN and the underlying disease. This seems particularly likely in patients with the more obvious clinical signs who also have more definite pathologic changes. However, the increased frequency of mesangial IgA in conjunction with diseases identified as associated with IgAN compared with the general population, and the tendency for such underlying disease to involve mucosae or lymphoid cells, suggest that these conditions do predispose to glomerular IgA deposits.

Clinical Outcome

Most cases of secondary IgAN are diagnosed serendipitously or at autopsy, are not associated with clinically apparent renal disease, and do not manifest an increased incidence of glomerular sclerosis. Hence, from a renal standpoint, most secondary IgAN is benign. On the other hand, patients with clinically manifest disease can progress to renal insufficiency. There is no evidence at present to suggest that the renal prognosis varies according to the underlying disease, nor is there anything to suggest that any single underlying disease (or group of diseases) appears to predispose to more overt clinical glomerular disease. These perceptions must, however, be qualified, since the aggregate experience with such patients is still limited.

SCHÖNLEIN-HENOCH SYNDROME

Schönlein reported the association of arthritis with a purpuric skin eruption in 1832 [548*a*]. Henoch recognized gastrointestinal and renal components of this syndrome in the late 19th century [269]. The nephritic component represents the major portent of prognosis [119,252,253,371,476].

Clinical Features

Schönlein-Henoch syndrome is a multi-organ system disease that may include purpura, arthralgia, acute enteritis, and nephritis [10,33,55,77,79, 80,85,90,95,102,118,120,121,145,150,221,253, 260,287,328,329,335,364,371,372,379,399,438, 475,476,488,492,512,522,581,584,591,596,618, 650,681]. It is thought to be a vasculitis with variable clinical manifestations consequent on IgA-rich immune complexes depositing within affected tissues and causing inflammation. The clinical signs and lesions associated with the nephritis closely resemble those of primary IgAN. However, acute renal failure, crescentic and necrotizing glomerular lesions, diffuse endocapillary proliferation, and fibrin deposits are more typically encountered in Schönlein-Henoch syndrome. Many investigators consider it a systemic form of IgAN [176,411,600,603,654]. Properly, it is perhaps better to consider primary IgAN (Berger's disease) a limited form of Schönlein-Henoch syndrome, since both appear to be immune complex diseases characterized by predominance of the IgA class among the antibody constituents.

DEMOGRAPHICS

Children, typically 5 to 15 years of age, make up the principal population (>80 percent), although patients range in age from 2 to 89 years [6,28,34, 55,75,86,121,141,196,203,277,290,309,322,353, 360,410,427,461,462,519,569,574,592]. Males account for 55 to 60 percent of patients. The disease has been described worldwide. Although the nephritis associated with the syndrome is a relatively uncommon cause of glomerular disease, it accounted for 7 to 8 percent of both glomerular disease and end-stage kidney disease in children in one large series from Paris [371]. As is the case with IgAN, policies regarding urinalysis and biopsy influence the frequency with which nephritis is recognized in Schönlein-Henoch syndrome, as well as the manifestations of renal involvement [63,79,254,399,512]. Among patients with Schönlein-Henoch syndrome, renal involvement is reported in 10 to 100 percent; a weighted mean of several series indicates that 35 percent of Schönlein-Henoch syndrome patients overall have nephritis [10,77,80,95,121,145,328,329, 335,364,438,475,476,488,492,512,522,581,584, 618,650].

MANIFESTATIONS OF DISEASE

The clinical constellation of Schönlein-Henoch syndrome encompasses any or all of the elements of vasculitis in general and may mimic or be mimicked by such conditions as polyarteritis, Wegener's granulomatosis, and systemic lupus erythematosus. It can be distinguished from these by lack of antineutrophil cytoplasmic antibodies (ANCA) and/or antinuclear antibodies so prevalent in polyarteritis, Wegener's granulomatosis, or lupus and by the prominence of IgA in its lesions. All combinations of dermal, gastrointestinal, articular, hepatic, pulmonary, neural, renal, and other soft-tissue inflammation or hemorrhage occur in Schönlein-Henoch syndrome. Generalized fever, lassitude, discomfort, and weight loss are common. The individual components are often episodic; they develop in concert or independently over several days or even weeks and resolve over many days to a few weeks. Notably, the combination of lung involvement (purpura or hemorrhage) and nephritis prompts confusion with anti-GBM antibody disease [67,123,162,272,297,303, 374,375,387,390,482,483,552,644,679].

Skin

The most common presenting element, which is observed in half the patients at onset, is the characteristic purpuric rash, beginning as wheals on the extensor surfaces of the limbs and lower trunk [221]. The wheals evolve into pink macropapules and can be exacerbated by pressure. After a day or so, the lesions appear as dusky red macules that do not blanch on pressure. Edema, independent of protein loss in the urine, is often encountered. Generally, these lesions wax and wane to resolution over weeks, but they may persist for years [203,252,287,371,372,399].

Gut

Abdominal pain is usually mild and spasmodic in nature [247]. In addition to colic and vomiting, hematochezia and hematemesis are reported in many patients. In some instances, the pain can be so severe as to mimic surgical emergencies, such as intussusception, infarction, perforation, and stricture of the gut [200,229,247,384,653]. Acute pancreatitis has been recognized as a presentation for Schönlein-Henoch syndrome as well [226].

Joints

Arthralgia without objective arthritis is reported and occurs mainly in the large joints of the leg [10, 121,141,203,221,253,329,438]. The joint pain is transient and often migratory but is distinguished from the joint involvement of rheumatic fever by the lack of redness and swelling.

Kidneys

The overall clinical manifestations of renal involvement are varied, but hematuria is the hallmark [86]. Gross or microscopic asymptomatic hematuria occurs in nearly all patients, but it is difficult to estimate the proportion of patients in each of the two categories, since detailed information is often not provided in the large series. Variable degrees of proteinuria are encountered in up to 95 percent of patients. While proteinuria is generally mild, nephrotic-range proteinuria or frank nephrotic syndrome may be encountered with variable frequency, especially in large referral centers [371,372,399]. Acute renal insufficiency and fluid retention are seen in as many as 40 percent of patients, and nephrosis is superimposed on nephritis in some 16 percent. Hypertension is perhaps more frequent than in age-matched populations lacking Schönlein-Henoch syndrome and nephritis and may be the presenting sign of disease [102,161]. Although oliguria is described, it is rare.

Pathologic Changes

GROSS APPEARANCE

The kidneys of patients with Schönlein-Henoch syndrome are likely to appear grossly normal, but little information is available.

MICROSCOPIC FINDINGS

Glomeruli

Like IgAN, the morphologic expression of glomerular injury in Schönlein-Henoch syndrome is variable, even within a single patient at a particular time. Classification of the pathologic changes in Schönlein-Henoch syndrome is based on the endocapillary and extracapillary components of the glomerulus (Table 6-3). Lesions center on mesangial and focal and segmental endocapillary proliferation, but extracapillary proliferation is generally much more prominent and frequent in Schönlein-Henoch syndrome nephritis than in IgAN (Fig. 6-32). Focal and segmental prolifera-

TABLE 6-3. *Classification of glomerular lesions in Schönlein-Henoch syndrome**

I. No crescents, minimal glomerular alteration
II. No crescents
    A. Pure mesangial proliferation
    B. Focal-segmental endocapillary proliferation
    C. Diffuse endocapillary proliferation
III. Crescents in some glomeruli (<50 percent)
    A. Focal endocapillary proliferation
    B. Diffuse endocapillary proliferation
IV. Crescents in many glomeruli (50 to 75 percent)
    A. Focal endocapillary proliferation
    B. Diffuse endocapillary proliferation
V. Crescents in most glomeruli (>75 percent)
    A. Focal endocapillary proliferation
    B. Diffuse endocapillary proliferation
VI. Pseudomembranoproliferative glomerulonephritis

*This scheme is slightly modified from Heaton's classification [265]; the modification relates to a distinction in group II between patients with only mesangial proliferation (A) and those with occlusion of some glomerular capillaries by cells in some glomeruli (B) or most glomeruli (C). The other categories do not distinguish purely mesangial hypercellularity or matrix expansion from endocapillary proliferation because the number of crescents seems to be the critical determinant of clinical course and outcome. This is in contrast to the classification proposed for IgA nephritis (Table 6-1), for which the critical histopathologic portents of clinical outcome remain controversial.

tion (Fig. 6-33) is observed in the majority of patients (75 to 90 percent) [22,29,54,55,75,126,203, 265,270,271,309,329,372,399,438,569,622,634]. In many affected glomeruli, the segments with proliferation show adhesion of the tuft to parietal epithelium [271,634]. Segmental lesions, especially at sites of adhesion of tuft to Bowman's capsule, may show splitting and duplication of basement membranes, and in a minority of patients, this is very widespread. Indeed, it often may be associated with conspicuous mesangial-cell interposition; a pattern closely resembling membranoproliferative glomerulonephritis type I can be seen [75,119,265,372]. Diffuse endocapillary proliferation, usually with, but perhaps without crescent formation, is also encountered. Focal fibrinoid necrosis is often present at onset (Fig. 6-34), but patients biopsied at a later time manifest segmental "disorganized" sclerosis that may well represent healed fibrinoid necrosis. Intracapillary thrombi are noted in some glomeruli. Small crescents are present in 20 to 30 percent of glomeruli in many cases, and in a few patients, more than half the glomeruli have crescents [75,265,372,399,569].

Diffuse extracapillary proliferation superimposed on changes similar to those just mentioned, affecting nearly all glomeruli, is the next most frequent appearance of glomeruli in Schönlein-Henoch syndrome [29,265,372,399,569]. In patients with this pattern (Fig. 6-35), numerous and severe extracapillary lesions are present. Often, mesangial or endocapillary proliferation is more severe in glomeruli with diffuse crescents, and either segmental fibrinoid necrosis (acutely) or segmental "disorganized" sclerosis (subacutely) is usually conspicuous under the light microscope [29,75,203, 220,353,368,371,372,399,438,501,648]. Expansion of mesangial matrix and proliferation confined to mesangial areas, involving all or some glomeruli, are an occasional pattern in Schönlein-Henoch syndrome. Although less frequent and less prominent, crescents are seen in some glomeruli in most biopsies from these patients. Rarely, patients with Schönlein-Henoch syndrome will have normal or equivocally abnormal glomeruli [29,203,371,372, 399,438,569].

Tubules

Degenerative changes, such as flattening, desquamation, vacuolization, and loss of microvillous brush borders, are encountered focally within the cortex in nearly all patients, a feature seen in only a minority of patients with IgAN. Tubular degeneration may be extensive (see Fig. 6-35). Tubular casts and/or atrophy are also encountered focally. These changes are consonant with the degree of glomerular injury, which tends on the whole to be more severe than in IgAN.

Blood Vessels

Medial hypertrophy and intimal fibroelastosis are present in small arteries in biopsies from some patients, although in most reported series details are scanty and an incidence of vascular sclerosis cannot be reliably estimated. Hyalin change and/or

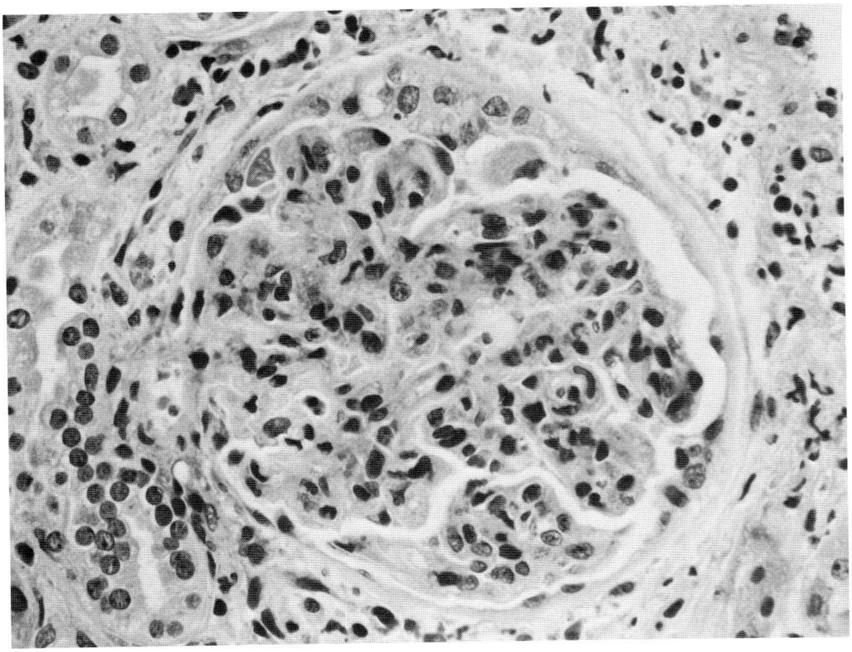

Fig. 6-32. *This glomerulus shows an increase in mesangial cells. At the top there is a small crescent. H&E; ×440.*

accumulations of fibrinoid material or frank necrosis may be present in afferent arterioles and interlobular arteries; an inflammatory component may accompany the more florid lesions (Fig. 6-36). These vascular changes, when present, may facilitate discrimination from IgAN, since arteritis is not a recognized component of IgAN.

Interstitium

The interstitium, like the tubules, is affected to a degree consonant with the severity of the glomerular injury. In the main, this is more severe in Schönlein-Henoch syndrome than in IgAN. Particularly in association with diffuse proliferative lesions and focal-segmental proliferation with numerous crescents, there may be edema and a leukocytic infiltrate consisting of lymphocytes, macrophages, and plasma cells. A definite acute interstitial component may be a helpful morphologic discriminator from IgAN. Although a well-developed acute interstitial reaction is observed in IgAN, it is unusual even among cases with severe glomerular disease.

Extrarenal Tissue

Prototypical leukocytoclastic vasculitis involving vessels in skin and gut is described [17,21,22,193, 203,239,240,268,368,369,371,578,582,599,614]. Arterioles, capillaries, and venules are surrounded by a mixed infiltrate of neutrophils and monocytes. Fibrinoid accumulation or necrosis of arterioles or venules is rarely encountered [648], although fibrin thrombi are seen focally in capillaries. Superficial capillaries in the reticular dermis and lamina propria appear affected more commonly than deep vessels. There is a paucity of information on histopathology of the joints in acute Schönlein-Henoch syndrome.

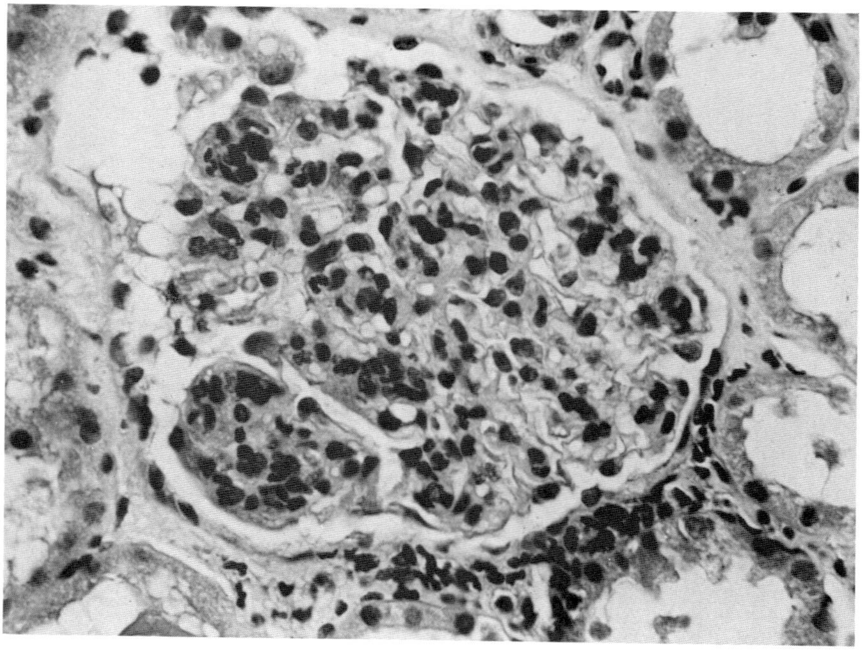

FIG. 6-33. *A glomerulus showing a localized area of cellular proliferation in the lobule at left of picture. This was taken from a 43-year-old man with Schönlein-Henoch syndrome with focal glomerulonephritis on biopsy. Half the glomeruli in the biopsy showed no changes. H&E; ×420.*

IMMUNOHISTOCHEMICAL FINDINGS

Glomeruli

The most characteristic feature by immunohistology is the deposition of IgA in glomeruli (Fig. 6-37). This was not recognized in work antedating the routine application of staining for IgA to renal biopsies but is now regarded as integral to the disease. Typically, there is diffuse granular mesangial deposition of IgA, sometimes associated with segmental or diffuse capillary wall staining. In rare instances, the staining of the capillary wall may predominate over that in the mesangium, and exceptionally, capillary wall deposits are present without associated mesangial deposits [265,372]. Capillary deposits are associated with endocapillary proliferation and may be segmental or diffuse. Extensive capillary deposits are associated with more severe diffuse endocapillary proliferation and/or extensive crescent formation. The predominant subclass of IgA deposited is IgA_1, and both light chain types are deposited equally [43–45, 51,344,350,382,383,432,605,625]. Regularly, J-chain is present in association with IgA, but secretory component is absent. Although staining for IgA is more intense than for other immunoglobulins, some staining for IgG and/or IgM is observed in 65 to 75 percent of cases [265,371, 372,472,569]. Fibrin-related antigen (Fig. 6-38) is associated with crescents but is also found in glomerular tufts—generally in a mixed mesangial and capillary pattern—in 65 to 75 percent of biopsies [265,371,372,472,569].

Complement component C3 is a frequent concomitant; it is present in 75 to 85 percent of cases,

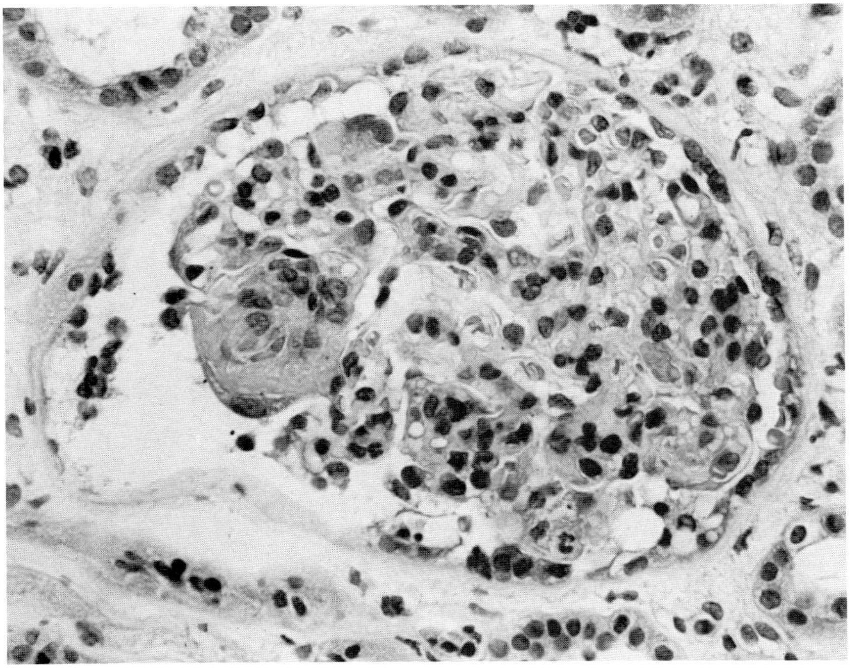

Fig. 6-34. *This glomerulus, with an area of necrosis in the lobule to left of picture, is from the same biopsy as in Fig. 6-33. H&E; ×400.*

as opposed to IgAN, where it is found in 95 percent of cases or more. Like IgAN, early classical pathway complement components C1 and C4 are present only rarely and stain with low intensity; in contrast, alternative pathway components and the membrane attack complex, including S-protein, are regularly present [23,51,52,98,157,189,224, 225,230,231,317,388,557,579,587,649].

Tubules

In those patients with frank interstitial nephritis, there are scattered focal deposits of IgA, C3, and sometimes IgG and/or IgM in tubular basement membranes [97,98,214]. This feature, if present, may help to distinguish Schönlein-Henoch syndrome nephritis from IgAN on strictly morphologic grounds. It should be emphasized that most cases do not reveal immune deposits in tubules.

Blood Vessels

Occasionally, there are granular deposits in arterioles and/or peritubular capillaries in the renal cortex [98,133,403,555]. These deposits contain IgA and C3, less often with admixed IgG and/or IgM. Such deposits are present in only a few of the many vessels in a microscopic field and are observed typically in those cases with severe glomerular changes by light microscopy and deposits in glomerular capillary walls.

Extrarenal Sites

Deposits of IgA and usually of C3 are present in capillaries in the papillary dermis both in areas of purpura and in normal skin [17,21,22,98,239,240, 268,369,582,599,614]. Codeposits of IgG and IgM are present in these sites in roughly 20 percent of patients, and linear deposits of IgA are pre-

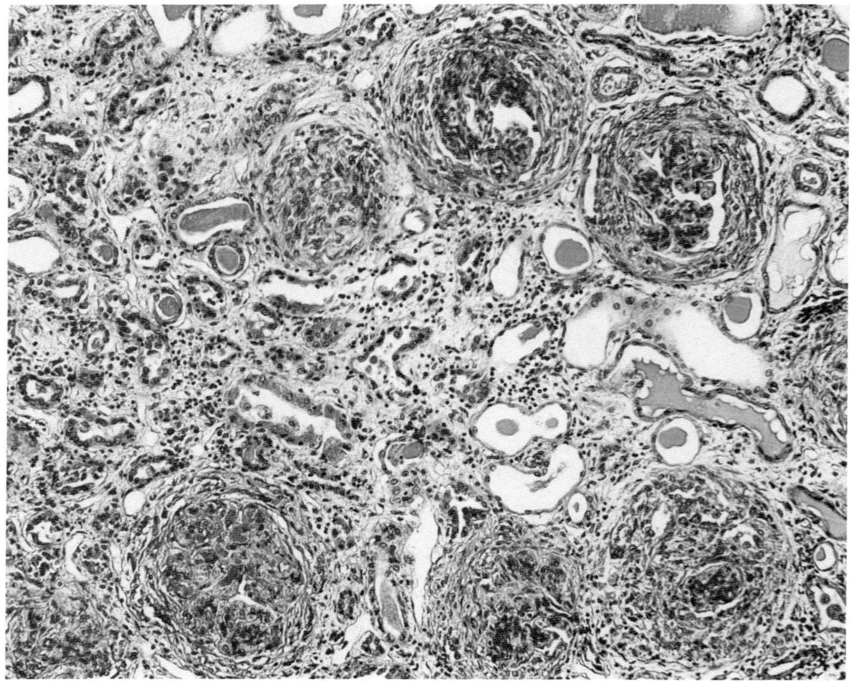

FIG. 6-35. *Plentiful crescent formation is evident in this florid form of glomerulonephritis in Schönlein-Henoch syndrome. There is extensive tubular loss. The specimen is from the 10-year-old girl described by Watson [648] (autopsy no. 1699, Johns Hopkins Hospital, in 1901). H&E; ×130.*

sent at the dermal-epidermal junction of normal and purpuric skin in 15 to 25 percent of patients.

ELECTRON MICROSCOPIC FINDINGS

Mesangial matrix expansion and cellular hypertrophy and hyperplasia are uniformly evident ultrastructurally [29,75,193,241,265,309,323,329, 478,504,569,621,622] (Fig. 6-39). Mesangial cells show accentuation of organelles, particularly rough endoplasmic reticulum, and long-spaced collagen is evident in the matrix. Electron-dense deposits are also uniformly encountered; in milder cases, the deposits are present primarily in the paramesangium and are small (100–200 nm), discrete, and osmiophilic. In more severe cases, deposits are larger (up to 800 nm), more coalescent and variegated in density, and lie deeper in the mesangial matrix. Patients with endocapillary proliferation evident by light microscopy frequently show foci of interposition of mesangial cells between layers of basement-membrane matrix in capillary walls. In these more severely involved kidneys, irregular subendothelial deposits are also observed (Fig. 6-40). Subepithelial deposits are frequent, even in the less severe cases [265, 323,392,423,622,674,680]. Electron-dense deposits reminiscent of humps are seen [623], but more characteristically they are festooned, scallop-shaped or garland-shaped, variable in staining, and often appear "fluffy" (Fig. 6-41). They are situated in the lamina rara externa, principally in the peripheral portions of the capillary loops, and are delimited by a thin area of new basement

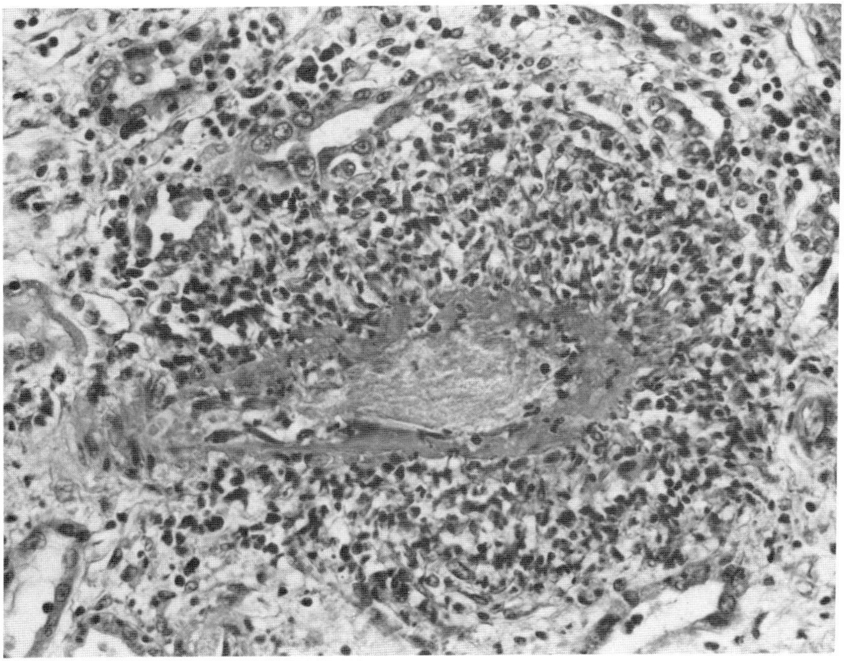

FIG. 6-36. *A small artery in the kidney shows necrosis and intense inflammatory changes. From same case as in Fig. 6-35. H&E; ×350.*

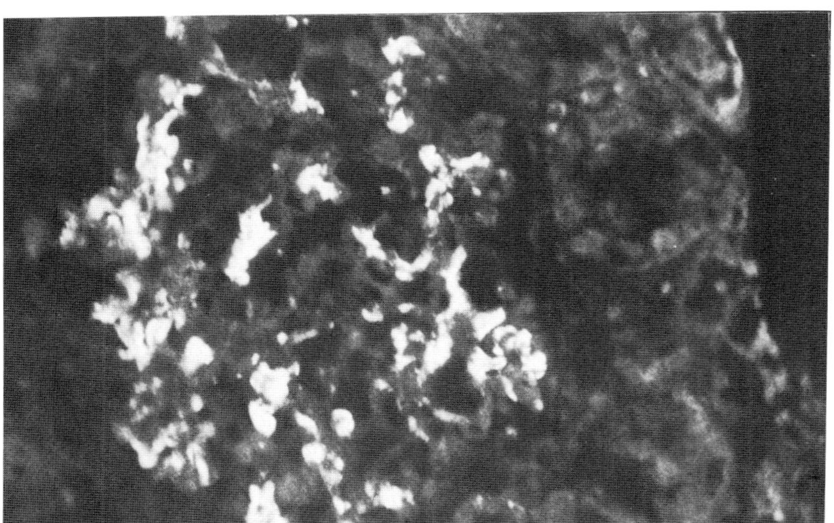

FIG. 6-37. *This immunofluorescence micrograph reveals the mesangial distribution of IgA in a child with Schönlein-Henoch syndrome. ×365.*

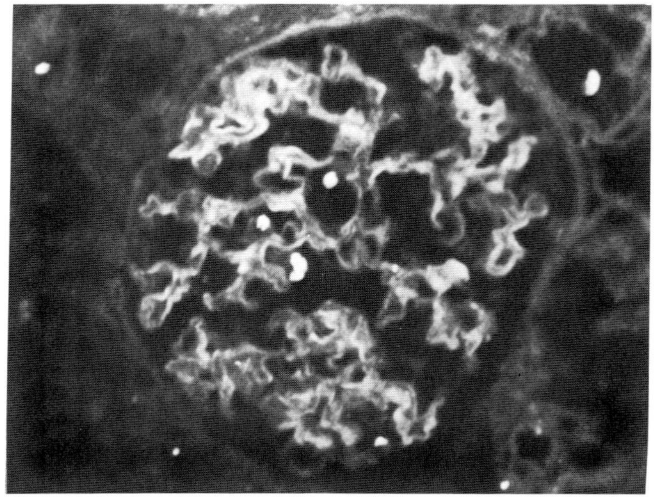

FIG. 6-38. *Fibrin-related antigen is localized in a mixed mesangial and peripheral capillary loop pattern in this glomerulus. A similar pattern was present for IgG, IgM, IgA, and C3 in this patient.* ×343.

membrane. As in IgAN, thinning, splitting, and splintering of the lamina densa have been described, especially in relation to the fluffy dome- or garland-shaped deposits just mentioned.

Etiology and Pathogenesis

Schönlein-Henoch syndrome is most likely a systemic vasculitis instigated by immune complexes of IgA antibody and exogenous antigens. Like IgAN, this syndrome is associated with increased circulating immune complexes and cryoglobulins containing IgA [88,110,112,126,134,138,152,257, 312,319,367,397,656,663]. Impaired clearance of immune complexes by the mononuclear phagocyte system and increased production of IgA immune complexes are both possible, and their relative importance is still debated [138,173]. Abnormalities in lymphocyte function parallel those already described in IgAN and include elevated serum IgA levels [31,38,45,89,167,173,338,386,469,533, 560,595,615]. Likewise, selected major histocompatibility complex genes may increase the risk for Schönlein-Henoch syndrome and/or the severity of the associated nephritis. The validity of these studies, particularly those related to relative risk of the syndrome, remains controversial [216, 381,452,467,472,505,550]. The only uncontested genetic association, as for IgAN, is an increased frequency of C4 null genotype [407].

Antigens derived from foodstuffs [6] or infectious organisms [419–421], drugs [190,242,402], and venoms [634] have been implicated in well-documented studies of limited numbers of patients. Mucosal infections, particularly of the upper respiratory tract, and chronic inflammation are also frequently noted in association with disease onset [20,29,121,209,220,228,252,259,329, 377, 393, 399, 408, 422, 454, 500, 521, 547, 587]. There is no clear evidence to support the earlier concept of anaphylactoid purpura as an allergic consequence to streptococci [20,80,634]. Elevated levels of rheumatoid factor and antinuclear antibodies in the patients' sera with Schönlein-Henoch syndrome suggest a potential autoimmune/ connective-tissue etiology of the disease. The titers of these antibodies are comparatively low in

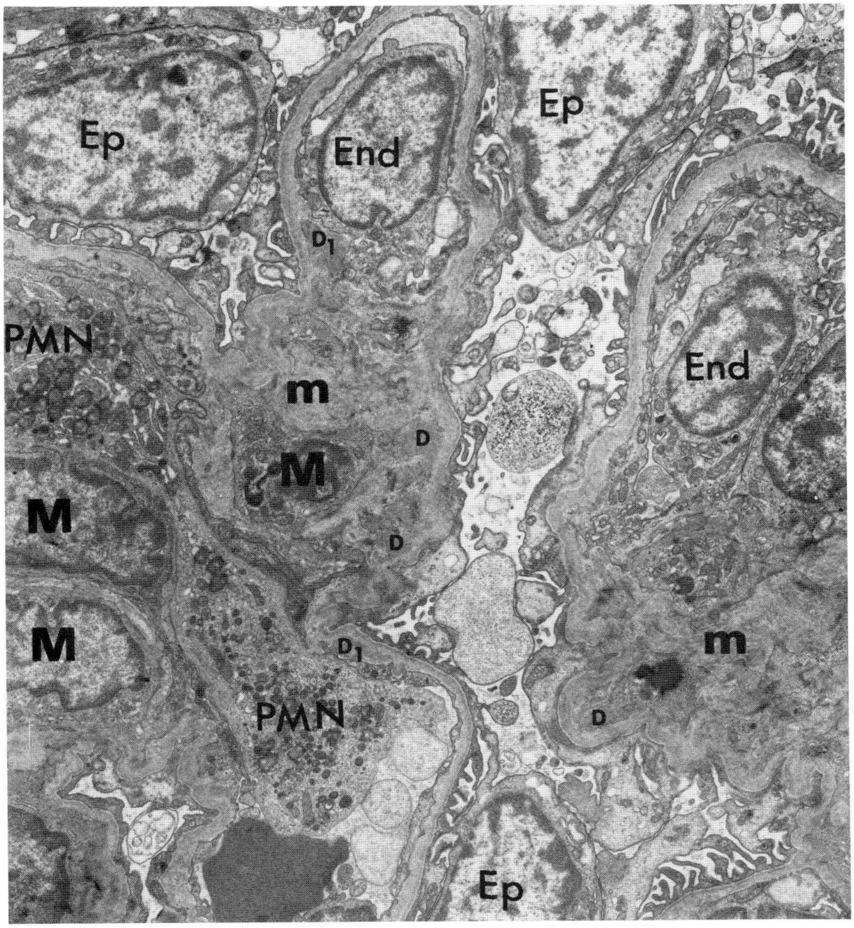

Fig. 6-39. A portion of a glomerulus from a patient with Schönlein-Henoch syndrome shows the mesangial region (M) of a lobule in which there is an increase in mesangial matrix (m) and numerous electron-dense deposits (D). Deposits (D_1) are also prominent at the base of loops near the mesangium. A polymorphonuclear leukocyte (PMN) has extended a long process into the mesangial region on the left. End, endothelial cell nucleus; Ep, epithelial cell nucleus. ×5800. (From Urizar, R. E., et al. Lab. Invest. *19: 437, 1968. Copyright 1968 by the U.S.–Canadian Division of the International Academy of Pathology. Used by permission.)*

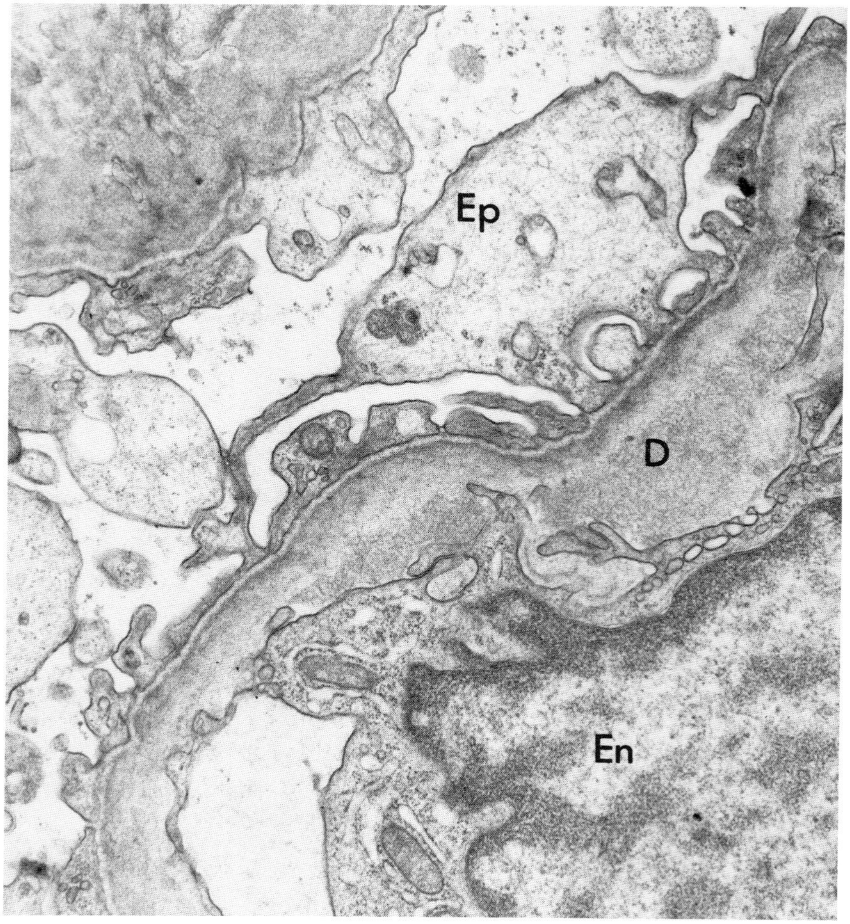

FIG. 6-40. *The base of a capillary shows substructural details of the electron-dense deposits (D) in the subendothelial space in a case of Schönlein-Henoch syndrome. En, endothelium, Ep, epithelium.* × *18,000. (From Urizar, R. E., et al.* Lab. Invest. *19: 437, 1968. Copyright 1968 by the U.S.–Canadian Division of the International Academy of Pathology. Used by permission.)*

the former condition, and the significance of such autoantibodies remains questionable [542,543].

Fibrin is very frequently part of the glomerular deposits in the nephritis accompanying Schönlein-Henoch syndrome, and intravascular coagulation has been proposed as an initiator of glomerular lesions [91,621,622]. The deposition of fibrin and/or fibrinopeptides, as in glomerulonephritis in general, appears related to necrosis of glomerular tufts.

From the foregoing considerations, it is apparent that both the pathogenesis and pathophysiology of Schönlein-Henoch syndrome share many features with primary IgAN. The spectra of glomerular pathology and clinical expression of the two entities overlap considerably, but the likeli-

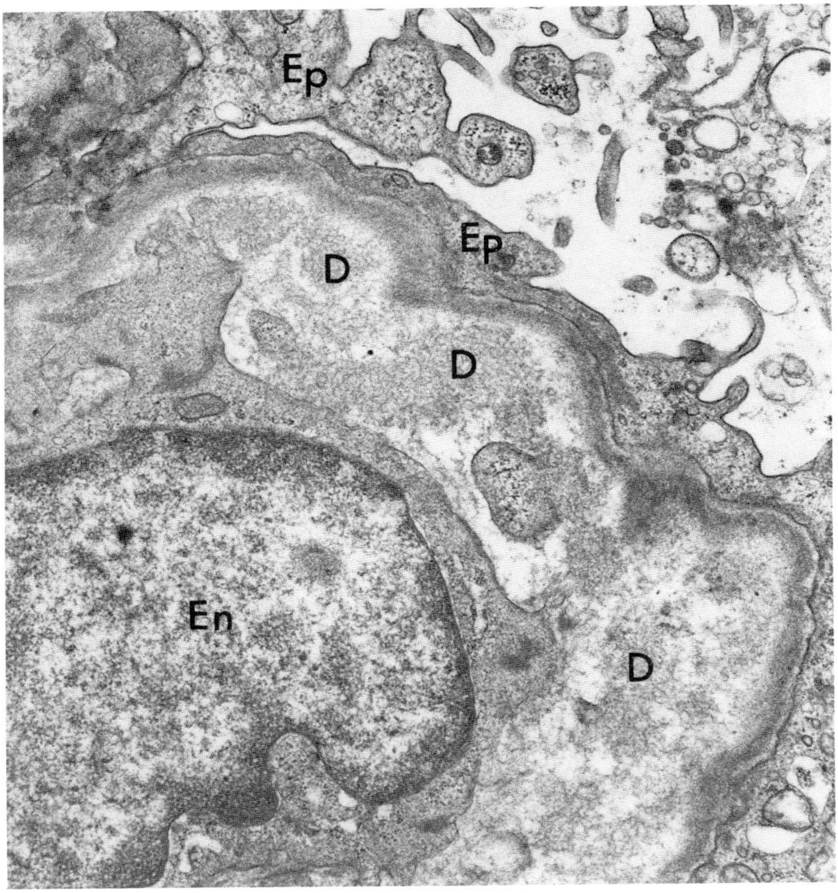

Fig. 6-41. *A portion of a glomerular capillary wall from a patient with Schönlein-Henoch syndrome shows extensive fluffy granular and fibrillar deposits (D) in the subendothelial space. Foot processes of the epithelial cell (EP) are extensively effaced. En, endothelial cell.* ×16,000. *(From Urizar, R. E., et al.* Lab. Invest. *19: 437, 1968. Copyright 1968 by the U.S.–Canadian Division of the International Academy of Pathology. Used by permission.)*

hood of more severe glomerular injury and the association of nephritis with systemic disease suggest that Schönlein-Henoch syndrome is indeed somehow different from IgAN. The first clues to identifying this difference are just now emerging from Rifai's laboratory (A. Rifai, personal communication). Injection of bacterial cell-wall antigen preparations from *S. pneumoniae* strains, followed by specific IgA antibody into mice, can elicit purpuric rash, gastrointestinal hemorrhage, and nephritis characterized by a necrotizing glomerulitis with IgA deposits. The propensity for each of these components—dermal, intestinal, and renal—to develop depends on the strain of bacteria used to prepare the polysaccharide and on the strain of mouse to which the complexes are given.

Thus some interaction between selected bacterial products and specific host factors under genetic control must account for the development of purpuric disease in these laboratory animals and the involvement of the various end-organs.

Although it is premature to define these interactions, it is reasonable to speculate along two broad lines. First, as already demonstrated by Rifai and associates [94], the antigenic component of immune complexes can dramatically influence nephritogenicity by influencing complement fixation by the complexes. Particularly if the antigen is a complex multimacromolecular structure, its complement-fixing ability could be associated with direct alternative pathway activation by virtue of complex carbohydrates and/or polyanions suitable as "activating surfaces" or with classical pathway activation by means of the action of immunoglobulin-binding factors. Many bacteria, particularly those which are gram-positive, produce factors that bind to the Fc regions of IgG, IgA, and IgM [177]. These factors, associated with the cell wall, are specific for selected species and strains of organisms, can aggregate immunoglobulin regardless of its antigen specificity, and can promote classical pathway complement activation and hypersensitivity. These features may determine the propensity for injury in each end-organ in the model of Schönlein-Henoch syndrome induced by immune complexes containing bacterial cell walls. The ratio of immunoglobulins to complement and alternative versus classical pathway components most likely influence the pattern of injury in the different combinations of mouse and bacterial strains.

A second possible pathway parallels earlier discussions of lectin-based binding of IgA to mesangium, particularly to fibronectin, as related to the pathogenesis of primary IgAN. Bacterial cell walls bear numerous organ- and species-specific attachment molecules, mostly lectin-like, which determine their pathogenicity. These molecules, present in cell walls and cell-wall preparations, may be the basis for the end-organ selectivity encountered in the murine model described above and also in Schönlein-Henoch syndrome. They may serve as well to promote aggregation of IgA and other immunoglobulin classes and complement activation either as antigens or by bridging glycosylation sites on the IgA component of complexes with tissue glycosylation sites.

Both these speculations presuppose infection as the inciting event in Schönlein-Henoch syndrome. There is ample circumstantial evidence in support of this notion, although other mechanisms are not excluded. Moreover, bacterial products can in some instances persist well after the acute infection resolves, and the tissue injury, once initiated, may progress independent of immunologic factors.

Clinical Outcome

The degree of renal involvement largely predicts patient outcome in nearly all cases of Schönlein-Henoch syndrome [119,252,253,371,372]. The disease is an important cause of chronic renal failure, accounting for 3 percent of children with terminal renal failure in Europe [253]. The vast majority of patients in most studies enjoy resolution of disease with few mild or no sequelae. While one study from a large referral center recorded a poor outcome in 20 percent of patients [253], several large series of unselected patients suggest that fewer than 8 percent of afflicted children die or develop end-stage kidney after a prolonged follow-up period [19,30,119,243,320,328,329,334,409,410,516,632]. A few died from acute renal failure.

More than half of all patients (52 percent) undergo complete spontaneous remission, usually within a year of onset. Another 15 percent have prolonged macroscopic hematuria and/or proteinuria exceeding 500 μg daily but normal GFR, and 18 percent of all patients have stable persistent microhematuria or microproteinuria without impaired filtration. Moreover, most children with normal renal function 2 years after onset ultimately enjoy complete remission. Among those patients who develop chronic renal insufficiency and/or end-stage kidney, progression of the glomerular disease is slow, requiring 5 to 10 years to reach that point [119,329,372].

Clinical premonitors of poor prognosis include proteinuria, macroscopic hematuria, and hypertension. Isolated hematuria and symptomless hematuria with proteinuria less than 1 g daily are associated with a good outcome; less than 5 percent of the patients with these initial clinical signs developed chronic renal failure after prolonged follow-up periods of up to 12 years [88,119,260, 329,371,399,438,673,681]. Moderately proteinuric patients (>1 g daily), patients with nephritic syndrome, and nephrotic patients have an intermediate long-term prognosis; 12 percent progress to terminal renal failure or death over a 10-year span. In this group, severity of the nephrotic syndrome and initial GFR are important predictors. Patients with acute nephritic syndrome and evolving early nephrosis have a poor prognosis; 25 percent of such patients progress to end-stage kidney within 10 years and another 25 percent develop chronic renal insufficiency. Severe nephrosis or renal insufficiency with nephrosis portends a grave prognosis, with 50 to 75 percent of patients progressing to end-stage renal failure or death; in contrast, less than 10 percent of patients with moderate nephrosis and normal GFR at onset developed chronic renal insufficiency. The number of recurrences does not seem to have predictive value for development of end-stage kidney in one series of patients [119], although another suggested that recurrences were predictive of poor outcome [253].

Pathologic features that are valuable portents of prognosis are histologic grade and percentage of glomeruli with crescents [119,260,329,372,399, 438,673,681]. Among patients with terminal renal failure, 80 percent had more than 50 percent crescents. Forty percent of patients with greater than 50 percent crescents developed end-stage kidney disease or died, but only 3 to 4 percent of patients with 50 percent or fewer glomeruli with crescents developed chronic renal failure. Repeat biopsies document that in this disease, histologic and clinical parameters resolve and exacerbate in parallel [248].

The number of patients who have received allografts is too small to allow any generalizations, but recurrence of disease is documented [24,27, 53,251,655]. IgA deposits without overt renal disease appear to be common among such patients, however.

GLOMERULAR INVOLVEMENT IN HEPATOBILIARY DISEASE

Renal complications of liver disease assume several different patterns [174,459]. Derangements in hemodynamics associated with acute liver failure may lead to acute renal failure (so-called hepatorenal syndrome, discussed in Chap. 18), and fluid and electrolyte abnormalities consequent to liver dysfunction, particularly hyponatremia and hyperkalemia, may lead to defective renal function as well. Many agents are both hepato- and nephrotoxins. The liver is a major target for several infectious diseases, notably viral hepatitis, schistosomiasis, and malaria, that may be associated with several different patterns of glomerular disease. These conditions are discussed in Chapters 5 and 28, which consider postinfectious glomerulonephritis and glomerulonephritides secondary to miscellaneous infections, respectively.

The final category, mesangiopathic glomerulopathy associated with cirrhosis, biliary atresia, or severe fatty metamorphosis of the liver, bears a particular relationship to IgAN and hence is discussed here. Recognition of glomerular disease in patients with liver cirrhosis dates back to the late 1940s, when the emphasis was on glomerular sclerosis [37,64,124,207,281,302,355,484]. Mild proliferative glomerulonephritis was added as another lesion associated with cirrhosis in 1959 [64,207], but series of patients without cirrhosis were first included for comparison in 1961 [302]. The significance of the lesions occurring in these descriptive reports was difficult to interpret because poststreptococcal glomerulonephritis, a known contributor to mesangiopathic lesions and perhaps to sclerosis, was so prevalent, and the causes of the cirrhosis were manifold. Hepatitis B antigenemia and alcohol intake were prevalent in these patients, and their contributions to the development of glomerular disease is uncertain [174,248,459, 530]. The advent of immunohistologic examination of kidneys in the 1960s prompted recognition that immunoglobulins and complement were present in glomeruli from cirrhotic individuals; IgA was recognized as a major constituent of the immune deposits soon thereafter [52,84,219,284, 395,398,431,433,455,464,561,586,630,651].

Clinical Features

DEMOGRAPHICS

Several series considering renal disease in association with cirrhosis of the liver collectively suggest that approximately 61 percent of patients manifest some evidence of glomerular injury [3,4,41,52, 64,69,84,124,125,185,207,219,302,310,455,465, 466,529,530,566,662]. Similar overall incidences seem appropriate for the association with biliary atresia, fatty change, and, to a lesser extent, alcoholic and viral hepatitis. Although there is a suggestion that alcoholic cirrhosis is more likely to result in hepatorenal syndrome or glomerular sclerosis, this seems unfounded, as does a predilection for renal disease among female patients with cirrhosis. The data regarding glomerular injury associated with cirrhosis and other liver diseases are heavily dependent on postmortem examination, a limitation to interpreting the data and in predicting outcome of patients. Cirrhosis secondary to viral hepatitis, hepatotoxicity, cystic fibrosis, hypersensitivity biliary disease, and cholangitis, as well as biliary atresia and fatty metamorphosis, have all been implicated extensively. Older cirrhotic patients and those with long-standing cirrhosis seem to be at higher risk for glomerular involvement.

MANIFESTATIONS OF DISEASE

Hematuria is the most conspicuous clinical manifestation. Although episodic macrohematuria has been described, microhematuria with some degree of proteinuria is most typical [3,4,37,41,52,84, 174,208,233,248,284,395,431,433,455,464,490, 529,530,535,561,586]. Proteinuria without hematuria is reported; sometimes it is in the nephrotic range, and hypoalbuminemia may be present. Acute renal insufficiency has been reported, but rapid progression is rare. Those patients with a rapid course reveal crescents, but many others who ultimately recover from their bouts of acute renal failure have only hemoglobin casts in their biopsies. The frequency of these clinical manifestations depends on whether autopsy series or biopsy series are considered [52,395,464]. The latter, requiring an invasive procedure, would clearly select patients with more severe functional derangement. Roughly 10 percent of patients studied at autopsy and 60 percent of patients recognized by renal biopsy have hematuria, and 1.6 and 14 percent, respectively, have heavy nephrotic-range proteinuria [52,64,84,124,174,207,219, 248,302,455,529,530,566,662]. Most patients from biopsy series have some degree of proteinuria. These clinical signs correlate well with severity of glomerular injury. It is clear, however, that most cirrhotic patients lack urinary abnormalities and therefore lack serious histopathologic changes in the kidney.

Pathologic Changes

GROSS APPEARANCE

The kidneys of these patients are likely to appear grossly normal, and to have no striking features.

MICROSCOPIC FINDINGS

Glomeruli

Two patterns of glomerular involvement predominate [3,4,37,41,52,64,84,124,207,208,233,281, 284,395,431,433,455,464,484,490,499,529,530, 535,561,566,586]. The first pattern described consisted essentially of an axial sclerosis. In the less severe examples of this form—now recognized to be more prevalent than the fully developed axial sclerosis—the glomeruli show expansion of mesangial matrix by fibrillar accumulations of periodic acid–Schiff–positive material, either segmentally or diffusely, perhaps with segmental collapse of capillaries (Fig. 6-42). In more advanced lesions, thickening and occasional segmental tortuousity of capillary walls are evident. Some 15 percent of patients with this form of renal disease have moderate or marked mesangial matrix expansion that is diffuse yet variable in severity from glomerulus to glomerulus; it may be associated with conspicuous capillary wall thickening (Fig. 6-43). The most severely affected of these kidneys can be confused with nodular diabetic glomerulosclerosis [281,499]. Approximately 5 percent of patients reveal focal and global glomerular sclerosis and obsolescence in more than 20 percent of their glomeruli, but many patients have fewer sclerotic

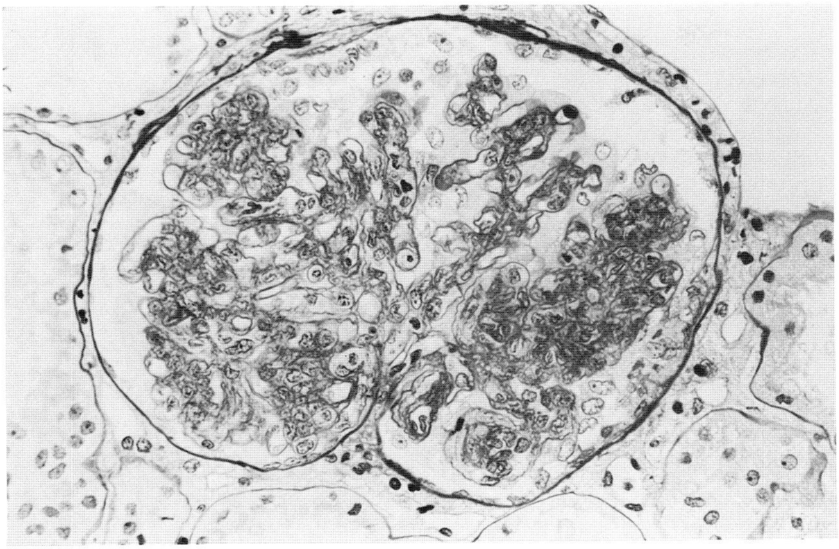

Fig. 6-42. *This glomerulus, from a patient with chronic alcoholic cirrhosis, microhematuria, and 500 μg per day proteinuria reveals mild to moderate mesangial hypercellularity associated with moderate expansion of the mesangial matrix. In addition, there is thickening of glomerular capillary walls and collapse and compression of glomerular capillary tufts. Rarely, tortuosity of capillary walls is evident.* PAS; ×450.

glomeruli. Endothelial swelling and lipid accumulation are frequently described in many patients, but they may be artefactual. Most samples in studies of cirrhosis-associated renal disease were obtained postmortem, and autolysis in the interval between death and autopsy may account for this change. Dilation of Bowman's space, often with proteinaceous coagula, is often seen in such patients, and glomeruli are frequently enlarged. Interestingly, marked enlargement of the juxtaglomerular apparatus is observed, especially in association with axial glomerular sclerosis [503].

The second major pattern, apparently more prevalent, is a mesangial proliferative glomerulonephritis. Patients with this form of involvement reveal mesangial hypercellularity, typically variable among glomeruli and within a given glomerulus (Fig. 6-44). Usually the degrees of proliferation and matrix expansion correlate well and are mild; moderate proliferation is sometimes encountered, but severe mesangial proliferation is rare. In instances where matrix and cellularity are disproportionate, matrix expansion usually predominates. Segmental endocapillary proliferation is unusual, and diffuse endocapillary proliferation is apparently unrecognized to date. Mixed patterns in which mild mesangial hypercellularity is associated with "hepatic sclerosis" sometimes occur. Finally, a lesion superficially resembling membranoproliferative glomerulonephritis is sometimes seen (Fig. 6-45). This pattern, which appears similar to the "mixed" pattern just mentioned, shows splitting of capillary walls and interposition of mesangial cells superimposed on the other features described. Splitting and mesangial interposition are much more frequently encountered in association with cirrhosis and biliary atresia than in primary IgAN [455]. Normal glomeruli are also re-

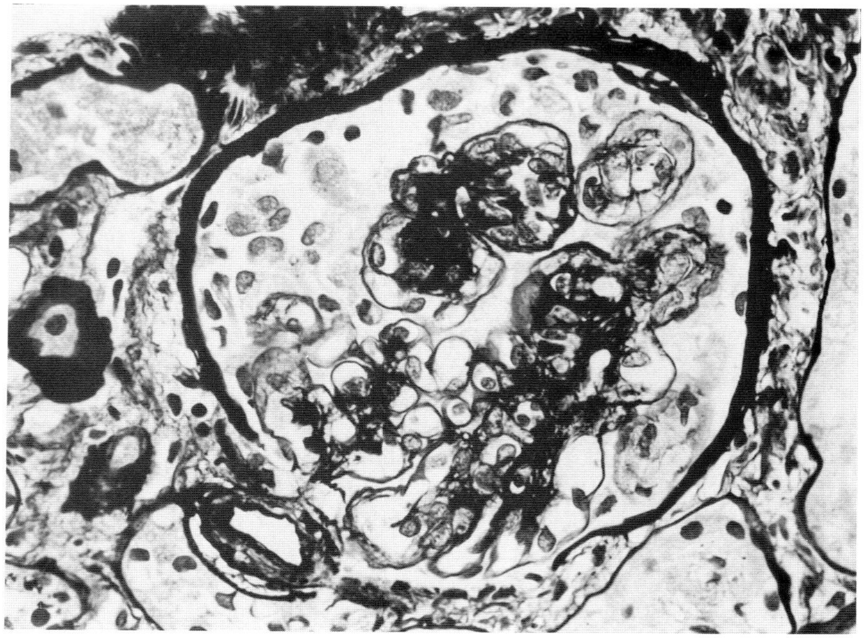

FIG. 6-43. *This glomerulus, from a patient with postnecrotic cirrhosis, reveals dense, somewhat nodular expansion of mesangial matrix. In this glomerulus, capillary walls are not thickened, but similar lesions in other patients are described in association with capillary wall thickening. Silver-methenamine;* $\times 500$.

ported in patients with cirrhosis, even if immune deposits are detected by immunofluorescence or electron microscopy. Crescents are described in association with cirrhosis but are rare; they are generally small. When crescents are present, rapid progression to renal failure can occur.

Tubules

There are few cases in which significant changes in tubules are emphasized. Nonetheless, experience at Case Western Reserve University and carefully reported series do indicate that flattening, vacuolization, and atrophy of tubules may develop in a focal pattern in patients with cirrhosis of the liver. Particularly, vacuoles that are positive with the Jones stain and focal atrophy are reported in patients with cirrhosis related to cystic fibrosis. However, it is clear that such changes are not limited to those cirrhotic patients with cystic fibrosis. Tubular casts are often seen.

Blood Vessels

Medial hypertrophy of arterioles, even in the absence of clinical hypertension, is almost a *sine qua non* in cirrhotic patients with glomerular abnormalities. Leukocytoclastic vasculitis is occasionally seen in association with cryoglobulinemia and a membranoproliferative-like pattern of glomerular injury.

Interstitium

Focal interstitial fibrosis occurs both in patients with hepatic glomerular sclerosis and with mesangial proliferative glomerulonephritis associated with cirrhosis but is much less frequent than in IgAN patients. Again, patients with cirrhosis sec-

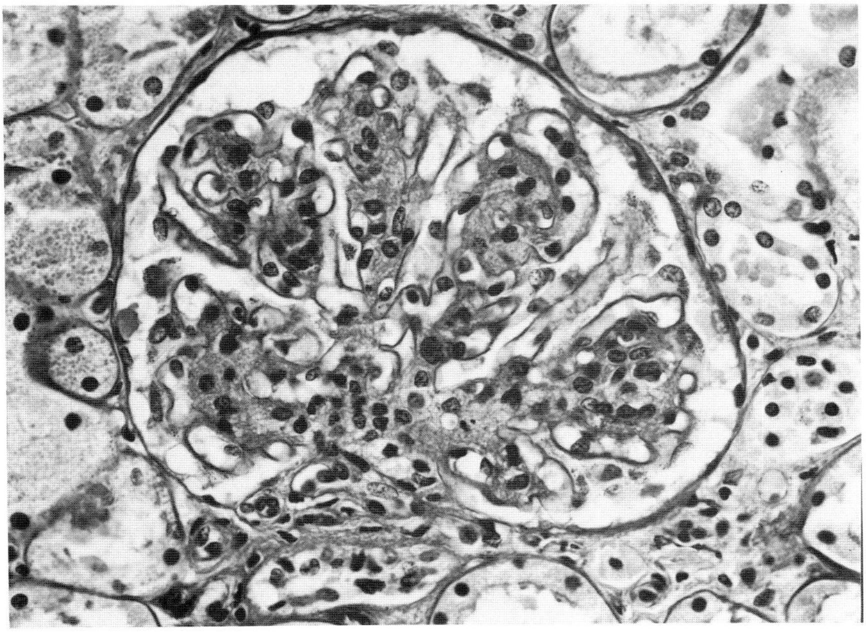

Fig. 6-44. *There is moderate to marked mesangial hypercellularity and associated matrix expansion in this glomerulus from a patient with biliary atresia and nephrotic syndrome. Although capillaries are patent, capillary walls are occasionally thickened with lucent areas, evident within the PAS-positive GBM. PAS; ×400. (Photographed from autopsy material kindly provided by Dr. R. Edwards.)*

ondary to cystic fibrosis are those with the best examples of interstitial fibrosis, but other series report small foci of fibrosis in some patients. Interstitial edema and/or leukocyte infiltrates are apparently not seen.

IMMUNOHISTOCHEMICAL FINDINGS

Glomeruli

Granular mesangial deposits of IgA are seen in approximately 70 percent of patients [3,4,37,41,52, 64,84,124,207,208,233,281,284,395,431,433, 455,464,484,490,499,529,530,535,561,566,586]. In many reports, less prominent codeposits of IgG and/or IgM and C3 are observed in some patients. Immune deposits are present in the mesangium even in patients with normal glomeruli or mild mesangial matrix expansion. These codeposits are more frequently present in patients recognized by biopsy rather than by autopsy; this is not surprising given the association with clinical expression of disease in biopsied patients. Extension of deposits to the capillary wall is seen in roughly 10 percent of patients; as expected, this takes place in those most severely affected. IgG and IgM each predominate in approximately 7 percent of cases, and 10 to 15 percent of cases reveal glomerular sclerosis without immunoglobulin deposits [52].

Fibrin is rarely encountered, but J-chain is usual. Secretory component—usually absent in cases of cirrhosis or fatty metamorphosis of the liver—is present in many patients with biliary atresia [3]. This observation suggests that in biliary atresia some of the IgA deposited represents "regurgitated" secretory IgA that reentered the circulation after secretion into the bile. Most depos-

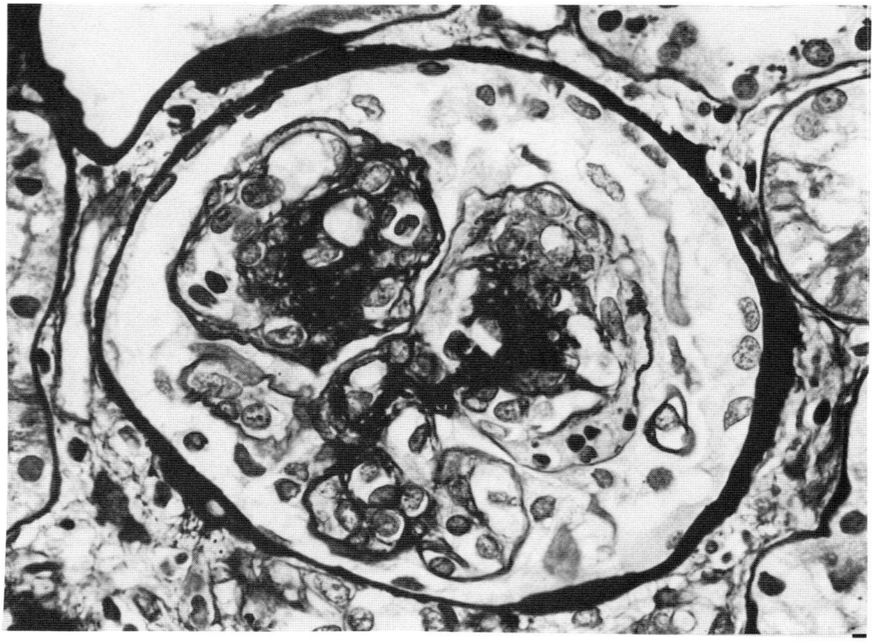

FIG. 6-45. *Hypersegmentation of glomerular capillary tufts associated with variable degrees of mesangial proliferation and splitting and duplication of glomerular capillary walls is evident in this glomerulus, from a patient with postnecrotic cirrhosis, azotemia, and microhematuria. The resemblance to membranoproliferative glomerulonephritis by light microscopy notwithstanding, this patient had marked mesangial and capillary deposition of IgA and C3 without other immunoglobulin or C1q deposits. By ultrastructural examination, extensive mesangial deposits were present in association with subendothelial and intramembranous deposits. Silver;* ×650.

its in all forms of these conditions can bind added free secretory component, suggesting that J-chain–linked dimer and multimer IgA is present. As in primary IgAN, the IgA_1 subclass predominates over IgA_2 in glomerular deposits of secondary IgAN; both light chains are present [663]. Little is known regarding deposition of other proteins, such as the membrane attack complex of complement. It is noteworthy, however, that capillary wall deposits and IgG/IgM codeposits are more frequent in clinically overt patients with histologically more severe disease; IgA deposits are equally evident in most patients, regardless of clinical status. Deposits of C1q are more frequent and conspicuous in cases of secondary IgAN than in primary IgAN [663].

Extraglomerular Sites

Deposits of immunoglobulin or complement in nonglomerular sites in the kidney or in skin are not reported. However, sinusoidal and perisinusoidal deposition of IgA in liver and occasionally IgA deposits outlining individual hepatocytes are described in alcoholic liver disease [588]. These deposits, considered specific for alcoholic liver disease, may be associated with glomerular IgA deposits, at least in patients who abuse ethanol.

ELECTRON MICROSCOPIC FINDINGS

Glomeruli

Ultrastructural examination of glomeruli corroborates the changes seen by light microscopy [52,84, 208,219,248,455,530,566,662]. Mesangial, endocapillary and/or extracapillary proliferation, mesangial matrix expansion, and capillary wall thickening may be seen. There is increased organelle content in mesangial cells in patients with mesangial hypertrophy, and long-spaced collagen is present in mesangial matrix (Fig. 6-46A). Polymerized fibrin is encountered exceptionally. Endothelial swelling may be present. Electron-dense deposits are observed in approximately 90 percent of patients (Fig. 6-46*B*). Mesangial deposits are typical, generally scattered throughout the matrix, and similar to those encountered in primary or secondary IgAN; they are found whether IgA deposits are evident by immunohistology or not. Subendothelial deposits are noted in perhaps one-fifth of cases, and intramembranous deposits are seen in one-tenth. These extramesangial deposits are generally present in glomeruli of patients with clinically evident glomerular disease. Round or ovoid lucencies (50–100 nm in diameter) containing fine osmiophilic granules have been described within the mesangial matrix by a number of investigators [208,248,530]. These symmetrical lu-

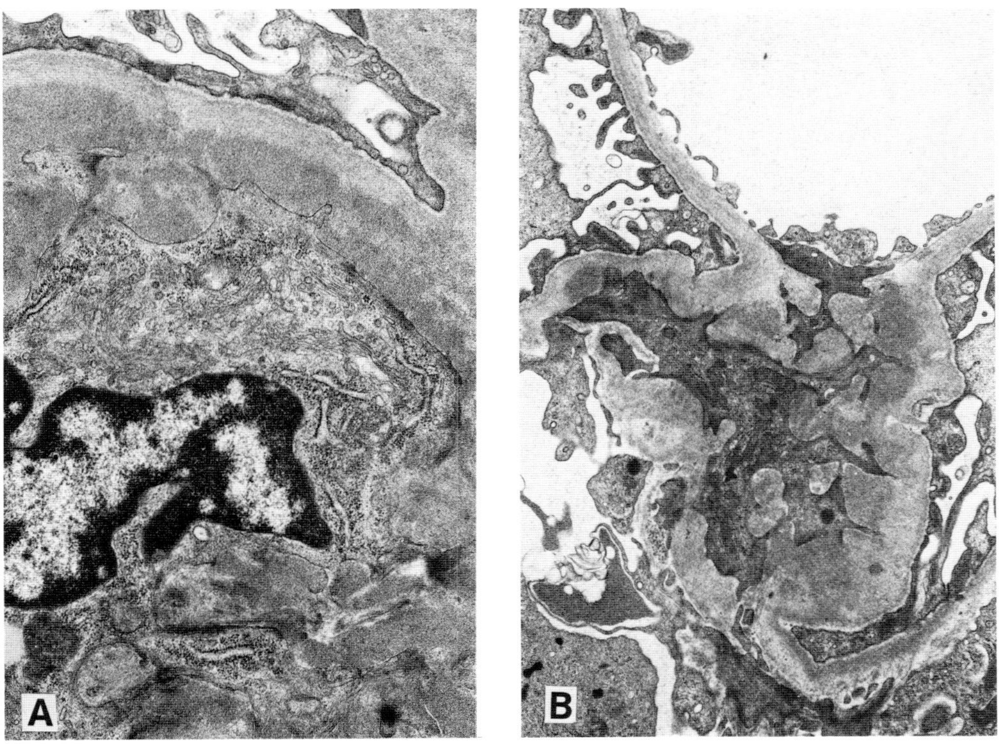

Fig. 6-46. *(A) Paramesangial electron-dense deposits and mesangial-cell hypertrophy with increased organelles, notably Golgi and rough endoplasmic reticulum, are seen with epithelial foot-process fusion. (B) Mesangial matrix expansion and paramesangial electron-dense deposits are present in association with electron-dense deposits deeper within the mesangial matrix. Podocytes are discrete, and the lamellated GBM is devoid of deposits. (A) ×15,050; (B) ×8325.*

cencies are an unusual feature encountered in patients with cirrhosis, and despite the fact that their proposed specificity for cirrhosis has been challenged, they may be of help in morphologically distinguishing these glomerular abnormalities from similar cases of IgAN or axial glomerular sclerosis.

Splitting, lamellation, and etching of glomerular capillaries, interposition of mesangial cells between layers of capillary basement membranes, duplication of the lamina densa, and irregular segmental widening of the lamina rara interna are also described in these patients (cf. Figs. 6-25 to 6-29), but none of these changes is specific.

Etiology and Pathogenesis

Much of the known etiology and pathogenesis of hepatic glomerular involvement has already been discussed in relation to secondary IgAN, and it is likely to be related to glomerular deposition of immune complexes. The liver plays a central role in the clearance of immune complexes from the circulation and in the secretion of polymeric IgA [508–510]. Although, as already discussed, impaired clearance of IgA immune complexes does not appear to be central to primary IgAN, such defects may well be the essential feature in the glomerular lesions associated with profound and protracted liver disease. Interestingly, instances in which glomerular IgA deposits precede cirrhosis are documented [69].

A substantial majority of cirrhotic patients with glomerulonephritis have circulating immune complexes rich in IgA. The immunoglobulin content of circulating immune complexes parallels glomerular deposits, and the levels of such complexes correlate with disease activity. The cryoglobulinemia so prevalent in patients with cirrhosis [52, 84,160,233,341,431,433,455,464,663] may reflect impaired immune complex clearance and serve as an indicator of mononuclear phagocyte function. Liver failure also may impair extrahepatic mononuclear phagocyte function by promoting accumulation of noxious substances; increased risk of infection in such patients, particularly alcoholics, may be evidence of this effect.

The hypocomplementemia frequently seen in patients with liver failure may be consequent to consumption of complement by fixation mediated by the accumulated immune complexes [12,84, 336,433,455,464,586,663]. On the other hand, since the liver is a major synthetic source of complement components, hypocomplementemia also may arise directly from liver failure. Since complement is an important element in the "detoxification" and clearance of immune complexes by several mechanisms (reviewed in ref. 181), hypocomplementemia may be a cause of cryogobulinemia and increased levels of immune complexes in the circulation. Functional portocaval shunts in cirrhotics may, furthermore, allow intestine-derived immune complexes or antigens to bypass normal hepatic clearance mechanisms. Immune complexes forming in the gut and entering the portal circulation might therefore escape hepatic surveillance.

Although hepatocyte-mediated transport of polymeric immunoglobulins in man is minimal, significant biliary transport is well documented [74,508–510]. Although believed minor compared with enteric transport, biliary transport of dimeric and oligomeric IgA may be important, and failure of this system may underlie accumulations of polymeric IgA in serum and kidneys [179,245,413]. In addition, sustained severe liver injury is likely to elicit heightened hepatic production of transforming growth factor β [15]. This potent cytokine is the most powerful known stimulus for IgA synthesis and secretion by plasma cells and can increase production of polymeric IgA dramatically [103]. As already discussed (under IgA as an Epiphenomenon), increased polymeric IgA can promote accentuated glomerular immune complex deposition by several distinct but related mechanisms.

In addition to impaired hepatic and extrahepatic clearance of immune complexes, diminished transport of polymeric IgA, and potentially enhanced polyclonal IgA production, it is likely that cirrhosis and the other hepatic diseases discussed here may promote increased penetration of the gut by a variety of commensal microorganisms and dietary antigens [137,536,541,669]. Increased production of antibodies to dietary and intestinal flora antigens is well documented in patients. The levels of these antibodies correlate with the severity of clinical disease. Cirrhosis or the underlying disease, such as alcoholism, also may promote penetration of immune complexes from the gut back into the systemic circulation. This does not appear to be a major factor in the associated glomerulopathies, however, because such complexes would contain secretory IgA, which is rarely deposited in glomeruli. An exception is biliary atresia, wherein the secretory IgA is likely to reflux from the chylous ducts rather than the gut [3].

A final curiosity is the potential contribution of abnormal lipid metabolism to glomerular disease [284]. Lucent mesangial deposits with punctate osmiophilic granules, similar to those which occur in cirrhotic patients, are seen in patients with lecithin : cholesterol acyltransferase (LCAT) deficiency (see Chap. 29). The potential relationship is intensified by cognizance that the propensity for membranoproliferative-like changes in glomeruli from patients with chronic liver disease mirrors the membranoproliferative-like lesion that develops in patients with familial (type II) hyperlipidemia. Obviously, we are as yet too ignorant of lipid-mesangial interactions to move beyond speculation in this regard.

Clinical Outcome

In part because of the severity of the underlying liver disease and the dominance of liver function in determining prognosis, little information is available regarding the renal disease. Few patients have evidence of glomerular dysfunction, and although progression to renal insufficiency is rare, it does occur [52,234,464]. In contrast to the more severe involvement encountered in Schönlein-Henoch syndrome patients, clinical and pathologic expression of glomerular IgA deposits in patients with hepatobiliary disease is milder than in patients with IgAN. Most patients who have any signs of illness at all have intermittent microhematuria and sometimes low-grade proteinuria.

Estimates suggest that in a relatively unselected (autopsy) population, 75 percent of patients with severe liver disease are clinically silent in terms of renal involvement, whereas among patients undergoing renal biopsy for clinically overt glomerular disease, 55 percent have impairment of renal function, which is generally mild. Most have normal glomeruli or mild expansion of mesangial matrix histologically. Although Berger reported no correlation between renal function and glomerular morphology, a membranoproliferative pattern and/or more severe glomerular changes were associated with renal insufficiency by others [52, 124,219,233,431,433,464,490,561,586]. Moreover, IgA deposits and capillary wall immune deposits are significantly more frequent in patients with hematuria and/or proteinuria. Long-term follow-up of patients with glomerulonephritis secondary to hepatobiliary disease is limited, partly because clinical signs are seldom apparent.

In summary, since it appears that the clinical and pathologic features in cirrhosis-associated glomerulopathy are very similar—if not identical—to primary and secondary IgAN, the overall prognosis would be expected to be similar. Since the clinical course is one of slow progression over 20 years, with only a small percentage of patients developing renal failure each year, the patient's outcome is generally determined by the hepatic disease. As Newell [459] admonished, however, recognition of glomerulonephritis associated with cirrhosis, biliary atresia, and severe fatty metamorphosis of the liver is important because it may spare the patient renal biopsy or other invasive procedures. This must not, however, be construed as contraindication to renal biopsy of cirrhotic patients with renal disease.

REFERENCES

1. Abe, S., Anagasaki, Y., Iyori, S., Konishi, K., Kato, E., and Sakaguchi, H. Significance of tubulointerstitial lesions in biopsy specimens of glomerulonephritic patients. *Am. J. Nephrol.* 9: 30, 1989.
2. Abe, T., Kida, H., Yoshimura, M., Yokoyama, H., Koshino, Y., Tomosugi, N., and Hattori, N. Participation of extracapillary lesions in progression of IgA nephropathy. *Clin. Nephrol.* 25:37, 1986.
3. Abramowsky, C. R., and Christiansen, D. M. Secretory immunoglobulin deposits in renal glomeruli of children with extrahepatic biliary atresia: Studies in a human counterpart of experimen-

tal ligation of the bile ducts. *Hum. Pathol.* 18: 1126, 1987.

4. Abramowsky, C. R., Dahms, B. B., and Swinehart, G. L. IgA-associated glomerular deposits in liver disease. *Hum. Pathol.* 16:1243, 1985.
5. Abuelo, J. G., Esparza, A. R., Matarese, R. A., Endreny, R. G., Carvalho, J. S., and Allegra, S. R. Crescentic IgA nephropathy. *Medicine (Baltimore)* 63:396, 1984.
6. Ackroyd, J. F. Allergic purpura, including purpura due to foods, drugs and infections. *Am. J. Med.* 14:605, 1953.
7. Adachi, M., Yodoi, J., Masuda, T., Takatsuki, T., and Uchino, H. Altered expression of lymphocyte Fcα receptor in selective IgA deficiency and IgA nephropathy. *J. Immunol.* 131:1246, 1983.
8. Alexander, F., Barabas, A. Z., and Jack, R. G. J. IgA nephropathy. *Hum. Pathol.* 8:173, 1977.
9. Alexopoulos, E., Seron, D., Hartley, R.B., Nolasco, F., and Cameron, J. S. The role of interstitial infiltrates in IgA nephropathy: A study with monoclonal antibodies. *Nephrol. Dial. Transplant.* 4:187, 1989.
10. Allen, D. M., Diamond, L. K., and Howell, D. A. Anaphylactoid purpura in children (Schönlein-Henoch syndrome): Review with a follow-up of the renal complications. *Am. J. Dis. Child.* 99:833, 1960.
11. Amore, A., Emancipator, S. N., Coppo, R., Roccatello, D., Quattrocchio, G., Maffei, S., Habib, R. B., Lamm, M. E., and Piccoli, G. Specific binding of gliadin to rat mesangial cells in culture (Abstract). *Nephrol. Dial. Transplant.* 16: 54, 1988.
12. André, F., and André, C. Cirrhotic glomerulonephritis and secretory immunoglobulin A. *Lancet* 1:197, 1976.
13. André, C., Berthoux, F. C., André, F., Gillon, J., Genin, C., and Sabatier, J. C. Prevalence of IgA_2 deposits in IgA nephropathies: A clue to their pathogenesis. *N. Engl. J. Med.* 303:1343, 1980.
14. Andreoli, S. P., Yum, M. N., and Bergstein, J. M. IgA nephropathy in children: Significance of basement membrane deposition of IgA. *Am. J. Nephrol.* 6:28, 1986.
15. Armendariz-Borunda, J., Seyer, J. M., Kang, A. H., and Raghow, R. Regulation of TGFβ gene expression in rat liver intoxicated with carbon tetrachloride. *FASEB J.* 4:215, 1990.
16. Arnaiz-Villena, A., Gonzalo, A., Mampaso, F., Teruel, J. L., and Ortunno, J. HLA and IgA nephropathy in Spanish population. *Tissue Antigens* 17:549, 1981.
17. Asamer, H., Wohlfarth, B., Schabel, F., Stühlinger, W., and Dittrich, P. Klinik und Immunologie des Schoenlein-Henoch Syndroms. *Schweiz. Med. Wochenschr.* 104:1188, 1974.
18. Aucouturier, P., Monteiro, R. C., Noel, L. H., Preud'homme, J. L., and Lesavre, P. Glomerular and serum immunoglobulin G subclasses in IgA nephropathy. *Clin. Immunol. Immunopathol.* 51: 338, 1989.
19. Austin, H. A., and Balow, J. E. Henoch-Schönlein nephritis: Prognostic features and the challenge of therapy. *Am. J. Kidney Dis.* 2:512, 1983.
20. Ayoub, E. M., and Hoyer, J. Anaphylactoid purpura: Streptococcal antibody titers and beta C1 globulin levels. *J. Pediatr.* 75:193, 1969.
21. Baart de la Faille-Kuyper, E. H., Kater, L., Kooiker, C. J., and Dorhout Mees, E. J. IgA deposits in cutaneous blood vessel walls and mesangium in Henoch-Schönlein syndrome. *Lancet* 1:892, 1973.
22. Baart de la Faille-Kuyper, E. H., Kater, L., Kuijten, R. H., Kooiker, C. J., Wagenaar, S. S., van der Zowen, P., and Dorhout Mees, E. J. Occurrence of vascular IgA deposits in clinically normal skin of patients with renal disease. *Kidney Int.* 9:424, 1976.
23. Baart de la Faille-Kuyper, E. H., Van der Meer, J. B., Kater, L., and Mul, N. Alternate-pathway complement activation of IgA in Schönlein-Henoch syndrome. *Neth. J. Med.* 17:5, 1974.
24. Bachman, U., Biava, C., Amend, W., Fedicska, N., Melzer, J., Salvatierra, O., and Vincenti, F. The clinical course of IgA nephropathy and Henoch-Schönlein purpura following renal transplantation. *Transplantation* 42:511, 1986.
25. Baehr, G., and Lande, H. Glomerulonephritis as a complication of subacute streptococcus endocarditis. *JAMA* 75:789, 1920.
26. Bailey, R. R., Burry, A. F., McGiven, A. R., Kirk, J. A., Laing, J. K., and Moller, P. A renal lesion in ankylosing spondylitis. *Nephron* 26:171, 1980.
27. Baliah, T., Kim, K. H., Anthone, S., Anthone, R., Montes, M., and Andres, G. A. Recurrence of Henoch-Schönlein purpura (HSP) glomerulonephritis in transplanted kidney. *Transplantation* 18:343, 1974.
28. Ballard, H. S., Eisinger, R. P., and Gallo, G. Renal manifestations of the Henoch-Schoenlein syndrome in adults. *Am. J. Med.* 49:328, 1970.
29. Ballardie, F. W., Brenchley, P. E., Williams, S., and O'Donoghue, D. J. Autoimmunity in IgA nephropathy. *Lancet* 2:588, 1988.
30. Bani, E., Bracci, M. A., Bertelli, L., Biver, P., and Federighi, F. Controllo a distanza di 62 bambini con sindrome de Schönlein-Henoch. *Minerva Pediatr.* 35:911, 1983.
31. Bannister, K. M., Drew, P. A., Clarkson, A. R., and Woodroffe, A. J. Immunoregulation in glomerulonephritis, Henoch-Schönlein purpura and lupus nephritis. *Clin. Exp. Immunol.* 53:384,

1983.

32. Barbiano di Belgiojoso, G. B., Mazzucco, G., Casanova, S., Radaelli, L., Monga, G., and Minetti, L. Steroid-sensitive nephrotic syndrome with mesangial IgA deposits: A separate entity? Observation of two cases. *Am. J. Nephrol.* 6:141, 1986.
33. Bardpare, M., Gaboardi, F., and Barbiano di Belgiojoso, G. Die glomerulonephritis beim Schoenlein-Henoch-Syndrom in Kindesalter. *Helv. Paediatr. Acta* 30:297, 1975.
34. Bar-on, H., and Rosenmann, E. Schoenlein-Henoch syndrome in adults: A clinical and histological study of renal involvement. *Isr. J. Med. Sci.* 8:1702, 1972.
35. Bartoli, E., Bosincu, L., Costanzi, G., Denti, S., Olmeo, N. A., and Soggia, G. IgA pseudo-linear deposits in glomerular basement membranes in dermatitis herpetiformis. *Am. J. Clin. Pathol.* 78:377, 1982.
36. Bates, R. C., Jennings, R. B., and Earle, D. P. Acute nephritis unrelated to group A hemolytic streptococcus infection: Report of 10 cases. *Am. J. Med.* 23:510, 1957.
37. Baxter, J. H., and Ashworth, C. T. Renal lesions in portal cirrhosis. *Arch. Pathol.* 41:476, 1946.
38. Beale, M. G., Nash, G. S., Bertovich, J., and MacDermott, R. P. Similar disturbances in B-cell activity and regulatory T-cell function in Henoch-Schönlein purpura and systemic lupus erythematosus. *J. Immunol.* 128:486, 1982.
39. Belman, A. L., Leicher, C. R., Moehé, S. L., and Mezey, A. P. Neurologic manifestations of Schönlein-Henoch purpura: Report of three cases and review of the literature. *Pediatrics* 75:687, 1985.
40. Belton, P., Carmody, M., Donohue, J., and O'-Dwyer, W. F. IgA nephropathy (Berger's disease): A clinical study of 32 cases. *Ir. J. Med. Sci.* 149:310, 1980.
41. Bene, M. C., De Korwin, J. D., Hurault de Ligny, B., Aymard, B., Kesler, M., and Faure, G. G. IgA nephropathy and alcoholic liver cirrhosis. *Am. J. Clin. Pathol.* 89:769, 1988.
42. Bene, M. C., and Faure, G. G. Composition of mesangial deposits in IgA nephropathy: Complement factors. *Nephron* 46:219, 1987.
43. Bene, M. C., and Faure, G. G. Berger's disease: Recent advances in immunology and genetics. *Adv. Nephrol.* 16:281, 1987.
44. Bene, M. C., Faure, G., and Duheille, J. IgA nephropathy: Characterization of the polymeric nature of mesangial deposits by in vitro binding of free secretory component. *Clin. Exp. Immunol.* 47:527, 1982.
45. Bene, M. C., Hurault de Ligny, B., Faure, G., Kessler, M., and Duheille, J. Histochemical discrepancies in primary IgA nephropathy and anaphylactoid purpura sustain relationships between mucosa and kidney. *Nephron* 43:214, 1986.
46. Bennett, W. M., and Kincaid-Smith, P. Macroscopic hematuria in mesangial IgA nephropathy: Correlation with glomerular crescents and renal dysfunction. *Kidney Int.* 23:393, 1983.
47. Bennett, W. M., Nicholls, K., and Kincaid-Smith, P. Clinicopathological associations in mesangial IgA nephropathy. *Am. J. Nephrol.* 7: 166, 1987.
48. Bennett, W. M., Walker, R. G., and Kincaid-Smith, P. Treatment of IgA nephropathy with eicosapentanoic acid: A two-year prospective trial. *Clin. Nephrol.* 31:128, 1989.
49. Berger, J. IgA glomerular deposits in renal disease. *Transplant. Proc.* 1:939, 1969.
50. Berger, J., and Hinglais, N. Les dépôts intercapillaires d'IgA-IgG. *J. Urol. Nephrol.* 74:694, 1968.
51. Berger, J., Yaneva, H., and Hinglais, N. Immunochemistry of glomerulonephritis. *Adv. Nephrol.* 1:11, 1971.
52. Berger, J., Yaneva, H., and Nabarra, B. Glomerular changes in patients with cirrhosis of the liver. *Adv. Nephrol.* 7:3, 1978.
53. Berger, J., Yaneva, H., Nabarra, B., and Barbanel, C. Recurrence of mesangial deposition after renal transplantation. *Kidney Int.* 7:232, 1975.
54. Bergstrand, A., Bergstrand, C. G., and Bucht, H. Kidney lesions associated with anaphylactoid purpura in children. *Acta Paediatr. (Stockh.)* 49:57, 1960.
55. Bernhardt, J. P., Chatelanat, F., and Veyrat, R. Le syndrome de Schönlein-Henoch chez l'adulte: Étude clinique de 16 cas, examen histologique du rein dans 7 cas. *Schweiz. Med. Wochenschr.* 37: 1228, 1966.
56. Berthoux, F. C., Genin, C., Gagne, A., Le Petit, J. C., and Sabatier, J. C. HLA-Bw35 antigen and mesangial IgA glomerulonephritis: A poor prognosis marker? *Proc. Eur. Dial. Transplant. Assoc.* 16:551, 1979.
57. Berthoux, F. C., Laurent, B., le Petit, J. C., Genin, C., Broutin, F., Touraine, F., Hassan, A. A., and Champailler, A. Immunogenetics and immunopathology of human primary membranous glomerulonephritis: HLA-A, B, DR antigens; functional activity of splenic macrophage Fc-receptors and peripheral blood T-lymphocyte subpopulations. *Clin. Nephrol.* 22:15, 1984.
58. Berthoux, F. C., Sabatier, J. C., Genin, C., Gonthier, R., and Toulon, J. Comparative Renal Status at Time of Initial and Five-Years-Later Renal Biopsies in Mesangial IgA Glomerulonephritis. In *Abstracts of the International Congress of Nephrology.* 1984. P. 71.
59. Beukhof, J. R., Kardaun, O., Ockhuizen, T., and

van der Hem, G. K. Kidney survival in IgA nephropathy: Multiple regression analysis of genetically differing subpopulations; is IgA nephropathy a real disease entity? *Semin. Nephrol.* 7:367, 1987.
60. Beukhof, J. R., Kardaun, O., Schaafsma, W., Poortema, K., Donker, A. J. M., Hoedemaeker, P. J., and van der Hem, G. K. Toward individual prognosis of IgA nephropathy. *Kidney Int.* 29:549, 1986.
61. Beukhof, J. R., Ockhuizen, T., Halie, L. M., Westra, J., Beelen, J. M., Donker, A. J. M., Hoedemaeker, P. J., and van der Hem, G. K. Subentities within adult primary IgA-nephropathy. *Clin. Nephrol.* 22:195, 1984.
62. Bignon, J. D., Houssin, A., Soulillon, J. P., Denis, J., Guimbretiere, J., and Guenel, J. HLA antigens and Berger's disease. *Tissue Antigens* 16:108, 1980.
63. Blazer, S., Alon, U., Berant, M., and Korman, S. H. Henoch-Schönlein syndrome—Paucity of renal disease. *Isr. J. Med. Sci.* 17:41, 1981.
64. Bloodworth, J. M. B., and Sommers, S. C. "Cirrhotic glomerulosclerosis," a renal lesion associated with hepatic cirrhosis. *Lab. Invest.* 8:962, 1959.
65. Bodian, M., Black, J. A., Kobayashi, N., Lake, B. D., and Shuler, S. E. Recurrent haematuria in childhood. *Q. J. Med.* 34:359, 1965.
66. Border, W. A. Nephrology forum: Distinguishing minimal-change disease from mesangial disorders. *Kidney Int.* 34:419, 1988.
67. Border, W. A., Baehler, R. W., Bhathena, D., and Glassock, R. J. IgA anti-basement membrane nephritis with pulmonary hemorrhage. *Ann. Intern. Med.* 91:21, 1979.
68. Border, W. A., Okuda, S., Languino, L. R., and Ruoslahti, E. Transforming growth factor β regulates production of proteoglycans by mesangial cells. *Kidney Int.* 37:689, 1990.
69. Borglin, M., and Pecchini, F. IgA nephropathy preceding liver cirrhosis. *Clin. Nephrol.* 24:213, 1985.
70. Boyce, N. W., Holdsworth, S. R., Thomson, N. M., and Atkins, R. C. Clinicopathological associations in mesangial IgA nephropathy. *Am. J. Nephrol.* 6:246, 1986.
71. Braden, G., Rastegar, A., Hession, J., Garb, J., Siegel, N., Fitzgibbons, J., and Kashgarian, M. Predictors of progression to chronic renal failure (CRF) in idiopathic membranous glomerulonephritis (MG) (Abstract). *Kidney Int.* 33:183, 1988.
72. Brettle, R., and Peters, D. K. Mesangial IgA glomerulonephritis and HLA antigens. *N. Engl. J. Med.* 299:200, 1978.
73. Brown, A. M., Lally, E. T., Frankel, A., Harwick, R., Davis, L. W., and Rominger, C. J. The association of the IgA levels of serum and whole saliva with the progression of oral cancer. *Cancer* 35:1154, 1975.
74. Brown, T. A., Russell, M. W., and Mestecky, J. Hepatobiliary transport of IgA immune complexes: Molecular and cellular aspects. *J. Immunol.* 128:2183, 1982.
75. Brun, D., Bryld, C., Fenger, L., and Jørgensen, F. Glomerular lesions in adults with the Schönlein-Henoch syndrome: A light and electron microscopy study. *Acta Pathol. Microbiol. Scand.* [A] 79:569, 1971.
76. Bruneau, C., Villiaumey, J., Avouac, B., Martigny, J., Laurent, J., Pichot, A., Belghiti, D., and Lagrue, G. Seronegative spondyloarthropathies and IgA glomerulonephritis: A report of four cases and a review of the literature. *Semin. Arthritis Rheum.* 15:179, 1986.
77. Burke, E. C., Mills, S. D., and Stickler, G. B. Nephritis associated with anaphylactoid purpura in childhood: Clinical observations and prognosis. *Proc. Mayo Clin.* 35:641, 1960.
78. Burkholder, P. M., Zimmerman, S. W., and Moorthy, A. V. A Clinicopathologic Study of the Natural History of Mesangial IgA Nephropathy. In Y. Yoshitoshi and Y. Ueda (Eds.), *Glomerulonephritis: Progression and Regression: Proceedings of the International Symposium on Glomerulonephritis.* Baltimore: University Park Press, 1978. P. 143.
79. Byrn, J. R., Fitzgerald, J. F., Northway, J. D., Anand, S. K., and Scott, J. R. Unusual manifestations of Henoch-Schönlein syndrome. *Am. J. Dis. Child.* 130:1335, 1976.
80. Bywaters, E. G. L., Isdale, I., and Kempton, J. J. Schönlein-Henoch purpura: Evidence for a group A beta-haemolytic streptococcal aetiology. *Q. J. Med.* 26:161, 1957.
81. Cagnoli, L., Beltrandi, E., Pasquali, S., Biasi, R., Casadei-Maldini, M., Rossi, L., and Zucchelli, P. B and T cell abnormalities in patients with primary IgA nephropathy. *Kidney Int.* 28:646, 1985.
82. Cairns, S. A., London, A., and Mallick, N. P. Circulating immune complexes following food: Delayed clearance in idiopathic glomerulonephritis. *J. Clin. Lab. Immunol.* 6:121, 1981.
83. Cairns, S. A., Mallick, N. P., Lawler, W., and Williams, G. Squamous carcinoma of the bronchus presenting with Henoch-Schönlein purpura. *Br. Med. J.* 2:474, 1978.
84. Callard, P., Feldmann, G., Prandi, D., Belair, M. F., Mandet, C., Weiss, Y., Druet, P., Benhamou, J. P., and Bariety, J. Immune complex type glomerulonephritis in cirrhosis of the liver. *Am. J. Pathol.* 80:329, 1975.
85. Callis, L., Vilalta, R., Fortuny, G., Castello, F., and Guardia, I. Long-term control of 55 children with nephropathy secondary to Schönlein-

Henoch purpura. *Bol. Med. Hosp. Infant Mex.* 41:219, 1984.
86. Cameron, J. S. Henoch-Schönlein purpura: Clinical presentation. *Contrib. Nephrol.* 40:246, 1984.
87. Cameron, J. S., and Turner, D. R. Recurrent glomerulonephritis in allografted kidneys. *Clin. Nephrol.* 7:47, 1977.
88. Camerone, G., Garelli, S., Valbonesi, M., and Mosconi, L. Plasma exchange treatment in a patient with severe Schönlein-Henoch purpura. *Minerva Med.* 18:1185, 1982.
89. Casanueva, B., Rodriguez-Valverde, V., Merino, J., Arias, M., and Garcia-Fuentes, M. Increased IgA-producing cells in the blood of patients with active Henoch-Schönlein purpura. *Arthritis Rheum.* 26:854, 1983.
90. Case records of the Massachusetts General Hospital. Weekly cliniopathological exercises: Case 14—1980. *N. Engl. J. Med.* 302:853, 1980.
91. Chan, M. K., Kwan, S. Y. C., Chan, K. W., and Yeung, C. K. Controlled trial of antiplatelet agents in mesangial IgA glomerulonephritis. *Am. J. Kidney Dis.* 9:417, 1987.
92. Chan, S. H., Ku, G., and Sinniah, R. HLA and Chinese IgA mesangial glomerulonephritis. *Tissue Antigens* 17:351, 1981.
93. Chatenoud, L., and Bach, M. A. Abnormalities of T-cell subsets in glomerulonephritis and systemic lupus erythematosus. *Kidney Int.* 20:267, 1981.
94. Chen, A., Wong, S. S., and Rifai, A. Glomerular immune deposits in experimental IgA nephropathy: A continuum of circulating and in situ formed immune complexes. *Am. J. Pathol.* 130: 216, 1988.
95. Chiappo, G. F., Mignone, F. Oggero, R., Licata, D., and Cordero, A. Complicanze renali nella sindrome di Schoenlein-Henoch in età pediatrica. *Minerva Pediatr.* 30:1933, 1978.
96. Chida, Y., Tomura, S., and Takeuchi, J. Renal survival rate of IgA nephropathy. *Nephron* 40:189, 1985.
97. Clarkson, A. R. (Ed.). *IgA Nephropathy.* Boston: Martinus Nijhoff, 1987.
98. Clarkson, A. R., Seymour, A. E., Thompson, A. J., Haynes, W. D. G., Chan, Y.-L., and Jackson, B. IgA nephropathy: A syndrome of uniform morphology, diverse clinical features, and uncertain prognosis. *Clin. Nephrol.* 8:459, 1977.
99. Clarkson, A. R., Seymour, A. E., Woodroffe, A. J., McKenzie, P. E., Chan, Y.-L., and Wooton, A. M. Controlled trial of phenytoin therapy in IgA nephropathy. *Clin. Nephrol.* 13:215, 1980.
100. Clarkson, A. R., and Woodroffe, A. J. Therapeutic perspectives in mesangial IgA nephropathy. *Contrib. Nephrol.* 40:187, 1984.
101. Clarkson, A. R., Woodroffe, A. J., Bannister, K. M., Lomax-Smith, J. D., and Aarons, I. The syndrome of IgA nephropathy. *Clin. Nephrol.* 21:7, 1984.
102. Cockrell, J. L., Steffe, L. A., and Chan, J. C. M. Anaphylactoid purpura: Hypertension with minimal urinary abnormalities. *Int. J. Pediatr. Nephrol.* 5:167, 1974.
103. Coffman, R. L., Lebman, D. A., and Shrader, B. Transforming growth factor β specifically enhances IgA production by lipopolysaccharide-stimulated murine B lymphocytes. *J. Exp. Med.* 170:1039, 1989.
104. Cohen, A. J., and Rosenstein, E. D. IgA nephropathy associated with disseminated tuberculosis. *Arch. Intern. Med.* 145:554, 1985.
105. Cohen, R. S., Rissell, M. T., Dickey, L. E., Schwartz, M. M., and Roberts, J. L. Properties of IgA Isolated from Serum of Patients with IgA Glomerulopathy. In *Abstracts of the IXth International Congress of Nephrology.* 1984. P. 274.
106. Cole, B. R., Brockleband, J. T., Kienstra, R. A., Kissane, J. M., and Robson, A. M. "Pulse" methylprednisolone therapy in the treatment of severe glomerulonephritis. *J. Pediatr.* 88:307, 1976.
107. Conley, M. E., Cooper, M. D., and Michael, A. F. Selective deposition of IgA_1 in IgA nephropathy, anaphylactoid purpura nephritis, and systemic lupus erythematosus. *J. Clin. Invest.* 66: 1432, 1980.
108. Conley, M. E., and Delacroix, D. L. Intravascular and mucosal immunoglobulin A: Two separate but related systems of immune defense? *Ann. Intern. Med.* 106:892, 1987.
109. Copley, J. B., and Hasbargen, J. A. "Idiopathic" hematuria: A prospective evaluation. *Arch. Intern. Med.* 147:434, 1987.
110. Coppo, R., Basolo, B., Martina, G., Rollino, C., DeMarchi, M., Giacchino, F., Mazzucco, G., Messina, M., and Piccoli, G. Circulating immune complexes containing IgA, IgG, and IgM in patients with primary IgA nephropathy and with Henoch-Schönlein nephritis. Correlation with clinical and histologic signs of activity. *Clin. Nephrol.* 18:230, 1982.
111. Coppo, R., Basolo, B., Mazzucco, G., Bulzomi, M. R., Roccatello, D., Messina, M., Barbiano, G., Martina, G., Rollino, C., and Piccoli, G. IgA_1 and IgA_2 in circulating immune complexes and in renal deposits of Berger's and Schönlein-Henoch glomerulonephritis. *Proc. Eur. Dial. Transplant. Assoc.* 19:648, 1982.
112. Coppo, R., Basolo, B., Piccoli, G., Mazzucco, G., Bulzomi, M. R., Roccatello, D., De Marchi, M., Carbonara, A. O., and Barbiano di Belgiojoso, G. IgA_1 and IgA_2 immune complexes in

primary IgA nephropathy and Henoch-Schönlein nephritis. *Clin. Exp. Immunol.* 57:583, 1984.
113. Coppo, R., Basolo, B., Rollino, C., Roccatello, D., Martina, G., Amore, A., Bongiorno, G., and Piccoli, G. Mediterranean diet and primary IgA nephropathy. *Clin. Nephrol.* 26:72, 1986.
114. Coppo, R., De Marchi, M., Aprato, A., Roccatello, D., Messina, M., Segoloni, G., Camussi, G., Alloatti, S., Giacchino, F., Carbonara, A. D., Vercellone, A., and Piccoli, G. A new test for IgA containing immune complexes or aggregated IgA: Its application to Berger and Schönlein-Henoch nephritis. *Proc. Eur. Dial. Transplant. Assoc.* 17:667, 1980.
115. Coppo, R., Roccatello, D., Basolo, B., Giachino, O., Lajolo, D., Martina, G., Rollino, C., Amore, A., Costa, M., and Piccoli, G. Immunological monitoring of plasma exchange in primary IgA nephropathy. *Artif. Organs* 9:351, 1985.
116. Cosio, F. G., Lam, S., Folami, A. O., Conley, M. E., and Michael, A. F. Immune regulation of immunoglobulin production in IgA nephropathy. *Clin. Immunol. Immunopathol.* 23:430, 1982.
117. Costa, R. A., Droz, D., and Noel, L. H. Long-standing spontaneous clinical remission and glomerular improvement in primary IgA nephropathy (Berger's disease). *Am. J. Nephrol.* 7:440, 1987.
118. Counahan, R., and Cameron, J. S. Henoch-Schönlein nephritis. *Contrib. Nephrol.* 7:143, 1977.
119. Counahan, R., Winterborn, M. H., White, R. H. R., Heaton, J. M., Meadow, S. R., Bluett, N. H., Swetschin, H., Cameron, J. S., and Chantler, C. Prognosis of Henoch-Schönlein nephritis in children. *Br. Med. J.* 2:11, 1977.
120. Cream, J. J. Cryoglobulins in vasculitis. *Clin. Exp. Immunol.* 10:117, 1972.
121. Cream, J. J., Gumpel, J. M., and Peachey, R. D. G. Schönlein-Henoch purpura in the adult: A study of 77 adults with anaphylactoid or Schönlein-Henoch purpura. *Q. J. Med.* 39:461, 1970.
122. Croker, B. P., Dawson, D. V., and Sanfilippo, F. IgA nephropathy: Correlation of clinical and histologic features. *Lab. Invest.* 48:19, 1983.
123. Crosnier, J., Mery, J. P., de Montera, J., Zaltman, S., and Rueff, B. Sur un syndrome associant une glomérulite segmentaire nécrotique at une pneumopathie hémoptoïque avec alvéolite hémorrhagique. *J. Urol. Nephrol. (Paris)* 68:569, 1962.
124. Crowson, C. N., and More, R. H. Glomerulotubular nephrosis correlated with hepatic lesions: II. Incidence and morphology of associated kidney and liver lesions in human autopsy material. *Arch. Pathol.* 60:73, 1955.
125. Cutz, E., Moroz, S. P., Balfe, J. W., and Sass-Kortsak, A. Glomerulonephritis in patients with cirrhosis of liver associated with alpha-1-antitrypsin (AIAT) deficiency. *Am. J. Pathol.* 74:12a, 1974.
126. Czerkinsky, C. M., Koopman, W. J., Jackson, S., Collins, J. S., Crago, S. S., Schrohenloer, R. E., Julian, B. A., Galla, J. H., and Mestecky, J. Circulating immune complexes and immunoglobulin A rheumatoid factor in patients with mesangial immunoglobulin A nephropathies. *J. Clin. Invest.* 77:1931, 1986.
127. D'Amico, G. Idiopathic Mesangial IgA Nephropathy. In T. Bertani and G. Remuzzi (Eds.), *Glomerular Injury 300 Years After Morgagni.* Milano: Wichtig Editore, 1983. P. 205.
128. D'Amico, G. The commonest glomerulonephritis in the world: IgA nephropathy. *Q. J. Med.* 64:709, 1987.
129. D'Amico, G., Colasanti, G., Ferrario, F., Ragni, A., Cantu, P., and Giangrande, A. La glomerulonefrite a depositi mesangiali di IgA. *Minerva. Nefrol.* 24:541, 1977.
130. D'Amico, G., Ferrario, F., Colasanti, G., Ragni, A., and Bosisio, M. B. IgA-mesangial nephropathy (Berger's disease) with rapid decline in renal function. *Clin. Nephrol.* 16:251, 1981.
131. D'Amico, G., Imbasciati, E., Barbiano di Belgioioso, G., Bertoli, S., Fogazzi, G., Ferrario, F., Fellin, G., Ragni, A., Colasanti, G., Minetti, L., and Ponticelli, C. Idiopathic IgA mesangial nephropathy: Clinical and histological study of 374 patients. *Medicine (Baltimore)* 64:49, 1985.
132. D'Amico, G., Minetti, L., and Ponticelli, C. (Eds.). IgA Mesangial Nephropathy. Volume 40 in G. M. Berlyne and S. Giovannetti (Eds.), *Contributions to Nephrology.* New York: Karger, 1984.
133. D'Amico, G., Minetti, L., Ponticelli, C., Fellin, G., Ferrario, F., Barbiano di Belgioioso, G., Imbasciati, E., Ragni, A., Bertoli, S., Fogazzi, G., and Duca, G. Prognostic indicators in idiopathic IgA mesangial nephropathy. *Q. J. Med.* 59:363, 1986.
134. Danielson, H., Eriksen, E. F., Johansen, A., and Solling, J. Serum immunoglobulin sedimentation patterns and circulating immune complexes in IgA GN and Schönlein-Henoch nephritis. *Acta Med. Scand.* 215:435, 1984.
135. Davies, D. R., Tighe, J. R., Jones, N. F., and Brown, G. W. Recurrent haematuria and mesangial IgA deposition. *J. Clin. Pathol.* 26:672, 1973.
136. Davin, J. C., Foidart, J. B., and Mahieu, P. R. Relation between biological IgA abnormalities and mesangial IgA deposits in isolated hematuria in childhood. *Clin. Nephrol.* 28:73, 1987.
137. Davin, J. C., Forget, P., and Mahieu, P. R. Increased intestinal permeability to ^{51}Cr EDTA is correlated with IgA immune complex plasma levels in children with IgA-associated nephropathies. *Acta Paediatr. Scand.* 77:118, 1988.

138. Davin, J. C., Vandenbroeck, M. C., Foidart, J. B., and Mahieu, P. R. Sequential measurements of the reticulo-endothelial system function in Henoch-Schönlein disease of childhood: Correlations with various immunological parameters. *Acta Paediatr. Scand.* 74:201, 1985.
139. Davison, A. M. The United Kingdom Medical Research Council's glomerulonephritis registry. *Contrib. Nephrol.* 48:24, 1985.
140. Day, N. K., Geiger, H., McLean, R., Resnick, J., Michael, A. F., and Good, R. A. The association of respiratory infection, recurrent hematuria and focal glomerulonephritis with activation of the complement system in the cold. *J. Clin. Invest.* 52:1698, 1973.
141. Debray, J., Krulik, M., and Giorgi, M. Le purpura rhumatoïde (syndrome de Schönlein-Henoch) de l'adulte. A propos de 22 observations. *Sem. Hop. Paris* 47:1805, 1971.
142. De Coteau, W. E., Gerrard, J. W., and Cunningham, T. A. Glomerulonephritis in dermatitis herpetiformis. *Lancet* 2:679, 1973.
143. Degli-Esposti, E., Zucchelli, P., Chiarini, C., Santoro, A., Sturani, A., Zuccala, A., Cagnoli, L., Donini, U., Mandreoli, M., and Pasquali, S. Berger's nephropathy: Relationship between histological pattern, blood pressure and renin. *Proc. Eur. Dial. Transplant. Assoc.* 19:696, 1982.
144. Demaine, A. G., Rambausek, M., Knight, J. F., Williams, D. G., Welsh, K. I., and Ritz, E. Relation of mesangial IgA glomerulonephritis to polymorphism of immunoglobulin heavy chain switch region. *J. Clin. Invest.* 81:611, 1988.
145. Derham, R. J., and Rogerson, M. M. The Schönlein-Henoch syndrome with particular reference to renal sequelae. *Arch. Dis. Child.* 31:364, 1956.
146. Deteix, P., Gebuhrer, L., Arkouche, W., Ducret, F., Betuel, H., and Traeger, J. HLA Antigens and Mesangial IgA Nephropathy. In *Abstracts of the IXth International Congress of Nephrology.* 1984. P. 276.
147. de Werra, P., Morel-Maroger, L., Leroux-Robert, C., and Richet, G. Glomérulites à dépôts d'IgA diffus dans le mésangium: Etude de 96 cas chez l'adulte. *Schweiz. Med. Wochenschr.* 103:761, 1973.
148. Dobrin, R. S., Hoyer, J. R., Nevins, T. E., Sharp, H., Gentry, W. C., and Vernier, R. L. The association of familial liver disease, subepidermal immunoproteins, and membranoproliferative glomerulonephritis. *J. Pediatr.* 90:901, 1977.
149. Dobrin, R. S., Knudson, F. E., and Michael, A. F. The secretory immune system and renal disease. *Clin. Exp. Immunol.* 21:318, 1975.
150. Dodge, W. F., Daeschner, C. W., Jr., Brennan, J. C., Rosenberg, H. S., Travis, L. B., and Hopps, H. C. Percutaneous renal biopsy in children: II. Acute glomerulonephritis, chronic glomerulonephritis, and nephritis of anaphylactoid purpura. *Pediatrics* 30:297, 1962.
151. Doi, T., Kanatsu, K., Nagai, H., Kohrogi, N., and Hamashima, Y. Immunoelectron microscopic studies of IgA nephropathy. *Nephron* 36: 246, 1984.
152. Doi, T., Kanatsu, K., Sekita, K., Yoshida, H., Nagai, H., and Hamashima, Y. Circulating immune complexes of IgG, IgA, and IgM classes in various glomerular diseases. *Nephron* 32:335, 1982.
153. Donadio, J. V., Jr., Holman, R. T., Holub, B. J., and Bergstralh, E. J. Effects of omega-3 polyunsaturated fatty acids (PUFA) in mesangial IgA nephropathy. *Kidney Int.* 37:255, 1990.
154. Donini, U., Casanova, S., Zini, N., and Zucchelli, P. The presence of J-chain in mesangial immune deposits of IgA nephropathy. *Proc. Eur. Dial. Transplant. Assoc.* 19:655, 1982.
155. Dosa, S., Cairns, S. A., Mallick, N. P., Lawler, W., and Williams, G. Relapsing Henoch-Schönlein syndrome with renal involvement in a patient with an IgA monoclonal gammopathy. *Nephron* 26:145, 1980.
156. Doyle, G. D., O'Dwyer, W. F., Carmody, M., Campbell, E., and Browne, O. IgA nephropathy—An immunopathological study. *Ir. J. Med. Sci.* 145:292, 1976.
157. Droz, D. Natural history of primary glomerulonephritis with mesangial deposits of IgA. *Contrib. Nephrol.* 2:150, 1976.
158. Droz, D., Noel, L. H., Barbanel, C. I., and Leibowitch, J. Glomérulonéphrite à depots intercapillaires d'IgA lors d'une gammapathie monoclonale bénigne. *Nouv. Presse Med.* 10:3652, 1981.
159. Druet, P., Bariety, J., Bernard, D., and Lagrue, G. Les glomérulopathies primitives a dépots mésangiaux d'IgA et d'IgG: Étude clinique et morphologique de 52 cas. *Presse. Med.* 78:583, 1970.
160. Druet, P., Letonturier, P., Contet, A., and Mandet, C. Cryoglobulinemia in human renal diseases: A study of 26 cases. *Clin. Exp. Immunol.* 15:483, 1973.
161. Dubois, D. R. Severe hypertension in Schönlein-Henoch purpura without hematuria. *J. Pediatr.* 75:731, 1969.
162. Duncan, D. A., Drummond, K. N., Michael, A. F., and Vernier, R. L. Pulmonary hemorrhage and glomerulonephritis: Report of six cases and study of the renal lesion by the fluorescent antibody technique and electron microscopy. *Ann. Intern. Med.* 62:920, 1965.
163. Dysart, N. K., Sisson, S., and Vernier, R. L. Immunoelectron microscopy of IgA nephropathy. *Clin. Immunol. Immunopathol.* 29:254, 1983.

164. Egido, J., Blasco, R., Lozano, L., Sancho, J., and Garcia-Hoyo, R. Immunological abnormalities in the tonsils of patients with IgA nephropathy: Inversion in the ratio of IgA : IgG bearing lymphocytes and increased polymeric IgA synthesis. *Clin. Exp. Immunol.* 57:101, 1984.
165. Egido, J., Blasco, R., and Sancho, J. Immunoregulation abnormalities in patients with IgA nephropathy. *Ann. N.Y. Acad. Sci.* 409:817, 1983.
166. Egido, J., Blasco, R., Sancho, J., Illescas, M., and Hernando, L. Abnormalities of immune regulation in patients with IgA mesangial glomerulonephritis (Berger's disease). *Proc. Eur. Dial. Transplant. Assoc.* 19:642, 1982.
167. Egido, J., Blasco, R., Sancho, J., and Lozano, L. T-cell dysfunctions in IgA nephropathy: Specific abnormalities in the regulation of IgA synthesis. *Clin. Immunol. Immunopathol.* 26:201, 1983.
168. Egido, J., Blasco, R., Sancho, J., Lozano, L., and Gutierrez-Millet, V. Immunological studies in a familial IgA nephropathy. *Clin. Exp. Immunol.* 54:532, 1983.
169. Egido, J., Blasco, R., Sancho, J., Lozano, L., Sanchez-Crespo, M., and Hernando, L. Increased rates of polymeric IgA synthesis by circulating lymphoid cells in IgA mesangial glomerulonephritis. *Clin. Exp. Immunol.* 47:309, 1982.
170. Egido, J., Rivera-Hernandez, F., Sancho, J., Moreno, M., Kreisler, M., and Hernando, L. Estudio del sistema HLA y factores de riesgo para la insufficiencia renal en la glomerulonephritis mesangial IgA. *Nefrologia* 1:21, 1981.
171. Egido, J., Sanchez-Crespo, M., Sancho, J., Kreisler, M., and Hernando, L. Phenytoin in the treatment of IgA mesangial glomerulonephritis (Berger's disease). *Clin. Nephrol.* 15:164, 1981.
172. Egido, J., Sancho, J., Lorente, F., and Fontar, G. Inhibition of neutrophil migration by serum IgA from patients with IgA nephropathy. *Clin. Exp. Immunol.* 49:709, 1982.
173. Egido, J., Sancho, J., Mampaso, F., Lopez-Trascasa, M., Sanchez-Crespo, M., Blasco, R., and Hernando, L. A possible common pathogenesis of the mesangial IgA glomerulonephritis in patients with Berger's disease and Schönlein-Henoch syndrome. *Proc. Eur. Dial. Transplant. Assoc.* 17:660, 1980.
174. Eknoyan, G. Glomerular Abnormalities in Liver Disease. In M. Epstein (Ed.), *The Kidney in Liver Disease.* Baltimore: Williams & Wilkins, 1988. P. 154.
175. Ellis, A. Natural history of Bright's disease: Clinical, histological and experimental observations. *Lancet* 1:1, 1942.
176. Elyouki, A. Y., Hijazi, Z. M., Tungekai, F., Qurtom, H. A., and Majeed, H. Berger's disease : Henoch-Schönlein syndrome—One disease entity. *Clin. Nephrol.* 31:53, 1989.
177. Emancipator, S. N. Nephrology forum: Immunoregulatory factors in the pathogenesis of IgA nephropathy. *Kidney Int.* 38:1216, 1990.
178. Emancipator, S. N., Gallo, G. R., and Lamm, M. E. Experimental IgA nephropathy induced by oral immunization. *J. Exp. Med.* 157:572, 1983.
179. Emancipator, S. N., Gallo, G. R., Razaboni, R., and Lamm, M. E. Experimental cholestasis promotes the deposition of glomerular IgA immune complexes. *Am. J. Pathol.* 113:19, 1983.
180. Emancipator, S. N., and Lamm, M. E. Biology of disease: IgA nephropathy: Pathogenesis of the most common form of glomerulonephritis. *Lab. Invest.* 60:168, 1989.
181. Emancipator, S. N., and Lamm, M. E. IgA nephropathy: Overproduction or decreased clearance of immune complexes? *Lab. Invest.* 61:365, 1989.
182. Emancipator, S. N., Ovary, Z., and Lamm, M. E. The role of mesangial complement in the hematuria of experimental IgA nephropathy. *Lab. Invest.* 57:269, 1987.
183. Emancipator, S. N., and Schena, F. P. (Eds.). *Immunoglobulin A Nephropathy.* Volume 7 in N. A. Kurtzman (Ed.), *Seminars in Nephrology.* Philadelphia: Grune & Stratton, 1987.
184. Endo, Y., and Hara, M. Glomerular IgA deposition in pulmonary diseases. *Kidney Int.* 29:557, 1986.
185. Endo, Y., Matsushita, H., Nozawa, Y., Nishikage, S., Matsuya, S., and Hara, M. Glomerulonephritis associated with liver cirrhosis. *Acta Pathol. Jpn.* 33:333, 1983.
186. Endoh, M., Sakai, H., Suga, T., Miura, M., Tomino, Y., and Nomoto, Y. Increase of peripheral blood B cells with Fc receptor for IgA in patients with IgA nephropathy. *Scand. J. Immunol.* 17:437, 1983.
187. Endoh, M., Suga, T., Miura, M., Tomino, Y., Nomoto, Y., and Sakai, H. In vivo alteration of antibody production in patients with IgA nephropathy. *Clin. Exp. Immunol.* 57:564, 1984.
188. Esparza, A. R., Abuelo, J. G., Matarese, R. A., Endreny, R. G., Carvahlo, J. S., and Allegra, S. R. Rapidly progressive IgA nephropathy (RPIGAN). *Kidney Int.* 23:122, 1983.
189. Evans, D. J., Williams, D. G., Peters, D. K., Sissons, J. G. P., Boulton-Jones, J. M., Ogg, C. S., Cameron, J. S., and Hoffbrand, B. I. Glomerular deposition of properdin in Henoch-Schönlein syndrome and idiopathic focal nephritis. *Br. Med. J.* 3:326, 1973.
190. Fagan, J. E. Henoch-Schönlein purpura and gamma-benzene hexachloride (Letter). *Pediatrics* 67:310, 1981.
191. Falk, R. J., Dalmasso, A. P., Kim, Y., Tsai, C. H.,

Sheimann, J. I., Gewurz, H., and Michael, A. F. Neoantigen of the polymerized ninth component of complement: Characterization of a monoclonal antibody and immunohistochemical localization in renal disease. *J. Clin. Invest.* 72:560, 1983.

192. Falk, R. J., Podack, E., Dalmasso, A. P., and Jennette, J. C. Localization of S-protein and its relationship to the membrane attack complex of complement in renal tissue. *Am. J. Pathol.* 127: 182, 1987.

193. Falls, W. F., Jr., Ford, K. L., Ashworth, C. T., and Carter, N. W. Renal vasculitis in a nonfatal case of Henoch-Schönlein purpura. *Ann. Intern. Med.* 64:1276, 1966.

194. Farhangi, M., Luger, A. M., and Morris, A. D. Pathogenic role of a monoclonal IgA (kappa) anti-IgG paraprotein associated with hemorrhagic diathesis, rheumatoid arthritis, vascular purpura, and acute membranoproliferative glomerulonephritis. *J. Clin. Immunol.* 2:75, 1982.

195. Fauchet, R., Gueguen, M., Genetet, B., Le Pagamp, P., Ramee, M.-P., Chevet, D., and Simon, P. HLA-DR antigen and IgA nephropathy (Berger's disease). *N. Engl. J. Med.* 302:1033, 1980.

196. Faull, R. J., Aarons, I., Woodroffe, A. J., and Clarkson, A. R. Adult Henoch-Schönlein nephritis. *Aust. N.Z. J. Med.* 47:396, 1987.

197. Feehally, J., Beattie, T. J., Brenchley, P. E. C., Coupes, B. M., Mallick, N. P., and Postlethwaite, R. J. Sequential study of the IgA system in relapsing IgA nephropathy. *Kidney Int.* 30:924, 1986.

198. Feehally, J., O'Donoghue, D. J., and Ballardie, F. W. Current nephrological practice in the investigation of haematuria: Relationship to incidence of IgA nephropathy. *J. R. Coll. Physicians Lond.* 23:228, 1989.

199. Feiner, H. D., Cabili, S., Baldwin, D. S., Schacht, R. G., and Gallo, G. R. Intrarenal vascular sclerosis in IgA nephropathy (BN). *Clin. Nephrol.* 18:183, 1982.

200. Feldt, R., and Stickler, G. B. The gastrointestinal manifestations of anaphylactoid purpura in children. *Mayo Clin. Proc.* 37:465, 1962.

201. Fellström, B., Klareskog, L., Heldin, C. H., Larsson, E., Rönnstrand, L., Terracio, L., Tufveson, G., Wahlberg, J., and Rubin, K. Platelet-derived growth factor receptors in the kidney—Upregulated expression in inflammation. *Kidney Int.* 36:1099, 1989.

202. Feltis, J. T., Churg, J., Holley, K. M., Feiner, H., Gallo, G., and Ackad, A. S. Active and chronic phases of Berger's disease (IgA nephropathy). *Am. J. Kidney Dis.* 3:349, 1984.

203. Fillastre, J.-P., Morel-Maroger, L., Ducroiset, B., and Richet, G. Atteinte rénale du purpura rhumatoïde chez l'adulte: Étude de 20 biopsies rénales. Intérêt de l'examen glomérulaire en immunofluorescence. *Presse Med.* 78:2375, 1970.

204. Finlayson, G., Alexander, R., Juncos, L., Schlein, E., Teague, P., Waldman, R., and Cade, R. Immunoglobulin A glomerulonephritis: A clinicopathologic study. *Lab. Invest.* 32:140, 1975.

205. Fiorini, G., Fornasieri, A., Sinico, R., Colasanti, G., Gibelli, A., Corneo, R., and D'Amico, G. Lymphocyte populations in the peripheral blood from patients with IgA nephropathy. *Nephron* 31:354, 1982.

206. Fishberg, A. M. *Hypertension and Nephritis,* 4th Ed. Philadelphia: Lea & Febiger, 1939.

207. Fisher, E. R., and Hellstrom, H. R. The membranous and proliferative glomerulonephritis of hepatic cirrhosis. *Am. J. Clin. Pathol.* 32:48, 1959.

208. Fisher, E. R., and Perez-Stable, E. Cirrhotic (hepatic) lobular glomerulonephritis: Correlation of ultrastructural and clinical features. *Am. J. Pathol.* 52:869, 1968.

209. Flatau, E., Kohn, D., Schitter, D., Lurie, M., and Levy, E. Schönlein-Henoch's syndrome in patients with familial Mediterranean fever. *Arthritis Rheum.* 25:42, 1982.

210. Fletcher, P., Al-Khader, A. A., Parsons, V., and Aber, G. M. The pathology of intrarenal vascular lesions associated with the loin-pain–hematuria syndrome. *Nephron* 24:150, 1979.

211. Fornasieri, A., Sinico, R., Fiorini, G., Goldaniga, D., Colasanti, G., Vendemia, F., Gibelli, A., and D'Amico, G. T-lymphocyte subsets in primary and secondary glomerulonephritis. *Proc. Eur. Dial. Transplant. Assoc.* 19:635, 1982.

212. Fornasieri, A., Sinico, R. A., Maldifassi, P., Bernasconi, P., Vegni, M., and D'Amico, G. IgA antigliadin antibodies in IgA mesangial nephropathy (Berger's disease). *Br. Med. J.* 295:78, 1987.

213. Forsstrom, J., Viander, M., Lehtonen, A., and Ekfors, T. *Yersinia enterocolitica* infection complicated by glomerulonephritis. *Scand. J. Infect. Dis.* 9:253, 1977.

214. Frasca, G. M., Vangelista, A., Biagini, G., and Bonomini, V. Immunological tubulointerstitial deposits in IgA nephropathy. *Kidney Int.* 22:184, 1982.

215. French, M. A. H., Shortland, J. P., Coward, R. A., and Brown, C. B. Glomerulonephritis and IgA deficiency. *Clin. Nephrol.* 27:199, 1987.

216. Freycon, M. T., Parchoux, B., Dechelette, E., Sellem, C., Lepetit, J. C., Betuel, H., and Gebuhrer, L. HLA et purpura rhumatoide avec ou sans néphropathie. *Pediatrie* 39:525, 1984.

217. Friedberg, M., Larsen, S., and Denneberg, T. *Yersinia enterocolitica* and glomerulonephritis. *Lancet* 1:498, 1978.

218. Fujimoto, T., Dohi, K., and Ishikawa, H. Inter-

stitial abnormalities in Sjögren's syndrome. *Nippon Jinzo Gakkai Shi* 25:932, 1983.

219. Fukuda, Y. Renal glomerular changes associated with liver cirrhosis. *Acta Pathol. Jpn.* 32:561, 1982.
220. Gaboardi, F., Perletti, L., Cambie, M., and Mihatsch, J. J. Dermatitis herpetiformis and nephrotic syndrome. *Clin. Nephrol.* 20:49, 1983.
221. Gairdner, D. The Schönlein-Henoch syndrome (anaphylactoid purpura). *Q. J. Med.* 17:95, 1948.
222. Galla, J. H., Kohaut, E. C., Alexander, R., and Mestecky, J. Racial differences in the prevalence of IgA-associated nephropathies. *Lancet* 2:522, 1984.
223. Gallo, G. R., Katafuchi, R., Neelakantappa, K., and Baldwin, D. S. Prognostic pathologic markers in IgA nephropathy. *Am. J. Kidney Dis.* 12:362, 1988.
224. Garcia-Fuentes, M., Chantler, C., and Williams, D. G. Cryoglobulinaemia in Henoch-Schönlein purpura. *Br. Med. J.* 2:163, 1977.
225. Garcia-Fuentes, M., Martin, A., Chantler, C., and Williams, D. G. Serum complement components in Henoch-Schönlein purpura. *Arch. Dis. Child.* 53:417, 1978.
226. Garner, J. A. Acute pancreatitis as a complication of anaphylactoid (Henoch-Schönlein) purpura. *Arch. Dis. Child.* 52:971, 1977.
227. Gärtner, H. V., Vetter, W., and Bohle, A. IgA Nephritis—Prognostic Relevance of Glomerular Focal-Segmental Lesions. In *Abstracts of the IXth International Congress of Nephrology.* 1984. P. 281.
228. Garty, B. Z. Schönlein-Henoch purpura associated with hepatitis A infection (Letter). *Am. J. Dis. Child.* 139:547, 1985.
229. Gaskell, H., Searle, M., and Dathan, J. R. Henoch-Schönlein purpura with severe ileal involvement responding to plasmapheresis. *Int. J. Artif. Organs* 8:163, 1985.
230. Geiger, H., Good, R. A., and Day, N. K. A study of complement components C3, C5, C6, C7, C8 and C9 in chronic membranoproliferative glomerulonephritis, systemic lupus erythematosus, poststreptococcal nephritis, idiopathic nephrotic syndrome and anaphylactoid purpura. *Z. Kinderheilk.* 119:269, 1975.
231. Gelfand, E. W., Clarkson, J. E., and Minta, J. O. Selective deficiency of the second component of complement in a patient with anaphylactoid purpura. *Clin. Immunol. Immunopathol.* 4:269, 1975.
232. Genin, C., Laurent, B., Sabatier, J. C., Colon, S., and Berthoux, F. C. IgA mesangial deposits in C3H/HeJ mice after oral immunization with ferritin or bovine serum albumin. *Clin. Exp. Immunol.* 63:385, 1986.
233. Genin, C., Sabatier, J. C., Laurent, P., Gunthier, R., Laurent, B., and Berthoux, F. C. Efficiency of High Dose Steroids and Plasma Exchanges in Severe Mesangial IgA Glomerulonephritis. In *Abstracts of the IXth International Congress of Nephrology.* 1984. P. 89.
234. Genin, C., Sabatier, J. C., Laurent, B., Laurent, P., Gunthier, R., and Berthoux, F. C. The Membranoproliferative Glomerulonephritis Associated with Cirrhosis: Good Evolution After Steroids and Plasma Exchange. In *Abstracts of the IXth International Congress of Nephrology.* 1984. P. 89.
235. Germuth, F. G., and Rodriguez, E. Focal mesangiopathic glomerulonephritis: Prevalence and pathogenesis. *Kidney Int.* 7:216, 1975.
236. Gesualdo, L., Sedor, J. R., Lamm, M. E., and Emancipator, S. N. Glomerular thromboxane but not prostaglandin or interleukin-1 is augmented in IgA nephropathy in rats (Abstract). *Kidney Int.* 35:347, 1989.
237. Gesualdo, L., Lamm, M. E., and Emancipator, S. N. Defective oral tolerance promotes nephritogenesis in experimental IgA nephropathy induced by oral immunization. *J. Immunol.* 145:3684, 1990.
238. Gesualdo, L., Ranier, E., Di Cillo, M., Marfella, C., Aventaggiato, L., Scivittaro, V., Lamm, M. E., Schena, F. P., and Emancipator, S. N. Defective Mucosal Immunoregulation as a Factor in the Pathogenesis of IgA Nephropathy. In H. Sakai, O. Sakai, and Y. Nomoto (Eds.), *Pathogenesis of IgA Nephropathy.* Tokyo: Harcourt Brace Jovanovitch, 1990. P. 111.
239. Giangiacomo, J., and Tsai, C. C. Dermal and glomerular deposition of IgA in anaphylactoid purpura. *Am. J. Dis. Child.* 131:981, 1977.
240. Giannetti, A., Serri, F., and Bernasconi, C. Immunofluorescent studies of the skin in mixed cryoglobulinemia and Schönlein-Henoch purpura. *Acta Derm. Venereol. (Stockh.)* 56:211, 1976.
241. Glasgow, E. F. Renal changes in Henoch-Schönlein purpura. *Arch. Dis. Child.* 45:151, 1970.
242. Goebel, K. M. Reversible overt nephropathy with Henoch-Schönlein purpura due to piroxicam. *Br. Med. J.* 284:311, 1982.
243. Gomez-Capdera, F. J., Niembro, E., Gomez-Capdera, J. A., Lopez-Gomez, J. M., and Luque de Pablos, A. La nefropatia en la purpura de Schönlein-Henoch en la infancia: Incidencia, aspectos clinicos y evolutivos a propisito de 151 observaciones. *Rev. Clin. Esp.* 168:333, 1983.
244. Goodyer, P. R., de Chadaverian, J. P., and Kaplan, B. S. Acute poststreptococcal glomerulonephritis mimicking Henoch-Schönlein purpura. *J. Pediatr.* 93:412, 1978.
245. Gormly, A. A., Smith, P. S., Seymour, A. E., Clarkson, A. R., and Woodroffe, A. J. IgA glomerular deposits in experimental cirrhosis. *Am. J. Pathol.* 104:50, 1981.

246. Gregory, M. C., Hammond, M. E., and Brewer, E. D. Renal deposition of cytomegalovirus antigen in immunoglobulin-A nephropathy. *Lancet* 1:11, 1988.
247. Grossman, H., Berdon, W. E., and Baker, D. H. Abdominal pain in Schönlein-Henoch syndrome. *Am. J. Dis. Child.* 108:67, 1964.
248. Guillan, R. A., Zelman, S., and Alonso, D. R. Hepatic glomerulosclerosis (an analysis of 60 cases). *Am. J. Gastroenterol.* 49:499, 1968.
249. Gutierrez-Millet, V., Navas-Palacios, J. J., Prieto, C., Ruilope, L. M., Usera, G., Barrientos, A., Alcazar, J. M., Perez, A. J., Jarillo, M. D., and Rodicio, J. L. Glomerulonephritis mesangial idopatica: Estudio clinico e immunopatologico de 40 casos y revision de la literatura. *Nefrologia* 2:1, 1982.
250. Habib, R. Périartérite Noueuse et Angéites Nécrosantes. In P. Royer, R. Habib, H. Mathieu, and M. Broyer (Eds.), *Néphrologie Pédiatrique.* Paris: Flammarion Medecine-Sciences, 1983. P. 368.
251. Habib, R., Antignac, C., Hinglais, N., Gagnedoux, M.-F., and Broyer, M. Glomerular lesions in the transplanted kidney in children. *Am. J. Kidney Dis.* 10:198, 1987.
252. Habib, R., Broyer, M., and Levy, M. Schönlein-Henoch Purpura Glomerulonephritis in Children. In J. Strauss (Ed.), *Pediatric Nephrology,* Vol. 4. New York: Garland Press, 1977. P. 155.
253. Habib, R., and Cameron, J. S. Schönlein-Henoch Purpura. In P. A. Bacon and N. M. Hadler (Eds.), *The Kidney and Rheumatic Disease.* London: Butterworth, 1982. P. 178.
254. Habib, R., and Levy, M. Les néphropathies du purpura rhumatoide chez l'enfant. Etude clinique et anatomique de 60 observations. *Arch. Fr. Pédiatr.* 29:305, 1972.
255. Hale, G. M., Howarth, G. S., Aarons, I., Clarkson, A. R., and Woodroffe, A. J. Quantitation of glomerular angiotensin II receptors in IgA nephropathy. *Clin. Nephrol.* 32:5, 1989.
256. Hale, G. M., McIntosh, S. L., Hiki, Y., Clarkson, A. R., and Woodroffe, A. J. Evidence for IgA-specific B-cell hyperactivity in patients with IgA nephropathy. *Kidney Int.* 29:718, 1986.
257. Hall, R. P., Lawley, T. J., Heck, J. A., and Katz, S. I. IgA-containing immune complexes in dermatitis herpetiformis, Henoch-Schönlein purpura, systemic lupus erythematosus and other diseases. *Clin. Exp. Immunol.* 40:431, 1980.
258. Hall, R. P., Stachura, I., Cason, J., Whiteside, T. L., and Lawley, T. J. IgA-containing circulating immune complexes in patients with IgA nephropathy. *Am. J. Med.* 74:56, 1983.
259. Halle, C. J. Henoch-Schönlein purpura after chickenpox (Letter). *Arch. Dis. Child.* 54:166, 1979.
260. Hamada, K. IgA nephropathy and Henoch-Schönlein purpura nephritis: Clinicopathological, histopathological, immunohistological, and electron-microscopical characteristics. *Hokkaido Igaku Zasshi* 59:456, 1984.
261. Hamazaki, T., Tateno, S., and Shishido, H. Eicosapentanoic acid and IgA nephropathy. *Lancet* 1:1017, 1984.
262. Hara, M., Endo, Y., Hara, S., Fukushima, O., and Mimura, N. IgA nephropathy with subendothelial deposits. *Virchows Archiv. [Pathol. Anat.]* 386:249, 1980.
263. Hattori, S., Karashima, S., Furuse, A., Terashima, T., Kiramatsu, M., Marakami, M., and Matsuda, I. Clinicopathological correlation of IgA nephropathy in children. *Am. J. Nephrol.* 5:182, 1985.
264. Hayat, P., Sonsino, E., Bompard, Y., Stora-Castaing, N., and Weisgerber, G. Sténose ischémique de l'uretère au cours d'un purpura rhumatoide. *Nouv. Presse Med.* 7:3913, 1978.
265. Heaton, J. M., Turner, D. R., and Cameron, J. S. Localization of glomerular "deposits" in Henoch-Schönlein nephritis. *Histopathology* 1:93, 1977.
266. Heironimus, J. D., and Perry, E. L. Dermatitis herpetiformis and glomerulonephritis: Case report and review of the literature. *Am. J. Med.* 80:508, 1986.
267. Helin, H., Mustonen, J., Reunala, T., and Pasternack, A. IgA nephropathy associated with celiac disease and dermatitis herpetiformis. *Arch. Pathol. Lab. Med.* 107:324, 1983.
268. Hené, R. J., Velthuis, P., Van de Wiel, A., Klepper, D., Dorhout Mees, E. J., and Kater, L. The relevance of IgA deposits in vessel walls of clinically normal skin: A prospective study. *Arch. Intern. Med.* 146:745, 1986.
269. Henoch, E. *Vorlesungen über Kinderkrankheiten,* 10th Ed. Berlin: Hirschwald, 1899, P. 839.
270. Heptinstall, R. H., and Joekes, A. M. Focal glomerulonephritis: A study based on renal biopsies. *Q. J. Med.* 28:329, 1959.
271. Heptinstall, R. H., and Joekes, A. M. Focal Glomerulonephritis. In G. E. W. Wolstenholme and M. P. Cameron (Eds.), *Ciba Foundation Symposium on Renal Biopsy.* Boston: Little, Brown, 1961. P. 194.
272. Heptinstall, R. H., and Salmon, M. V. Pulmonary haemorrhage with extensive glomerular disease of the kidney. *J. Clin. Pathol.* 12:272, 1959.
273. Hernando, P., Egido, J., de Nicolas, R., and Sancho, J. Clinical significance of polymeric and monomeric IgA complexes in patients with IgA nephropathy. *Am. J. Kidney Dis.* 8:410, 1986.
274. Hernando, P., González, E., Egido, J., de Nicolas, R., Gómez, C., Gómez-Chiarri, M., and Hernando, L. Release of platelet-activating factor and oxygen radicals by mesangial cells stimulated

with IgA and IgG immune aggregates (Abstract). *Nephrol. Dial. Transplant.* 4:427, 1989.
275. Higgins, M. R., Randall, R. E., and Still, W. J. S. Nephrotic syndrome with oat-cell carcinoma. *Br. Med. J.* 3:450, 1974.
276. Hiki, Y., Kobayashi, Y., Tateno, S., Sada, M., and Kashiwagi, N. Strong association of HLA-DR4 with benign IgA nephropathy. *Nephron* 32: 222, 1982.
277. Hillion, D., Mignon, F., Ramée, M. P., Morel-Maroger, L., and Richet, G. Critères de pronostic et evolution de la néphropathie du purpura rhumatoide de l'adulte: A propos de 28 cas. *Ann. Med. Interne (Paris)* 129:505, 1978.
278. Hinglais, N., Kazatchkine, M. D., Bhakdi, S., Appay, M.-D., Mandet, C., Grossetete, J., and Bariety, J. Immunohistochemical study of the C5b-9 complex of complement in human kidneys. *Kidney Int.* 30:399, 1986.
279. Honkanen, E., Tornroth, T., Rettersson, E., and Kuhlback, B. Glomerulonephritis in renal allografts: Results of 18 years of transplantations. *Clin. Nephrol.* 21:210, 1984.
280. Hood, S. A., Velosa, J. A., Holley, K. E., and Donadio, J. V. IgA-IgG nephropathy: Predictive indices of progressive disease. *Clin. Nephrol.* 16: 55, 1981.
281. Horn, R. C., and Smetana, H. Intercapillary glomerulosclerosis. *Am. J. Pathol.* 18:93, 1942.
282. Hotta, O., Yoshizawa, N., Oshima, S., Takeuchi, A., Kawamura, O., Kondo, S., Kubota, T., and Niwa, H. Significance of renal hyaline arteriolosclerosis and tubulointerstitial change in IgA glomerulonephritis and focal glomerulosclerosis. *Nephron* 47:262, 1987.
283. Houssin, A., Riberi, P., and Hurez, D. Incidence de la phénytoïne sur les immunoglobulines au cours de la maladie de Berger. *Presse Med.* 12:2001, 1983.
284. Hovig, T., Blomhoff, J. P., Holme, R., Flatmark, A., and Gjone, E. Plasma lipoprotein alterations and morphologic changes with lipid deposition in the kidney of patients with hepatorenal syndrome. *Lab. Invest.* 38:540, 1978.
285. Hubert, D., Beaufils, M., and Meyrier, A. Néphropathie glomérulaire à immunoglobulines A associée à une colite inflammatoire. A propos de deux observations. *Presse Med.* 13:1083, 1984.
286. Hughson, M. D., Megill, D. M., Smith, S. M., Tung, K. S. K., Miller, G., and Hoy, W. E. Mesangiopathic glomerulonephritis in Zuni (New Mexico) Indians. *Arch. Pathol. Lab. Med.* 113: 148, 1989.
287. Hurley, R. M., and Drummond, K. N. Anaphylactoid purpura nephritis: Clinicopathological correlations. *J. Pediatr.* 81:904, 1972.
288. Hyman, L. R., Wagnild, J. P., Beirne, G. J., and Burkholder, P. M. Immunoglobulin A distribution in gomerular disease: Analysis of immunofluorescence localization and pathogenic significance. *Kidney Int.* 3:397, 1973.
289. Imai, H., Nakamoto, Y., Miki, K., Miyakuni, T., and Miura, A. B. Pseudo-thrombocytopenia and IgA-related platelet agglutinin in a patient with IgA nephritis. *Nephron* 34:154, 1983.
290. Imai, I., and Matsumoto, S. Anaphylactoid purpura with cardiac involvement. *Arch. Dis. Child.* 45:727, 1970.
291. Imbasciati, E., Colasanti, G., Barbiano di Belgioioso, G., Banfi, G., Durante, A., Ragni, A., Ponticelli, C., Minetti, L., and D'Amico, G. Long-term follow-up of IgA mesangial deposits glomerulonephritis. *Proc. Eur. Soc. Dial. Transplant.* 14:472, 1977.
292. Inenagu, T., Nanishi, F., Harada, A., Onoyama, K., and Omae, T. Reticuloendothelial Function in Patients with IgA Nephropathy. In *Abstracts of the IXth International Congress of Nephrology.* 1984. P. 284.
293. Isaacs, K. L., and Miller, F. Role of antigen size and charge in immune complex glomerulonephritis: I. Active induction of disease with dextran and its derivatives. *Lab. Invest.* 47:198, 1982.
294. Isaacs, K., Miller, F., and Lane, B. Experimental model for IgA nephropathy. *Clin. Immunol. Immunopathol.* 20:419, 1981.
295. Jackson, S. Immunoglobulin–anti-immunoglobulin interactions and immune complexes in IgA nephropathy. *Am. J. Kidney Dis.* 12:425, 1988.
296. Jackson, S., Montgomery, R. I., Mestecky, J., Julian, B. A., Galla, J. H., and Czerkinsky, C. Antibodies directed at Fab of IgA in the sera of normal individuals and IgA nephropathy patients. *Adv. Exp. Biol. Med.* 216:1537, 1987.
297. Jacome, A. F. Pulmonary haemorrhage and death complicating anaphylactoid purpura. *South. Med. J.* 60:1003, 1967.
298. Jennette, J. C. The immunohistochemistry of IgA nephropathy. *Am. J. Kidney Dis.* 12:348, 1988.
299. Jennette, J. C., Ferguson, A. L., Moore, M. A., and Freeman, D. G. IgA nephropathy associated with seronegative spondyloarthropathies. *Arthritis Rheum.* 25:144, 1982.
300. Jennette, J. C., Newman, W. J., and Diaz-Buxo, J. A. Overlapping IgA and membranous nephropathy. *Am. J. Clin. Pathol.* 88:74, 1987.
301. Jennette, J. C., Wall, S. D., and Wilkman, A. S. Low incidence of IgA nephropathy in blacks. *Kidney Int.* 28:944, 1985.
302. Jones, W. T., Rao, D. R. G., and Braunstein, H. The renal glomerulus in cirrhosis of the liver. *Am. J. Pathol.* 39:393, 1961.

303. Joseph M. Nephritis with lung haemorrhage. *Lancet* 1:1160, 1963.
304. Julian, B. A. (Ed.) First national symposium on IgA nephropathy. *Am. J. Kidney Dis.* 7:337, 1988.
305. Julian, B. A., Phillips, J. A., III, Orlando, P. J., Wyatt, R. J., and Butler, M. G. Analysis of immunoglobulin heavy chain restriction fragment length polymorphisms in IgA nephropathy. *Semin. Nephrol.* 7:306, 1987.
306. Julian, B. A., Quiggins, P. A., Thompson, J. S., Woodford, S. Y., Gleason, K., and Wyatt, R. J. Familial IgA nephropathy: Evidence of an inherited mechanism of disease. *N. Engl. J. Med.* 312:202, 1985.
307. Julian, B. A., Woodford, S. Y., Baehler, R. W., McMorrow, R. G., and Wyatt, R. J. Familial clustering and immunogenetic aspects of IgA nephropathy. *Am. J. Kidney Dis.* 12:366, 1988.
308. Julian, B. A., Wyatt, R. J., McMorrow, R. G., and Galla, J. H. Serum complement proteins in IgA nephropathy. *Clin. Nephrol.* 20:251, 1983.
309. Kalowski, S., and Kincaid-Smith, P. Glomerulonephritis in Henoch-Schönlein Syndrome. In P. Kincaid-Smith, T. H. Mathew, and E. L. Becker (Eds.), *Glomerulonephritis: Morphology, Natural History, and Treatment.* New York: Wiley, 1973. P. 1123.
310. Kalsi, J., Delacroix, D. L., and Hodgson, H. J. F. IgA in alcoholic cirrhosis. *Clin. Exp. Immunol.* 52:499, 1983.
311. Kanayama, Y., Shiota, K., Kotumi, K., Ikuno, Y., Yasumoto, R., Ishii, M., and Inoue, T. *Mycoplasma pneumoniae* pneumonia associated with IgA nephropathy. *Scand. J. Infect. Dis.* 14:231, 1982.
312. Kasai, N., Parbtani, A., Cameron, J. S., Yewdall, V., Shepherd, P., and Verroust, P. Platelet-aggregating immune complexes and intraplatelet serotonin in idiopathic glomerulonephritis and systemic lupus. *Clin. Exp. Immunol.* 43:64, 1981.
313. Kashiwabara, H., Shishido, H., Tomura, S., Tuchida, H., and Miyajima, T. Strong association between IgA nephropathy and HLA-DR4 antigen. *Kidney Int.* 22:377, 1982.
314. Katafuchi, R., Takebayashi, S., Taguchi, T., and Harada, T. Structural-functional correlations in serial biopsies from patients with glomerulonephritis. *Clin. Nephrol.* 28:169, 1987.
315. Katz, A., Dyck, R. F., and Bear, R. A. Celiac disease associated with immune complex glomerulonephritis. *Clin. Nephrol.* 11:39, 1979.
316. Katz, A., Karanicolas, S., and Falk, J. A. Family study of IgA nephritis: The possible role of HLA antigens. *Transplantation* 29:505, 1980.
317. Katz, A., Underdown, B. J., Minta, J. O., and Lepow, I. H. Glomerulonephritis with mesangial deposits of IgA unassociated with systemic disease. *J. Can. Med. Assoc.* 114:209, 1976.
318. Katz, A., Walker, J. F., and Landy, P. J. IgA nephritis with nephrotic range proteinuria. *Clin. Nephrol.* 20:67, 1983.
319. Kauffmann, R. M., Hermann, W. A., Meyer, C. J., Daha, M. R., and Van Es, L. A. Circulating IgA immune complexes in Henoch-Schönlein purpura. *Am. J. Med.* 69:859, 1980.
320. Kauffman, R. H., and Honwert, D. A. Plasmapheresis in rapidly progressive Henoch-Schönlein glomerulonephritis and the effect on circulating IgA immune complexes. *Clin. Nephrol.* 16:155, 1981.
321. Kauffmann, R. H., Van Es, L. A., and Daha, M. R. The specific detection of IgA immune complexes. *J. Immunol. Methods* 40:117, 1981.
322. Kher, K. K., Kumudchandra, J. S., and Makker, S. P. Stenosing ureteritis in Henoch-Schönlein purpura. *J. Urol.* 129:1040, 1983.
323. Kim, C. K., Aikawa, M., and Makker, S. P. Electron-dense subepithelial glomerular deposits in Henoch-Schönlein purpura syndrome. *Arch. Pathol. Lab. Med.* 103:595, 1979.
324. Kincaid-Smith, P., Bennett, W. M., Dowling, J. P., and Ryan, G. B. Acute renal failure and tubular necrosis associated with hematuria due to glomerulonephritis. *Clin. Nephrol.* 19:206, 1983.
325. Kincaid-Smith, P., and Nicholls, K. Mesangial IgA nephropathy. *Am. J. Kidney Dis.* 3:102, 1983.
326. Kincaid-Smith, P., Nicholls, K., and Birchall, I. Polymorphs infiltrate glomeruli in mesangial IgA glomerulonephritis. *Kidney Int.* 36:1108, 1989.
327. Klotman, P. E., Bruggeman, L., Hassell, J., Horigan, E., Martin, G., and Yamada, Y. Regulation of extracellular matrix by thromboxane (Abstract). *Kidney Int.* 35:294, 1989.
328. Kobayashi, O., Wada, H., Kanasawa, M., and Kamiyama, T. The anaphylactoid purpura-nephritis in childhood. *Acta Med. Biol. (Niigata)* 13:181, 1965.
329. Kobayashi, O., Wada, H., Okawa, K., and Takeyama, I. Schönlein-Henoch's syndrome in children. *Contrib. Nephrol.* 4:48, 1977.
330. Kobayashi, Y., Tateno, S., Hiki, Y., and Shigematsu, H. IgA nephropathy: Prognostic significance of proteinuria and histological alterations. *Nephron* 34:146, 1983.
331. Komatsu, N., Nagura, H., Watanabe, K., Nomoto, Y., and Kobayashi, K. Mesangial deposition of J-chain–linked polymeric IgA in IgA nephropathy. *Nephron* 33:61, 1983.
332. Komori, K., Nose, Y., Inone, H., Tsuji, K., Nomoto, Y., and Sakai, H. Study on HLA system in IgA nephropathy. *Tissue Antigens* 14:32, 1979.
333. Koni, I., Nakashima, A., Kawai, M., Miyazaki, R., Otani, I., Tofuku, Y., Kuroda, M., and Takeda, R. Decreased Fcα Receptor Function in

Polymorphonuclear Leukocytes in IgA Nephropathy Patients. In *Abstracts of the IXth International Congress of Nephrology*. 1984. P. 287.
334. Koskimies, O., Mir, S., Rapola, J., and Vilska, J. Henoch-Schönlein nephritis: Long-term prognosis of unselected patients. *Arch. Dis. Child.* 56:482, 1981.
335. Koskimies, O., Rapola, J., Savilahti, E., and Vilska, J. Renal involvement in Schönlein-Henoch purpura. *Acta Paediatr. Scand.* 63:57, 1974.
336. Kourilsky, O., Leroy, C., and Peltier, A. P. Complement and liver cell function in 53 patients with liver disease. *Am. J. Med.* 55:783, 1973.
337. Krothapalli, R., Neeland, B., Small, S., Duffy, W. B., and Senekjian, H. O. IgA nephropathy in a patient with ankylosing spondylitis and a solitary kidney. *Clin. Nephrol.* 21:134, 1984.
338. Kuno-Sakai, H., Sakai, H., Nomoto, Y., Takakura, I., and Kimura, M. Increase of IgA-bearing peripheral blood lymphocytes in children with Henoch-Schönlein purpura. *Pediatrics* 64:918, 1979.
339. Kupor, L. R., Mullins, J. D., and McPhaul, J. J. Immunopathologic findings in idiopathic renal hematuria. *Arch. Intern. Med.* 135:1204, 1975.
340. Kusumoto, Y., Takebayashi, S., Taguchi, T., Harada, T., and Naito, S. Long-term prognosis and prognostic indices of IgA nephropathy in juvenile and adult Japanese. *Clin. Nephrol.* 28:118, 1987.
341. Kutteh, W. H., Prince, S. J., Phillips, J. O., Spenney, J. G., and Mestecky, J. Properties of immunoglobulin A in serum of individuals with liver disease and in hepatic bile. *Gastroenterology* 82:184, 1982.
342. Lagrue, G., Hirbec, G., Fournel, M., and Intrator, L. Glomérulonéphrite mésangiale à dépôts d'IgA: étude des immunoglobulines sériques. *J. Urol. Nephrol. (Paris)* 80:385, 1974.
343. Lagrue, G., Robeva, R., and Laurent, J. Antiproteinuric effect of captopril in primary glomerular diseases. *Nephron* 46:99, 1987.
344. Lai, K. N., Chan, K. W., Lai, F. M., Ping, C., Yan, K. W., Lam, C. W. K., and Vallance-Owen, J. The immunochemical characterization of the light chains in the mesangial IgA deposits in IgA nephropathy. *Am. J. Clin. Pathol.* 85:548, 1986.
345. Lai, K. N., Lai, F. M., Chan, K. W., Ho, C. P., Leung, A. C. T., and Vallance-Owen, J. An overlapping syndrome of IgA nephropathy and Lipoid nephrosis. *Am. J. Clin. Pathol.* 86:716, 1986.
346. Lai, K. N., Lai, F. M., Chiu, S. H., Chan, Y. M., Tsao, G. S. W., Leung, K. N., and Lam, C. W. K. Studies of lymphocyte subpopulations and immunoglobulin production in IgA nephropathy. *Clin. Nephrol.* 28:281, 1987.
347. Lai, K. N., Lai, F. M., Ho, C. P., and Chan, K. W. Corticosteroid therapy in IgA nephropathy with nephrotic syndrome: A long-term controlled trial. *Clin. Nephrol.* 26:174, 1986.
348. Lai, K. N., Lai, F. M., Leung, A. C. T., Ho, C. P., and Vallance-Owen, J. Plasma exchange in patients with rapidly progressive idiopathic IgA nephropathy: A report of two cases and review of literature. *Am. J. Kidney Dis.* 10:66, 1987.
349. Lai, K. N., Lai, F. M., Li, P. K., and Vallance-Owen, J. Cyclosporin treatment of IgA nephropathy: A short-term controlled trial. *Br. Med. J.* 295:1165, 1987.
350. Lai, K. N., Lai, F. M., Lo, S. T. H., and Lam, C. W. K. Light chain composition of IgA in IgA nephropathy. *Am. J. Kidney Dis.* 11:425, 1988.
351. Lai, K. N., Lai, F. M., and Vallance-Owen, J. The clinical use of serum beta-2-microglobulin and fractional beta-2-microglobulin excretion in IgA nephropathy. *Clin. Nephrol.* 25:260, 1986.
352. Lamm, M. E. Cellular aspects of immunoglobulin A. *Adv. Immunol.* 22:223, 1976.
353. Lampen, H. Akute Nephritis als Komplikation der anaphylaktoiden Purpura Schönlein-Henoch. *Medizinische* 48:1604, 1954.
354. Lamperi, S., and Carozzi, S. Skin-muscle biopsy in patients with various nephropathies. *Nephron* 24:46, 1979.
355. Laube, H., Norris, H. T., and Robbins, S. L. The nephromegaly of chronic alcoholics with liver disease. *Arch. Pathol.* 84:290, 1967.
356. Laurent, J., Belghiti, D., Bruneau, C., and Lagrue, G. Diclofenac, a nonsteroidal anti-inflammatory drug, decreases proteinuria in some glomerular diseases: A controlled study. *Am. J. Nephrol.* 7:198, 1987.
357. Laurent, J., Branellec, A., Heslan, J.-M., Rostoker, G., Bruneau, C., Andre, C., Intrator, L., and Lagrue, G. An increase in circulating IgA antibodies in gliadin in IgA mesangial glomerulonephritis. *Am. J. Nephrol.* 7:718, 1987.
358. Lawrence, S., Pussell, B. A., and Charlesworth, J. A. Mesangial IgA nephropathy: Detection of defective reticulophagocytic function in vivo. *Clin. Nephrol.* 16:280, 1983.
359. Lee, G. S. L., Woo, K. T., and Lin, C. H. Controlled trial of dipyridamole and low-dose warfarin in patients with IgA nephritis with renal impairment. *Clin. Nephrol.* 31:276, 1989.
360. Lee, H. S., Koh, H. I., Kim, M. J., and Rah, H. Y. Henoch-Schönlein nephritis in adults: A clinical and morphological study. *Clin. Nephrol.* 26: 125, 1986.
361. Lee, H. S., Koh, H. I., Lee, H. B., and Park, H. C. IgA nephropathy in Korea: A morphological and clinical study. *Clin. Nephrol.* 27:131, 1987.
362. Lee, S. M. K., Rao, V. M., Franklin, W. A., Schiffer, M. S., Aronson, A. J., Spargo, B. H., and Katz, A. I. IgA nephropathy: Morphologic

predictors of progressive renal disease. *Hum. Pathol.* 13:314, 1982.
363. Leinikki, P. O., Mustonen, J., and Pasternack, A. Immune response to oral polio vaccine in patients with IgA glomerulonephritis. *Clin. Exp. Immunol.* 68:33, 1987.
364. Lelong, M., and Deroibaix, P. Le purpura rhumatoïde de Schönlein-Henoch: Étude de 36 observations. *Lille Med.* 13:307, 1968.
365. Le Petit, J. C., Cazes, M. H., Berthoux, F. C., van Loghem, E., Goguen, J., Seger, J., Chapius-Cellier, C., Marcelin, M., De Lange, G., Garovon, M. R., Serre, J. L., Brizars, C. P., and Carpentier, C. B. Genetic investigation in mesangial IgA nephropathy. *Tissue Antigens* 19:108, 1982.
366. Lesavre, P. H., Digeon, M., and Bach, J. F. Analysis of circulating IgA and detection of immune complexes in primary IgA nephropathy. *Clin. Exp. Immunol.* 48:61, 1982.
367. Levinsky, R. J., and Barratt, T. M. IgA immune complexes in Henoch-Schönlein purpura. *Lancet* 2:1100, 1979.
368. Levitt, L. M., and Burbank, B. Glomerulonephritis as a complication of the Schönlein-Henoch syndrome. *N. Engl. J. Med.* 248:530, 1953.
369. Levy, M., Bacri, J. L., Dommergues, J. P., Gonzales, G., and Beziau, A. IgA deposition along dermal capillaries in anaphylactoid purpura. *Int. J. Pediatr. Nephrol.* 2:223, 1981.
370. Levy, M., Beaufils, H., Gubler, M. C., and Habib, R. Idiopathic recurrent macroscopic hematuria and mesangial IgA-IgG deposits in children (Berger's disease). *Clin. Nephrol.* 1:63, 1973.
371. Levy, M., Broyer, M., Arsan, A., Levy-Bentolila, D., and Habib, R. Anaphylactoid Purpura Nephritis in Childhood: Natural History and Immunopathology. In J. Hamburger, J. Crosnier, and M. H. Maxwell (Eds.), *Advances in Nephrology,* Vol. 6. Chicago: Year Book Medical, 1976. P. 183.
372. Levy, M., Broyer, M., and Habib, R. Pathology and Immunopathology of Schönlein-Henoch Nephritis. In P. Kincaid-Smith, A. J. F. d'Apice, and R. Atkins (Eds.), *Progress in Glomerulonephritis.* New York: Wiley, 1979. P. 261.
373. Levy, M., Gonzales-Burchard, C., Broyer, M., Dommergues, J. P., Foulard, M., Sorez, J. P., and Habib, R. Berger's disease in children: Natural history and outcome. *Medicine (Baltimore)* 64:157, 1985.
374. Lewis, E. J., Schur, P. H., Busch, G. J., Galvanek, E., and Merrill, J. P. Immunopathologic features of a patient with glomerulonephritis and pulmonary hemorrhage. *Am. J. Med.* 54:507, 1973.
375. Lexow, P., and Sigstad, H. Glomerulonephritis with initial lung purpura. *Acta Med. Scand.* 168: 405, 1960.
376. Li, H.-L., Hancock, W. W., Hooke, D. H., Dowling, J. P., and Atkins, R. C. Mononuclear cell activation and decreased renal function in IgA nephropathy with crescents. *Kidney Int.* 37:1552, 1990.
377. Liew, S. W., and Kessel, I. Mycoplasmal pneumonia preceding Henoch-Schönlein purpura. *Arch. Dis. Child.* 49:912, 1974.
378. Linné, T., Aperia, A., Broberger, O., Bergstrand, A., Bohman, S. O., and Rekola, S. Course of renal function in IgA glomerulonephritis in children and adolescents. *Acta Paediatr. Scand.* 71: 735, 1982.
379. Linné, T., Aperia, A., Broberger, O., Bergstrand, A., Bohman, S. O., and Wasserman, J. Renal function and biopsy changes during the course of Henoch-Schönlein glomerulonephritis. *Acta Paediatr. Scand.* 72:104, 1983.
380. Linné, T., and Wasserman, J. Lymphocyte subpopulations and immunoglobulin production in IgA nephropathy. *Clin. Nephrol.* 23:109, 1985.
381. Lofters, W. S., Pineo, G. F., Luke, K. H., and Yaworsky, R. G. Henoch-Schönlein purpura occurring in three members of a family. *Can. Med. Assoc. J.* 109:46, 1973.
382. Lomax-Smith, J. D., Woodroffe, A. J., Clarkson, A. R., and Seymour, A. E. IgA nephropathy—Accumulated experience and current concepts. *Pathology* 17:219, 1985.
383. Lomax-Smith, J. D., Zabrowarny, L. A., Howarth, G. S., Seymour, A. E., and Woodroffe, A. J. The immunochemical characterization of mesangial IgA deposits. *Am. J. Pathol.* 113:359, 1983.
384. Lombard, K. A., Shah, P. C., Thrasher, T. V., and Grill, B. B. Ileal structure as a late complication of Henoch-Schönlein purpura. *Pediatrics* 77:396, 1986.
385. Lopez-Trascasa, M., Egido, J., Sancho, J., and Hernando, L. Evidence of high polymeric IgA levels in serum of patients with Berger's disease and its modification with phenytoin treatment. *Proc. Eur. Dial. Transplant. Assoc.* 16:513, 1979.
386. Lopez-Trascasa, M., Egido, J., Sancho, J., and Hernando, L. IgA glomerulonephritis (Berger's disease): Evidence of high serum levels of polymeric IgA. *Clin. Exp. Immunol.* 42:247, 1980.
387. Loughlin, G. M., Taussig, L. M., Murphy, S. A., Strunk, R. C., and Kohnen, P. W. Immune-complex–mediated glomerulonephritis and pulmonary hemorrhage simulating Goodpasture syndrome. *J. Pediatr.* 93:181, 1978.
388. Lowance, D. C., Mullins, J. D., and McPhaul, J. J. Immunoglobulin A (IgA) associated glomerulonephritis. *Kidney Int.* 3:167, 1973.

389. MacDonald, I. M., Dumble, L. J., and Kincaid-Smith, P. HLA-Bw35, circulating immune complexes and IgA deposits in mesangial proliferative glomerulonephritis. *Aust. N.Z. J. Med.* 10:480, 1980.
390. MacGregor, C. S., Johnson, R. S., and Turk, K. A. D. Fatal nephritis complicating idiopathic pulmonary haemosiderosis in young adults. *Thorax* 15:198, 1960.
391. Mackensen-Haen, S., Eisele, R., and Bohle, A. Contribution on the correlation between morphometric parameters gained from the renal cortex and renal function in IgA nephritis. *Lab. Invest.* 59:239, 1988.
392. Maeda, H., Wada, H., Higuchi, A., Tanizawa, T., Okada, T., Suzuki, Y., Sato, H., Takada, T., Yanagihara, T., Okawa, K., and Kobayashi, O. Henoch-Schönlein's syndrome in childhood: Renal histopathology: II. Electron microscopic study. *Acta Med. Biol.* 31:151, 1984.
393. Maggiore, G., Martini, A., Grifeo, S., de Giacomo, C., and Scotta, H. S. Hepatitis B virus infection and Schönlein-Henoch purpura. *Am. J. Dis. Child.* 188:681, 1984.
394. Makdassy, R., Beaufils, M., Meyrier, A., Mignon, F., Moulonguet-Doleris, L., and Richet, G. Pathologic conditions associated with IgA mesangial nephropathy: Preliminary results. *Contrib. Nephrol.* 40:292, 1984.
395. Manigand, G., Morel-Maroger, L., Simon, J., and Deparis, M. Lésions rénales glomérulaires et cirrhose du foie. Note préliminaire sur les lésions histologique du rein au cours des cirrhoses hépatiques, d'apres 20 prélèvements biopsiques. *Rev. Eur. Etud. Clin. Biol.* 15:989, 1970.
396. Martini, A., Magrini, U., Scelsi, M., Capelli, V., and Barberis, L. Chronic mesangioproliferative IgA glomerulonephritis complicated by a rapidly progressive course in a 14-year-old boy. *Nephron* 29:164, 1981.
397. Martini, A., Ravelli, A., Notarangelo, L. D., Burgio, V. L., and Plebani, A. Henoch-Schönlein syndrome and selective IgA deficiency. *Arch. Dis. Child.* 60:160, 1985.
398. Masugi, Y., Ishizaki, M., Fukuda, Y., Sano, J., Kogoshi, T., Maekawa, A., and Sugisaki, Y. Immunopathologic studies of renal glomerular change in liver cirrhosis with special reference to its pathogenesis. *Acta Pathol. Jpn.* 29:571, 1979.
399. Mathew, T. H., Mathews, D. C., Hobbs, J. B., and Kincaid-Smith, P. Glomerular lesions after renal transplantation. *Am. J. Med.* 59:177, 1975.
400. Mathews, D. C., Bell, J. A., Dowling, J. P., and Kincaid-Smith, P. S. Immunoelectron microscopic localization of glomerular IgA deposits using a postembedding method with a protein A–colloidal gold probe. *Ultrastruct. Pathol.* 8:43, 1985.
401. Maurice, T. R. Carcinoma of the bronchus presenting with Henoch-Schönlein purpura. *Br. Med. J.* 2:831, 1978.
402. McCombs, R. P., Patterson, J. F., and MacMahon, H. E. Syndromes associated with "allergic" vasculitis. *N. Engl. J. Med.* 225:251, 1956.
403. McCoy, R. C., Abramowsky, C. R., and Tisher, C. C. IgA nephropathy. *Am. J. Pathol.* 76:123, 1974.
404. McEnery, P. T., McAdams, A. J., and West, C. D. Glomerular Morphology, Natural History and Treatment of Children with IgA-IgG Mesangial Nephropathy. In P. Kincaid-Smith, T. H. Mathew, and E. L. Becker (Eds.), *Glomerulonephritis: Morphology, Natural History, and Treatment.* New York: Wiley, 1973. P. 305.
405. McKenzie, P. E., Gormly, A. A., Clarkson, A. R., Seymour, A. E., Kwitko, A. O., Shearman, D. J. C., and Woodroffe, A. J. Gut-derived antigens and immune complexes in IgA nephropathy. *Aust. N.Z. J. Med.* 10:126, 1980.
406. McKenzie, P. E., Taylor, A. E., Woodroffe, A. J. Seymour, A. E., Cahn, Y. L., and Clarkson, A. R. Plasmapheresis in glomerulonephritis. *Clin. Nephrol.* 12:97, 1979.
407. McLean, R. H., Wyatt, R. J., and Julian, B. A. Complement phenotypes in glomerulonephritis: Increased frequency of homozygous null C4 phenotypes in IgA nephropathy and Schönlein-Henoch purpura. *Kidney Int.* 26:855, 1984.
408. Meadow, S. R. Henoch-Schönlein syndrome after chickenpox (Letter). *Arch. Dis. Child.* 54:564, 1979.
409. Meadow, S. R. The prognosis of Henoch-Schönlein nephritis. *Clin. Nephrol.* 9:87, 1978.
410. Meadow, S. R., Glasgow, E. F., White, R. H. R., Moncrieff, M. W., Cameron, J. S., and Ogg, C. S. Schönlein-Henoch nephritis. *Q. J. Med.* 41:241, 1972.
411. Meadow, S. R., and Scott, D. G. Berger disease: Henoch-Schönlein syndrome without the rash. *J. Pediatr.* 106:27, 1985.
412. Meenakshi, M., Allen, I. V., and Hill, C. M. Possible Stewart's nasal granuloma with dissemination to meninges, peripheral nerves and muscle and renal glomerular IgA deposition. *J. Pathol.* 141:1, 1983.
413. Melvin, T., Burke, B., Michael, A. F., and Kim, Y. Experimental IgA nephropathy in bile duct ligated rats. *Clin. Immunol. Immunopathol.* 27: 369, 1983.
414. Mené, P., Simonson, M. S., and Dunn, M. J. Physiology of the mesangial cell. *Physiol. Rev.* 69:1347, 1989.

415. Mery, J. P., Kenouch, S., and Dard, S. More on IgA nephropathy in a patient with ankylosing spondylitis and a solitary kidney. *Clin. Nephrol.* 22:267, 1984.
416. Mestecky, J., and McGhee, J. R. Immunoglobulin A (IgA): Molecular and cellular interactions involved in IgA biosynthesis and immune response. *Adv. Immunol.* 40:153, 1987.
417. Mestecky, J., Tomana, M., Czerkinsky, C., Tarkowski, A., Matsuda, S., Waldo, F. B., Moldoveanu, Z., Julian, B. A., Galla, J. H., Russell, M. W., and Jackson, S. IgA-associated renal diseases: Immunochemical studies of IgA_1 proteins, circulating immune complexes, and cellular interactions. *Semin. Nephrol.* 7:332, 1987.
418. Michalk, D., Waldherr, R., Seelig, H. P., Webe, H. P., and Scharer, K. Idiopathic mesangial IgA-glomerulonephritis in childhood. *Eur. J. Pediatr.* 134:13, 1980.
419. Miescher, P. A. Bakteriell-allergische Vasculitiden als Ursache von Organerkrankungen. *Schweiz. Med. Wochenschr.* 87:1339, 1957.
420. Miescher, P. A., Paronetto, F., and Koffler, D. Immunofluorescent Studies in Human Vasculitis. In P. Graber and P. A. Miescher (Eds.), *Fourth International Symposium on Immunopathology.* Basel: Schwabe, 1965. P. 446.
421. Miescher, P. A., Reymond, A., and Ritter, O. Le rôle de l'allergie bactérienne dans la pathogénèse de certaines vasculites. *Schweiz. Med. Wochenschr.* 86:799, 1956.
422. Mignone, F., Bona, F., and Ciravegna, P. Incidenza della infezione streptococcica nella sindrome di Schönlein-Henoch's con complicanza renale. *Minerva Pediatr.* 35:499, 1983.
423. Mihatsch, M. J., Imbasciati, E., Fogazzi, G., Giani, M., Ghio, L., and Gaboardi, F. Ultrastructural lesions of Henoch-Schönlein syndrome and IgA nephropathy: Similarities and differences. *Contrib. Nephrol.* 40:255, 1984.
424. Miki, K., Nakamoto, Y., Imai, H., and Yasuda, T. Enhancement of Murine IgA Nephritis by Reticuloendothelial System (RES) Blocking and Failure to Induce It by Oral Immunization. In *Abstracts of the IXth International Congress of Nephrology.* 1984. P. 252.
425. Mina, S. N., and Murphy, W. M. IgA nephropathy: A comprehensive study of the clinicopathologic features in children and adults. *Am. J. Clin. Pathol.* 83:669, 1985.
426. Mita, S., Sakai, O., Matsumoto, A., Kitajima, T., and Miyahara, T. Clinicopathological Study on Renal Involvement in Patients with Sjögren's Syndrome. In *Abstracts of the IXth International Congress of Nephrology.* 1984. P. 292.
427. Mitrofanoff, P. Urétérite sténosante et purpura rhumatoide. *Ann. Chir. Infant* 18:343, 1977.
428. Miyazaki, R., Kuroda, M., Akiyama, T., Tofuku, Y., and Takeda, R. Glomerular deposition and serum levels of complement control proteins in patients with IgA nephropathy. *Clin. Nephrol.* 21:335, 1984.
429. Monteiro, R. C., Halbwachs-Mecarelli, L., Berger, J., and Lesavre, P. Characteristics of eluted IgA in primary IgA nephropathy. *Contrib. Nephrol.* 40:107, 1984.
430. Monteiro, R. C., Noel, L. H., Halbwachs-Mecarelli, L., Berger, J., and Lesavre, P. Charge restriction of mesangial IgA in primary IgA nephropathy. (Abstract) *Kidney Int.* 27:218, 1985.
431. Montoliu, J., Darnell, A., Grau, J. M., Torras, A., and Revert, L. Renal involvement in a syndrome of vasculitis complicating HB_sAg negative cirrhosis of the liver. *Proc. Eur. Dial. Transplant. Assoc.* 21:677, 1984.
432. Montoliu, J., Darnell, A., Torras, A., Ercilla, G., Valles, M., and Revert, L. Familial IgA nephropathy: Report of two cases and brief review of the literature. *Arch. Intern. Med.* 140:1374, 1980.
433. Montoliu, J., Darnell, A., Torras, A., and Revert, L. Glomerular disease in cirrhosis of the liver: Low frequency of IgA deposits. *Am. J. Nephrol.* 6:199, 1986.
434. Moorthy, A. V., Zimmerman, S. W., and Maxim, P. E. Dermatitis herpetiformis and celiac disease: Association with glomerulonephritis, hypocomplementemia and circulating immune complexes. *JAMA* 239:2019, 1978.
435. Morel-Maroger, L., Leathem, A., and Richet, G. Glomerular abnormalities in nonsystemic diseases: Relationship between findings by light microscopy and immunofluorescence in 433 renal biopsy specimens. *Am. J. Med.* 53:170, 1972.
436. Morel-Maroger, L., Mery, J. P., Robert, C. L., and Richet, G. Mesangial IgA Deposits. In P. Kincaid-Smith, T. H. Mathew, and E. L. Becker (Eds.), *Glomerulonephritis: Morphology, Natural History and Treatment.* New York: Wiley, 1973. P. 301.
437. Morzycka, M., Croker, B. P., Jr., Seigler, H. F., and Tisher, C. C. Evaluation of recurrent glomerulonephritis in kidney allografts., *Am. J. Med.* 72:588, 1982.
438. Mota-Hernandez, F., Valbuena-Paz, R., and Gordillo-Paniagua, G. Long-term prognosis of anaphylactoid purpura nephropathy. *Paediatrician* 4:52, 1975.
439. Murakami, T., Furuse, A., Hattori, S., Kobayashi, K., and Matsuda, I. IgA_1 and IgA_2 deposits in IgA nephropathies. *Nephron* 35:120, 1983.
440. Murray, F. E., Lombard, M. G., Donohoe, J. F., Doyle, G. D., Campbell, E., and Alton, B. G.

Simultaneous presentation of IgA nephropathy and sarcoidosis. *Sarcoidosis* 4:134, 1987.
441. Mustonen, J., Helin, H., and Pasternack, A. IgA nephropathy associated with bronchial small-cell carcinoma. *Am. J. Clin. Pathol.* 76:652, 1981.
442. Mustonen, J., Pasternack, A., and Helin, H. IgA mesangial nephropathy in neoplastic diseases. *Contrib. Nephrol.* 40:283, 1984.
443. Mustonen, J., Pasternack, A., Helin, H., and Nikkila, M. Clinicopathologic correlations in a series of 143 patients with IgA glomerulonephritis. *Am. J. Nephrol.* 5:150, 1985.
444. Mustonen, J., Pasternack, A., Helin, H., Rilua, A., Penttinen, K., Wager, O., and Harmoinen, A. Circulating immune complexes, the concentration of serum IgA and the distribution of HLA antigens in IgA nephropathy. *Nephron* 29:170, 1981.
445. Nagy, J., Brasch, H., Sule, T., Hamori, A., Deak, G., and Ambrus, M. IgA glomerulonephritis: Mesangial IgA deposition without systemic signs (Berger's disease). *Int. Urol. Nephrol.* 11:367, 1979.
446. Nagy, J., Brasch, H., Trinn, C., and Burger, T. Clinical features and course of IgA glomerulonephritis. *Acta Med. Acad. Sci. Hung.* 39:201, 1982.
447. Nagy, J., Hamori, A., Ambus, M., and Hernadi, E. More on IgA glomerulonephritis and HLA antigens. *N. Engl. J. Med.* 300:92, 1979.
448. Nagy, J., Miltenyi, M., Dobos, M., and Burger, T. Tubular proteinuria in IgA glomerulonephritis. *Clin. Nephrol.* 27:76, 1987.
449. Nagy, J., Scott, H., and Brandtzaeg, P. Antibodies to dietary antigens in IgA nephropathy. *Clin. Nephrol.* 30:182, 1988.
450. Nagy, J., Trinn, C., Deak, G., Schmelzer, M., and Burger, T. The role of the tubulointerstitial changes in the prognosis of IgA glomerulonephritis. *Klin. Wochenschr.* 62:1094, 1984.
451. Nagy, J., Uj, M., Szÿcs, G., Trinn, C., and Burger, T. Herpesvirus antigens and antibodies in kidney biopsies and sera of IgA glomerulonephritis. *Clin. Nephrol.* 21:259, 1984.
452. Naito, S., Kohara, M., and Arakawa, K. Association of class II antigens of HLA with primary glomerulopathies. *Nephron* 45:111, 1987.
453. Nakajima, M., Hirota, T., Kusumoto, K., Taira, K., and Kamitsuji, H. Immunoelectron microscopic study of glomerular lesions using a post-embedding method with a protein A–gold complex. *Nephron* 46:182, 1987.
454. Nakamoto, Y., Asano, Y., Dohi, K., Fujioka, M., Iida, H., Keda, H., Kibe, Y., Hattori, N., and Takeuchi, S. Primary IgA glomerulonephritis and Schönlein-Henoch purpura nephritis: Clinicopathological and immunohistological characteristics. *Q. J. Med.* 47:495, 1978.
455. Nakamoto, Y., Iida, H., Kobayashi, K., Dohi, K., Kida, H., Hattori, N., and Takeuchi, J. Hepatic glomerulonephritis: Characteristics of hepatic IgA glomerulonephritis as the major part. *Virchows Arch.* [A] 392:45, 1981.
456. Nakamoto, Y., Miki, K., Miura, A. B., Doki, K., and Nomura, G. Hypertension and intrarenal small-vessel lesions in patients with IgA nephritis. *Nippon Jinzo Gakkai Shi* 28:1211, 1986.
457. Navas-Palacios, J. J., Gutierrez-Millet, L. V., Usera-Sarraga, G., and Garzon-Martin, A. IgA nephropathy: An ultrastructural study. *Ultrastruct. Pathol.* 2:151, 1981.
458. Neelakantappa, K., Gallo, G. R., and Baldwin, D. S. Proteinuria in IgA nephropathy. *Semin. Nephrol.* 7:344, 1987.
459. Newell, G. C. Cirrhotic glomerulonephritis: Incidence, morphology, clinical features, and pathogenesis. *Am. J. Kidney Dis.* 9:183, 1987.
460. Ng, W. L., Chan, C. W., Yeung, C. K., and Hua, S. P. The pathology of primary IgA glomerulonephritis—A renal biopsy study. *Pathology* 13:137, 1981.
461. Niaudet, P., Lenoir, G., and Habib, R. La Néphropathie du Purpura Rhumatoide. In *Journées Parisienens de Pédiatrie.* Paris: Flammarion Médecine-Sciences, 1986. P. 145.
462. Niaudet, P., Levy, M., Broyer, M., and Habib, R. Clinicopathologic correlations in severe forms of Henoch-Schönlein purpura nephritis based on repeat biopsies. *Contrib. Nephrol.* 40:250, 1984.
463. Nicholls, K., and Kincaid-Smith, P. Defective in vivo Fc- and C3b-receptor function in IgA nephropathy. *Am. J. Kidney Dis.* 4:128, 1984.
464. Nochy, D., Callard, P., Bellon, B., Bariety, J., and Druet, P. Association of overt glomerulonephritis and liver disease: A study of 34 patients. *Clin. Nephrol.* 6:422, 1976.
465. Nochy, D., and Druet, P. Les glomérulopathies au cours des maladies hépatiques. *Nouv. Presse. Med.* 8:1595, 1979.
466. Nochy, D., Druet, P., and Bariety, J. IgA nephropathy in chronic liver disease. *Contrib. Nephrol.* 40:268, 1984.
467. Noël, L. H., Descamps, B., Jungers, P., Bach, J. F., Busson, M., Suet, C., Hors, J., and Dausset, J. HLA antigen in three types of glomerulonephritis. *Clin. Immunol. Immunopathol.* 10:19, 1973.
468. Nolasco, F. E., Cameron, J. S., Hartley, B., Coelho, A., Hildreth, G., and Reuben, R. Intraglomerular T cells and monocytes in nephritis: Study with monoclonal antibodies. *Kidney Int.* 31:1160, 1987.
469. Nomoto, Y., Sakai, H., and Aimori, S. Increase of IgA-bearing lymphocytes in peripheral blood from patients with IgA nephropathy. *Am. J. Clin.*

Pathol. 71:158, 1979.

470. Nunan, T. O., Eykyn, S. J., and Jones, N. F. Brucellosis with mesangial IgA nephropathy: Successful treatment with doxycycline and rifampicin. *Br. Med. J.* 288:1802, 1984.
471. Nussenzveig, V., Saldanha, L. B., and Marcondos, M. Primary mesangial IgA nephropathy in Sao Paolo, Brazil. *Nephron* 52:198, 1989.
472. Nyulassy, S., Buc, M., Sasinka, M., Pavlovic, M., Slugen, I., Hirschova, V., Kaiserova, M., Menkyna, R., and Stefanovic, J. The HLA system in glomerulonephritis. *Clin. Immunol. Immunopathol.* 7:319, 1977.
473. Okada, K., Kawakami, K., Yano, I., Funai, M., Kagami, S., Kuroda, Y., and Oite, T. Ultrastructural alterations of glomerular anionic sites in IgA nephropathy. *Clin. Nephrol.* 31:96, 1989.
474. Okada, M., Okamura, K., Ohmura, N., and Kitaoka, T. Clinicopathological Study of IgA Nephropathy in Comparison with Mesangial Proliferative Glomerulonephritis Without IgA Deposits. In *Abstracts of the IXth International Congress of Nephrology.* 1984. P. 117.
475. Oliver, T. K., Jr., and Barnett, H. L. The incidence and prognosis of nephritis associated with anaphylactoid (Schönlein-Henoch) purpura in children. *Am. J. Dis. Child.* 90:544, 1955.
476. Osler, W. On the visceral manifestations of the erythema group of skin diseases. *Am. J. Med. Sci.* 127:1, 1904.
477. Paller, M. S., Daniels, B. S., and Hostetter, T. H. Severe flank pain as the predominant symptom of IgA nephropathy. *Am. J. Kidney Dis.* 13:494, 1989.
478. Panner, B. Nephritis of Schönlein-Henoch syndrome: Electron microscopic study of the glomerular lesion in an adult. *Arch. Pathol.* 74:230, 1962.
479. Pape, J. F., Mellbye, O. J., Oystese, B., and Brodwall, E. K. Glomerulonephritis in dermatitis herpetiformis. *Acta Med. Scand.* 203:445, 1978.
480. Parai, S. K., and Ghose, T. IgA nephropathy in adults: Immunohistologic findings and clinical course. *Can. Med. Assoc. J.* 132:1381, 1985.
481. Pardo, V., Pardo, T., Clerch, A., Strauss, J., and Esquenazy, V. HLA-Bw35 antigen as a marker for segmental sclerosis and progressive disease in IgA mesangial glomerulonephritis. *Kidney Int.* 19:134, 1981.
482. Parkin, T. W., Rusted, I. E., Burchell, H. B., and Edwards, J. E. Hemorrhagic and interstitial pneumonitis with nephritis. *Am. J. Med.* 18:220, 1955.
483. Pasternack, A., Linder, E., and Kuhlbäck, B. Glomerulonephritis with initial pulmonary haemorrhage. *Acta Med. Scand.* 177:601, 1955.
484. Patek, A. J., Seegal, D., and Bevans, M. The coexistence of cirrhosis of the liver and glomerulonephritis. Report of 14 cases. *Am. J. Med. Sci.* 221:77, 1951.
485. Payne, W. W., and Illingworth, R. S. Acute nephritis in childhood, with special reference to the diagnosis of focal nephritis. *Q. J. Med.* 9:37, 1940.
486. Payton, C. D., McLay, A., and Boulton Jones, J. M. Progressive IgA nephropathy: The role of hypertension. *Nephrol. Dial. Transplant.* 2: 183, 1988.
487. Perez-Fontan, M., Miguel, J. L., Picazo, M. L., Martinez-Ara, J., Selgas, R., and Sicilia, L. S. Idiopathic IgA nephropathy presenting as malignant hypertension. *Am. J. Nephrol.* 6:482, 1986.
488. Philpott, M. G. The Schönlein-Henoch syndrome in childhood with particular reference to the occurrence of nephritis. *Arch. Dis. Child.* 27:480, 1952.
489. Pierucci, A., Simonetti, B. M., Pecci, G., Mavrikakis, G., Feriozzi, S., Cinotti, G. A., Patrignani, P., Ciabattoni, G., and Patrono, C. Improvement of renal function with selective thromboxane antagonism in lupus nephritis. *N. Engl. J. Med.* 320:421, 1989.
490. Praga, M., Costa, J. R., Shandas, G. J., Martinez, M. A., Mirandi, B., and Rodicio, J. L. Acute renal failure in cirrhosis associated with macroscopic hematuria of glomerular origin. *Arch. Intern. Med.* 147:173, 1987.
491. Praga, M., Millet, V. G., Navas, J., Morles, J. M., Ruilope, L. M., Alcazar, J. M., and Rodicio, J. L. Acute worsening of renal function during episodes of macroscopic hematuria in IgA nephropathy. *Kidney Int.* 28:69, 1985.
492. Pratesi, G., and Rizzuto, A. Le glomerulonefrite nel corso della sindrome di Schönlein-Henoch. *Rass. Fisiopat. Clin. Ter.* 28:443, 1956.
493. Propper, D. J., Power, D. A., Simpson, J. G., Edward, N., and Catto, G. R. D. The incidence, mode of presentation, and prognosis of IgA nephropathy in northeast Scotland. *Semin. Nephrol.* 7:363, 1987.
494. Rajaraman, S., Goldblum, R. M., and Cavallo, T. IgA-associated glomerulonephritides: A study with monoclonal antibodies. *Clin. Immunol. Immunopathol.* 39:514, 1986.
495. Rambausek, M., Schuhmacher, R., Spitzenberg, R., Rother, U., and Ritz, E. Genetic Polymorphism of C3 and Mesangial IgA Glomerulonephritis. In *Abstracts of the IXth International Congress of Nephrology.* 1984. P. 120.
496. Rambausek, M., Seelig, H. P., Andrassy, K., Waldherr, R., Kehry, I., Lenhard, V., and Ritz, E. Mesangiale IgA-glomerulonephritis. *Dtsch. Med. Wochenschr.* 108:125, 1983.
497. Rambausek, M., Seelig, H. P., Andrassy, K., Waldherr, R., Lenhard, V., and Ritz, E. Clinical and

serological features of mesangial IgA glomerulonephritis. *Proc. Eur. Dial. Transplant. Assoc.* 19: 663, 1982.

498. Ramirez, G., Stinson, J. B., Zawada, E. T., and Moatamed, F. IgA nephritis associated with mycosis fungoides. *Arch. Intern. Med.* 141:1287, 1981.

499. Raphael, S. S., and Lynch, M. J. G. Kimmelstiel-Wilson glomerulopathy: Its occurrence in diseases other than diabetes mellitus. *Arch. Pathol.* 65:420, 1958.

500. Rasmussen, H. Henoch-Schönlein syndrome after yersiniosis (Letter). *Arch. Dis. Child.* 57:322, 1982.

501. Rathery, F., and Dérot, M. Étude clinique biologique et anatomo-pathologique d'un cas de néphrite subaiguë apparue après un purpura rhumatoïde. *Bull. Soc. Med. Hop. Paris* 50:1430, 1934.

502. Rauterberg, E. W., Lieberknecht, H.-M., Wingen, A.-M., and Ritz, E. Complement membrane attack complex (MAC) in idiopathic IgA-glomerulonephritis. *Kidney Int.* 31:820, 1987.

503. Reeves, G., Lowenstein, L. M., and Sommers, S. C. The macula densa and juxtaglomerular body of cirrhosis. *Ann. Intern. Med.* 112:708, 1963.

504. Régnier, C., and Bouissou, H. Apport de la microscopie électronique dans les néphropathies du syndrome des Schönlein-Henoch. *Arch. Fr. Pediatr.* 17:384, 1960.

505. Richman, A. V., Mahoney, J. J., and Fuller, T. J. Higher prevalence of HLA-B12 in patients with IgA nephropathy. *Ann. Intern. Med.* 90:201, 1979.

506. Rifai, A. Experimental models for IgA-associated nephritis. *Kidney Int.* 31:1, 1987.

507. Rifai, A., Chen, A., and Imai, H. Complement activation in experimental IgA nephropathy: An antigen-mediated process. *Kidney Int.* 32:838, 1987.

508. Rifai, A., and Mannik, M. Clearance kinetics and fate of mouse IgA immune complexes prepared with monomeric or dimeric IgA. *J. Immunol.* 130:1826, 1983.

509. Rifai, A., and Mannik, M. Clearance of circulating IgA immune complexes is mediated by a specific receptor on Kupffer cells in mice. *J. Exp. Med.* 160:125, 1984.

510. Rifai, A., Schena, F. P., Montinaro, V., Mele, M., D'Addabbo, A., Nitti, L., and Pezzullo, J. C. Clearance kinetics and fate of macromolecular IgA in patients with IgA nephropathy. *Lab. Invest.* 61:381, 1989.

511. Rifai, A., Small, P. A., Teague, P. O., and Ayoub, E. M. Experimental IgA nephropathy. *J. Exp. Med.* 150:1161, 1979.

512. Roberts, F. B., Slater, R. J., and Laski, B. The prognosis of Henoch-Schönlein nephritis. *Can. Med. Assoc. J.* 87:49, 1962.

513. Roccatello, D., Coppo, R., and Piccoli, G. IgA-containing monocytes from patients with IgA nephropathy. *Nephron* 38:213, 1984.

514. Roccatello, D. Coppo, R., Piccoli, G., Martina, G., Rollino, C., Picciotto, G., Sena, L. M., and Amoroso, A. Circulating Fc-receptor blocking factors in IgA nephropathies. *Clin. Nephrol.* 23: 159, 1985.

515. Roccatello, D., Picciotto, G., Coppo, R., Piccoli, G., Molino, A., Cacace, G., Amore, A., Amoroso, A., Quattrocchio, G., and Sena, L. M. Clearance of polymeric IgA aggregates in humans. *Am. J. Kidney Dis.* 14:354, 1989.

516. Rose, G. M., Cole, B. R., and Robson, A. M. The treatment of severe glomerulopathies in children using high dose intravenous methylprednisolone pulses. *Am. J. Kidney Dis.* 1:148, 1981.

517. Ross, J. H. Recurrent focal nephritis. *Q. J. Med.* 29:391, 1960.

518. Rostoker, G., Pech, M.-A., del Prato, S., Petit-Phar, M., Maadi, A., Dubert, J.-M., Lang, P., Weil, B., and Lagrue, G. Serum IgG subclasses and IgM imbalances in adult IgA mesangial glomerulonephritis and idiopathic Henoch-Schoenlein purpura. *Clin. Exp. Immunol.* 75:30, 1989.

519. Roth, D. A., Wilz, D. A., and Theil, G. B. Schönlein-Henoch syndrome in adults. *Q. J. Med.* 55:145, 1985.

520. Roy, L. P., Fish, A. J., Vernier, R. L., and Michael, A. F. Recurrent macroscopic hematuria, focal nephritis, and mesangial deposition of immunoglobulin and complement. *J. Pediatr.* 82: 767, 1973.

521. Roza, M., Galbe, C., Gonzales-Baschwitz, C., Fernandez, M., and Miguel, M. A. Henoch-Schönlein purpura after shigellosis (Letter). *Clin. Nephrol.* 20:269, 1983.

522. Rubin, M. (Discussion following presentation "The incidence and prognosis of nephritis associated with anaphylactoid (Schönlein-Henoch) purpura in children" by T. K. Oliver, Jr., and H. L. Barnett). *AMA J. Dis. Child.* 90:545, 1955.

523. Rusby, N. L., and Wilson, C. Lung purpura with nephritis. *Q. J. Med.* 29:501, 1960.

524. Russell, M. W., and Mansa, B. Complement-fixing properties of human IgA antibodies: Alternative pathway complement activation by plastic-bound, but not specific antigen-bound, IgA. *Scand. J. Immunol.* 30:175, 1989.

525. Russell, M. W., Mestecky, J., Julian, B. A., and Galla, J. H. IgA-associated renal diseases: Antibodies to environmental antigens in sera and deposition of immunoglobulins and antigen in glomeruli. *J. Clin. Immunol.* 6:74, 1986.

526. Russell, M. W., Reinholdt, J., and Kilian, M. Anti-inflammatory activity of human IgA anti-

bodies and the Fabα fragments: Inhibition of IgG-mediated complement activation. *Eur. J. Immunol.* 19:2243, 1989.
527. Sabadini, E., Castiglione, A., Colasanti, G., Ferrario, F., Civardi, R., Fellin, G., and D'Amico, G. Characterization of interstitial infiltrating cells in Berger's disease. *Am. J. Kidney Dis.* 12:307, 1988.
528. Sabatier, J. C., Genin, C., Assenat, H., Colon, S., Ducret, F., and Berthoux, F. C. Mesangial IgA nephritis in HLA-identical brothers. *Clin. Nephrol.* 11:35, 1979.
529. Sakaguchi, H. Hepatic glomerulosclerosis—Light microscopic study of autopsy cases. *Acta Pathol. Jpn.* 18:407, 1968.
530. Sakaguchi, H., Dachs, S., Grishman, E., Paronetto, F., Salomon, M., and Churg, J. Hepatic glomerulosclerosis: An electron microscopic study of renal biopsies of liver disease. *Lab. Invest.* 14:533, 1965.
531. Sakai, H., Endoh, M., Tomino, Y., and Nomoto, Y. Increase of IgA specific helper T cells in patients with IgA nephropathy. *Clin. Exp. Immunol.* 50:77, 1982.
532. Sakai, H., Kitajima, T., Kawamura, K., and Ueda, Y. Clinicopathological Studies on IgA Glomerulonephritis. In Y. Yoshitoshi (Ed.), *Glomerulonephritis: Proceedings of the International Symposium on Glomerulonephritis.* Baltimore: University Park Press, 1979. P. 167.
533. Sakai, H., Nomoto, Y., and Arimori, S. Decrease of IgA specific suppressor T-cell activity in patients with IgA nephropathy. *Clin. Exp. Immunol.* 38:243, 1979.
534. Sakai, H., Nomoto, Y., Arimori, S., Komori, K., Inouye, H., and Tsuji, K. Increase of IgA bearing peripheral blood lymphocytes in families of patients with IgA nephropathy. *Am. J. Clin. Pathol.* 72:452, 1979.
535. Salomon, M., Sakaguchi, H., Churg, J., Dachs, S., Grishman, E., Mautner, W., Paronetto, F., and Rosenthal, W. S. Renal lesions in hepatic disease: A study based on kidney biopsies. *Arch. Intern. Med.* 115:704, 1965.
536. Sancho, J., Egido, J., Rivera, F., and Hernando, L. Immune complexes in IgA nephropathy: Presence of antibodies against diet antigens and delayed clearance of specific polymeric IgA immune complexes. *Clin. Exp. Immunol.* 54:194, 1983.
537. Sancho, J., Gonzalez, E., and Egido, J. Handling of IgA immune aggregates by liver cell. *Contrib. Nephrol.* 40:93, 1984.
538. Sanfilippo, F., Croker, B. P., and Bollinger, R. R. Fate of four cadaveric donor renal allografts with mesangial IgA deposits. *Transplantation* 33:370, 1982.
539. Sato, M., Idewa, T., and Koshikawa, S. Experimental IgA nephropathy in mice. *Lab. Invest.* 54:377, 1986.
540. Sato, M., Jakajima, Y., and Koshikawa, S. Effect of sodium cromoglycate on an experimental model of IgA nephropathy. *Clin. Nephrol.* 27:141, 1987.
541. Sato, M., Takayama, K., Wakasa, M., and Koshikawa, S. Estimation of circulating immune complexes following oral challenge with cow's milk in patients with IgA nephropathy. *Nephron* 47:43, 1987.
542. Saulsbury, F. T. Case report: Antinuclear antibody in Henoch-Schönlein purpura. *Am. J. Med. Sci.* 291:180, 1986.
543. Saulsbury, F. T. IgA rheumatoid factor in Henoch-Schönlein purpura. *J. Pediatr.* 108:71, 1986.
544. Savi, M., Neri, T. M., Silvestri, M. G., Allegri, L., and Migone, L. HLA antigens and IgA mesangial glomerulonephritis. *Clin. Nephrol.* 12:45, 1979.
545. Schena, F. P., Mastrolitti, G., Fracasso, A. R., Pastore, A., and Ladisa, N. Increased immunoglobulin-secreting cells in the blood of patients with active idiopathic IgA nephropathy. *Clin. Nephrol.* 26:163, 1986.
546. Schena, F. P., Pastore, A., Sinico, R. A., Montinaro, V., and Fornasieri, A. Polymeric IgA decreases the capacity of serum to solubilize circulating immune complexes in patients with primary IgA nephropathy. *J. Immunol.* 141:125, 1988.
547. Schlesinger, M., Vardy, P. A., and Rubinow, A. Henoch-Schönlein purpura and familial Mediterranean fever. *Isr. J. Med. Sci.* 21:83, 1985.
548. Schmekel, B., Soalade, C., Bacht, H., and Westberg, N. G. Mesangial IgA glomerulonephritis in adults. *Acta Med. Scand.* 210:363, 1981.
548a. Schönlein, J. L. *Allgemeine und Specielle Pathologie und Therapie.* (2nd ed.) Würzburg: Etlinger, 1832. Vol. 2., P. 68.
549. Seedat, Y. K., Nathoo, B. C., Parag, K. B., Naiker, I. P., and Ramsaroop, R. IgA nephropathy in Blacks and Indians of Natal. *Nephron* 50:137, 1988.
550. Sengar, D. P., Acharya, C. D., and Wolfish, N. M. HLA specificities, lymphocyte subsets, and mitogenic response in HSP nephritis. *Int. J. Pediatr. Nephrol.* 5:197, 1984.
551. Shand, B. I., Barley, R. R., and Simpson, L. O. Blood rheology in IgA nephropathy. *Clin. Nephrol.* 29:288, 1988.
552. Shichiri, M., Tsutsumi, K., Yamamoto, I., Ida, T., and Iwamoto, H. Diffuse intrapulmonary hemorrhage and renal failure in adult Henoch-Schönlein purpura. *Am. J. Nephrol.* 7:140, 1987.
553. Shigematsu, H., Kobayashi, Y., Tateno, S., Hiki, Y., and Kwao, S. Ultrastructural glomerular loop abnormalities in IgA nephritis. *Nephron* 30:1, 1982.

554. Shigematsu, H., Kobayashi, Y., Tateno, S., and Tsukada, M. Ultrastructure of acute glomerular injury in IgA nephritis. *Arch. Pathol. Lab. Med.* 104:303, 1980.
555. Shirai, T., Tomino, Y., Sato, M., Yoshiki, T., and Itoh, T. IgA nephropathy: Clinicopathology and immunopathology. *Contrib. Nephrol.* 9:88, 1978.
556. Shu, K. H., Lian, J. D., Yang, Y. F., Lu, Y. S., Wang, J. Y., Lan, J. L., and Chou, G. Glomerulonephritis in ankylosing spondylitis. *Clin. Nephrol.* 25:169, 1986.
557. Shulman, S. Y., Barratt, T. M., and Soothill, J. F. Immunoconglutinin and complement studies in congenital nephrotic syndrome and nephritis of Henoch-Schönlein purpura in children. *Arch. Dis. Child.* 46:838, 1971.
558. Silva, F. G., Chander, P., Pirani, C. L., and Hardy, M. A. Disappearance of glomerular mesangial IgA deposits after renal allograft transplantation. *Transplantation* 33:214, 1982.
559. Silver, B. J., Jaffer, F. E., and Abboud, H. E. Platelet-derived growth factor (PDGF) synthesis in mesangial cells: Induction by multiple peptide mitogens. *Proc. Natl. Acad. Sci. USA* 86:1056, 1989.
560. Simila, S., Kouvalainen, K., and Lannin, M. Serum immunoglobulin levels in the course of anaphylactoid purpura in children. *Acta Paediatr. Scand.* 66:537, 1977.
561. Singhal, P. C., and Scharschmidt, L. A. Membranous nephropathy associated with primary biliary cirrhosis and bullous pemphigoid. *Ann. Allergy* 5:484, 1985.
562. Sinico, R. A., Fornasieri, A., Maldifassi, P., Colasanti, G., and D'Amico, G. The clinical significance of IgA rheumatoid factor in idiopathic IgA mesangial nephropathy (Berger's disease). *Clin. Nephrol.* 30:182, 1988.
563. Sinico, R. A., Fornasieri, A., Oreni, N., Benuzzi, S., and D'Amico, G. Polymeric IgA rheumatoid factor in idiopathic IgA mesangial nephropathy (Berger's disease). *J. Immunol.* 137:536, 1986.
564. Sinnassamy, P., and O'Regan, S. Mesangial IgA deposits with steroid responsive nephrotic syndrome: Probable minimal lesion nephrosis. *Am. J. Kidney Dis.* 5:267, 1985.
565. Sinniah, R. Mucin-secreting cancer with mesangial IgA deposits. *Pathology* 14:303, 1982.
566. Sinniah, R. Heterogeneous IgA glomerulonephropathy in liver cirrhosis. *Histopathology* 8:947, 1984.
567. Sinniah, R. IgA mesangial nephropathy: Berger's disease. *Am. J. Nephrol.* 5:73, 1985.
568. Sinniah, R., and Churg, J. Effect of IgA deposits on the glomerular mesangium in Berger's disease. *Ultrastruct. Pathol.* 4:9, 1983.
569. Sinniah, R., Feng, P. H., and Chen, B. T. M. Henoch-Schönlein syndrome: A clinical and morphological study of renal biopsies. *Clin. Nephrol.* 9:219, 1978.
570. Sinniah, R., Javier, A. R., and Ku, G. The pathology of IgA nephritis with clinical correlation. *Histopathology* 5:469, 1981.
571. Sissons, J. G. P., Woodrow, D. F., Curtis, J. R., Evans, D. J., Gower, P. E., Sloper, J. C., and Peters, D. K. Isolated glomerulonephritis with mesangial IgA deposits. *Br. Med. J.* 3:611, 1975.
572. Smith, S. M., Hoy, W. E., Pathak, D., Megill, D. M., Tung, K. S. K., and Hughson, M. D. Pathologic findings in mesangiopathic glomerulonephritis in Navajo Indians. *Arch. Pathol. Lab. Med.* 113:158, 1989.
573. Solomon, L. R., Rowlinson, V. I., Howarth, S., and Mallick, N. P. Reticuloendothelial function in glomerulonephritis. *Nephron* 37:54, 1984.
574. Somekh, E., Fried, D., and Hanukogly, A. Muscle involvement in Schönlein-Henoch syndrome. *Arch. Dis. Child.* 58:919, 1983.
575. Sonoda, E., Matsumoto, R., Hitoshi, Y., Ishii, T., Sugimoto, M., Araki, S., Tominaga, A., Yamaguchi, N., and Takatsu, K. Transforming growth factor β induces IgA production and acts additively with interleukin 5 for IgA production. *J. Exp. Med.* 170:1415, 1989.
576. Southwest Pediatric Nephrology Study Group. A multicenter study of IgA nephropathy in children: A report of the Southwest Pediatric Nephrology Study Group. *Kidney Int.* 22:643, 1982.
577. Southwest Pediatric Nephrology Study Group. Association of IgA nephropathy with steroid-responsive nephrotic syndrome. *Am. J. Kidney Dis.* 5:157, 1985.
578. Spiegel, R. Clinical aspects of periarteritis nodosa. *Arch. Intern. Med.* 58:993, 1936.
579. Spitzer, R. E., Urmson, J. R., Farnett, M. L., Stitzel, A. E., and Post, E. M. Alteration of the complement system in children with Henoch-Schönlein purpura. *Clin. Immunol. Immunopathol.* 11:52, 1978.
580. Stachura, I., Singh, G., and Whiteside, T. L. Immune abnormalities in IgA nephropathy (Berger's disease). *Clin. Immunol. Immunopathol.* 20:373, 1981.
581. Sterky, G., and Thilén, A. A study on the onset and prognosis of acute vascular purpura (the Schönlein-Henoch syndrome) in children. *Acta Paediatr. (Stockh.)* 49:217, 1960.
582. Stevenson, J. A., Leong, L. A., Cohen, A. H., and Border, W. A. Henoch-Schönlein purpura. Simultaneous demonstration of IgA deposits in involved skin, intestine and kidney. *Arch. Pathol. Lab. Med.* 106:192, 1982.
583. Striker, L. M.-M., Killen, P. D., Chi, E., and

Striker, G. E. The composition of glomerulosclerosis: I. Studies in focal sclerosis, crescentic glomerulonephritis, and membranoproliferative glomerulonephritis. *Lab. Invest.* 51:181, 1984.

584. Striker, G. E., Quadracci, L. J., Larter, W., Hickman, R. O., Kelly, M. R., and Schaller, J. The Nephritis of Henoch-Schönlein Purpura. In P. Kincaid-Smith, T. H. Mathew, and E. L. Becker (Eds.), *Glomerulonephritis: Morphology, Natural History and Treatment.* New York: Wiley, 1973. P. 1105.
585. Subais, R., Botey, A., Darnell, A., Montoliu, J., and Revert, L. Malignant or accelerated hypertension in IgA nephropathy. *Clin. Nephrol.* 27:1, 1987.
586. Suga, T., Endoh, M., Miura, M., Tomino, Y., Nomoto, Y., and Sakai, H. Hepatic glomerulosclerosis with IgA deposition—Report of three cases. *Tokai J. Exp. Clin. Med.* 8:317, 1983.
587. Sussman, M., Jones, J. H., Almeida, J. D., and Lachman, P. J. Deficiency of the second component of complement associated with anaphylactoid purpura and presence of mycoplasma in the serum. *Clin. Exp. Immunol.* 14:531, 1973.
588. Swerdlow, M. A., Chowdhury, L. N., and Horn, T. Patterns of IgA deposition in liver tissues in alcoholic liver disease. *Am. J. Clin. Pathol.* 77: 259, 1982.
589. Syre, G. IgA mesangial glomerulonephritis: Significance and pathogenesis of segmental-focal glomerular lesions. *Virchows Arch.* [A] 402:11, 1983.
590. Syre, G. IgA Glomerulonephritis: An Additional Pathogenic Factor Responsible for an Unfavorable Outcome. In *Abstracts of the IXth International Congress of Nephrology.* 1984. P. 262.
591. Takada, T., Yanigihara, T., Yoshizumi, A., Wada, H., Maeda, H., Suzuki, Y., Okada, T., Tanizawa, T., Okawa, K., and Kobayashi, O. Henoch-Schönlein's syndrome in childhood: Renal histopathology: I. Light microscopic study. *Acta Med. Biol.* 30:101, 1983.
592. Talwalkar, Y. B., Tamanaha, K., and Ashimine, K. A rare complication of Schönlein-Henoch syndrome. *Int. J. Pediatr. Nephrol.* 5:179, 1984.
593. Tamura, T., Muso, E., Kuwabara and Kawai, T. The Pathogenesis of Hypertension in IgA Nephropathy. In *Abstracts of the IXth International Congress of Nephrology.* 1984. P. 227.
594. Tanaka, M. Immunoelectron microscopic studies of IgA nephropathy in children. *Hokkaido Igaku Zasshi* 61:83, 1986.
595. Tanaka, M., Fuzisawa, S., and Okuda, R. Anaphylactoid purpura in childhood: III. Follow-up study of serum levels of immunoglobulins (G, M, A). *Ann. Paediatr. Jpn.* 15:19, 1969.
596. Tanizawa, T., Okada, T., Uenoyama, F., Maeda, H., Wada, H., Takada, T., Yanigihara, T., Okawa, K., and Kobayashi, O. Henoch-Schönlein's syndrome in childhood: Renal histopathology: III. Immunofluorescent microscopic study. *Acta Med. Biol.* 31:153, 1984.
597. Tateno, S., and Kobayashi, Y. Quantitative analysis of mesangial areas in serial biopsied patients within IgA nephropathy. *Nephron* 46:28, 1987.
598. Terasaki, T., Sano, M., Narita, M., and Tojo, S. Ultrastructural study of gaps of the glomerular basement membrane in IgA nephropathy. *Am. J. Nephrol.* 6:443, 1986.
599. Thompson, A. J., Chan, Y. L., Woodroffe, A. J., Clarkson, A. R., and Seymour, A. E. Vascular IgA deposits in clinically normal skin of patients with renal disease. *Pathology* 12:407, 1980.
600. Thorner, P. S., Farine, M., Arbus, G. S., Poucell, S., and Baumal, R. IgA nephropathy: Henoch-Schönlein purpura and Berger's disease in one patient. *Int. J. Pediatr. Nephrol.* 7:131, 1986.
601. Tolkoff-Rubin, N. E., Cosimi, A. B., Fuller, T., Rubin, R. H., and Colvin, R. B. IgA nephropathy in HLA-identical siblings. *Transplantation* 26:430, 1978.
602. Tomino, Y. Complement system in IgA nephropathy. *Tokai J. Exp. Clin. Med.* 5:15, 1980.
603. Tomino, Y., Endoh, M., Miura, M., Nomoto, Y., and Sakai, H. Immunopathological similarities between IgA nephropathy and Henoch-Schönlein purpura nephritis. *Acta Pathol. Jpn.* 33:122, 1983.
604. Tomino, Y., Endoh, M., Nomoto, Y., and Sakai, H. Activation of complement by renal tissues from patients with IgA nephropathy. *J. Clin. Pathol.* 34:35, 1981.
605. Tomino, Y., Endoh, M., Nomoto, Y., and Sakai, H. Immunoglobulin A_1 in IgA nephropathy. *N. Engl. J. Med.* 305:1159, 1981.
606. Tomino, Y., Endoh, M., Nomoto, Y., and Sakai, H. Specificity of eluted antibody from renal tissues of patients with IgA nephropathy. *Am. J. Kidney Dis.* 1:276, 1982.
607. Tomino, Y., and Sakai, H. Exacerbating factors in patients with IgA nephropathy. *Semin. Nephrol.* 7:315, 1987.
608. Tomino, Y., Sakai, H., Endoh, M., Kaneshige, H., and Nomoto, Y. Detection of immune complexes in polymorphonuclear leukocytes by double immunofluorescence in patients with IgA nephropathy. *Clin. Immunol. Immunopathol.* 24:63, 1982.
609. Tomino, Y., Sakai, H., Endoh, M., Suga, T., Miura, M., Kaneshige, H., and Nomoto, Y. Cross-reactivity of IgA antibodies between renal mesangial areas and nuclei of tonsillar cells in patients with IgA nephropathy. *Clin. Exp. Immunol.* 51:605, 1983.

610. Tomino, Y., Sakai, H., Hashimoto, K., and Tanaka, S. Antigenic heterogeneity in patients with IgA nephropathy. *Semin. Nephrol.* 7:294, 1987.
611. Tomino, Y., Sakai, H., Miura, M., Endoh, M., and Nomoto, Y. Detection of polymeric IgA in glomeruli from patients with IgA nephropathy. *Clin. Exp. Immunol.* 49:419, 1982.
612. Tomino, Y., Sakai, H., Suga, T., Miura, M., Kaneshige, H., Endoh, M., and Nomoto, Y. Impaired solubilization of glomerular immune deposits by sera from patients with IgA nephropathy. *Am. J. Kidney Dis.* 3:48, 1983.
613. Tomino, Y., Yagami, M., Eguchi, K., Nomoto, Y., and Sakai, H. Immunofluorescent studies on S-protein in glomeruli from patients with IgA nephropathy. *Am. J. Pathol.* 129:402, 1987.
614. Touchard, G., Maire, P., Beauchant, M., Doevre, P., Babin, P., Pecheur, H., Becq-Giraudon, B., and Matuchansky, C. Vascular IgA and C3 deposition in gastrointestinal tract of patients with Henoch-Schönlein purpura (Letter). *Lancet* 1: 771, 1983.
615. Trygstad, C. W., and Stiehm, E. R. Elevated serum IgA in anaphylactoid purpura. *Pediatrics* 47:1023, 1971.
616. Tsai, C. C., Giangiancomo, J., and Zuckner, J. Dermal IgA deposits in Henoch-Schönlein purpura and Berger's nephritis. *Lancet* 1:347, 1975.
617. Tung, K. S. K., Woodroffe, A. J., Ahlin, T. D., Williams, R. C., Jr., and Wilson, C. B. Application of the solid phase C1q and Raji cell radioimmune assays for the detection of circulating immune complexes in glomerulonephritis. *J. Clin. Invest.* 62:61, 1978.
618. Tveterås, E. Anaphylactoid purpura (Schönlein-Henoch's syndrom) med nefrit sóm komplikation. *Sven. Lakartidn.* 53:1434, 1956.
619. Ueda, Y., Sakai, O., Yamagata, M., Kitajima, T., and Kawamura, K. IgA glomerulonephritis in Japan. *Contrib. Nephrol.* 4:36, 1977.
620. Underdown, B. J., and Schiff, J. M. Immunoglobulin A: Strategic defense initiative at the mucosal surface. *Annu. Rev. Immunol.* 4:389, 1986.
621. Urizar, R. E., and Herdman, R. C. Anaphylactoid purpura: III. Early morphologic glomerular changes. *Am. J. Clin. Pathol.* 53:258, 1970.
622. Urizar, R. E., Michael, A., Sisson, S., and Vernier, R. L. Anaphylactoid purpura: II. Immunofluorescent and electron microscopic studies of the glomerular lesions. *Lab. Invest.* 19:437, 1968.
623. Urizar, R. E., Singh, J. K., Muhjamad, T., and Hines, O. Henoch-Schönlein anaphylactoid purpura nephropathy: Electron microscopic lesions mimicking acute post-streptococcal nephritis. *Hum. Pathol.* 9:223, 1978.
624. Valdes, A. J., and Germuth, F. G. The significance of mesangial alterations in immune complex disease. *Fed. Proc.* 27:246, 1968.
625. Valentjin, R. M. J., Kauffmann, R. H., Brutel de la Riviere, G., Daha, M. R., and Van Es, L. A. Presence of circulating macromolecular IgA in patients with hematuria due to primary IgA nephropathy. *Am. J. Med.* 74:375, 1983.
626. van den Wall Bake, A. W. L., Daha, M. R., Radl, J., Haaijman, J. J., van der Ark, A., Valentijn, R. M., and van Es, L. A. The bone marrow as production site of the IgA deposited in the kidneys of patients with IgA nephropathy. *Clin. Exp. Immunol.* 72:321, 1988.
627. van de Putte, L. B. A., Burtel del la Riviere, G., and Vriesman, P. J. C. B. Recurrent or persistent hematuria. *N. Engl. J. Med.* 290:1165, 1974.
628. van der Peet, J., Arisz, L., Brentjens, J. R. H., Marrink, J., and Hoedemaeker, P. J. The clinical course of IgA nephropathy in adults. *Clin. Nephrol.* 8:335, 1977.
629. van der Woude, F. J., Hoedemaeker, P. J., van der Giessen, M., de Graeff, P. A., de Monchy, J., The, T. H., and van der Hem, G. K. Do food antigens play a role in the pathogenesis of some cases of human glomerulonephritis? *Clin. Exp. Immunol.* 51:587, 1983.
630. van de Wiel, A., Schuurman, H. J., and Kater, L. Immunoglobulin A in alcoholic liver disease. *Contrib. Nephrol.* 40:276, 1984.
631. van de Wiel, A., Schuurman, H. J., van Riesen, D., Haaijman, J. J., Radl, J., Delacroix, D. L., van Hattum, J., Blok, A. P., and Kater, L. Characteristics of IgA deposits in liver and skin of patients with liver disease. *Am. J. Clin. Pathol.* 86:724, 1986.
632. Vernier, R. L., Farquhar, M. G., Brunson, J. G., and Good, R. A. Chronic renal disease in children: Correlation of clinical findings with morphologic characteristics seen by light and electron microscopy. *Am. J. Dis. Child.* 96:306, 1958.
633. Vernier, R. L., Resnick, J. S., and Mauer, S. M. Recurrent hematuria and focal glomerulonephritis. *Kidney Int.* 7:224, 1975.
634. Vernier, R. L., Worthen, H. G., Peterson, R. D., Colle, E., and Good, R. A. Anaphylactoid purpura: I. Pathology of the skin and kidney and frequency of streptococcal infection. *Pediatrics.* 27: 181, 1961.
635. Vialtel, P., Dechelette, E., Hachache, T., Colomb, H., Cordonnier, D., Roux, O., Dumas, G., et al. Role de l'amygdalectomie sur l'évolution des symptomes de la glomérulonéphrite a dépots mésangiaux d'IgA. In R. Kuss and M. Legrain (Eds.), *Seminaires d'uro-nephrologie.* Paris: Masson, 1981. P. 173.
636. Volhard, F., and Fahr, T. *Die Brightsche Nierenkrankheit.* Berlin: Springer, 1914.
637. Waldherr, R., Rambausek, M., Rauterberg, W.,

Andrassy, K., and Ritz, E. Immunohistochemical features of mesangial IgA glomerulonephritis. *Contrib. Nephrol.* 40:99, 1984.

638. Waldherr, R., Seelig, H. P., Rambausek, M., Andrassy, K., and Ritz, E. Deposition of polymeric IgA in idiopathic mesangial IgA glomerulonephritis. *Klin. Wochenschr.* 61:911, 1983.

639. Waldo, F. B., Alexander, R., Wyatt, R. J., and Kohaut, E. C. Alternate-day prednisone therapy in children with IgA-associated nephritis. *Am. J. Kidney Dis.* 13:55, 1989.

640. Waldo, F. B., Beischel, L., and West, C. C. IgA synthesis by lymphocytes from patients with IgA nephropathy and their relatives. *Kidney Int.* 29: 1229, 1986.

641. Waldo, F. B., Britt, W. J., Tomana, M., Julian, B. A., and Mestecky, J. Nonspecific mesangial staining with antibodies against cytomegalovirus in immunoglobulin-A nephropathy. *Lancet* 1:129, 1989.

642. Waldo, F. B., and Cochran, A. M. Systemic immune response to oral polio immunization in patients with IgA nephropathy. *J. Clin. Lab. Immunol.* 28:109, 1987.

643. Waldo, F. B., and Cochran, A. M. Mixed IgA-IgG aggregates as a model of immune complexes in IgA nephropathy. *J. Immunol.* 142:3841, 1989.

644. Walker, J. M., and Joekes, A. M. Survival after haemoptysis and nephritis. *Lancet* 2:1199, 1963.

645. Wallace, A. C. IgA nephropathy. *Pathology* 13:401, 1981.

646. Walshe, J. J., Brentjens, J. R., Costa, G. G., Andres, G. A., and Venuto, R. G. Abdominal pain with IgA nephropathy. *Am. J. Pediatr.* 77: 765, 1984.

647. Ward, D. M., Spiegelberg, H. L., and Wilson, C. B. Persistence of IgA aggregates in the glomerular mesangium in mice. *Kidney Int.* 16:801, 1979.

648. Watson, W. T. A fatal case of Schönlein's disease. *Md. Med. J.* 46:141, 1903.

649. Wedgewood, R. J. P., and Janeway, C. A. Serum complement in children with "collagen diseases." *Pediatrics* 11:569, 1953.

650. Wedgewood, R. J. P., and Klaus, M. H. Anaphylactoid purpura (Schönlein-Henoch syndrome): A long-term follow-up study with special reference to renal involvement. *Pediatrics* 16:196, 1955.

651. Wehner, H., and Andler, D. Uber die intercapilläre glomerulosklerose bei lebercirrhose. *Virchows Arch.* [*Pathol. Anat.*] 360:265, 1973.

652. Wehrmann, M., Bohle, A., Bogenschütz, O., Eissele, R., Freislederer, A., Öhlschlegel, C., Schumm, G., Batz, C., and Gärtner, H.-V. Long-term prognosis of chronic idiopathic membranous glomerulonephritis: An analysis of 334 cases with particular regards to tubulointerstitial changes. *Clin. Nephrol.* 31:67, 1989.

653. Weisgerber, G., Sonsino, E., Hayat, P., Bourillon, A., Lecointre, C., and Boureau, M. Nécrose aiguë de l'oesophage thoracique et de l'iléon au cours d'un purpura rhumatoïde. *Arch. Fr. Pediatr.* 36:194, 1979.

654. Weiss, J. H., Bhathena, D. B., and Curtis, J. J. A possible relationship between Henoch-Schönlein syndrome and IgA nephropathy (Berger's disease). *Lancet* 1:347, 1975.

655. Weiss, J. H., Bhathena, D. B., Curtis, J. J., Lucas, B. A., and Luke, R. G. A possible relationship between Henoch-Schönlein syndrome and IgA nephropathy (Berger's disease): An illustrative case. *Nephron* 22:582, 1978.

656. Wenner, N. P., and Safai, B. Circulating immune complexes in Henoch-Schönlein purpura. *Int. J. Dermatol.* 22:383, 1983.

657. Westberg, N. G., Bakhei, K., Schmekel, B., Gillberg, R., and Brandtzaeg, P. Quantitation of immunoglobulin-producing cells in small intestinal mucosa of patients with IgA nephropathy. *Clin. Immunol. Immunopathol.* 26:442, 1983.

658. Whitworth, J. A., Leibowitz, S., Kennedy, M. C., Cameron, J. S., and Chantler, C. IgA and glomerular disease. *Clin. Nephrol.* 5:33, 1976.

659. Woo, K. T., Edmondson, R. P. S., Wu, A. Y. T., Chiang, G. S. C., Pwee, H. S., and Lim, C. H. The natural history of IgA nephritis in Singapore. *Clin. Nephrol.* 25:15, 1986.

660. Woo, K. T., Edmondson, R. P. S., Yap, H. K., Wu, A. Y. T., Chiang, G. S. C., Lee, E. J. C., Pwee, H. S., and Lim, C. H. Effects of triple therapy on the progression of mesangial proliferative glomerulonephritis. *Clin. Nephrol.* 27:56, 1987.

661. Woo, K. T., Tan, Y. O. Lau, Y. K., Ng, S. L., Chew, T. S., Chan, S. H., and Lim, C. H. Suppressor cell function in IgA nephritis. *Aust. N.Z. J. Med.* 12:208, 1982.

662. Woodroffe, A. J. IgA, glomerulonephritis and liver disease. *Aust. N.Z. J. Med.* 11 (Suppl. 1):109, 1981.

663. Woodroffe, A. J., Gormly, A. A., McKenzie, P. E., Wootton, A. M., Thompson, A. J., Seymour, A. E., and Clarkson, A. R. Immunologic studies in IgA nephropathy. *Kidney Int.* 18:366, 1980.

664. Woodroffe, A. J., Thomson, N. M., Meadows, R., and Lawrence, J. R. IgA-associated glomerulonephritis. *Aust. N.Z. J. Med.* 5:97, 1975.

665. Wu, G., Katz, A., Cardella, C., and Oreopoulos, D. G. Spontaneous remission of nephrotic syndrome in IgA glomerular disease. *Am. J. Kidney Dis.* 6:96, 1985.

666. Wyatt, R. J., and Julian, B. A. Activation of complement in IgA nephropathy. *Am. J. Kidney Dis.* 12:437, 1988.

667. Wyatt, R. J., Julian, B. A., Woodford, S. Y., McLean, R. H., and Thompson, J. S. Immunogenetic markers as prognostic features in patients with IgA nephropathy. *Semin. Nephrol.* 7:389, 1987.
668. Yap, H. K., Sakai, R. S., Bahn, L., Rappaport, V., Woo, K. T., Ananthuraman, V., Lim, C. H., Chiang, G. J. C., and Jordan, S. C. Antivascular endothelial cell antibodies in patients with IgA nephropathy: Frequency and clinical significance. *Clin. Immunol. Immunopathol.* 49:450, 1988.
669. Yap, H. K., Sakai, R. S., Woo, K. T., Lim, C. H., and Jordan, S. C. Detection of bovine serum albumin in the circulating IgA immune complexes of patients with IgA nephropathy. *Clin. Immunol. Immunopathol.* 43:395, 1987.
670. Yokoska, H., Nagase, M., Maeda, T., and Koide, K. Mesangial IgA glomerulonephritis: Clinicopathological study of 85 cases. *Contrib. Nephrol.* 9:101, 1978.
671. Yoshikawa, N., Cameron, A. H., and White, R. H. R. Glomerular morphometry: II. Familial and nonfamilial haematuria. *Histopathology* 5:251, 1981.
672. Yoshikawa, N., Ito, H., Iijima, K., Nakahara, C., Maehara, K., Hasegawa, O., Okada, S., and Matsuo, T. Macroscopic hematuria in childhood IgA nephropathy. *Clin. Nephrol.* 28:217, 1987.
673. Yoshikawa, N., White, R. H. R., and Cameron, H. H. Prognostic significance of the glomerular changes in Henoch-Schönlein nephritis. *Contrib. Nephrol.* 16:223, 1981.
674. Yoshikawa, N., Yoshiara, S., Yoshiya, K., Matsuo, T., and Okada, S. Lysis of the glomerular basement membrane in children with IgA nephropathy and Henoch-Schönlein nephritis. *J. Pathol.* 150:119, 1986.
675. Yoshimura, M., Kida, H., Abe, T., Takeda, S., Katagiri, M., and Hattori, N. Significance of IgA deposits on the glomerular capillary walls in IgA nephropathy. *Am. J. Kidney Dis.* 9:404, 1987.
676. Yum, M. N., Lampton, L. M., Bloom, P. M., and Edwards, J. L. Asymptomatic IgA nephropathy associated with pulmonary hemosiderosis. *Am. J. Med.* 64:1056, 1978.
677. Zimmerman, S. W., and Burkholder, P. M. Immunoglobulin A nephropathy. *Arch. Intern. Med.* 135:1217, 1975.
678. Zollinger, H. U., and Gaboardi, F. Verzögerte Heilung einer diffusen intra- und extracapillaren Glomerulonephritis mit IgA-Depots: Klinische, licht-, elektronen-, und immunofluorescenz mikroskopische Untersuchungen on Sequenzbiopsien. *Virchows Arch. [Pathol. Anat.]* 354:349, 1971.
679. Zollinger, H. U., and Hegglin, R. Die idiopathische Lungenhämosiderose als pulmonale Form der Purpura Schönlein-Henoch. *Schweiz. Med. Wochenschr.* 88:439, 1958.
680. Zollinger, H. U., Mihatsch, M. J., Gaboardi, F., Banfi, G., Edefonti, A., Bardare, M., and Gudat, F. Schönlein-Henoch glomerulonephritis: Characteristic ultrastructural changes in the glomerular basement membrane and localisation of osmiophilic deposits. *Virchows Arch. [Pathol. Anat.]* 388:155, 1980.
681. Zurowska, A. M., Wrzolkowa, T., and Uszycka-Karcz, M. Henoch-Schönlein nephritis in children—A clinicopathological study. *Int. J. Pediatr. Nephrol.* 6:183, 1985.

Fred G. Silva

7
Membranoproliferative Glomerulonephritis

Membranoproliferative glomerulonephritis (MPGN) is a histologically distinct form or pattern of chronic glomerulonephritis in which, as the name implies, there is thickening of the glomerular capillary wall (*membrano-*) as well as an increase in the number of cells in the glomerular tuft (*-proliferative*). Because the hypercellularity is predominantly in the mesangium (centrilobular region), there is often accentuation of the lobules of the glomeruli. Because of the extensive involvement of the mesangium, this pattern is also referred to as *mesangiocapillary glomerulonephritis*, a term used first by Churg et al. [70] and now by a number of European and British authors. This pattern also has a number of other synonyms, such as *hypocomplementemic persistent* (or *chronic*) *glomerulonephritis* [369] or *lobular glomerulonephritis;* however, most publications have used the designation *membranoproliferative glomerulonephritis* (MPGN).

Earlier authors described this form as a mixed proliferative and membranous glomerulonephritis, and it is probably what Fahr [115] called the "intracapillary form" of subchronic glomerulonephritis. This glomerular pattern has probably been in existence for a long time, and Cameron [50] believes that at least two of the patients originally studied by Richard Bright at Guy's Hospital in the 1820s indeed represented a form of membranoproliferative glomerulonephritis. Three of the original kidneys in the Gordon museum at Guy's Hospital were sectioned, and two of the kidneys had the features of membranoproliferative glomerulonephritis. As Cameron [50] states, it is remarkable that this pattern can still be recognized 150 years later, after preservation first with brandy and then with formalin.

MacCallum in 1934 [213] and Ellis in 1942 [112] described patients with chronic progressive glomerulonephritis showing membranoproliferative (glomerular hypercellularity) and lobular features. Bell [24,25] also described a series of patients having a "latent chronic glomerulonephritis" or "chronic azotemic glomerulonephritis" that also probably represents what we now call membranoproliferative glomerulonephritis. Allen [3] used the term *chronic lobular glomerulonephritis* and noted that there was a tendency for the "periphery of each lobule to be laminated by two or three layers of endothelial cells" and for splitting of the basement membranes. Churg and Grishman [69] described 28 patients with subacute glomerulonephritis with mesangial-cell interposition (i.e., between the glomerular endothelium and the glomerular basement membrane). They also noted that with time the cellularity of the glomerular lesions decreased and central nodular scars developed. Habib et al. [145] in 1961 in a Ciba Foundation Symposium presented 108 nephrotic patients. Fifteen patients had "endocapillary proliferative glomerulitis associated with hyalin nodules" ("lobular glomerulitis"). Seven additional patients had complex or unclassified forms of glomerular disease with thick glomerular capillary walls and endocapillary hypercellularity. The light and electron microscopic findings described at this benchmark symposium that launched renal biopsy conform to what we now accept as membranoproliferative glomerulonephritis type I.

David Jones, using an elegant staining method (periodic acid–methenamine silver stain) on thin, paraffin-embedded and plastic-embedded sections, defined the characteristic glomerular capillary wall lesions in membranoproliferative glomerulonephritis type I [169–172]. He demonstrated the formation of a new basement membrane internal to the original glomerular basement membrane and described the continuity of the mesangial (stalk) region with the peripheral capillary wall lesion. Arakawa and Kimmelstiel [14] described the histologic and ultrastructural appearance of circumferential mesangial-cell interposition in a series of patients with diffuse (and often lobular) glomerulonephritis. They concluded that circumferential mesangial-cell interposition can be regarded as a distinct form of mesangial proliferation in glomerulonephritis; it corresponds to lobular glomerulonephritis.

West et al. [369] and Gotoff and coworkers [137], almost simultaneously first noted depletion of serum complement in children with chronic renal disease and so named it *hypocomplementemic persistent,* or *chronic, glomerulonephritis.* The glomerular pathology in these patients was manifest by increased cellularity, thickening of the glomerular capillary walls, argyrophilic splitting of the basement membranes by nonargyrophilic material, and prominent lobulation of the tuft with some central hyalin zones [137,369]. Subsequent studies showed similar glomerular lesions. With later studies showing that hypocomplementemia was not invariably present in patients with this pattern, the morphologic appearance became the sole criterion for the identification or diagnosis of this disease entity.

Several forms or presumed variants of membranoproliferative glomerulonephritis have been described. Berger and Galle [27] described cases in which extremely dense deposits were present in the glomerular capillary basement membranes by electron microscopy. Although there were many similarities between this pattern and the one referred to earlier, there were sufficient differences from morphologic and immunologic points of view to suggest that they indeed represented separate and distinct entities. For the first form mentioned, the term *membranoproliferative glomerulonephritis type I with massive subendothelial deposits* (or the *classic form*) seems the most appropriate. The form with the glomerular intramembranous dense deposits is referred to as *dense deposit disease* or by some as *membranoproliferative glomerulonephritis type II*. Glomeruli with accentuated lobules and solidification of the centrilobular or mesangial areas may be found in both the type I and type II forms of membranoproliferative glomerulonephritis, and in the past, cases with this feature were termed *lobular glomerulonephritis*. I agree with Heptinstall [150] that it is confusing to retain this term *lobular* except as a qualifying adjective for certain cases of types I or II with this histologic pattern. It is a term used to describe hyalin areas in the center of glomerular lobules and is now recognized as a late manifestation of membranoproliferative glomerulonephritis. Prominent lobules also can be present in other renal diseases.

Further variations or types of the membranoproliferative pattern have been noted by a number of investigators. A type with many of the features of MPGN type I but with the added presence of electron-dense deposits on the subepithelial side of the glomerular capillary basement membranes was designated "type III" by Burkholder et al. [45,47,48]. This pattern had some glomerular capillaries that were indistinguishable from type I, yet other segments of the glomerular tuft showed changes similar to classic membranous glomerulonephritis. Although this terminology did not find much favor, the issue is now complicated by the use of the term *type III* to describe a form of membranoproliferative glomerulonephritis described by two other groups of workers [8,326]. This form has complex GBM formations and electron-dense deposits on both the subepithelial and subendothelial sides of the basement membranes. In addition, some intramembranous deposits bridge the GBM and connect the subendothelial and the subepithelial deposits. Silver staining of ultrathin sections and subsequent ultrastructural studies are needed to render this diagnosis. Still other forms of membranoproliferative glomerulonephritis have been described and will be detailed later.

Much of the early confusion over the diagnosis of membranoproliferative glomerulonephritis was due either to the early suggestion that the diagnosis was always linked to the presence of hypocomplementemia or to the inability of authors to distinguish between the several types. It also should be noted that some of these patterns (especially type I) can occur either as a primary, apparently isolated disease, or be associated with or secondary to a wide variety of well-defined disease states such as infective endocarditis, sickle cell disease, hepatitis B infection, and systemic lupus erythematosus. Although the etiology and pathogenetic mechanisms might not be identical in all patients, most authors believe that membranoproliferative glomerulonephritis is likely a result of chronic antigenemia. The list of diseases associated with membranoproliferative glomerulonephritis is constantly growing.

MEMBRANOPROLIFERATIVE GLOMERULONEPHRITIS TYPE I (WITH MASSIVE SUBENDOTHELIAL DEPOSITS), CLASSIC TYPE

Clinical Features

Membranoproliferative glomerulonephritis type I has been recorded in patients of all ages, although it is described most commonly in children [7,15, 86,98,140–142,182,206,216,283,352,369,371]. It has been described in patients before the age of 2 years [141,206,330], but most patients present after the age of 8 years [206]. Although it can occur in adults of all ages [56,99,216,220,233], only a few cases beyond the seventh decade have been recorded [58,216,333]. There does not appear to be a male or female predominance, although a few series suggest that there may be a slight male preponderance. There also may be a predilection for Caucasians.

The clinical presentation is varied. Patients may present clinically with either a nephritic or a nephrotic syndrome. Some patients have a clinical picture resembling acute glomerulonephritis with macroscopic hematuria and red blood cell casts [206]. Dysmorphic or distorted red blood cells may be found in the urine. On average, approximately 10 to 20 percent of patients present with the acute nephritic syndrome [206] and have oliguria, edema, hematuria, hypertension, and renal insufficiency. Hypertension is commonly present at the clinical onset (noted in about a third of patients) but is usually of mild degree. Some series note it more commonly [216], and occasionally, it may be severe [82,99,149,216,360]. It is usually only transient and decreases to normal levels within several weeks in most patients [206]. Hypertension is commonly observed as the renal disease progresses and is more common in adults than in children [58]. Most patients have microscopic hematuria. Recurrent attacks of gross hematuria occur in a minority of patients and are more common in children than in adults [58]. Persistent microscopic hematuria is a frequent finding.

Proteinuria is almost uniformly present; the nephrotic syndrome is a frequent mode of presentation and was noted in over half of patients [99,142,182,216]. Membranoproliferative glomerulonephritis is one of the most common histopathologic patterns noted in children with idiopathic nephrotic syndrome; it accounted for approximately 7.5 percent of pediatric patients with idiopathic nephrotic syndrome in the International Study of Kidney Disease in Children report [162]. Among the 39 patients with membranoproliferative glomerulonephritis in this series, 30 had type I and 9 had dense deposit disease. If the 9 patients with dense deposit disease are excluded, then the percentage drops to 5.8 percent.

With regard to steroid therapy for idiopathic nephrotic syndrome in children with presumed minimal change lesions, Hogg [154] has stated, "The renal biopsy has been very important in defining pediatric patients with membranoproliferative glomerulonephritis prior to therapy because children with membranoproliferative glomerulonephritis who receive high doses of daily prednisone often encounter significant problems with hypertension. It is relevant, therefore, to seriously consider the performance of a renal biopsy in any child with idiopathic nephrotic syndrome who has features that are suggestive of membranoproliferative glomerulonephritis before proceeding to a therapeutic trial with steroids. Such features include hypocomplementemia, persistent hematuria, hypertension or decreased renal function." Although several formulas have been proposed (based on clinical and laboratory findings) to establish the diagnosis of membranoproliferative glomerulonephritis without renal biopsy [162,345], biopsy is obviously the only way to determine with certainty the exact nature of the glomerular disease in the individual patient. If the nephrotic syndrome is not present at clinical presentation, it often develops during the course of the disease. The nephrotic syndrome was found in over 80 percent of patients in one series in children [141]. However, in this series and others, the definition of nephrotic syndrome did not require edema or hyperlipidemia; thus the incidence of the nephrotic syndrome depends on its definition. Heavy proteinuria is very common and, when studied, is generally of moderately or poorly selective type [54]. Patients with proteinuria generally also have accompanying microscopic hematuria. Some patients may not have overt clinical symptomatology, and the proteinuria is simply discovered on routine or incidental urinalysis. This occurred in almost half the children in one study [206].

Blood urea nitrogen (BUN) and serum creatinine levels are elevated at clinical onset in about a fourth of patients. These values may stay elevated (presaging the onset of permanent renal failure) or return to normal over a few weeks in about half the patients. Depression of glomerular filtration rate (GFR) is more commonly noted in adults than in children [58]. The clinical onset is not uncommonly preceded by a history of a respiratory infection; this is noted in about half the patients [182]. Although group A streptococcal infections are not thought to play a role in the genesis of this pattern of renal disease, some studies have shown elevated ASO titers in 38 percent [54] and 25 percent [206] of patients. It is likely that these figures differ little from the prevalence rate in the general population [182]. As noted before, it may be difficult to distinguish membranoproliferative glomerulonephritis from acute postinfectious glomerulonephritis on clinical and morphologic grounds in some patients. Renal tubular dysfunction or injury has been described in patients with membranoproliferative glomerulonephritis type I, as evidenced by increased urinary excretion of *N*-acetyl-beta-glucosaminidase [158], defects in the maximal urinary concentration and urinary acidification, and elevated levels of the fractional excretion of sodium [126]. Potassium-losing nephropathy, generalized aminoaciduria, and glycosuria (reversible with steroid therapy) have also been described [212].

The commonly encountered feature of hypocomplementemia was recognized (and was the impetus for the discovery of this type of glomerulonephritis) by West et al. [369] and Gotoff et al. [137]. There is usually a decrease in the C3 levels in the serum [56,99,150,151,205,216,220], although the levels tend to fluctuate. Depressed levels of serum C3 were found at the time of diagnosis in approximately a third to half the patients [141,144,182,268]. In most patients, serial determinations usually reveal hypocomplementemia some time during the course of the renal disease. A certain number of patients do not appear to have depression of the serum complement level, and a normal level may persist throughout the course of the illness or, as mentioned earlier, show depression at a later time [56,205]. In the series of Habib et al. [142,145] as many as 40 percent of patients with membranoproliferative glomerulonephritis did not have depressed serum complement. Serum concentrations of the early components of the classical pathway of complement activation (i.e., C1q, C4, and C2) and components of the alternative pathway (i.e., factor B, properdin) are also frequently decreased. More will be said later about serum complement and the C3-nephritic factor.

Circulating immune complexes (CIC) have been searched for utilizing a number of different techniques and have been present in about 20 percent or more of patients with membranoproliferative glomerulonephritis; this percentage depends on the sensitivity of the technique employed for identifying the complexes [36,90,329,379]. Davis et al. [90] demonstrated CICs when the renal disease was mild or silent, but CICs were almost always absent when renal impairment was incipient or had developed. This suggested to the authors that the CICs detected were either not nephritogenic or they programmed subsequent renal events that augment renal parenchymal injury in the absence of CICs. These workers also suggested that the measurement of CICs was of minimal value in the diagnosis or prognosis of patients with membranoproliferative glomerulonephritis. Some groups have failed to find evidence of CICs altogether [379]. IgM-rheumatoid factors (i.e., autoantibodies to IgG) have been noted [113], as has cryoglobulinemia [276], in patients with membranoproliferative glomerulonephritis type I.

There have been some suggestions that the frequency of this type of membranoproliferative glomerulonephritis is decreasing [19], and its prevalence is low [342]. Renal vein thrombosis can occur; in one series, membranoproliferative glomerulonephritis was the most frequent nephropathy associated with renal vein thrombosis [354]. Successful pregnancies are common in affected patients [21], although Surian et al. [331] noted a high incidence of complications.

Clinical Course

The renal disease is generally progressive, and the overall renal prognosis is poor (Fig. 7-1). The clinical course of patients can be quite variable [55,99,141,150,151,206,366]. The nephrotic syndrome persists in some, while others have intermittent nephrotic or nephritic episodes with abnormal urinalysis between the episodes. Rarely, patients may become entirely asymptomatic with normal renal function and urinary findings [54,150,151,264]. This clinically silent phase may

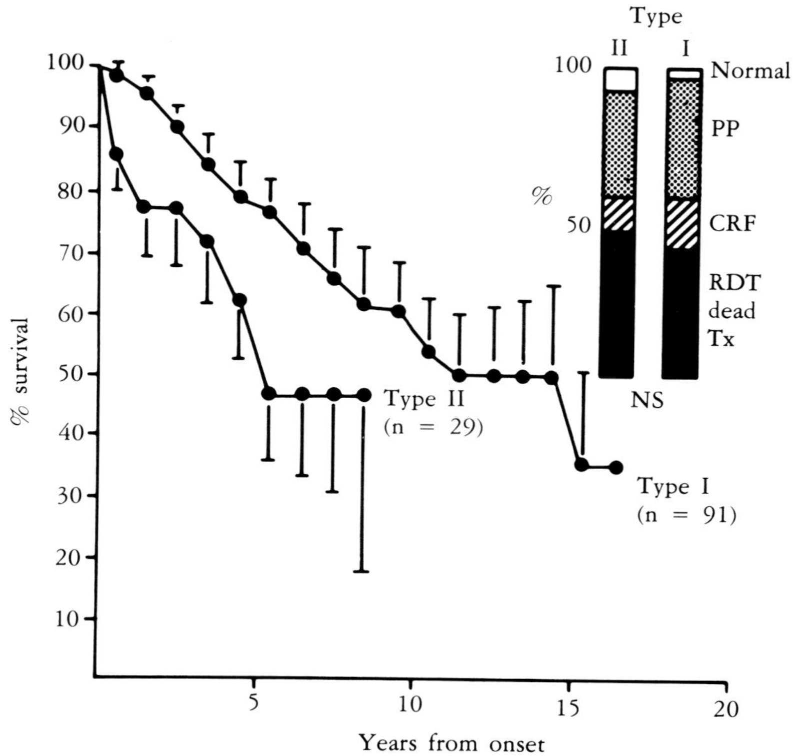

FIG. 7-1. *Survival of patients with type I and type II MPGN calculated by the method of Cutler and Ederer [78a]. For the purposes of this analysis, death and the need for regular dialysis or transplantation have been taken as equivalent. Survival therefore refers to survival of renal function. The insert bar graphs (top right) show the status of patients in the two groups at last follow-up (type I, mean 6.4 years from onset; type II, 4.2 years from onset). PP, persistent proteinuria with or without a nephrotic syndrome and with normal renal function (GFR > 80 ml/min/1.73 m²); CRF, chronic renal failure in which GFR is less than 80 ml/min/1.73 m²; RDT, regular dialysis therapy; Tx, transplanted. (Modified from Cameron, J. S. In J. Strauss (Ed.),* Pediatric Nephrology, Vol. 5: Nephrotic Syndrome: Current Concepts in Diagnosis and Management. *New York: Garland, 1978. P. 153, Fig. 7; used by permission.)*

last for many years despite persistence of the renal morphologic abnormalities.

Clinical remission is noted in 5 to 20 percent of patients [87,103,142,225,229]. Complete remission occurs in only a few patients in whom there has been long-term follow-up [50,58,206]. The series of Levy et al. [206] showed complete remission in only 4 of 84 children. In this study, 17 children went into remission, but relapse occurred in 13; in only 4 patients was the remission maintained for periods of up to 4 years [206]. Kim et al. [182] noted complete clinical remission in 5 of 63 patients.

A large number of patients develop end-stage renal disease (ESRD) [50,58,87,99,150,151,206, 216,220]. Survival rates from study to study are not uniform, not only because of inclusion of patients with different severities of renal disease, but also because of different starting points for calculating the time course of the patients (i.e., from the clinical onset or from the point of the diagnostic renal biopsy). In Cameron's study [50,58], the actuarial survival was 50 percent at 11 years (see Fig. 7-1), which was similar to that of Habib et al. [141]. (Death and the need for chronic dialysis or renal transplantation were regarded as equivalent.) In the large series of children from Paris, referred to earlier [206], 84 were followed for periods of up to 18 years; one-fourth were dead from renal insufficiency or on chronic hemodialysis, 11 percent were in chronic renal failure, 21 percent had persistent nephrotic syndrome, 38 percent had isolated proteinuria, and only 5 percent appeared to be in spontaneous renal remission. Repeat renal biopsies sometimes showed decrease in mesangial cellularity or disappearance of double contours, but these were not always related to clinical improvement. Donadio et al. [99] studied mainly adults and showed that 40 percent developed end-stage renal disease during their period of follow-up; the mean time of onset of renal failure was just over 5 years. It is likely in most of the series reported that other patients will progress to end-stage renal disease. Droz et al. [103] reported on 10-year survival rates in (mostly) adult patients with membranoproliferative glomerulonephritis type I; they found a survival rate of 60 percent.

A number of patients have persistent proteinuria (with or without the nephrotic syndrome) with no renal insufficiency. In three series [50,99,206], the patients in this category accounted for 27 percent of patients.

Certain features have been considered to influence the outcome of the disease, and these are listed in Table 7-1. There is debate as to whether membranoproliferative glomerulonephritis has a worse renal prognosis in children than in adults. There appears to be no major difference in clinical outcome between children and adults, although the data are often difficult to interpret because of possible differences in biopsy policies between children and adults; that is, the entry criteria or decision to perform renal biopsy may be different for children and adults. The study of Magil et al. [216] found that the 50 percent survival time in children was 76 months, whereas the 50 percent survival time in adults was 44 months. Adult

Table 7-1. *Indicators of poor renal prognosis in patients with MPGN type I and dense deposit disease**

Strong association:
Hypertension [99]
Impaired renal function [99,141,142,333]
Nephrotic syndrome [11,50,141,142,333]
Crescents (>20%) [52,242,333]
Sclerosis; mesangial deposits [310,317]
Less strong association:
Macroscopic hematuria [141,142]
Male gender [216]
Adults [58]
No correlation:
Serum C [104,117,141,142,268,367]
C3NeF [104,117,141,142,268,367]
Circulating immune complexes [90,316]

*Considered together here since most publications include both membranoproliferative glomerulonephritis type I and dense deposit disease.

males tended to develop renal failure in a relatively shorter time than women and children.

The presence of the nephrotic syndrome at clinical onset has been thought to be indicative of a poor prognosis [50,58,206,216,265,360], but others have not found this to be so [87]. Other features suggestive of a poor prognosis include the absence of clinical remission during the course of the disease, initial depression of renal function, persistent hypertension [149,165,273,360], and the presence of gross hematuria [55,56,99,142,187, 206], although Watson et al. [360] did not find that gross hematuria was a sign of a poor prognosis. Patients with hypocomplementemia do not fare worse than those with normal levels of complement [55,56]. Although some have suggested that depression of C1q and C4 [391]—in addition to depression of C3—indicated a poor renal prognosis, others do not agree.

Morphologic indicators of a poor renal prognosis are also not absolute. Patients with large numbers of crescents [58,142,182,206,242] do not do well; in one series [142], all patients with crescents developed end-stage renal disease within a 4-year period of follow-up. Glomerular sclerosis is also thought to signal a poor prognosis [58]. As noted in other renal diseases, increase in the renal interstitial volume correlated directly with the level of serum creatinine [119]. Watson et al. [360] suggested three subtypes with different outcomes: (1) those with focal segmental duplication of the GBM, (2) those with diffuse duplication of the GBM, and (3) mixed segmental and global duplication of the GBM. Those patients with focal and segmental duplication had a favorable renal outcome compared with the others with more diffuse disease. Other authors have noted similar findings [324]. Clinical remission accompanied by morphologic evidence of regression on repeat renal biopsy has been noted by a few investigators [103,142, 225,229].

Effect of Treatment on Clinical Course

The response to therapy is quite controversial. No specific therapy has yet to be shown to definitively alter the natural course of membranoproliferative glomerulonephritis. Most published studies with steroid or cytotoxic therapy (cyclophosphamide and/or azathioprine) have not shown improvement in the clinical course of the renal disease [56,99,139,141,142,303], although treatment with corticosteroids, cytotoxic agents, and anticoagulants in largely uncontrolled series has been somewhat promising [62,97,147,188,225,228,271,365, 370].

Because of the evidence of increased platelet activation and consumption [174], a number of studies have been performed utilizing platelet inhibitors. Kincaid-Smith [187,188] reported favorable responses to combined treatment with cyclophosphamide, dipyridamole, and anticoagulants in membranoproliferative glomerulonephritis. Two randomized clinical trials have been performed with cyclophosphamide, dipyridamole, and warfarin [60,343]. Because of the small number of patients studied [60], the high rate of drug toxicity [343], and the lack of benefit after 3 years of therapy [343], neither study confirms the efficacy of this therapy [60,343].

Two prospective studies using platelet inhibitors have been performed [97,390]. Although there was a beneficial effect on renal function, a high complication rate related to the drugs was noted in one of the investigations [390]. In the other, Donadio et al. [97] reported stabilization of both renal function and structure in patients treated with the platelet-inhibitor drugs aspirin and dipyridamole. Chapman et al. [62] reported a favorable response in a small number of children with a combination of immunosuppressive drugs and anticoagulation.

West et al. [225,228–230,365,370] reported that long-term alternate-day prednisone was beneficial in children with membranoproliferative glomerulonephritis and successfully stabilizes the renal parenchymal damage. This experience was gained over a 17-year period, and some patients were followed on the regimen for an average of 6.5 years [229]. Although glomerular sclerosis was apparently increased with therapy, the glomerular capillary walls appeared thinner with more patent glomerular capillaries; moreover, there was less mesangial hypercellularity in the second renal biopsy following therapy.

The International Study of Kidney Disease in Children, (ISKDC) [109,163], in a randomized, controlled clinical trial in 37 children with membranoproliferative glomerulonephritis, suggested that an alternate-day regimen of steroid therapy could slow the progression rate of the renal disease. However, there was no statistical improvement in GFR, and there were substantial side effects to the drugs. Warady et al. [359] reported a diminution in proteinuria and normalization of the creatinine clearance with prednisone therapy in six children. Others [253] also have suggested that prednisone therapy may retard the development of end-stage renal disease (ESRD) in children with membranoproliferative glomerulonephritis.

Lagrue et al. [196] and Laurent et al. [199] suggested a role of long-term treatment of membranoproliferative glomerulonephritis with nonsteroidal anti-inflammatory drugs. Plasmapheresis also has been suggested as a form of therapy [232,248]. Well-controlled, prospective studies involving large numbers of patients are needed because of the prolonged and variable natural history of the disease.

Pathologic Changes

GROSS APPEARANCE

Both kidneys are equally involved. By the time the kidneys are studied, either at nephrectomy prior to transplantation or at autopsy following death due to renal failure, they are usually pale. Yellow flecking may be seen in the cortex. With advancing disease, they become small and have a granular surface. There is a firm consistency, and the arteries may be prominent.

MICROSCOPIC FINDINGS

The light microscopic findings have been well described on numerous occasions [34,54,87,99,141, 151,173,206,220,233,256,352,369].

Glomeruli

The glomeruli typically show characteristic and uniform changes. They are all enlarged and show a diffuse increase in glomerular tuft hypercellularity (Figs. 7-2 through 7-4). The hypercellularity is generally global (i.e., involving all portions of each glomerular tuft to about the same degree). The increase in cellularity within each glomerular lobule creates an accentuation of the lobular pattern, or "lobulation" (Figs. 7-5 and 7-6). The increase in cells in the mesangial regions and increase in amount of mesangial matrix create a much larger mesangial or centrilobular area, with the lobules sometimes assuming a club shape. In some patients there is widespread glomerular hypercellularity with little accentuation of the lobular pattern. It has been suggested that the severity of the mesangial lesion relates to the presence and

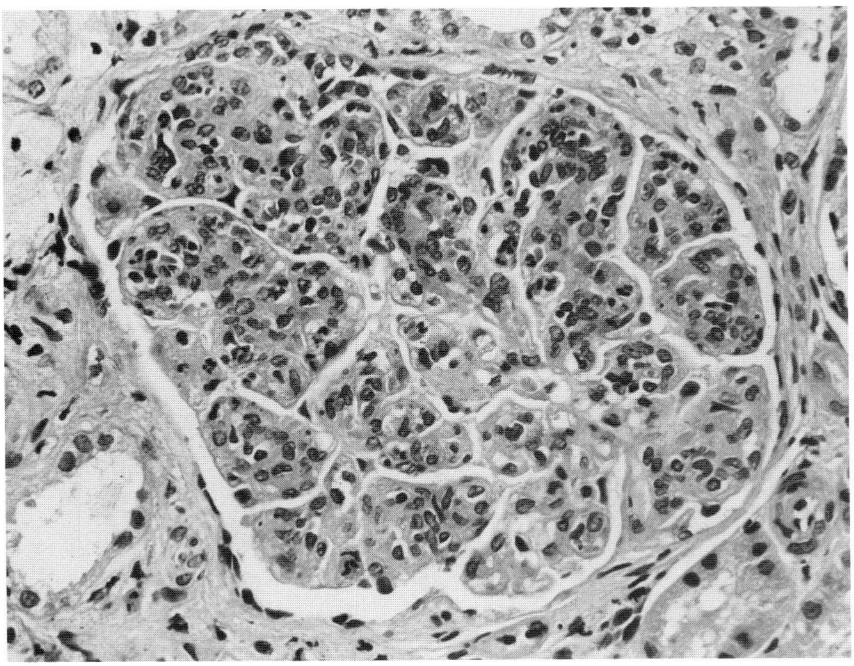

FIG. 7-2. *Glomerulus from patient with MPGN type I. There is increased lobulation, hypercellularity in the mesangium, and thickening of the capillary walls. H&E; ×315.*

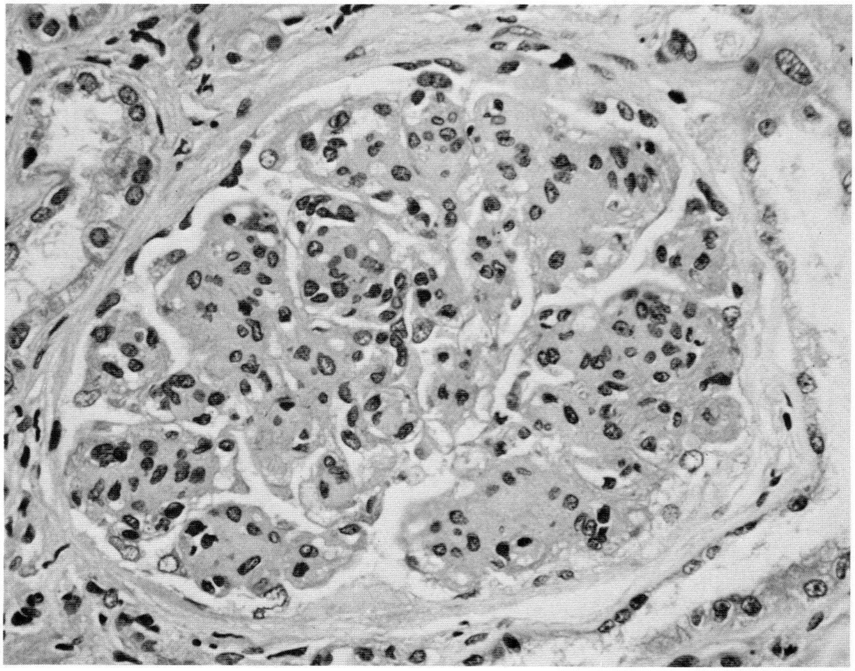

FIG. 7-3. *Glomerulus from patient with MPGN type I to show increase in mesangial substance. Also seen are localized capillary wall thickenings, increased cellularity, and pronounced lobulation. H&E; ×450.*

duration of renal disease. As the lobular lesion progresses, the cellularity tends to diminish and is replaced by an increase in mesangial matrix (sclerosis). In approximately a fourth of cases there is a marked polymorphonuclear leukocytic infiltration (exudative form) [173]. In contrast to several other forms of glomerulonephritis, however, infiltration by monocytic cells was not found in the mesangial areas utilizing nonspecific esterase as a monocyte cellular marker [118,245]. Cases of primary mixed or essential cryoglobulinemic glomerulonephritis with a membranoproliferative glomerular pattern, however, did show a marked number of infiltrating monocytic cells [118,215, 245]. In contrast, Laohapand et al. [198], using α_1-antitrypsin as a marker for mononuclear leukocytes, noted an abundance of monocytes in severe cases of membranoproliferative glomerulonephritis; the highest numbers of monocytes were noted in renal biopsies with the greatest glomerular hypercellularity and the largest number of glomerular subendothelial and subepithelial deposits.

There is marked diffuse thickening of the glomerular capillary walls; the thickening can be more prominent in some glomeruli and in some capillary loops than in others. PAS and silver methenamine stains show that the thickened glomerular capillary walls often have two basement membranes with a clear or nonargyrophilic region between them. This double contour is sometimes termed *tram-tracking, splitting,* or *reduplication* of the GBM (Fig. 7-7). The double contour is brought about by the outward migration of mesangial cells along the inside of the capillary walls. Because mesangial cells produce basement membrane–like material, the cytoplasm of these cells is covered on the outside by the original basement membrane and on the inside by the newly formed

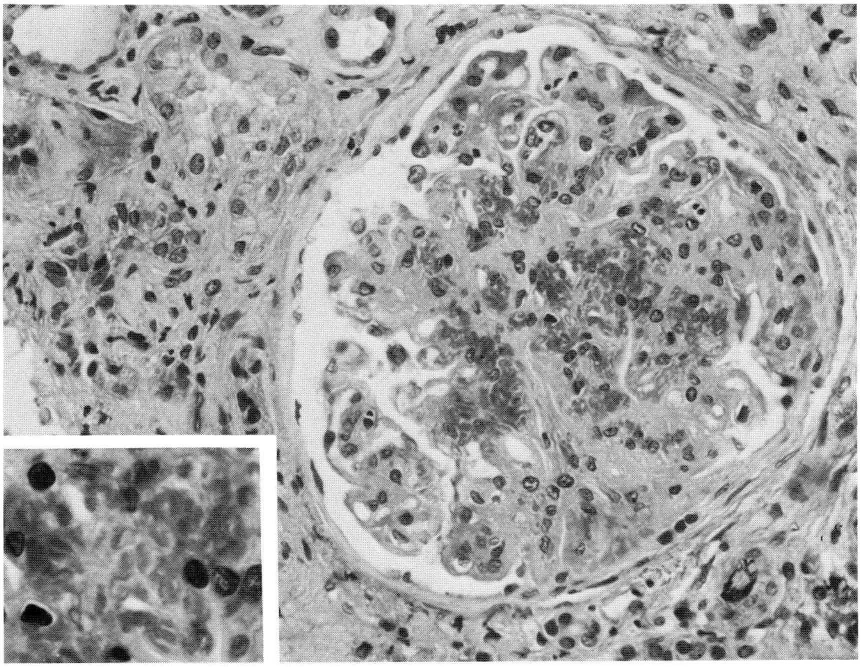

Fig. 7-4. *Glomerulus from MPGN type I which, in addition to usual features, shows basophilic worm-like structures in the mesangium. Trichrome; ×475. Inset is a higher-power view of worm-like structures. Trichrome; ×800.*

"membrane." Both the membranes stain positively with silver and so give rise to the double contour. The newly formed basement membrane–like material—the inner contour—may be thin, incomplete, and at times difficult to discern because of extreme glomerular hypercellularity. In certain cases, capillary loops show the "spiking" phenomenon noted in membranous glomerulonephritis [141,142,206].

The glomerular capillary lumens are often diffusely and globally reduced by the increase in matrix and cellularity in the mesangial regions, as well as by the thickening of the capillary walls. Generally, the subendothelial deposits contribute little to this luminal narrowing. In addition to the increased endocapillary cellularity, migrant inflammatory cells also may contribute to this capillary lumen closure.

Discrete glomerular subendothelial deposits may be identified with the use of trichrome preparations, although, as will be seen later, they are better demonstrated using electron microscopy. Mesangial deposits are generally small and difficult to identify. In some cases, scattered glomerular fuchsinophilic subepithelial humps may be detected with trichrome stains and oil immersion.

Bohle et al. [33] have suggested that "hyperperfusion injury" can be seen with great frequency in membranoproliferative glomerulonephritis; this is defined as the presence of glomerular adhesions (synechiae), glomerular subendothelial hyalinosis, and the presence of fat droplets in the hyalin material.

Crescents also may be noted and occur in about 10 percent of patients [182]. These crescents may be small and focal [99], or they may be larger,

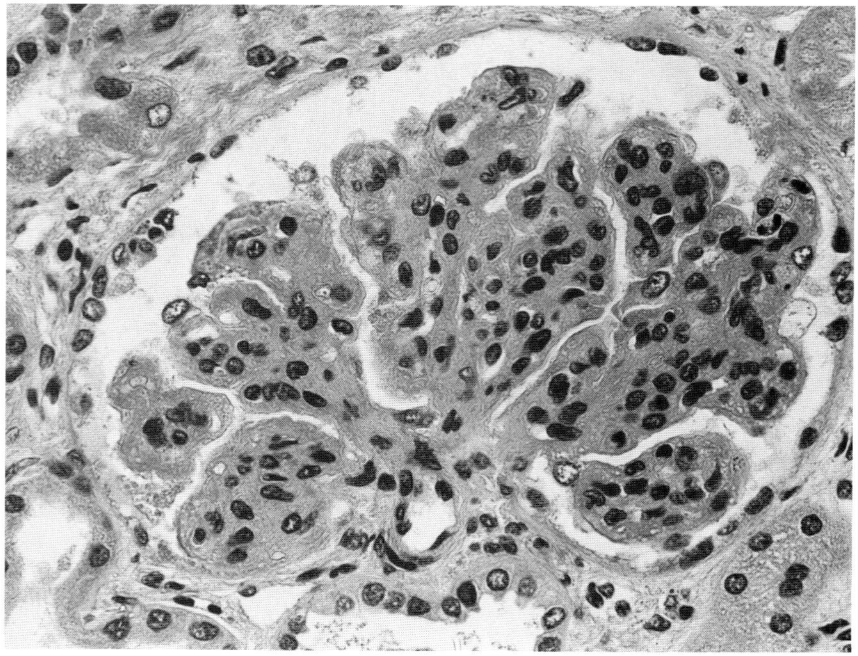

FIG. 7-5. *Representative glomerulus from a patient with MPGN type I. There was a diffuse and global increase in glomerular cellularity with expansion of the lobules and accentuation of the lobular pattern. H&E; ×450.*

affecting most of the glomeruli [141]. They are often indicative of a poor prognosis [58,142, 182,206,242]. Crescentic glomerulonephritis superimposed on classic membranoproliferative glomerulonephritis has been known to develop within weeks of an initial biopsy being diagnosed as uncomplicated membranoproliferative glomerulonephritis [194]. Parietal epithelial cells may be prominent without the presence of obvious crescents [127].

Serial biopsies are not commonly performed, but in those few patients in whom they have been done, the glomerular tuft hypercellularity may become less pronounced with an increase in the amount of mesangial matrix (sclerosis). End-stage sclerotic glomeruli may develop later still.

There are reports of focal or segmental membranoproliferative glomerulonephritis [206,324,360, 384]. In these reports, in which only some glomeruli show lesions while others do not, it is not always clear whether the glomeruli that are normal by light microscopy contain deposits by electron microscopic and immunofluorescence studies. Most authors require diffuse and global changes to warrant the diagnosis of membranoproliferative glomerulonephritis.

In renal biopsies with membranoproliferative glomerulonephritis, it is important for the pathologist to look for refractile eosinophilic hyalin globules in the glomerular capillary lumens suggestive of cryoglobulin deposits. More will be said about this in the section dealing with cryoglobulinemia (in Chap. 24).

Tubules

Morphologic changes in the tubules and interstitium are generally thought to reflect the changes

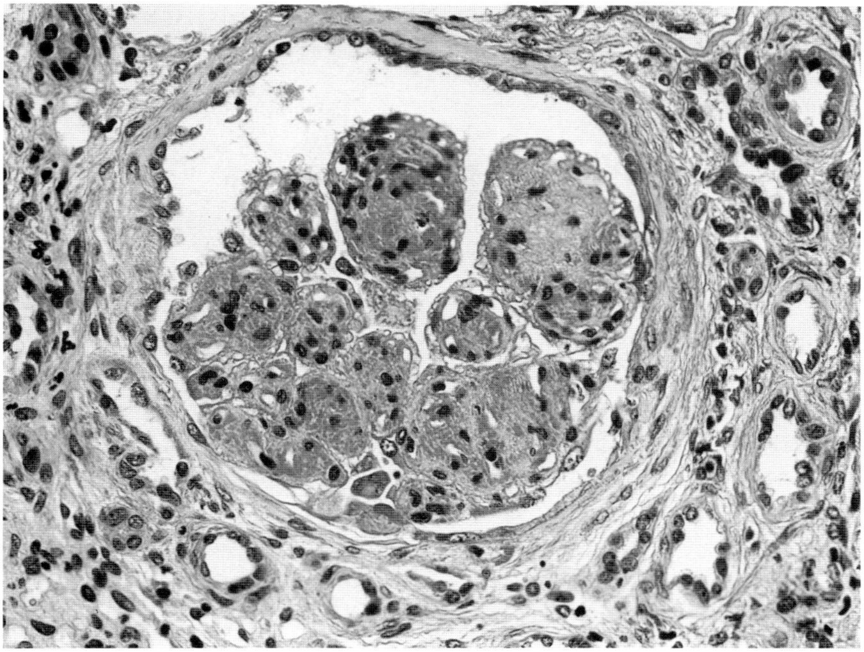

FIG. 7-6. *Accentuation of the lobular pattern in MPGN type I. H&E; ×325. (Courtesy of Drs. Conrad L. Pirani and Vivette D'Agati.)*

noted in the glomeruli [182]. The tubules may contain hyalin droplets (so-called hyalin degeneration); these are protein resorption droplets (phagolysosomes) and are related to the glomerular loss of proteins. Tubules may contain red blood cells. With evolution of the disease toward more severe renal parenchymal damage, tubular atrophy and interstitial inflammation, edema, and fibrosis may occur. Foam cells may be noted in the interstitium and/or tubular epithelium. Clefts—sometimes noted in the lumina of tubules—probably represent cholesterol ester. The study by Schmitt et al. [306], however, suggests that the tubulointerstitial findings are unrelated to the severity of the glomerular alterations. Severe glomerular lesions can be seen in the absence of tubulointerstitial disease; conversely, severe tubulointerstitial disease can be seen with mild glomerular disease. These authors suggest that the tubulointerstitial changes result in many of the renal functional disturbances.

Blood Vessels

Arteries and arterioles are affected in those patients in whom renal failure with hypertension develops. Severe arterial intimal thickening occurs in patients with long-standing renal disease and in those in whom dialysis has been instituted. If vasculitis is identified, then a cryoglobulinemia or HB_sAg-related membranoproliferative glomerulonephritis should be explored.

Interstitium

Interstitial inflammation with scattered chronic inflammatory cells may occur, as may cholesterol granulomas. There is a good correlation between the volume of interstitium and the level of serum creatinine [119].

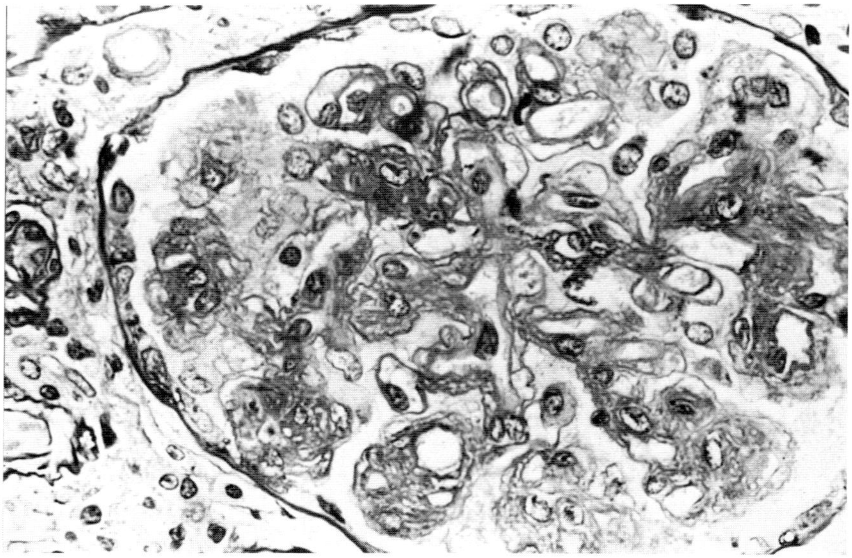

FIG. 7-7. *Glomerulus with silver stain showing tram-tracking or reduplication of the glomerular basement membrane at 11 to 12 o'clock. Jones silver methenamine; ×250. (Courtesy of Dr. Gene Moore.)*

ELECTRON MICROSCOPIC FINDINGS

The electron microscope has helped to separate and distinguish this pattern from other glomerular lesions with membranoproliferative features and has helped clarify what is noted by light microscopy [9,47,54,99,141,152,206,216,220,256,391]. Ultrastructural studies have shown a native GBM of normal thickness accompanied by large subendothelial deposits (Figs. 7-8 and 7-9) and other glomerular deposits. There is hypercellularity and increased mesangial matrix, both of which are often present between the normal-appearing GBM and the glomerular endothelium (mesangial interposition) (Fig. 7-10). As described earlier, the new mesangial matrix–like material produced by the migrating mesangial cells produces an inner "basement membrane." The thickened capillary wall is therefore composed of two or more layers of basement membrane–like material, interposed mesangial cells, and electron-dense, discrete "immune type" deposits (see Fig. 7-10).

The electron-dense deposits are generally described as "subendothelial" but are really nearer the inner aspect of the original basement membrane. Their exact position is somewhat obscured because of the migrating mesangial cells and the new "layers" of basement membrane–like material. The deposits range from small and discrete to large and elongated; they are found both along the periphery of the "filtering" glomerular capillary walls and just under the GBM as it overlies the mesangium. Discrete electron-dense deposits also may be

FIG. 7-8. *Low-magnification electron micrograph of a portion of a glomerulus from a patient with typical MPGN type I. Note the presence of a large number of discrete electron-dense osmiophilic deposits throughout the glomerular structures. There are numerous large subendothelial deposits and scattered mesangial deposits. Some of the glomerular capillaries are closed, and others are patent. Uranyl acetate and lead citrate; ×4785.*

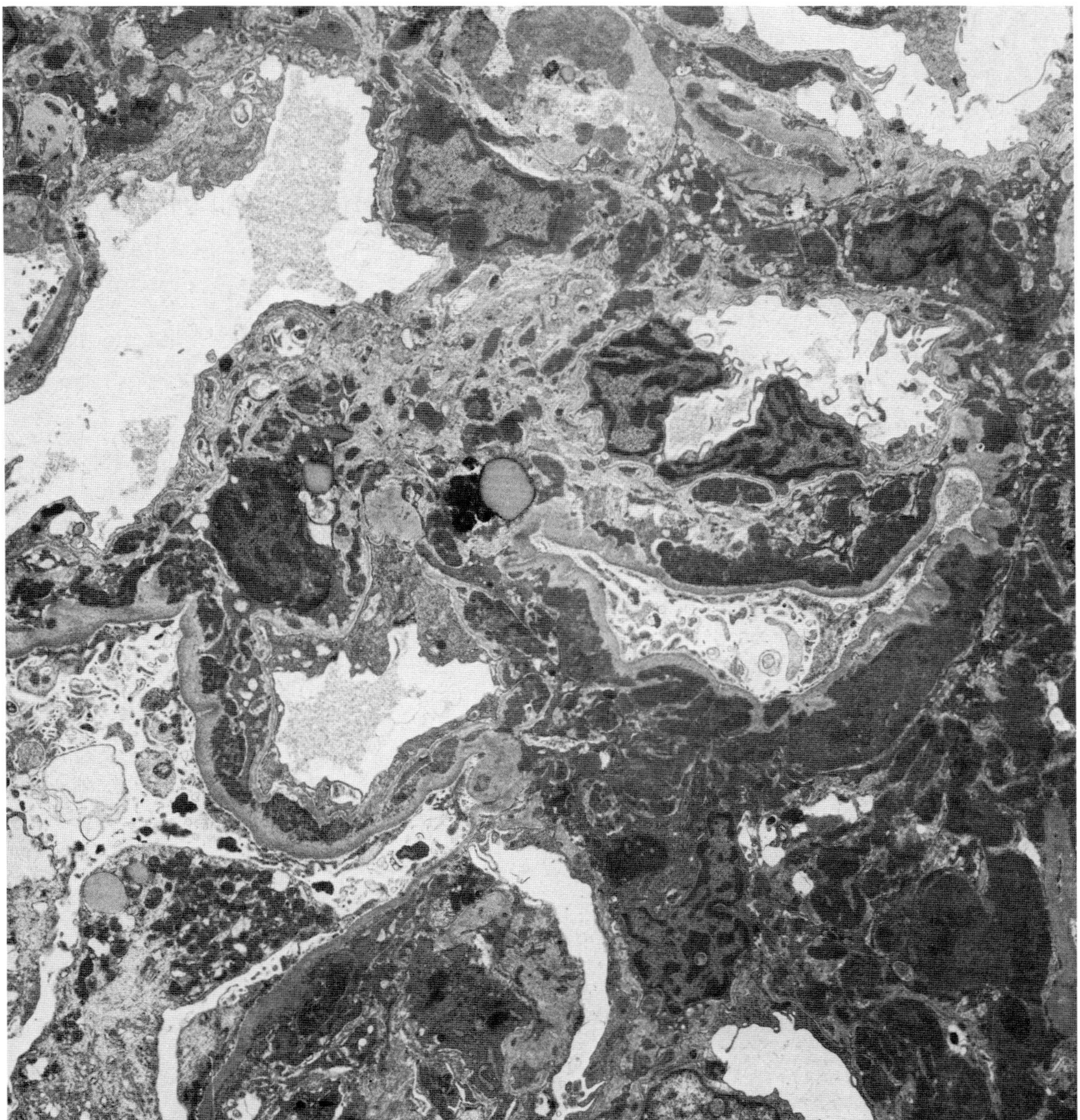

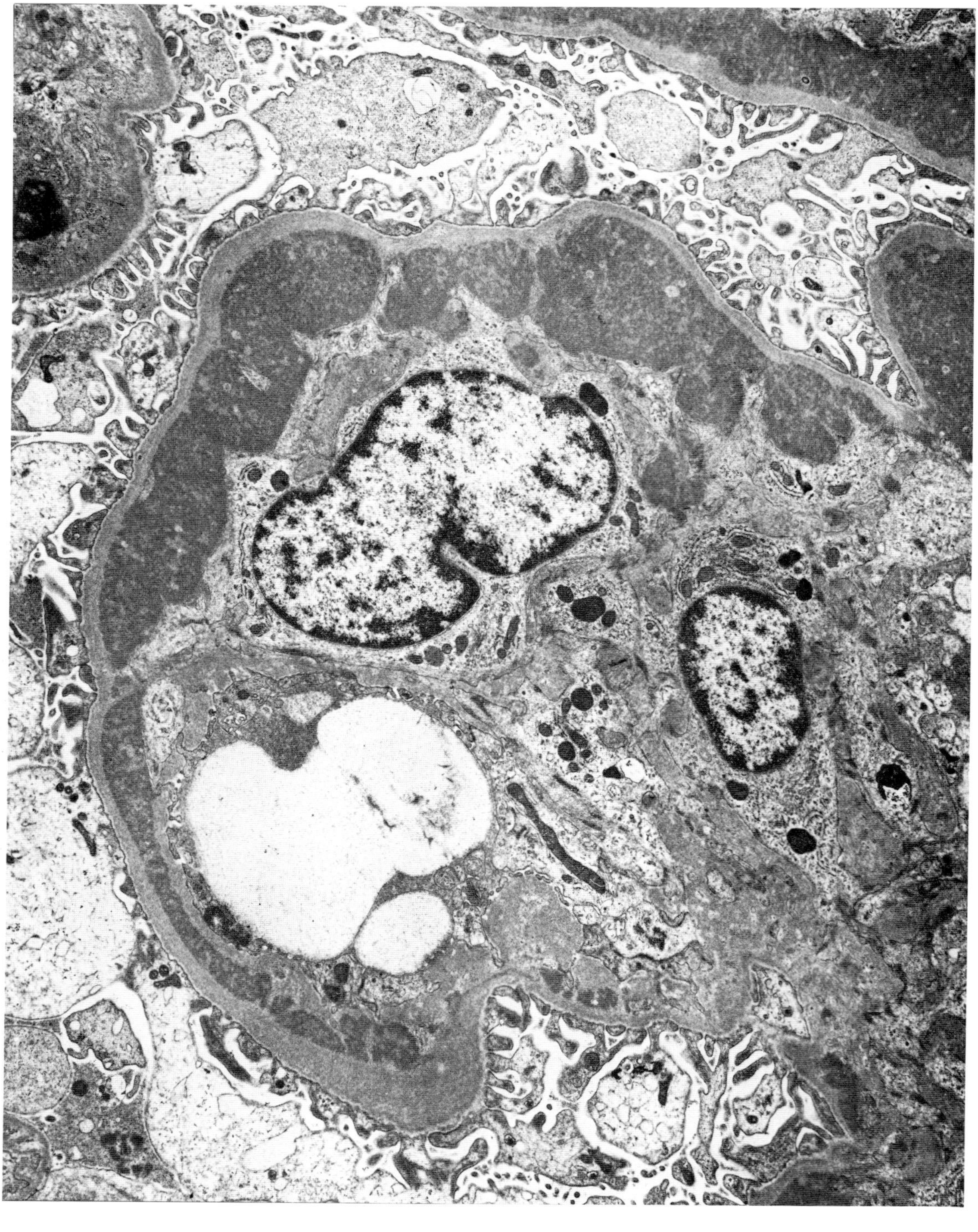

found within the mesangium; in this site they are usually small and discrete, but sometimes they are more bulky. They are associated with an increase in intracapillary hypercellularity (Fig. 7-11). Mesangial deposits may be especially common in biopsy specimens obtained early in the course of the disease. Some patients have scattered, small glomerular subepithelial deposits quite similar to the humps noted in classic acute postinfectious (poststreptococcal) glomerulonephritis [141,216,333,391]. They are found in as many as 30 percent [216] or 50 percent [206] of cases studied. Rarely, these small subepithelial deposits may have accompanying protruding spikes of GBM-like material similar to that noted in membranous glomerulonephritis. As described later, the presence of larger numbers of glomerular subepithelial deposits forms part of the pattern of membranoproliferative glomerulonephritis type III. Occasionally, intramembranous deposits are noted in membranoproliferative glomerulonephritis type I, and fragmentation of the GBM can occur [333]. The application of silver impregnation to renal electron microscopy is particularly important in the various patterns of membranoproliferative glomerulonephritis [101]. It also may be important to perform the ultrastructural studies at high magnification (e.g., 30,000 ×) to determine if the deposits have a substructure such as one sees with cryoglobulinemia [276].

There is increase in mesangial cellularity and matrix formation, the latter being especially prominent in the lobular variant of membranoproliferative glomerulonephritis type I. Hypercellularity, production of matrix (sclerosis), and movement or extension of mesangial cells around the glomerular capillary wall are all manifestations of the great activity on the part of the mesangial cells. Collagen is only rarely demonstrated in the mesangium by electron microscopy [220]. Platelets and/or fibrin tactoids may be found in one-fourth of biopsies studied by electron microscopy. Glomerular visceral epithelial-cell foot-process effacement is often noted. Bonsib [35] has utilized special enzymatic digestion techniques to remove cellular elements and deposits, coupled with scanning electron microscopy, to study the three-dimensional aspects of the glomerulus. The picture seen in membranoproliferative glomerulonephritis type I is illustrated in Figure 7-12.

Fig. 7-9. *Electron micrograph showing a segment of a glomerular capillary with large, discrete electron-dense deposits in the subendothelial space. Uranyl acetate and lead citrate; ×5844. (Courtesy of Dr. Edith Hawkins.)*

IMMUNOFLUORESCENCE FINDINGS

Immunofluorescence staining is generally quite typical [20,28,87,89,132,141,151,206,216,220,250,252,373,391]. The most consistent finding is strongly positive staining for C3 in a fine to coarse granular pattern along the glomerular capillaries (Figs. 7-13 and 7-14). A characteristic picture is produced, with the glomerular capillaries around the periphery of the expanded lobules being predominantly, and often solely, affected so that the lobules stand out quite clearly, cloaked by strongly positive immunofluorescence. In some instances, the peripheral glomerular capillaries show coarse, somewhat elongated areas of immunofluorescence that may impart a broken, wide, linear pattern. C3 also may be noted in the glomerular mesangium, a finding that is somewhat inconsistent. When there is a great increase in the amount of mesangial matrix, mesangial deposits are often obscured or absent [150]. Mesangial C3 is less frequent than in dense deposit disease (membranoproliferative glomerulonephritis type II). Early components of the classical pathway of complement activation (C1q and C4) are sometimes noted and are present in about one-half to two-thirds of patients [89,391]. Yamashina et al. [381], using an avidin-biotin-peroxidase complex method and proteolytic digestion of formalin-fixed paraffin-embedded sections, noted the presence of all complement components. Properdin is virtually always present [182] (Fig. 7-15); properdin deposits were found in 90 percent of cases in one series [99] and in 100 percent in another [373]. There is no correlation between the immunofluorescence pattern and the serum complement profile [391]. Kazatchkine et al. [176] found normal staining of the glomerular visceral epithelial-cell

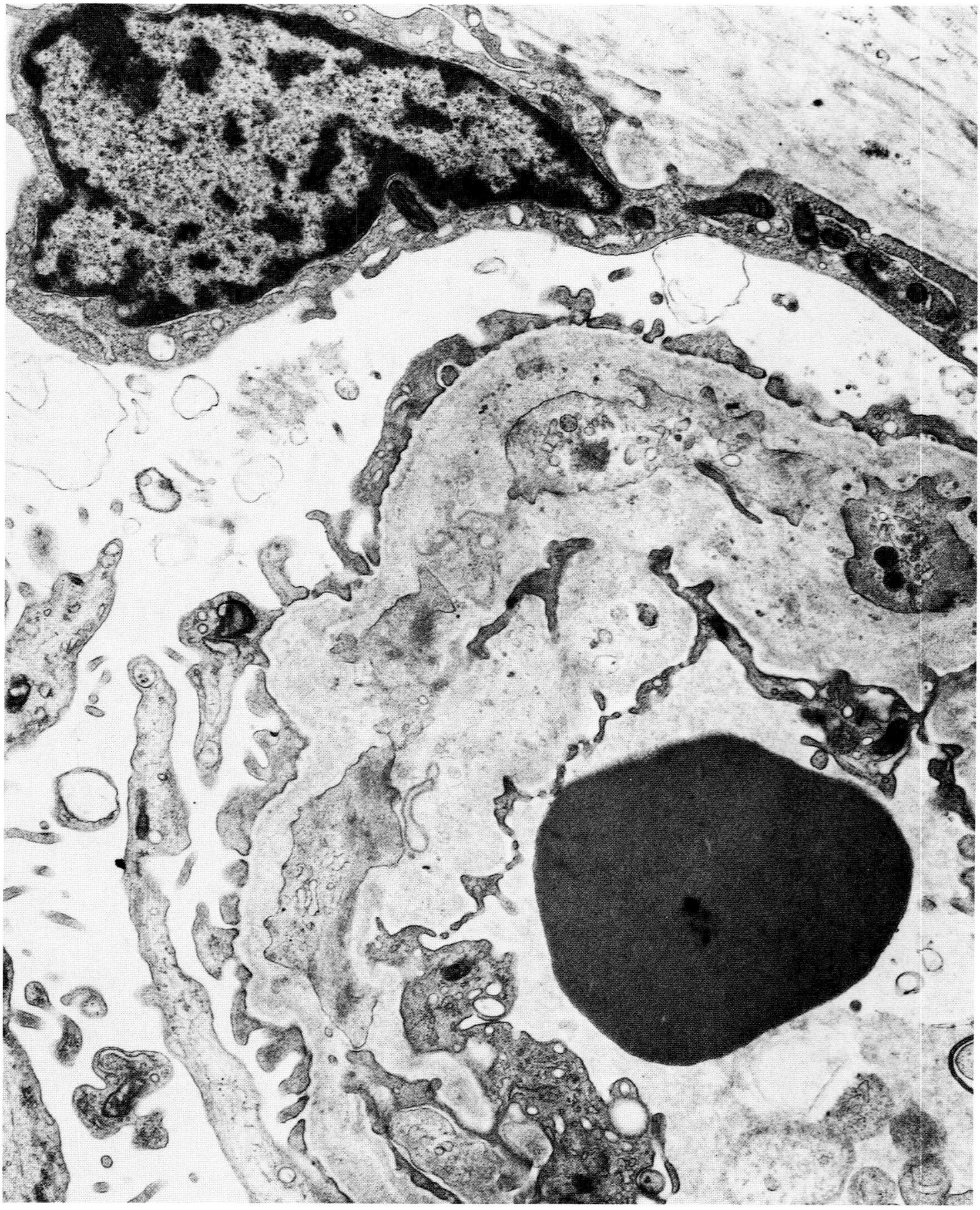

podocytes with antibodies to C3b receptor in renal biopsies with membranoproliferative glomerulonephritis type I or type II.

Immunoglobulins are noted in many, if not most, patients [89,391], but although the immunofluorescent staining is generally present in regions similar to that of C3, it is generally fainter than with C3. IgG is the immunoglobulin most commonly found, noted in some two-thirds of biopsies (Fig. 7-16); the staining for IgG is thought to decrease as the disease progresses and the deposits become replaced or obscured by the increase in mesangial matrix [151]. Doi et al. [96] demonstrated all four IgG subclasses in renal biopsies showing membranoproliferative glomerulonephritis, but in contrast, Bannister et al. [18] noted an excess of IgG_3 compared with the other classes. IgM is less commonly noted than IgG but was present in 86 percent of patients in one series [391], 73 percent of patients in another series [250], and 60 percent in yet another [99] (Fig. 7-17). IgA is found even less commonly but was present in one-third of patients in some studies [99,391]. It is important to determine whether the IgA is the predominant or codominant immunoreactant present in order to diagnose a membranoproliferative form of IgA nephritis [148]. IgD has been recorded but is usually accompanied by other immunoglobulins. Orfila et al. [270] noted the presence of both kappa and lambda light chains in membranoproliferative glomerulonephritis. Serial renal biopsy studies have shown that some patients had IgG deposits during the early stages of the disease, with subsequent (later) biopsies showing only deposits of complement [205].

Subtypes of membranoproliferative glomerulonephritis type I have been suggested by Levy et al. [205,206] on the basis of the immunofluorescence pattern. In their study of 38 children, group 1 (26 patients) exhibited C3 and immunoglobulins; 15 of these had immunofluorescent staining along the glomerular capillary walls, but *not* in the mesangial regions [205]. In these 15 patients, IgG and IgM were the most common immunoglobulins, and C1q and C4 also were present. The other 11 patients in group 1 had C3 and immunoglobulins (mainly IgG) along the glomerular capillaries but also had mesangial deposits of C3. C1q and C4 were noted in a location similar to that of the immunoglobulins in all these patients studied. Group 2 (10 patients) consisted of the presence of C3 only, without any other immunoreactants; C3 was noted along the glomerular capillary walls and in the mesangial regions. No early complement components were found in group 2. Barbiano di Belgiojoso et al. [20] suggested a different grouping by immunofluorescence findings, but the findings are somewhat in agreement. In their study, C3 was demonstrated in all 80 biopsies. In 59 of the 80 (group 1), C3 and immunoglobulins (IgG and IgM) were present in a granular pattern along the glomerular capillary wall and sometimes in the mesangial areas. IgA was infrequently present (<10 percent of biopsies). Group 2 (16 patients) showed predominant C3 in a distribution similar to group 1; however, immunoglobulin deposition (IgG and IgM) was focal and segmental. In 5 patients (group 3), isolated C3 was noted in the capillary walls and mesangial areas. The early components of the classic complement pathway (C1q, C4) were present in groups 1 and 2. Properdin was noted in two-thirds or more of the biopsies in each group in a similar pattern to that of C3 (see Fig. 7-15). There did not appear to be any major difference in the distribution of immunoreactants between membranoproliferative glomerulonephritis with or without lobular accentuation. Fibrin(ogen)-related antigens also can be identified.

In summary, C3 is demonstrated in virtually all biopsies with membranoproliferative glomerulonephritis type I, and it is usually localized to the glomerular capillary walls and mesangial areas. The intensity and distribution of immunofluorescent staining can vary from patient to patient. Immunoglobulins may often accompany complement components, but there is a group of patients with only complement deposition. Thus, when C3 is the only reactant noted in the glomeruli, there is

Fig. 7-10. *Electron micrograph of portions of the glomerular capillary wall showing "double" basement membrane-like material. The mesangial cell has interposed itself between the endothelium and the basement membrane and in so doing has also produced mesangial matrix-basement membrane-like material. Uranyl acetate and lead citrate; ×13,475. (Courtesy of Drs. Srinivasan Rajaraman and Tito Cavallo.)*

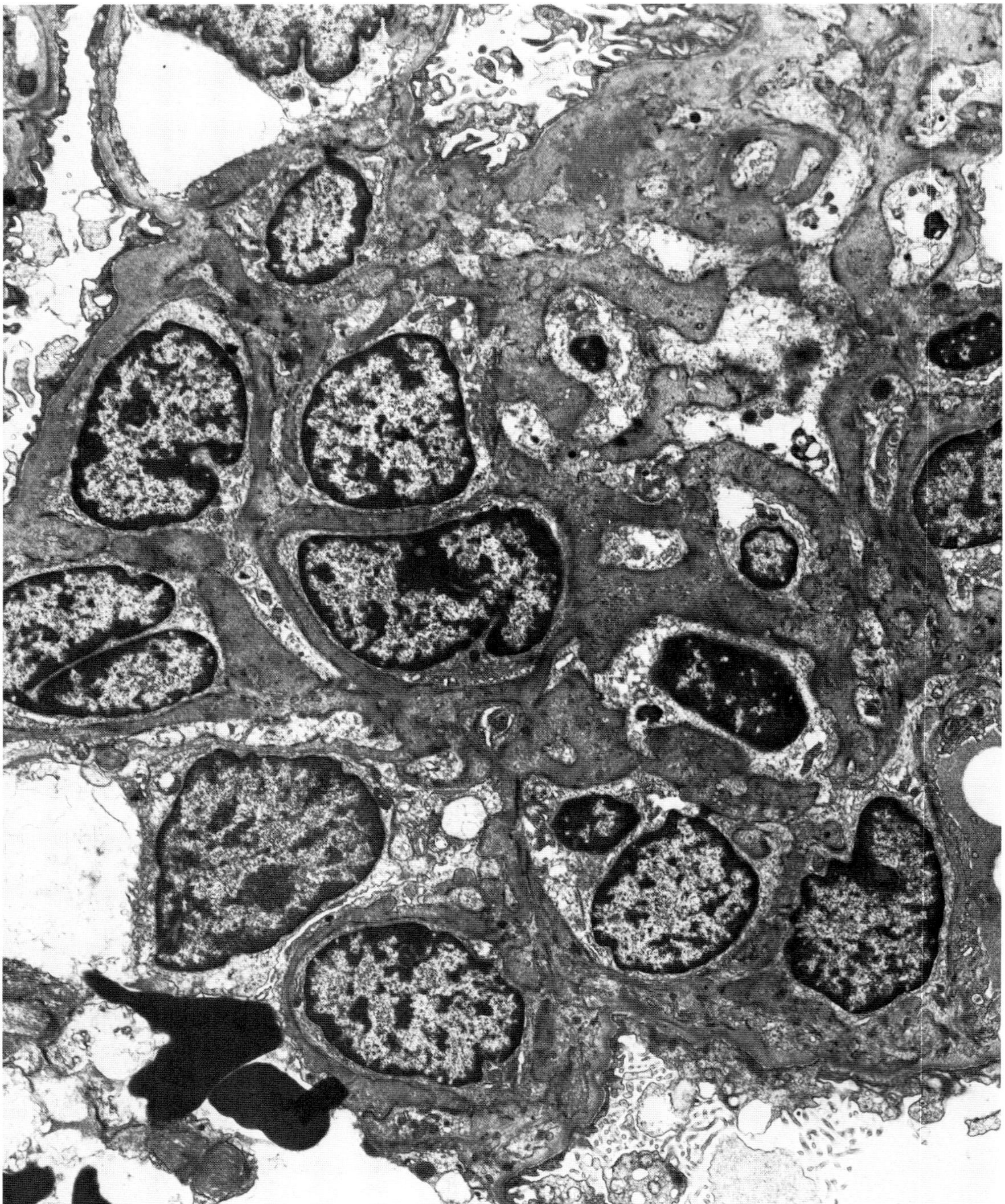

no C1q and C4, whereas when immunoglobulins are noted in addition to C3, C1q and C4 can usually be demonstrated.

Although immunofluorescence findings along the tubular basement membranes are generally negative, some authors have noted immune complexes along them [201]. Immunofluorescence techniques also have been utilized to search for the presence of other antigens. Murphy and d'Apice [255] and Nakamura et al. [258] studied kidneys with membranoproliferative glomerulonephritis with a variety of monoclonal antibodies to human glomerular antigens and demonstrated fibronectin in both the GBM and mesangium. Fibronectin was noted with a global distribution in the glomerular tufts in another study [161] and appeared to correspond to expansion of the mesangial matrix. Hara et al. [146], utilizing antisera to human GBM, type IV collagen, and P3 antigen, a rat nephritogen, noted that in membranoproliferative glomerulonephritis, the expanded mesangium and thickened glomerular capillary walls reacted positively with anti-GBM and anti-type IV collagen antibodies; only the outer portion of the capillary walls was positive with anti-P3. Using monoclonal antibodies specific for type III and IV collagen, Striker et al. [328] noted that all the synechiae in renal tissues with membranoproliferative glomerulonephritis consisted exclusively of extracellular matrix material. Crescents had interstitial collagen only when there were breaks or gaps in Bowman's capsule.

DENSE DEPOSIT DISEASE (MEMBRANOPROLIFERATIVE GLOMERULONEPHRITIS TYPE II)

In 1963, Berger and Galle [27] described a type of glomerulonephritis in which the major identifying characteristic was the presence of unique, extremely osmiophilic electron-dense deposits in the glomerular basement membranes. Since that time, many additional reports of what is referred to as *dense deposit disease* have appeared [7,11,15,46,47,68,87,98,128,130,139,141,173,197,205,206]. Since it has many of the features of membranoproliferative glomerulonephritis, it is also called *membranoproliferative glomerulonephritis type II.* It is much less common in biopsy reports than membranoproliferative glomerulonephritis type I, and in studies of consecutive patients with both types of membranoproliferative glomerulonephritis, dense deposit disease accounted for 15 to 33 percent of the total [58,99,139].

Fig. 7-11. *A portion of a glomerulus from a patient with typical MPGN type I showing increased numbers of cells in the mesangial or centrilobular regions. Although a number of these cells may represent native mesangial cells, it is also possible that many of them are mononuclear cells. Uranyl acetate and lead citrate; ×5850.*

Clinical Features

This condition affects males and females equally and is primarily a disease of children and young adults [58]. Older patients have been reported [310], and I have seen a man who was 80 years old at the time of diagnosis by renal biopsy. However, the vast majority are under the age of 20 years at the time of presentation, and patients under the age of 5 years of age have been described [11,139,206]. The clinical picture is quite similar to that of membranoproliferative glomerulonephritis type I, and it is impossible to distinguish one from the other on clinical grounds alone [11,87,99,104,139,197,206,353].

A number of patients present with the acute nephritic syndrome; this presentation is found in from 16 percent [353] to 38 percent [11] of patients. There may be acute glomerulonephritis-like episodes (gross hematuria, edema, hypertension) and/or episodes of renal insufficiency that are reversible and show complete clinical subsidence [11]; at other times the acute nephritic episodes and renal insufficiency may presage chronic renal failure [99]. In the study of Sibley and Kim [310], five of six patients with a focal and segmental necrotizing glomerulonephritis due to dense deposit disease presented with signs and symptoms of the acute nephritic syndrome. Macroscopic or gross hematuria is a common feature at the time of clinical presentation, and one or the other is present in from 11 percent [353] to 57 percent [87] of patients. Gross hematuria may develop later in the

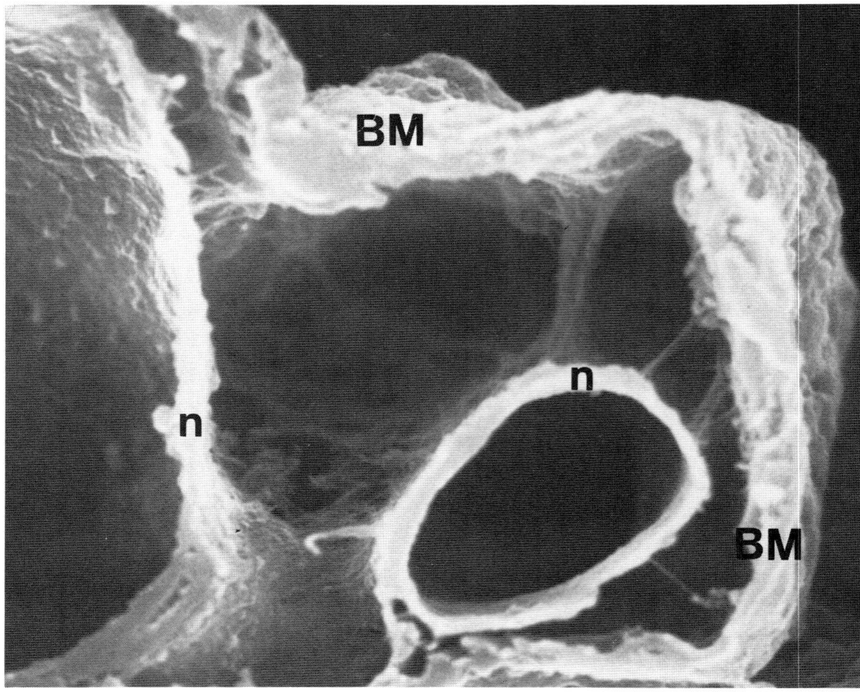

A

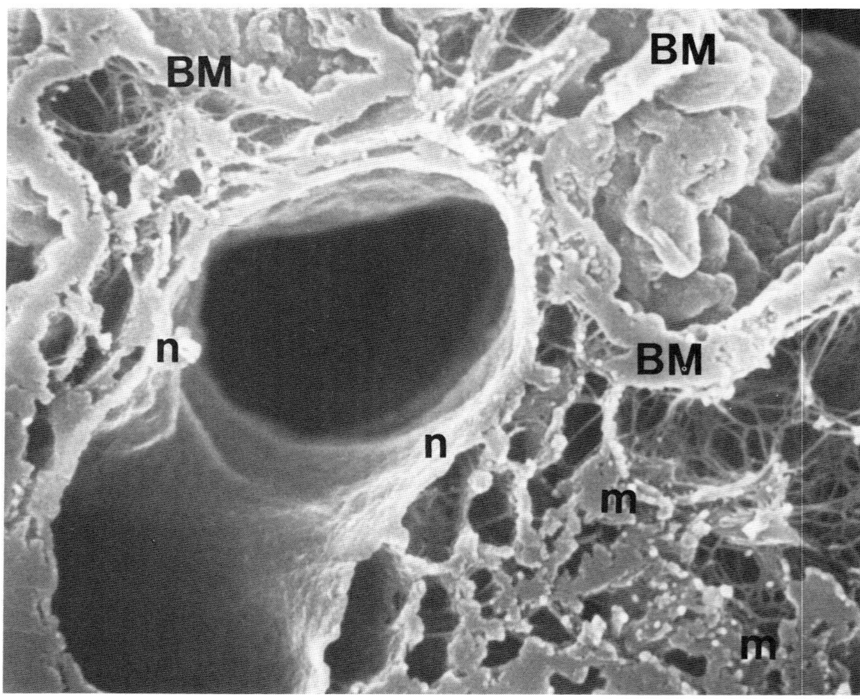

B

course of the disease; recurrent bouts of gross hematuria are encountered in a minority of patients [205,206]. Microscopic hematuria is found in most patients either at the time of clinical presentation or during the course of the disease [87,130,139]. Sterile pyuria is sometimes a feature [11].

Proteinuria is common; it was found at one time or another in all patients in two series [87,139]. It is almost invariably accompanied by microscopic hematuria. The nephrotic syndrome is a common mode of presentation, although the figures for its prevalence vary, probably because of the different criteria used to define nephrotic syndrome. It was present at the time of clinical presentation in 12 percent [11], 42 percent [353], and 50 percent [87] of patients. If not present initially, it may appear during the course of the disease, so it affected as many as 84 percent of patients at one time or another [139].

Elevations in BUN and/or serum creatinine levels are often noted initially, especially in those patients presenting with the acute nephritic syndrome. In the large series of Habib et al. [139], renal insufficiency was noted in 17 of 44 patients at clinical onset, and 4 more were affected within a few weeks. In only 6 patients was there a return of the BUN or serum creatinine levels to normal, the others progressing to end-stage renal disease over varying periods of time. Thus clinical remissions are uncommon [58,139].

Hypertension is commonly noted either at clinical onset or during the course of the disease. It is

Fig. 7-12. *Scanning electron microscopic technique of Bonsib [35] in which the cellular elements and deposits have been removed by enzymatic digestion, leaving behind only extracellular basement membranes and basement-membrane–like material from a renal biopsy with MPGN type I. (A) Enlarged subendothelial space is clearly seen. (B) Greater complexity of new basement-membrane–like material is present within the subendothelial space as compared with (A). Also demonstrated is the continuity of the enlarged subendothelial space with the mesangial matrix. BM, original or native glomerular basement membrane; n, new basement-membrane–like material; m, mesangial matrix. ×12,000. (Courtesy of Dr. Stephen M. Bonsib.)*

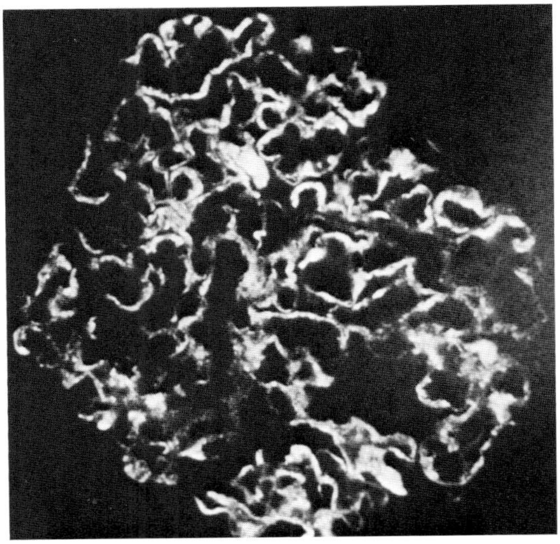

Fig. 7-13. *Glomerulus from a case of MPGN type I to show distribution of C3 seen by immunofluorescence microscopy. The pattern is a coarse, broken-linear type, with some areas of coarse granularity along capillary loops. (Courtesy Dr. George Bannayan.)*

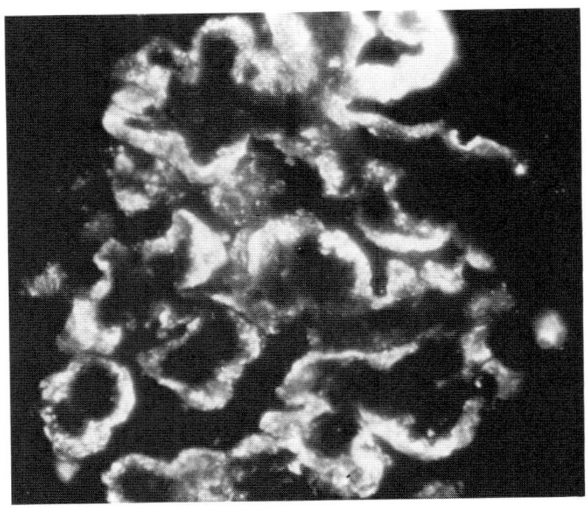

Fig. 7-14. *Immunofluorescence shows intense staining along all glomerular capillary walls for C3. The granular staining is quite broad in this instance. ×315.*

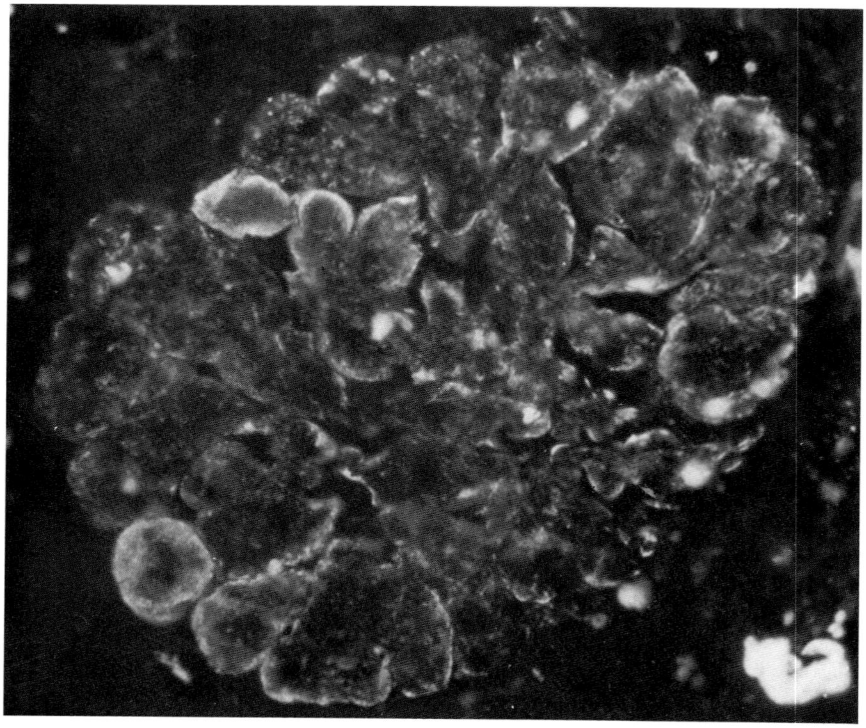

FIG. 7-15. *Glomerulus from 12-year-old boy with MPGN type I stained with fluorescein-labeled antibody to human properdin. Distribution along peripheral capillaries in a granular and interrupted linear pattern.* ×402. *(Courtesy Dr. Robert Vernier.)*

usually transient initially [139] but becomes permanent in those patients developing end-stage renal disease.

The clinical onset of dense deposit disease is often preceded by an upper respiratory tract infection. Evidence of this type of infection is noted in approximately one half of patients [11,87,139, 353]. Elevated ASO titers were noted in 21 to 45 percent of patients with infective episodes [87, 139,353]; therefore, some were undoubtedly related to group A streptococcal infection. Partial lipodystrophy is present in some patients with dense-deposit disease, and this association is discussed later in a separate section. Occasionally, there may be associations with other disease processes, but they are rare and probably unrelated to the etiology/pathogenesis of dense deposit disease. These processes include Alport's syndrome [12], narcotic addiction [191], acquired cutis laxa [347], and systemic lupus erythematosus [124]. Pregnancy may lead to exacerbation of dense deposit disease [203].

Depressed levels of serum C3 are commonly found, although this is not an invariable feature. Persistently low serum levels of C3 are found in most patients (approximately 80 percent) [139, 144,182,268], whereas fluctuating levels are found in others. A minority of patients have normal levels of serum C3 [87,139,353]. In contrast with membranoproliferative glomerulonephritis type I, serum levels of the early components of the classical pathway (C1q and C4) are usually normal, and C3-nephritic factor (C3NeF) is commonly detected. Serum concentrations of factor B and pro-

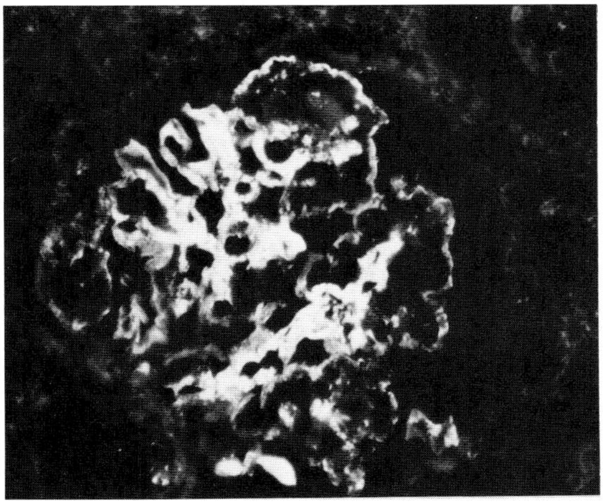

FIG. 7-16. *Immunofluorescence from a patient with MPGN type I showing intense glomerular mesangial and capillary wall staining with anti-IgG antiserum.* ×315.

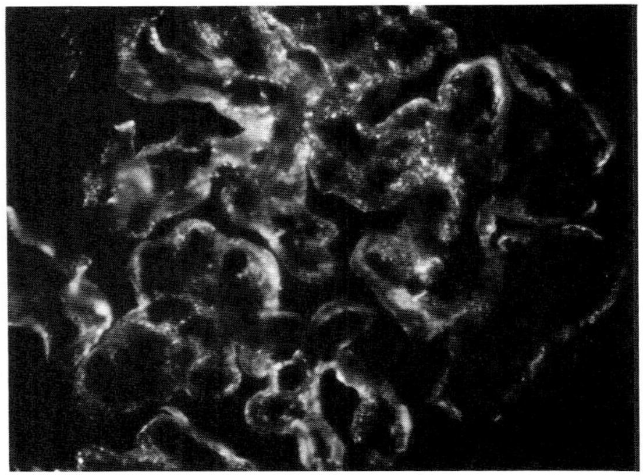

FIG. 7-17. *Immunofluorescence showing moderately intense staining for IgM along the glomerular capillary walls in a granular pattern from a patient with MPGN type I.* ×283.

perdin of the alternative pathway are decreased. These complement profiles suggest that complement is activated in dense deposit disease primarily through the alternative pathway, whereas membranoproliferative glomerulonephritis type I occurs through the classical and alternative pathways. These various aspects of complement activation will be discussed in the section dealing with pathogenesis.

Clinical Course

The overall long-term prognosis for patients with dense deposit disease is poor [58]. Although temporary remissions may occur, it is unusual for them to be permanent. In a large series of 44 children [139], only 1 patient was found to have remission; it was maintained for 5 years. End-stage renal disease occurs in most patients, although the time period over which this develops varies widely. In the large series of children just noted [139], 10 of the 44 went into end-stage renal disease over a 20-month period from clinical onset of the illness, and a further 5 patients did so over a 2½- to 10-year period. Those patients with the rapid course had crescents on renal biopsy. In the study by Vargas et al. [353], 8 of 33 children developed terminal renal failure over a mean of 33 months. Galle and Mahieu [130] noted that 20 of their 40 children and adults followed up to 21 years had developed end-stage renal disease. While 4 of these patients developed renal failure in less than 1 year, others took up to 13 years to do so. In 3 patients in this series, proteinuria persisted, but renal failure did not develop during follow-up periods of 19, 20, and 21 years. Similar findings have been noted by a number of other investigators [87,197].

As with other renal diseases, the presence of the nephrotic syndrome is thought to be a harbinger of a poor renal prognosis [139,197,206] (see Table 7-1). However, this is not an invariable experience [87]. Other clinical features thought to be indicative of a poor renal prognosis in dense deposit disease include the absence of clinical remission during the course of the renal disease, an initial decrease in renal function, and the presence of gross hematuria [139,206]. Davis et al. [87] failed to identify any single clinical or laboratory feature that was indicative of a poor renal prognosis. Hypertension has been suggested as a cause of deterioration of renal function [197].

The prognosis for children with dense deposit

disease is not uniform, and certain renal biopsy findings, rather than clinical or laboratory features, can be helpful in determining which patients are most likely to develop progressive renal insufficiency. These histologic indicators include the presence of mesangial deposits, glomerular sclerosis, and crescents [58,139,206,353]. In an analysis of factors potentially responsible for differences in outcome, the Southwest Pediatric Nephrology Study Group [317] noted that whereas the initial clinical and/or laboratory features were not useful indicators of outcome, certain pathologic findings on renal biopsy did appear to be helpful. Increased glomerular lobulation, mesangial sclerosis, and hypercellularity with glomerular capillary loop obliteration and glomerular mesangial deposits were all associated with a poor outcome. Sibley and Kim [310] reached similar conclusions. Thus morphologic features are not merely the only way to make a definitive diagnosis of dense deposit disease but are also helpful in determining which patients will proceed to end-stage renal failure.

The overall renal prognosis of dense deposit disease is thought not to be significantly different from membranoproliferative glomerulonephritis type I by some authors [87]. In contrast, others [139] noted that at the end of a mean follow-up of 4¾ years, 41 percent of patients with dense deposit disease had developed end-stage renal disease, whereas at the end of a longer follow-up period (5 11/12 years), only 25 percent of patients with membranoproliferative glomerulonephritis type I were in a similar state. In the same series, 50 percent mortality occurred between the ninth and tenth year for patients with dense deposit disease compared with the seventeenth and eighteenth years for membranoproliferative glomerulonephritis type I [139]. This 50 percent end-stage renal disease rate at approximately the ninth to twelfth years has been noted in other series [11,58]. Ten of 21 patients of Habib et al. [139] with dense deposit disease in which the GFR was decreased at the time of clinical onset had a rapidly progressive course ending in end-stage renal disease within 2 years of clinical onset. These authors attributed the worse prognosis in dense deposit disease to the greater frequency of crescents. Klein et al. [190] reported that 56 percent of their patients developed end-stage renal disease within 2.9 years of clinical presentation. In the 16 patients studied by the Southwest Pediatric Nephrology Study Group (SPNSG) [317] who had dense deposit disease, a rapid course was observed in only 2 patients. Klein and colleagues [190] observed a more benign course in 5 of their 18 patients during a period of 11 years of follow-up; the SPNSG [317] noted a similar relatively benign course in 10 of 16 patients, 6 of whom were followed for more than 7 years (mean 10 years). Mild forms of dense deposit disease do exist [190,317]. In the series of Klein et al. [190], some patients with dense deposit disease had a benign clinical course; these patients had normal levels of C3 and factor B and low levels of C3NeF.

Effect of Treatment on Clinical Course

The treatment of dense deposit disease is controversial, and varying regimens of alternate-day steroids and anticoagulants or antiplatelet drugs have been suggested. Large, prospective, well-controlled studies have not been forthcoming. In the study by Habib et al. [139], 28 patients received steroid therapy but showed no remission of proteinuria. Four of 10 patients in the series of Lamb et al. [197] developed chronic renal failure; 9 of 10 patients received corticosteroid or immunosuppressive therapy or both. These authors concluded that dense deposit disease is largely unresponsive to conventional steroid therapy.

However, West and colleagues [370] have suggested that as in type I membranoproliferative glomerulonephritis, benefit may be observed in dense deposit disease when alternate-day high-dose steroids are administered. McEnery and McAdams [227] described regression of dense deposit disease in six children treated continuously with an alternate-day prednisone regimen. All showed reduction of glomerular mesangial hypercellularity and widening of the glomerular capillary lumens. A change in the position of the dense deposits was noted from the lamina densa to the lamina rara interna of the GBM in four patients; there was a reduction in the prevalence of deposits in three children, with a virtual absence of deposits in two.

Kher et al. [178] likewise noted regression of the dense deposits in a child treated with immunosuppression and anticoagulant therapy. Although most of the patients in the SPNSG study [317] who maintained normal renal function for long periods had received alternate-day prednisone, and most of those not receiving steroids did develop end-stage renal disease, no conclusions could be drawn regarding the efficacy of such treatment in an uncontrolled, short-term, retrospective study.

Such discordance among reports might be due to variations in the dosages of steroids used or to the inclusion of different degrees of morphologic severity of dense deposit disease itself. Clearly, large-scale, prospective studies on biopsy-defined dense deposit disease utilizing different therapeutic regimens need to be undertaken.

Pathologic Changes

GROSS APPEARANCE

Our knowledge of dense deposit disease is based almost solely on renal biopsy material, and for this reason, there is little information on the gross appearance of the kidneys with this disease pattern. Although whole kidneys may become available upon nephrectomy before renal transplantation, the changes are obscured by those caused by dialysis, a matter that is considered in Chapter 11.

MICROSCOPIC FINDINGS

The light microscopic findings have been described by many investigators [27,46,47,59,68,87, 130,139,142,167,173,197,205,206].

Glomeruli

Although the term *membranoproliferative glomerulonephritis type II* suggests that this entity is similar to membranoproliferative glomerulonephritis type I, the former can have a number of glomerular light microscopic appearances [310] (Figs. 7-18 through 7-22). There is no constant glomerular finding by light microscopy, and a variety of light microscopic patterns are noted [310,317] (Table 7-2). The basic feature is the presence of deposits in the glomerular capillary wall (GBM to be specific), and a variable degree of mesangial hypercellularity and/or sclerosis may be seen, although often less than that noted in membranoproliferative glomerulonephritis type I [182]. At one extreme are glomeruli that appear almost normal by light microscopy with little glomerular hypercellularity but with some glomerular capillary wall thickening. This thickening, according to Heptinstall [150], usually affects more glomerular capillary loops than are seen in membranoproliferative glomerulonephritis type I, yet is not usually so widespread as in membranous glomerulonephritis. Other renal biopsies show a more pronounced glomerular tuft hypercellularity. Leukocytes may be more common when the lesions are diffuse than when they are focal and segmental. The mesangium may show differing degrees of matrix increase (mesangial sclerosis), and at the end of the spectrum there are sclerotic nodules with an accentuated lobular pattern (so-called lobular glomerulonephritis). Focal and segmental necrotizing glomerular lesions also may be noted occasionally [310], although this is not common in my experience; it is in patients with this pattern that light microscopic identification of dense deposit disease is difficult and open to misinterpretation [310]. Electron microscopy is needed to establish the diagnosis.

The thickening of the glomerular capillary walls is caused by elongated, irregular intramembranous deposits. These deposits are often ribbon-like, stain strongly with eosin, and appear somewhat refractile. They are intensely PAS positive, and the trichrome stain shows them to be fuchsinophilic (red) (Fig. 7-23). These glomerular intramembranous deposits appear dark blue with toluidine blue

Table 7-2. *Light microscopic patterns noted in patients with dense deposit disease*

1. Membranoproliferative glomerulonephritis
2. Lobular glomerulonephritis or glomerular sclerosis
3. Pure mesangial hypercellularity (focal and segmental or diffuse)
4. Membranous glomerulonephritis–like pattern
5. Crescentic glomerulonephritis
6. Minimal changes
7. Focal and segmental necrotizing glomerulonephritis

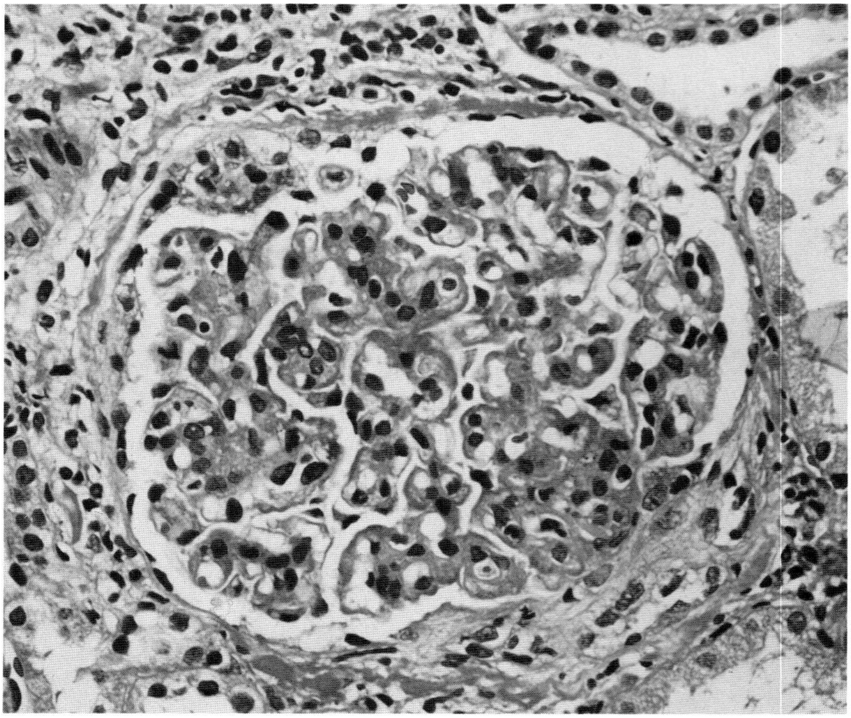

FIG. 7-18. *Glomerulus showing widespread thickening of capillary walls with mild increase in cellularity. From patient with dense deposit disease. H&E; ×375.*

in 0.5 or 1.0-μm plastic-embedded sections. With methenamine silver staining the intramembranous deposits are not as argyrophilic as the GBM and are somewhat brownish [87,139] (Fig. 7-24). Thus the intramembranous nonstaining deposit is often bordered on each side by a thin, silver-positive GBM [130]. A double-contour appearance of the glomerular capillary wall is noted in approximately half of patients [182] (see Fig. 7-24). The glomerular intramembranous deposits may stain with the fluorochrome dye thioflavine-T [68,84].

Date et al. [84] studied 50 patients with various forms of membranoproliferative glomerulonephritis by thioflavine-T and electron microscopy. All renal biopsies with dense deposit disease stained brightly with thioflavine-T; however, some staining also was noted in certain cases of membranoproliferative glomerulonephritis type I and membranoproliferative glomerulonephritis type III. These authors concluded that the staining corresponded to the extent of the glomerular deposit rather than its location or nature.

The glomerular intramembranous deposits vary greatly in size and number, and it is this that determines the extent of the glomerular capillary wall thickening. Although some authors believe that dense deposit disease can and should be diagnosed by light microscopy, in some cases electron microscopy may be needed to reveal the presence of deposits with certainty [150]. This is also true for the demonstration of mesangial deposits. In some biopsies, PAS- and trichrome-positive mesangial deposits can be demonstrated, although in my experience this is often difficult. Deposits are also noted in the basal lamina of Bowman's capsule and tubular basement membranes; the ex-

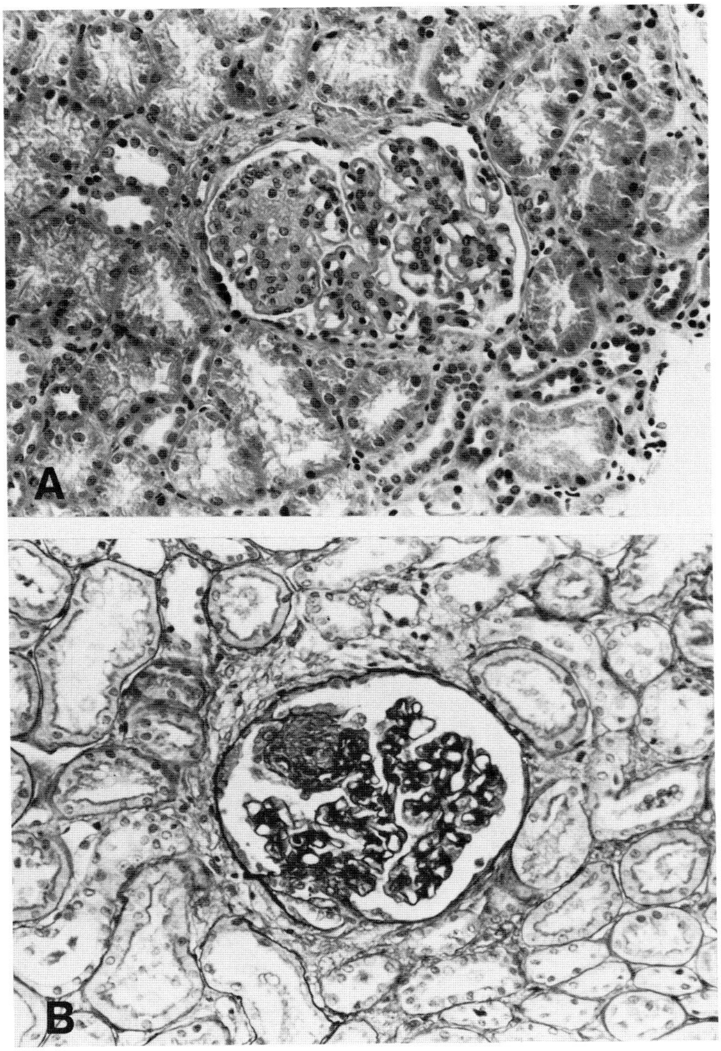

Fig. 7-19. (A, B) Focal and segmental (intracapillary) proliferative glomerulonephritis may be one of several patterns noted in dense deposit disease. (A) H&E and (B) PAS; ×250. (Courtesy of Drs. Edith Hawkins and Regina Verani.)

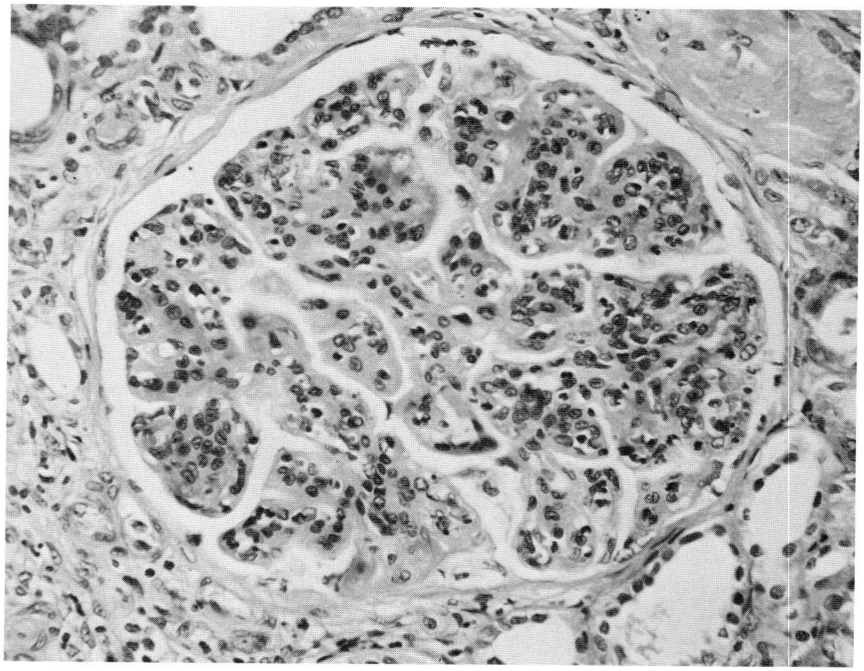

FIG. 7-20. *Glomerulus from patient with dense deposit disease. There is pronounced mesangial hypercellularity in addition to extensive—although not diffuse—thickening of the capillary walls. H&E; ×450.*

tent of this extraglomerular involvement is quite variable.

Glomerular subepithelial electron-dense discrete deposits similar to the subepithelial humps noted in classic acute postinfectious (poststreptococcal) glomerulonephritis may be seen in dense deposit disease [333]. Rarely, spikes of GBM-like material (as seen in classic stage 3 of membranous glomerulonephritis) may be noted around the subepithelial humps [139]. Double contours with methenamine silver staining, however, are more common [139]; this is due to the nonargyrophilia of the intramembranous deposits. Polymorphonuclear leukocytes may be noted, occasionally giving an exudative glomerulonephritic appearance.

Crescents may be present in large or small numbers. The frequency with which they are found varies from about 7 percent [87] to almost a third of cases [139]. In the series of dense-deposit disease by Sibley and Kim [310], 9 of their 16 patients had a membranoproliferative glomerulonephritis–like pattern, 5 had a focal and segmental intracapillary and extracapillary necrotizing glomerulonephritis, and 2 had a focal and segmental proliferative glomerulonephritis. Characteristic deposits could be recognized by light microscopy in most of their patients.

As the renal disease progresses, the glomeruli undergo sclerosis, although even in advanced cases it is usually still possible to demonstrate the characteristic intramembranous dense deposits by electron microscopy [130].

Tubules

The tubular epithelium may show either hyalin droplets (evidence of glomerular filtration of protein) or vacuolization. The same type of deposit noted in the GBM may be identified along the tubular basement membranes (Fig. 7-25). With pro-

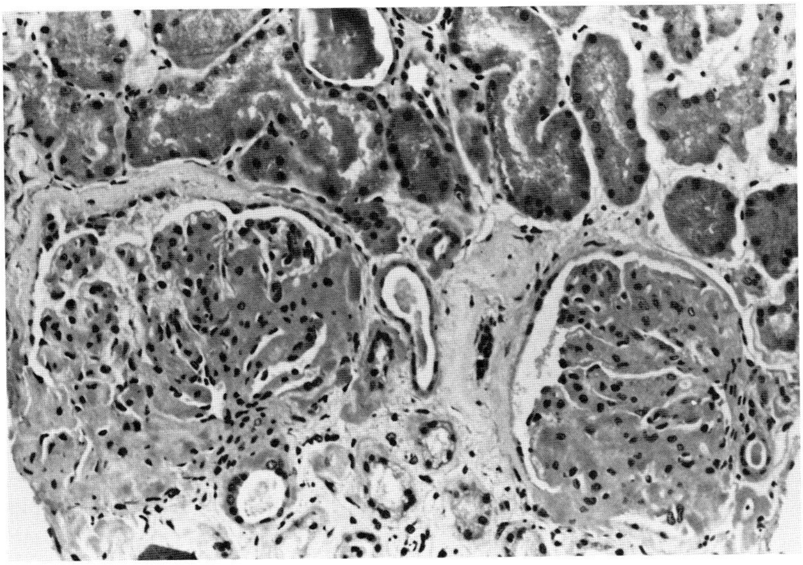

FIG. 7-21. *Glomerulus from a patient with dense deposit disease showing a progressing stage of the disease. Note the narrowing or closure of the glomerular capillary lumens by amorphous acellular material (dense deposits). This pattern is somewhat reminiscent of amyloid or an advanced membranous glomerulonephritis. H&E; ×200. (Courtesy of Dr. Conrad Pirani.)*

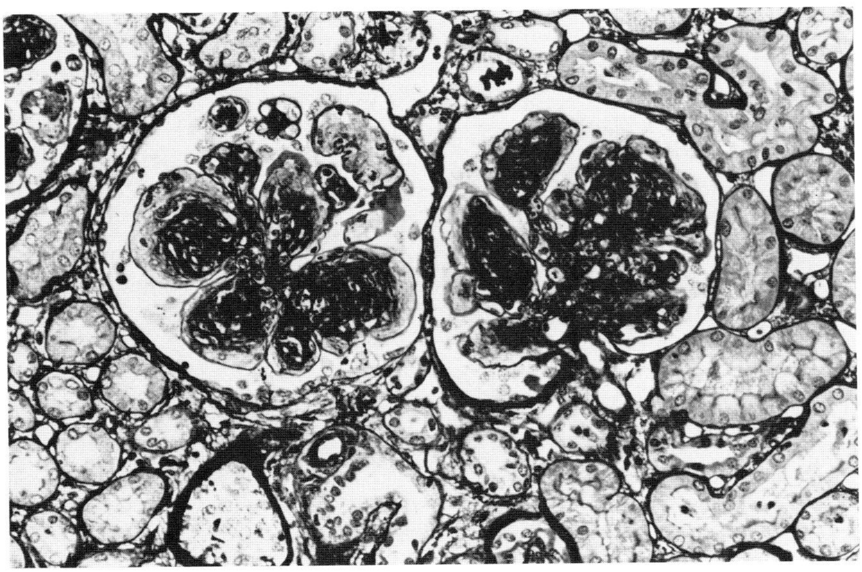

FIG. 7-22. *A lobular form of dense deposit disease may be seen. Note the accentuation of the lobular pattern by increase both in the amount of mesangial matrix and cells. Jones silver methenamine; ×200. (Courtesy of Drs. Tito Cavallo and Srinivasan Rajaraman.)*

gression of the glomerular sclerosis, there is tubular atrophy and interstitial fibrosis.

Blood Vessels

There is intimal thickening of the arteries as the disease progresses, probably secondary to the accompanying hypertension. Electron-dense deposits may be identified in occasional interstitial capillaries and arterioles [139,167].

Interstitium

There may be interstitial inflammation, mostly by chronic inflammatory cells (i.e., lymphocytes). Foam cells are sometimes present, predictive of the nephrotic syndrome. Interstitial fibrosis occurs as renal failure develops. A tubulointerstitial nephritis may be seen [310].

ELECTRON MICROSCOPIC FINDINGS

It was the use of electron-microscopy that led to the discovery of this condition, which is uniquely different from all other forms of renal disease [27]. It is from the characteristic ultrastructural appearance of the glomerular intramembranous deposits that the disease takes its name (Figs. 7-26 and 7-27). There have been many reports on the electron microscopic findings [47,58,68,87,130,139,173,197], and there is generally good agreement on the ultrastructural findings. Confirmation of the diagnosis of dense deposit disease requires electron microscopy, in my opinion, although this opinion is not shared by all.

The hallmark of the disease is the presence of dense osmiophilic deposits in the glomerular basement membranes, basal lamina of Bowman's capsule, tubular basement membranes (probably mostly proximal), and mesangial regions (Figs. 7-28 through 7-30). Involvement of the glomerular capillary walls is variable and may show a variety of patterns. The lamina densa is most often uniformly thickened by the deposits. The deposit may replace the entire width of the lamina densa, whereas in some patients with less extensive involvement it only occupies part of the width. In the latter instances, the remnant or native GBM can be identified on one or both sides of the dense deposits. There may be fusiform segmental thickening of regions of the GBM or large, irregular masses of the dense deposits that cause considerable distortion of the GBM.

The elongated or ribbon-like deposits in the GBM usually involve long stretches of many loops. In less involved cases, only a few loops are involved by shorter and narrower dense deposits. In some cases of mild involvement, the glomerular capillary wall deposits appear toward the inner (subendothelial) aspect of the GBM. Large glomerular subendothelial deposits are scanty or rare. I have seen one biopsy from a patient with dense deposit disease in which the deposits in one glomerular capillary were distinctly and solely subendothelial; however, they were intramembranous in all the other glomerular capillaries.

The electron-dense deposits lack a substructure, even at very high magnification. Although the deposits are quite dense without staining of any sort, their density is accentuated several orders of magnitude after staining with lead or uranyl salts [130]. Because their osmiophilia is so much greater than that of the lamina densa of the GBM, the deposits can readily be identified and distinguished from the lamina densa of the GBM, even if they are only focal and small. It has been suggested that the ultrastructural deposits are different from the finely granular discrete deposits that characterize the various forms of immune complex glomerulonephritis. At the ultrastructural level, the deposits have the same affinity for silver as the lamina densa when impregnated with methenamine silver [182].

It should be noted that although the term *deposit* is extensively used, a transformation of the lamina densa is just as likely an explanation [47,130]. Muda et al. [254] studied these densities by means of ultrastructural histochemical techniques using thin sections from formaldehyde fixed, OsO_4 postfixed, and epon-embedded specimens collected for diagnostic electron microscopy. The dense deposits had a higher osmium affinity than the normal lamina densa of the GBM; it was found that the electron density was strictly an osmium-dependent phenomenon, suggesting the presence of a lipid component. Further extraction studies for lipids confirmed this suggestion [254].

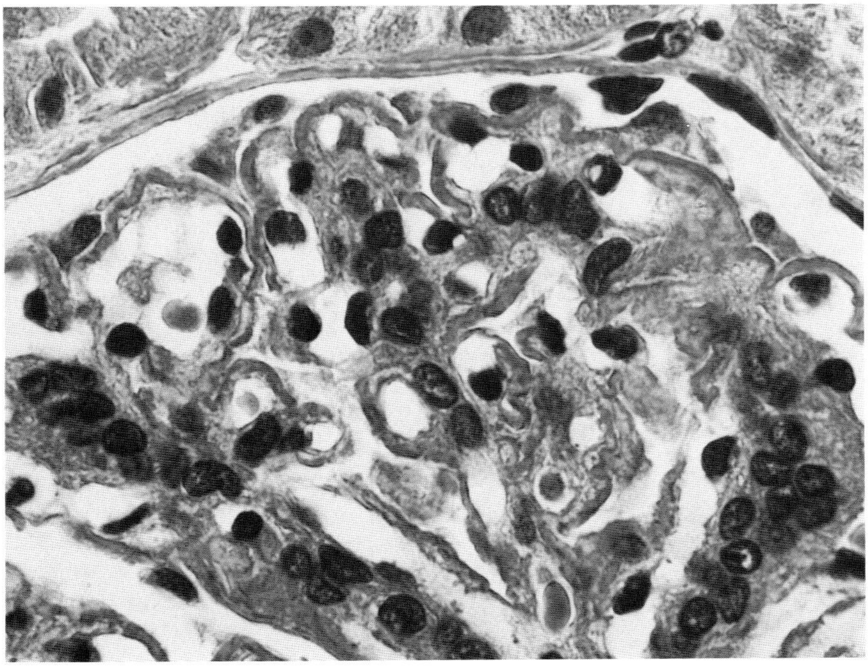

Fig. 7-23. *A glomerulus from a patient with dense deposit disease. There is ribbon-like staining along all of the glomerular capillary walls with trichrome stain. Masson's trichrome; × 1425. (Courtesy of Dr. Edith Hawkins.)*

A granular variant of the dense deposit has been described [189], but the significance of this is not clear, and it may actually represent a plasma-cell dyscrasia–induced glomerular disease. Mild or early forms have been described [86,190,219]. Sato et al. [302] described an 8-year-old girl whose initial renal biopsy showed a membranoproliferative and lobular glomerulonephritis in which only lamellation of the lamina densa was found by electron microscopy; no dense deposits were noted. Repeat renal biopsy 5½ years later showed typical ultrastructural features of dense deposit disease. This suggested to the authors [302] that the lamellation of the lamina densa was the first morphologic manifestation of dense deposit disease. Regression of glomerular intramembranous dense deposits has been reported in a few children treated with immunosuppressive and anticoagulant therapy [178,227].

The mesangial regions may show several changes. There may be an increase in the number of cells in the mesangial regions, either endocapillary or inflammatory cells or both. There also may be an increase in the amount of mesangial matrix, which may be so severe as to produce nodules (lobular glomerulonephritis variant). Electron-dense deposits may occur in the mesangial regions (see Fig. 7-28). Sibley and Kim [310] noted in cases of dense deposit disease with a focal necrotizing glomerulonephritis that the glomerular intramembranous dense deposits were localized to the paramesangial glomerular basement membranes and the mesangial regions. Mesangial deposits are typically nongranular and quite dense (like those of the GBM); they may be well circumscribed or be large with vague margins.

Other glomerular ultrastructural changes include crescent formation and the glomerular sub-

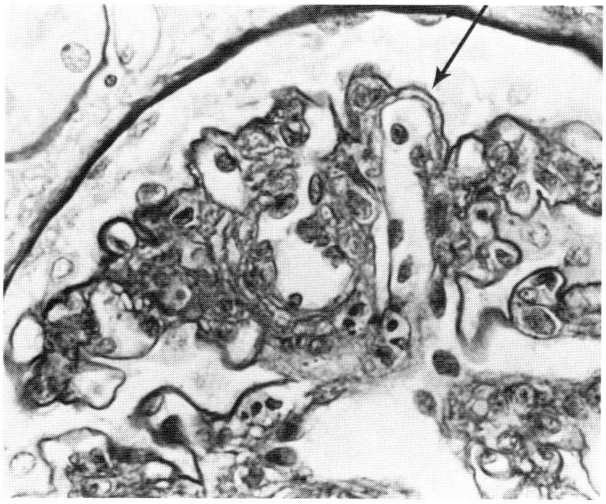

FIG. 7-24. *Glomerulus from a patient with dense deposit disease to show splitting of the glomerular capillary wall. The explanation for this appearance with silver staining is that the nonargyrophilic dense deposit is flanked by thin layers of argyrophilic surviving capillary basement membrane. Silver impregnation; ×344. (Courtesy of Drs. Tito Cavallo and Srinivasan Rajaraman.)*

epithelial humps noted before (Fig. 7-31). This latter change was noted in many series [87, 139,167,168] and was present in 10 of 14 cases studied in one of them [139]. It has been suggested that these glomerular subepithelial deposits are more finely granular and lack the extreme electron density of the classic intramembranous deposits. They are found more frequently in dense deposit disease than in membranoproliferative glomerulonephritis type I. Other ultrastructural changes include an increase in mesangial matrix and mesangial interposition, although this is seen less frequently than in patients with membranoproliferative glomerulonephritis type I.

Electron-dense deposits may be noted along the basal lamina of Bowman's capsule (see Fig. 7-30), along the tubular basement membranes (see Fig. 7-30), and in interstitial capillaries, arterioles, and small arteries [139,167]. Dense deposits are almost always found in Bowman's capsule, although they may be quite focal and segmental. These deposits may or may not expand Bowman's capsule. Campbell-Boswell et al. [59] noted typical dense deposits in six of nine renal biopsies in which an

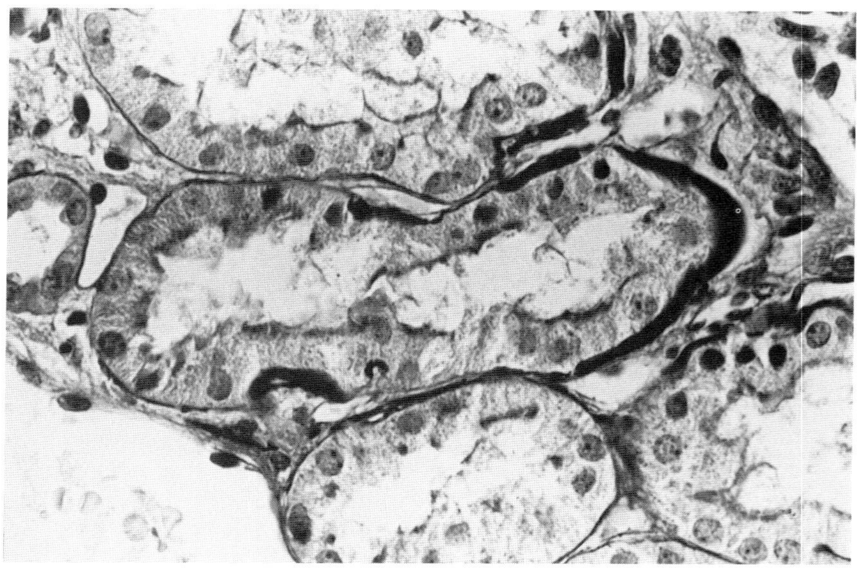

FIG. 7-25. *Dense deposits in tubular basement membrane. Periodic acid–Schiff technique; ×400. (Courtesy of Dr. Edith Hawkins.)*

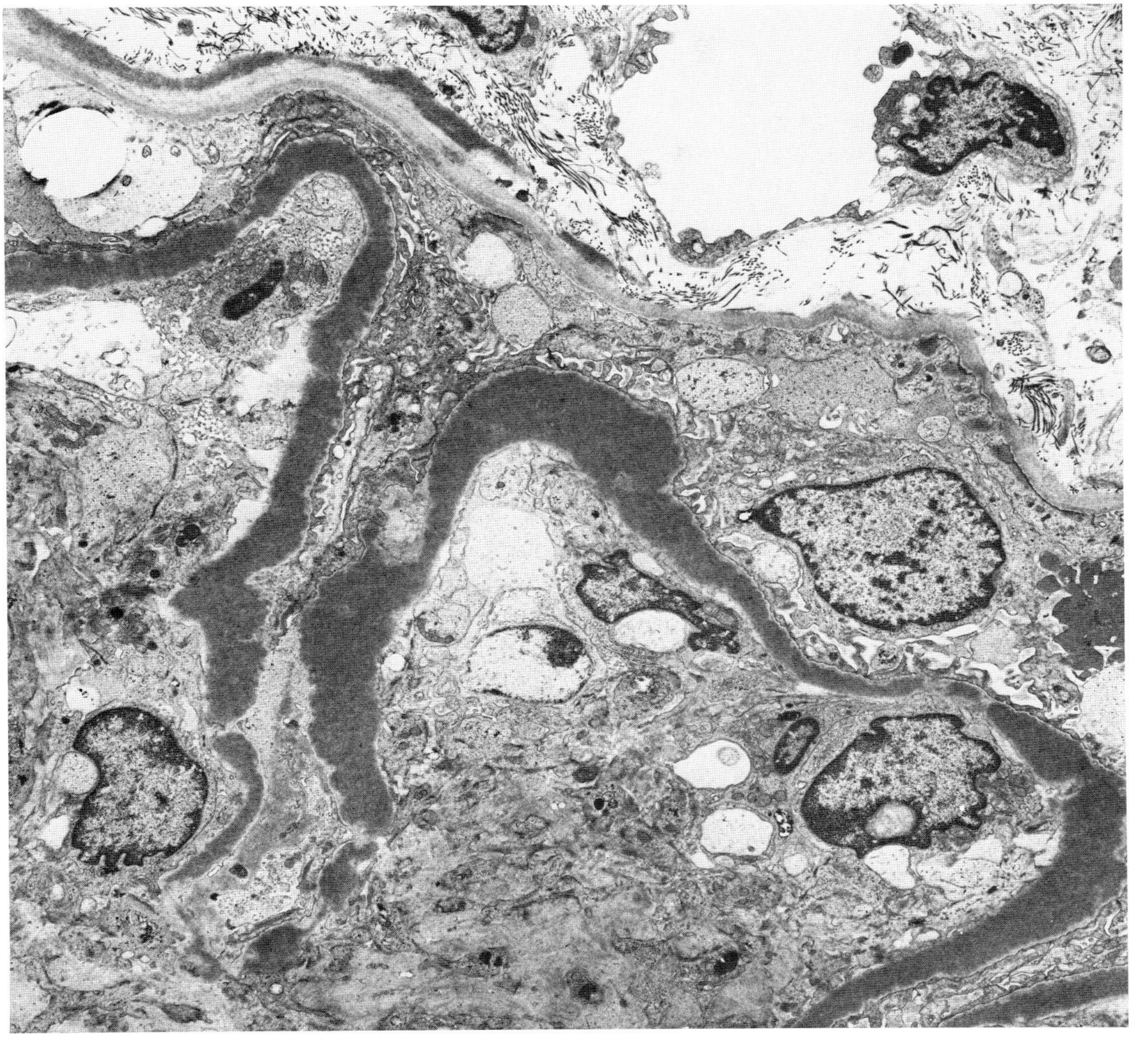

Fig. 7-26. *Dense deposits in the glomerular basement membranes. Note that the deposits are much more osmiophilic (or electron dense) than the normal-appearing GBM or mesangial matrix. Uranyl acetate and lead citrate;* ×4680. *(Courtesy of Dr. Edith Hawkins.)*

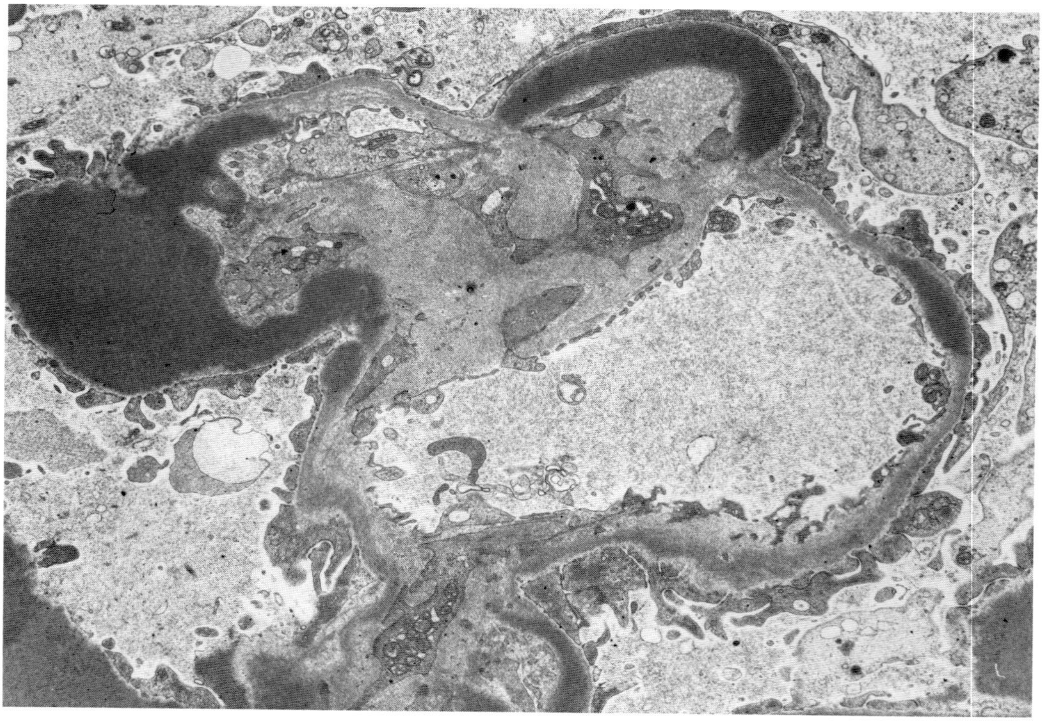

FIG. 7-27. *Dense deposits in the GBM. They are of a much greater density than the lamina densa and are usually elongated as in this picture.* ×3200. *(Courtesy Dr. T. Antonovych and Director of Armed Forces Institute of Pathology.)*

extensive search for tubular deposits was undertaken. The tubular basement membrane deposits were always less numerous and smaller than the intramembranous deposits in glomeruli. Using scanning electron microscopy, Weidner and Lorentz [361] studied the three-dimensional appearance of GBMs rendered acellular by enzymatic digestion. When dense-deposit disease was compared with normal controls, the acellular GBM appeared "rigid" and thickened with a coarsely granular or undulating surface that was punctuated by single or clustered crater-like deformities. These authors thought that this three-dimensional appearance was unique for dense deposit disease.

Extrarenal dense deposits have been sought using thioflavine-T and electron microscopy in a number of patients with dense deposit disease, but they have only been noted in the basement membranes of the splenic sinusoids in two patients [272,340]. No other organ system (such as brain, heart, lung, liver, adrenal, or pancreas) was involved. Duvall-Young et al. [106] recently reported fundus changes in a patient with dense deposit disease; the deposits in Bruch's membrane of the fundus were histologically very similar to those noted in the kidney.

FIG. 7-28. *Dense deposits may be noted not only in the intramembranous portion of the glomerular basement membranes, but also in the mesangial regions (lower left and lower center). Some investigators believe that the presence of increased mesangial matrix and mesangial deposits indicates a poor prognosis. Uranyl acetate and lead citrate;* ×6545. *(Courtesy of Dr. Regina Verani.)*

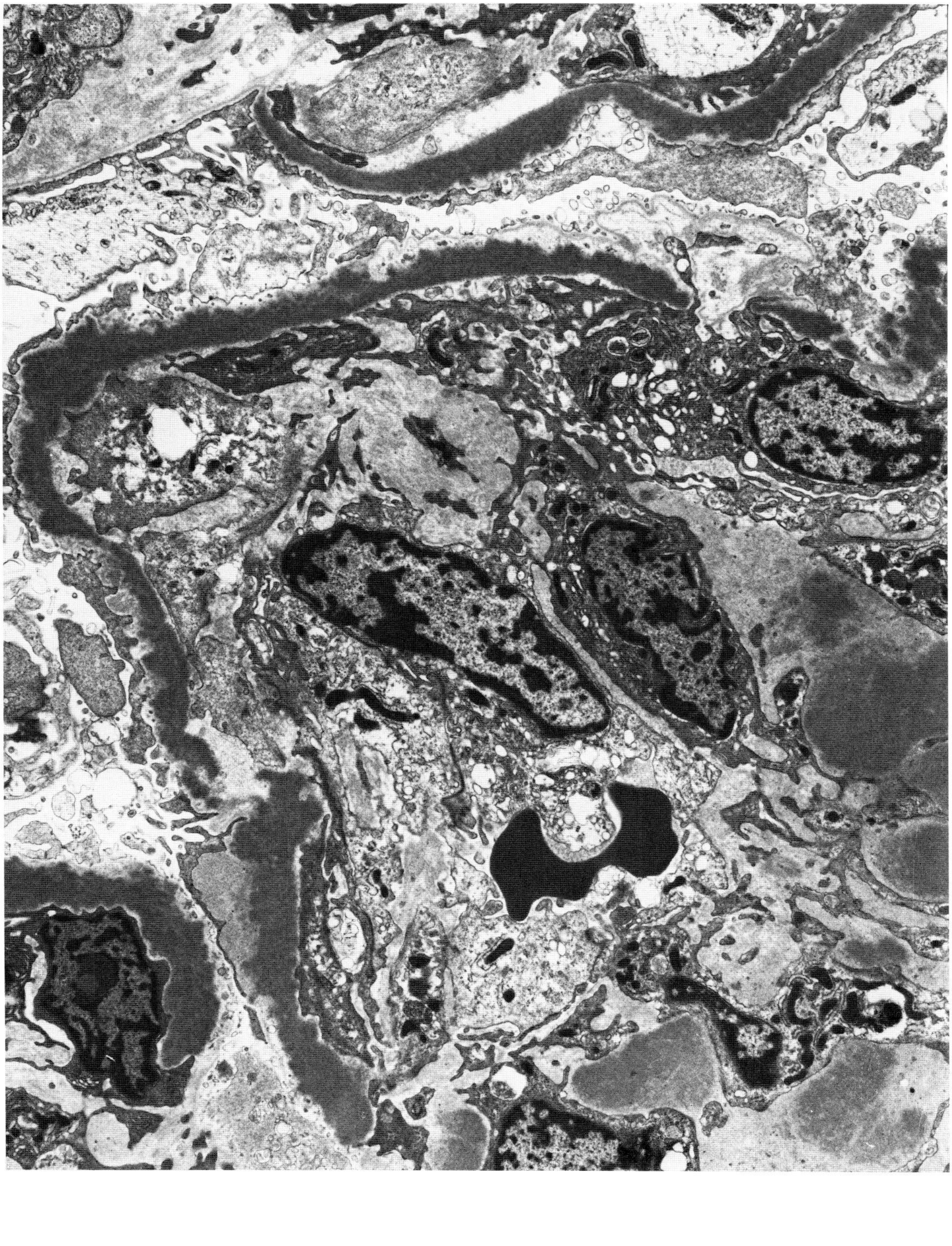

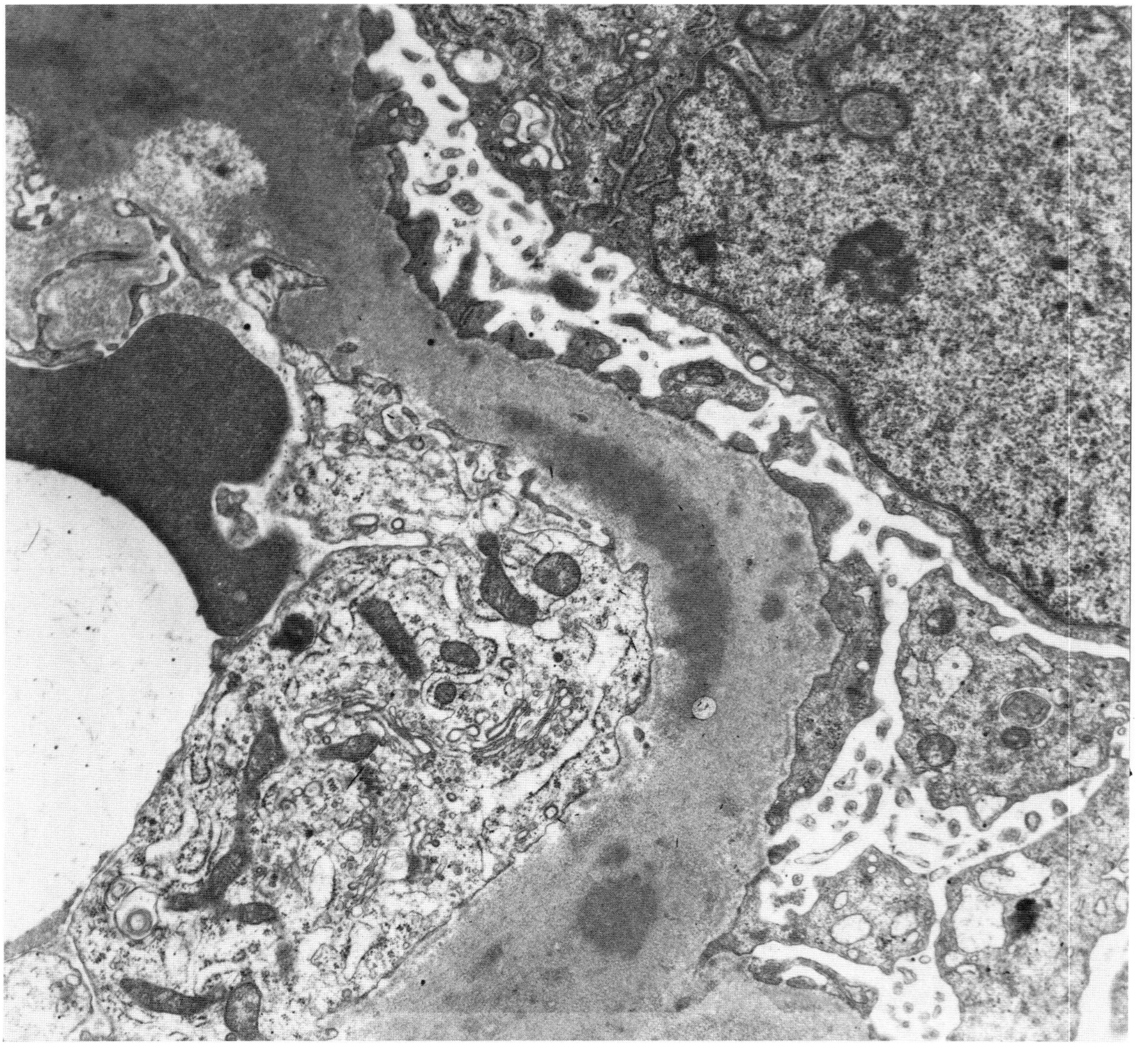

FIG. 7-29. *Glomerular subendothelial deposits or deposits in the inner (subendothelial) portion of the GBM may occasionally be noted to occur focally in patients with otherwise typical dense deposit disease. Uranyl acetate and lead citrate; × 13,680.*

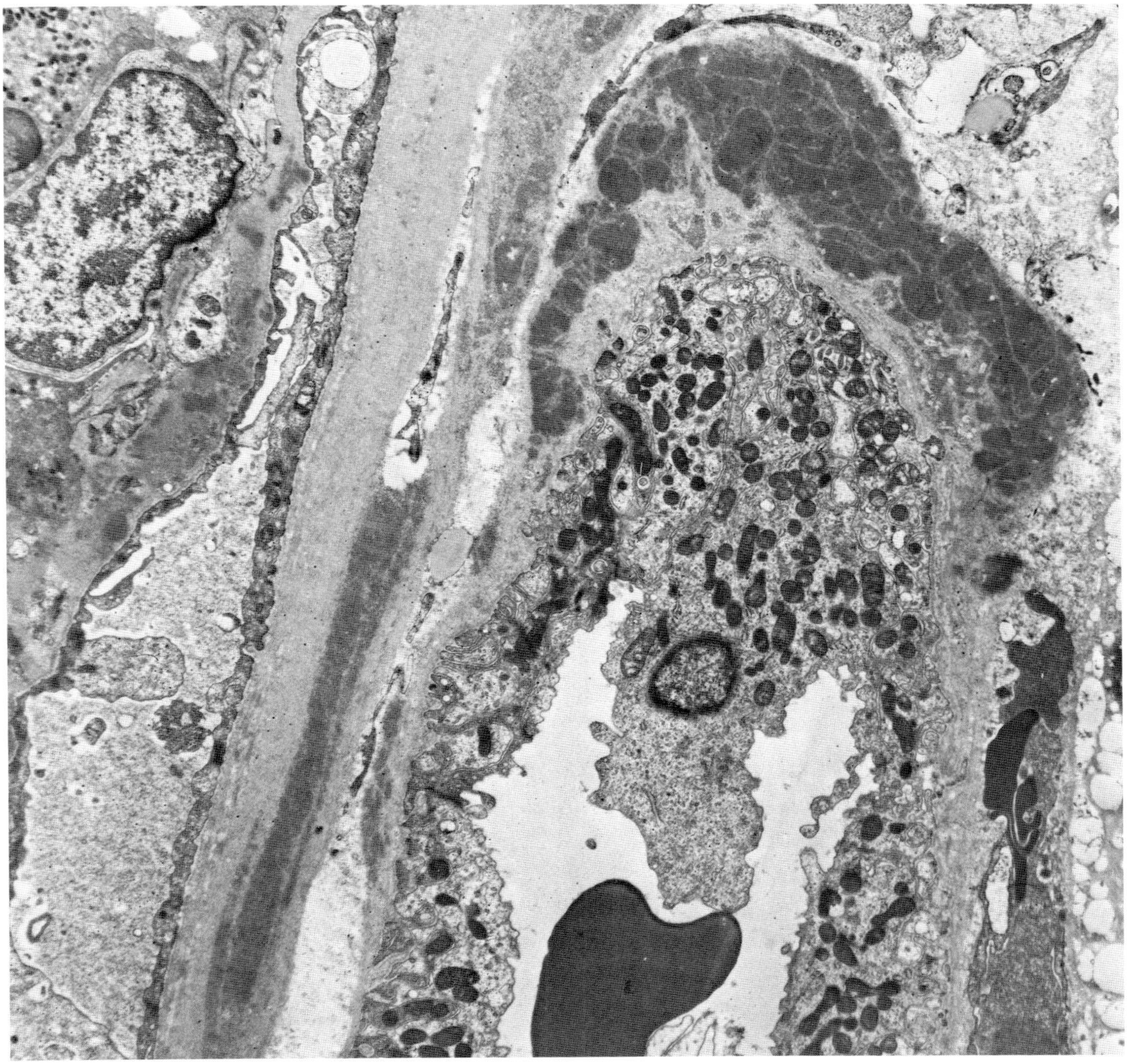

Fig. 7-30. *Extraglomerular deposits are frequently identified in biopsies showing dense deposit disease. Note the discrete and large electron-dense osmiophilic deposits in the basal lamina of Bowman's capsule (left) as well as in the tubular basement membrane. Uranyl acetate and lead citrate;* ×*4620. (Courtesy of Dr. Conrad L. Pirani.)*

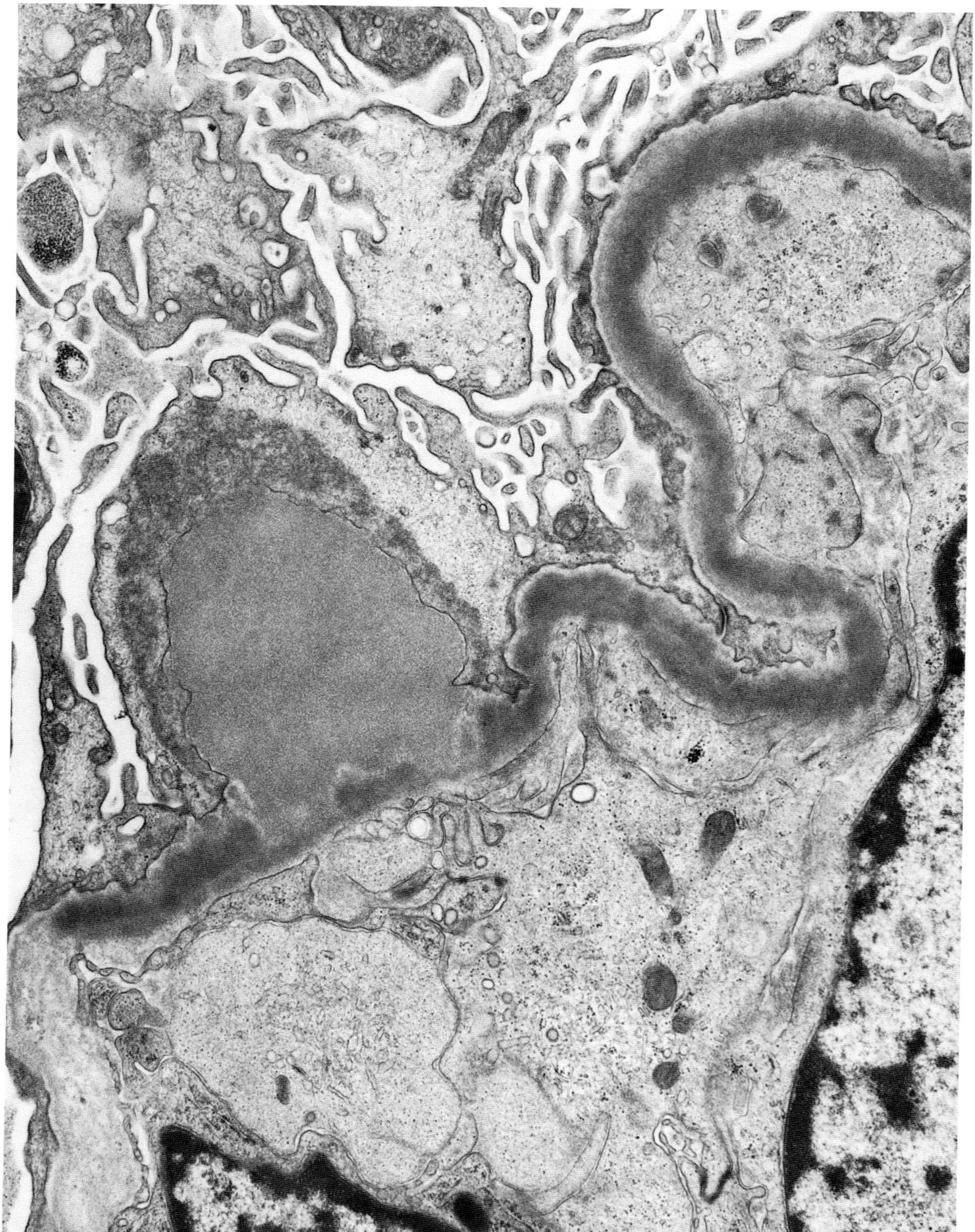

IMMUNOFLUORESCENCE FINDINGS

Immunofluorescence microscopy has been performed in many cases of dense deposit disease [20, 28,46,47,87,139,167,185,250,380]. Intense staining for C3 is noted along the glomerular capillary walls and often in the glomerular mesangial regions (Figs. 7-32 and 7-33). The immunofluorescence patterns have been variously described as linear, pseudolinear, smooth, ribbon-like, granular, or nodular [20,87,139,141,142,168,185,197, 268,310,353]. The intensity of the immunofluorescent staining varies considerably. The staining may be continuous or discontinuous (interrupted). The mesangial deposits may stain either as scattered granules or as heavy, coarse granules. The early components of complement, C1q and C4, are usually absent, although occasionally C1q is noted [380]. One study [310] reported C4 in 9 of 13 patients when glomerular granular capillary wall staining was present. C3 is also noted in Bowman's capsule and along the tubular basement membranes (see Fig. 7-33).

Immunoglobulins are usually absent or seen only in a segmental form. If they are noted, they are usually IgM with a segmental distribution; IgG and especially IgA are less common but not unheard of [185,317]. The study of Sibley and Kim [310] showed staining of IgM in 12 of 13 patients, IgG in 6 of 13, and IgA in only 2 of 13. The study of the Southwest Pediatric Nephrology Study Group [317] recorded IgM (70 percent), IgG (20 percent), and IgA (10 percent). Properdin is usually demonstrated [47,167,185,197,317].

Kim et al. [185] have noted a special staining characteristic for C3 (and to lesser extent for C4 and properdin). A double linear appearance, referred to as "railroad tracks," was noted in the glomerular capillary walls, while numerous circular, unevenly stained structures termed *mesangial rings* were noted in the mesangial areas. Using phase-contrast and electron microscopy with a double-labeling antibody technique (rhodamine-conjugated anti-GBM and fluoresceinated anti-C3), these authors felt that the railroad tracks and the mesangial rings represented the deposition of C3 along the margin but not within the central portions of the large intramembranous or mesangial deposits [185]. No similar staining was noted in any of their patients with membranoproliferative glomerulonephritis type I. The authors further suggested that the complement system was activated at the edge of the intramembranous deposits rather than within the material itself. C4 was noted within the railroad tracks and the mesangial rings in about one-half of biopsies with dense deposit disease [185].

Using a monoclonal antibody (poly C9-MA) to a neoantigen of the C9 portion of the membrane attack complex (MAC) of complement, Falk et al. [116] performed immunofluorescence and immunoelectron microscopy to study the antigen distribution in renal biopsies with dense deposit disease.

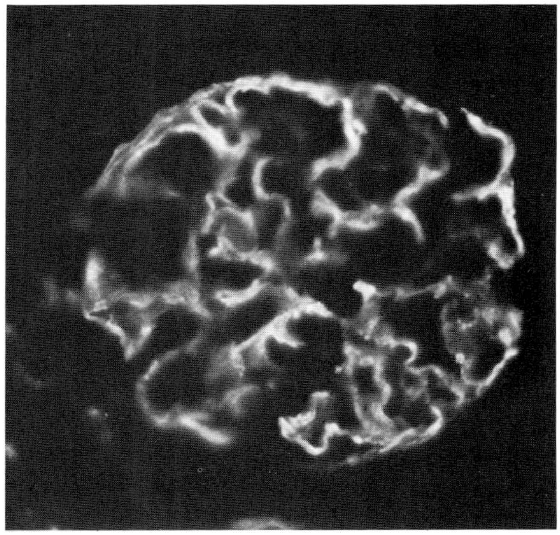

Fig. 7-32. *Immunofluorescence with antiserum to C3 in a patient with dense deposit disease. Staining is present along the glomerular capillary walls. Few mesangial deposits are noted.*

Fig. 7-31. *Electron micrograph of a glomerulus from a patient with dense deposit disease. This segment of a glomerulus shows a large, discrete, subepithelial deposit (hump) in addition to the dense intramembranous deposits. There is marked effacement of the glomerular visceral epithelial-cell foot processes over the hump. × 15,516. (Courtesy of Dr. Richard Sibley.)*

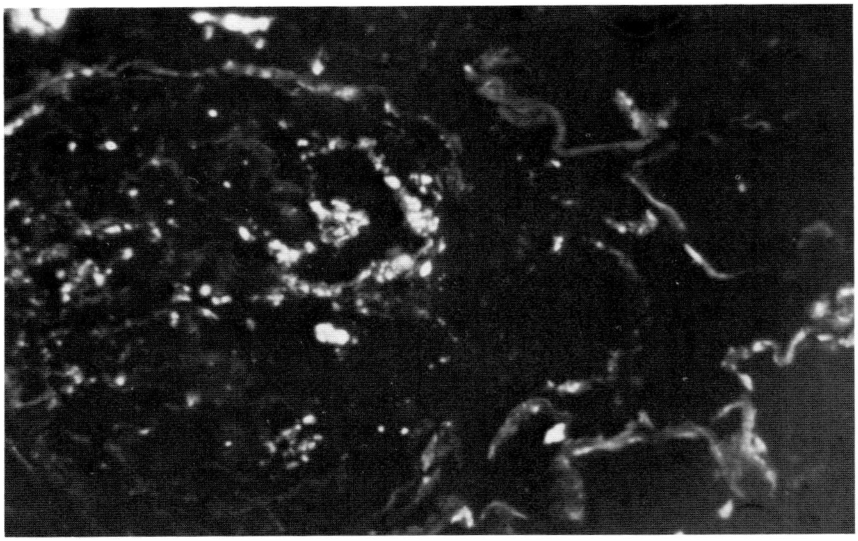

FIG. 7-33. *Immunofluorescence with antiserum to C3 in a patient with dense deposit disease. Glomerulus (left) shows a granular pattern, and tubules (right) also give a positive reaction. (Courtesy Dr. L. Morel-Maroger.)*

Poly C9-MA and C3 were distributed along either side of the dense deposits within the glomerular basement membranes and tubular basement membranes, around the circular mesangial deposits, and within the subepithelial deposits. It is therefore apparent from these studies that electron microscopic and immunofluorescence studies show major differences in the pattern and composition of the deposits between dense-deposit disease and membranoproliferative glomerulonephritis type I. However, as Kim et al. [182] stated, granular deposits of immunoglobulins similar to those noted in typical membranoproliferative glomerulonephritis type I also can be noted in dense deposit disease, although to a lesser extent.

Comparisons Between Membranoproliferative Glomerulonephritis Type I and Dense Deposit Disease

Although it is not possible to determine on clinical or laboratory grounds whether an individual patient has membranoproliferative glomerulonephritis type I or dense deposit disease, there do appear to be differences between the two when large numbers of patients are studied [182,223] (Table 7-3). Asymptomatic proteinuria and hematuria at clinical onset of the renal disease are more common in membranoproliferative glomerulonephritis type I. Patients with dense deposit disease tend to be younger at clinical onset [139,206] and more commonly have persistent nephrotic syndrome, gross hematuria, and acute nephritic episodes [11,58,139]. Severe and persistent depression of serum complement level [58,87,99, 139,141,142,353] and the presence of C3NeF are more frequent in patients with dense deposit disease [58,81,307,339,375,376]. C3NeF is more commonly noted in children than in adults [58]. Partial lipodystrophy with hypocomplementemia and C3NeF [159,278], as well as recurrence in renal transplants [51,78,139], is more frequently noted in dense deposit disease. The prognosis of dense deposit disease is said to be worse than that of membranoproliferative glomerulonephritis type

Table 7-3. *Comparisons between membranoproliferative glomerulonephritis type I and dense deposit disease*

Feature	Membranoproliferative glomerulonephritis type I	Dense deposit disease	References
Age (at clinical onset)	Older	Younger	[139,206]
Asymptomatic urinary findings (at clinical onset)	Asymptomatic proteinuria and hematuria	Less common	[182]
Nephrotic syndrome	Less common	More common	[11,58,139]
Acute nephritic syndrome	Less common	More common	[11,58,139]
Gross hematuria	Less common	More common	[11,58,139]
Low serum complement	Less common (less severe, less persistent)	Common (severe, persistent)	[58,87,99,139,141,142,353]
C3NeF (C3-nephritic factor)	Less common	Common	[58,81,307,339,375,376]
Partial lipodystrophy (with hypocomplementemia and C3NeF)	Uncommon	More common	[159,278]
Recurrence in renal transplants	Less common	More common	[51,78,139]
Renal prognosis	Better	Worse	[11,50,58,139]
" "	Same	Same	[52,87,141,142,333]

(possibly related in part to the more frequent presence of crescents in dense deposit disease) [11,50,58,139], although not all agree [52,87,141,142,333].

Many of the major morphologic differences between these two patterns have been referred to and are summarized in Tables 7-4, 7-5, and 7-6. Many investigators believe that a complete distinction should be made between dense deposit disease and membranoproliferative glomerulonephritis type I; they regard dense deposit disease as a separate entity and do not consider it a subtype of membranoproliferative glomerulonephritis [223]. Differentiation between dense deposit disease and membranoproliferative glomerulonephritis type I is generally straightforward if light, electron, and immunofluorescence microscopy are all performed. It can be a problem when the characteristic and diagnostic dense deposits are focal or segmental and when the light microscopic features are those of focal and segmental necrotizing or crescentic glomerulonephritis. Use of thioflavine-T is helpful. Transformation of membranoproliferative glomerulonephritis type I into dense deposit disease, or vice versa, is virtually unknown.

Partial Lipodystrophy

Several patients with dense deposit disease have been noted to have partial lipodystrophy, a condition with symmetrical loss of adipose tissue from the face, arms, and upper portions of the trunk [111,143,278,295,314,353]. Partial lipodystrophy is often accompanied by low levels of serum C3, normal serum levels of the early components of complement, and the presence of C3-nephritic factor (C3NeF) in the serum [26,209,314]. All the serologic features just noted suggest activation of complement by the alternative pathway, and it has been suggested that this activation somehow predisposes to the development of the commonly present glomerulonephritis [278,314]. Patients with partial lipodystrophy may have no recognizable complement deficiencies, and dense deposit disease need not be present [143,314]; some lack C3NeF [314]. Méry et al. [236] described one pa-

TABLE 7-4. *Comparisons of histologic findings from renal biopsies of patients in the Southwest Pediatric Nephrology Study Group*

Histologic finding	MPGN type I	Dense deposit disease	*p* value
Male-female ratio	1:1	1:1	
Age (mean)	11 years	13 years	
Large glomeruli	28/33	12/16	0.449
Tuft lobulation	32/33	13/16	0.096
Tuft hypercellularity	33/33	15/16	0.327
Mesangial sclerosis	28/33	14/16	1.0
GBM thickening	32/33	12/16	0.034
GBM splitting	32/33	7/16	0.001
Neutrophils	12/33	3/16	0.324
Loop obliteration	31/33	13/16	0.313
Crescents	2/33	4/16	0.08
Karyorrhexis	8/33	0/16	0.041
Tubular atrophy	15/33	10/16	0.364
Interstitial edema	17/33	4/16	0.124
Interstitial fibrosis	17/33	7/16	0.762
Intimal fibrosis	6/33	2/16	0.705
Intramural hyalin	2/33	3/16	0.313

TABLE 7-5. *Comparisons of ultrastructural findings from patients in the Southwest Pediatric Nephrology Study Group*

Electron microscopic findings	MPGN type I	Dense deposit disease	*p* value
Interposed mesangial cytoplasm	30/33	3/16	0.001
GBM thickening	31/33	15/16	1.0
"Fusion" of foot processes	31/33	14/16	0.588
Subendothelial deposits	30/33	1/16	0.001
Intramembranous deposits	29/33	9/16	0.025
Mesangial deposits	24/33	3/16	0.001
Subepithelial deposits	22/33	8/16	0.351
GBM spikes	12/33	3/16	0.324

TABLE 7-6. *Comparison of iummunofluorescence findings in patients from the Southwest Pediatric Nephrology Study Group*

Immunofluorescence findings	MPGN type I	Dense deposit disease	*p* value
IgA	8/22	1/10	0.210
IgG	14/24	2/10	0.063
IgM	16/24	7/10	1.0
C1q	5/7	3/6	0.59
C3	24/24	10/10	1.00

Tables 7-4, 7-5, and 7-6 from the studies of Drs. T. Cavallo, S. Guggenheim, F. Silva, R. Hogg, and the Southwest Pediatric Nephrology Study Group.

tient with typical partial lipodystrophy and dense deposit disease without any recognizable complement deficiencies. Partial lipodystrophy has been described in an older patient with dense deposit disease [286]. Membranoproliferative glomerulonephritis type I also has been described in patients with partial lipodystrophy [26,314], as has membranoproliferative glomerulonephritis type III [65].

MEMBRANOPROLIFERATIVE GLOMERULONEPHRITIS TYPE III

Burkholder et al. [45,47,48] described a form or type of membranoproliferative glomerulonephritis under the name of *mixed membranous and proliferative glomerulonephritis.* This pattern had some of the features of typical membranoproliferative glomerulonephritis type I, such as thickening of the glomerular capillary walls, double contours, mesangial interposition, and subendothelial deposits. In addition, however, there were silver-positive spikes along the GBM and trichrome-positive subepithelial humps such as are seen in stage II membranous glomerulonephritis. Ultrastructural studies confirmed the presence of glomerular electron-dense deposits, and immunofluorescent staining showed a heavy granular pattern along the glomerular capillary walls and mesangium for C3 and sometimes for IgG and IgM. The clinical features were similar to those of membranoproliferative glomerulonephritis type I and dense deposit disease; serum C3 was depressed in two of five patients. This pattern was described subsequently in a patient with both HB_eAg and HB_sAg [6].

Another form also has been designated as membranoproliferative glomerulonephritis type III by workers in Cincinnati [166,225,321,326] and independently by workers in Mainz [8] (Figs. 7-34 and 7-35). This form of membranoproliferative

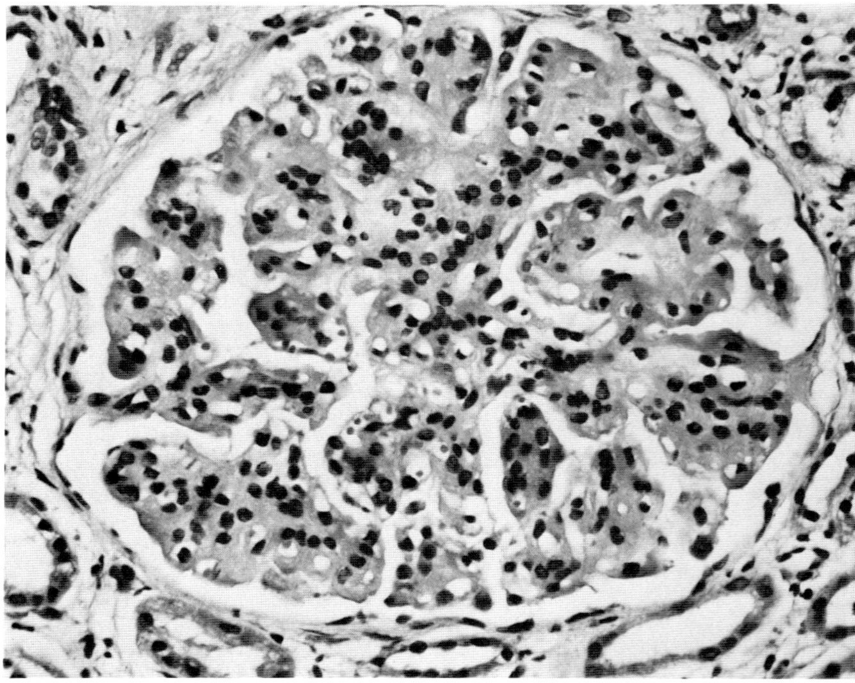

FIG. 7-34. *Glomerulus from a patient with membranoproliferative glomerulonephritis type III. This representative glomerulus shows a global increase in cellularity in the tuft. There is accentuation of the lobular pattern, and the light microscopic pattern is similar (if not identical) to membranoproliferative glomerulonephritis type I. H&E; ×540. (From Strife, C. F., et al.* Clin. Nephrol. *7: 65, 1977.)*

glomerulonephritis (type III) is the most commonly accepted form of type III, and it will now be considered in detail.

Clinical Features

The clinical and laboratory findings are generally thought to be similar to those of patients with classic membranoproliferative glomerulonephritis type I and dense deposit disease. In a comparison of membranoproliferative glomerulonephritis types I and III, Jackson et al. [166] noted that type III was more frequently detected by the chance discovery of hematuria and proteinuria in otherwise healthy individuals; this suggests that the onset is insidious and remains subclinical for some time. The nephrotic syndrome is also a common mode of presentation.

Serum C3, C5, and properdin levels are low in about half of patients, but the early classical pathway complement components (C1q and C4) are generally normal, suggesting an alternative pathway activation. There is no evidence of classical pathway activation. Serum C3 levels do not correlate with renal prognosis, and C3NeF is absent or present in very low levels [166]. The cause of the complement perturbation is unknown.

Clinical Course

Nephrotic syndrome, hypertension, and impaired renal function at the time of renal biopsy are har-

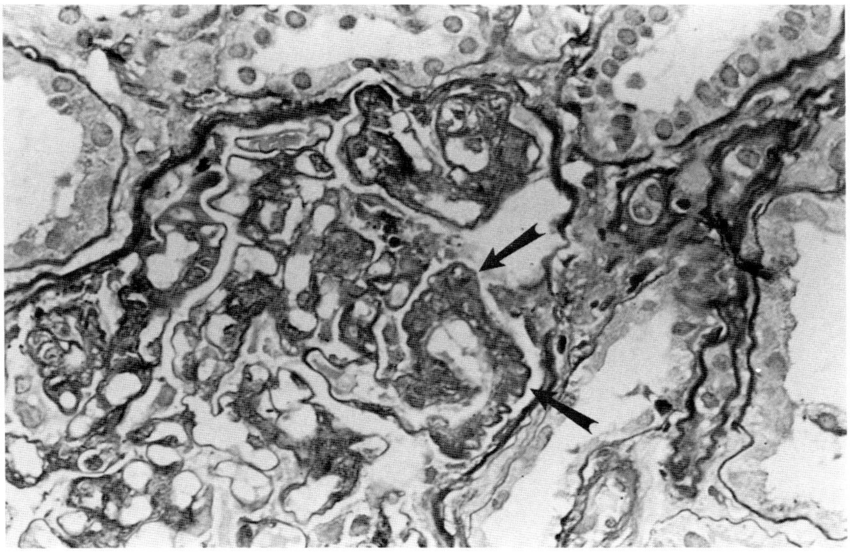

Fig. 7-35. *Silver staining of a glomerulus from a patient with membranoproliferative glomerulonephritis type III. Note that there is marked thickening of the glomerular capillary wall at 3 o'clock and tortuosity of the GBM (arrows). Jones silver methenamine;* ×600. *(Courtesy of Dr. Victor Saldivar.)*

bingers of a poor prognosis [321]. Progression to end-stage renal failure is variable but similar to the experience with type I, although some studies have suggested that type III will stabilize or improve following treatment with alternate-day prednisone [321].

Pathologic Changes

MICROSCOPIC FINDINGS

Light microscopic findings include varying degrees of accentuation of the glomerular lobular pattern, mesangial hypercellularity, more diffuse glomerular capillary wall thickening than in membranoproliferative glomerulonephritis type I and dense deposit disease, and occasional spiking with the silver methenamine stain (see Figs. 7-34 and 7-35). Anders et al. [8], in comparing membranoproliferative glomerulonephritis type I, type II, and type III, found less pronounced glomerular hypercellularity and enlargement in type III as compared with type I; hypercellularity was greater in type III than in dense deposit disease. Jackson et al. [166] noted less glomerular hypercellularity in type III than in type I. Subepithelial spikes were more commonly noted in type III than the other types. The pattern may be focal and segmental by light microscopy [324].

ELECTRON MICROSCOPIC FINDINGS

There are glomerular subendothelial and subepithelial deposits, which are often contiguous or connect through the lamina densa of the GBM [8,9,142,326] (Fig. 7-36). These deposits sometimes have a washed out appearance (see Fig. 7-37). There is often a layering of the lamina densa–like material. This pattern was initially described on the basis of ultrathin silver-impregnated plastic-embedded sections studied with the electron microscope [101] (Figs. 7-37 and 7-38). There is a complex disruption of the glomerular basement membrane (lamina densa), often with thickening and expansion of the basement membrane and lay-

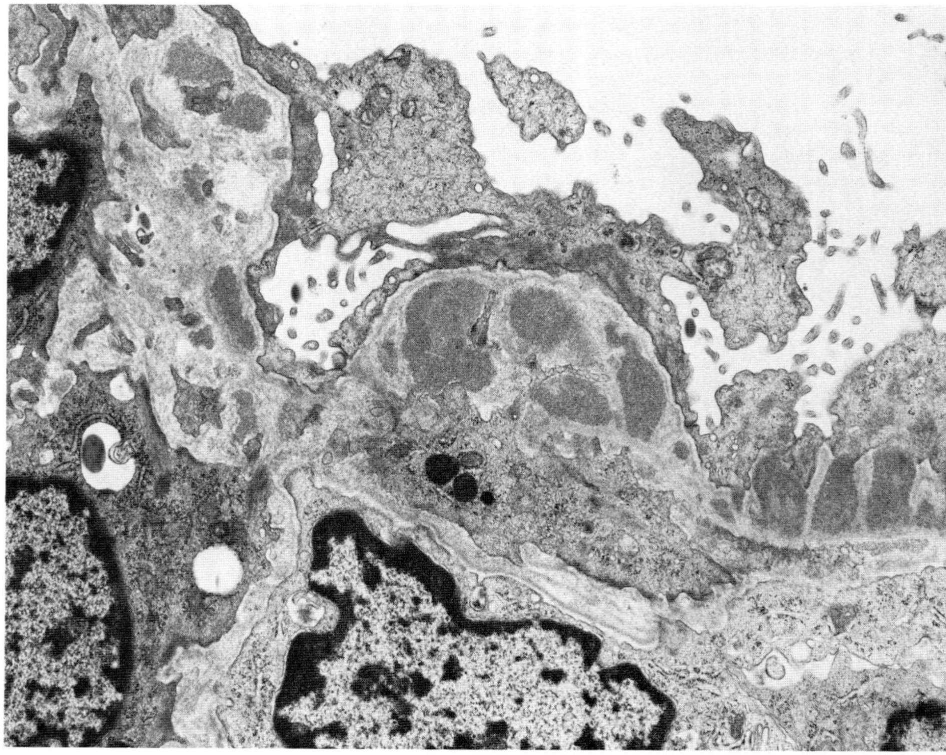

FIG. 7-36. *Electron micrograph of a portion of a glomerulus showing numerous large electron-dense deposits. There are large intramembranous and subepithelial deposits and spikes of GBM-like material.* × *15,000. (Courtesy of Dr. A. James McAdams.)*

ering by a silver-negative basement membrane–like material. In contrast with membranoproliferative glomerulonephritis type III of Burkholder [45,47,48], subepithelial deposits and spikes were less frequent [326]. Strife et al. [326] also considered that their type III differed from that of Burkholder in the presence of disruption and extensive duplication of the GBM, features not commented on by Burkholder. They concluded that although some features were similar to those seen in patients with type I, their type III was distinctive. Bonsib [35], using scanning electron microscopy of acellular glomeruli (after treatment with osmotic lysis, detergents, and DNase), noted alterations of the glomerular subepithelial portions of the GBM surface.

IMMUNOFLUORESCENCE FINDINGS

Immunofluorescence techniques [321,326] show C3 in a finely granular fashion along the glomerular capillaries and in the mesangial regions (Fig. 7-39). IgG and IgM are noted in some patients. Properdin is often present and prominent and, like C3, occurs in a granular pattern along the glomerular capillary walls and in the mesangial regions.

Relationship to Membranoproliferative Glomerulonephritis Type I

Because the suggested technologies to demonstrate the GBM abnormalities in type III of Strife et al. [321,326] are seldom used, some authors believe

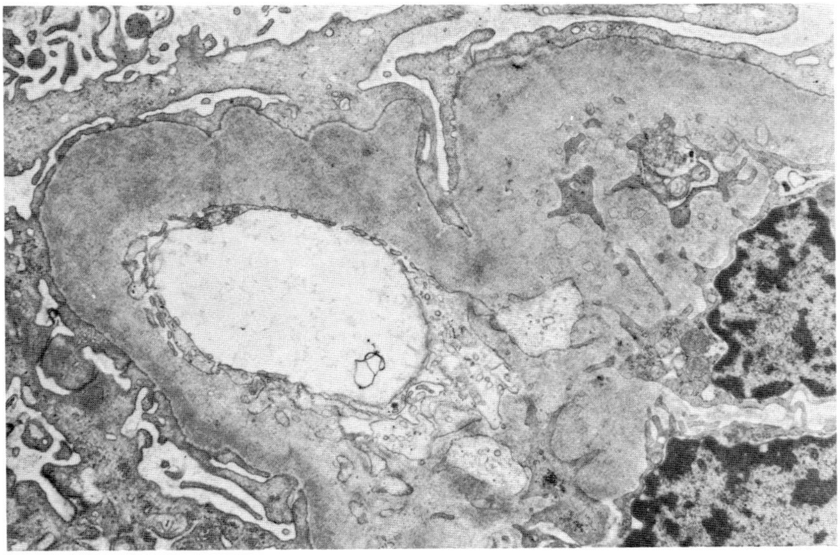

A

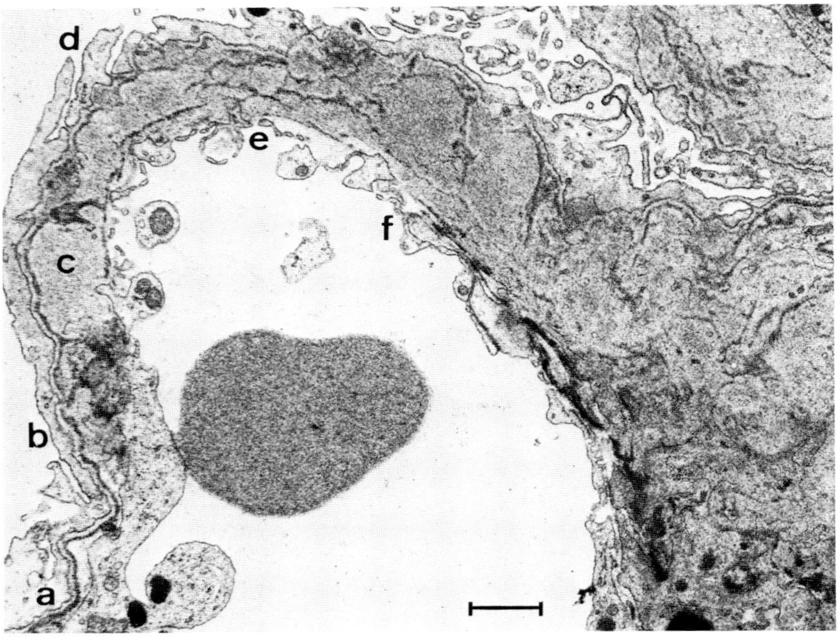

B

FIG. 7-37. *(A) Electron micrograph (not impregnated with silver) showing diffuse, ill-defined basement membrane thickening. (B) Silver-impregnated material allows resolution of basement membrane thickening. Several stages are shown starting from lower left: a, intact lamina densa; b, disrupted and distorted argyrophilic material; c, subendothelial deposits; d, subepithelial and subendothelial argyrophilic layer; e, multifold layering; f, complete loss of argyrophilic linear structure or replacement of lamina densa, respectively, by accumulating masses of nonargyrophilic material in places reminiscent of subepithelial deposits.* ×9000. *(From Anders, D., Agricola, B., Sippel, M., and Thoenes, W.* Virchows Arch. [A] *376: 1, 1977, Figs. 4A and 4B; used by permission.)*

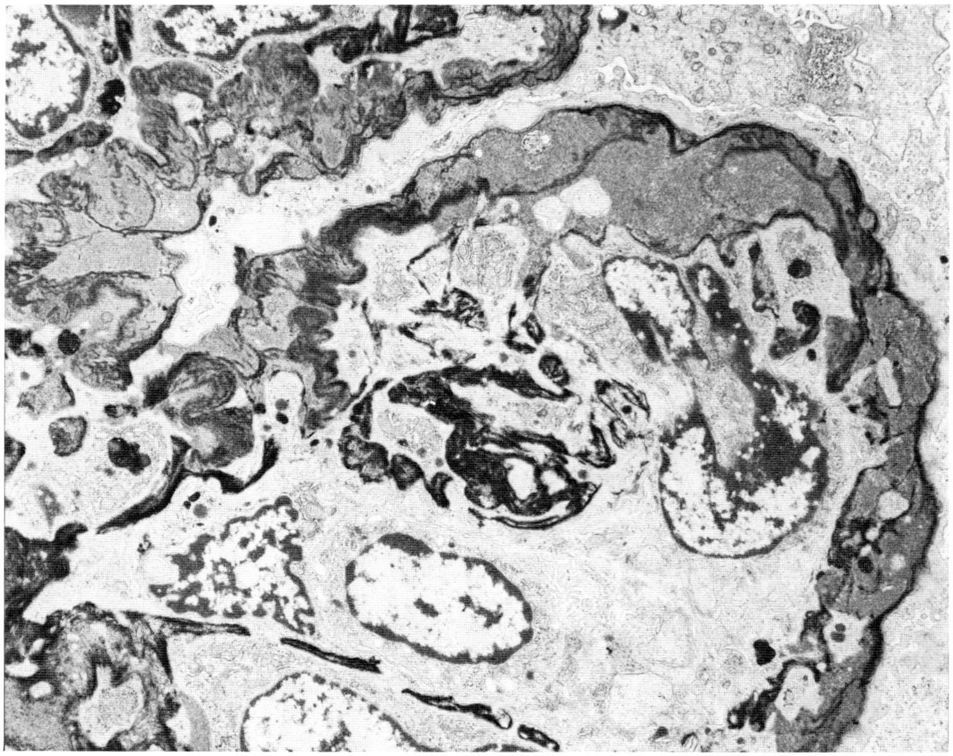

FIG. 7-38. *Higher magnification of the silver impregnation of the plastic-embedded sections for transmission electron microscopy; a segment of a glomerulus from a patient with membranoproliferative glomerulonephritis type III. The remnant GBM is quite argyrophilic (electron dense) but contains numerous large (and sometimes confluent), less argyrophilic regions representing deposits. These large deposits are contiguous throughout the GBM and lead to complex disruptions of the lamina densa.* ×10,000. *(Courtesy of Dr. A. James McAdams.)*

that type III may simply be a variant of type I [166,182]. Others believe that membranoproliferative glomerulonephritis type III needs to be recognized as an established and distinct clinicopathologic entity [1]. Jackson et al. [166] consider that although light microscopy, electron microscopy, immunofluorescence observations, and laboratory findings suggest that membranoproliferative glomerulonephritis type III is distinct from membranoproliferative glomerulonephritis type I, there is evidence from other studies that a predisposition to both may be inherited and that similar genetic factors may play a role. Although the majority of clinical findings (presentation and prognosis) do not allow ready distinction between type I and type III, C3NeF is rarely detectable in membranoproliferative glomerulonephritis type III. The absence of transition (by electron microscopy) of a type III lesion to another type, and the presence of a different immunofluorescence pattern and serum complement findings, also suggest that this is a somewhat unique form of membranoproliferative glomerulonephritis. This pattern also has been described in a homosexual patient

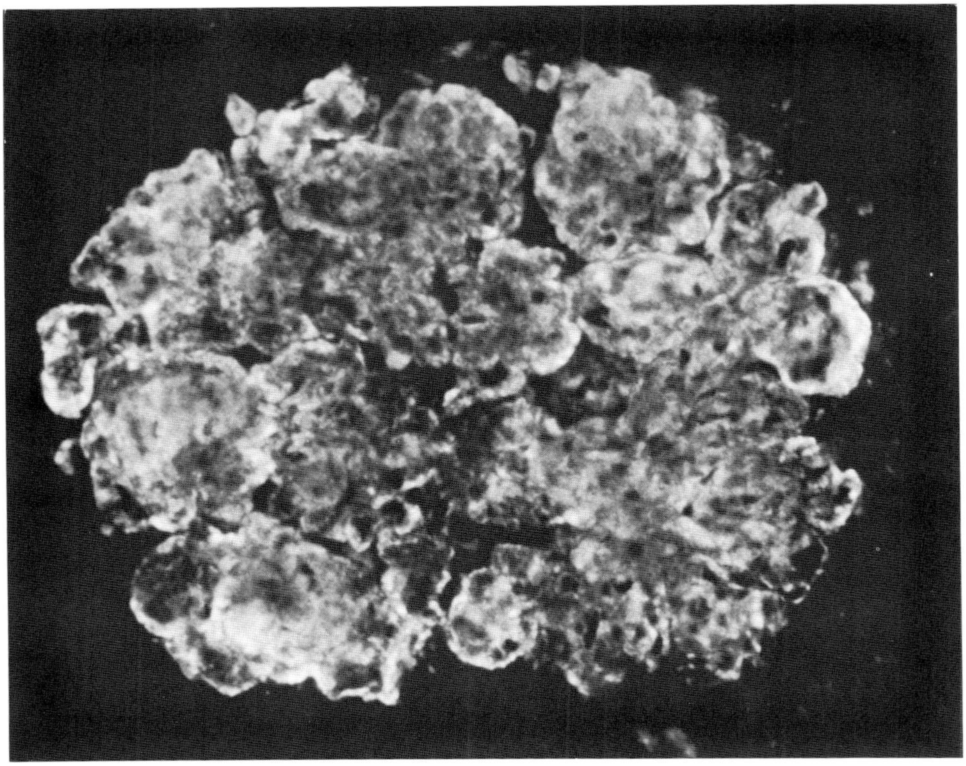

FIG. 7-39. *Immunofluorescence demonstrating C3 in a patient with type III membranoproliferative glomerulonephritis. Note the intense glomerular capillary wall and mesangial staining. (Courtesy of Dr. A. James McAdams.)*

with plexogenic pulmonary arteriopathy and AIDS [180].

LOBULAR GLOMERULONEPHRITIS

Lobular glomerulonephritis is the term that was used in the past to describe a light microscopic picture in which the glomerular mesangial regions contained rounded or nodular eosinophilic areas that were intensely PAS positive (Fig. 7-40). These glomerular nodules are generally not hypercellular, although nuclei may be found at their periphery; the mesangial nodules are generally diffuse and present within all mesangial regions of all glomeruli. This pattern needs to be distinguished from nodular diabetic glomerulosclerosis and light chain deposition [152,193]. Lobular glomerulonephritis differs from classic nodular diabetic glomerulosclerosis in that more nodules are noted in each glomerulus and that all nodules are approximately of the same size. The glomerular capillaries around the nodules are often collapsed or compressed, but localized thickening of the glomerular capillary walls may be present and needs to be evaluated by electron microscopy. In diabetes, the glomerular basement membranes are more severely and diffusely thickened, and in addition, there is severe accompanying vascular disease. Light chain

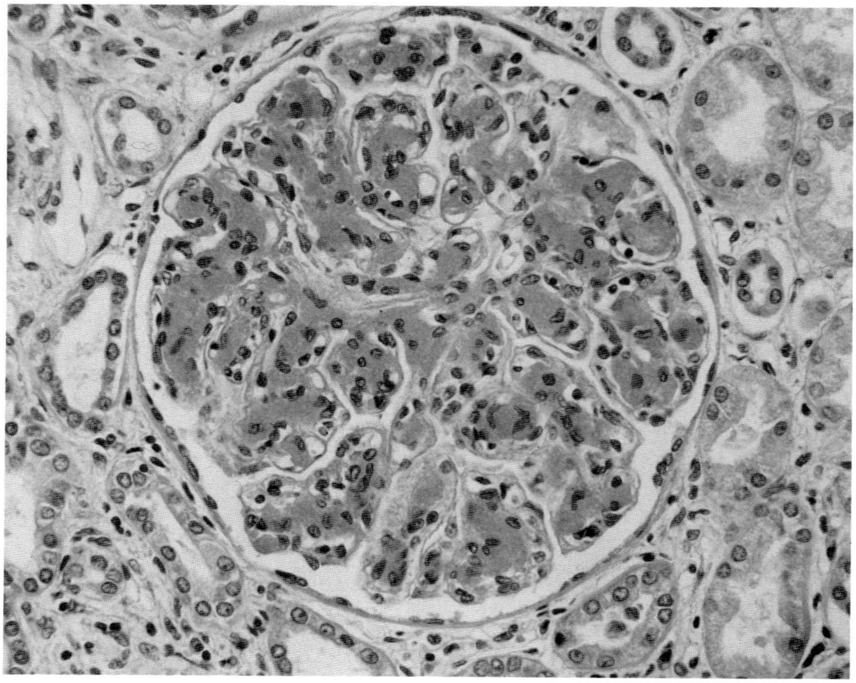

FIG. 7-40. *Glomerulus from lobular variant of membranoproliferative glomerulonephritis showing solid areas at centers of lobules with increased lobulation and mild increase in cellularity. H&E; ×290.*

deposition in glomeruli also needs to be excluded (Fig. 7-41), and immunofluorescence staining with both kappa and lambda light chain antisera needs to be performed. Ultrastructural studies are also useful in separating these entities.

As noted earlier, lobular glomerulonephritis may occur in both membranoproliferative glomerulonephritis type I and dense deposit disease [139,140,141,173]. I believe that it is preferable to use the term *lobular variant* of either of these two patterns rather than *lobular glomerulonephritis* because of its uncertain meaning. Transition from glomerular hypercellularity to the relatively acellular lobular variant of membranoproliferative glomerulonephritis type I has been described [220]. In this patient, well-formed glomerular mesangial nodules were present in a renal biopsy taken 2 years after the demonstration of a very cellular glomerular lesion with minimal nodule formation; thus this lobular variant may represent "healing" or progressive sclerosis of the mesangial lesion. It is likely that the lobular variant represents a "final common pathway" of glomerular reaction to a number of injuries with excessive production of mesangial matrix. Heptinstall [150] has noted that similar pictures may be seen in certain patients who have had poststreptococcal glomerulonephritis and who still have persistent proteinuria (Fig. 7-42).

Recently, a type of lobular glomerulonephritis has been described that does not seem to represent membranoproliferative glomerulonephritis type I, dense deposit disease, light chain deposition, or diabetes. The cause of this pattern is unclear. The outcome appears to be slowly progressive renal failure [5] (Fig. 7-43).

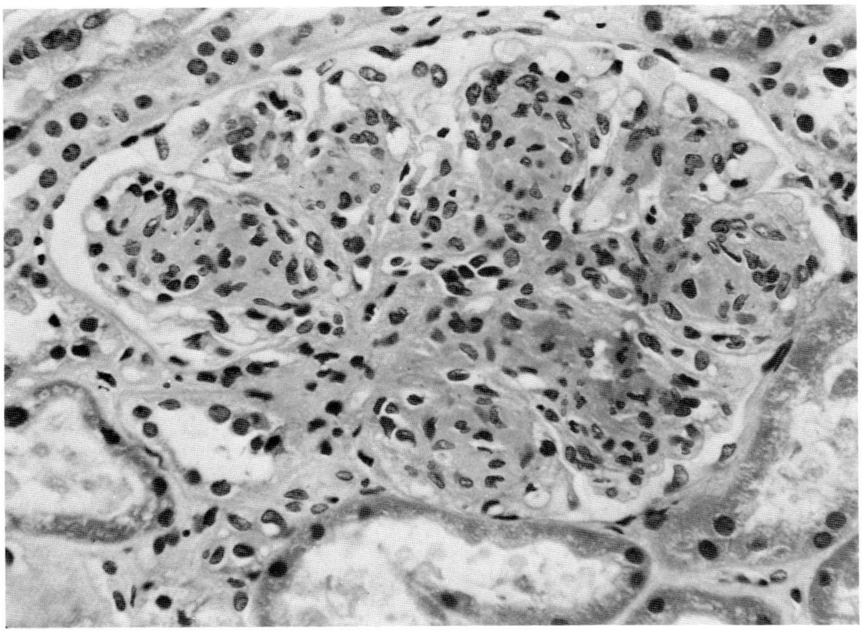

Fig. 7-41. *Glomerulus from patient with light chain deposition. There is early solidification in mesangial areas that also show increased numbers of cells. Lobulation is accentuated. H&E; ×340.*

RECURRENCE OF DISEASE FOLLOWING RENAL TRANSPLANTATION

There are numerous reports of recurrence of the original disease in kidneys grafted into patients with end-stage renal disease due to either membranoproliferative glomerulonephritis type I or dense deposit disease [23,32,59,102,129,130,138,197, 222,348]. As will be noted in Chapter 27, it may be difficult to determine the true frequency of recurrence of membranoproliferative glomerulonephritis type I because of its similar clinical and histologic findings to those of chronic allograft rejection [138,175,288,388,389]. Some series are marred because the diagnosis of recurrence is based on clinical rather than morphologic evidence. Thus strict morphologic criteria (including light microscopy, electron microscopy, and immunofluorescence) must be applied and knowledge of the primary disease leading to renal failure must be available.

The percentages of reported recurrence of *membranoproliferative glomerulonephritis type I* range from 18 to 50 percent [234]. These wide differences may be due to dissimilar patient populations or selection, changing criteria for the morphologic diagnosis, and heterogeneity of patients with membranoproliferative glomerulonephritis [182]. Katz [175] has described the major differences in the morphologic patterns between transplant rejection and membranoproliferative glomerulonephritis. The presence of large, discrete, glomerular electron-dense subendothelial "immune type" deposits by electron microscopy accompanied by broad glomerular capillary wall deposits of C3 suggests recurrence of membranoproliferative glomerulonephritis type I rather than rejection, although others feel that this differential diagnosis may be difficult even with the aid of the electron micro-

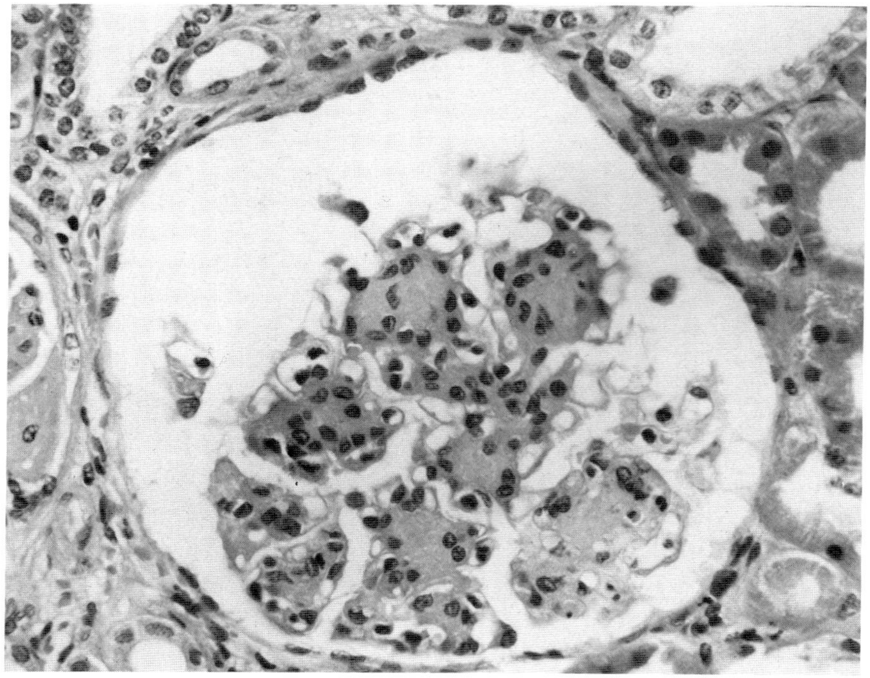

FIG. 7-42. *Glomerulus showing mesangial solidification and no apparent change in capillary walls, with mild cellular increase. A repeat biopsy on a young woman with renal failure 18 months after an attack of biopsy proven poststreptococcal glomerulonephritis. H&E;* ×*370.*

scope [346]. It is uncertain whether the level of serum complement at the time of renal transplantation has any bearing on the likelihood of recurrence [32,234]. Membranoproliferative glomerulonephritis type I has been reported to recur in successive renal transplants [135]. The clinical manifestations of recurrence of membranoproliferative glomerulonephritis type I may be absent following renal transplantation, although proteinuria, the nephrotic syndrome, hypertension, and renal insufficiency may develop [182]. Of interest are two renal allograft recipients with the electron microscopic picture of MPGN type I transmitted with the donor kidneys [43]; the glomerular subendothelial deposits initially present resolved over a period of 6 to 9 months following transplantation.

Dense deposit disease almost invariably recurs in the renal allograft. Because the renal morphologic changes in this condition are so unique, it is generally easy to recognize recurrence in the renal transplant. The lesion in dense deposit disease can recur along the glomerular basement membranes, mesangial regions, basal lamina of Bowman's capsule, and/or tubular basement membranes, but this is not constant, and the deposits may be primarily localized to the glomerular basement membranes at the vascular pole of the glomerulus [102]. The glomerular subepithelial humps also may recur. Recurrences may be quick and have been noted in as short a time as 2 weeks following renal transplantation [41,57,102,129,173,348]. Although it has been claimed that the glomerular cellularity tends to be mild in recurrent dense deposit disease [41,129], I have seen considerable glomerular hypercellularity in this situation. There may not be

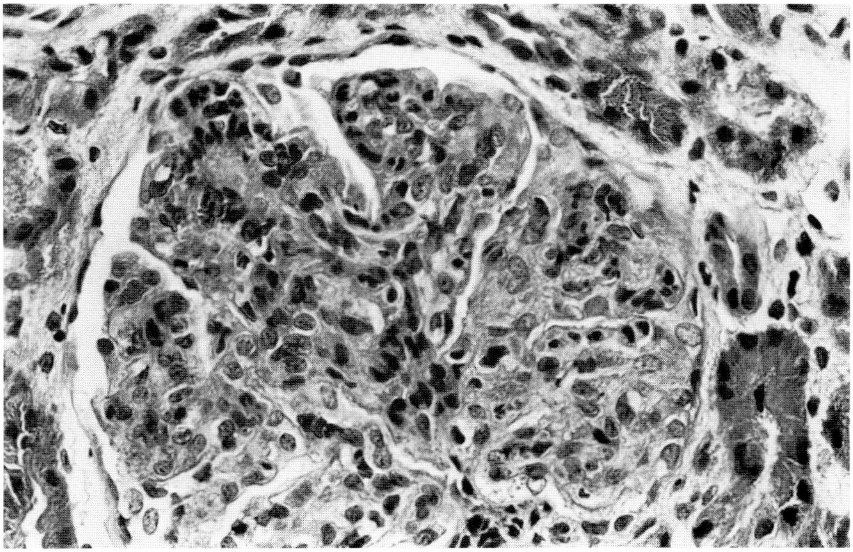

Fig. 7-43. *This form of lobular glomerulonephritis was not associated with deposits by either electron microscopic or immunofluorescence studies. The patient (an elderly man with moderate proteinuria and renal failure) did not have diabetes mellitus or plasma-cell dyscrasia. This "pure" form of lobular glomerulonephritis (i.e., independent of MPGN types I, II, or III, diabetes, or myeloma) is described by Alpers [5]. H&E; ×250.*

any clinical manifestations of renal disease when recurrence occurs [51,57,102,129,348].

Droz et al. [102] and others [7,8] studied serial renal biopsies and noted that the lesions could remain unchanged, progress, or regress in the transplanted kidney. However, as various authors [41, 52,78,138] have suggested, renal failure is usually the consequence of rejection rather than being secondary to recurrence. Kim et al. [182], though, have noted recurrence of such severity that nephrectomy was necessary. Others also have suggested that recurrent dense deposit disease may lead directly to loss of the allograft [108]. It has been observed that transplantation of the crescentic form of dense deposit disease is followed by recurrent glomerulonephritis of a similar nature sufficient to cause renal allograft failure [39,51, 78,108]. Although C3NeF levels and serum complement concentrations are often reduced after renal transplantation, possibly as a result of steroid therapy [349], the levels of serum complement (either pre- or postoperatively) do not predict or recognize recurrence of dense deposit disease [1,202,348]. Regression of recurrent dense deposit disease has been described in a transplanted kidney after plasmapheresis therapy [266].

ETIOLOGY AND PATHOGENESIS OF MEMBRANOPROLIFERATIVE GLOMERULONEPHRITIS AND DENSE DEPOSIT DISEASE

Infection and Chronic Antigenemia

Information on the etiologic agents in all types of membranoproliferative glomerulonephritis (types I, II, and III) is scanty, and the pathogenesis is not completely understood. It has been suggested [173] that type I represents a chronic antigenemia (chronic serum sickness–like response). The exact nature of the putative antigen(s) in membranoproliferative glomerulonephritis type I is unknown. The etiology of dense deposit disease is obscure at this time. Elevated ASO titers are noted in some patients with both type I [54,206] and dense deposit disease [86,87,139,353]; however, most authors are not impressed with the importance of this. In the early days of renal pathology, several investigators described patients with "chronic proliferative or chronic membranous and proliferative glomerulonephritis" [107], with a certain percentage of these patients having antibodies to type 12 streptococcal organisms, but the lack of immunofluorescence and electron microscopic studies precludes any interpretation of these data. It is noteworthy that in the West et al. account [369] of what is now termed *membranoproliferative glomerulonephritis,* two of their three patients had ASO titers of over 250 units. Most publications emanating from the United States have not supported a possible link with streptococcal infections, but a few British authors have made this suggestion. It should be added, however, that a variety of bacterial organisms have been associated with and implicated in the genesis of the forms of membranoproliferative glomerulonephritis that are found with infective endocarditis and infected ventriculoatrial shunts (see Chap. 5).

The role of viruses in the induction of membranoproliferative glomerulonephritis is uncertain, but antibodies to certain viruses such as BK papovavirus have common antigenic determinants present on human immunoglobulins and are known to give a false-positive immunofluorescence reaction because of this cross-reactivity [100]. Thus caution must be exercised in the interpretation of the presence of viral antigens as the putative cause of membranoproliferative glomerulonephritis.

Much of the older literature is confusing because of the failure to distinguish between the different types or forms of membranoproliferative glomerulonephritis, and many authors talk of the three types as though they were a homogeneous entity. Electron microscopy and immunofluorescence studies are often missing from these publications.

Role of Complement Activation

Membranoproliferative glomerulonephritis was initially described by a series of authors in the context of its association with hypocomplementemia [137, 369]. The term coined by West et al. [369] was *hypocomplementemic persistent glomerulonephritis.* Depression of serum C3 level has been found in both membranoproliferative glomerulonephritis type I and dense deposit disease [55,56,86,87, 139,205,216,252,353,377], but most authors find that the depression is more persistent and the levels lower in dense deposit disease than in membranoproliferative glomerulonephritis type I [56,75,268,280,377]. Serum levels of the early components of the classical pathway of complement activation (e.g., C1q and C4) are not as commonly or severely depressed in dense deposit disease as in membranoproliferative glomerulonephritis type I [206,268,280,377].

Several possible explanations have been advanced to account for the decreased levels of serum C3. They include (1) decreased synthesis, (2) increased consumption of C3 in the glomerular lesions, (3) extravascular sequestration of C3, and finally, (4) the presence in the serum of a factor that leads to breakdown of C3. There is little direct evidence of decreased synthesis [4,75, 281,298], although Charlesworth et al. [64] found reduced rates of C3 synthesis in patients with hypocomplementemia. Increased consumption of C3 in the glomerular lesions is considered unlikely because of the absence of correlations between the disease activity in the glomerulus and the levels of serum complement [280]; it is noteworthy that removal of both kidneys does not restore serum complement levels to normal [239,350]. There is also little evidence at this time of extravascular sequestration of C3 [64].

The concept of enhanced breakdown of C3 received initial support from the classic studies of West et al. [372], who noted C3d, a breakdown product of C3, in patients with membranoproliferative glomerulonephritis type I. C3-activating factor was noted in similar patients [318]. Much investigation has been performed on characterizing and determining the role of C3-activating factor, which is now referred to as *C3-nephritic factor (C3NeF)* or, simply, *nephritic factor* [85,88,117, 280,318,351,367,370,375]. C3NeF acts by means of the alternative pathway of complement activation. This system depends on a positive-feedback mechanism that leads to the generation of a C3-splitting enzyme referred to as *C3bBb,* the production of which requires C3b, factor B, and factor D. Under normal circumstances, C3bBb is formed in small amounts and does not lead to breakdown of C3 because two control proteins, C3b inactivator and B1H, tend to inactivate it. C3NeF stabilizes C3bBb so that it becomes resistant to C3b inactivator and B1H and yet at the same time retains the ability to cleave additional C3 molecules. It is now known that C3NeF is an IgG autoantibody with specificity directed against the newly formed determinants on C3bBb (C3 convertase) [308]. It activates the alternative pathway by stabilizing C3bBb [79,80,86,87,280,308]. Both C3NeF and properdin bind to and stabilize C3 convertase. The differences between these two is that properdin is a physiologic protein normally present in the serum, whereas C3NeF is apparently only found in serum in pathologic conditions. C3NeF has been found in the serum of 40 to 70 percent of patients with dense deposit disease and 20 to 30 percent of patients with membranoproliferative glomerulonephritis type I; it has been demonstrated in half the patients with membranoproliferative glomerulonephritis and associated cryoglobulinemia [40,49,134,323], SLE [2], and shunt nephritis [16,93,114,292,382,392]. Although the stabilizing function of properdin on C3 convertase is reversible by the action of B1H, the stabilizing action of C3NeF is not; this allows continuous activation of the alternative complement pathway (the so-called amplification loop mechanism by amplification of C3 convertase). C3NeF is almost always present in patients with dense deposit disease [205,268,304,353,377], but inconstantly in patients with membranoproliferative glomerulonephritis type I (less than a third). The level of C3NeF is also lower in patients with membranoproliferative glomerulonephritis type I than in patients with dense deposit disease [182,185, 205,268,377]. C3NeF also has been identified in patients with "secondary" membranoproliferative glomerulonephritis [304].

The origin of C3NeF is unknown, but it is not apparently of renal origin, since it persists in the circulation (accompanied by low levels of C3 and CH50) after bilateral nephrectomy [104,117,350]. This factor is not by itself nephritogenic because some patients with partial lipodystrophy and high levels of C3NeF and severe hypocomplementemia do not have renal disease [26,279,314]. Kim et al. [184] reported an infant (born to a mother with dense deposit disease and high levels of C3NeF) who was hypocomplementemic during the newborn period because of placental transfer of the IgG-C3NeF; the child's serum complement returned to normal adult levels in 7 months, and no renal disease developed.

It has been suggested that complement deficiency induced by C3NeF could predispose to viral or other infections that might cause partial lipodystrophy and/or glomerulonephritis [314]. There is little evidence that C3NeF is either the cause of the disease or related to progression of the glomerular lesions [367], although some authors suggest that the presence of C3NeF is associated with a more rapid deterioration of renal function [304]. McLean and Nilson [235] and others have provided evidence for activation of the classical complement pathway in patients with C3NeF and partial lipodystrophy or dense deposit disease. Ng and Peters [262] described a group of patients with membranoproliferative glomerulonephritis or partial lipodystrophy and hypocomplementemia who had an unusual C3NeF; this C3NeF stabilized cell-bound C3 convertase but caused such weak fluid-phase C3 conversion that the standard fluid-phase screening test for C3NeF was negative. Serum concentrations of C5 in these patients was low. Other novel C3-nephritic–activating factors (some not immunoglobulins) have been noted in patients with membranoproliferative glomerulonephritis type I [77,296]. Some of these factors have been demonstrated in renal tissue from patients with membranoproliferative glomerulonephritis, suggesting a pathogenetic role for these factors [296]. Hiramatsu et al. [153] noted that C3NeF could be produced in vitro by Epstein-Barr–transformed B cell lines derived from a patient with dense deposit disease; this C3NeF was functionally identical to the conventional C3NeF in serum. Other inherited defects in the various components controlling the complement pathway in patients with membranoproliferative glomerulonephritis have been reported [221]. Kim et al. [182] have identified an interesting abnormality in patients with dense deposit disease. There appeared to be a discrepancy between the results of the functional total hemolytic assay (the so-called Meyer's CH50) and the immunochemical determinations of serum complement concentrations. While these authors found a good correlation between serum C3 levels (measured immunochemically) and the total hemolytic complement titers (CH50) in membranoproliferative glomerulonephritis type I, CH50 titers were inappropriately high compared with C3 levels in eight of nine patients with dense deposit disease, all of whom had very low serum C3 levels. It is uncertain if this discrepancy is secondary to the stabilizing effect of C3NeF on C3 convertase of the complement pathway [120,235]. In addition to the increased catabolism of C3 noted earlier, increased turnover of factor B has been found in patients with membranoproliferative glomerulonephritis who had decreased levels of serum C3 [64]. There does not appear to be a generalized deficiency in the modulation of complement activation; three proteins involved in the control of the complement cascade (C1 inhibitor, C3b inactivator, and B1H) were found in appropriate levels in the serum and renal tissue of patients with membranoproliferative glomerulonephritis in two studies [252,380].

Terminal complement pathway activation in plasma has been studied, and elevated levels of terminal complement complexes (C5, C7, and C9) identified in the sera of patients with membranoproliferative glomerulonephritis [155]. Clardy et al. [71] measured serum levels of C3 through C9 in the hypocomplementemic glomerulonephritides and noted that the late terminal components were activated to a greater extent in membranoproliferative glomerulonephritis type III than in other forms. Levels of C5 and terminal components were normal in patients with dense deposit disease. Fractions other than C3NeF have been noted to activate components of the complement cascade in the sera of patients with membranoproliferative glomerulonephritis [72]. Clardy et al. [72] identified an IgG fraction of serum from patients with membranoproliferative glomerulonephritis types I and III that contained a nephritic factor different from C3NeF in that it converted C5 and C9, as well as C3, and was dependent on properdin. C3 conversion occurred in the absence of an intact classical pathway, and like C3NeF, this factor correlated with the serum C3 level but did not clearly correlate with the clinical course.

Role of Complement Deficiency

As noted earlier, membranoproliferative glomerulonephritis has been associated with a number of complement deficient states such as partial lipodystrophy (considered elsewhere in this chapter) and genetic deficiencies of C1q [30], C2 [73,181, 205,210,315], C3 [73,289,297], C6 [73,74], C7 [73], C8 [73], factor B [73] and C1 inhibitor [284]. Some investigators have suggested that complement depletion represents an immune-deficiency state that predisposes the individual to chronic bacterial and viral infections and subsequent immune complex formation [73]. Other investigators suggest that complement deficiency impairs the solubilization, disaggregation, and clearance of deposited immune complexes [22,73,240,335–337,364]. Coleman et al. [73] noted complement deficiencies with significantly higher frequency (23 percent) in patients with membranoproliferative glomerulonephritis types I and III than among normal subjects (7 percent) or among patients with other types of glomerulonephritis (5 percent). These complement deficiencies in patients with membranoproliferative glomerulonephritis were partial in nine patients and virtually unmeasurable in another. They were present for long periods of time and were found in family members. The deficiencies in six patients were thought to be the result of null structural genes, and in two were associated with a structurally abnormal component. Welch et al. [364] noted inhibition of immune complex solubilization by sera of patients with membranoproliferative glomerulonephritis; the inhibition was more dramatic in those with active disease but did not correlate with the therapy, proteinuria, level of circulating immune complexes, or serum level of complement.

However, prolonged hypocomplementemia induced by chronic administration of zymosan [355] or cobra venom factor [312] has failed to induce a chronic glomerulonephritis. There are no experimental models of immune complex nephritis or of nephritis mediated by indirect activation of the complement pathway that closely resemble membranoproliferative glomerulonephritis, except for the model that has been described in young Finnish Landrace lambs, which are C3 deficient [10]. The early lesions in these lambs consist of a predominant deposition of C3 that later develops into a more generalized immune complex renal disease with the deposition of immunoglobulins (IgM, IgA, and later IgG). Other evidence that activation of complement and hypocomplementemia per se are not injurious to the kidneys includes the lack of renal disease in some patients with partial lipodystrophy, hypocomplementemia, and the presence of C3NeF [314]. As noted earlier, a case is also on record of a mother with dense deposit disease who delivered a baby without renal disease [184].

Role of Circulating Immune Complexes and Humoral Immunity

There is much evidence to suggest that membranoproliferative glomerulonephritis type I is an immune complex–mediated glomerulonephritis. This includes the demonstration of immunoreactants in the glomeruli, the presence of cryoglobulins [376], the presence of circulating immune complexes in the serum in about one-half of patients [90,92, 237,269,290,316,329,379], and the occurrence of morphologically similar patterns of membranoproliferative glomerulonephritis type I in patients with known immune complex diseases such as SLE [13,311], shunt nephritis, chronic bacteremia [87,99] and chronic hepatitis B infections [44,94, 148,160]. However, the value of the demonstration of circulating immune complexes (by whatever assay) can be questioned because circulating immune complexes can be found in conditions in which glomerulonephritis is not present and does not develop later. Waldo and West [356] only rarely identified circulating immune complexes in patients with membranoproliferative glomerulonephritis types I, II, and III. The proportion of B lymphocyte subsets with surface immunoglobulin G in one study was found to be increased in a number of primary glomerular diseases which included membranoproliferative glomerulonephritis [338].

Role of Cellular Immunity

Lymphocytotoxic antibodies were commonly found and were present in high titers in patients with membranoproliferative glomerulonephritis [257]; these antibodies are thought to play an important role in the regulation of lymphocyte subsets (specifically, T gamma cells) that leads to a modulation of the immunologic network. They may play a role in the pathogenesis of this form and possibly other types of glomerulonephritis. Other investigators [63] also found evidence of lymphocytotoxic activity. Some authors have noted depression of natural killer activity and antibody-dependent cell-mediated cytotoxicity in patients with membranoproliferative glomerulonephritis [95,156,301, 327]. These lymphocyte defects may be important in the pathogenesis of the disease or may be just an epiphenomenon secondary to the nephrotic state.

It is also unclear at the present time as to whether there is a significant alteration in T lymphocyte immunoregulation in patients with membranoproliferation. Brando et al. [38] noted a decrease in the $CD4^+$-$CD8^+$ ratio and in the suppressor-cell function in hypocomplementemic nonnephrotic patients with membranoproliferative glomerulonephritis who had normal renal function. However, two other studies [66,121] failed to find alterations in the $CD4^+$-$CD8^+$ ratio of peripheral T cells.

Role of Clearance of Immune Products

As noted earlier, a number of investigators have suggested that complement deficiency impairs the solubilization and clearance of deposited immune complexes [22,73,240,335–337,364]. McGinley et al. [231] studied the splenic reticuloendothelial function in patients with membranous glomerulonephropathy and membranoproliferative glomerulonephritis and found that clearance rates of heat-damaged RBCs were normal or enhanced. The clearance rates of RBCs in patients with the membranoproliferative form correlated with the degree of hypocomplementemia but not with disease activity or the HLA haplotype.

Role of Platelet Activation

Platelets may participate in the pathogenesis of glomerular injury in various experimental forms of immune complex or anti-GBM–induced glomerulonephritis [52,53,174]. Platelets contain potent mitogenic proteins such as platelet-derived growth factor (PDGF) that can recruit and mitogenically stimulate mesenchymal cells [259]. PDGF (and other platelet factors) have chemotactic activity for neutrophils and monocytes [91]. Although ultrastructural identification of platelets is quite difficult because of their evanescence, platelet antigens have been identified, utilizing antiplatelet antibodies, in both the glomerular capillaries and the arterial walls of the kidneys from patients with membranoproliferative glomerulonephritis type I and dense deposit disease [105,241].

Patients with membranoproliferative glomerulonephritis have been found to show increased platelet activation, such as decreased intraplatelet concentrations of serotonin, increased free plasma serotonin, and nonthrombin platelet-aggregating material [174,274]. Although there was some correlation with disease activity, there was considerable overlap between normal and abnormal values, and several types of glomerulonephritis seemed to be involved. George et al. [133] found selective platelet consumption in patients with different types of glomerulonephritis, including membranoproliferative glomerulonephritis. Donadio et al. [97] provided evidence of decreased platelet survival in over two-thirds of their patients; the GFR stabilized or improved after treatment with antiplatelet drugs (dipyridamole and aspirin). The actual role and importance of in vivo platelet activation are still not totally clarified.

Genetic Factors

Complement activation or deficiency may not be a cause, but merely a marker of disease. There may be an impairment of closely linked B cell alloantigens (also called Ia antigens) that are concerned with the genetic control of specific immunologic responses. This could be related to antigen recognition or to the ability to respond to that antigen.

Some authors have suggested that a specific B lymphocyte determinant (or surface antigen) is associated with membranoproliferative glomerulonephritis [125]. Immunoglobulin-bearing lymphocytes were studied in another investigation, and an increase in the number of those bearing IgM was found in patients with type I and dense deposit disease and in certain family members of patients who had no renal disease [300]. These studies suggest that some familial predisposition to membranoproliferative glomerulonephritis may occur.

Rashid et al. [294] noted an association between membranoproliferative glomerulonephritis and Bw44 antigens. Welch et al. [362] searched for genetic markers within the major histocompatibility complex in 34 patients and their families and in 29 normal families. They found the extended haplotype HLA-B8, DR3, SCO1, GLO2 more frequently in patients with membranoproliferative glomerulonephritis (compared to normal subjects) and noted a higher incidence of renal insufficiency than in those without it. They theorized that a specific extended haplotype of the major histocompatibility complex is associated with a susceptibility to the development of membranoproliferative glomerulonephritis and that patients who have this extended haplotype have a poorer renal prognosis. Wank et al. [358] studied the association between membranoproliferative glomerulonephritis and HLA markers. They phenotyped patients with a variety of primary forms of glomerulonephritis for alleles of the MHC-linked complement genes *C4A*, *C4B*, and *BF*. A rare variant of the *C4B* locus, *C4B*2.9*, was significantly associated with the membranoproliferative glomerulonephritis form [358]. Other studies [363] of C3 genetic polymorphisms in membranoproliferative glomerulonephritis failed to show any relationship.

Berry et al. [31] described membranoproliferative glomerulonephritis in two sibships. In one, the sister had type I and the brother had type III. The second family had two brothers; both had type I with similar manifestations. Stutchfield et al. [330] described two related males with membranoproliferative glomerulonephritis inherited as an X-linked disorder.

Experimental Approaches

Experimental work in rabbits shows that chronic immunization with egg albumin produces a type I pattern [195]; in this model of chronic serum sickness, rabbits producing precipitating antibodies of high avidity develop a membranoproliferative glomerulonephritic pattern. There are other experimental animal models of membranoproliferative glomerulonephritis [164,263], and Isaacs and Miller [164] produced this type of pattern by the administration of polycationic dextran-antidextran immune complexes. All the human and experimental scenarios suggest a common pathogenesis secondary to chronic antigen exposure (to infections or tissue antigens). Thus different antigens may be responsible for this pattern in different patients. However, there is no direct evidence that the glomerular deposits contain antibody combined with antigen. Membranoproliferative glomerulonephritis has been found to occur spontaneously in dogs [61,211,214], horses [299], sheep [385], mice [217], and, as mentioned, Finnish Landrace cross lambs [122]; these naturally occurring models may in the future be useful in the determination of the etiology and pathogenesis of this glomerular pattern.

In summary, recognizable etiologic agents are generally lacking in all forms of membranoproliferative glomerulonephritis. The role of streptococcal organisms has not been well pursued. Complement activation by means of the classical pathway, with a contribution from the alternative pathway in some, has been noted in patients with type I. There is also good evidence for an immune complex pathogenesis in this type.

The data suggest that hypocomplementemia is the result of increased catabolism of the various components of the complement pathway [64]. As noted earlier, however, despite severe abnormalities of the complement pathway, there is no correlation between the levels of serum complement or C3NeF and the clinical picture or outcome [54,349,367,368]. The pathologic events are complicated, and the mechanisms of complement activation are not yet completely understood.

The Special Nature of Dense Deposit Disease

The nature of dense deposit disease is totally obscure. The characteristic glomerular intramembranous deposits are unlike those found in any other established human or experimental immune complex disease. Immune complexes may play a role, as evidenced by the demonstration of immunoreactants in renal tissue [185] and by the demonstration of cryoglobulins [376] and immune complexes [269] in the sera of patients with dense deposit disease. The presence of glomerular subepithelial deposits in some patients suggests that immune complexes may sometimes be present and play a role.

The composition of the dense deposit material is unknown. Ganter and Berger [131] believed that the deposit was composed of glycoproteins based on certain histochemical staining characteristics. Jenis et al. [167] described the presence of properdin and suggested that it was the glycoprotein that caused the histochemical staining reactions noted above.

Galle and Mahieu [130] noted the absence of gamma globulins and questioned the idea that the changes in the basement membranes of dense deposit disease represent true "immune type" deposits. They suggested that the dense deposit change was due to an alteration of the GBM, with accumulation of a biochemically modified glycoprotein-membrane substance that had a greater amount of sialic acid and less cystine content than normal GBMs. It is possible that there is a primary alteration of the GBM that generates substances able to activate the complement system. Neither immunoglobulins nor complement have been found in the dense deposits themselves using phase-contrast and electron microscopy with double-labeling antibody techniques. Complement and immunoglobulin appear to be localized at the margins or edge of the dense deposit, that is, between the deposit and the adjacent lamina densa of the GBM [182,185]. The deposit also lacks C3NeF. Kim et al. [182] were unable to produce an antibody to the dense deposits by immunization of rabbits with glomerular basement membranes containing these deposits. This was thought to be consistent with the findings of Galle and Mahieu [130] and suggested that the biochemically modified glycoproteins had lost antigenic determinants. In the double-labeling studies of Kim et al. [185] there was loss of the endothelial-GBM antigen(s) in the segments of the GBM that contained the dense deposits. Kidneys from patients with dense deposit disease have been stained with antibodies from the serum of Goodpasture's syndrome [305]. The GBM showed splitting and a double or bilaminar distribution of the Goodpasture antigen adjacent to the intramembranous deposit (just like C3). The mesangial deposits did not stain with the Goodpasture antibody. It appeared that the glomerular intramembranous dense deposit had split the area of the GBM that contained the Goodpasture antigen(s). This selective splitting of the Goodpasture antigenic zone has not been demonstrated in any other renal disease thus far studied, including membranoproliferative glomerulonephritis type I. It was proposed that these findings suggest that dense deposit disease represents an accumulation of basement-membrane–like material in the GBM and mesangial matrix. Nevins [261] performed a study of dense deposit disease with various lectins and antibodies. It was found that wheat germ agglutinin and its succinylated derivative bound selectively to the glomerular intramembranous dense deposits; neither normal GBM nor the immunoreactants stained in this way. Eight other lectins and antisera to renal antigen did not bind to dense deposits. The author suggested that this lectin reactivity indicates that these deposits contain large amounts of internally linked *N*-acetylglucosamine.

Inevitable recurrence of dense deposit disease in the renal allograft is compelling evidence that a circulating systemic factor plays a role in its pathogenesis. Dense deposit disease could result from the accumulation of serum protein(s) or other materials in either their native or denatured state [182]. As noted before, however, antisera to human serum proteins (including immunoglobulins and complement components) do not react with the dense deposits. Kim et al. [182] have been unable to demonstrate any reactivity to the deposits with antisera to normal GBM, collagen, immunoglobulins, complement components, or antisera raised to glomerular basement membranes from patients with dense deposit disease. Despite strong reactivity in dense deposit disease to thioflavine-T (which stains amyloid intensely), antisera to amyloid proteins fail to react with the deposits [182], and studies utilizing antibodies to kappa and lambda light chains also have provided negative results. Dense deposit disease could represent deposition of a host protein that has lost its antigenic epitopes and is no longer immunologically recognizable by standard immunofluorescence techniques [182].

Dense deposit disease is frequently associated with C3NeF in the serum and is considered to be associated with activation of the alternative pathway. There is also a strong association between dense deposit disease and partial lipodystrophy.

MEMBRANOPROLIFERATIVE GLOMERULONEPHRITIS WITH RECOGNIZABLE ETIOLOGIC AGENTS OR OCCURRING IN ASSOCIATION WITH OTHER DISEASES

Morphologic pictures referred to as membranoproliferative glomerulonephritis have been described in a number of specific clinical settings (Table 7-7). In some of the reports the membranoproliferative glomerulonephritis apparently corresponds well to the accepted forms just described, but in other reports there appear to be differences despite the terminology used. In most instances the morphologic pattern resembles membranoproliferative glomerulonephritis type I, but in others there are certain atypical morphologic or immunofluorescence patterns. For example, mesangial interposi-

Table 7-7. *Membranoproliferative glomerulonephritis associated with known conditions*

I. Systemic immune disorders
 A. Mixed cryoglobulinemia [40,49,76,134,224,246,276,376]
 B. Systemic lupus erythematosus [2,13,124,277,311]
 C. Sjögren syndrome [177,309]
 D. Hereditary deficiencies of complement components [30,31,37,73,74, 148,181,210,221,279,289,297,315]
II. Infectious disease
 A. Bacterial [16,77,93,114,150,292,325,378,382,392]
 B. Viral [17,44,100,157,192,332]
 C. Protozoal [83]
 D. Empyema [123]
 E. Schistosomiasis (see Chapt. 28)
 F. Tuberculosis [238]
 G. Candida endocrinopathy [67]
III. Neoplasms
 A. Light chain disease and plasma-cell dyscrasia [42,152,193]
 B. Leukemias and lymphomas [134]
 C. Carcinomas [357]
 D. Wilms tumor [341]
 E. Malignant melanoma [267]
IV. Chronic liver disease
 A. Chronic active hepatitis [44,94,148,160,192,200,320,334]
 B. Cirrhosis [29,249,251,313]
 C. α_1-Antitrypsin deficiency [251,322]
V. Miscellaneous
 A. Acquired cutis laxa [347]
 B. AIDS [180]
 C. Alveolar hemorrhage and anti–smooth-muscle antibody [387]
 D. Celiac disease and sprue [334]
 E. Coexisting glomerulonephropathies
  1. Amyloidosis [243]
  2. Diabetes mellitus [319]
 F. Drug abuse [191,199]
 G. Familial [31,94,289,295]
 H. H deficiency (B1H globulin deficiency) [207]
 I. Hemolytic uremic syndrome [183]
 J. Hereditary angioedema [285]
 K. Immunoglobulin deficiency [293]
 L. Kartagener's syndrome [110]
 M. Partial lipodystrophy (mainly dense deposit disease) [26,65,111,143,159,209,236, 278,282,286,295,314]
 N. Nephropathy–gonadal dysgenesis type II [186]
 O. Polyarteritis [247,291]
 P. Pregnancy-related [203,331]
 Q. Psoriasis vulgaris [179]
 R. Renal artery dysplasia [204]
 S. Renal vein thrombosis [354]
 T. Rheumatoid arthritis [344]
 U. Sarcoidosis [244]
 V. Sickle cell disease [226,275]
 W. Takayasu's arteritis [383]
 X. "Toxic oil epidemic syndrome" [260]
 Y. Turner's syndrome [136]
 Z. X-linked [330]
VI. Renal allografts
 A. Transplant glomerulopathy and recurrence [32,39,41,43,51,57,102,108,117,129,135, 138,202,222,234,266,288,346,348,388,389]
 B. De novo glomerulonephritis [287,346]

tion may be infrequent, noncircumferential, or nonuniform, and glomerular tuft hypercellularity may not be uniform. In some cases, renal biopsy may provide evidence of additional features such as characteristic ultrastructural deposits in patients with cryoglobulinemia. In certain cases, the criteria for membranoproliferative glomerulonephritis type I are not met at the light, electron, and immunofluorescence microscopic levels, and the lesion is better termed a *diffuse intracapillary glomerulonephritis of immune complex origin.* Low serum C3 and C3NeF levels are frequently noted in patients with "secondary" membranoproliferative glomerulonephritis [304].

Hepatitis B Antigenemia

Membranous glomerulonephropathy is the best known renal complication of hepatitis B antigenemia, which may occur with or without chronic hepatitis. A number of reports of membranoproliferative glomerulonephritis in the setting of hepatitis B antigenemia have been forthcoming. In one series of 15 children diagnosed as having membranoproliferative glomerulonephritis, HB_sAg was identified in the glomeruli in 12; 10 of the children had HB_sAg in the blood and 12 had circulating antibodies to HB_cAg [44]. None of these children had clinically apparent liver disease. Ultrastructural studies showed glomerular subendothelial and/or mesangial deposits. Immunofluorescence findings consisted of mesangial IgG, IgM, IgA, and C3 in all glomeruli. Such cases had several of the features of membranoproliferative glomerulonephritis type I, but the immunofluorescence was somewhat dissimilar. Stratta et al. [320] described an adult patient with chronic active hepatitis with several anomalous features; these included electron microscopic deposits confined to the mesangial regions and C3 restricted to the mesangium by immunofluorescence techniques. IgG and IgM were noted in a glomerular subendothelial position. Hepatitis B antigen was demonstrated in the mesangial regions. Other cases [192] have pathologic features quite consistent with membranoproliferative glomerulonephritis type I. Hepatitis B antigen can be found in the glomeruli and the blood, and one patient had chronic active hepatitis [192]. Some of the hepatitis B–related cases are characteristic of membranoproliferative glomerulonephritis type I, whereas others are not.

Shunt Nephritis and Endocarditis

This is detailed in Chapter 5. *Staphylococcus epidermidis* is the most common organism responsible for glomerulonephritis associated with infected ventriculoatrial shunts. The histologic picture resembles that of membranoproliferative glomerulonephritis type I. The major difference from the classic idiopathic form of membranoproliferative glomerulonephritis type I is that there is disappearance of the clinical abnormalities when the infected shunts are replaced, in contrast to the inexorable progression of the idiopathic form of type I.

Schistosomiasis

This is considered in Chapter 28.

Sickle Cell Disease and Trait

This is considered in detail in Chapter 30. The patterns described appear to have features quite similar to classic idiopathic membranoproliferative glomerulonephritis type I [275].

Candidiasis

Dense deposit disease has been described in a 16-year-old boy with the *Candida endocrinopathy syndrome* [67]. The patient exhibited mucocutaneous candidiasis, hypoparathyroidism, hypoadrenalism, and hypocomplementemia. Renal biopsy showed changes similar to dense deposit disease. *Candida albicans* antigen was demonstrated in the glomeruli and tubules. Antifungal therapy led to a rise in the level of serum complement as well as normalization of renal function tests. No repeat biopsy was performed.

α_1-Antitrypsin Deficiency

Three children with α_1-antitrypsin deficiency (protease inhibitor type ZZ) have been described who died from cirrhosis and at autopsy were found to have membranoproliferative glomerulonephritis [322]. Oliguria, hematuria, and abnormal renal function tests were noted during life. Light microscopic examination showed a membranoproliferative glomerulonephritis–like pattern. Electron and immunofluorescence microscopy were performed on only one patient in this series; glomerular subendothelial and mesangial deposits were noted by electron microscopy. Immunofluorescence studies showed granular capillary wall staining for IgG, IgA, IgM, C3, and C4. α_1-antitrypsin was detected in the glomerular capillaries; it was not detected in the glomeruli of patients with membranoproliferative glomerulonephritis who did not have this deficiency, nor in children with chronic liver disease and no deficiency.

Liver Disease

Membranoproliferative glomerulonephritis has been used to describe the renal lesion in patients with liver disease [200,249,313,334]. IgA nephritis may also have this pattern, so the codominant/predominant staining of the glomerular mesangial regions for IgA (Berger's disease) must be excluded.

Whether this represents a form of IgA nephritis or membranoproliferative glomerulonephritis with IgA is uncertain. Dobrin et al. [94] reported membranoproliferative glomerulonephritis type I as a familial disease in two patients with splenomegaly/hypersplenism and biochemical evidence of hepatic excretory dysfunction. Glomerular manifestations of hepatobiliary disease are treated more extensively in Chapter 6.

Chronic Lymphocytic Leukemia

Cases of membranoproliferative glomerulonephritis type I have been reported in this condition [134]. They were accompanied by single-component IgG cryoglobulinemia, and immune complexes were detected in the sera and cryoglobulins. It was suggested that the complexes were of IgG–anti-IgG type and that they played a major role in the pathogenesis of the renal disease.

Inherited Deficiency of C2

Membranoproliferative glomerulonephritis has been described in patients with an apparently inherited C2 deficiency [181]. The pattern resembled type I except that no glomerular capillary wall deposits were noted for C3, which was confined to the mesangial regions. Ultrastructural studies showed glomerular subendothelial and mesangial deposits. The authors commented that the classical pathway of activation of complement was not necessary for the development of the glomerular injury.

Polyarteritis Nodosa

Montes et al. [247] described a patient with polyarteritis confirmed at autopsy in whom there was membranoproliferative glomerulonephritis type I. C1q was identified in the glomeruli (as were IgG, IgA, and C3), suggesting that the classical pathway of complement activation had been activated by immune complexes. However, although membranoproliferative glomerulonephritis–like patterns have been noted in patients with polyarteritis, most authors do not find evidence of immune deposits in this condition.

Malignancy

Olson et al. [267] described a patient with malignant melanoma who had many of the features of dense deposit disease. It differed somewhat from the classic form in that immunoglobulins were present and that C1q and C4, as well as C3, were present. Tumor antigen and antimelanoma antibody were present in kidney eluates and serum. Thus a putative inciting antigen was present along with the features of dense deposit disease.

Summary

Several of the secondary forms of membranoproliferative glomerulonephritis do not conform to the generally accepted and well-defined types described earlier in this chapter. Other cases do, and they provide possible clues as to the etiology and pathogenesis of the idiopathic forms. The presence of immune complexes in shunt nephritis, hepatitis B–related lesions, and α_1-antitrypsin deficiency in association with membranoproliferative glomerulonephritis type I strengthens the role of immune-complex mechanisms in the genesis of the idiopathic form.

REFERENCES

1. Abreo, K., and Moorthy, A. V. Type 3 membranoproliferative glomerulonephritis: Clinicopathologic correlations and long-term follow-up in nine patients. *Arch. Pathol. Lab. Med.* 106:413, 1982.
2. Adu, D., Williams, D. G., Taube, D., Vilches, A. R., Turner, D. R., Cameron, J. S., and Ogg, C. S. Late onset systemic lupus erythematosus and lupus-like disease in patients with apparent idiopathic glomerulonephritis. *Q. J. Med.* 52:471, 1983.
3. Allen, A. C. *The Kidney: Medical and Surgical Disease.* New York: Grune & Stratton, 1951.
4. Alper, C. A., and Rosen, F. S. Studies of the in vivo behavior of human C3 in normal subjects and patients. *J. Clin. Invest.* 46:2021, 1967.
5. Alpers, C. E. Idiopathic lobular glomerulonephritis. *Clin. Nephrol.* 32:68, 1989.
6. Amemiya, S., Ito, H., Kato, H., Hasegawa, H., and Hajikano, H. A case of membranous proliferative glomerulonephritis type III (Burkholder)

with the deposition of both HB_eAg and HB_sAg. *Int. J. Pediatr. Nephrol.* 4:267, 1983.
7. Anders, D. Cooperative Long Term Follow-Up Study of Children with Membranoproliferative Glomerulonephritis (MPGN, 3 Types). In K. Murakami, T. Kitagawa, K. Yabuta, and T. Sakai (Eds.), *Recent Advances in Pediatric Nephrology.* New York: Excerpta Medica, 1987. P. 253.
8. Anders, D., Agricola, B., Sippel, M., and Thoenes, W. Basement membrane changes in membranoproliferative glomerulonephritis: II Characterization of a third type by silver impregnation of ultrathin sections. *Virchows Arch.* [A] 376:1, 1977.
9. Anders, D., and Thoenes, W. Basement membrane changes in membranoproliferative glomerulonephritis: A light and electron microscopic study. *Virchows Arch.* [A] 369:87, 1975.
10. Angus, K. W., Gardiner, A. C., Mitchell, B., and Thomson, D. Mesangiocapillary glomerulonephritis in lambs: The ultrastructure and immunopathology of diffuse glomerulonephritis in newly born Finnish lambs. *J. Pathol.* 131:65, 1980.
11. Antoine, B., and Faye, C. The clinical course associated with dense deposits in the kidney basement membranes. *Kidney Int.* 1:420, 1972.
12. Antonovych, T. T. Personal communication.
13. Appel, G. B., Silva, F. G., Pirani, C. L., Meltzer, J. I., and Estes, D. Renal involvement in SLE: A study of 56 patients emphasizing histologic classification. *Medicine (Baltimore)* 57:371, 1978.
14. Arakawa, M., and Kimmelstiel, P. Circumferential mesangial interposition. *Lab. Invest.* 21: 276, 1969.
15. Arbus, G., Getu, H., Baumal, R., Mraz, V., Jabs, D., and Eddy, A. Long-Term Follow-Up Including Renal Transplantation, of Children with Membranoproliferative Glomerulonephritis. In J. Murakami, T. Kitagawa, K. Yabuta, and T. Sakai (Eds.), *Recent Advances in Pediatric Nephrology.* New York: Excerpta Medica, 1987. P. 241.
16. Arze, R. S., Rashid, H., Morley, R., Ward, M. K., and Kerr, D. N. Shunt nephritis: Report of two cases and review of the literature. *Clin. Nephrol.* 19:48, 1983.
17. Austin, T. W., and Ray, C. G. Coxsackie virus group B infections and the hemolytic-uremic syndrome. *J. Infect. Dis.* 127:698, 1973.
18. Bannister, K. M., Howarth, G. S., Clarkson, A. R., and Woodroffe, A. J. Glomerular IgG subclass distribution in human glomerulonephritis. *Clin. Nephrol.* 19:161, 1983.
19. Barbiano di Belgiojoso, G., Baroni, M., Pagliari, B., Lavagni, M. G., Porri, M. T., Banfi, G., Colasanti, G., and Confalonieri, R. Is membranoproliferative glomerulonephritis really decreasing? *Nephron* 40:380, 1985.
20. Barbiano di Belgiojoso, G., Tarantino, A., Bazzi, C., Colasanti, G., Guerra, L., and Durante, A. Immunofluorescence patterns in chronic membranoproliferative glomerulonephritis (MPGN). *Clin. Nephrol.* 6:303, 1976.
21. Barceló, P., Lopez-Lillo, J., Cabero, L., and Del Rio, G. Successful pregnancy in primary glomerular disease. *Kidney Int.* 30:914, 1986.
22. Bartolotti, S. R., and Peters, D. K. Complement fixation in acute serum sickness: Assembly of glomerular-bound C3 convertase. *Clin. Exp. Immunol.* 37:391, 1979.
23. Beaufils, M., Gubler, M. C., Karam, J., Gluckman, J. C., Legrain, M., and Küss, R. Dense-deposit disease: Long-term follow-up of three cases of recurrence after transplantation. *Clin. Nephrol.* 7:31, 1977.
24. Bell, E. T. *Renal Diseases,* 2nd Ed. Philadelphia: Lea & Febiger, 1950.
25. Bell, E. T. A clinical and pathological study of subacute and chronic glomerulonephritis, including lipoid nephrosis. *Am. J. Pathol.* 14:691, 1938.
26. Bennett, W. M., Bardana, E. J., Wuepper, K., Houghton, D., Border, W. A., Götze, O., and Schreiber, R. Partial lipodystrophy, C3 nephritic factor and clinically inapparent mesangiocapillary glomerulonephritis. *Am. J. Med.* 62:757, 1977.
27. Berger, J., and Galle, P. Dépôts denses au sein des membranes basales du rein: Étude en microscopies optique et électronique. *Presse Med.* 71: 2351, 1963.
28. Berger, J., Yaneva, H., and Hinglais, N. Immunohistochemistry of Glomerulonephritis. In J. Hamburger, J. Crosnier, and M. H. Maxwell (Eds.), *Advances in Nephrology.* Chicago: Year Book Medical, 1971. P. 11.
29. Berger, J., Yaneva, H., and Nabarra, B. Glomerular changes in patients with cirrhosis of the liver. *Adv. Nephrol.* 7:3, 1977.
30. Berkel, A. I., Loos, M., Sanal, O., Mauff, G., Gungen, Y., Ors, U., Ersoy, F., and Yegin, O. Clinical and immunological studies in a case of selective complete C1q deficiency. *Clin. Exp. Immunol.* 38:52, 1979.
31. Berry, P. L., McEnery, P. T., McAdams, A. J., and West, C. D. Membranoproliferative glomerulonephritis in two siblings. *Clin. Nephrol.* 16:101, 1981.
32. Berthoux, F. C., Ducret, F., Colon, S., Blanc-Brunat, N., Zech, P. Y., and Traeger, J. Renal transplantation in mesangioproliferative glomerulonephritis (MPGN): Relationship between the high frequency of recurrent glomerulonephritis

and hypocomplementemia. *Kidney Int.* 7(Suppl. 3):S323, 1975.

33. Bohle, A., Biwer, E., and Christensen, J. A. Hyperperfusion injury of the human kidney in different glomerular diseases. *Am. J. Nephrol.* 8:179, 1988.
34. Bohle, A., Gärtner, H. V., Fischbach, H., Bock, K. D., Edel, H. H., Frötscher, U., Kluthe, R., Mönninghoff, W., and Scheler, F. The morphological and clinical features of membranoproliferative glomerulonephritis in adults. *Virchows Arch.* [A] 363:213, 1974.
35. Bonsib, S. M. Segmental subepithelial deposits in primary glomerulonephritis: Scanning electron microscopic examination of acellular glomeruli. *Hum. Pathol.* 16:1115, 1985.
36. Border, W. A. Immune complex detection in glomerular diseases. *Nephron* 24: 105, 1979.
37. Borzy, M. S., and Houghton, D. Mixed pattern immune deposit glomerulonephritis in a child with inherited deficiency of the third complement. *Am. J. Kidney Dis.* 5:54, 1985.
38. Brando, B., Busnach, G., Bertoli, S., Nova, M. L., and Minetti, L. T-suppressor cell abnormalities in type I membranoproliferative glomerulonephritis. *Proc. Eur. Dial. Transplant. Assoc.* 19:669, 1983.
39. Briner, J. Glomerular Lesions in Renal Allografts. In P. Frick, G. A. von Harnack, K. Kochsiek, G. A. Martini, and A. Prader (Eds.), *Advances in Internal Medicine and Pediatrics.* Berlin: Springer-Verlag, 1982. P. 1.
40. Brouet, J. C., Clauvel, J. P., Danon, R., Klein, M., and Seligmann, M. Biologic and clinical significance of cryoglobulins: A report of 86 cases. *Am. J. Med.* 57:775, 1974.
41. Broyer, M., Gagnadoux, M. F., Guest, G., Buerton, D., Niaudet, P., Habib, R., and Busson, M. Kidney transplantation in children: Results of 383 grafts performed at Enfants Malades Hospital from 1973 to 1984. *Adv. Nephrol.* 16:307, 1987.
42. Bruneval, P., Foidart, J. M., Nochy, D., Camilleri, J. P., and Bariety, J. Glomerular matrix proteins in nodular glomerulosclerosis in association with light chain deposition disease and diabetes mellitus. *Hum. Pathol.* 16:477, 1985.
43. Brunt, E. M., Kissane, J. M., Cole, B. R., and Hanto, D. W. Transmission and resolution of type I membranoproliferative glomerulonephritis in recipients of cadaveric renal allografts. *Transplantation* 46:595, 1988.
44. Brzosko, W. J., Krawczynski, K., Nazarewicz, T., Morzycka, M., and Nowoslawski, A. Glomerulonephritis associated with hepatitis B surface antigen immune complexes in children. *Lancet* 2:477, 1974.
45. Burkholder, P. M. *Atlas of Human Glomerular Pathology.* New York: Harper & Row, 1974.
46. Burkholder, P. M., and Bradford, W. D. Proliferative glomerulonephritis in children: A correlation of varied clinical and pathologic patterns utilizing light, immunofluorescence, and electron microscopy. *Am. J. Pathol.* 56:423, 1969.
47. Burkholder, P. M., Hyman, L. R., and Krueger, R. P. Characterization of Mixed Membranous and Proliferative Glomerulonephritis: Recognition of Three Varieties. In P. Kincaid-Smith, T. H. Mathew, and E. L. Becker (Eds.), *Glomerulonephritis: Morphology, Natural History, and Treatment.* New York: Wiley, 1973. P. 557.
48. Burkholder, P. M., Marchand, A., and Krueger, R. P. Mixed membranous and proliferative glomerulonephritis: A correlative light, immunofluorescence and electron microscopic study. *Lab. Invest.* 23:459, 1970.
49. Cacciatore, L., Coto, V., Giardina, M. G., Lucariello, A., Usberti, M., and Stanziale, P. Idiopathic cryoglobulinemia, membranoproliferative glomerulonephritis, hypogammaglobulinemia and nucleoprotein turnover. *Panminerva Med.* 26:199, 1984.
50. Cameron, J. S. The Natural History of Glomerulonephritis. In P. Kincaid-Smith, A. d'Apice, and R. Atkins (Eds.), *Progress in Glomerulonephritis.* New York: Wiley, 1979. P. 1.
51. Cameron, J. S. Glomerulonephritis in renal transplants. *Transplantation* 34:237, 1982.
52. Cameron, J. S. The Pathogenesis of Glomerulonephritis. In T. Bertani and G. Remuzzi (Eds.), *Glomerular Injury 300 Years After Morgagni.* Milano: Wichtig Editore, 1983. P. 18.
53. Cameron, J. S. Platelets in glomerular disease. *Annu. Rev. Med.* 35:175, 1984.
54. Cameron, J. S., Glasgow, E. F., Ogg, C. S., and White, R. H. R. Membranoproliferative glomerulonephritis and persistent hypocomplementaemia. *Br. Med. J.* 4:7, 1970.
55. Cameron, J. S., Ogg, C. S., White, R. H. R., and Glasgow, E.F. The clinical features and prognosis of patients with normocomplementemic mesangiocapillary glomerulonephritis. *Clin. Nephrol.* 1:8, 1973.
56. Cameron, J. S., Ogg, C. S., Turner, D. R., Weller, R. O., White, R. H. R., Glasgow, E. F., Peters, D. K., and Martin, A. Mesangiocapillary Glomerulonephritis and Persistent Hypocomplementemia. In P. Kincaid-Smith, T. H. Mathew, and E. L. Becker, (Eds.), *Glomerulonephritis: Morphology, Natural History, and Treatment,* Part 1. New York: Wiley, 1973. P. 541.
57. Cameron, J. S., and Turner, D. R. Recurrent glomerulonephritis in allografted kidneys. *Clin.*

Nephrol. 7:47, 1977.

58. Cameron, J. S., Turner, D. R., Heaton, J., Williams, D. G., Ogg, C. S., Chantler, C., Haycock, G. B., and Hicks, J. Idiopathic mesangiocapillary glomerulonephritis: Comparison of types I and II in children and adults and long-term prognosis. *Am. J. Med.* 74:175, 1983.
59. Campbell-Boswell, M. V., Linder, D., Naylor, B. R., and Brooks, R. E. Kidney tubule basement membrane alterations in type II membranoproliferative glomerulonephritis. *Virchows Arch.* [A] 382:49, 1979.
60. Cattran, D. C., Cardella, C. J., Roscoe, J. M., Charron, R. C., Rance, P. C., Ritchie, S. M., and Corey, P. N. Results of a controlled drug trial in membranoproliferative glomerulonephritis. *Kidney Int.* 27:436, 1985.
61. Center, S. A., Smith, C. A., Wilkinson, E., Erb, H. N., and Lewis, R. M. Clinicopathologic, renal immunofluorescent, and light microscopic features of glomerulonephritis in the dog: 41 cases (1975–1985). *J. Am. Vet. Med. Assoc.* 190:81, 1987.
62. Chapman, S. J., Cameron, J. S., Chantler, C., and Turner, D. Treatment of mesangiocapillary glomerulonephritis in children with combined immunorepression and anticoagulation. *Arch. Dis. Child.* 55:446, 1980.
63. Charlesworth, J. A., Bowman, C., Perl, S. I., Yasmeen, D., and Pussell, B. A. Lymphocytotoxic activity in primary glomerulonephritis: Evidence for immune complex–mediated cytotoxicity. *J. Clin. Lab. Immunol.* 6:233, 1981.
64. Charlesworth, J. A., Williams, D. G., Sherington, E., Lachmann, P. J., and Peters, D. K. Metabolic studies of the third component of complement and the glycine-rich beta glycoprotein in patients with hypocomplementemia. *J. Clin. Invest.* 53:1578, 1974.
65. Chartier, S., Buzzanga, J. B., and Paquin, F. Partial lipodystrophy associated with a type 3 form of membranoproliferative glomerulonephritis. *J. Am. Acad. Dermatol.* 16:201, 1987.
66. Chatenoud, L., and Bach, M. A. Abnormalities of T-cell subsets in glomerulonephritis and systemic lupus erythematosus. *Kidney Int.* 20:267, 1981.
67. Chesney, R. W., O'Regan, S., Guyda, H. J., and Drummond, K. N. *Candida* endocrinopathy syndrome with membranoproliferative glomerulonephritis: Demonstration of glomerular *Candida* antigen. *Clin. Nephrol.* 5:232, 1976.
68. Churg, J., Duffy, J. L., and Bernstein, J. Identification of dense deposit disease: A report for the International Study of Kidney Diseases in Children. *Arch. Pathol. Lab. Med.* 103:67, 1979.
69. Churg, J., and Grishman, E. Subacute glomerulonephritis. *Am. J. Pathol.* 35:25, 1959.
70. Churg, J., Habib, R., and White, R. H. Pathology of the nephrotic syndrome in children: A report for the International Study of Kidney Disease in Children. *Lancet* 1:1299, 1970.
71. Clardy, C. W., Forristal, J., Strife, C. F., and West, C. D. Serum terminal complement component levels in hypocomplementemic glomerulonephritides. *Clin. Immunol. Immunopathol.* 50: 307, 1989.
72. Clardy, C. W., Forristal, J., Strife, C. F., and West, C. D. A properdin dependent nephritic factor slowly activating C3, C5, and C9 in membranoproliferative glomerulonephritis, types I and III. *Clin. Immunol. Immunopathol.* 50:333, 1989.
73. Coleman, T. H., Forristal, J., Kosaka, T., and West, C. D. Inherited complement component deficiencies in membranoproliferative glomerulonephritis. *Kidney Int.* 24:681, 1983.
74. Coleman, T. H., Forristal, J., and West, C. D. Hereditary C6 deficiency in membranoproliferative glomerulonephritis (MPGN) type I. *Pediatr. Res.* 13:446, 1979.
75. Colten, H. R., Levey, R. H., Rosen, F. S., and Alper, C. A. Decreased synthesis of C3 in membranoproliferative glomerulonephritis (Abstract). *J. Clin. Invest.* 52:20a, 1973.
76. Cordonnier, D., Vialtel, P., Renversez, J. C., Chenais, F., Favre, M., Tournoud, A., Barioz, C., Bayle, F., Dechelette, E., Denis, M. C., and Couderc, P. Renal diseases in 18 patients with mixed type II IgM-IgG cryoglobulinemia: Monoclonal lymphoid infiltration (2 cases) and membranoproliferative glomerulonephritis (14 cases). *Adv. Nephrol.* 12:177, 1983.
77. Craddock, C. F., Richards, N. P., Powell, R. J., and Morgan, A. G. Novel C3 nephritic factor activity in the glomerulonephritis of staphylococcal endocarditis. *Q. J. Med.* 65:895, 1987.
78. Curtis, J. J., Wyatt, R. J., Bhathena, D., Lucas, B. A., Holland, N. H., and Luke, R. G. Renal transplantation for patients with type I and type II membranoproliferative glomerulonephritis: Serial complement and nephritic factor measurements and the problem of recurrence of disease. *Am. J. Med.* 66:216, 1979.
78a. Cutler, S. J., and Ederer, F. Maximum utilization of the life-table method in analyzing survival. *J. Chronic Dis.* 8:699, 1958.
79. Daha, M. R., Austen, K. F., and Fearon, D. T. Heterogeneity, polypeptide chain composition and antigenic reactivity of C3 nephritic factor. *J. Immunol.* 120:1389, 1978.
80. Daha, M. R., Fearon, D. T., and Austen, K. F. C3 nephritic factor (C3NeF): Stabilization of fluid phase and cell bound alternative pathway conver-

tase. *J. Immunol.* 116:1, 1976.

81. Daha, M. R., and van Es, L. A. Further evidence for the antibody nature of C3 nephritic factor (C3NeF). *J. Immunol.* 123:755, 1979.
82. Danielsen, H., Kornerup, H. J., Olsen, S., and Posborg, V. Arterial hypertension in chronic glomerulonephritis: An analysis of 310 cases. *Clin. Nephrol.* 19:284, 1983.
83. Date, A., Neela, P., and Shastry, J. C. Membranoproliferative glomerulonephritis in a tropical environment. *Ann. Trop. Med. Parasitol.* 77:279, 1983.
84. Date, A., Neela, P., and Shastry, J. C. Thioflavin T fluorescence in membranoproliferative glomerulonephritis. *Nephron* 32:90, 1982.
85. Davis, A. E., Gelfand, E. W., Schur, P. H., Rosen, F. S., and Alper, C. A. IgG subclass studies of C3 nephritic factor. *Clin. Immunol. Immunopathol.* 11:98, 1978.
86. Davis, A. E., Schneeberger, E. E., and Grupe, W. E. Mesangial proliferative glomerulonephritis with irregular intramembranous deposits: Another variant of hypocomplementemic nephritis. *Am. J. Med.* 63:481, 1977.
87. Davis, A. E., Schneeberger, E. E., Grupe, W. E., and McCluskey, R. T. Membranoproliferative glomerulonephritis (MPGN type 1) and dense-deposit disease (DDD) in children. *Clin. Nephrol.* 9:184, 1978.
88. Davis, A. E., Ziegler, J. B., Gefland, E. W., Rosen, F. S., and Alper, C. A. Heterogeneity of nephritic factor and its identification as an immunoglobulin. *Proc. Natl. Acad. Sci. USA* 74:3980, 1977.
89. Davis, B. K., and Cavallo, T. Membranoproliferative glomerulonephritis: Localization of early components of complement in glomerular deposits. *Am. J. Pathol.* 84:283, 1976.
90. Davis, C. A., Marder, H., and West, C. D. Circulating immune complexes in membranoproliferative glomerulonephritis. *Kidney Int.* 20:728, 1981.
91. Deuel, T. F., Senior, R. M., Huang, J. S., and Griffin, G. L. Chemotaxis of monocytes and neutrophils to platelet derived growth factor. *J. Clin. Invest.* 69:1046, 1982.
92. Digeon, M., Laver, M., Riza, J., and Black, J. F. Detection of circulating immune complexes in human sera by simplified assays with polyethylene glycol. *J. Immunol. Methods* 16:165, 1977.
93. Dobrin, R. S., Day, N. K., Quie, P. G., Moore, H. L., Vernier, H. L., Michael, A. F., and Fish, A. J. The role of complement, immunoglobulin and bacterial antigen in coagulase-negative staphylococcal shunt nephritis. *Am. J. Med.* 59:660, 1975.
94. Dobrin, R. S., Hoyer, J. R., Nevins, T. E., Sharp, H., Gentry, W. C., and Vernier, R. L. The association of familial liver disease, subepidermal immunoproteins, and membranoproliferative glomerulonephritis. *J. Pediatr.* 90:901, 1977.
95. Dohi, K., Yamada, H., Takai, M., Fujii, Y., and Ishikawa, H. Natural killer activity and antibody-dependent cell-mediated cytotoxicity in primary glomerular diseases. *Clin. Nephrol.* 27:11, 1987.
96. Doi, T., Mayumi, M., Kanatsu, K., Suehiro, F., and Hamashima, Y. Distribution of IgG subclasses in membranous nephropathy. *Clin. Exp. Immunol.* 58:57, 1984.
97. Donadio, J. V., Jr., Anderson, C. F., Mitchell, J. C., III, Holley, K. E., Ilstrup, D. M., Fuster, V., and Chesebro, J. H. Membranoproliferative glomerulonephritis: A prospective clinical trial of platelet-inhibitor therapy. *N. Engl. J. Med.* 310:1421, 1984.
98. Donadio, J. V., and Holley, K. E. Membranoproliferative glomerulonephritis. *Semin. Nephrol.* 2:204, 1982.
99. Donadio, J. V., Jr., Slack, T. K., Holley, K. E., and Ilstrup, D. M. Idiopathic membranoproliferative (mesangiocapillary) glomerulonephritis: A clinicopathologic study. *Mayo Clin. Proc.* 54:141, 1979.
100. Donini, U., Rossi, L., Palanchetti, F., Zucchelli, P., Poli, F., Altavilla, G., Corallini, A., and Barbanti-Brodano, G. BK papovavirus immune complexes in glomerulonephritis. *Proc. Eur. Dial. Transplant. Assoc.* 17:637, 1980.
101. Dowling, J. P., and Mathews, D. C. Silver methenamine impregnation: A useful adjunct to renal electron microscopy. *Pathology* 19:410, 1987.
102. Droz, D., Nabarra, B., Noel, L. H., Leibowitch, J., and Crosnier, J. Recurrence of dense deposits in transplanted kidneys: I. Sequential survey of the lesions. *Kidney Int.* 15:386, 1979.
103. Droz, D., Noel, L. H., Barbanel, C., and Grünfeld, J. P. Evolution à long terme des glomérulonéphrites membranoprolifératives de l'adulte: Rémission spontanée durable chez 13 malades avec étude de biopsies rénales itérative dans 5 cas. *Nephrologie* 3:6, 1982.
104. Droz, D., Zanetti, M., Noel, L. H., and Leibowitch, J. Dense deposit disease. *Nephron* 19:1, 1977.
105. Duffus, P., Parbtani, A., Frampton, G., and Cameron, J. S. Glomerular localization of platelet related antigens, platelet factor 4 and beta-thromboglobulin in glomerulonephritis. *Clin. Nephrol.* 17:288, 1982.
106. Duvall-Young, J., MacDonald, M. K., and McKechnie, N. M. Fundus changes in (type II) mesangiocapillary glomerulonephritis simulating

drusen: A histopathological report. *Br. J. Ophthalmol.* 73:297, 1989.
107. Earle, D. P., and Jennings, R. B. Poststreptococcal Glomerulonephritis. In G. E. W. Wolstenholme and M. P. Cameron (Eds.), *Ciba Foundation Symposium on Renal Biopsy.* Boston: Little, Brown, 1961. P. 156.
108. Eddy, A., Sibley, R., Mauer, S. M., and Kim, Y. Renal allograft failure due to recurrent dense intramembranous deposit disease. *Clin. Nephrol.* 21:305, 1984.
109. Edelmann, C. M., Jr. Long-term low-dose prednisone ameliorates the course of membranoproliferative glomerulonephritis (MPGN): A report of the International Study of Kidney Disease in Children. *Pediatr. Res.* 21:474, 1987.
110. Egbert, B. M., Schwartz, E., and Kempson, R. L. Kartagener syndrome: Report of a case with mesangiocapillary glomerulonephritis. *Arch. Pathol. Lab. Med.* 101:95, 1977.
111. Eisinger, A. J., Shortland, J. R., and Moorhead, P. J. Renal disease in partial lipodystrophy. *Q. J. Med.* 41:343, 1972.
112. Ellis, A. Natural history of Bright's disease: Clinical, histological and experimental observations. *Lancet* 1:1, 1942.
113. Endoh, M., Suga, T., and Sakai, H. IgG, IgA, and IgM rheumatoid factors in patients with glomerulonephritis. *Nephron* 39:330, 1985.
114. Ernst, A., Radonic, M., and Belicza, M. The syndrome of long-standing *Staphylococcus albus* bacteremia, bacterial endocarditis and diffuse membranoproliferative glomerulonephritis complicating ventriculoatrial shunt infection: Case report and review of literature. *Acta Med. Iugosl.* 34:137, 1980.
115. Fahr, T. Pathologische Anatomie des Morbus Brightii. In F. Henke and O. Lubarsch (Eds.), *Handbuch der Speziellen Pathologischen Anatomie und Histologie,* Vol. 6, Part 1. Berlin: Springer, 1925. P. 156.
116. Falk, R. J., Sisson, S. P., Dalmasso, A. P., Kim, Y., Michael, A. F., and Vernier, R. L. Ultrastructural localization of the membrane attack complex of complement in human renal tissues. *Am. J. Kidney Dis.* 9:121, 1987.
117. Fearon, D. T., Daha, M. R., Strom, T. B., Weiler, J. M., Carpenter, C. B., and Austen, K. F. Pathways of complement activation in membranoproliferative glomerulonephritis and allograft rejection. *Transplant. Proc.* 9:729, 1977.
118. Ferrario, F., Castiglione, A., Colasanti, G., Barbiano di Belgiojoso, G., Bertoli, S., and D'Amico, G. The detection of monocytes in human glomerulonephritis. *Kidney Int.* 28:513, 1985.
119. Fischbach, H., Mackensen, S., Grund, K. E., Kellner, A., and Bohle, A. Relationship between glomerular lesions, serum creatinine and interstitial volume in membranoproliferative glomerulonephritis. *Klin. Wochenschr.* 55:603, 1977.
120. Fontaine, M., Daveau, M., and Lebreton, J. P. A common antigenic determinant on human C4b and C3b. *Mol. Immunol.* 17:1075, 1980.
121. Fornasieri, A., Sinico, R., Fiorini, G., Goldaniga, D., Colasanti, G., Vendemia, F., Gibelli, A., and D'Amico, G. T-lymphocyte subsets in primary and secondary glomerulonephritis. *Proc. Eur. Dial. Transplant. Assoc.* 19:635, 1983.
122. Frelier, P. F., Pritchard, J., Armstrong, D. L., Nagge, W. T., and Lewis, R. M. Spontaneous mesangiocapillary glomerulonephritis in Finn cross lambs from Alberta. *Can. J. Comp. Med.* 48:215, 1984.
123. Frew, A. J., and Higgins, R. M. Empyema and mesangiocapillary glomerulonephritis with nephrotic syndrome. *Br. J. Dis. Chest.* 82:93, 1988.
124. Friedman, A. L., Chesney, R. W., Oberley, T. D., and McEnery, P. T. Clinical systemic lupus erythematosus with dense-deposit disease. *Int. J. Pediatr. Nephrol.* 4:171, 1983.
125. Friend, P. S., Yunis, E. J., Noreen, H. J., and Michael, A. F. B-cell alloantigen associated with chronic mesangiocapillary glomerulonephritis. *Lancet* 1:562, 1977.
126. Futrakul, P., Kullavanijaya, P., Watana, D., and Sensidivatana, R. Tubular functions in glomerulonephropathies in childhood. *Int. J. Pediatr. Nephrol.* 2:17, 1981.
127. Gaffney, E. F. Prominent parietal epithelium: A common sign of renal glomerular injury. *Hum. Pathol.* 13:651, 1982.
128. Galle, P. Mise en évidence au microscope électronique d'une lésion singulière des membranes basales due rein et de la substance hyaline. Thesis in Medicine, University of Paris, 1962 (cited in ref. 130).
129. Galle, P., Hinglais, N., and Crosnier, J. Recurrence of an original glomerular lesion in three renal allografts. *Transplant. Proc.* 3:368, 1971.
130. Galle, P., and Mahieu, P. Electron-dense alteration of kidney basement membranes: A renal lesion specific of a systemic disease. *Am. J. Med.* 58:749, 1975.
131. Ganter, P., and Berger, J. Néphropathie associant une glomérulite proliférative et des dépôts au sein des basales: II. Étude histochimique de trois cas. *J. Urol. Nephrol (Paris)* 69:96, 1963.
132. Gärtner, H. V., Wehner, H., and Bohle, A. The immunohistological findings in various forms of glomerulonephritis: A comparative investigation based on 335 renal biopsies. Part II: Minimal proliferating intercapillary glomerulonephritis (with

nephrotic syndrome), focal sclerosing, epi-extra-perimembranous, membranoproliferative and extracapillary (rapidly progressive) glomerulonephritis. *Pathol. Res. Pract.* 162:198, 1978.
133. George, C. R., Slichter, S. J., Quadracci, L. J., Striker, G. E., and Harker, L. A. A kinetic evaluation of hemostasis in renal disease. *N. Engl. J. Med.* 291:1111, 1974.
134. Gilboa, N., Durante, D., Guggenheim, S., Lacher, J., Holman, R., Schorr, W., Garfield, D., and McIntosh, R. M. Immune deposit nephritis and single-component cryoglobulinemia associated with chronic lymphocytic leukemia: Evidence for a role of circulating IgG–anti-IgG immune complexes in the pathogenesis of the renal lesion. *Nephron* 24:223, 1979.
135. Glickich, D., Matas, A. J., Sabley, L. B., Senitzer, D., Tellis, V. A., Soberman, R., and Veith, F. J. Recurrent membranoproliferative glomerulonephritis type I in successive renal transplants. *Am. J. Nephrol.* 7:143, 1987.
136. Goodyer, P. R., Fong, J. S., and Kaplan, B. S. Turner's syndrome, 46X, del (X) (p 11), persistent complement activation and membranoproliferative glomerulonephritis. *Am. J. Nephrol.* 2:272, 1982.
137. Gotoff, S. P., Fellers, F. X., Vawter, G. F., Janeway, C. A., and Rosen, F. S. The beta 1C globulin in childhood nephrotic syndrome: Laboratory diagnosis of progressive glomerulonephritis. *N. Engl. J. Med.* 273:524, 1965.
138. Habib, R., Antignac, C., Hinglais, N., Gagnadoux, M. F., and Broyer, M. Glomerular lesions in the transplanted kidney in children. *Am. J. Kidney Dis.* 10:198, 1987.
139. Habib, R., Gubler, M. C., Loirat, C., Maiz, H. B., and Levy, M. Dense-deposit disease: A variant of membranoproliferative glomerulonephritis. *Kidney Int.* 7:204, 1975.
140. Habib, R., and Kleinknecht, C. The Primary Nephrotic Syndrome of Childhood: Classification and Clinicopathologic Study of 406 Cases. In S. C. Sommers (Ed.), *Pathology Annual,* Vol. 6. New York: Appleton-Century-Crofts, 1971. P. 417.
141. Habib, R., Kleinknecht, C., Gubler, M. C., and Levy, M. Idiopathic membranoproliferative glomerulonephritis in children: Report of 105 cases. *Clin. Nephrol.* 1:194, 1973.
142. Habib, R., Kleinknecht, C., Gubler, M. C., and Maiz, H. B. Idiopathic Membranoproliferative Glomerulonephritis:' Morphology and Natural History. In P. Kincaid-Smith, T. H. Mathew, and E. L. Becker (Eds.), *Glomerulonephritis: Morphology, Natural History, and Treatment,* Part 1. New York: Wiley, 1973. P. 491.
143. Habib, R., Levy, M., Gubler, M. C., Broyer, M., and Habib, M. Lipodystrophie partielle, hypocomplementémie et glomérulonéphrite. *Arch. Fr. Pediatr.* 34:197, 1977.
144. Habib, R., Loirat, C., Gubler, M. C., and Levy, M. Morphology and serum complement levels in membranoproliferative glomerulonephritis. *Adv. Nephrol.* 4:109, 1974.
145. Habib, R., Michielsen, P., DeMontera, E., Hinglais, N., Galle, P., and Hamburger, J. Clinical, Microscopic and Electron Microscopic Data in the Nephrotic Syndrome of Unknown Origin. In G. E. W. Wolstenholme and M. P. Cameron (Eds.), *Renal Biopsy: Clinical and Pathological Significance.* London: Churchill, 1961. P. 70.
146. Hara, M., Mase, D., Inaba, S., Higuchi, A., Tanizawa, T., Yamanaka, N., Sugisaki, Y., Sado, Y., and Okada, T. Immunohistochemical localization of glomerular basement membrane antigens in various renal diseases. *Virchows Arch.* [A] 408:403, 1986.
147. Hasegawa, O., and Ito, H. Methylprednisone Pulse Therapy (MPT) for Children with Type 1 Membranoproliferative Glomerulonephritis (MPGN): Significance of Complement Profile on the Therapy. In K. Murakami, T. Kitagawa, K. Yabuta, and T. Sakai (Eds.), *Recent Advances in Pediatric Nephrology.* New York: Excerpta Medica, 1987. P. 247.
148. Hawkins, E., and Berry, P. L. Membranoproliferative glomerulonephritis with significant IgA deposits (Abstract). *Lab. Invest.* 46:6P, 1982.
149. Heidbreder, E., Hüller, U., Schäfer, B., and Heidland, A. Severe hypertensive retinopathy: Increased evidence in renoparenchymal hypertension. *Am. J. Nephrol.* 7:394, 1987.
150. Heptinstall, R. H. *Pathology of the Kidney,* 3rd Ed. Boston: Little, Brown, 1983.
151. Herdman, R. C., Pickering, R. J., Michael, A. F., Vernier, R. L., Fish, A. J., Gewurz, H., and Good, R. A. Chronic glomerulonephritis associated with low serum complement activity (chronic hypocomplementemic glomerulonephritis) *Medicine (Baltimore)* 49:207, 1970.
152. Hill, G. S. Multiple Myeloma, Amyloidosis, Waldenström's Macroglobulinemia, Cryoglobulinemias, and Benign Monoclonal Gammopathies. In R. H. Heptinstall (Ed.), *Pathology of the Kidney,* 3rd Ed. Boston: Little, Brown, 1983. P. 993.
153. Hiramatsu, M., Balow, J. E., and Tsokos, G. C. Production of nephritic factor of the alternative complement pathway by Epstein-Barr virus transformed B-cell lines derived from a patient with membranoproliferative glomerulonephritis. *J. Immunol.* 136:4451, 1986.
154. Hogg, R. J. Diagnostic, prognostic and therapeutic implications of renal biopsy in children with renal disease. *Semin. Nephrol.* 5:240, 1985.

155. Horigome, I., Seino, J., Sudo, K., Kinoshita, Y., Saito, T., and Yoshinaga, K. Terminal complement complex in plasma from patients with systemic lupus erythematosus and other glomerular diseases. *Clin. Exp. Immunol.* 70:417, 1987.
156. Hruby, Z., Kopec, W., and Szewczyk, Z. Activity of circulating monocytes in patients with chronic glomerulonephritis. *Int. Urol. Nephrol.* 17:379, 1985.
157. Huang, T. W., and Wiegenstein, L. M. Mesangiolytic glomerulonephritis in an infant with immune deficiency and echovirus infection. *Arch. Pathol. Lab. Med.* 101:125, 1977.
158. Hultberg, B., and Ravnskov, U. The excretion of *N*-acetyl-beta-glucosaminidase in glomerulonephritis. *Clin. Nephrol.* 15:33, 1981.
159. Hunter, A. M., Lawson, A. A., and Thomson, D. Partial lipodystrophy with nephrotic syndrome. *Postgrad. Med. J.* 54:286, 1978.
160. Iada, H., Izumino, K., Asaka, M., Kameyama, T., Takata, M., Mizumura, Y., and Sasayama, S. Membranoproliferative glomerulonephritis associated with chronic hepatitis B in adults: Pathogenic role of HB_sAg. *Am. J. Nephrol.* 7:319, 1987.
161. Ikaya, M., Nagase, M., and Honda, N. Intraglomerular distribution of fibronectin in primary glomerular diseases. *Clin. Nephrol.* 24:53, 1985.
162. International Study of Kidney Disease in Children. Nephrotic syndrome in children: Prediction of histopathology from clinical and laboratory characteristics at time of diagnosis. *Kidney Int.* 13:159, 1978.
163. International Study of Kidney Disease in Children. Alternate-day steroid therapy in membranoproliferative glomerulonephritis: A randomized controlled clinical trial. *Kidney Int.* 21:150, 1982.
164. Isaacs, K. L., and Miller, F. Antigen size and charge in immune complex glomerulonephritis, part II. *Am. J. Pathol.* 111:298, 1983.
165. Ito, Y., Kinoshita, S., Yoshimoto, M., Shindou, S., and Yamashita, F. Hypertension and renal insufficiency in children with chronic glomerulonephritis. *Int. J. Pediatr. Nephrol.* 7:187, 1986.
166. Jackson, E. C., McAdams, A. J., Strife, C. F., Forristal, J., Welch, T. R., and West, C. D. Differences between membranoproliferative glomerulonephritis types I and III in clinical presentation, glomerular morphology, and complement perturbation. *Am. J. Kidney Dis.* 9:115, 1987.
167. Jenis, E. H., Sandler, P., Hill, G. S., Knieser, M. R., Jensen, G. E., and Roskes, S. D. Glomerulonephritis with basement membrane dense deposits. *Arch. Pathol.* 97:84, 1974.
168. Jenis, E. H., and Lowenthal, D. T. Renal Basement Membrane Dense-Deposit Disease. In E. H. Jenis and D. T. Lowenthal, (Eds.), *Kidney Biopsy Interpretation.* Philadelphia: Davis, 1977. P. 63.
169. Jones, D. B. Inflammation and repair of the glomerulus. *Am. J. Pathol.* 27:991, 1951.
170. Jones, D. B. Glomerulonephritis. *Am. J. Pathol.* 29:33, 1953.
171. Jones, D. B. Nephrotic glomerulonephritis. *Am. J. Pathol.* 33:313, 1957.
172. Jones, D. B. The nature of scar tissue in glomerulonephritis. *Am. J. Pathol.* 42:185, 1963.
173. Jones, D. B. Membranoproliferative glomerulonephritis: One or many diseases? *Arch. Pathol. Lab. Med.* 101:457, 1977.
174. Kasai, N., Parbtani, A., Cameron, J. S., Yewdall, V., Shepherd, P., and Verroust, P. Platelet aggregating immune complexes and intraplatelet serotonin in idiopathic glomerulonephritis and systemic lupus. *Clin. Exp. Immunol.* 43:64, 1981.
175. Katz, S. M. Reduplication of the glomerular basement membrane: A study of 110 cases. *Arch. Pathol. Lab. Med.* 105:67, 1981.
176. Kazatchkine, M. D., Fearon, D. T., Appay, M. D., Mandet, C., and Bariety, J. Immunohistochemical study of the human glomerular C3b in normal kidney and in 75 cases of renal diseases. *J. Clin. Invest.* 69:900, 1982.
177. Khan, M. A., Akhtar, M., and Taher, S. M. Membranoproliferative glomerulonephritis in a patient with primary Sjögren's syndrome. *Am. J. Nephrol.* 8:235, 1988.
178. Kher, K. K., Makker, S. P., Aikawa, M., and Kirson, I. J. Regression of dense deposits in type II membranoproliferative glomerulonephritis: Case report of clinical course in a child. *Clin. Nephrol.* 17:100, 1982.
179. Kida, H., Asamoto, T., Abe, T., Tomosugi, N., and Hattori, N. Psoriasis vulgaris associated with mesangiocapillary glomerulonephritis. *Clin. Nephrol.* 23:255, 1985.
180. Kim, K. K., and Factor, S. M. Membranoproliferative glomerulonephritis and plexogenic pulmonary arteriopathy in a homosexual man with acquired immunodeficiency syndrome. *Hum. Pathol.* 18:1293, 1987.
181. Kim, Y., Friend, P. S., Dresner, I. G., Yunis, E. J., and Michael, A. F. Inherited deficiency of the second component of complement (C2) with membranoproliferative glomerulonephritis. *Am. J. Med.* 62:765, 1977.
182. Kim, Y., Michael, A. F., and Fish, A. J. Idiopathic Membranoproliferative Glomerulonephritis. In B. Brenner and J. Stein (Eds.), *Nephrotic Syndrome.* New York: Churchill-Livingstone: 1982. P. 237.
183. Kim, Y., Miller, K., and Michael, A. F. Breakdown products of C3 and factor B in hemolytic-uremic syndrome. *J. Lab. Clin. Med.* 89:845, 1977.
184. Kim, Y., Shvil, Y., and Michael, A. F. Hypo-

complementemia in a newborn infant caused by placental transfer of C3 nephritic factor. *J. Pediatr.* 92:88, 1978.

185. Kim, Y., Vernier, R. L., Fish, A. J., and Michael, A. F. Immunofluorescence studies of dense-deposit disease: The presence of railroad tracks and mesangial rings. *Lab. Invest.* 40:474, 1979.
186. Kinberg, J. A., Angle, C. R., and Wilson, R. B. Nephropathy–gonadal dysgenesis, type 2: Renal failure in three siblings with XY dysgenesis in one. *Am. J. Kidney Dis.* 9:507, 1987.
187. Kincaid-Smith, P. The Natural History and Treatment of Mesangiocapillary Glomerulonephritis. In P. Kincaid-Smith, T. L. Mathew, and E. L. Becker, (Eds.), *Glomerulonephritis: Morphology, Natural History and Treatment.* New York: Wiley, 1973. P. 591.
188. Kincaid-Smith, P. The treatment of chronic mesangiocapillary (membranoproliferative) glomerulonephritis with impaired renal function. *Med. J. Aust.* 2:587, 1972.
189. King, J. T., Valenzuela, R., McCormack, L. J., and Osborne, D. G. Granular dense deposit disease. *Lab. Invest.* 39:591, 1978.
190. Klein, M., Poucell, S., Arbus, G. S., McGraw, M., Rance, C., Yoon, S., and Baumal, R. Characteristics of a benign subtype of dense deposit disease: Comparison with the progressive form of this disease. *Clin. Nephrol.* 20:163, 1983.
191. Kleinknecht, D., Kourilsky, O., Morel-Maroger, L., Adhemar, J. P., Droz, D., Masselot, J. P., and Adam, C. Dense deposit disease with rapidly progressive renal failure in a narcotic addict. *Clin. Nephrol.* 14:309, 1980.
192. Knieser, M. R., Jenis, E. H., Lowenthal, D. T., Bancroft, W. H., Burns, W., and Shalhoub, R. Pathogenesis of renal disease associated with viral hepatitis. *Arch. Pathol.* 97:193, 1974.
193. Knobler, H., Kopolovic, J., Kleinman, Y., Rubinger, D., Silver, J., Friedlaender, M. M., and Popovtzer, M. M. Multiple myeloma presenting as dense deposit disease: Light chain nephropathy. *Nephron* 34:59, 1983.
194. Korzets, Z., Bernheim, J., and Bernheim, J. Rapidly progressive glomerulonephritis (crescentic glomerulonephritis) in the course of type I idiopathic membranoproliferative glomerulonephritis. *Am. J. Kidney Dis.* 10:56, 1987.
195. Kuriyama, R. Chronic glomerulonephritis induced by prolonged immunization in the rabbit. *Lab. Invest.* 28:224, 1973.
196. Lagrue, G., Laurent, J., and Belghiti, D. Renal survival in membranoproliferative glomerulonephritis (MPGN): Role of long-term treatment with nonsteroid anti-inflammatory drugs (NSAID). *Int. Urol. Nephrol.* 20:669, 1988.
197. Lamb, V., Tisher, C. C., McCoy, R. C., and Robinson, R. R. Membranoproliferative glomerulonephritis with dense intramembranous alterations: A clinicopathologic study. *Lab. Invest.* 36:607, 1977.
198. Laohapand, T., Cattell, V., and Gabriel, J. R. Monocyte infiltration in human glomerulonephritis. *Clin. Nephrol.* 19:309, 1983.
199. Laurent, J., Belghiti, D., Bruneau, C., and Lagurue, G. Diclofenac, a nonsteroidal anti-inflammatory drug, decreases proteinuria in some glomerular diseases: A controlled study. *Am. J. Nephrol.* 7:198, 1987.
200. Lee, H. S., Choi, Y., Yu, S. H., Koh, H. I., Kim, M. J., and Ko, K. W. A renal biopsy study of hepatitis B virus–associated nephropathy in Korea. *Kidney Int.* 34:537, 1988.
201. Lehman, D. H., Wilson, C. B., and Dixon, F. J. Extraglomerular immunoglobulin deposits in human nephritis. *Am. J. Med.* 58:765, 1975.
202. Leibowitch, J., Halbwachs, L., Wattel, S., Gaillard, M. H., and Droz, D. Recurrence of dense deposits of transplanted kidney: II. Serum complement and nephritic factor profiles. *Kidney Int.* 15:396, 1979.
203. Leichter, H. E., Jordan, S. C., Cohen, A. H., Ettenger, R. B., Salusky, I. B., and Fine, R. N. Postpartum renal failure in a patient with membranoproliferative glomerulonephritis type II. *Am. J. Nephrol.* 6:382, 1986.
204. Leslie, B. R., Hamburger, R. J., Stilmant, M. M., and Flamenbaum, W. Renal artery dysplasia in a patient with membranoproliferative glomerulonephritis. *Am. J. Med.* 66:528, 1979.
205. Levy, M., Gubler, M. C., Sich, M., Beziau, A., and Habib, R. Immunopathology of membranoproliferative glomerulonephritis with subendothelial deposits (type 1 MPGN). *Clin. Immunol. Immunopathol.* 10:477, 1978.
206. Levy, M., Gubler, M. C., and Habib, R. New Concepts in Membranoproliferative Glomerulonephritis. In P. Kincaid-Smith, A. J. F. d'Apice, and R. C. Atkins (Eds.), *Progress in Glomerulonephritis.* New York: Wiley, 1979. P. 177.
207. Levy, M., Halbwachs-Mecarelli, L., Gubler, M. C., Kohout, G., Bensenouci, A., Niaudet, P., Hauptmann, G., and Lesavre, P. H deficiency in two brothers with atypical dense intramembranous deposit disease. *Kidney Int.* 30:949, 1986.
208. Lewy, J. E., Salinas-Madrigal, L., Herdson, P., Pirani, C., and Metcoff, J. Clinicopathologic correlations in acute poststreptococcal glomerulonephritis. *Medicine (Baltimore)* 50:453, 1971.
209. Ljunghall, S., Fjellström, K. E., and Wibell, L. Partial lipodystrophy and chronic hypocomplementemic glomerulonephritis. *Acta Med. Scand.* 195:493, 1974.
210. Loirat, C., Levy, M., Peltier, A. P., Broyer, M.,

Checoury, A., and Mathieu, H. Deficiency of the second component of complement: Its occurrence with membranoproliferative glomerulonephritis. *Arch. Pathol. Lab. Med.* 104:467, 1980.

211. Ludders, J. W., Grauer, G. F., Dubielzig, R. R., Ribble, G. A., and Wilson, J. W. Renal microcirculatory and correlated histologic changes associated with dirofilariasis in dogs. *Am. J. Vet. Res.* 49:826, 1988.

212. Luder, A. S., Cohen, S. L., and Fisher, C. Nephrotic syndrome complicated by tubular dysfunction: Case report and review of possible mechanisms. *Postgrad. Med. J.* 56:282, 1980.

213. MacCallum, W. G. Glomerular changes in nephritis. *Bull. Johns Hopkins Hosp.* 55:416, 1934.

214. MacDougall, D. F., Cook, T., Steward, A. P., and Cattell, V. Canine chronic renal disease: Prevalence and types of glomerulonephritis in the dog. *Kidney Int.* 29:1144, 1986.

215. Magil, A. B. Monocytes and glomerulonephritis associated with remote visceral infection. *Clin. Nephrol.* 22:169, 1984.

216. Magil, A. B., Price, J. D., Bower, G., Rance, C. P., Huber, J., and Chase, W. H. Membranoproliferative glomerulonephritis type 1: Comparison of natural history in children and adults. *Clin. Nephrol.* 11:239, 1979.

217. Maggio-Price, L., Russell, R., Wolf, N. S., Alpers, C. E., and Engel, D. Clinicopathologic features of young and old *sphha/sphha* mice: Mutants with congenital hemolytic anemia. *Am. J. Pathol.* 132:461, 1988.

218. Mahieu, P. Biochemical structure of glomerular basement membrane in chronic glomerulonephritis: I. Lobular and membranoproliferative glomerulonephritis. *Kidney Int.* 1:115, 1972.

219. Mampaso, F., Levya-Cobian, F., Marginez-Montero, J. C., Gonzalo, A., Bellas, C., Moneo, I., and Junquera, E. Mesangial proliferative glomerulonephritis with unusual intramembranous granular dense deposits. *Clin. Nephrol.* 19:92, 1983.

220. Mandalenakis, N., Mendoza, N., Pirani, C. L., and Pollack, V. E. Lobular glomerulonephritis and membranoproliferative glomerulonephritis: A clinical and pathologic study based on renal biopsies. *Medicine (Baltimore)* 50:319, 1971.

221. Marder, H. K., Coleman, T. H., Forristal, J., Beischel, L., and West, C. D. An inherited defect in the C3 convertase, C3b, Bb, associated with glomerulonephritis. *Kidney Int.* 23:749, 1983.

222. Mathew, T. H. Recurrence of disease following renal transplantation. *Am. J. Kidney Dis.* 12:85, 1988.

223. Mazzucco, G., Barbiano di Belgiojoso, G., Confalonieri, R., Coppo, R., and Monga, G. Glomerulonephritis with dense deposits: A variant of membranoproliferative glomerulonephritis or a separate morphological entity? Light, electron microscopic and immunohistochemical study of eleven cases. *Virchows Arch.* [A] 387:17, 1980.

224. Mazzucco, G., Mongà, G., Casanova, S., and Cagnoli, L. Cell interposition in glomerular capillary walls in cryoglobulinemic glomerulonephritis (CRYGN): Ultrastructural investigation of 23 cases. *Ultrastruct. Pathol.* 10:355, 1986.

225. McAdams, A. J., McEnery, P. T., and West, C. D. Mesangiocapillary glomerulonephritis: Changes in glomerular morphology with long-term alternate-day prednisone therapy. *J. Pediatr.* 86:23, 1975.

226. McCoy, R. C. Ultrastructural alterations in the kidney of patients with sickle cell disease and the nephrotic syndrome. *Lab. Invest.* 21:85, 1969.

227. McEnery, P. T., and McAdams, A. J. Regression of membranoproliferative glomerulonephritis type II (dense deposit disease): Observations in six children. *Am. J. Kidney Dis.* 12:138, 1988.

228. McEnery, P. T., McAdams, A. J., and West, C. D. Membranoproliferative glomerulonephritis: Improved survival with alternate-day prednisone therapy. *Clin. Nephrol.* 13:117, 1980.

229. McEnery, P. T., McAdams, A. J., and West, C. D. The effect of prednisone in a high-dose, alternate-day regimen on the natural history of idiopathic membranoproliferative glomerulonephritis. *Medicine (Baltimore)* 64:401, 1985.

230. McEnery, P. T., West, C. D., and McAdams, A. J. Membranoproliferative glomerulonephritis (MPGN): Clinical follow-up of 36 children 1957 through 1977. (Astract). *Kidney Int.* 12:470, 1977.

231. McGinley, E., Martin, W., Henderson, N., and Boulton-Jones, J. M. Defective splenic reticuloendothelial function in idiopathic membranous nephropathy. *Clin. Exp. Immunol.* 56:295, 1984.

232. McGinley, E., Watkins, R., McLay, A., and Boulton-Jones, J. M. Plasma exchange in the treatment of mesangiocapillary glomerulonephritis. *Nephron* 40:385, 1985.

233. McGovern, V. J. Persistent nephrotic syndrome: A renal biopsy study. *Australas. Ann. Med.* 13:306, 1964.

234. McLean, R. H., Geiger, H., Burke, B., Simmons, R., Najarian, J., Vernier, R. L., and Michael, A. F. Recurrence of membranoproliferative glomerulonephritis following kidney transplantation: Serum complement component studies. *Am. J. Med.* 60:60, 1976.

235. McLean, R. H., and Nilson, S. H. C3 nephritic factor stabilization of the classic C3 convertase: A role for C2 in C3 nephritic factor activity. *Proc. Soc. Exp. Biol. Med.* 161:358, 1979.

236. Méry, J. Ph., Kourilsky, O., Morel-Maroger, L.,

and Adam, C. Partial lipodystrophy and glomerulonephritis without complement activation. *N. Engl. J. Med.* 298:1034, 1978.
237. Meyer, O., and Descamps, B. Detection of soluble immune complexes by the technique of ADCC inhibition in human diseases. *J. Clin. Lab. Immunol.* 2:311, 1979.
238. Meyrier, A., Valensi, P., and Sebaoun, J. Mesangiocapillary glomerulonephritis and the nephrotic syndrome in the course of disseminated tuberculosis. *Nephron* 49:341, 1988.
239. Michael, A. F., Westberg, N. G., Fish, A. J., and Vernier, R. L. Studies on chronic membranoproliferative glomerulonephritis with hypocomplementemia. *J. Exp. Med.* 134:208, 1971.
240. Miller, G. W., and Nussenzweig, V. A new complement function: Solubilization of antigen-antibody aggregates. *Proc. Natl. Acad. Sci. USA* 72:418, 1975.
241. Miller, K., Dresner, I. G., and Michael, A. F. Localization of platelet antigens in human kidney disease. *Kidney Int.* 18:472, 1980.
242. Miller, M. N., Baumal, R., Poucell, S., and Steele, B. T. Incidence and prognostic importance of glomerular crescents in renal diseases of childhood. *Am. J. Nephrol.* 4:244, 1984.
243. Miller, R. R. Membranoproliferative glomerulonephritis and amyloidosis. *Hum. Pathol.* 15: 1185, 1984.
244. Molle, D., Baumelou, A., Beaufils, H., Vannier, R., and Legrain, M. Membranoproliferative glomerulonephritis associated with pulmonary sarcoidosis. *Am. J. Nephrol.* 6:386, 1986.
245. Monga, G., Mazzucco, G., Barbiano di Belgiojoso, G., and Busnach, G. The presence and possible role of monocyte infiltration in human chronic proliferative glomerulonephritides: Light microscopic, immunofluorescence, and histochemical correlations. *Am. J. Pathol.* 94:271, 1979.
246. Monga, G., Mazzucco, G., Casanova, S., Boero, R., Cagnoli, L., Barbiano di Belgiojoso, G., and Confalonieri, R. Ultrastructural glomerular findings in cryoglobulinemic glomerulonephritis. *Appl. Pathol.* 5:108, 1987.
247. Montes, M., Andres, G. A., Elwood, C. M., Sepulveda, M. R., and DeCoteau, W. E. Membranoproliferative glomerulonephritis with polyarteritis: A case report. *Hum. Pathol.* 6:391, 1975.
248. Montoliu, J., Bergada, E., Botey, A., Torras, A., Darnell, A., Arrizabalaga, P., Lopez-Pedret, J., and Revert, L. Plasmapheresis induced recovery from renal failure in mesangiocapillary glomerulonephritis of acute onset. *Proc. Eur. Dial. Transplant. Assoc.* 19:794, 1983.
249. Montoliu, J., Darnell, A., Torras, A., and Revert, L. Glomerular disease in cirrhosis of the liver: Low frequency of IgA deposits. *Am. J. Nephrol.* 6:199, 1986.
250. Morel-Maroger, L., Leathem, A., and Richet, G. Glomerular abnormalities in nonsystemic diseases: Relationship between findings by light microscopy and immunofluorescence in 433 renal biopsy specimens. *Am. J. Med.* 53:170, 1972.
251. Moroz, S. P., Cutz, E., Balfe, J. W., and Sass-Kortsak, A. Membranoproliferative glomerulonephritis in childhood cirrhosis associated with alpha-1-antitrypsin deficiency. *Pediatrics* 57:232, 1976.
252. Moseley, H. L., and Whaley, K. Control of complement activation in membranous and membranoproliferative glomerulonephritis. *Kidney Int.* 17:535, 1980.
253. Mota-Hernandez, F., Gordillo-Paniagua, G., Munoz-Arizpe, R., Lopez-Arriaga, J., and Barboza-Madueno, L. Prednisone versus placebo in membranoproliferative glomerulonephritis: Long-term clinicopathological correlations. *Int. J. Pediatr. Nephrol.* 6:25, 1985.
254. Muda, A. D., Barsotti, P., and Marinozzi, V. Ultrastructural histochemical investigations of "dense deposit disease." *Virchows Arch.* [A] 413:529, 1988.
255. Murphy, B. F., and d'Apice, A. J. Identification of components of glomerular immune deposits using monoclonal antibodies. *Pathology* 20:130, 1988.
256. Nagi, A. H. Histological, ultrastructural and immunofluorescence studies in membranoproliferative glomerulonephritis. *J. Pathol.* 106:151, 1972.
257. Nakabayashi, K., Arimura, Y., Yoshida, M., and Nagasawa, T. Anti-T cell antibodies in primary glomerulonephritis. *Clin. Nephrol.* 23:74, 1985.
258. Nakamura, T., Oite, T., Kazama, T., Suzuki, S., Orikasa, M., Arakawa, M., and Shimizu, F. Monoclonal antibodies to human glomerular antigens. *Virchows Arch.* [A] 412:573, 1988.
259. Nakashima, Y., Hirose, S., and Hamashima, Y. Proliferation of cultured rabbit renal glomerular cells stimulated by platelet factor. *Acta Pathol. Jpn.* 30:1, 1980.
260. Navas-Palacios, J. J., Usera-Sarraga, G., Gil-Margin, R., and Gutierrez-Millet, V. Pathology of the kidney in "toxic oil epidemic syndrome." *J. Toxicol. Environ. Health* 13:1, 1984.
261. Nevins, T. E. Lectin binding in membranoproliferative glomerulonephritis: Evidence for *N*-acetylglucosamine in dense intramembranous deposits. *Am. J. Pathol.* 118:325, 1985.
262. Ng, Y. C., and Peters, D. K. C3 nephritic factor (C3NeF): Dissociation of cell-bound and fluid phase stabilization of alternative pathway C3 convertase. *Clin. Exp. Immunol.* 65:450, 1986.
263. Noble, B., Olson, K. A., Milgrom, M., and Albini, B. Tissue deposition of immune complexes in mice receiving daily injections of bovine serum

albumin. *Clin. Exp. Immunol.* 42:255, 1980.
264. Northway, J. D., McAdams, A. J., Forristal, J., and West, C. D. A "silent" phase of hypocomplementemic persistent nephritis detectable by reduced serum beta-1c-globulin levels. *J. Pediatr.* 74:28, 1969.
265. Nyberg, M., Petterson, E., Tallqvist, G., and Pasternack, A. Survival in idiopathic glomerulonephritis. *Acta Pathol. Microbiol. Scand.* [A] 88:319, 1980.
266. Oberkircher, O. R., Enama, J., West, J. C., Campbell, P., and Moran, J. Regression of recurrent membranoproliferative glomerulonephritis type II in a transplanted kidney after plasmapheresis therapy. *Transplant. Proc.* 20(Suppl. 1):418, 1988.
267. Olson, J. L., Philips, T. M., Lewis, M. G., and Solez, K. Malignant melanoma with renal dense deposits containing tumor antigens. *Clin. Nephrol.* 12:74, 1979.
268. Ooi, Y. M., Vallota, E. H., and West, C. D. Classical complement pathway activation in membranoproliferative glomerulonephritis. *Kidney Int.* 9:46, 1976.
269. Ooi, Y. M., Vallota, E. H., and West, C. D. Serum immune complexes in membranoproliferative and other glomerulonephritides. *Kidney Int.* 11:275, 1977.
270. Orfila, C., Rakotoarivony, J., Manuel, Y., and Suc, J. M. Immunofluorescence characterization of light chains in human nephropathies. *Virchows Arch.* [A] 412:591, 1988.
271. Orlowski, T., Rancewicz, Z., Lao, M., Juskowa, J., Klepacka, J., Gradowska, L., Morzycka-Michalik, M., and Glyda, J. Long-term immunosuppressive therapy of idiopathic membranoproliferative glomerulonephritis. *Klin. Wochenschr.* 66: 1019, 1988.
272. Ormos, J., Mágori, A., Sonkodi, S., and Streitmann, K. Type 2 membranoproliferative glomerulonephritis with electron-dense basement membrane alteration in the spleen. *Arch. Pathol. Lab. Med.* 103:265, 1979.
273. Orofino, L., Quereda, C., Lamas, S., Orte, L., Gonzalo, A., and Mampaso, F. Hypertension in primary chronic glomerulonephritis: Analysis of 288 biopsied patients. *Nephron* 45:22, 1987.
274. Parbtani, A., Frampton, G., and Cameron, J. S. Platelet and plasma serotonin concentrations in glomerulonephritis II. *Clin. Nephrol.* 14:112, 1980.
275. Pardo, V., Strauss, J., Kramer, H., Ozawa, T., and McIntosh, R. W. Nephropathy associated with sickle cell anemia: An autologous immune complex nephritis: II. Clinicopathologic study of seven patients. *Am. J. Med.* 59:650, 1975.
276. Perez, G. O., Pardo, V., and Fletcher, M. Renal involvement in essential mixed cryoglobulinemia. *Am. J. Kidney Dis.* 10:276, 1987.
277. Perrin, L. H., Lambert, P. H., and Miescher, P. A. Complement breakdown products in plasma from patients with systemic lupus erythematosus and patients with membranoproliferative or other glomerulonephritis. *J. Clin. Invest.* 56:165, 1975.
278. Peters, D. K., Charlesworth, J. A., Sissons, J. G., Williams, D. G., Boulton-Jones, J. M., Evans, D. J., Kourilsky, O., and Morel-Maroger, L. Mesangiocapillary nephritis, partial lipodystrophy, and hypocomplementaemia. *Lancet* 2:535, 1973.
279. Peters, D. K., and Lachmann, P. J. Immunity deficiency in pathogenesis of glomerulonephritis. *Lancet* 1:58, 1974.
280. Peters, D. K., and Lachmann, P. J. The Complement System in Renal Disease. In D. Black and N. F. Jones (Eds.), *Renal Disease,* 4th Ed. Oxford: Blackwell, 1979. P. 169.
281. Peters, D. K., Martin, A., Weinstein, A., Cameron, J. S., Barratt, T. M., Ogg, C. S., and Lachmann, P. J. Complement studies in membranoproliferative glomerulonephritis. *Clin. Exp. Immunol.* 11:311, 1972.
282. Peters, D. K., and Williams, D. G. Complement and mesangiocapillary glomerulonephritis: Role of complement deficiency in the pathogenesis of nephritis. *Nephron* 13:189, 1974.
283. Pickering, R. J., Herdman, R. C., Michael, A. F., Vernier, R. L., Gewurz, H., Fish, A. J., and Good, R. A. Chronic glomerulonephritis associated with low serum complement activity (chronic hypocomplementemic glomerulonephritis). *Medicine (Baltimore)* 49:207, 1970.
284. Pickering, R. J., Michael, A. F., and Herdman, R. C. The complement system in chronic glomerulonephritis: Three newly associated observations. *J. Pediatr.* 78:30, 1971.
285. Plaza, J., Malasit, P., and Kerr, D. N. Hereditary angio-oedema with mesangiocapillary glomerulonephritis. *Postgrad. Med. J.* 53:627, 1977.
286. Pollock, J., Wood, B., and Kelly, J. P. Membranoproliferative glomerulonephritis type II and partial lipodystrophy in an adult. *Am. J. Kidney Dis.* 8:274, 1986.
287. Pommer, W., Schultze,G., Bohl, D., and Krause, P. H. De novo membranoproliferative glomerulonephritis in a renal allograft. *Int. Urol. Nephrol.* 15:359, 1983.
288. Porter, K. A., Dossetor, J. B., Marchioro, T. L., Peart, W. S., Rendall, J. M., Starzl, T. E., and Terasaki, P. I. Human renal transplants: I. Glomerular changes. *Lab. Invest.* 16:153, 1976.
289. Pussell, B. A., Bourke, E., Nayef, M., Morris, S., and Peters, D. K. Complement deficiency and

nephritis: A report of a family. *Lancet* 1:675, 1980.
290. Pussell, B. A., Lockwood, C. M., Scott, D. M., Pinching, A. J., and Peters, D. K. Value of immune-complex assays in diagnosis and management. *Lancet* 2:359, 1978.
291. Rajarajeswari, G., Manivannan, T., Radhakrishnan, S., and Viswanathan, J. Systemic angiitis with membranoproliferative glomerulonephritis. *J. Assoc. Physicians India* 26:1185, 1978.
292. Rames, L., Wise, B., Goodman, J. R., and Piel, C. F. Renal disease with *Staphylococcus albus* bacteremia: A complication in ventriculoatrial shunts. *JAMA* 212:1671, 1970.
293. Rashid, H. U., Biswas, C. K., Morley, A. R., and Kerr, D. N. Mesangiocapillary glomerulonephritis type I associated with immunoglobulin deficiency. *Br. Med. J.* 283:407, 1981.
294. Rashid, H. U., Papiha, S. S., Agroyannis, B., Morley, A. R., Ward, M. K., Roberts, D. F., and Kerr, D. N. The associations of HLA and other genetic markers with glomerulonephritis. *Hum. Genet.* 63:38, 1983.
295. Reichel, W., Köbberling, J., Fischbach, H., and Scheler, F. Membranoproliferative glomerulonephritis with partial lipodystrophy: Discordant occurrence in identical twins. *Klin. Wochenschr.* 54:75, 1976.
296. Roberts, J. L., Levy, M., Chioros, P. G., Bartlow, B. G., Forristal, J., West, C. D., Habib, R., and Lewis, E. J. A serum C3-activating factor: Its characterization and its presence in glomerular deposits. *J. Immunol.* 127:1131, 1981.
297. Roord, J. J., van Diemen-van Steenvoorde, R. A., Schuurman, H. J., Rijkers, G. T., Zegers, B. J., Gmelig Meyling, F. H., and Stoop, J. W. Membranoproliferative glomerulonephritis in a patient with congenital deficiency of the third component of complement. *Am. J. Kidney Dis.* 13:413, 1989.
298. Ruddy, S., Carpenter, C. B., Chin, K. W., Knostman, J. N., Sorter, N. A., Götze, O., Müller-Eberhard, H. J., and Austen, K. F. Human complement metabolism: An analysis of 144 studies. *Medicine (Baltimore)* 54:165, 1975.
299. Sabnis, S. G., Gunson, D. E., and Antonovych, T. T. Some unusual features of mesangioproliferative glomerulonephritis in horses. *Vet. Pathol.* 21:374, 1984.
300. Sakai, H., Nomoto, Y., Arimori, S., Itoh, H., and Hasegawa, O. Increase of IgM-bearing peripheral blood lymphocytes in patients with idiopathic membranoproliferative glomerulonephritis (MPGN) and their family members. *Clin. Nephrol.* 12:210, 1979.
301. Sasdelli, M., Cagnoli, L., Candi, P., Mandreoli, M., Beltrandi, E., and Zucchelli, P. Cell-mediated immunity in idiopathic glomerulonephritis. *Clin. Exp. Immunol.* 46:27, 1981.
302. Sato, H., Sato, T., Seino, J., Ootaka, T., Kyogoku, Y., Furuyama, T., and Yoshinaga, K. Dense deposit disease: Its possible pathogenesis suggested by an observation of a patient. *Clin. Nephrol.* 27:41, 1987.
303. Schena, F. P., and Cameron, J. S. Treatment of proteinuric idiopathic glomerulonephritides in adults: A retrospective survey. *Am. J. Med. Sci.* 17:119, 1988.
304. Schena, F. P., Pertosa, G., Stanziale, P., Vox, E., Percoraro, C., and Andreucci, V. E. Biological significance of the C3 nephritic factor in membranoproliferative glomerulonephritis. *Clin. Nephrol.* 18:240, 1982.
305. Schiffer, M. S., Michael, A. F., Kim, Y., and Fish, A. J. Distribution of glomerular basement membrane antigens in diseased human kidneys. *Lab. Invest.* 44:234, 1981.
306. Schmitt, H., Cavalcanti de Oliveira, V., and Bohle A. Tubulointerstitial alterations in type I membranoproliferative glomerulonephritis: An investigation of 259 cases. *Pathol. Res. Pract.* 182:6, 1987.
307. Schreiber, R. D., Götze, O., and Müller-Eberhard, H. J. Nephritic factor: Its structure and function and its relationship to initiating factor of the alternative pathway. *Scand. J. Immunol.* 5:705, 1976.
308. Scott, D. M., Amos, N., Sissons, J. G. P., Lachmann, P. J., and Peters, D. K. The immunoglobulin nature of nephritic factor (NeF). *Clin. Exp. Immunol.* 32:12, 1978.
309. Siamopoulos, K. C., Mavridis, A. K., Elisaf, M., Drosos, A. A., and Moutsopoulos, H. M. Kidney involvement in primary Sjögren's syndrome. *Scand. J. Rheumatol.* 61:156, 1986.
310. Sibley, R. K., and Kim, Y. Dense intramembranous deposit disease. *Kidney Int.* 25:660, 1984.
311. Silva, F. G. The Nephropathies of Systemic Lupus Erythematosus. In S. Rosen (Ed.), *Pathology of Glomerular Disease.* New York: Churchill-Livingstone, 1983. P. 79.
312. Simpson, I. J., Moran, J., Evans, D. J., and Peters, D. K. Prolonged complement activation in mice. *Kidney Int.* 13:467, 1978.
313. Sinniah, R. Heterogeneous IgA glomerulonephropathy in liver cirrhosis. *Histopathology* 8:947, 1984.
314. Sissons, J. G. P., West, R. J., Fallows, J., Williams, D. G., Boucher, B. J., Amos, N., and Peters, D. K. The complement abnormalities of lipodystrophy. *N. Engl. J. Med.* 294:461, 1976.
315. Sobel, A. T., Moisy, M., Hirbrec, G., Tournesac, A., Berry, J. P., Mannoni, P., Peltier, A. P., and Lagrue, G. Hereditary C2 deficiency associated with nonsystemic glomerulonephritis. *Clin. Ne-*

phrol. 12:132, 1979.
316. Solling, J. Circulating immune complexes in glomerulonephritis: A longitudinal study. *Clin. Nephrol.* 20:177, 1983.
317. Southwest Pediatric Nephrology Study Group. Dense deposit disease in children: Prognostic value of clinical and pathologic indicators. *Am. J. Kidney Dis.* 6:161, 1985.
318. Spitzer, R. E., Vallota, E. H., Forristal, J., Sudora, E., Stitzel, A., Davis, N. C., and West, C. D. Serum C3 lytic system in patients with glomerulonephritis. *Science* 164:436, 1969.
319. Srikanta, S., Malaviya, A. N., Rajagopalan, P., Bhuyan, U. N., and Ahuja, M. M. Association of type I (insulin-dependent) diabetes mellitus, autoimmunity, antinuclear antibody, and membranoproliferative glomerulonephritis. *Diabetes Care* 6:71, 1983.
320. Stratta, P., Camussi, G., Ragni, R., and Vercellone, A. Hepatitis B antigenaemia associated with active chronic hepatitis and mesangioproliferative glomerulonephritis. *Lancet* 2:179, 1975.
321. Strife, C. F., Jackson, E. C., and McAdams, A. J. Type III membranoproliferative glomerulonephritis: Long-term clinical and morphologic evaluation. *Clin. Nephrol.* 21:323, 1984.
322. Strife, C. F., Hug, G., Chuck, G., McAdams, A. J., Davis, C. A., and Kline, J. J. Membranoproliferative glomerulonephritis and alpha-1-antitrypsin deficiency in children. *Pediatrics* 71:88, 1983.
323. Strife, C. F., Leahy, A. E., and West, C. D. Antibody to a cryptic, solid phase C1q antigen in membranoproliferative nephritis. *Kidney Int.* 35: 836, 1989.
324. Strife, C. F., McAdams, A. J., and West, C. D. Membranoproliferative glomerulonephritis characterized by focal, segmental proliferative lesion. *Clin. Nephrol.* 18:9, 1982.
325. Strife, C. F., McDonald, B. M., Ruley, E. J., McAdams, A. J., and West, C. D. Shunt nephritis: The nature of the serum cryoglobulins and their relation to the complement profile. *J. Pediatr.* 88:403, 1976.
326. Strife, C. F., McEnery, P. T., McAdams, A. J., and West, C. D. Membranoproliferative glomerulonephritis with disruption of the glomerular basement membrane. *Clin. Nephrol.* 7:65, 1977.
327. Strife, C. F., and Ruley, E. J. Reduction of phagocyte adherence by nephritic sera: Relation to complement activation. *Pediatr. Res.* 18:637, 1984.
328. Striker, L. M.-M., Killen, P. D., Chi, E., and Striker, G. E. The composition of glomerulosclerosis I: Studies in focal sclerosis, crescentic glomerulonephritis, and membranoproliferative glomerulonephritis. *Lab. Invest.* 51:181, 1984.
329. Stuhlinger, W. D., Verroust, P. J., and Morel-Maroger, L. Detection of circulating soluble immune complexes in patients with various renal diseases. *Immunology* 30:43, 1976.
330. Stutchfield, P. R., White, R. H., Cameron, A. H., Thompson, R. A., Mackintosh, P., and Wells, L. X-linked mesangiocapillary glomerulonephritis. *Clin. Nephrol.* 26:150, 1986.
331. Surian, M., Imbasciati, E., Cosci, P., Banfi, G., Barbiano di Belgiojoso, G., Brancaccio, D., Minetti, L., and Ponticelli, C. Glomerular disease and pregnancy. *Nephron.* 36:101, 1984.
332. Sutherland, J. C., Olweny, C. L. M., Levine, P. H., and Mardiney, M. R., Jr. Epstein-Barr virus immune complexes in postmortem kidneys from African patients with Burkitt's lymphoma and American patients with and without lymphoma. *J. Natl. Cancer Inst.* 60:941, 1978.
333. Swainson, C. P., Robson, J. S., Thomson, D., and MacDonald, M. K. Mesangiocapillary glomerulonephritis: A long-term study of 40 cases. *J. Pathol.* 141:449, 1983.
334. Swarbrick, E. T., Fairclough, P. D., Campbell, P. J., Levison, D. A., Greenwood, R. H., and Baker, L. R. Coeliac disease, chronic active hepatitis, and mesangiocapillary glomerulonephritis in the same patient (Letter). *Lancet* 2:1084, 1980.
335. Takahashi, M., Czop, J., Ferreira, A., and Nussenzweig, V. Mechanism of solubilization of immune aggregates by complement: Implications for immunopathology. *Transplant. Rev.* 32:121, 1976.
336. Takahashi, M., Tack, B. F., and Nussenzweig, V. Requirements for the solubilization of immune aggregates by complement: Assembly of a factor B-dependent C3-convertase on the immune complexes. *J. Exp. Med.* 145:86, 1977.
337. Takahashi, M., Takahashi, S., Brade, V., and Nussenzweig, V. Requirements for the solubilization of immune aggregates by complement: The role of the classical pathway. *J. Clin. Invest.* 62:349, 1978.
338. Tani, Y., Kida, H., Abe, T., Tomosugi, N., Saito, Y., Asamoto, T., and Hattori, N. B-lymphocyte subset patterns and their significance in idiopathic glomerulonephritis. *Clin. Exp. Immunol.* 48:201, 1982.
339. Thompson, R. A. C3 inactivating factor in the serum of a patient with chronic hypocomplementaemic proliferative glomerulonephritis. *Immunology* 22:147, 1972.
340. Thorner, P., and Baumal, R. Extraglomerular dense deposits in dense deposit disease. *Arch. Pathol. Lab. Med.* 106:628, 1982.
341. Thorner, P., McGraw, M., Weitzman, S., Balfe, J. W., Klein, M., and Baumal, R. Wilms tumor and glomerular disease: Occurrence with features

of membranoproliferative glomerulonephritis and secondary focal, segmental glomerulosclerosis. *Arch. Pathol. Lab. Med.* 108:141, 1984.

342. Tiebosch, A. T., Wolters, J., Frederik, P. F., and van der Wiel, T. W. Epidemiology of idiopathic glomerular disease: A prospective study. *Kidney Int.* 32:112, 1987.

343. Tiller, D. J., Clarkson, A. R., Mathew, T., Thompson, N., Row, G., Lauer, C., Hobbs, J., and Seymour, A. A Prospective Randomized Trial in the Use of Cyclophosphamide, Dipyridamole and Warfarin in Membranous and Mesangiocapillary Glomerulonephritis. In W. Zurukzoglu, M. Papadimitriou, M. Pyrapasopoulos, M. Sion, and C. Zamboulis (Eds.), *Proceedings of the 8th International Congress of Nephrology. (Advances in Basic and Clinical Nephrology)*. Basel: Karger, 1981. P. 345.

344. Ting, H. C., and Wang, R. Mesangiocapillary (membranoproliferative) glomerulonephritis and rheumatoid arthritis. *Br. Med. J.* 1:270, 1977.

345. Tomura, S., Tsutani, K., Sakuma, A., and Takeuchi, J. Discriminant analysis in renal histological diagnosis of primary glomerular diseases. *Clin. Nephrol.* 23:55, 1985.

346. Tornroth, T. Recurrent and de novo glomerulonephritis in allografted kidneys: Aspects of ultrastructural diagnosis. *Appl. Pathol.* 5:88, 1987.

347. Tsuji, T., Imajo, Y., Sawabe, M., Kuniyuki, S., Ishii, M., Hamada, T., Ishimura, E., Hamada, N., Nishisawa, Y., and Morli, H. Acquired cutis laxa concomitant with nephrotic syndrome. *Arch. Dermatol.* 123:1211, 1987.

348. Turner, D. R., Cameron, J. S., Bewick, M., Sharpstone, P., Melcher, P., Ogg, C. S., Evans, D. J., Trafford, A. J. P., and Leibowitz, S. Transplantation in mesangiocapillary glomerulonephritis with intramembranous dense "deposits": Recurrence of disease. *Kidney Int.* 9:439, 1976.

349. Vallota, E. H., Forristal, J., Davis, N. C., and West, C. D. The C3 nephritic factor and membranoproliferative nephritis: Correlation of serum levels of the nephritic factor with C3 levels, with therapy and with progression of the disease. *J. Pediatr.* 80:947, 1972.

350. Vallota, E. H., Forristal, J., Spitzer, R. E., Davis, N. C., and West, C. D. Continuing C3 breakdown after bilateral nephrectomy in patients with membranoproliferative glomerulonephritis. *J. Clin. Invest.* 50:522, 1971.

351. Vallota, E. H., Götze, O., Spiegelberg, H. L., Forristal, J., West, C. D., and Müller-Eberhard, H. J. A serum factor in chronic hypocomplementemic nephritis distinct from immunoglobulins and activating the alternate pathway of complement. *J. Exp. Med.* 139:1249, 1974.

352. van Acker, K. J., van den Brande, J., and Vincke, H. Membranous-proliferative glomerulonephritis. *Helv. Paediatr. Acta* 25:204, 1970.

353. Vargas, A. R., Thomson, K. J., Wilson, D., Cameron, J. S., Turner, D. R., Gill, D. Chantler, C., and Ogg, C. S. Mesangiocapillary glomerulonephritis with dense "deposits" in the basement membranes of the kidney. *Clin. Nephrol.* 5:73, 1976.

354. Velasquez Forero, F., Garcia Prugue, N., and Ruiz Morales, N. Idiopathic nephrotic syndrome of the adult with asymptomatic thrombosis of the renal vein. *Am. J. Nephrol.* 8:457, 1988.

355. Verroust, P. J., Wilson, C. B., and Dixon, F. J. Lack of nephrogenicity of systemic activation of the alternate complement pathway. *Kidney Int.* 6:157, 1974.

356. Waldo, F. B., and West, C. D. Quantitation of $(C1INH)_2$ C1r-C1s complexes in glomerulonephritis as an indicator of C1 activation. *Clin. Immunol. Immunopathol.* 42:239, 1987.

357. Walker, J. F., O'Neil, S., Campbell, E., Browne, O., Doyle, G., Carmody, M., and O'Dwyer, W. F. Carcinoma of the oesophagus associated with membranoproliferative glomerulonephritis. *Postgrad. Med. J.* 57:592, 1981.

358. Wank, R., Schendel, D. J., O'Neill, G. J., Riethmüller, G., Held, E., and Feucht, H. E. Rare variant of complement C4 is seen in high frequency in patients with primary glomerulonephritis. *Lancet* 1:872, 1984.

359. Warady, B. A., Guggenheim, S. J., Sedman, A., and Lum, G. M. Prednisone therapy of membranoproliferative glomerulonephritis in children. *J. Pediatr.* 107:702, 1985.

360. Watson, A. R., Poucell, S., Thorner, P., Arbus, G. S., Rance, C. P., and Baumal, R. Membranoproliferative glomerulonephritis type I in children: Correlation of clinical features with pathologic subtypes. *Am. J. Kidney Dis.* 4:141, 1984.

361. Weidner, N., and Lorentz, W. B., Jr. Three-dimensional studies of acellular glomerular basement membranes in dense-deposit disease. *Virchows Arch.* [A] 409:595, 1986.

362. Welch, T. R., Beischel, L., Balakrishnan, K., Quinlan, M., and West, C. D. Major histocompatibility complex extended haplotypes in membranoproliferative glomerulonephritis. *N. Engl. J. Med.* 314:1476, 1986.

363. Welch, T. R., and Berry, A. C3 alleles in diseases associated with C3 activation. *Dis. Markers* 5:81, 1987.

364. Welch, T. R., Kleesattel, A., and Beischel, L. Inhibition of immune complex solubilization by sera of patients with membranoproliferative glomerulonephritis. *Clin. Exp. Immunol.* 72:103, 1988.

365. West, C. D. Childhood membranoproliferative

glomerulonephritis: An approach to management (clinical conference). *Kidney Int.* 29:1077, 1986.
366. West, C. D. Membranoproliferative hypocomplementemic glomerulonephritis. *Nephron* 11:134, 1973.
367. West, C. D. Pathogenesis and approaches to therapy of membranoproliferative glomerulonephritis. *Kidney Int.* 9:1, 1976.
368. West, C. D., and McAdams, A. J. Serum beta-1c globulin levels in persistent glomerulonephritis with low serum complement: Variability unrelated to clinical course. *Nephron* 7:193, 1970.
369. West, C. D., McAdams, A. J., McConville, J. M., Davis, N. C., and Holland, N. H. Hypocomplementemic and normocomplementemic persistent (chronic) glomerulonephritis: Clinical and pathologic characteristics. *J. Pediatr.* 67:1089, 1965.
370. West, C. D., McEnery, P. T., and McAdams, A. J. Experience with Alternate-Day Prednisone in the Management of Forty-Five Children with Membranoproliferative Glomerulonephritis (MPGN). In K. Murakami, T. Kitagawa, K. Yabuta, and T. Sakai (Eds.), *Recent Advances in Pediatric Nephrology.* New York: Excerpta Medica, 1987. P. 81.
371. West, C. D., Ruley, E. J., Spitzer, R. E., and Davis, N. C. The Natural History of Membranoproliferative Glomerulonephritis: Its Relation to the Hypocomplementemia. In P. Kincaid-Smith, T. H. Mathew, and E. L. Becker (Eds.), *Glomerulonephritis: Morphology, Natural History, and Treatment,* Part 1. New York: Wiley, 1973. P. 531.
372. West, C. D., Winter, S., Forristal, J., McConville, J. M., and Davis, N. C. Evidence for in vivo breakdown of beta-1c-globulin in hypocomplementemic glomerulonephritis. *J. Clin. Invest.* 46:539, 1967.
373. Westberg, N. G., Naff, G. B., Boyer, J. T., and Michael, A. F. Glomerular deposition of properdin in acute and chronic glomerulonephritis with hypocomplementemia. *J. Clin. Invest.* 50:642, 1971.
374. Whaley, K., Ward, D., and Ruddy, S. Modulation of the properdin amplification loop in membranoproliferative and other forms of glomerulonephritis. *Clin. Exp. Immunol.* 35:101, 1979.
375. Williams, D. G., Bartlett, A., and Duffus, P. Identification of nephritic factor as an immunoglobulin. *Clin. Exp. Immunol.* 33:425, 1978.
376. Williams, D. G., Garcia-Fuentes, M., and Losito, A. Cryoglobulinemia in mesangiocapillary glomerulonephritis (Abstract). In *Proceedings of the Seventh International Congress on Nephrology, Montreal, Canada, June 18–23, 1978.* P. G-11.
377. Williams, D. G., Peters, D. K., Fallows, J., Petrie, A., Kourilsky, O., Morel-Maroger, L., and Cameron, J. S. Studies of serum complement in the hypocomplementaemic nephritides. *Clin. Exp. Immunol.* 18:391, 1974.
378. Williams, R. C., Jr., and Kunkel, H. G. Rheumatoid factor, complement and conglutinin aberrations in patients with subacute bacterial endocarditis. *J. Clin. Invest.* 41:666, 1962.
379. Woodroffe, A. J., Border, W. A., Theofilopoulos, A. N., Götze, O., Glassock, R. J., Dixon, F. J., and Wilson, C. B. Detection of circulating immune complexes in patients with glomerulonephritis. *Kidney Int.* 12:268, 1977.
380. Wyatt, R. J., McAdams, A. J., Forristal, J., Snyder, J., and West, C. D. Glomerular deposition of complement-control proteins in acute and chronic glomerulonephritis. *Kidney Int.* 16:505, 1979.
381. Yamashina, M., Takami, T., Kanemura, T., Orii, T., and Ojima, A. Immunohistochemical demonstration of complement components in formalin-fixed and paraffin embedded renal tissues. *Lab. Invest.* 60:311, 1989.
382. Yen, B. P., Young, H. F., Schatzki, P. F., and Bear, E. S. Immune complex disease associated with an infected ventriculojugular shunt: A curable form of glomerulonephritis. *South. Med. J.* 70: 1141, 1977.
383. Yoshikawa, N., Truong, L. D., Mattioli, C. A., and Lederer, E. Membranoproliferative glomerulonephritis in Takayasu's arteritis. *Am. J. Nephrol.* 8:240, 1988.
384. Yoshikawa, N., Yoshiara, S., Yoshiya, K., Matsuo, T., Matsuyama, S., and Okada, S. Focal and diffuse membranoproliferative glomerulonephritis in children. *Am. J. Nephrol.* 8:102, 1988.
385. Young, G. B., Sales, D. I., Waddington, D., Angus, K. W., and Gardiner, A. C. Genetic aspects of mesangiocapillary glomerulonephritis in Finnish sheep. *Br. Vet. J.* 137:368, 1981.
386. Zamurovic, D., and Churg, J. Idiopathic and secondary mesangiocapillary glomerulonephritis. *Nephron* 38:145, 1984.
387. Zell, S. C., Duxbury, G., and Shankel, S. W. Alveolar hemorrhage associated with a membranoproliferative glomerulonephritis and smooth muscle antibody. *Am. J. Med.* 82:1073, 1987.
388. Zhang, P. F., Rao, K. V., and Anderson, W. R. An ultrastructural study of the membranoproliferative variant of transplant glomerulopathy. *Ultrastruct. Pathol.* 12:185, 1988.
389. Zimmerman, S. W., Hyman, L. R., Uehling, D. T., and Burkholder, P. M. Recurrent membranoproliferative glomerulonephritis with glomerular properdin deposition in allografts. *Ann. Intern. Med.* 80:169, 1974.

390. Zimmerman, S. W., Moorthy, A. V., Dreher, W. H., Friedman, A., and Varanasi, U. Prospective trial of warfarin and dipyridamole in patients with membranoproliferative glomerulonephritis. *Am. J. Med.* 75:920, 1983.
391. Zucchelli, P., Sasdelli, M., Cagnoli, L., Donini, U., Casanova, S., and Rovinetti, C. Membranoproliferative glomerulonephritis: Correlations between immunological and histological findings. *Nephron* 17:449, 1976.
392. Zunin, C., Castellani, A., Olivetti, G., Marini, G., and Gabriele, P. W. Membranoproliferative glomerulonephritis associated with infected ventriculoatrial shunt: Report of two cases recovered after removal of the shunt. *Pathologica* 69:297, 1977.

Melvin M. Schwartz

8 Membranous Glomerulonephritis

BACKGROUND

Membranous glomerulonephritis (MGN) is a morphologic diagnosis that describes a glomerular disease characterized by a spectrum of changes in the glomerular basement membrane (GBM) initiated by the formation of subepithelial immune aggregates. This pathologic picture is usually not accompanied by glomerular proliferation or infiltration by inflammatory cells. Although the etiology of MGN is unknown in most cases, the immunopathology of the human disease and its congruence with several forms of immunologically mediated experimental glomerulonephritis (GN) support the notion of an immunologic pathogenetic mechanism. If the immune deposits are large and bulky, or the underlying basal lamina of the glomerular capillary wall is increased in thickness, the changes are readily appreciated by light microscopy using the methenamine silver–periodic acid–Schiff stain (Jones). However, if the deposits are small and the basal lamina is relatively normal, electron and/or immunofluorescence microscopy may be required to make the diagnosis. The frequent subtlety of the light microscopic diagnosis of MGN explains much of the confusion that surrounded the concept of MGN during its evolution as a discrete pathologic entity [14]. Until its histopathology was established, the natural history, outcome, and therapeutic responsiveness of MGN remained unknown. Since the clinical presentation of MGN is frequently indistinguishable from other glomerular lesions, a careful pathologic description of the lesion using light, immunofluorescence, and electron microscopy is the starting point for any rational discussion of prognosis, natural history, or therapy.

MGN is the most common cause of the nephrotic syndrome in adults, and although it occurs less frequently in children, many cases in childhood also have been reported [92,93,236,237]. MGN is most common in a primary or idiopathic form. It also occurs secondary to other conditions, and the medical literature is replete with case reports detailing its anectdotal associations. It is tempting to construct an encyclopedic list of associated conditions, but the variety of diagnoses linked to MGN minimizes the fact that in most instances the relationship is tentative and the etiologic implication is unproven. The negative aspect of casually and uncritically linking diseases and agents to MGN is that purely chance associations, along with genuine misinformation, are promulgated in the medical literature, where they develop a life of their own.

The alleged causal relationship between MGN and the angiotensin-converting enzyme inhibitor captopril is particularly instructive. Following the initial report from the State University of Groningen in Holland [198] of immune complex glomerulopathy occurring in a captopril-treated patient, other reports of an association between captopril therapy and MGN soon appeared. Hoorntje et al. [110] followed their original report with a series of renal biopsies from 13 nonproteinuric hypertensive patients treated for variable periods of time with captopril. Although this series was weighted by the inclusion of the two index cases of captopril-associated MGN, it also contained two other previously unreported patients with regular, granular GBM deposits of immunoglobulins and subepithelial electron-dense deposits. The other 9 patients had "small, sparse, subepithelial, spherical dense bodies" that did not have the usual appearance of immune aggregates. Although the 9 patients were nonproteinuric and had negative immunofluorescence, the authors concluded that in the context of the cases of MGN in the series, the ultrastructural findings supported an etiologic role for captopril in MGN. A subsequent study of patients from the same institution attempted to evaluate the effect of captopril on the pathology of hypertensive patients in a controlled fashion by comparing renal biopsies from hypertensive patients being considered for captopril therapy with those of patients who were treated with captopril for at least 6 months [254]. The authors found that "spherical dense bodies" were equally frequent in both groups, and the absence of a consistent relation with immunofluorescence findings indicated that they were not immune aggregates. Both groups of hypertensive patients had comparable mesangial and arteriolar C3, which was attributed to hypertension. Although the two index cases were confirmed to have MGN and two other treated patients had asymptomatic immune complex disease with mesangial and GBM electron-dense deposits, two of the untreated patients also had preexisting immune complex disease—IgA nephritis (asymptomatic) and MGN (with proteinuria). The authors concluded that renal biopsies from hypertensive patients may reveal ultrastructural and immunopathologic abnormalities that cannot be ascribed to captopril or any other drugs. Because of the real possibility that subclinical glomerular lesions due to preexisting renal disease may be present in the hypertensive population, caution was advised before attributing glomerular disease to drugs in patients in whom the pretreatment status of the kidney is not carefully and completely defined.

Secondary Forms of MGN

Well-established secondary causes of MGN include the autoimmune diseases systemic lupus erythematosus and rheumatoid arthritis, chronic infections (such as secondary syphilis and hepatitis B), drugs (such as penicillamine, gold compounds, and mercury), and miscellaneous conditions, including sarcoidosis, Sjögren syndrome, and carcinoma. MGN secondary to penicillamine and gold is of special pathogenetic interest because the period of exposure to the etiologic agent is historically defined. These disorders are covered in this chapter along with MGN secondary to hepatitis B, sarcoidosis, Sjögren syndrome, carcinoma, and transplantation. MGN associated with SLE is covered in Chapter 13, and the uncommon secondary forms, such as syphilis and mercury, are discussed in Chapters 28 and 31, respectively. However, most cases of MGN remain in a primary or idiopathic form, which will be the primary focus of this chapter.

Nosology

The nosology of MGN is complicated by the preference of some pathologists for such synonymous terms as *membranous nephropathy, epimembranous nephropathy,* and *perimembranous nephropathy.* The designation of MGN is not without problems itself, for the term was originally used to describe a progressive form of glomerular disease distinct from the more obviously inflammatory glomerulonephritides. Early investigators believed the pathology resided in the GBM rather than in the inflammatory nature of the process. Available histologic techniques did not allow the differentiation of MGN and several other pathologic conditions, including minimal change glomerulonephropathy and its variants and certain forms of chronic glomerulonephritis. The presence of immunoglobulin and complement components in the glomerular deposits and the C5b-9 membrane attack complex in the glomeruli and urine of patients with MGN [47,220] is convincing evidence implicating the inflammatory process. Thus the central role of inflammation in the pathogenesis of MGN is acknowledged by retaining the designation MGN throughout this chapter.

IDIOPATHIC MEMBRANOUS GLOMERULONEPHRITIS

Clinical Features

MGN is seen throughout adult life, with a peak incidence in the fourth and fifth decades [21,43, 64,65,82,85,106,111,126,158,172,179,194,215], and males are more commonly afflicted in both adults [21,53,64,65,73,78,82,85,106,111,126, 158,172,179,193,194,201,215] and children [37, 93,263].

The most common clinical presentation of MGN is the *nephrotic syndrome,* with most series reporting a prevalence of from 60 to 100 percent, but in fact, a significant percentage of patients with MGN present with *asymptomatic proteinuria* or *abnormal urinalysis,* reported in various series to range from 7 to 54 percent [15,37,65,73,78,82, 85,93,105,107,126,172,180,193,200,201,263]. In our series of 64 adults with idiopathic MGN, we found that 37.5 percent presented with asymptomatic proteinuria [279]. Obviously, the proportion of patients with asymptomatic proteinuria varies with the intensity of screening for renal disease. Beregi and Varga [15] utilized extensive screening of children and adults for renal disease and found that almost 50 percent of patients with MGN had only proteinuria or hematuria. Kida et al. [126] reported that 40.4 percent of their patients with MGN were not initially nephrotic. They attributed this high incidence to a nationwide screening program and a government-controlled medical insurance system. Of 50 children reported by Habib et al. [93], 27 had proteinuria discovered by routine urinalysis. These observations suggest that a large pool of patients with MGN exists that comes to clinical attention accidentally, if at all. This has important implications for the natural history of MGN, because prognosis, histologic healing of the GBM, resolution of proteinuria, and response to therapy have all been related to the level of proteinuria at the time of diagnosis. Epidemiologic considerations led Mallick et al. [157] to suggest that the prevalence of MGN is much greater than that derived from biopsy reports and transplantation registries. The existence of many patients with asymptomatic MGN implies that we only know about the patients with the most severe proteinuria and progressive forms of MGN, and we must be prepared to temper our conclusions about the clinical course of MGN with the knowledge that more inclusive series may have a different prognosis related to a more benign clinical course.

Much of the clinical literature on MGN is devoted to the search for the constellation of clinical and laboratory features that will unequivocally separate MGN from the other glomerular lesions that cause the idiopathic nephrotic syndrome. *Microscopic hematuria* accompanies proteinuria in the majority of patients (range 25 to 85 percent) [70,42,82,85,93,107,172,180,191,199,201,215], but *gross hematuria* is less common (1 to 17 percent) [42,102,201,215]. In contrast, hematuria, either gross or microscopic, is a very uncommon presenting feature (2 to 18 percent) [93,102,172]. *Renal function,* measured as the serum creatinine level, is abnormal in approximately one-half of patients when MGN is initially detected [53,70, 78,81,85,93,126,191,201,215], but renal failure is the presenting problem in only occasional patients (1 to 10 percent) [37,172,263]. Shemesh et al. [227], using inulin clearances, found decreased GFR in 75 percent of patients with MGN (GFR < 80 ml/min/1.73 m^2). It was depressed to approximately one-half the value of normal controls (58 $\pm$ 7 versus 109 $\pm$ 3 ml/min/1.73 m^2, $p < 0.001$). From 17 to 50 percent of adult patients have *hypertension* when MGN is initially diagnosed [21,42,64,65,70,78,83,85,107,111,172,180, 191,193,194,200,201,215]. When a patient with MGN presents to a physician, he or she has clinical evidence of glomerular disease, and the hypertension and loss of renal function suggest that it is chronic. The nonspecific nature of these features has led to a more critical evaluation of urinary protein excretion.

The relative excretion of albumin and larger serum proteins is called *selectivity,* and diseases with greater anatomic distortion of the GBM are expected to have a *nonselective* type of proteinuria in which the large serum proteins are found in the urine along with albumin. In fact, several studies have shown a loss of selectivity in patients with MGN [37,43,93,193,215], and this is different from patients with minimal-change disease, who retain selectivity in the face of massive proteinuria [34]. Shemesh et al. [227] determined the fractional clearances of neutral dextrans (radius 28–48 Å) and glomerular filtration data in patients with MGN and in controls and applied the results to a heteroporous model of the glomerular capillary wall. This model assumes that most of the glomerular capillary wall is perforated by identical small pores that do not filter macromolecules and that there is a "shunt" pathway (nonselective) that does not discriminate among macromolecules on the basis of size. The authors found that the fraction of the filtrate permeating the shunt pathway was three to four times greater than in controls, and that it correlated strongly in individual patients with elevations of the fractional clearances of both IgG and albumin. This study supports the contention that selectivity is lost in MGN, although the same authors have shown expansion of the nonselective shunt pathway in other glomerular diseases. Thus selectivity appears to separate minimal-change disease from MGN, but since loss of selectivity is a feature of other causes of the nephrotic syndrome, its presence does not uniquely identify the patient with MGN.

CLINICAL IMMUNOLOGY

The immunopathology of MGN has prompted a search for serologic evidence of immune dysfunction. *Serum complement* levels are usually normal [78,85,93,215]. *Circulating immune complexes* are present in some patients with MGN [2,24], but attempts to identify a specific antigen have, in general, been unsuccessful (see below). A number of case reports and short series have demonstrated circulating immune complexes in individual patients with MGN, often in association with hepatitis B antigenemia [132,277]. On the other hand, Collins et al. [44] were unable to detect circulating immune complexes (Raji cell assay) in six patients with idiopathic MGN. In a larger study, Zager et al. [282] found circulating immune complexes in 6 of 26 patients with MGN (Raji cell assay), but 5 of the 6 had another medical condition that might also have explained the immune complex activity (malignancy, 2; renal vein thrombosis, 1; transplantation, 1; SLE, 1). Abrass et al. [2] found circulating immune complexes by any of three assays (fluid- and solid-phase C1q binding and Raji cell assays) in 26 of 55 patients with idiopathic MGN ($p < 0.001$ compared with controls), but the presence of complexes did not predict remission of the nephrotic syndrome or decline of renal function, and did not differentiate MGN from minimal change disease or focal glomerular disease. Cairns et al. [30] found circulating immune complexes at some time in 94 percent of MGN patients using any one of four assays, but the presence of circulating immune complexes did not separate MGN from other forms of idiopathic glomerular disease, including minimal change disease, Schönlein-Henoch syndrome, and mesangial proliferative glomerulonephritis. Although one early report failed to demonstrate circulating immune complexes in patients with MGN, the same authors did find circulating immune complexes in a subpopulation with renal vein thrombosis [185]. Finally, Cairns et al. [29] observed that there was no correlation, either quantitative or qualitative, between circulating immune complexes and glomerular immune deposits.

Other abnormalities of the immune system in patients with MGN include prolongation of the half-life of sensitized erythrocytes that correlates with exacerbation of proteinuria and declines during remission [18], various alterations in T cell subsets and $CD4^+$-$CD8^+$ ratios (reviewed by Honkanen et al. [108]), decreased synthesis of IgG and IgM by peripheral blood lymphocytes when stimulated by pokeweed mitogen [185], defective in vitro T cell colony formation [160], and impaired lymphocyte and suppressor-cell function [251]. Rocatello et al. [210] demonstrated Fc receptor dysfunction of splenic macrophages in 7 of 19 patients with idiopathic MGN. Although HLA-B8 and DR3 antigens were significantly more frequent in patients than in controls, the authors found no relationship between Fc receptor dysfunction and any HLA antigen tested. Although this catalog of immune dysfunction is not diagnostically helpful at present, it does raise the possibility that in idiopathic MGN there is an underlying immunologic defect based on genetic susceptibility.

GENETIC ASPECTS

The importance of the individual's genetic composition is supported by reports of family members with MGN [219,229], and more definitive evidence is derived from population studies that have shown an increased incidence of discrete HLA antigens in patients with MGN. In England, Klouda et al. [128] found HLA-DR3 in 75 percent of patients with MGN compared with 20 percent of controls ($p = 0.000014$). Subsequently, the same group of investigators reported that HLA-B18 [29] and the rare properdin factor B allotype Bf1 [67] also were associated with MGN, and patients with the superphenotype HLA-B18, DR3, and Bf1 progressed rapidly to renal failure [228]. In France, Berthoux et al. [18] found a similar association between MGN and DR3, and while not finding an association with HLA-B18, 65.38 percent of MGN patients had the HLA-B8 antigen compared with 27 percent of the local controls. Müller et al. [170] from Germany found an association with DR3, but like the French group, they found no association with HLA-B18 or Bf1. In Japan, Tomura et al. [257] have reported an association between DR2 and MT1 B cell alloantigens in patients with MGN, and Abe et al. [1] concluded that the better prognosis reported for MGN in Japanese patients is related to genetic differences. In northeast England, Papiha et al. [188] found a preponderance of HLA-B8 and DR3 antigens in patients with idiopathic MGN, and the occurrence of the superphenotype DR3 B8 alleles in the BfSS homozygotes also was more common in MGN than in controls. The authors identified 6 of 55 patients with DR3-B8 and common Bf*S alleles who had a significantly worse course. They concluded that idiopathic MGN is not a single disease but a lesion that results from several combinations of genetic predispositions and environmental stimuli.

Demaine et al. [55] showed an association between immunoglobulin (Gm) allotype frequencies and MGN. Using restriction fragment length polymorphism analysis with probes for the T cell antigen receptor constant beta-chain genes and immunoglobulin heavy chain switch region genes, they also demonstrated that HLA-DR–typed MGN patients have specific polymorphisms associated with these loci [56].

None of these genetic findings explains the susceptibility to develop MGN, but the variability documented among different populations suggests that genetic susceptibility is unique in each and supports the concept that the genetic makeup of the individual is an important determinant in the pathogenesis of MGN. Genetic studies should be considered when family members are affected with MGN, and the possibility of a genetic susceptibility also should be considered in patients with secondary forms of MGN in whom presumably similar antigenic stimuli are associated with the glomerular lesion in only a small proportion of the cases (e.g., carcinoma, hepatitis B antigenemia, gold, and penicillamine). Furthermore, in evaluating the results of therapeutic trials, it must be recognized that genetically homogeneous populations may have a unique natural history.

Despite the intriguing possibilities raised by the clinical features of the patient with MGN, the renal biopsy remains the definitive technique for differentiating MGN from the other causes of the idiopathic nephrotic syndrome. In children, a therapeutic trial with steroids is useful as a diagnostic maneuver because steroid-responsive minimal change glomerulopathy causes most of the cases of the nephrotic syndrome. However, the risk-benefit ratio is reversed in adults, in whom MGN and other nonresponsive lesions comprise 75 percent of the lesions, and a trial is no longer a tenable therapeutic approach [148].

Clinical Course

MGN is a morphologic pattern of glomerular injury seen with different diseases, and its natural history may be affected by several factors, including the underlying disease, therapy, and the severity of the glomerular pathology of the cases included in the study. In the secondary forms, the underlying disease affects the clinical outcome. In lupus MGN, an indolent renal course is the rule unless there is superimposed glomerular proliferation and activity, in which case the patient will have a much more acute and unfavorable outcome [222]. In MGN secondary to drugs and infections, removal of the etiologic agent frequently leads to resolution of the clinical signs of MGN as well as the morphologic lesion. These examples emphasize that the diagnosis of MGN covers a heterogeneous group of diseases. Thus, in idiopathic MGN, morphologic homogeneity should not be equated with etiologic identity, and the various outcomes seen may be a function of as yet unrecognized differences in etiology rather than individual variability in response to a single stimulus.

Although the therapeutic efficacy of steroids is controversial (see below), their clinical introduction coincided with the recognition of MGN as a separate morphologic entity, and most series contain a mixture of treated and untreated patients. The possibility that therapy has an effect on outcome cannot be totally ignored. The method of case finding also may have profound effects on the natural history of the patients in a series (see above). When patients are identified by screening asymptomatic individuals, it is possible that an entirely different spectrum of disease will be selected compared with studies dominated by the symptomatic nephrotic patient. With these caveats in mind, we may turn to the published series. Row et al. [215] reviewed 12 series published before 1975 containing 435 adults (greater than 15 years old) and 82 children. These are included in references 37, 70, 73, 76, 78, 85, 93, 182, and 194. Since some of these patients were treated with steroids, the results are not strictly comparable with those of later reports of untreated adults (see below). Male preponderance was present in both adults (61 percent) and children (70 percent), and nephrotic syndrome was the most common presentation (adults, 85 percent; children, 79 percent). Adults with MGN had a worse outcome than children. Two-hundred and seven adults and 29 children were followed for 5 years or until death, and 82 adults (19 percent) and only 4 children (4 percent) died of renal failure. Remissions with complete loss of proteinuria were more frequent in children (49 percent) than in adults (16 percent), and 50 percent of the adult remissions and 67 percent of the remissions in children were spontaneous.

A graphic presentation of the progressive nature of MGN is given in Figure 8-1, which is constructed from various series reported up to 1976 [32]. Survival in the figure includes the patients who are alive with or without persistent proteinuria and/or renal insufficiency but are not maintained on dialysis or by renal transplantation. With the exception of one series [93], these are

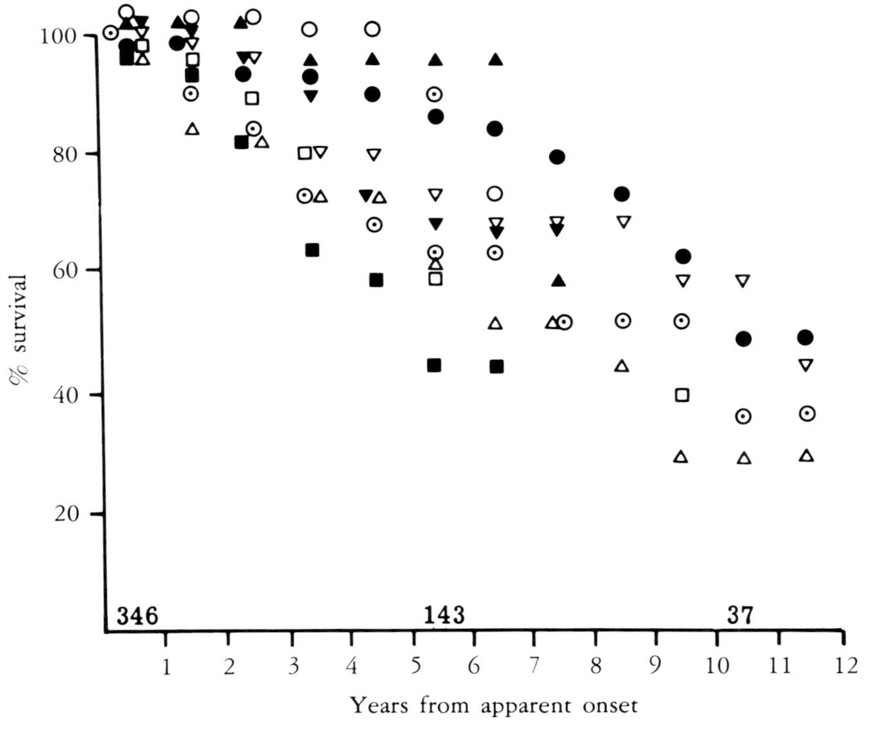

Fig. 8-1. *Survival of patients with biopsies showing membranous glomerulonephritis. The figures at the bottom of the diagram show the number of patients still being followed at that point. The following series of patients have been included, and for each series, the survival has been calculated using the life-table method:* ▲ [93]; ○ [194]; ▼ [76]; ▽ [73]; ⊙ [85]; ● [215]; ■ [97]; □ [70]; △ [78]. *(From Cameron, J. S. In D. Black, and N. F. Jones (Eds.),* Renal Disease, *4th Ed. Oxford: Blackwell, 1979; used by permission.)*

predominantly adults. The progressive nature of MGN is indicated by the substantial proportion of patients in all series who are dead, on dialysis, or have received a transplant by 10 years. Figure 8-2 is an actuarial survival curve of 35 of Cameron's patients followed for more than 10 years. Despite the chronic course, after 10 years, the number of deaths attributable to renal failure remains low and constant, while a significant proportion of the patients have achieved a complete or partial remission by the same time.

COURSE OF UNTREATED MGN

The natural history of idiopathic MGN may be determined definitively from the studies that have followed large numbers of untreated patients, frequently as the control arm of a clinical trial. Davison et al. [53] followed 64 untreated adult patients (male-to-female ratio 47 : 17) with MGN to terminal renal failure or for a minimum of 2 years (range 2–15 years). During follow-up, there was no deterioration of renal function in 30 patients (48 percent). In 27 patients (43.5 percent) there was a steady decline in renal function, taking an average of 30 months (range 5–60) for the serum creatinine level to reach 400 μmol/liter. None of the 14 patients whose serum creatinine level was normal 5 years after biopsy demonstrated any deterioration of renal function during subsequent follow-up.

Noël et al. [180] reported 116 patients (only 7 were less than 16 years old) with a mean age of 37.6 years. There were 60 males and 56 females. At the time of diagnosis, 75.8 percent had the nephrotic syndrome and 24.2 percent had asymptomatic proteinuria. Microscopic hematuria was frequent (55 percent), but none had gross hematuria. Twenty-nine patients had hypertension diagnosed during the course of MGN, but only 17 where hypertensive when MGN was originally diagnosed. Five of the initially hypertensive patients

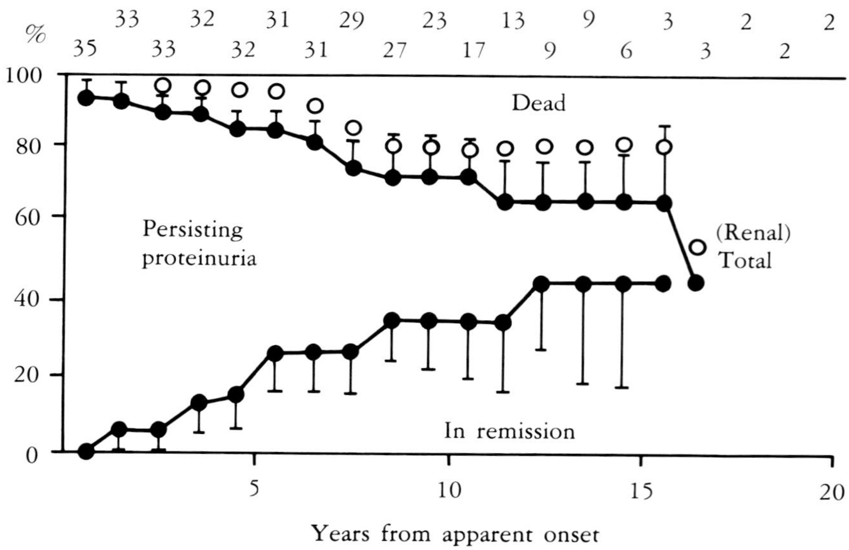

FIG. 8-2. *Actuarial curve of 35 patients with membranous glomerulonephritis. Open circles represent deaths from renal failure; closed circles on upper line, the total deaths; and closed circles on lower line, the patients in remission. Figures at top represent numbers of patients still being followed at various time intervals. (Courtesy of Dr. J. S. Cameron.)*

also had renal insufficiency at the time of diagnosis, and 3 more developed renal insufficiency over the following 12 to 18 months. Despite the implication that hypertension is an adverse prognostic sign, 9 hypertensive patients did not develop renal insufficiency during 2 to 6 years of follow-up, and clinical remission occurred in 3. There was a mean follow-up of 4.5 years, and the actuarial survival at 10 years was 76 percent. In this group, none of whom received corticosteroids or immunosuppressive therapy, 23.4 percent went into remission with normal renal function and urine sediment. The remissions occurred from 1 to 20 years after the diagnosis of MGN (mean 5.5 years). Twenty-one of the 27 patients who went into remission had the nephrotic syndrome initially, while 6 had asymptomatic proteinuria. Seventeen of the initially nephrotic patients improved so that they lost edema but remained proteinuric. Improvement occurred a mean of 1.9 years after the onset and was stable without recurrence for 1 to 6 years of follow-up. Renal function decreased ($S_{Cr} > 1.5$ mg/100 ml, or 133 μmol/liter) in 22 patients (17 percent), of whom 20 had the nephrotic syndrome at the onset. Three of 7 with renal insufficiency initially went into terminal renal failure in from 1 to 4 years. Renal insufficiency also developed within 2 months to 6 years after the diagnosis of MGN in 15 patients who initially had normal renal function, and 8 reached end-stage kidney disease 1 to 6 years after the development of chronic renal insufficiency. Overall, 50 percent of the patients presenting with renal insufficiency reached end-stage renal failure, but they comprised only 9.5 percent of all patients. Fifty patients with initially normal renal function were unchanged at the end of follow-up. Nineteen nephrotic and 13 proteinuric patients were followed a mean of 5.5 years (range 1–19 years), and 18 patients were followed less than 1 year.

Donadio et al. [65] reported the natural histories of 89 adult patients with MGN who were not treated with corticosteroids or immunosuppressive drugs. Their age at diagnosis was 50.8 ± 17 (mean ± SD) years, and the male-to-female ratio was 56 : 33. Actuarial survival was 85 percent at 5 years and 75 percent at 10 years, which was not different from a normal control Midwestern population. Survival without death or renal failure was 71 percent at 5 years and 58 percent at 10 years. The follow-up was for a mean of 6.2 years. The outcome of renal function by serum creatinine level showed 60 patients (57 percent) with a stable level (within 0.3 mg/100 ml or 27 μmol/liter of baseline), 16 (18 percent) with a serum creatinine level greater than 5 mg/100 ml or 442 μmol/liter, and 13 (15 percent) with renal insufficiency (S_{Cr} = 2–5 mg/100 ml or 177–442 μmol/liter). The outcome of proteinuria at last follow-up found 41 of 72 (57 percent) in partial or complete remission, 7 (10 percent) with persistent proteinuria, and 24 (33 percent) with persistent nephrotic syndrome. The 16 patients who developed end-stage kidney disease took 3.9 ± 1.4 years (mean ± SD). A subgroup of 11 patients who went into renal failure in 2.5 years or less was identified. Multivariate analysis showed that progression in this group was significantly associated with initial level of serum creatinine, initial 24-hour urinary protein excretion, and serum triglyceride concentration. The 89 untreated patients were compared with a prednisone-treated group, and there were no differences in any of the outcome parameters.

Cattran et al. [36] conducted a prospective, randomized study in patients with biopsy-confirmed MGN who received either no specific therapy or 6 months of alternate-day prednisone. The untreated control group had an interval of 16.8 ± 1.0 months (mean ± SEM) from the time of detection of a renal abnormality to study entry, and the interval from renal biopsy to entry into the study was 9.3 months. Although these intervals suggest the disease was present for a relatively long time before study entry, there was no difference between the untreated controls (n = 77) and the prednisone-treated patients (n = 81). The period of observation after study entry was 48 ± 3.2 months (mean ± SEM). The actuarial survival of renal function of the untreated controls, in whom a creatinine clearance of less than 0.16 ml/s was used as the end point, showed 94 percent at 5 years and 91 percent at 8 years, and this was not different from the prednisone-treated patients. Nineteen control patients (25 percent) achieved complete remission by 3 years, but 5 subsequently relapsed. Nineteen patients (25 percent) had a sustained increase in S_{Cr} of 25 percent or greater after 5 years, and 4 patients had developed end-stage renal failure. The controls and the prednisone-treated patients were analyzed for the different outcomes of increase in the initial S_{Cr} of 25 percent or greater, mean annual change in the slope of the C_{Cr}, median annual change in the slope of the C_{Cr}, and differences in the percentage of patients with complete or partial remission; no significant differences were found between the two groups. Although not specifically stated, approximately 50 percent of the untreated patients showed no change in function during the study.

A number of points emerge from this wealth of data concerning the natural history of MGN. As seen by nephrologists in medical centers, MGN is an indolent disease that progresses slowly in most cases so that even when renal insufficiency develops it takes years to reach end stage. However, there is a subpopulation that progresses more rapidly (see below under Prognostic Indicators). Approximately 25 percent of patients will experience a complete or partial spontaneous remission, but this may take many years to occur. The chronic nature of MGN is further evidenced by the relapses that are part of the course. Manos et al. [158] reported 8 patients in a series of 60 patients with idiopathic MGN who relapsed after remissions of 25 months to 30 years. Although 3 of these patients remained nephrotic and 1 had mild renal insufficiency at the end of the study, 3 others had gone back into remission. Compared with the patients in the rest of the series, the overall prognosis was not affected by the relapses. Finally, as many as 50 percent of the patients will suffer no significant loss of renal function. The variability of the natural history of MGN, the chronicity of its course, its propensity for spontaneous remissions, and the occurrence of relapses complicate the interpretation of results of clinical trials that have been developed to test various therapeutic regimens. The implications of these observations for the design of clinical therapeutic trials are long follow-up because of the prolonged course to renal failure and/or remission, large differences in outcome between treated and control groups to counter the variability of the course, a homogeneous population (see Prognostic Indicators), and large groups of patients to provide statistical power to the conclusions.

EFFECTS OF THERAPY

Therapy has the potential to affect outcome, shorten the course, and alter the histologic appearance of MGN. It is beyond the scope of this chapter to exhaustively review therapy, but a number of points deserve emphasis. The role of renal biopsy in the current morphologic definition of MGN coincided with the introduction of corticosteroids in the treatment of MGN. Given the natural history of MGN, it is not surprising that uncontrolled trials recorded the occurrence of remissions in treated patients. Despite early optimism for steroid therapy [70], the therapy of MGN remains controversial [203]. Of the first four controlled trials of prednisone used by itself in the treatment of MGN, two [19,163] had insufficient patients to support the essentially negative conclusions. The positive result of the adult collaborative study [43] appears to have occurred because of the very poor outcome obtained by the control group rather than as a real benefit of therapy. In contrast, Cattran et al. [36], Donadio et al. [65], and Cameron et al. [34*a*] reported that prednisone has essentially no effect on the outcome of MGN. The question remains open whether prednisone alters the course of MGN by decreasing the time to remission, but the long-term benefits in terms of preservation of renal function and percentage of patients who achieve remission are not obvious.

Immunosuppressive therapy for MGN had an equally ambiguous history until controlled trials were begun [64]. Recently, an optimistic note has been sounded by Ponticelli et al. [196], who reported their experience with a combination of methylprednisolone and chlorambucil in biopsy-proven adult MGN patients with the nephrotic syndrome followed for a median of 5 years. Forty-two randomly selected patients were given methylprednisolone (0.4 mg/kg of body weight per day) for a month at a time, alternating with a monthly course of chlorambucil (0.2 mg/kg per day) for a total of 6 months. Thirty-nine controls received supportive therapy only. At follow-up, significantly more treated patients had complete or partial remissions compared with untreated controls (67 percent compared with 23 percent). The treated patients had better preservation of renal function when analyzed by the percentage achieving a 50 percent increase in serum creatinine (10 percent compared with 49 percent) or by plotting the reciprocal of the serum creatinine value over time. The treatment group significantly decreased its protein excretion after 6 months of therapy and sustained the decrease for 24 months, while protein excretion remained unchanged in the controls. Four of 41 patients (10 percent) did not tolerate the regimen and had to be taken off the protocol. Although this report leaves little doubt that therapy altered the course of MGN and was effective in inducing early remissions of the nephrotic syndrome, this optimism must be balanced with the realization that the cumulative doses of chlorambucil are in the range that causes gonadal toxicity and neoplasia [148]. Others have tried modifications of the Ponticelli et al. regimen and have found more toxicity and less success in altering the course of MGN [272]. In view of the real and potential toxicity of steroids and immunosuppressive drugs, the controversy that still surrounds the response to therapy, and the natural history of the disease, it is imperative that all therapeutic trials begin with a biopsy-confirmed diagnosis.

Pathologic Changes

GROSS APPEARANCE

The prolonged clinical course and successful medical management of intercurrent illnesses have made the gross examination of the early case of MGN a rare event. In cases reported prior to the histopathologic definition of MGN [70,119], there was sufficient confusion between MGN and other causes of the nephrotic syndrome to cast a shadow of doubt on all the gross descriptions. Ehrenreich and Churg [70] described 10 autopsied cases of histologically confirmed MGN. In patients dying at the height of the nephrotic syndrome without renal insufficiency, the kidneys were large and white with combined weights from the upper limit of normal (300 g) to 450 g or more. Although the opportunity to see such cases seldom presents itself, I have seen the kidneys of a middle-aged woman with MGN who died of metastatic breast cancer. At autopsy, the kidneys weighed 175 g each and had smooth, unscarred surfaces and a pale cortex. When MGN runs its course to end-stage renal failure, there is frequently, but not invariably, contraction of the parenchyma, sometimes with granularity of the surface and prominent corticomedullary arteries. These changes are accentuated in the individual with hypertension. Since the glomerular lesions progress at approximately the same rate in all glomeruli, the hypertrophied nephrons that are characteristic of other forms of chronic glomerular disease are not seen in MGN. This may explain the relatively smooth cortical surface sometimes described even in advanced cases.

MICROSCOPIC FINDINGS

Glomeruli

The pathology of MGN is primarily within the GBM, and the glomerular changes within a biopsy are very homogeneous, showing little variation from one glomerulus to another. On the other hand, because the GBM undergoes evolutionary pathologic changes, its appearance may vary from patient to patient and from one biopsy to another from the same patient, depending on the time at which the sample is taken. An awareness of the spectrum of GBM pathology that falls under the rubric of MGN is essential for the diagnosis, and the interrelationships provide the basis for the pathogenetic theories that will be discussed later (see Evolution of the Glomerular Lesion, below). The changes in the GBM may be subtle, and even with optimally stained thin sections, there are a significant number of biopsies in which diagnostic changes will not be obvious by light microscopy alone. Gärtner [82] found single, scattered, barely visible spikes in 21 percent of 472 cases of MGN, and in 25 cases the changes were so minimal the diagnosis could only be established after immunohistology and/or electron microscopy. The necessity of performing immunofluorescence and electron microscopy is reinforced by the ease with which the diagnosis may be established using these modalities.

The glomerular architecture is usually preserved

with widely patent capillary loops and normal mesangial matrix and cellularity. The normality of the glomeruli may be exaggerated, and the tuft may have a "stiff," perfused appearance (Fig. 8-3). Characteristically, the glomerular capillary wall appears thicker than normal in histologic sections using a variety of stains (Fig. 8-4). Although the GBM itself may appear thickened in hematoxylin and eosin–stained sections, this stain is not reliable for evaluating GBM thickness because it also stains cellular elements and protein deposits in the capillary wall. In most instances, there are demonstrable abnormalities of the GBM in sections stained with methenamine silver–PAS [70] or trichrome stain and viewed at high magnification.

The earliest abnormality is mottling of the GBM in en face sections stained with the methenamine silver–PAS (Fig. 8-5). Although these are the result of indentations in the GBM underlying the subepithelial electron-dense deposits in MGN, Tallqvist et al. [249] have demonstrated similar abnormalities in diseases that do not have electron-dense deposits. Thus they are not specific for MGN. Irregularities in the outer aspect of the GBM resolve into small projections of silver-positive material. Initially, these "spikes" may be small and segmental, and their demonstration may require a careful search under oil immersion. As the lesion progresses, the spikes become large and diffuse, and in some cases the ends of the spikes become enlarged and clubbed (Fig. 8-6). It has been suggested that cases with focal spikes represent either an earlier or a milder form of the disease [93]. This possibility has not been completely excluded, but it should be noted that the immune deposits that correspond to the segmental GBM changes are much more diffusely distributed than would be indicated by the light microscopic changes.

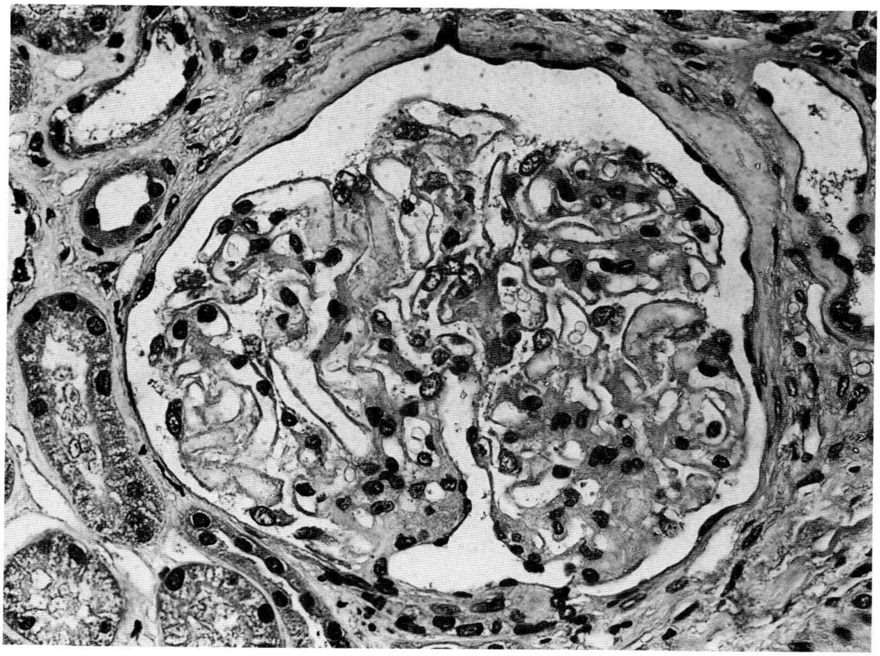

FIG. 8-3. *Early stage of idiopathic membranous glomerulonephritis. The light microscopic appearance is within normal limits, and the glomerular capillary walls are not appreciably thickened. H&E; ×400.*

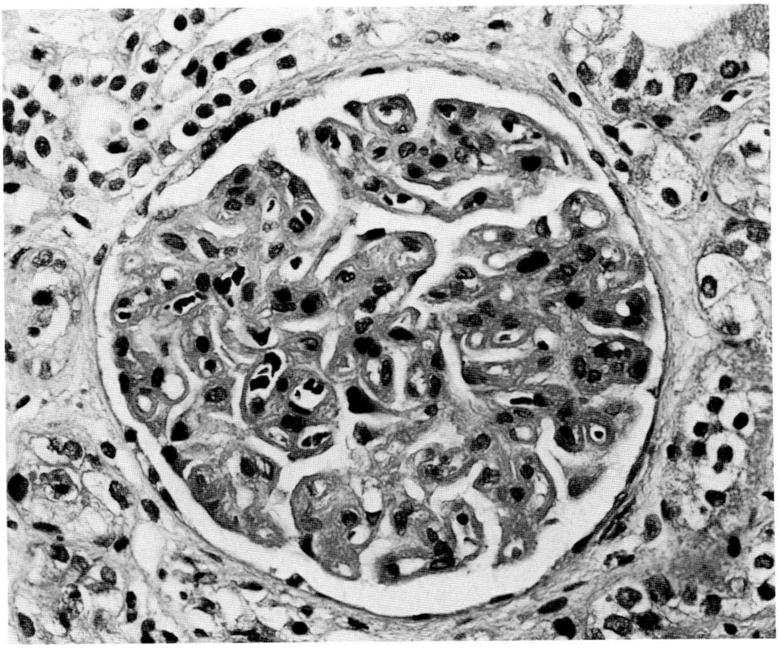

Fig. 8-4. *Diffuse thickening of the glomerular capillary walls becomes obvious by light microscopy in the more advanced stages of idiopathic MGN. Although the mesangial matrix is slightly increased, glomerular cellularity remains normal.* H&E; ×400.

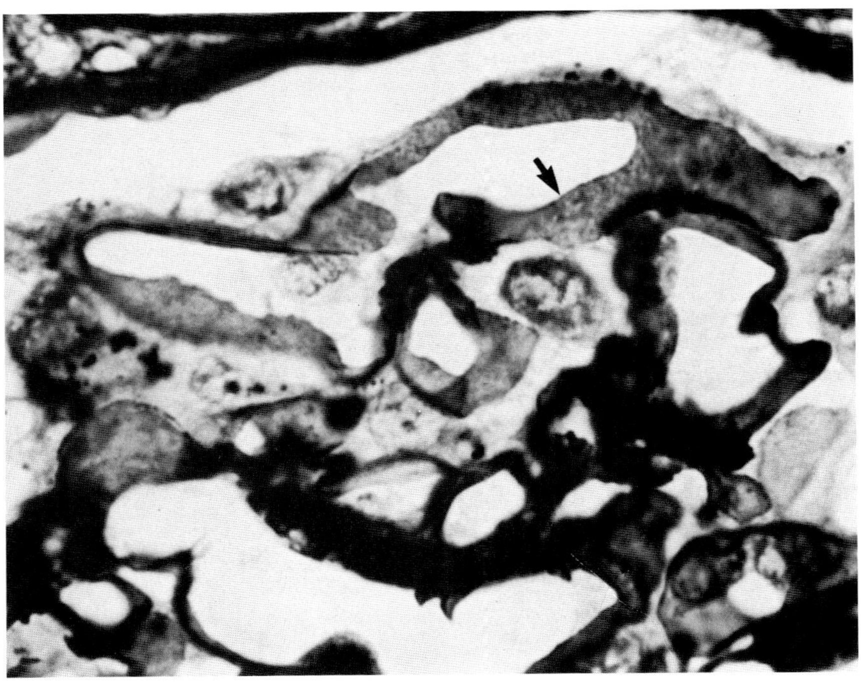

Fig. 8-5. *Early GBM changes in idiopathic MGN seen with a silver impregnation technique are indicated by arrows and include mottling of the staining and scattered pinholes in the en face areas. Methenamine silver–periodic acid–Schiff (Jones);* ×648.

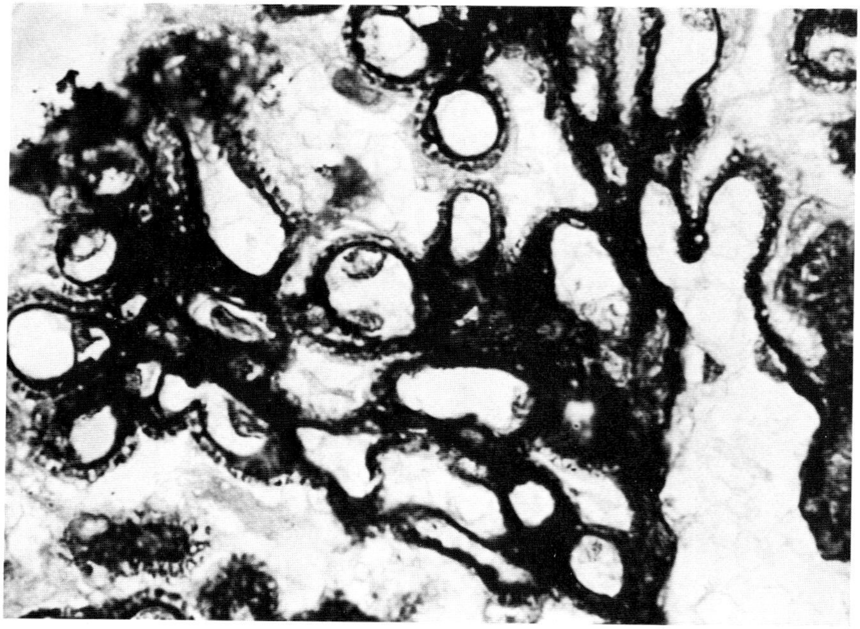

FIG. 8-6. *Light microscopy of a glomerulus from a patient with idiopathic MGN. The diffuse nature of the membranous pathology is indicated by the presence of spikes in every capillary loop. The distal ends of many of the spikes are expanded and club shaped. Methenamine silver–periodic acid–Schiff (Jones);* ×648.

The GBM is also increased in thickness by the inclusion of material that does not take up the silver stain. The nonargyrophilic "holes" are best seen in en face sections of the GBM (Fig. 8-7A), and in some examples their irregular shape imparts a reticular appearance to the tangential sections (Fig. 8-7B). Finally, combinations of these various abnormalities may be seen, with spikes, holes, and complex thickening of the GBM simultaneously present in the same biopsy. The nonargyrophilic material deposited within the GBM and on its epithelial side reacts with histochemical stains that differentiate basement membrane from other proteins. This material stains red with Heidenhain or trichrome stains in contrast to the GBM, which stains blue or green depending on the method used. The deposits also may be demonstrated in toluidine blue–stained 1-μm sections of plastic-embedded tissue (Fig. 8-8). Unfortunately, this helpful feature is not always demonstrable even in obvious cases of MGN, and appears to be related to the size of the protein deposits as well as to their state of aggregation. Thus the primary and consistent histologic abnormality in MGN is in the GBM, and there is no other general morphologic feature.

Other pathologic changes have been described in cases of MGN, and they include glomerular lobulation, mesangial hypercellularity, segmental scars or inflammation, and necrosis. However, these morphologic abnormalities are so unusual that finding them in a renal biopsy should suggest the presence of a systemic disease rather than a morphologic variant of the primary form of MGN. Recently, a few patients have been reported who presented with hematuria and proteinuria; their renal biopsies showed mesangial electron-dense deposits, mesangial deposits of IgA, and MGN

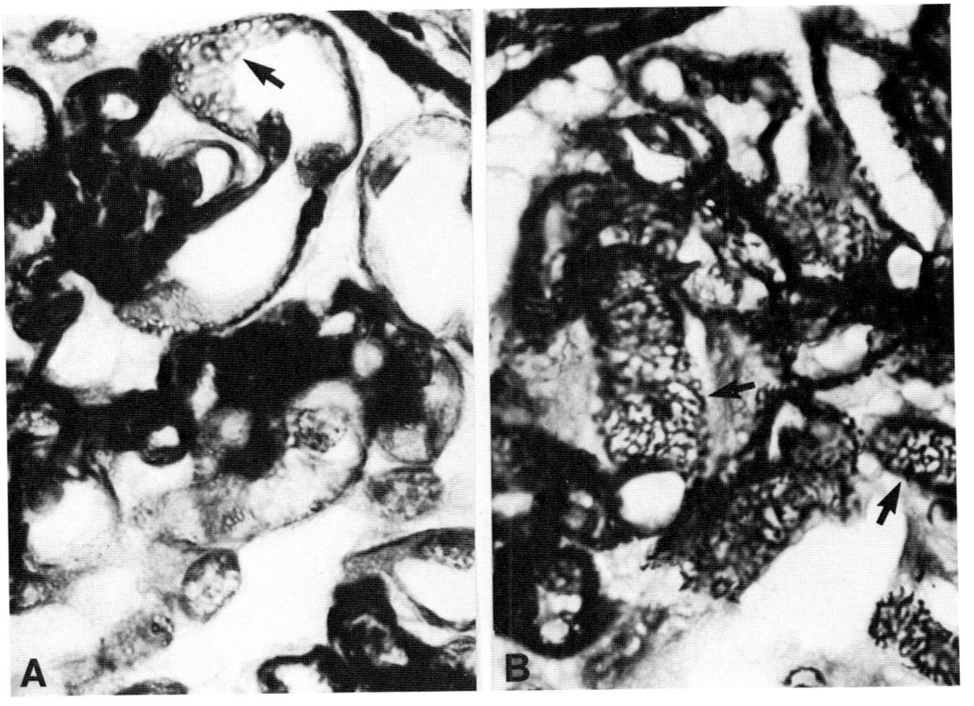

Fig. 8-7. *Light micrograph of a glomerulus from a patient with idiopathic MGN. The deposits of nonargyrophilic material contribute to the thickness of the glomerular basement membrane. (A) In en face sections of the GBM, indicated by arrows, they are seen as holes. In contrast to the minimal changes illustrated in Fig. 8-5, these definite abnormalities are much more suggestive of MGN. (B) Enlargement and confluence of the nonargyrophilic material deposited in the GBM produces a reticular pattern in en face sections (arrows). (A and B) Methenamine silver–periodic acid–Schiff (Jones);* ×720.

[62,117,131]. Since they had no clinical evidence of a systemic disease, the authors interpreted the morphologic findings as an overlap between IgA nephropathy and MGN. Multiple glomerular lesions including MGN were reported by Bertani et al. [17] in a patient with diabetes, amyloidosis, and MGN. In contrast to these sporadic reports, the association of diabetes mellitus with MGN is relatively common [70,130], and the association of MGN with either IgA nephritis in patients with chronic hepatitis B antigenemia or crescentic glomerulonephritis (see below) is well-documented.

The glomeruli in MGN appear larger than normal, and in a morphometric study, Gärtner et al. [83] showed a significant increase in the total glomerular area. Although they also demonstrated an absolute increase in mesangial cells and area, these features are probably related to the increase in glomerular size and are not signs of glomerular injury. In my experience with 64 cases of primary MGN, mesangial hypercellularity was apparent in 3 cases, and it was only moderately increased in the severest case (Fig. 8-9). Global glomerular scarring of a histologically nonspecific nature becomes prominent in advanced cases with renal insufficiency.

A more interesting diagnostic problem is the presence of segmental scars in biopsies from patients with relatively well-preserved renal function

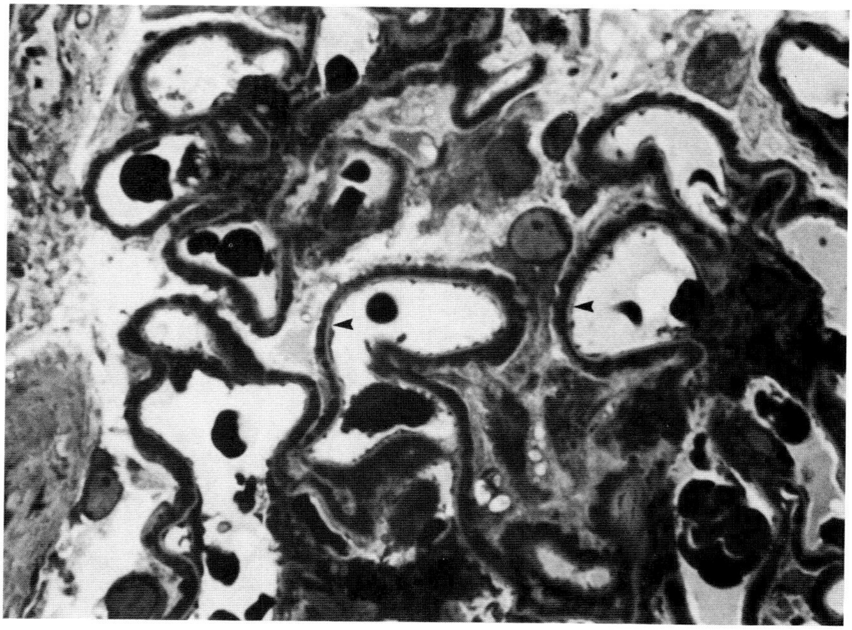

FIG. 8-8. *Light micrograph of a glomerulus from a patient with idiopathic MGN. Diffuse, dark, irregularly sized deposits lie outside the GBM (indicated by a pale continuous line) (arrowheads). Toluidine blue–stained, plastic-embedded, 1-μm section;* ×648.

(Fig. 8-10). In 64 patients with primary MGN [279], we found segmental scars in 12 biopsies, but 7 of the patients had hypertension with azotemia and 1 was uremic. One 18-year-old man presented with hypertension and an S_{Cr} value of 2.1 mg/100 mg (186 μmol/liter), and he progressed to end-stage renal failure in 2.5 years. Despite repeated serologic and clinical evaluations, he had no evidence of SLE until after he went into renal failure and was on maintenance hemodialysis. He then developed hypocomplementemia and a positive ANA test. Three patients had semental scars without hypertension or azotemia: One was a 71-year-old man with 15 g of proteinuria per 24 hours; one was a 40-year-old normotensive man with normal renal function; and one was a 4-year-old normotensive boy with normal renal function. Our results suggest that segmental glomerular scars are occasionally associated with uncomplicated MGN, but it is not known whether they have a prognostic significance separate from hypertension and azotemia (see Prognostic Indicators below). Although segmental lesions are characteristic of systemic diseases such as SLE, it is important to recognize that segmental scars also can occur in idiopathic MGN.

We did not systematically search for clinical or radiographic evidence of renal vein thrombosis (see Chapter 12 for a discussion of the relationship between renal vein thrombosis and MGN). However, it was diagnosed in four patients, and in two there were segmental glomerular capillary thrombi.

Tubules

The tubules are not the primary site of injury in idiopathic MGN. Until progression of glomerular disease results in tubular ischemia with ensuing

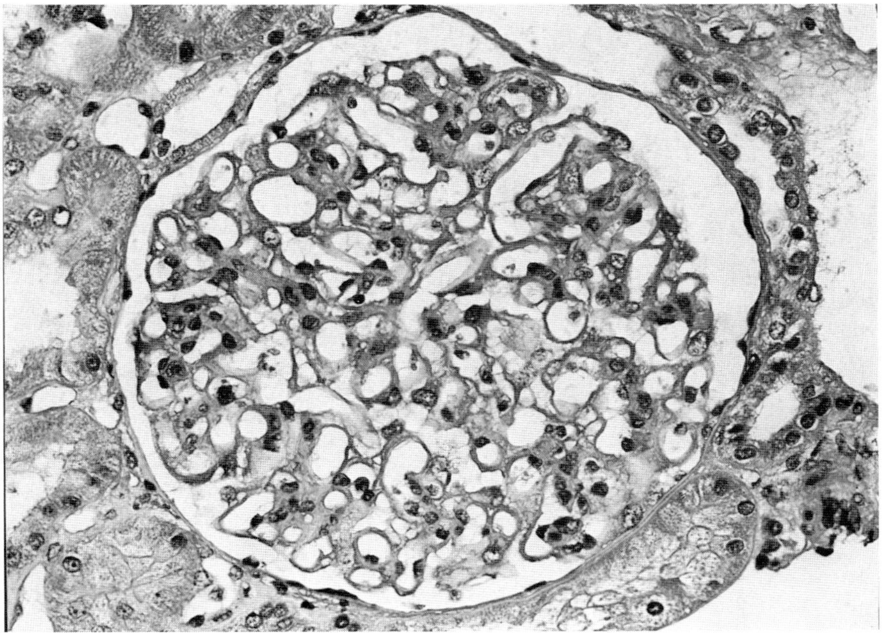

Fig. 8-9. *Light micrograph of a glomerulus from a patient with idiopathic MGN. There is diffuse, moderate mesangial hypercellularity (up to three to four cells per mesangial area) in this otherwise typical case of MGN. H&E;* ×325.

nephron loss, the tubular changes are mainly secondary to reabsorption of filtered plasma proteins and lipoproteins. Hyalin droplet changes represent reabsorption of filtered plasma proteins. Foam cells may be seen either in the interstitium or related to the tubules, and as in other causes of the nephrotic syndrome, they are associated with hyperlipidemia and the reabsorption of filtered lipoproteins. When functionally significant acute tubular injury is seen in MGN, it is usually iatrogenic and related to antibiotic or diuretic therapy. Although there is some evidence linking tubular injury to the pathogenesis of experimental MGN, there is little evidence to support this sequence of events in human beings (see below).

Blood Vessels

Reflecting the older age of the patients with MGN, arterial sclerosis may be seen in the larger arteries. Although hypertension does not always accompany MGN, when it is present, both arterial and arteriolar sclerosis may be prominent. In the absence of systemic disease, vascular inflammation is not seen in MGN.

Interstitium

In uncomplicated MGN, diffuse interstitial fibrosis tends to occur early without prominent interstitial inflammation or tubular atrophy. Although the development of interstitial fibrosis is not dependent on a comparable degree of glomerular obsolescence, it may reflect a generalized decrease in postglomerular perfusion associated with progression of the glomerular lesion. A different pathogenetic mechanism was suggested by Alexopoulos et al. [7], who showed that monocyte/macrophages and lymphocytes were the predominant interstitial cell types, helper/inducer lymphocytes ($CD4^+$) predominated ($CD4^+$-$CD8^+$ ratio 2.2 ± 1.5), and higher numbers of DR-expressing cells

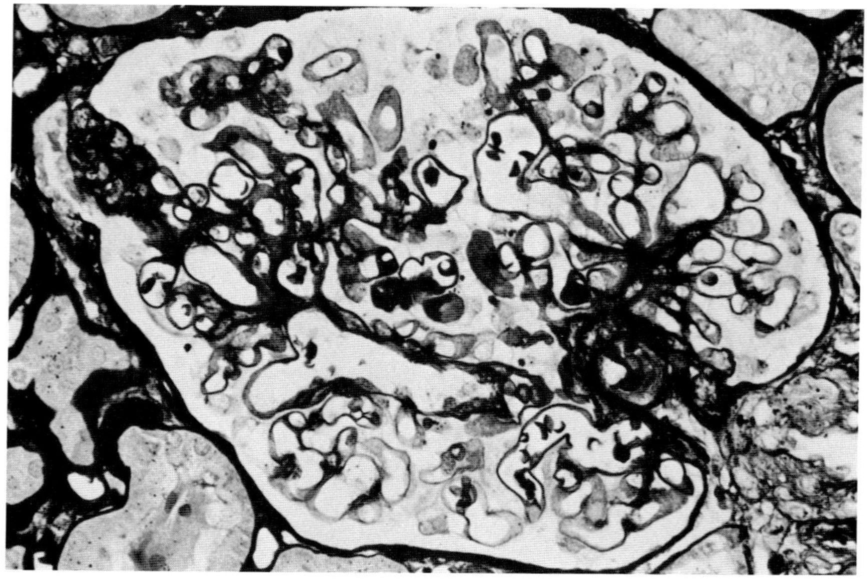

FIG. 8-10. *Light photomicrograph of segmental glomerular sclerosis from a patient with idiopathic MGN. The patient was a 69-year-old black man with a serum creatinine level of 123 μmol/liter and a history of hypertension (180/110 mmHg at the time of the biopsy). Methenamine silver–periodic acid–Schiff (Jones);* ×405

were present in the interstium of renal biopsies from patients with MGN than in controls. The number of cells correlated with the degree of renal impairment at the time of biopsy, but there was no correlation with the degree of tubulointerstitial nephritis. The authors concluded that interstitial monocyte/macrophages were important determinants in the pathogenesis of MGN. Stachura et al. [239] also showed a predominance of T helper/inducer lymphocytes ($CD4^+$) and a $CD4^+$-$CD8^+$ ratio of 2.5 ± 0.9. Honkanen et al. [108] used fine-needle aspiration biopsy of the kidney to show increased numbers of lymphocytes in 24 patients with MGN compared with 7 normal controls and a lowered $CD4^+$-$CD8^+$ ratio in patients (0.96 ± 0.07, mean ± SEM) compared with controls (1.49 ± 0.12, $p < 0.01$) due to a decreased number of $CD4^+$ lymphocytes. This abnormality in lymphocyte subsets in the aspirate was reflected by similar changes in the peripheral blood. In nine patients in whom renal biopsy was studied for the simultaneous presence of interstitial mononuclear cell infiltrates, there was concordance in only four. Although these results suggest a pathogenetic role for mononuclear cell infiltrates in the interstitial lesion of MGN analogous to that shown in Heymann nephritis [246], the absence of a role for renal tubular epithelial antigen in MGN (see below) and the paucity of interstitial infiltrates in most cases of MGN make the significance of these observations unknown.

Cholesterol granulomas have been described and attributed to the hyperlipiduria of the nephrotic syndrome, but this feature is unusual in my experience.

ELECTRON MICROSCOPIC FINDINGS

Electron microscopy clarified the diagnosis of MGN by definitively separating it from other nonproliferative forms of glomerulonephritis and suggesting that the pathogenesis of GBM thickening was related to the characteristic electron-dense deposits in the GBM [12,70,73,78,82,83,85,92, 93,194,197,211,215,238]. Awareness that the electron-dense deposits were present at different levels in the GBM and in different states of aggregation (suggested by variability of electron density of electron-dense deposits; see below) led to the hypothesis that there is a sequence of changes in the GBM following initial subepithelial deposition [70] (see Evolution of the Glomerular Lesion below). The electron-dense deposits in MGN are subepithelial and/or intramembranous. The subepithelial deposits are in contact with the glomerular epithelial cells (GECs), which have fibrillar condensation of the cytoplasm overlying the deposit and diffuse or focal effacement of the foot processes (Fig. 8-11). The subepithelial deposits lie between the GECs and the GBM, and they are accommodated by an indentation in the GEC cytoplasm. In some cases, the GECs appear very active, with increased cytoplasm, active organelles, lipid and protein reabsorption droplets, and microvillous transformation. It has been suggested that the accumulation of subepithelial electron-dense deposits is a sign of defective GEC function [225]. Despite its close proximity to the deposits, there is no convincing evidence that the GEC is capable of ingesting and removing the deposits, despite its considerable phagocytic potential [225]. The corresponding light microscopy may be completely normal or show only mottling of the silver-stained GBM, but scanning electron microscopy of acellular glomeruli shows shallow pits or indentations of the GBM [22,23] (Fig. 8-12).

The deposits vary in size, and although they are usually diffusely distributed along the GBM, some

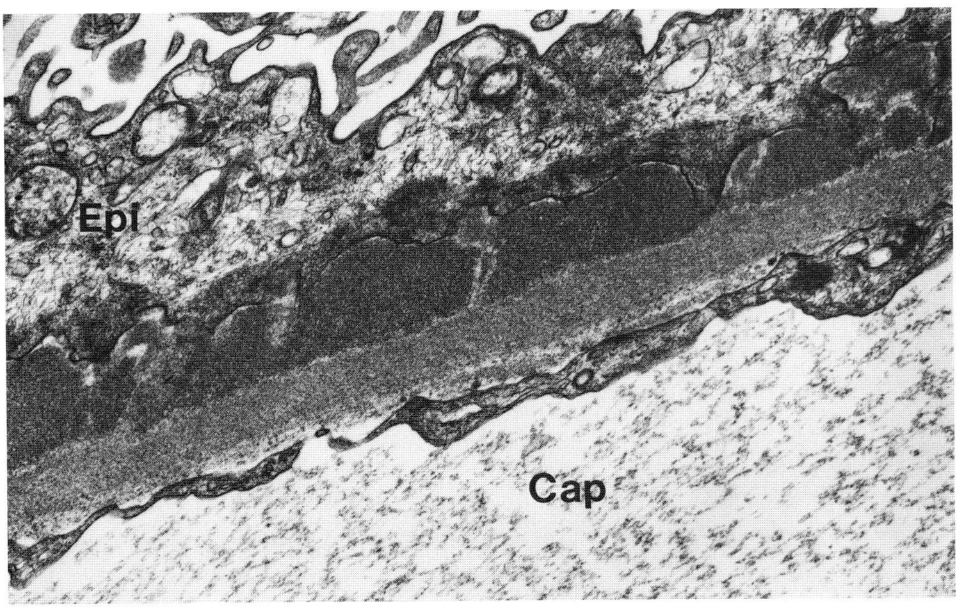

Fig. 8-11. *Electron micrograph from the renal biopsy of a 69-year-old woman with a 2-month history of the nephrotic syndrome. The closely packed subepithelial electron-dense deposits are accommodated by indentations in the cytoplasm of the glomerular epithelial cells (Epi) that show diffuse effacement of their foot processes and fibrillar condensation of the cytoplasm overlying the deposits. Cap, capillary lumen. Uranyl acetate and lead citrate;* ×28,000.

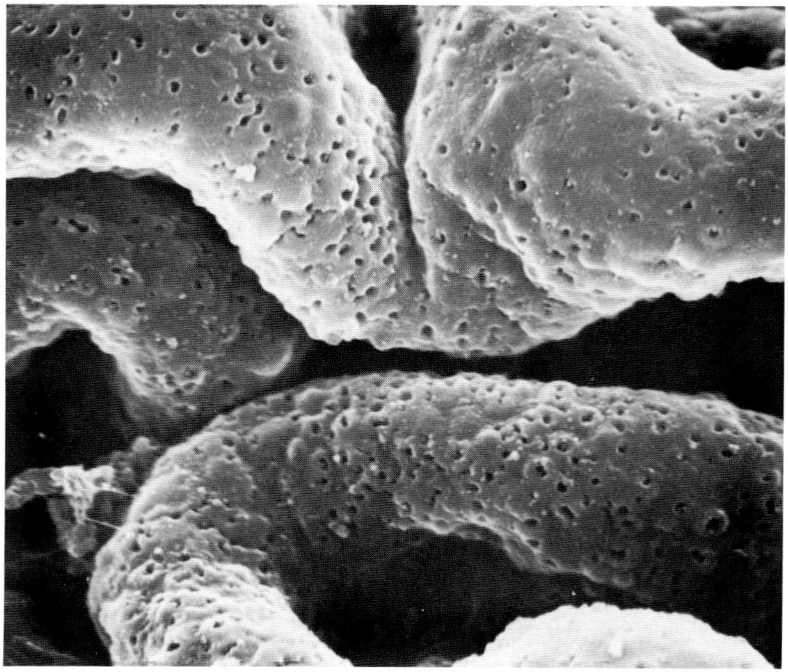

FIG. 8-12. *Scanning electron micrograph of an acellular glomerulus from a patient with idiopathic MGN. The cells were removed from the tissue by sequential treatment with detergents and deoxyribonuclease. The GBM contains scattered shallow pits representing the sites of electron-dense deposits removed in the preparation of the tissue.* ×5000. *(Courtesy of Dr. Stephen M. Bonsib.)*

cases have only focal subepithelial deposits with many capillary loops free of deposits (Fig. 8-13). Visualization of deposits by light microscopy is a function at least in part of their size, but when the deposits are sparse or focal, they may be difficult to see. The thin section examined by electron microscopy usually demonstrates more of the deposits than are apparent in the light or immunohistologic preparation. Still there are occasional cases of MGN in which the deposits are segmental by all morphologic techniques. I consider these examples of focal MGN as morphologic variants, and at present, I assign no special clinical significance to them. Graham and Nagle [86] have suggested that the distribution of subepithelial electron-dense deposits is useful in differentiating the primary from the secondary forms of MGN. By ultrastructural morphometry, they determined that the mean percentage of the GBM involved by subepithelial and/or intramembranous electron-dense deposits was 49 ± 15 percent (mean ± SD) in 23 cases of primary MGN and 16 ± 15 percent in 22 cases of secondary MGN that included 10 cases of SLE, 3 cases of gold nephropathy, 2 cases of penicillamine nephropathy, 1 with mixed connective-tissue disease, and 1 with malignancy. Although it is also my impression that the drug-related forms of MGN have sparse and small deposits, this is usually not a diagnostic problem because of the clinical history. However, when we [222] examined a group of patients with "pure" SLE MGN, the incidence of subepithelial deposits was higher (54 ± 22 percent) than reported by Graham and Nagle (16 ± 15 percent). Since our results were

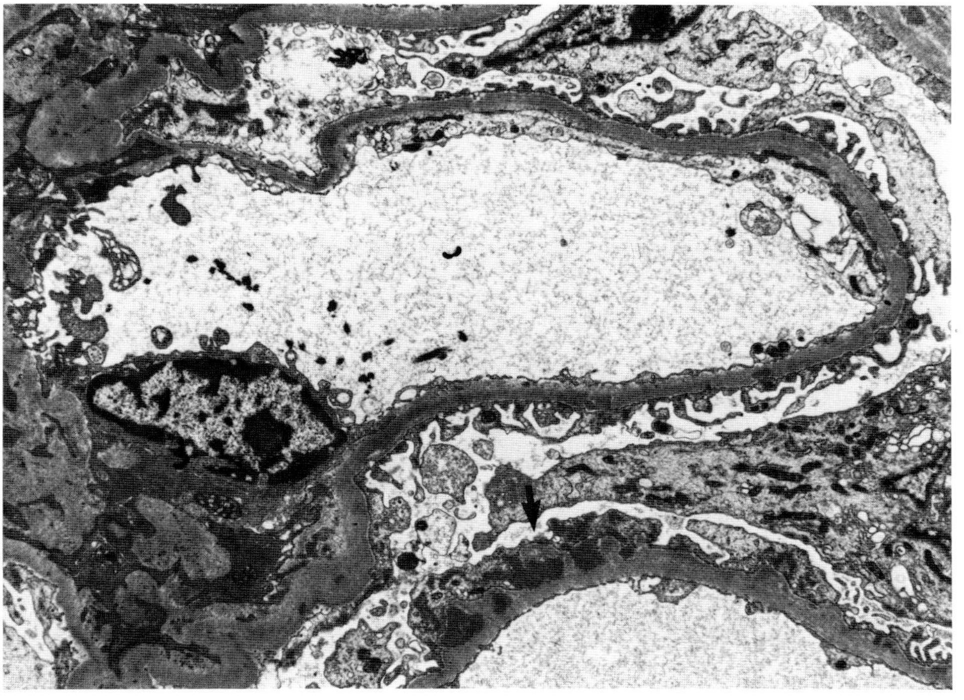

FIG. 8-13. *Electron micrograph showing segmental subepithelial electron-dense deposits (arrow) from a patient who had circulating anti–brush border antibody and Fx1A in the glomerular deposits (see section entitled Renal Tubular Antibodies). The segmental character of the deposits was confirmed by immunofluorescence microscopy. Uranyl acetate and lead citrate;* × *16,000.*

in the same range as their idiopathic group, quantitation of subepithelial deposits would not have been useful in differentiating our cases of SLE MGN from primary MGN. Shemesh et al. [227] found the ratio of the deposit area to GBM area was 0.23 ± 0.03 in 15 patients with MGN. This morphologic parameter did not correlate with either the GFR or the fractional clearances of albumin and IgG.

The electron-dense deposits have fine granularity that does not resolve into crystalline structures or microtubules. There are several reports of MGN in which the deposits appear as microtubules [87,183,213]. I think these are best classified as immunotactoid glomerulonephropathy [133] because the glomerular distribution of the deposits in the GBM and the mesangium is different from the usual case of MGN, and the diagnosis of immunotactoid glomerulonephropathy (see Chapter 24) carries a different prognosis and therapeutic implications from MGN.

A significant GBM reaction to deposits is indicated by irregular projections of basement-membrane–like material that surround and separate them. These are responsible for the spikes seen by light microscopy in methenamine silver–PAS–stained sections. This newly formed basement membrane cannot be assumed to be normal because Fukatsu et al. [79] have shown that type IV collagen and laminin are not homogeneously distributed in spikes and over the deposits. In these locations, laminin is preferentially deposited. It

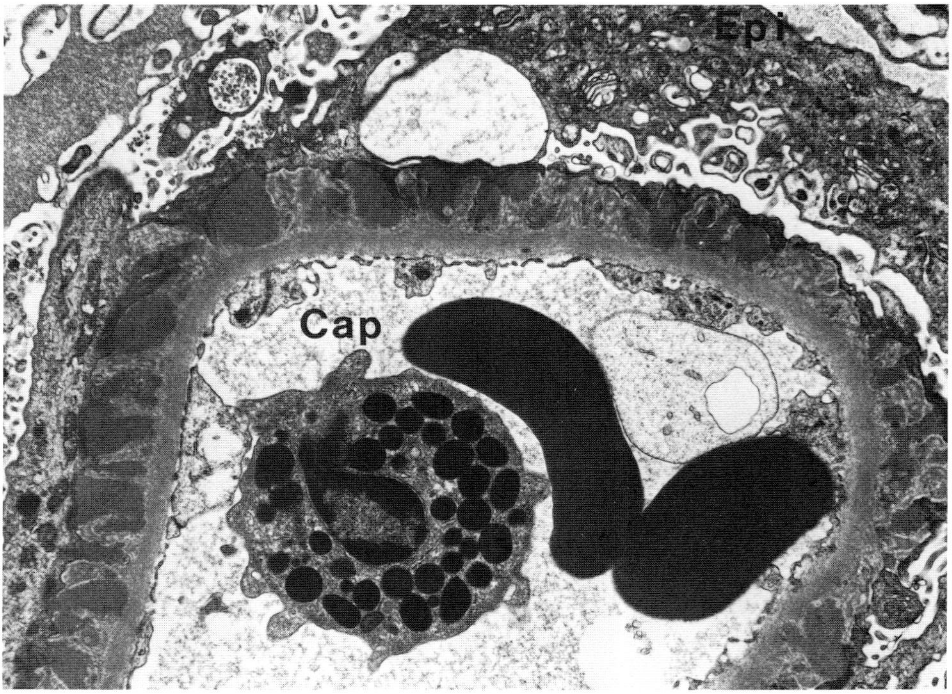

FIG. 8-14. *Electron micrograph from a patient with idiopathic MGN showing subepithelial electron-dense deposits separated by irregular projections of basement membrane–like material. The glomerular epithelial cell (Epi) has diffuse foot-process effacement, and there are microvillous structures in the urinary space. There are neither intramembranous nor subendothelial deposits, and the capillary lumen (Cap) is unremarkable. Uranyl acetate and lead citrate; ×11,000.*

was concluded that this abnormal distribution of the major collagenous and noncollagenous components of the GBM may have reflected either a biosynthetic abnormality or evidence of degradation by the GECs. Okada et al. [181] found that anionic sites in the lamina rara externa are decreased and disrupted by subepithelial electron-dense deposits early in the course of MGN. As the deposits are incorporated into the GBM, the anionic sites are restored to the lamina rara externa and the GEC surface coat. The authors interpreted this loss of charge as the result of immune complex deposition and related it to altered GBM permselectivity.

The spikes are of varying height and complexity (Fig. 8-14). By scanning electron microscopy of acellular glomeruli [22,23], these correspond to a complex reticular pattern (Fig. 8-15) that is mirrored in tangential sections of GBM seen in thin sections (Fig. 8-16) and in histologic sections stained with silver (see Fig. 8-7*B*). The length of the spikes and their distribution determine the

FIG. 8-16. *Transmission electron micrograph of an en face section of GBM from a patient with idiopathic MGN. Both the darker electron-dense deposits and the lighter projections of basement membrane–like material form complementary anastomosing patterns suggesting that the electron-dense deposits have an elongated configuration that is not appreciated in the usual ultrastructural representation. Uranyl acetate and lead citrate; ×4200.*

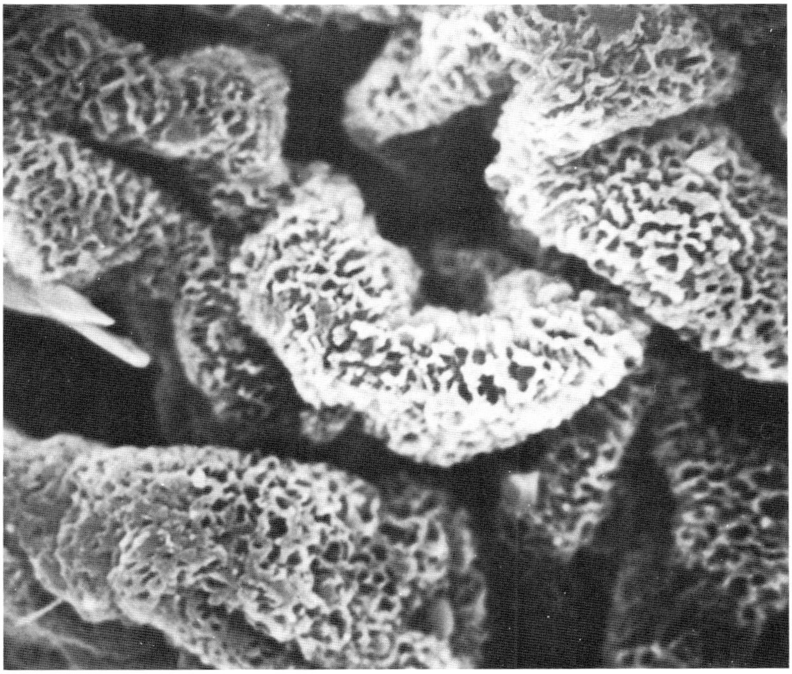

Fig. 8-15. *Scanning electron micrograph of an acellular glomerulus prepared as described in Fig. 8-12 from a patient with idiopathic MGN. The projections of basement membrane–like material are seen as a complex anastomosing network on the outer surface of the GBM. ×4000. (Courtesy of Dr. Stephen M. Bonsib.)*

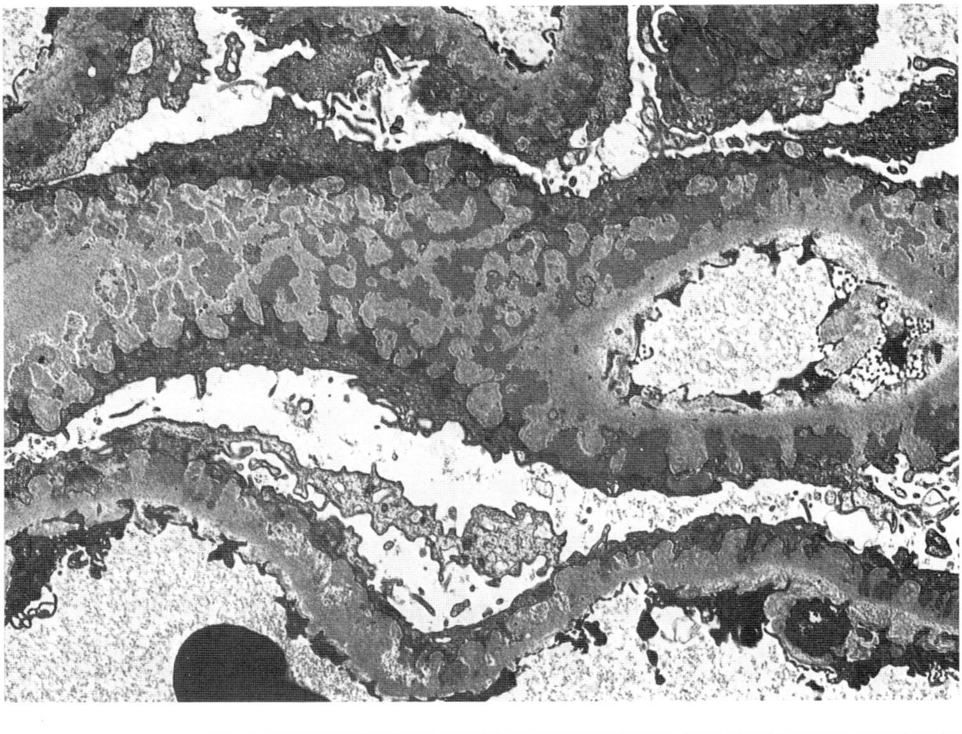

ease with which this feature is visualized by light microscopy. The inner aspect of the GBM and the endothelial cells are unremarkable. As noted earlier, the mesangium shows mild expansion [82,83], and hypercellularity, when present, is due to a proliferation of mesangial cells. The mesangial matrix may show some condensation, but electron-dense deposits are an unusual feature.

Mesangial electron-dense deposits are uncommon in MGN, even in the series in which they are specifically sought [106,226,237]. Their presence suggests that the patient has the membranous form of SLE glomerulonephritis, and when mesangial electron-dense deposits occur in the absence of clinical or serologic evidence, SLE may still become manifest after a latent period of several years [4,150,237]. I have seen two examples of this long latent period. One was a 28-year-old woman who carried the diagnosis of idiopathic MGN for 3 years before she had a clinical attack of lupus. The second was an 18-year-old man whose kidney disease progressed to end-stage failure over a 2.5-year period. Because of his functional deterioration, mesangial electron-dense deposits, and segmental glomerular scars, he was repeatedly evaluated for SLE with negative results. After 2.5 years on dialysis, he developed a positive ANA, anti-native DNA antibody in high titer, and hypocomplementemia. In our series of 64 patients with primary MGN, in whom the diagnosis of SLE was excluded clinically and serologically [279], 6 patients (9 percent) had small mesangial electron-dense deposits (Fig. 8-17). Shearn et al. [226] found them in 9 of 107 cases (8.5 percent)

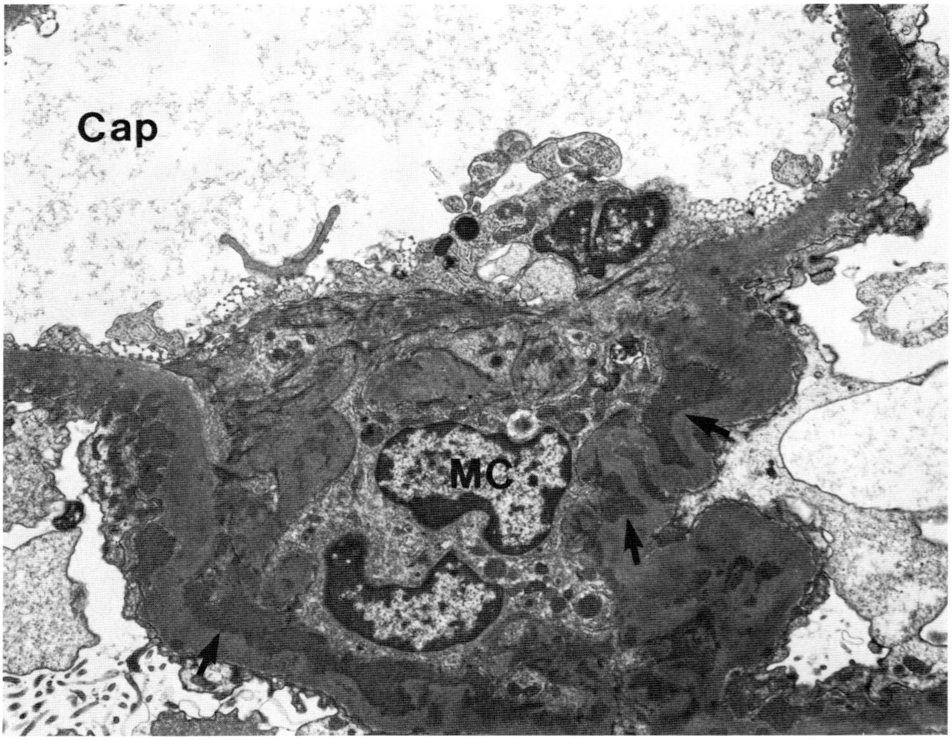

FIG. 8-17. *Electron micrograph of a glomerular capillary from a patient with idiopathic MGN. Note the diffuse subepithelial electron-dense deposits and GEC foot-process effacement. In addition, the mesangium is expanded by cells (MC) and electron-dense deposits (short arrows). Cap, capillary lumen. Uranyl acetate and lead citrate;* $\times 8400$.

of MGN in which SLE was specifically excluded and in which SLE was not detected during a follow-up period of 2 to 16.5 years (mean 9.8 years). In a series of 53 children with idiopathic MGN followed for a mean of 53 months (range 2–167 months) without evidence of SLE, the Southwest Pediatric Nephrology Study Group [237] reported an incidence of mesangial electron-dense deposits of 31 percent. This is a higher incidence than in adult series and is unexplained since lupus and hepatitis B antigenemia, two diagnoses associated with mesangial electron-dense deposits, were specifically excluded. Sixteen repeat biopsies revealed one patient who lost his mesangial deposits and none who developed them. Jennette et al. [116] critically compared the clinical and morphologic features in 148 patients with idiopathic MGN with those of 22 patients with SLE MGN. The morphologic features studied included glomerular cellularity, stage of subepithelial deposits, endothelial tubular reticular structures, tubular basement membrane deposits, mesangial electron-dense deposits, and glomerular and tissue immune deposits. The authors found mesangial deposits in 11 percent of the cases of idiopathic MGN compared with 96 percent in SLE MGN. The other morphologic features were less helpful in differentiating idiopathic from SLE MGN. Although the presence of mesangial electron-dense deposits was sensitive (96 percent) and specific (89 percent) for SLE, it was better at excluding the diagnosis (negative predictive value of 99 percent) than confirming it (positive predictive value of 63 percent). The authors concluded that the individual morphologic features studied were not sufficient to diagnose SLE, but when one morphologic feature with some degree of specificity for SLE was present, or especially when more than one was present, along with hypocomplementemia, the clinical suspicion was strongly supported.

Many cases have a much more complicated ultrastructural picture with marked thickening and distortion of the GBM. The key feature is the incorporation of electron-dense deposits into the GBM with or without simultaneous subepithelial deposits. In some instances the intramembranous deposits have only a tenuous layer of GBM enclosing them, while in others the deposits are deep within the substance of the GBM. The intramembranous deposits have a variable electron density, with the more fully enclosed deposits gradually losing their electron density (Fig. 8-18). This loss of electron density has been interpreted as dissolution of the deposits, or as suggested by the frequent inclusion of cell processes and cellular debris (Fig. 8-19), the deposits are being actively reabsorbed by cellular mechanisms. Intramembranous deposits have been associated with a variety of descriptions of the GBM in silver-stained histologic sections, including splitting, holes, reticular, and "twisted rope." The GBM is not actually split. The new layers of GBM laid down by the GECs over the deposits are responsible for this appearance. The presence within the silver-positive GBM of nonargyrophilic deposits and cell processes is responsible for the other appearances. Scanning electron microscopy of acellular glomeruli [22,23] shows bridging over the reticular arrays that surround the subepithelial deposits, and coalescence into broad, enlarging plaques as the deposits are incorporated into the GBM (Fig. 8-20). The ultrastructural features seen in remission are discussed below under Evolution of the Glomerular Lesion.

IMMUNOFLUORESCENCE FINDINGS

Immunofluorescence microscopy has shown that the structural changes seen in the GBM at the light and electron microscopic levels are due to a combination of deposition of immunoglobulin and complement components and the GBM reaction to these deposits [12,15,16,82,83,85,166,167,180, 215]. Although the antigen is not known in idiopathic MGN, analogy to experimental models and secondary causes of MGN identifies the granular deposits as immune complexes (see Etiology and Pathogenesis below) that correspond to the electron-dense deposits seen by electron microscopy. The typical immunofluorescence finding in MGN is the presence of granular deposits of immune reactants that follow the contour of the GBM (Fig. 8-21). Although they continue around and outline the mesangial areas, deposits within the mesangium are uncommon, in agreement with the ultrastructural findings. In one large series [82,83] that specifically reported mesangial deposits, the incidence was only 6 of 123 (5 percent), and in our series, 3 of 54 cases

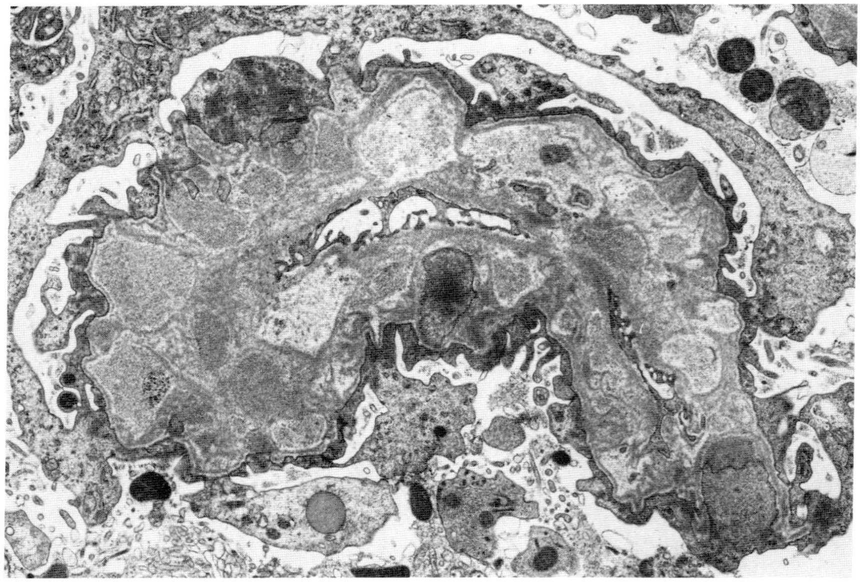

FIG. 8-18. *Electron micrograph of a glomerular capillary loop from a 10-year-old boy with nephrotic syndrome 18 months after onset. There is thickening of the basement membrane, which has many deposits incorporated into it. In some places the deposits have been partially resorbed and are seen as pale areas surrounded by basement membrane–like material.* ×6500. *Stage III* [70]. *(Courtesy of Dr. E. H. Jenis.)*

(6 percent) had mesangial deposits [279]. As noted by Jennette et al. [116], small mesangial deposits are difficult to differentiate from tangential sections of the capillary wall when there is heavy granular staining. The deposits are usually discrete and uniform, but in some cases they are small and very crowded. In these instances they may appear linear, but careful examination will almost always reveal focal granules or discontinuities that are not seen with linear staining. Occasionally, the deposits are either sparse or segmental.

The principal and invariable component of these deposits is IgG, and even when other immunoglobulin and complement components are present, they have a weaker staining reaction and/or are present in a segmental distribution (Fig. 8-22). C3 is more frequently found than either IgM or IgA [12,82,83,93,116,180,215,237]. Some of the variability in the reported incidence of IgM (range 1–58 percent) and IgA (range 17–54 percent) may be related to the reporting of low levels of staining. In our series [279], the incidence of staining for IgM, IgA, and C3 is 35, 20, and 78 percent, respectively, but the corresponding incidences fall to 20, 9, and 58 percent when only staining equal to or greater than 1^+ (on a scale from $0–4^+$) is reported. The presence of IgA and C1q in the deposits has been proposed as a marker for SLE MGN, but since they are also seen in some cases of idiopathic MGN, their diagnostic specificity is low when the issue is examined critically [116]. Kusonoki et al. [136], using the detection of C4d and C4-binding protein as more sensitive indicators of classical pathway complement activation, found these complement components in 11 of 12 patients (92 percent) with idiopathic MGN. This is consistent with the observation that proteinuria in experimental MGN is caused

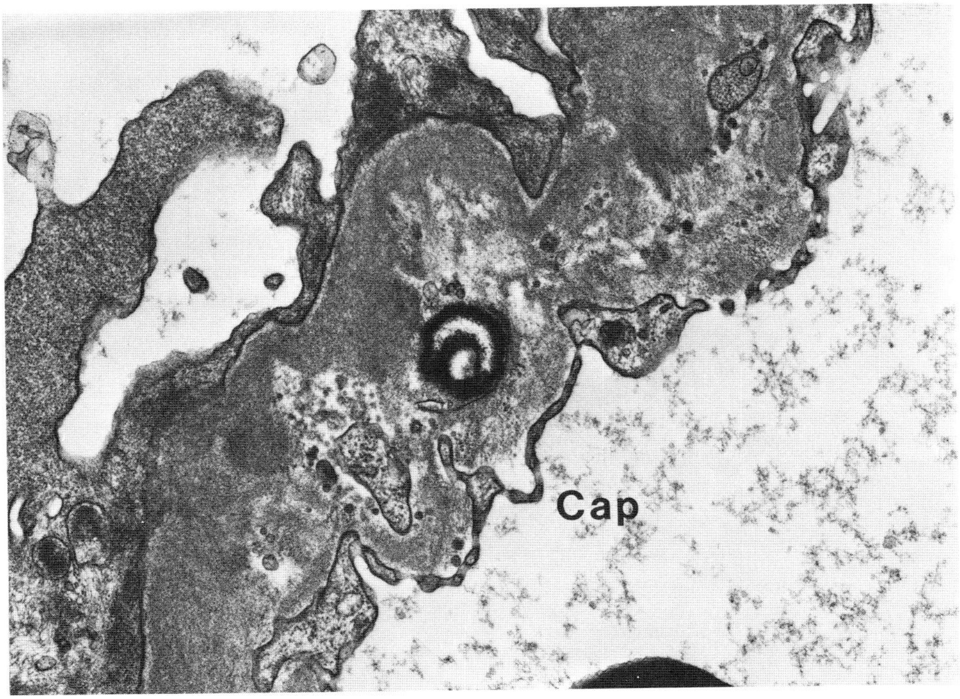

FIG. 8-19. *Electron micrograph at high magnification of a portion of a glomerular capillary wall from a 35-year-old man with a 4.5-year history of proteinuria and 3.9 g of proteinuria daily. The GBM is irregularly thickened by cellular debris and cytoplasmic processes. Although there are some ill-defined lacunae, there are no electron-dense deposits. Immunofluorescence microscopy showed diffuse, weak (1^+) granular deposits of IgG. Cap, capillary lumen. Uranyl acetate and lead citrate;* $\times 40,000$. *Stage III* [70].

by the cytolytic effects of the late complement components independent of inflammatory cells (see Etiology and Pathogenesis below). The preponderance in the immune deposits of MGN of the IgG_4 subgroup, which fixes complement poorly, has been suggested as the reason why the C3 deposits are weak and variable despite the large amounts of IgG [11,63,209]. Nöel et al. [179] observed a subgroup restriction in the serum and glomerular deposits of patients with idiopathic MGN with a predominance of IgG_4 (81 percent) and IgG_1 (75 percent). However, the authors could not determine whether the glomerular and serum IgG subclass imbalance was due to a clonally restricted antibody response to a particular antigen or to a host immune response defect or both. Other immune reactants have been reported in the glomerular deposits.

Extraglomerular deposits have been reported in only a few patients with idiopathic MGN [26, 66,82,116,144], and the presence of granular tubular basement membrane (TBM) deposits suggests the diagnosis of SLE MGN, where they have been reported in 30 to 50 percent of the cases (reviewed by Jennette et al. [116]). Our experience with 64 cases of idiopathic MGN [279], in which we found granular TBM deposits in only one case, appears similar to the experience of others [26,82,116,144]. We have reported this unique patient with idiopathic MGN because he had

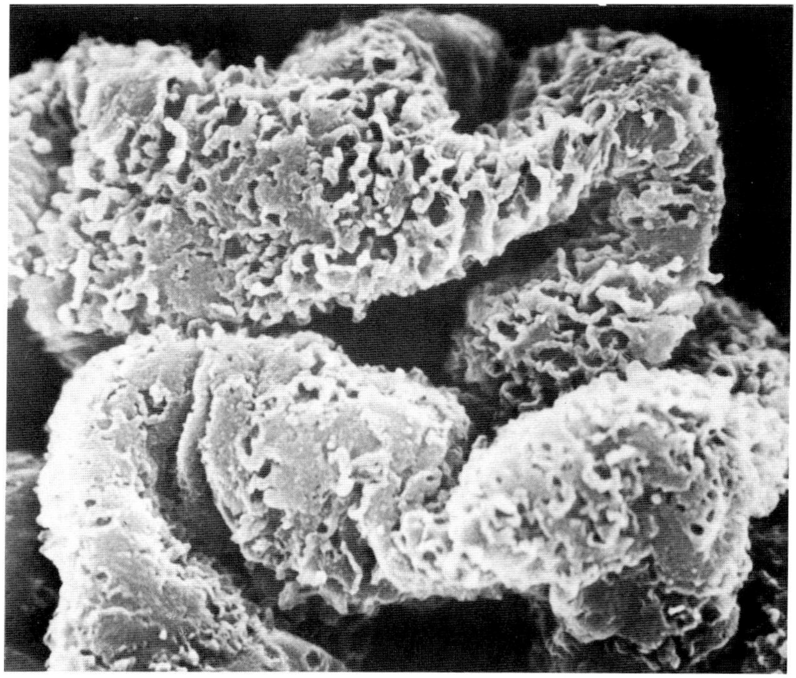

FIG. 8-20. *Scanning electron micrograph of acellular glomerulus prepared as described in Fig. 8-12 from a patient with idiopathic MGN. The anastomosing ridges of basement membrane–like material that surround and project above the electron-dense deposits (removed in this material by processing) show focal areas where they bridge over the deposits and present smooth plaques on the external surface of the GBM.* ×*5000.*

TBM deposits, anti-brush border antibodies, and Fx1A in the glomerular deposits [66] (see below). Gärtner [82] reported "peritubular" deposits in 8 of 124 patients, but since she did not illustrate this feature, it is not certain that she was reporting TBM deposits. Finally, there is a group of children with idiopathic MGN and granular or linear TBM deposits with anti-TBM activity [72,145,159, 266]. These children have a variety of immunopathologic abnormalities, including antialveolar antibodies [145] and antibodies against intestinal epithelium [72,159].

Evolution of the Glomerular Lesion

The different morphologic patterns seen in MGN have led to the hypothesis that they represent temporally related morphologic stages linking the initial GBM deposition of immune complexes, the glomerular reaction, and the ultimate fate of the glomerulus [12,70,82,258,260]. This concept is supported by the observation that an increase in the time interval between the onset of clinical evidence of renal disease and renal biopsy is correlated with more advanced morphologic changes in the GBM. Also, more advanced GBM pathology is associated with decreasing immunopathologic evidence of glomerular immune complexes and decreased protein excretion. Although there are differences among the various classifications of the glomerular pathology of MGN [12,70,82,258, 260], there is agreement about the basic observations. The classifications are all based on the ultrastructural appearance of the glomerulus, but many of the same features can be appreciated by

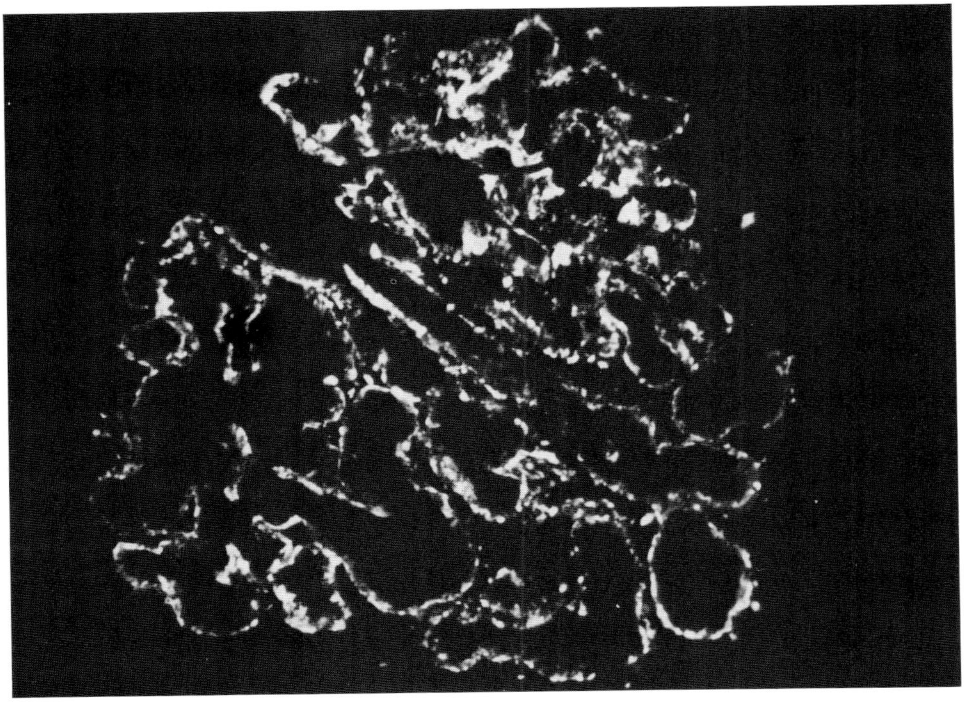

Fig. 8-21. *Immunofluorescence photomicrograph of a glomerulus stained for human IgG from a 45-year-old man with idiopathic MGN, a 2-week history of edema, and 23 g of proteinuria daily. IgG is present in a strong (3+) granular pattern. C3 is present in the same pattern but at lower intensity (1+), and IgM (illustrated in Fig. 8-22) is present in trace amounts.* ×450.

light and immunofluorescence microscopy. In 61 cases classified into stages [70] by both light and electron microscopy, we [279] found agreement between the two modalities in a majority of cases (90 percent). Frequently, the lesions were more complex when seen by electron microscopy, and multiple stages were present. The 6 cases in which light and electron microscopic diagnoses differed were biopsies in which spikes seen by electron microscopy (stage II) were not evident by light microscopy. The morphologic changes observed in MGN have been variously interpreted as evidence of an inexorably progressive course, healing, or episodic injury and healing. These differing dynamic interpretations of morphology reflect disagreement concerning the outcome of the pathologic process in the GBM.

STAGE I

These lesions are the same in all classifications. They consist of subepithelial electron-dense deposits with a relatively normal underlying GBM, which at most may have depressions related to the deposits (see Figs. 8-11 and 8-12). Since the demonstration of the deposits by light microscopy may be limited by their small size and patchy distribution, the sections must be examined at high magnification to find the small, focal spikes on silver stain and the small red deposits with Heidenhain or trichrome stains. Sections tangential to the GBM may show irregular mottling or bubbles (see Fig. 8-5) that correspond to the depressions in the GBM seen by transmission (see Fig. 8-11) and scanning (see Fig. 8-12) electron microscopy. Im-

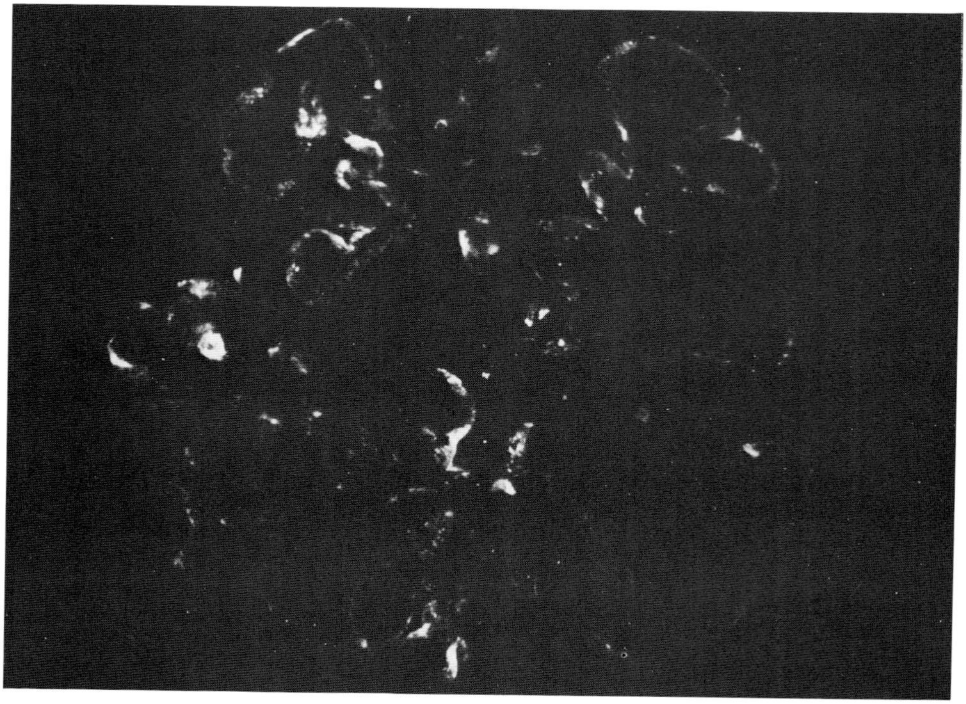

FIG. 8-22. *Immunofluorescence photomicrograph of a glomerulus stained for human IgM from the same patient illustrated in Fig. 8-21. Although there is some segmental accentuation, most of the deposits are stained much less intensely than for IgG.* ×450.

munofluorescence microscopy shows corresponding discrete granular GBM deposits.

STAGE II

This stage corresponds to the fully developed lesion in Ehrenreich and Churg's [70] original scheme. The electron-dense deposits lie under the glomerular epithelial cell in contact with or partially embedded within the substance of the GBM. They are surrounded by cup-like projections of GBM that are seen as spikes of basement-membrane–like material by transmission electron microscopy (see Fig. 8-14), as a reticular pattern of basement-membrane projection by scanning electron microscopy of acellular glomeruli (see Fig. 8-15), and as a similar reticular pattern in tangential sections of methenamine silver–stained sections seen by light microscopy (see Fig. 8-7*B*). At this stage the spikes of GBM begin to develop lateral extensions that occasionally bridge over the deposits. The visualization of these spikes by light microscopy depends on their length, and unless they exceed the thickness of the GBM, they may not be apparent [258]. Corresponding to the lateral GBM extensions are "clubbed" ends of the spikes seen by light microscopy [70]. The deposits are more diffusely distributed, and they appear larger by light microscopy with Heidenhain and trichrome stains and by immunofluorescence microscopy. At this stage, the GBM usually appears thickened by light microscopy.

STAGE III

Ehrenreich and Churg [70] described deposits incorporated into the GBM in stage III (see Figs. 8-18 and 8-19). This occurs when new layers of

GBM are laid down over the electron-dense deposits by the glomerular epithelial cell, and with time the deposits appear to sink deeper into the GBM as the GBM slowly reforms [260]. The intramembranous deposits have a variable electron density. Some are identical to subepithelial electron-dense deposits, but others show decreasing electron density, first in the periphery of the deposits and finally involving the entire deposit. Gärtner [82] divided the intramembranous deposits into an electron-dense stage and one in which the deposit can no longer be seen within its GBM lacunae. The GBM is obviously thickened as judged by light microscopy at this stage, and the nonstaining intramembranous deposits have a complex, variable appearance in silver-stained preparations. Corresponding to the loss of electron density, the deposits are not well seen with Heidenhain or trichrome stains, but although the staining intensity is reduced, they may still be recognized as discrete granular deposits by immunofluorescence microscopy. This sequence, especially the appearance of pure stage III, is seen only in cases where one generation of deposits, presumably due to limited exposure to antigenic stimulation, is followed by a healing sequence [258]. In fact, most cases of MGN present a mixed appearance, and classification into one stage requires that a judgment be made as to the dominant pattern. Most stage III cases will not only have intramembranous deposits of varying electron density, but also will have evidence of newly formed subepithelial deposits. We [279] found a mixture of stages II and III in 36 percent of 61 cases, compared with 34 percent that were in either pure stage II and 13 percent that were in pure stage III.

STAGE IV

The major point of contention concerning the evolution and fate of the intramembranous deposits is seen in the different attempts to define stage IV. As originally conceptualized by Ehrenreich and Churg [70], stage III MGN led to a stage IV in which the GBM was irregularly thickened without the presence of electron-dense deposits or lacunae. By light microscopy, the GBM was appreciably thickened, and with the silver stain some spikes and nonargyrophillic irregularities could be seen in the GBM. Based on their experience with three patients in stage III with decreased protein excretion who were rebiopsied and showed persistence or progression of the renal lesion, these authors suggested that stage IV was the morphologic equivalent of inexorable progression to end-stage renal disease. Ehrenreich and Churg described a stage V characterized by capillary collapse, adhesions, focal mesangial cellularity, crescents, and sclerosis. In these advanced cases of glomerulonephritis, MGN was identified as the underlying pathologic process because focal areas of typical MGN in stages II, III, or IV were present. As might be predicted from the evanescent ultrastructural appearance of the deposits, staining for immune reactants is irregular and decreased in stage IV [12].

Subsequent experience has shown that many patients with MGN do not develop progressive renal failure, and a significant number experience a complete or partial remission of proteinuria with stable, although sometimes reduced renal function. A few patients with MGN, usually in stage I or II, have shown complete or partial regression of the glomerular lesion on rebiopsy [12,76,82,85], but Gärtner [82] found that the reparative stage V in her terminology (corresponding to stage IV of Ehrenreich and Churg) could evolve from any preceding stage. Forland and Spargo [76] described and illustrated a patient with a stage II [70] lesion who went into remission, and a subsequent biopsy showed a virtually normal light and electron microscopic picture (Fig. 8-23). Other electron microscopic pictures of MGN in remission show a regular line of basement-membrane–like material on the epithelial side of the capillary wall with irregular electron-lucent areas on the somewhat uneven endothelial aspect [12,76,215,261] (Fig. 8-24). However, the most common finding in patients rebiopsied while in remission is either no change or evolution of the GBM changes without complete disappearance of the deposits [12,70,82, 85,180,202].

The progression from proliferative glomerulonephritis to MGN that occurs occasionally in SLE is unusual in MGN. The four cases reported by Richet et al. [204] began as diffuse proliferative glomerulonephritis and progressed to MGN. Kapur et al. [123] described a patient who had acute

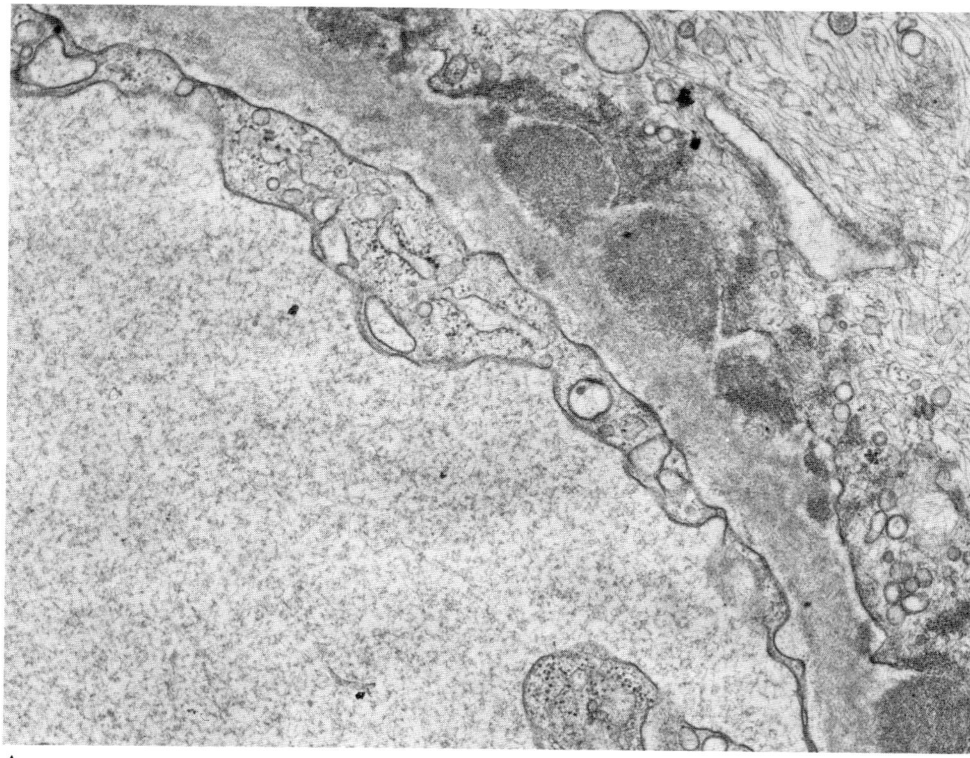

A

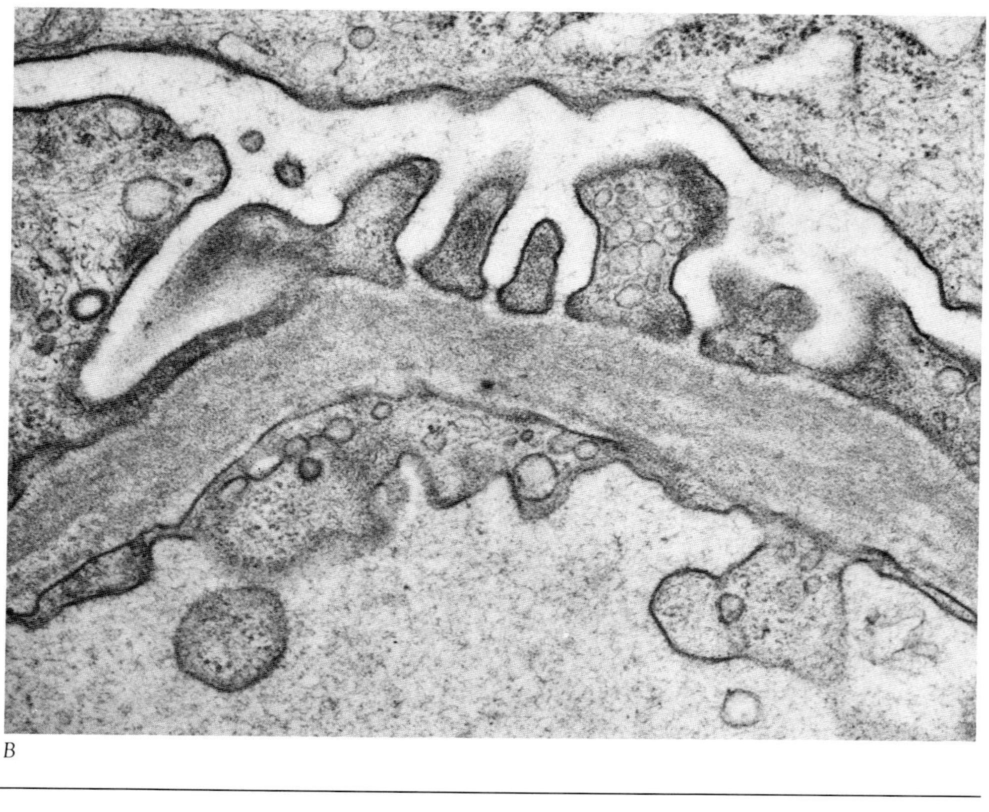

B

hypocomplementemic nephritis and the renal biopsy showed proliferative and exudative glomerulonephritis with subepithelial humps. In addition to granular immune deposits along the capillary wall, there also were mesangial deposits. SLE and hepatitis were ruled out by appropriate serologic tests, and there was no serologic evidence of an antecedent streptococcal infection. The patient was biopsied 19 and 28 months after the onset, and the glomeruli showed an evolution to typical MGN without evidence of mesangial immune deposits. Although the subepithelial location of deposits in poststreptococcal glomerulonephritis is morphologically similar to that of MGN, the infrequency of this transformation suggests that some factor other than the location of the deposits determines their pathogenetic consequences.

The dynamic and potentially reversible nature of the GBM pathology in MGN has both clinical and pathologic significance. Following subepithelial immune complex deposition in MGN, there is a sequence of changes that can have the different outcomes of healing or progression to renal failure. The factors that determine which outcome occurs are not apparent from the morphology, but Törnroth [258] has suggested that complete healing cannot occur as long as subepithelial deposits form continuously or intermittently in the glomerulus. Furthermore, thickening of the GBM is not the morphologic equivalent of glomerular dysfunction indicated by proteinuria. Rather, it suggests a prolonged disease course [260]. Since the molecular configuration of the immune complexes may be important in activating complement-mediated glomerular injury, their loss of integrity, indicated by decreased electron density and intensity of immunofluorescence staining, may explain why protein excretion is decreased in the later stages of MGN. Although reabsorption of immune aggregates may be a morphologic indication of healing, it takes a long time for the GBM to return to normal after membranous transformation has occurred, especially from the more advanced stages. Thus morphologic alterations in the GBM may be detected long after proteinuria has resolved and renal function has stabilized.

FIG. 8-23. *Serial biopsies on patient referred to in the text. (A) First biopsy taken during nephrotic syndrome. Electron-dense deposits on epithelial side of basement membrane with loss of foot processes.* ×22,000. *(B) Second biopsy taken during clinical remission. Restitution of basement membrane to normal and restoration of foot processes.* ×20,000. *(From Forland, M., and Spargo, B. H.* Nephron 6: 498, 1969.*)*

Prognostic Indicators

Many clinical and pathologic features have been examined in an attempt to separate the MGN patients who have a good prognosis from those who eventually develop progressive glomerular disease. These factors may be divided into those which are thought to be of importance in the progression of glomerular disease in general, and those which are uniquely related to the prognosis of MGN. There is controversy in the literature on each point, with some reports supporting and others denying the importance of the feature. This discussion will consider the data from larger series and emphasize points that have been examined statistically and found significant by multivariate analysis. Abnormal renal function, high-grade protein excretion, loss of selectivity of excreted protein, elevated arterial blood pressure, and the presence of tubular atrophy and interstitial fibrosis have been examined in a number of renal diseases; they may be considered as general indicators of adverse prognosis.

ABNORMAL RENAL FUNCTION

Renal function is almost always abnormal at the time of biopsy in patients who develop renal failure, require dialysis, die of renal or nonrenal causes, or fail to lose their proteinuria [53,65, 70,107,111,172,194,215,274]. Wehrmann et al. [274] found that of 260 of 334 patients (78 percent) with idiopathic MGN who had an initial creatinine level equal to or less than 1.3 mg/100 ml, 98 percent survived 5 years with normal renal function or "compensated renal insufficiency" (kidney survival rate) and 90 percent survived 10 years. In contrast, 74 (22 percent) of their patients presented with an initial S_{Cr} greater than 1.3 mg/100 ml, and they had 5- and 10-year kidney survival rates of 60 and 40 percent, respectively. This

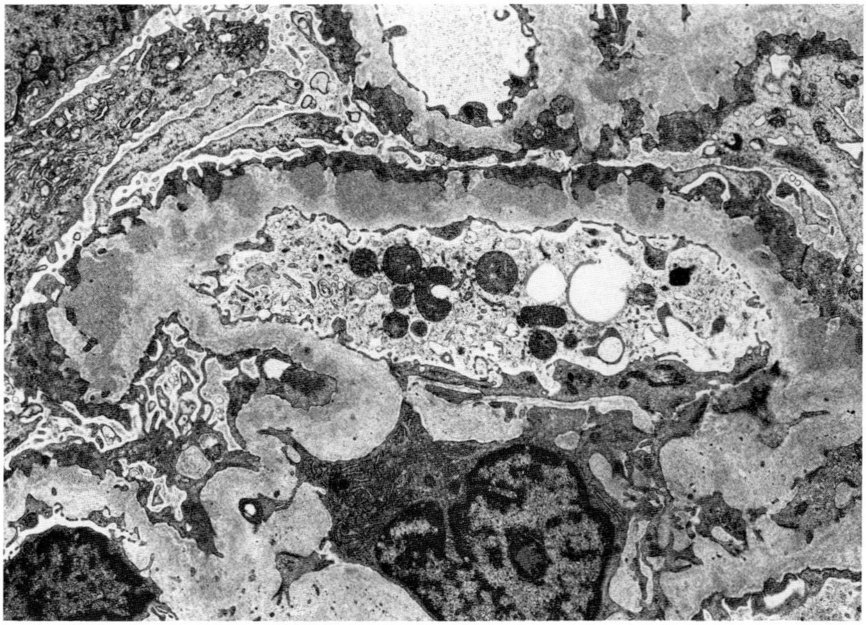

A

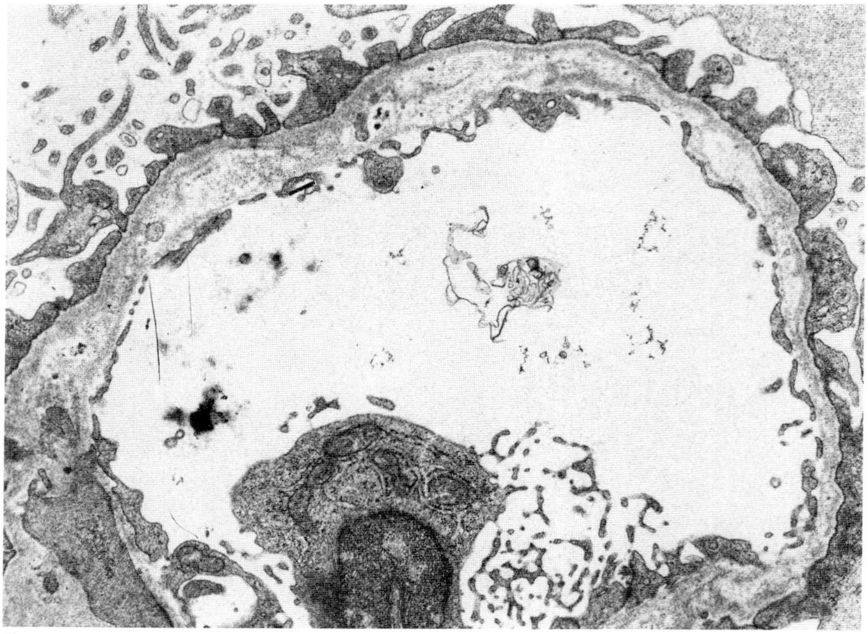

B

FIG. 8-24. *Sequence of two biopsies from a 50-year-old man with nephrotic syndrome caused by idiopathic membranous glomerulonephritis who went into remission; second biopsy was taken during remission. (A) Glomerular capillary loop with numerous subepithelial electron-dense deposits and spikes. ×5500. (B) Regular line of basement membrane–like material on epithelial side with electron-lucent scalloped endothelial aspect. Foot processes have been restored. ×13,300. (Courtesy of Dr. E. H. Jenis.)*

difference was highly significant by uni- and multivariate analysis ($p = 0.001$). In two dissenting series [65,201] there was no correlation with outcome when more sensitive indicators of renal function were used (C_{Cr} and $C_{Iothalamate}$). Franklin et al. [78] found that the initial S_{Cr} did not correlate with the occurrence of a clinical remission.

HIGH-GRADE PROTEIN EXCRETION

Evidence concerning the effect of high-grade protein excretion on the outcome of renal function is less straightforward. Davison et al. [53] found deterioration of renal function in 2 of 12 patients with asymptomatic proteinuria compared with 25 of 50 with nephrotic syndrome at the time of biopsy ($p < 0.05$). Donadio et al. [65] found an initial protein excretion of 14.8 ± 8 g/24 h (mean ± SD) in 17 patients who progressed to end-stage renal failure in under 2.5 years compared with 7.5 ± 4.5 g/24 h in 127 patients who maintained stable renal function ($p < 0.001$). Erwin et al. [73] found that their nonnephrotic MGN patients did not develop nephrotic syndrome or renal failure. Honkanen [107] found that patients with "slight" proteinuria never developed renal failure. Murphy et al. [172] found the nephrotic syndrome at the time of biopsy in 23 of 28 patients (82 percent) who developed decreased renal function and in 52 of 121 (43 percent) who maintained renal function. Pierides et al. [193] found that 8 of 28 patients with initial nephrotic syndrome developed renal failure, while none of 9 patients with nonnephrotic proteinuria developed renal failure. Row et al. [215] found that 54 patients with nephrotic syndrome did worse than 12 with nonnephrotic proteinuria, and progression of renal dysfunction did not occur in the absence of proteinuria. On the other hand, Wehrmann et al. [274], using a higher level of protein excretion (5.0 g/24 h) to define the nephrotic syndrome, found an incidence of 73 percent in 334 cases of MGN. The kidney survival rate in those with and without the nephrotic syndrome was 74 and 85 percent, respectively, which was not significantly different. Donadio et al. [65] found the nephrotic syndrome in all 28 patients who progressed to end-stage renal disease, and protein excretion exceeding 10 g/24 h was associated with rapid progression to end-stage kidney disease within 2.5 years. When they compared intervals of proteinuria by survival analysis, the probability of surviving without renal failure was significantly worse in the severely nephrotic range (10 g/24 h or more) compared with the nonnephrotic (less than 3.4 g/24 h, $p < 0.001$) and the midnephrotic range (3.5–9.9 g/24 h, $p < 0.0001$).

SELECTIVITY

Selectivity of proteinuria in glomerular disease in general correlates with the severity of the glomerular lesion, and patients with highly selective proteinuria have a good response to steroid therapy, while those with poorly selective proteinuria have a variable response that tends to be worse [34]. Although most patients with MGN have poorly selective proteinuria [34,43,201,202], a significant number do undergo remission. There are a few publications suggesting that patients with MGN and selective proteinuria respond well to prednisone therapy [43,263], but others disagree [201]. At the present time, the relation between selectivity and renal functional outcome remains unresolved.

HYPERTENSION

Because of the adverse effect of hypertension on the course of glomerular disease in general, it might be predicted that hypertension at the time of renal biopsy would identify patients with a poor prognosis. This point is the subject of some controversy, with certain investigators reporting an adverse effect of hypertension [111,182,194] and others reporting no effect [65,201,274]. In a series of 100 patients, Hopper et al. [111] reported that men had a higher incidence of renal death and a lower incidence of renal improvement than women. The men also had a much higher incidence of hypertension (54 percent) than women (26 percent). Wehrmann et al. [274] found hypertension in 117 (35 percent) of his series of 334 patients, and their kidney survival rate of 5 and 10 years was 80 and 60 percent, respectively. In contrast, the 200 normotensive patients had kidney survival rates at 5 and 10 years of 95 and 90 percent. However, sequential multivariate analysis failed to support a role for initial high blood pressure as an independent determinant of outcome.

INTERSTITIAL FIBROSIS AND TUBULAR ATROPHY

Interstitial pathology, whether qualitatively judged as significant [195,196,201,274] or semiquantitated by point counting [208], has a high predictive value for outcome. In fact, it correlates better than any other histologic feature of MGN, including glomerular stage [274]. When Wehrmann et al. [274] subjected the various clinical and pathologic features of MGN to multivariate analysis, the presence of interstitial fibrosis and the initial S_{Cr} were the only independent variables.

The clinical and pathologic features that have been proposed to be specifically related to the prognosis of MGN are also variable in their relevance to outcome. They include childhood onset, female sex, stages of membranous transformation, duration of symptoms prior to biopsy, and the course subsequent to the biopsy.

AGE

The prognosis for children and adults with MGN is very different. The initial studies that reported a dismal outlook for adults with MGN contained few children. However, when reports in children began to appear [37,93,182,200,201,215], it became obvious that children had a much better prognosis than adults. The question of whether older and younger adults have different prognoses is controversial. Donadio et al. [65] found no relation between rapid progression to end-stage renal disease and age in adult patients. Honkanen [107] found an older mean age in the patients with deterioration of renal function (49.9 years compared with 36.8 years, $p < 0.01$). Ramzy et al. [201] found that patients who went into remission were only slightly younger than those with persistent disease. Wehrmann et al. [274] found a mean age of 43 years in 334 patients with MGN, and 22 percent were less than 30 years of age. There was a higher incidence of end-stage renal disease and death due to renal-related causes after 10 years in patients older than 30 years (26 percent) than in younger patients (15 percent). Even though this series apparently contains children, who are known to have a better prognosis than adults [82], this difference was not found to be significant. Davison et al. [53] found that patients older than 60 years of age developed deterioration of renal function more frequently (89 percent) than patients less than 60 years old (45 percent). Although the age groups were admittedly small, discriminant analysis revealed that age was an independent variable with respect to outcome of renal function.

SEX

There is evidence that suggests that females have a better prognosis for preservation of renal function and achieving remission than males [53,65, 111,172], but other authors disagree [78,107, 215,274]. Hopper et al. [111] presented an influential series in which renal death, defined as end-stage kidney disease causing death or the need for dialysis, was more common in 65 men than 35 women (43 compared with 8.6 percent, $p = 0.0006$), and improvement with complete healing was more common in women (83 compared with 43 percent). However, the men had a greater incidence of proteinuria equal to or greater than 10 g/24 h (58 compared with 5.2 percent), initial S_{Cr} of 1.5 mg/100 ml or more (40 compared with 11.4 percent), and elevated diastolic blood pressure (54 compared with 25.7 percent). The benignity of the disease in women was apparent clinically, since almost all of them were not treated with steroids. The question naturally arises whether sex is an independent variable. Davison et al. [53] found that it was, and Wehrmann et al. [274] found that it was not. Considering the conflicting data, the independent role of sex as a determinant of outcome remains controversial.

STAGES OF MEMBRANOUS TRANSFORMATION

As described by Ehrenreich and Churg [70], the stages of membranous transformation were the morphologic representations of the progressive nature of MGN. Subsequently, the stage of the initial biopsy has been correlated with the outcomes of proteinuria [70,85,180,194,200,215] and renal function [70,73,178,195,199]. In both instances, favorable outcomes are generally related to early stages (I and II) of membranous transformation. Several studies have suggested that membranous transformation as outlined by Ehrenreich and Churg actually represents the reaction that the GBM undergoes when confronted with a single generation of deposits [82,258,260]. Factors other than membranous transformation that may lead to end-stage kidney disease include the length of time for which deposits are formed, the rapidity with which deposits form, their size, and the presence of more than one episode of deposit formation [258]. In fact, Ehrenreich and Churg [70] noted that resolution of proteinuria occurred in the presence of early and late pathologic changes. The former was interpreted as healing, but the latter was related to the apparently impermeable nature of the greatly thickened GBM and was seen as a prelude to terminal renal failure. The fact that several large studies have not found a relation between glomerular stage and outcome [65,208, 215,274] suggests that the morphologic stage has limited value as a prognostic indicator.

INTERVAL FROM FIRST SYMPTOMS TO BIOPSY

The duration of clinically apparent renal disease prior to biopsy has been found by some to have prognostic value [43,107], but lack of precision in determining this duration reduces its usefulness.

COURSE OF MGN SUBSEQUENT TO BIOPSY

There are several features in the clinical course of MGN subsequent to biopsy that appear to have prognostic value. The first is the outcome of proteinuria. In contrast to patients with persistent nephrotic syndrome or high-grade proteinuria, those who enter a clinical remission have a good prognosis for renal functional outcome [189,215] and complete or partial remission of proteinuria [189]. The presence of multiple indicators of an adverse outcome identifies patients who fare worse than MGN patients in general. Donadio et al. [65] identified a group of patients who went into renal failure within 2.5 years of biopsy. These patients, who declared their prognosis early in the course, had multiple clinical indicators of adverse outcome, including elevated initial S_{Cr}, tubulointerstitial changes, massive unresolving proteinuria, and hypertension. Patients with MGN usually enter renal failure late in the course [53,65], but when renal function remains normal after 5 years, a continued benign course with preservation of renal function has been demonstrated [53,126].

Renal Tubular Antibodies and Membranous Glomerulonephritis

Similarities between experimental autologous immune complex nephritis (Heymann nephritis) and MGN have suggested that they might arise by similar pathogenetic mechanisms. The active Heymann nephritis model is produced by immunizing rats with either a crude preparation of renal cortex or purified renal cortical antigens. The animals develop antibodies against the immunizing antigen(s) [89,156], and similar antibodies are identified in the glomerular immune deposits. These experimental observations have instigated attempts to identify Heymann nephritis antigens in the sera and glomerular immune deposits of patients with MGN. Naruse et al. [176] first reported the localization of tubular antigen in the immune deposits of patients with MGN. Using antisera prepared against an extract of human renal cortex (according to Edgington et al. [69]), they found positive staining with the same pattern as was found for IgG and C3 in 3 of 7 cases of MGN, but in none of 11 miscellaneous cases with glomerular deposits of IgG and C3. Subsequently, the same group [177] reported glomerular deposits that stained with their antibody preparation in 4 of 9 additional patients with MGN. They also purified the antigen preparation by gel filtration and DEAE chromatography and produced antibody against four separate fractions. Although all these antibodies stained proximal tubule brush border, only the one against the fraction identified as

0.07M localized to the immune deposits in MGN. Using the antibody raised against 0.07M, the authors developed a radioimmunoassay and demonstrated tubular antigen in the sera of normal subjects, anephric patients, and a control group with increased serum alkaline phosphatase activity. Tubular antigen also was present in concentrated urine specimens of all 13 normal subjects tested. This antigen was present in pronase extracts of other organs, and although distributed similarly to alkaline phosphatase in tissue, it was biochemically distinct from that enzyme. The ubiquitous distribution of antigens originally derived from tubular preparations also has been shown in Heymann nephritis [231], and this suggests that injury to other organs may initiate an immune response that eventuates in glomerular immune complex disease.

Other reports have implicated brush border antigens and/or anti–brush border antibodies in the pathogenesis of MGN. Makker [155] incubated rat kidney with normal human serum and demonstrated brush border antibody in 36 percent of 358 normal subjects by indirect immunofluorescence. Zanetti et al. [283] reported a patient who developed de novo MGN in a transplant. High-titer anti–brush border antibody activity in the patient's serum was demonstrated by indirect immunofluorescence using rat kidney as the substrate. The staining was abolished by absorption with rat Fx1A. In this patient, the antibodies were present prior to transplantation, and they decreased posttransplant, presumably as they were being deposited in the kidney. Deposition of immune complexes in the transplanted kidney was associated with clinically apparent proteinuria. Eluate of the renal biopsies weakly stained rat brush border. This suggested to the authors that this antibody was important in the pathogenesis of this disease. Douglas et al. [66] presented a patient with MGN and a circulating antibody that stained human, rat, rabbit, and mouse proximal tubule brush border. The brush border staining was blocked by absorption with human Fx1A and by prior exposure of the sections to rabbit anti-human Fx1A. High-titer rabbit anti-human Fx1A stained glomerular immune deposits after partial elution with 2.5 M potassium thiocyanate. Circulating immune complexes were not detected. The distribution of the immune deposits was atypical for MGN because they also were present in Bowman's capsule and focally in the TBM, but attempts to demonstrate SLE and other systemic diseases were negative. Although these reports are sporadic, they suggest a role for the Heymann antigen-antibody system in the pathogenesis of some cases of MGN.

Despite the above-mentioned immunopathologic evidence, attempts to systematically demonstrate anti–brush border antibodies in the serum or glomerular deposits of patients with MGN have been unsuccessful. Whitworth et al. [276] examined 24 renal biopsies from patients with MGN for the presence of autologous renal tubular epithelial antigen by indirect immunofluorescence. The antigen was isolated from normal human urine, was shown to be immunologically identical with one of the membrane-bound proximal tubular antigens, and localized to the proximal tubular brush border. It could not be detected in the serum. In the patients' kidneys, the antigen was detected in the brush border of all cases, but staining of the glomerular immune deposits was not observed. Whitworth et al. [276] suggested that the differences between their studies and those of Naruse et al. [176,177] were due to differences in either the antigen preparation or geographic differences in the pathogenesis of MGN between England and Japan. Thorpe and Cavallo [255] attempted to resolve these disparate results by preparing antibody according to the protocols of Naruse et al. [176,177] and Whitworth et al. [276], and studying the reaction of the two different antibody preparations with the immune deposits in 60 patients with MGN (50 were idiopathic). These authors were unable to demonstrate brush border antigens in the glomerular immune deposits with antisera either before or after acid elution of the tissue sections. They concluded that the observed discrepancies were not due to differences in the antigen preparations, but that putative geographic differences remained an open question. Collins et al. [44] examined renal tissue from 71 patients with MGN by indirect immunofluorescence using rabbit anti-human Fx1A. This antiserum reacted with antigens normally present in human and rat proximal tubular brush border and in the glomerular deposits of rats with Heymann nephritis but did not react with the glomerular deposits in any case of MGN before or after elution. In addition, sera from 6 patients and eluates from 5 renal specimens of MGN contained no activity against tubular antigen. Zager et al. [282] found no reactivity against human Fx1A (radioimmunoassay) in the sera of 29 MGN patients and 11 patients with other glomerular diseases.

Despite the facts that tubular brush border antigens are normally present in human urine [276], that antibody activity against tubular antigens has been reported in normal human sera [155], and that renal tubular antigens have been definitively identified in the immune deposits of isolated cases of idiopathic and secondary MGN [66,187], the bulk of evidence suggests that the antigen-antibody system involved in Heymann nephritis has little to do with the pathogenesis of idiopathic MGN. The cluster of reports in favor of a role for tubular antigens in MGN are all from the same Japanese group [167,176,177]. It is possible that some local factor has favored this antibody system in Japan, but when tested elsewhere, the Heymann antigen-antibody system does not appear to play a significant role in the pathogenesis of idiopathic MGN.

Etiology and Pathogenesis

The etiology of the idiopathic form of MGN is unknown. A variety of antigens have been implicated in the formation of subepithelial immune deposits, but so far, no single antigen has been implicated in the pathogenesis of idiopathic MGN. As more antigenic systems are identified in MGN, it appears that idiopathic MGN is the final morphologic pathway for many diseases. For example, if Blumberg had not described the Australia antigen, and if it had not subsequently been demonstrated in the glomerular immune deposits of some examples of MGN, the cases we now attribute to hepatitis B would still be classified as idiopathic MGN. Other antigenic systems implicated include SLE, tumors, gold, penicillamine and mercury compounds, and certain specific infections. As we have seen, it is unlikely that renal proximal tubular brush border antigens are involved in most cases.

The morphologic and immunopathologic similarities between MGN and the two experimental immunologic glomerular diseases, serum sickness nephritis [60,84] and autologous immune complex glomerulonephritis [69], support the conclusion that MGN is an immune complex–mediated disease. Couser [49] reviewed the possible mechanisms of subepithelial immune complex formation in MGN and found experimental evidence to support both in situ immune complex formation and trapping of circulating immune complexes. Since most of these data are derived from animal studies, the matter is reviewed in detail in Chapter 3. The strongest clinical evidence supporting a role for circulating immune complexes is their presence in some cases of MGN. They have been reported in cases of idiopathic MGN (see above), but in large series of patients with MGN, they are present in a minority regardless of the sensitivity of the assay used [44,282]. Border [24] summarized the results of several series in which various combinations of six different techniques had been used to detect circulating immune complexes in MGN. He found that complexes were present in only 23 percent of 235 patients. Using a more sensitive assay (solid-phase C1q binding), the Collaborative Study of Adult Nephrotic Syndrome [43] found immune complexes in 47 percent of 55 patients at the time of entry, and 66 percent had positive assay results on at least one occasion over the period of the study. In light of the inconstancy with which circulating immune complexes are demonstrable in clinical practice, Couser [49] has concluded from his appraisal of the clinical and experimental data that the subepithelial trapping of preformed immune complexes has not been convincingly shown to occur. On the other hand, he found considerable experimental support for the reaction of unbound antibody with antigen in situ in the subepithelial space. Although unproven in man, the weight of experimental evidence supports this mechanism in the pathogenesis of idiopathic MGN.

The mechanism of glomerular injury is a perplexing problem in MGN, a disease that characteristically has a paucity both of infiltrating inflammatory cells in the glomeruli and C3 in the immune deposits. In his review of glomerular injury in immune complex disease, Couser [49] discussed five mechanisms by which immune complexes can initiate tissue injury, and two seem relevant to MGN. The first is the reaction of antibody with intrinsic GBM and glomerular epithelial cell (GEC) antigens that causes proteinuria independent of cells and complement. There is no evidence that this mechanism is active in man. The second is seen in Heymann nephritis, where there is a complement-dependent mechanism of proteinuria that is independent of inflammatory cells [217]. The development of proteinuria in several forms of experimental glomerulonephritis with subepithelial immune deposits requires the later complement components [88]. In addition, the demonstration of the C5b-9 neoantigens of the membrane attack complex (MAC) in the glomerular immune deposits of MGN suggests the importance of a membranolytic role for complement in the pathogenesis of this disease [75]. Pruchno et al. [199] showed that urinary excretion of MAC, which distinguished passive Heymann nephritis from other experimental forms of MGN not involving GEC membrane antigens, correlated with the presence and quantity of glomerular antibody and C3 deposition. They concluded that the presence of MAC in the urine was an indicator of immunologic activity (distinct from the continued evidence of proteinuria and glomerular pathology) and a potential guide to therapy directed against the immune mechanism. When the same group [220] studied human urine for MAC by ELISA, they found no MAC in 40 normal urines. The values were higher in MGN urine than in nondiabetic, non-MGN proteinuric patients. In addition, the MGN patients with very high urinary MAC levels had more proteinuria and shorter duration from onset of proteinuria to renal biopsy than MGN patients with low levels. Coupes et al. [47] confirmed this observation, and in addition, they demonstrated that serial urinary MAC levels in patients correlated with the amount of proteinuria, serum creatinine level, and steroid therapy. This observation provides a rationale for treatment aimed at immunologic activity rather than the pathologic changes that are known to persist long after the etiologic agent is removed. Whether it identifies a therapeutically responsive subgroup of MGN patients remains to be proven.

Hepatitis B Antigen and Membranous Glomerulonephritis

The association of hepatitis B and MGN is a paradigm for secondary MGN. Epidemiologic studies suggest that hepatitis B is a major etiologic factor in MGN, and immunopathologic studies have implicated various hepatitis B antigens and antibodies in the pathogenesis of MGN. In addition, many of the reported cases are in children, and this has diagnostic implications. The initial report by Combes et al. [45] described a 53-year-old man with posttransfusion hepatitis who developed MGN. Subsequently, a number of similar cases have been reported (reviewed by Levy and Kleinknecht up to 1980 [146]). There are now several series that document the association between hepatitis B antigenemia and MGN in geographically and ethnically diverse populations [105,112,141, 146,166,175,234,236,247,277,281]. These observations implicate hepatitis B in the pathogenesis of MGN by virtue of the clinical association between the carrier state and MGN. By describing several morphologic patterns of glomerulonephritis in association with hepatitis B antigenemia, the reports also raise the possibility that hepatitis B virus carriers are predisposed to develop glomerular immune complex disease in general [175], as well as MGN in particular. Hepatitis B surface antigen (HB_sAg) remains the most frequently reported serum antigen in case reports of hepatitis B–associated MGN, as well as in series of patients with MGN examined for serologic evidence of hepatitis B antigens [105,141,146,166,175,234, 247,277,281].

Studies for other hepatitis B–associated antigens are less extensive, but both hepatitis B core antigen (HB_cAg) [105,139,234] and hepatitis B e antigens (HB_eAg) [99,139,141,166,247,281] and antibodies [105,141] have been reported in the serum of patients with MGN. Delta antigen has been the subject of only one negative report [166]. Circulating immune complexes that form in the presence of chronic hepatitis B antigenemia

[132,277] and hypocomplementemia in some patients with hepatitis B–associated MGN [236,281] also suggest immunologic activity.

The glomeruli contain large amounts of immunoglobulins and complement, but the demonstration of hepatitis B antigens and their specific antibodies in the glomerular deposits is not as consistent as the serologic association between hepatitis B antigenemia and MGN. The immune deposits in hepatitis B–associated MGN are invariably described as granular and localized along the GBM, and they always contain IgG and, less frequently, C3. IgM and IgA are occasionally present [105,129,247]. The demonstration of glomerular hepatitis B antigens is inconstant, even for HB_sAg. The early reports demonstrated antigens variously reported as HB_sAg, Australia antigen, and hepatitis B antigen in the glomerular immune deposits, but Levy and Kleinknecht [146] were unable to detect HB_sAg by direct immunofluorescence before and after elution. In their review of 54 positive patients among 123 patients studied up to 1980, they noted variation in technique and diversity of antisera in terms of source of antigen, immunization schedule, and titer. They suggested that some of the differences might be due to the uncontrolled nature of the studies. Subsequent to this review, some investigators have been unable to demonstrate HB_sAg in the glomeruli of patients with HB_sAg-associated MGN [105,141,247,277, 281]. However, Slusarcyzk et al. [234] found HB_sAg and HB_eAg in about a third each of 21 cases of hepatitis B–associated MGN. Elution studies in 4 patients demonstrated anti-HB_eAg in the eluate, while the eluted glomeruli demonstrated anti-HB_sAg activity by taking up the antigen. The observation was repeated with appropriate blocking and adsorption controls. Hsu et al. [112] found HB_eAg in the glomerular deposits of 95 percent of Taiwanese children with hepatitis B–associated childhood MGN. The deposits contained neither HB_sAg nor HB_cAg. Maggiore et al. [153] screened 136 consecutive patients with various glomerular lesions for HB_sAg in serum and kidney. None of the 11 patients who were seropositive for HB_sAg had demonstrable antigen in their glomerular immune deposits. However, 5 seronegative patients with glomerular deposits that stained for HB_sAg by the direct method also had IgM with antiglobulin activity in the glomerular deposits. The staining was not confirmed by direct immunofluorescence with anti-HB_sAg Fab′, and unconjugated IgM blocked the reaction. The authors concluded that the presence of IgM in the glomerular deposits confuses the interpretation of a positive staining reaction because of the nonspecific uptake of immunoglobulins by IgM antiglobulin activity.

The glomerular pathology of hepatitis B antigen–associated MGN is very similar to idiopathic MGN (Fig. 8-25). However, it has been suggested that several ultrastructural features have value as differential points (Fig. 8-26). These include the presence of tubuloreticular structures in the endothelium [71], viral particles in the deposits [129,139,247], subendothelial and mesangial electron-dense deposits, and glomerular proliferation of either mesangial or segmental nature. Yoshikawa et al. [281] studied 14 patients with hepatitis B–associated MGN and found mesangial electron-dense deposits in 13 and subendothelial electron-dense deposits in 4. In contrast, in 9 children with idiopathic MGN, there were mesangial deposits in 2, and none had subendothelial deposits. Since all these features have been described in idiopathic MGN, their presence does not allow the differentiation of hepatitis B–associated MGN on a morphologic basis.

Hepatitis B–associated MGN has been reported in adults and children, but the high incidence in children dictates that a child with MGN be evaluated for hepatitis B. Lee et al. [141] screened 732 consecutive Korean patients with glomerular diseases and found 87 who were HB_sAg carriers. Ten of 49 adults and 8 of 10 children with MGN, and 28 of 32 adults and 1 of 4 children with membranoproliferative glomerulonephritis were carriers. In contrast, only 15 of 192 adults and 1 of 22 children with IgA nephritis and sporadic patients with minimal change glomerulopathy (6 of 140), focal and segmental sclerosis (6 of 70), postinfectious glomerulonephritis (4 of 43), nonspecific glomerulonephritis (6 of 76), and SLE (1 of 56) had HB_sAg in their serum. In adults, various glomerular diseases have been associated with the hepatitis B carrier state, but a child with hepatitis B–

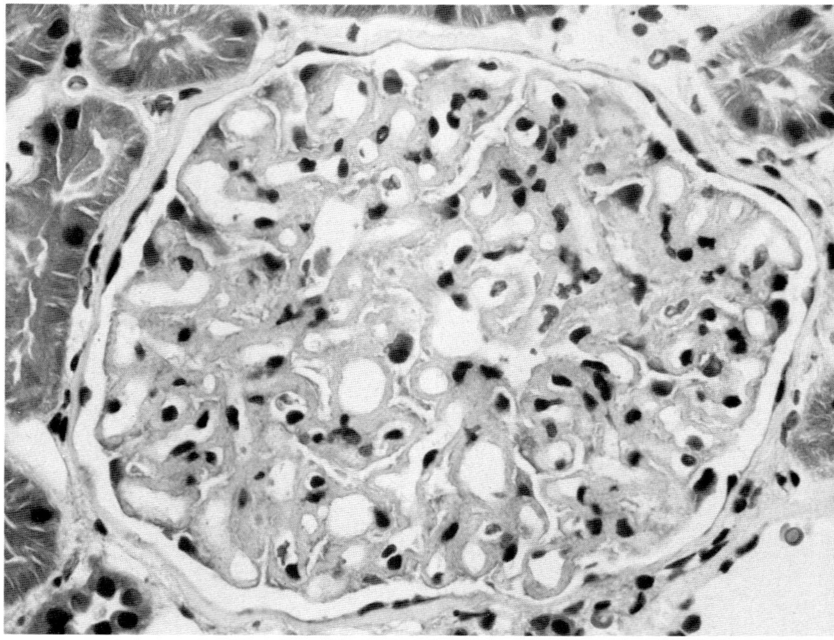

FIG. 8-25. *Glomerulus from a 24-year-old man with chronic active hepatitis, persistent Australia (hepatitis B) antigenemia, persistent proteinuria, and microscopic hematuria. There is diffuse thickening of the capillary walls with no cellular increase. H&E; ×450. (Courtesy of Drs. M. R. Knieser and E. H. Jenis.)*

associated glomerulonephritis is most likely to have MGN.

More than one glomerular disease may be seen simultaneously in patients with hepatitis B antigenemia, and these are most commonly MGN and IgA nephritis [117,154]. The liver disease in patients with the hepatitis B carrier state and MGN is usually asymptomatic. However, when the liver enzymes associated with acute hepatic injury are studied, they are frequently elevated [147,247]. Liver biopsy has shown a spectrum of hepatitic lesions, including acute hepatitis, chronic active hepatitis, and cirrhosis. The role of hepatitis B virus is also discussed on page 223 in Chapter 3.

Combined Membranous and Crescentic Glomerulonephritis

The association of MGN with crescents is a rare occurrence that has been reported approximately 20 times [3,5,40,134,135,178,190,192,224,250, 256]. The reported patients are all adults, and the majority is male (11 of 18). Since the combination of MGN and crescents can be seen in SLE, it should be excluded, as it was in all the reported cases. The association has a grim prognosis, and in the patients with follow-up, 8 went into end-stage renal disease, 3 had decreased but stable renal function, and 2 resolved the acute injury (although 1 had persistent hematuria). Gaffney and Panner [80] performed quantitative and semiquantitative analyses on 41 cases of idiopathic MGN and found glomerular hypercellularity in 24 cases and abnormal parietal epithelium in 25. These authors correlated the morphologic findings with an adverse outcome, but the features they illustrated are unimpressive and certainly are not sufficient for the diagnosis of crescentic glomerulonephritis. Even though it is unusual, superimposed crescentic glomerulonephritis should be included in the

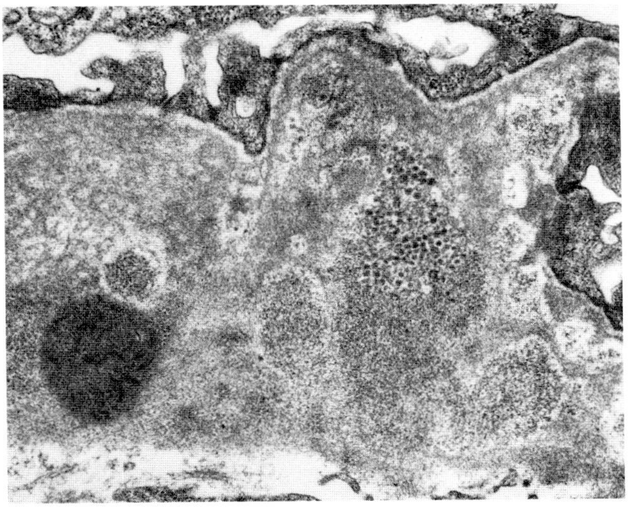

A

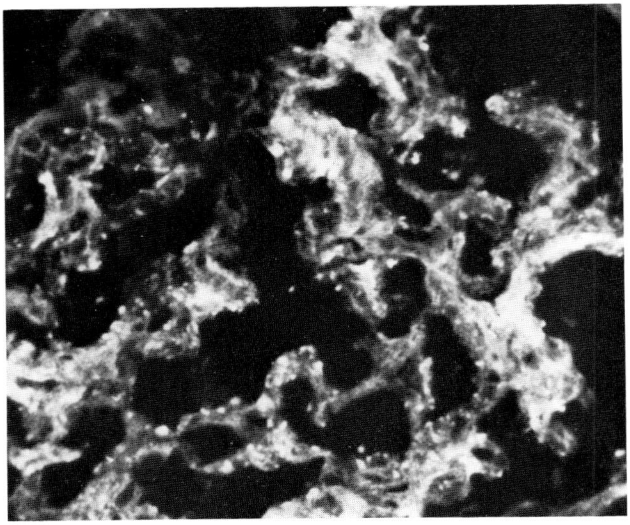

B

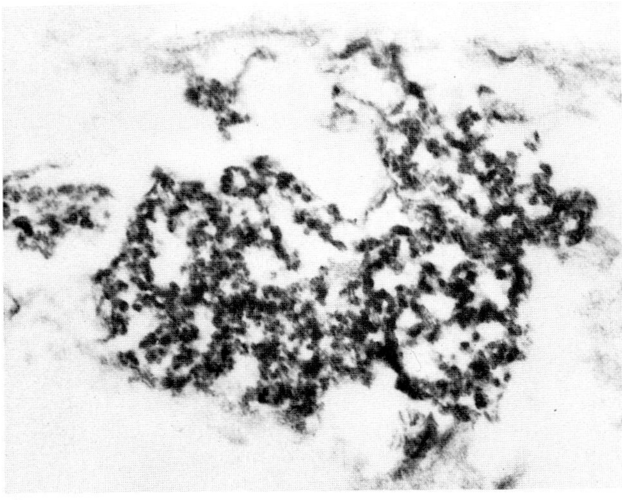

C

FIG. 8-26. *Same patient as in Fig. 8-25. (A) Electron micrograph to show electron-dense deposits and virus-like particles incorporated into a markedly thickened glomerular capillary basement membrane. ×13,000. (B) Immunofluorescence against IgG. ×800. (C) The way in which monospecific horseradish peroxidase–conjugated antiserum to Australia (hepatitis B) antigen stained the virus-like particles demonstrated in (A). ×32,000. (Courtesy of Drs. M. R. Knieser and E. H. Jenis.)*

differential diagnosis of the MGN patient who experiences a rapid loss of renal function.

The first case of combined membranous and crescentic glomerulonephritis, reported by Klassen et al. [127], was associated with pathogenic anti-GBM antibodies. The patient was a 49-year-old man with known MGN who developed a rapidly progressive renal course and died. At autopsy, he had crescentic glomerulonephritis superimposed on advanced MGN. Although anti-GBM antibodies were not present in the patient's serum, IgG eluted from the kidneys fixed to human and monkey kidney in a linear pattern in vitro, and when injected into two monkeys, it localized specifically to GBM and caused glomerular inflammation.

Pettersson et al., in a review of the literature [192], observed that the relationship between MGN and anti-GBM antibody fell into three patterns: primary anti-GBM disease followed by granular subepithelial deposits [5,240], primary MGN followed by anti-GBM disease [127,135,205], and simultaneous detection of both lesions [190,192,224,256]. Three of the four cases of subepithelial electron-dense deposits occurring in patients with Goodpasture's syndrome fell into the last category (Fig. 8-27). In two of them [190,224], the complex immunologic picture was indicated by the presence of a double contour on fluorescence microscopy, suggesting the presence of both subepithelial electron-dense deposits and anti-GBM antibody. However, the subepithelial deposits in these cases are very small and are not associated with membranous transformation (Fig. 8-28). In addition, one patient with Goodpasture's syndrome had very mild renal involvement, and the whole syndrome resolved without treatment [5]. Although Klassen et al. [127] suggested that MGN damaged the GBM and released antigens that then incited the anti-GBM disease, the converse mechanism may be operative in the cases of MGN associated with Goodpasture's syndrome, in which the anti-GBM antibodies are dominant and the immune complex component is minimal. The case presented by Hill et al. [104] is of a combined crescentic and membranous picture developing after an initial biopsy had shown pure MGN. The patient developed renal failure, and transplantation was performed following removal of the patient's native kidneys. It was not possible to demonstrate anti-GBM antibody in the patient's blood before or after transplantation, but the combined picture of MGN and crescents seen in the native kidneys developed in the transplant. The pathogenesis of MGN in a transplant will be discussed below, but the occurrence of crescentic glomerulonephritis in the absence of anti-GBM antibodies should come as no surprise, since many cases of crescentic glomerulonephritis occur without demonstrable anti-GBM antibodies [221]. Excluding the cases of Goodpasture's syndrome, 6 of 12 reported cases of MGN with crescents had no evidence of anti-GBM antibody.

Development of Membranous Glomerulonephritis in Transplanted Kidneys

MGN occurs in transplanted kidneys both in the context of a prior diagnosis of MGN in the native kidneys (recurrence) and when the patient's original renal disease is unrelated (de novo). Hume

FIG. 8-27. *Glomerulus from a 25-year-old man who presented with massive pulmonary hemorrhage and rapidly progressive glomerulonephritis. This photomicrograph is representative of the diffuse cellular crescents present in the renal biopsy. The cells in Bowman's space are compressing the glomerulus, which shows little intrinsic cellular proliferation. The patient had circulating anti-GBM antibodies that stained both the glomerular and alveolar basement membranes [224]. Methenamine silver–periodic acid–Schiff (Jones); ×450.*

FIG. 8-28. *Electron micrograph of a glomerular capillary from the same patient illustrated in Fig. 8-27. There are diffuse subepithelial (Epi) electron-dense deposits. When the glomerulus was stained for IgG and examined by fluorescence microscopy, there was a definite double contour, suggesting the presence of both anti-GBM antibody and granular immune aggregates. However, only subepithelial deposits are seen by electron microscopy. Uranyl acetate and lead citrate; ×25,000.*

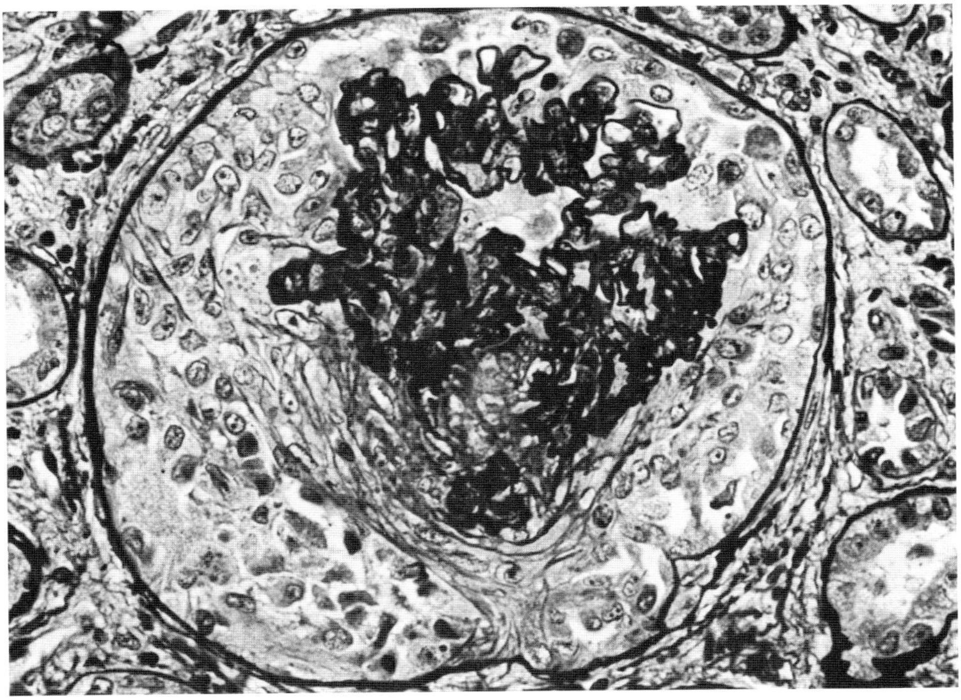

Fig. 8-27

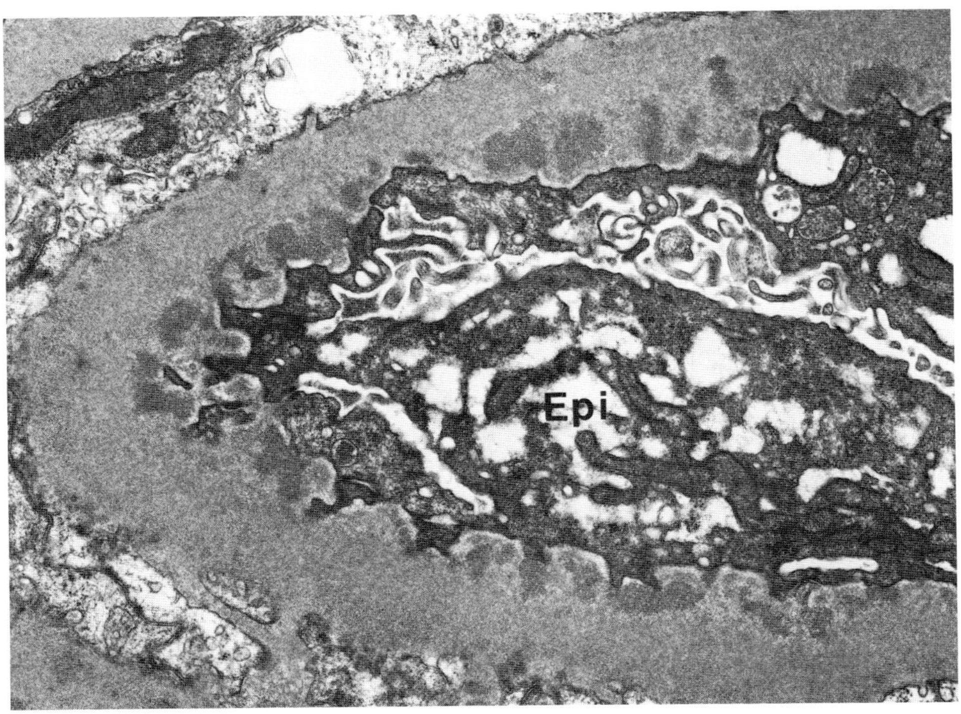

Fig. 8-28

and Bryant [113], in defining recurrent glomerulonephritis in a transplanted kidney, emphasized that the identity of the original disease and the absence of disease in the graft at the time of transplantation must be demonstrated. This is crucial, for currently there is no morphologic feature that differentiates recurrent from de novo MGN. Since transplanted kidneys are susceptible to all the known causes of MGN, the presence of this lesion should initiate a search to exclude the secondary forms (especially hepatitis B). Although MGN is the most frequent cause of nephrotic syndrome in adults, and progresses to end-stage renal disease in approximately 25 percent of the cases, Cameron [33] has estimated that only 2 percent of European patients requiring transplantation have a prior biopsy diagnosis of MGN. Given the small pool of patients who reach end-stage renal disease because of MGN, it is not surprising that there are only a few well-documented cases of recurrent MGN [104,151]. The etiology of these cases is unknown, and although they fulfill all the criteria listed above, until the antigen responsible for the original disease is identified and is demonstrated in the immune deposits of the graft, it can only be said that the patient has retained the ability to develop MGN. Whether these few cases represent recurrent or de novo MGN remains unresolved.

De novo MGN, in contrast, is a well-established entity that has been the subject of numerous case reports. In contrast to the infrequency of recurrent MGN, the incidence of de novo MGN is estimated to be from 2 to 4 percent [38,262,271]. Although most of the reported cases are in adults, de novo MGN also occurs in children. Habib et al. [91] reported an incidence of 9.3 percent in 310 grafts in children. In the largest series, Charpentier and Levy [38] reported 19 cases in 1550 renal transplants (1.2 percent). Proteinuria was detected at a mean time of 26 months after transplantation. None of the factors they investigated, including age, sex, donor-recipient HLA phenotypes, first graft versus second graft, cadaver versus related graft, HLA matching, recipient treatment, number of transfused blood units, lymphocytoxins, number of rejection episodes, number and length of ATN episodes, and viral or bacterial infection, seemed to be related to the development of de novo MGN. Truong et al. [262] found 95 well-documented cases of de novo MGN in the literature and presented the clinical and pathologic features of 10 cases of their own. In their literature review, 38 of 82 patients had either lost their grafts 4 to 82 months (mean 35 months) after transplantation or died a nonrenal death. The adverse prognosis of this lesion also was reflected in their patients, of whom 5 lost their grafts and 1 died a nonrenal death. Although the glomerular lesion is similar to idiopathic MGN in native kidneys, Truong et al. note that de novo MGN has distinct morphologic differences in that all their patients had histologic evidence of cellular and/or humoral rejection. In 6 patients the rejection process was documented by renal biopsy to precede de novo MGN. The authors found the presence of nephrotic syndrome and renal insufficiency to be ominous signs, with 5 of 6 patients presenting with the nephrotic syndrome losing their grafts 2 to 42 months after the diagnosis of MGN. The authors did not feel that graft failure was due to de novo MGN, which tended to be segmental and in an early stage, but when superimposed on an injured kidney with ongoing rejection, it identified a group of kidney transplant patients with a poor prognosis for graft survival.

Ward and Koyle [271] reviewed more than 40 cases of de novo MGN in the literature, but they concluded that the descriptive clinical and pathologic studies added no insights to the pathogenesis of the glomerular lesion. Thus they investigated the immunopathologic and physicochemical properties of the immune complexes or immune complex components in the sera of 7 patients with de novo MGN and compared them with 7 patients with untreated idiopathic MGN, 6 patients with normal functioning renal grafts, and 6 patients with recurrent focal and segmental glomerular sclerosis in their transplanted kidneys. The features that they tested have been experimentally implicated in the formation of subepithelial immune complexes. High-molecular-weight circulating immune complexes (19 S) were demonstrated by C1q binding in six of seven cases of de novo MGN, and low-molecular-weight (9 S) immune complexes were shown to be present by the rheumatoid factor inhibition assay in five of seven.

Strongly cationic IgG spectrotypes (PI 8.0–9.2) were seen in five of seven patients with de novo MGN, and the immune complexes themselves were cationic in three of four cases tested by isoelectric focusing. Indirect immunofluorescence demonstrated brush border and tubular epithelial/interstitial antibodies in five of seven cases. At least one of these factors was present in each patient with de novo MGN, and all four factors were seen in five patients. Although statistical comparisons between de novo MGN and the control groups were not done, the immunopathologic features were only sporadically present in the patients with recurrent focal and segmental glomerular sclerosis and normally functioning renal grafts, while the patients with idiopathic MGN had serologic similarities to those of de novo MGN. These findings are very provocative, since the authors also found HLA phenotypes associated with increased risk of developing MGN in either the donor or the recipient in six of seven de novo MGN cases. If confirmed, these results have implications for the pathogenesis of both de novo and native MGN, because they suggest that in both circumstances MGN occurs in a strongly nephritogenic internal milieu.

SECONDARY FORMS OF MEMBRANOUS GLOMERULONEPHRITIS

Gold Therapy and Membranous Glomerulonephritis

Because they are toxic, gold salts are almost exclusively limited as therapeutic agents to cases of rheumatoid arthritis that are severe and unresponsive to nonsteroidal anti-inflammatory drugs and prednisone. A variety of renal manifestations of gold therapy have been reported. These include oliguric renal failure [58], but by far the most common renal complication is proteinuria. This association was an early clinical observation that preceded the pathologic correlation with MGN, but it has made frequent urine testing mandatory prior to initiating therapy and before each subsequent dose. Although many patients were reported with proteinuria while receiving gold, the role of MGN in the underlying glomerular pathology was unknown until the application of renal biopsy to affected patients. The incidence of proteinuria in patients receiving gold is from 1 to 12.5 percent [98,165,230]. The onset of proteinuria is not related to the total amount of gold or to the length of time over which it is administered [39,82,259], and when tested, the blood and urine levels of gold fall in the therapeutic range [39,230]. Recently, it has been reported that oral gold is better tolerated than the standard parenteral preparations; not only is there a lower incidence of proteinuria (3 percent), but of eight patients whose gold therapy was discontinued because of proteinuria, seven were able to tolerate oral gold when rechallenged [125]. Despite the presence of nephrotic-range proteinuria, there is a remarkable incidence of clinical resolution when the drug is withdrawn [51,77,124,141,230,245].

Hall et al. [94] have recently reviewed the topic and have presented morphologic and clinical data on 21 patients of their own who developed proteinuria while being treated for rheumatoid arthritis with gold. Of the 21 patients studied, 15 had MGN, 2 had minimal-change disease, 2 had mesangial electron-dense deposits, and 2 had no pathologic changes. They developed proteinuria from 7 months to 2 years after the initiation of therapy, and after discontinuation of the drug, they reached a maximum protein excretion of 2.1 g/day (range 0.7–30.7 g/day) after a median interval of 2 months (range 1–13 months). Proteinuria resolved spontaneously in 18 patients over a 2-year period, and all patients were protein-free by 39 months. There was no change in the median first and last C_{Cr}, and no patient died from or needed therapy for renal failure. A few patients have been reported whose proteinuria did not resolve, but their follow-up was short [77,142]. It is important to note that not only does clinical proteinuria resolve, but the morphologic changes of MGN are also reversible [82,124,142,230,245,259,267].

MGN is the predominant glomerular pathologic change in proteinuric gold-treated patients, and it is indistinguishable from idiopathic MGN. The glomeruli are usually normal by light microscopy. Although the membranous changes are seen by light microscopy in some cases. Törnroth and Skrifvars [259] were only able to make the diagnosis in 1 of 10, and Gärtner [82] found that 9 of 14 cases had stage I changes detectable only by electron microscopy. Like idiopathic MGN, the immunofluorescence findings are invariably granular deposits of IgG along the GBM, with lesser amounts of C3 in the same location [82,124,280]. IgM and IgA have been reported occasionally in the deposits [51,77,82,124,233,259,264,269, 273,280]. Electron microscopy shows small subepithelial electron-dense deposits that usually have no associated membranous transformation. This explains the difficulty in seeing the lesions by light microscopy [51,124,142,230,233,245, 259,264,269,280] (Fig. 8-29). However, membranous transformation does occur, with cases presenting in all stages [82,259]. Törnroth and Skrifvars [260], in a study of serial biopsies in patients who had discontinued gold therapy after the onset of proteinuria, have suggested that this is an example of MGN with one generation of immune deposits, and some cases apparently heal without going through all the stages of membranous transformation. Without further injury caused by new generations of subepithelial deposits, the GBM heals with time by epithelial GBM synthesis and turnover.

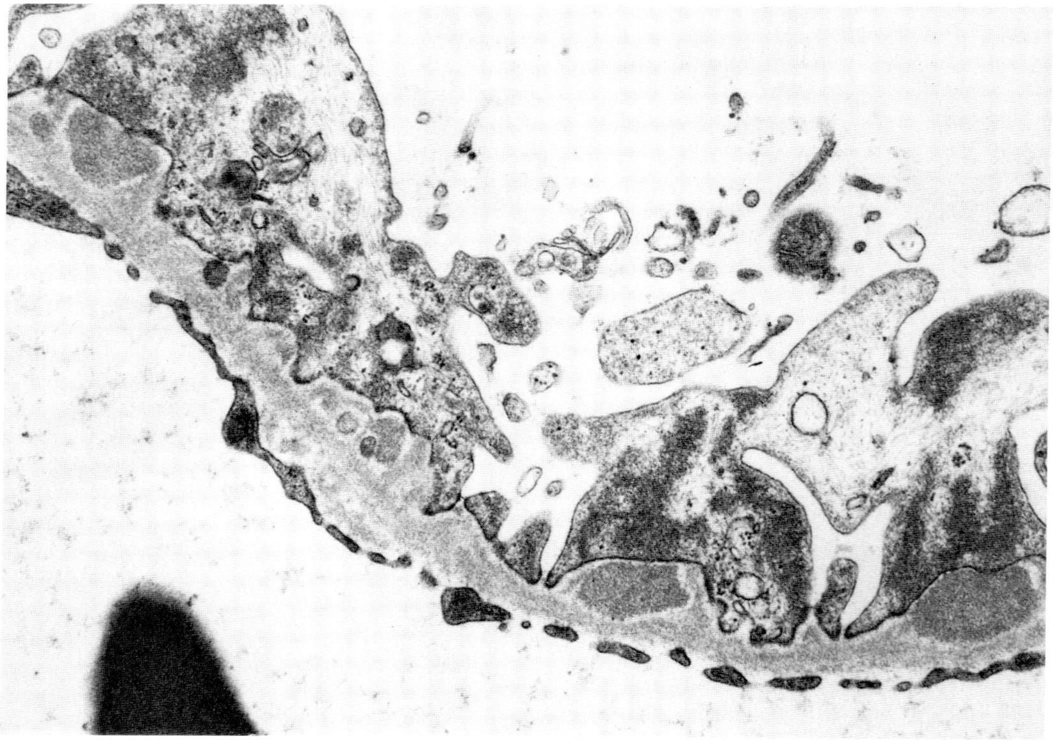

FIG. 8-29. *Electron micrograph of a glomerulus from a patient who developed proteinuria during a course of treatment with gold. Light microscopy revealed mild patchy thickening of the glomerular capillary walls, and IgG and IgM were present in a granular pattern. There are numerous deposits on the epithelial side of the GBM with small intervening spikes.* ×23,000. *(Courtesy of Dr. E. Jenis.)*

The presence of gold inclusions in the proximal convoluted tubule and the glomerular epithelial and mesangial cells is the unique morphologic finding in gold nephropathy. These are described as filamentous electron-dense strands with associated granules [6,82,124,230,245,264,269,273, 280] (Fig. 8-30). Gold has been demonstrated histochemically in the proximal convoluted tubule and the glomerular tuft, and has persisted for up to 28 years in interstitial macrophages after the last gold injection [28]. In addition, a number of electron microscopic x-ray dispersion techniques have demonstrated gold in the inclusions but not in the electron-dense deposits [6,264,269,273, 280]. Thus the relationship between the affinity of gold for the proximal convoluted tubule and the pathogenesis of MGN is the subject of considerable debate.

Pathogenetic insight is gained from clinical observations and experimental studies. Gold is toxic to the proximal tubule in experimental animals. Although the mechanism is not known, it localizes to the mitochondria in acutely intoxicated rats and causes tubular necrosis [81,244]. Given chronically in lower doses, it is associated with degenerating mitochondria that are extruded into the lumen of the proximal tubule. Nagi et al. [174] injected rats intramuscularly with sodium aurothiomalate on a weekly basis for 12 weeks. Those receiving 1 mg per week showed no glomerular changes, but there was tubular degeneration with histochemically demonstrable tubular gold. The rats receiving 0.025 mg per week showed lesser degrees of tubular damage, but in contrast to the previous group, they had diffuse thickening of the glomerular capillary wall with electron-dense deposits on the epithelial side of the GBM. IgG and C3 were present as small granules along the glomerular capillary wall. Gold was not demonstrable in the glomeruli. The authors concluded that gold damages the proximal tubule, releasing antigens that form complexes in the glomerulus in a manner analogous to that taking place in experimentally produced autologous immune complex disease (see Chap. 3). Tubular damage has been demonstrated in asymptomatic patients treated with gold by showing elevated excretion of leucine aminopeptidase, a brush border enzyme, and N-acetyl-beta-glucosaminidase, a lysosomal hydrolase, when compared with similar patients not treated with gold [164]. Tubular damage was associated with tubular dysfunction in 9 of 33 patients demonstrated by elevated urinary β_2-microglobulin. The authors concluded that gold at therapeutic levels causes sufficient tubular damage to cause dysfunction. Finally, patients with rheumatoid ar-

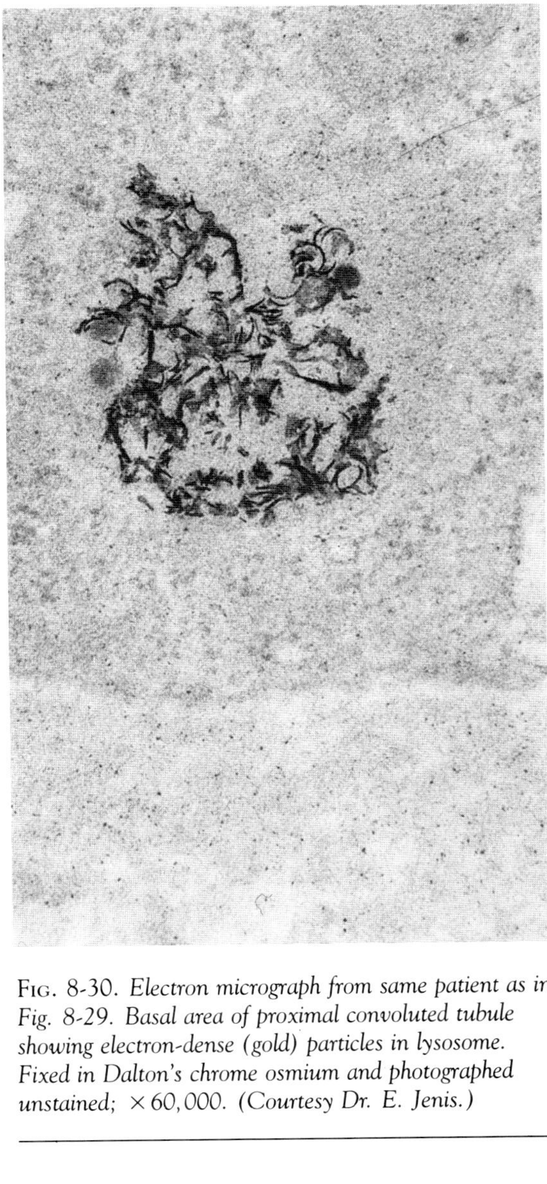

Fig. 8-30. *Electron micrograph from same patient as in Fig. 8-29. Basal area of proximal convoluted tubule showing electron-dense (gold) particles in lysosome. Fixed in Dalton's chrome osmium and photographed unstained;* $\times$ *60,000. (Courtesy Dr. E. Jenis.)*

thritis start with an abnormal immune system, and Hall et al. [94] found HLA-B8 and/or DR3 alloantigens in 7 of 21 proteinuric gold-treated rheumatoid arthritis patients. This supports the concept that in rheumatoid arthritis, as in idiopathic MGN and de novo MGN, the lesion of MGN occurs in a susceptible subgroup.

Thus gold affects the proximal convoluted tubule in patients and experimental animals in the same fashion, and similar glomerular lesions develop in both. Despite this congruity, the suggestion that a similar mechanism is involved will remain speculative until it is demonstrated that gold intoxication releases a tubular antigen capable of causing MGN. As indicated earlier, there is little evidence implicating tubular antigens in human MGN in general, and this has not been accomplished in the gold-associated form of MGN.

The unanswered question is whether all the cases are truly caused by gold, or do they represent an underlying relationship between MGN and rheumatoid arthritis? There are well-documented cases of MGN in patients with rheumatoid arthritis who have never been treated with gold [103,109,218]. Samuels et al. [218] are particularly critical of the primacy of gold in causing the lesion and have suggested that it merely augments the proteinuria. In this context, the study of Skrifvars et al. [232] is of considerable interest. They studied renal biopsies from 20 patients with rheumatoid arthritis by immunofluorescence microscopy, half of whom had never received gold. In this latter group, 4 patients showed glomerular granular deposits of IgG and C3. Although 2 patients had positive antinuclear antibodies, suggesting that an underlying SLE may have caused the lesion, and one had only segmental deposits, the remaining 2 patients seem to represent early cases of MGN. Despite the fact that rheumatoid arthritis, by itself, is occasionally associated with MGN, the temporal relationship between gold therapy and the onset of proteinuria, the presence of gold in the proximal tubules, and the prompt resolution of proteinuria with healing of the GBM when gold is discontinued strongly support an etiologic role for gold.

Other glomerular lesions have been described in patients receiving gold, including mesangial immune complex trapping, minimal change disease, focal segmental glomerulonephritis, and no changes. Davis et al. [52] described a case that showed mesangial expansion and hypercellularity by light microscopy, electron-dense deposits in a subepithelial and subendothelial position in the GBM as well as the mesangium, and IgG, IgM, C3, and C1q in a finely granular pattern along the glomerular capillary wall and in the mesangium. Sjögren syndrome and SLE were excluded. Skrifvars et al. [232] described a patient with rheumatoid arthritis who developed granulomatous glomerulonephritis while receiving gold therapy, but I have seen several cases [137] of necrotizing glomerulonephritis in rheumatoid arthritis patients who were not treated with gold. Thus all glomerular lesions occurring in gold-treated rheumatoid arthritis patients must be critically evaluated in the light of the known glomerular pathology of rheumatoid arthritis itself.

In summary, gold in the therapeutic range may cause mild tubular damage, although this is rarely associated with serious clinical problems. Various forms of glomerular injury have been recorded, but MGN is the most common. The fact that an identical lesion can occur in rheumatoid arthritis patients who are not treated with gold casts doubt on the hitherto unquestioned idea that gold is primarily responsible for the glomerular lesion. The various forms of glomerulonephritis described in rheumatoid arthritis are considered in Chapter 16.

Penicillamine Therapy and Membranous Glomerulonephritis

Among patients treated with penicillamine, proteinuria (frequently accompanied by the nephrotic syndrome) is a common complication. It occurs in from 7.4 to 33 percent of patients [54,59,171,243] and is the most frequent cause for permanent discontinuation of the drug. In contrast to gold, which is used almost exclusively in the treatment of rheumatoid arthritis, penicillamine is used to treat diseases not associated with MGN. It has been suggested that MGN is more likely to complicate autoimmune diseases such as rheumatoid arthritis treated with penicillamine [9,60,96,114, 171], but the occurrence of MGN in penicillamine-treated patients with such disparate diseases as Wilson's disease [54,138,241], scleroderma [54], and cystinuria [100] supports a separate role for the drug in the etiology of MGN. Originally, it was believed that the racemic form was responsible for the glomerular lesion [241], but almost all the subsequently reported cases have been associated with D-penicillamine therapy.

Dische [59] noted that subsequent to his initial report of four penicillamine-treated rheumatoid arthritis patients who developed MGN, he has rarely seen this association. He attributed the decreased incidence to the lower recommended dosage currently in use, and there are reports that support this contention [60,243]. Dixon et al. [60] reported a controlled clinical trial of the efficacy of low (600 mg/day) and high (1200 mg/day) doses of penicillamine in the control of rheumatoid arthritis. The low dose was just as effective as the high dose in controlling objective and subjective symptomatology, and the high dose had more adverse reactions. However, the only reaction requiring discontinuance of the drug was proteinuria, and this occurred in a patient receiving the lower dose. There are sporadic reports of the reaction occurring with low doses [241], and two large series have found no relationship between size of the daily dose or total dose of the drug and MGN [9,82]. The idiosyncratic association between penicillamine and proteinuria makes mandatory the testing of urine prior to initiation of therapy and frequently during the course of treatment.

The patient usually presents with asymptomatic proteinuria or symptoms of the nephrotic syndrome during the first year of penicillamine therapy [9,82,95,100,241,243]. Hematuria is an inconstant presenting finding. Despite the presence of massive proteinuria, renal function is usually normal at presentation [9,59,82,114,241,242, 243]. On the other hand, one of eight patients reported by Sternlieb [241] developed renal insufficiency and anuria. One of 13 proteinuric patients reported by Stockman et al. [243] had decreased renal function, but renal biopsy showed amyloidosis. In Gärtner's series of 51 patients [82], the C_{Cr} was less than 80 ml/min/1.73 m^2 in 42 percent. Although the immunopathology suggests an immune complex pathogenesis of the glomerular lesion, tests for circulating immune complexes are usually negative, and serum complement is normal [9].

The course of proteinuria after penicillamine is withdrawn is one of slow resolution with complete disappearance of proteinuria [95,100,138,171]. In a study of 33 patients, Hall et al. [95] reported that when treatment was stopped, the proteinuria reached a median peak of 4.2 g/24 h (range 0.3–15.0 g/24 h) at 1 month (range 0–7 months) before resolving spontaneously by 6 months (12 patients), 12 months (21 patients), or 18 months (29 patients). In all patients, except one with carcinoma of the renal pelvis, proteinuria resolved by 21 months, and the median duration of proteinuria was 8 months. The patients showed no deterioration of renal function (creatinine clearance), and no patient required treatment for renal failure. Bacon et al. [9] reported that 10 of 11 patients with the nephrotic syndrome initially had greatly reduced their level of protein excretion by 1 year or at the 6-month follow-up, but low levels of proteinuria persisted in 12 of 13 patients. In Gärtner's series [82], proteinuria disappeared completely in 29 of 46 patients (63 percent) after a mean of 13.6 ± 9.7 months. The 17 patients with persistent proteinuria had 2.2 ± 1.4 g/24 h after a mean of 20 ± 11 months off therapy. Those in whom it persisted had received a higher total dose of the drug and had a higher initial level of protein excretion. Interestingly, several patients have been rechallenged with the drug, usually at a reduced dose, after they were protein-free, and some have tolerated the drug without proteinuria or at a markedly reduced and clinically acceptable level [138].

The pathology is similar in all the reported cases irrespective of the original condition for which penicillamine was used. Although there may be mesangial expansion and hypercellularity, it has been emphasized that the light microscopy is remarkably normal [9]. In a few cases, trichrome stains have demonstrated red deposits on the basement membranes [114]. Gärtner [82], using semithin silver-stained sections, found no changes or only focal spikes in one-half of 51 patients and definite membranous changes in the others. Electron microscopy shows small, focal or diffuse, subepithelial electron-dense deposits, and when unaccompanied by basement-membrane changes, this ultrastructural appearance correlates with the minimal light microscopic changes [9,59,82,96, 100,243]. The absence of membranous transformation is most often seen early in the course (at the time of diagnosis or when penicillamine is discontinued). However, when biopsies are studied later in the course (when penicillamine is discontinued [9,82] or on repeat biopsy [82,96,114, 138]), the full range of membranous transformation has been described.

Bacon et al. [9] noted that biopsies performed at the time of diagnosis were characterized by subepithelial electron-dense deposits and diffuse foot-process effacement. In biopsies taken 6 months or more after discontinuation of penicillamine, the basement membrane had only focal subepithelial electron-dense deposits, and there was restoration of the foot processes. In the patients in whom proteinuria persisted at a high level after discontinuation of penicillamine, there were numerous deposits, but they were frequently surrounded by a clear halo and had loss of their electron density. Although the authors emphasized that proteinuria persisted in many patients, the three cases with persistent proteinuria had only 1.7 and 0.4 g/24 h at 12 months and 2.8 g/24 h at 6 months, respectively. In the renal biopsies from these patients, the description of reabsorbing deposits suggests that the lesions were actually healing.

Patients receiving penicillamine who do not develop proteinuria show no deposits on renal biopsy [100]. There are occasional patients who have mesangial or subendothelial electron-dense deposits, but this is not a general observation [95,243].

Immunofluorescence microscopy demonstrates diffuse granular deposits of IgG and C3 along the capillary wall [9,59,82,114,138,242,243]. IgM and/or IgA are described in a few instances [59,82,138,243], but it is always emphasized that these deposits stain less intensely than for IgG. Complement components other than C3 have not been reported in many cases, but C1q and C4 have been seen [59,82]. In repeat biopsies performed when proteinuria is lessened, the staining intensity is decreased and segmental [9,82,138], corresponding to reabsortion of the deposits seen by electron microscopy.

Other pathologic lesions described in penicillamine nephropathy are usually related to the underlying disease process. These include amyloidosis [82,243] and vasculitis [10,137] in patients with rheumatoid arthritis.

The pathology and immunopathology seen in penicillamine nephropathy suggest an immune complex mechanism, and patients with rheumatoid arthritis in general have circulating immune complexes. However, what distinguishes the majority from penicillamine-treated patients who develop MGN is unknown. Skrifvars et al. [232] have suggested that the presence of rheumatoid factor prevents immune complex deposition, and penicillamine causes either a decrease in or disappearance of the circulating immune complexes. Since penicillamine can dissociate macroaggregates, the drug may act by removing immune complexes from the circulation and by making the antibody available in a form that more readily localizes to the kidney. It also has been suggested that the susceptibility to develop this lesion might be under genetic control. There is also the possibility that penicillamine might have a more direct action, either by acting as a hapten or by injuring the tubules and causing glomerular lesions as in the Heymann-Edgington model of autologous immune complex glomerulonephritis. At present, there is no proof for any of these mechanisms.

Several other glomerular lesions have been reported in association with penicillamine therapy, and necrotizing glomerulonephritis, with or without crescents, is the most frequent. Hayslett et al. [100] described three patients with cystinuria who developed proteinuria while taking penicillamine. Renal biopsy in all three showed focal and segmental glomerulonephritis, but the illustrations suggest that these were very segmental and minimally destructive. There also were subepithelial electron-dense deposits without membranous transformation. Withdrawal of the drug led to resolution of proteinuria, and after 6 months rebiopsy showed some segmental scarring with persistence of the deposits. Sternlieb et al. [242] presented three patients with Wilson's disease treated with penicillamine who developed crescentic glomerulonephritis and pulmonary hemorrhage. Immunologic studies performed in one patient showed interrupted staining for IgG and C3 in the kidneys but not in the lungs. Although the immunologic relationship between the lung and kidney lesions was not established in the one patient studied, the presence of crescentic lesions is illustrated in all three patients. Falck et al. [74] described a patient with seronegative rheumatoid arthritis and features of SLE who developed proteinuria and terminal renal failure after 6 months of penicillamine therapy. Renal biopsy showed early MGN and vasculitis of the renal blood vessels. Banfi et al. [10] reported a similar patient with rheumatoid arthritis who developed proteinuria and rapidly progressive glomerulonephritis after 3 months on penicillamine. Renal biopsy showed crescentic glomerulonephritis with vasculitis. Immunofluorescence microscopy showed mesangial and granular IgA and C3, and electron microscopy revealed only subendothelial deposits. Withdrawal of the drug and institution of prednisone therapy led to diuresis and stable chronic renal failure. Kuznetsky et al. [137] described four patients with rheumatoid arthritis and necrotizing glomerulonephritis, one of whom had MGN and a history of penicillamine therapy. Finally, there are several case reports in which the proteinuria was associated with "normal" renal biopsies [241]. Since most of these were studied by light microscopy only, the diagnosis of MGN cannot be excluded under these circumstances. Sternlieb [241] did describe one patient who had a normal biopsy by electron microscopy, and two patients have been reported who had minimal change disease [95].

Epithelial Neoplasia and Membranous Glomerulonephritis

Proteinuria, frequently of sufficient magnitude to present as the nephrotic syndrome, has been reported in association with neoplasms arising within the kidney and far removed from it. When processes associated with malignancy and known to cause proteinuria (amyloidosis, renal vein thrombosis, and direct invasion of the renal parenchyma by tumor) are excluded, there remains a group of patients with proteinuria and a neoplasm who have the glomerulopathy of neoplasia [68]. Lee et al. [143], in the first clinicopathologic study of this association, reported malignant tumors in 11 adults in a series of 111 patients with the nephrotic syndrome (10.9 percent). The expected incidence of cancer in this group (from life insurance tables) was 1 percent, and in a closely age-matched control group with coronary artery disease, only 1 case of MGN was found. In other reports, the incidence has been comparable. Brueggemeyer and Ramirez [27] found 4 malignancies within 14 months of the diagnosis of MGN in 128 patients. Row et al. [215] found 7 patients with a simultaneous neoplasm in a series of 66 patients (10.9 percent) with MGN. In addition, a large number of case reports continue to appear describing the temporal association of MGN in a wide variety of malignant epithelial tumors, hematologic neoplasms, and benign tumors (reviewed in refs 68 and 278). The most common tumors are from lung and the gastrointestinal tract, but case reports cite the association with tumors of breast, pancreas, kidney, prostate, cervix, skin, Hodgkin's disease, lymphosarcoma, chronic lymphocytic leukemia, melanoma, Wilms tumor, neuroblastoma, and pheochromocytoma. In 8 of the 11 cases reported by Lee et al. [143], the glomerular lesion was MGN, but carcinomas also were associated with two other glomerular diseases: lobular glomerulonephritis and minimal change disease. In their review, Eagen and Lewis [68] emphasized the striking association between carcinomas and MGN. Whereas, among 134 patients selected from the literature for the nephrotic syndrome and a tumor, the incidence of MGN was only 24 percent, it was 70 percent among 48 patients with carcinoma and the nephrotic syndrome. Other glomerular lesions associated with the nephrotic syndrome and a neoplasm included minimal change disease, membranoproliferative glomerulonephritis, amyloidosis, extracapillary glomerulonephritis, proliferative sclerosing glomerulonephritis, proliferative glomerulonephritis, unclassified glomerulonephritis, renal dysplasia, and thrombotic microangiography.

The glomerular pathology of MGN of neoplasia is identical to that of idiopathic MGN. Light microscopy shows normal cellularity or mild, segmental mesangial proliferation. The glomerular basement membranes are usually thickened, and with the silver stain, spikes, holes, and complexity may be seen. Red GBM deposits may be seen in trichrome preparations [46,48,50,143,215,278]. The characteristic ultrastructural features are subepithelial and intramembranous electron-dense deposits and diffuse epithelial-cell foot-process effacement. In some early cases associated with low-grade proteinuria, the deposits may be small and sparse, while in biopsies taken long after the onset of the nephrotic syndrome, especially during remissions following resection of the tumor, the deposits are intramembranous, show loss of their electron density, and appear to be in the process of reabsorption [46,102,143,215,278]. Subendothelial and mesangial electron-dense deposits and tubuloreticular structures in the endothelium are either not specifically mentioned or are stated to be absent. Immunofluorescence microscopy almost always finds diffuse granular deposits of IgG and C3 along the glomerular capillary walls [46,48,50,102,215]. Other immunoglobulins and complement components [46,48] and mesangial deposits are only occasionally mentioned, and they are usually less intense and/or segmentally distributed. Thus the renal pathology and immunopathology in the majority of patients with nephrotic syndrome and carcinoma suggests an immune complex pathogenesis.

Patients with this syndrome usually present with symptomatic proteinuria and a malignant tumor diagnosed simultaneously or within 1 year. Although there are published reports with the nephrotic syndrome occurring 3 and 4 years after the diagnosis of malignancy, most authors believe that a causal relationship exists only if the former sequence is observed. Since cancer patients may have elevated levels of soluble circulating immune complexes early in the course of their disease [214], the presentation of patients with proteinuria due to immune complex glomerulopathy is consistent with current knowledge of host response to neoplasia. As would be expected with this spectrum of carcinomas, Eagen and Lewis [68] recorded a grave prognosis: 77 percent died with a median survival of 12 months from presentation, and only 7 of 34 survived for more than 2 years. After recognition of the tumor, median survival was only 3 months. Most of the patients developed carcinomatosis and died of their malignancy. In all but 2, the nephrotic syndrome persisted. There are several reports in which the patient has gone into remission of proteinuria following successful removal of the tumor. These include a patient who was alive and in remission of both cancer and proteinuria 10 years after removal of a gastric cancer [35] and two cases of long-term remissions of the nephrotic syndrome following resection of a malignant tumor [278]. One of the latter patients presented with the nephrotic syndrome, and the diagnosis of MGN was documented by renal biopsy. A carcinoma of the breast was resected during the same admission. Fourteen months after resection of the tumor, proteinuria had almost disappeared. Nine years later, a renal-cell carcinoma was resected, and renal tissue examined at that time showed complete healing of the membranous lesion by electron microscopy. The patient remained free of proteinuria. This well-documented example of healing of the membranous lesion suggests that removal of the source of antigen and cessation of antibody deposition in immune complexes in the kidney allowed the basement membrane to undergo healing [260].

The association between MGN and carcinoma is supported by the clinical course, the immunobiology of host tumor response, and the glomerular pathology. Proof of a causal relationship between the tumor and the glomerular lesion, however, requires demonstration that the glomerular immune aggregates contain an antigen related to the tumor and its specific antibody. Eagen and Lewis [68] have discussed the possible antibody-antigen systems that might be relevant to the pathogenesis of MGN associated with carcinoma. They include tumor-associated antigens, reexpressed fetal antigens, viral antigens, and autologous nontumor antigens, along with their respective specific antibodies. Although both tumor-related antigen and its specific antibody have not been demonstrated in any single case of MGN, immunopathologic studies have provided evidence for a tumor-related antigen or antibodies in several instances of carcinoma-related MGN.

Using indirect immunofluorescence techniques, several investigators have shown carcinoembryonic antigen (CEA) in the same glomerular distribution as the patient's own deposits of IgG in cases of adenocarcinoma of the colon, stomach, and palate [25,46,270]. Similarly, melanoma-associated antigen has been demonstrated in the glomerular deposits of a patient with melanoma [275]. In several other reports, antibody eluted from the kidney was shown to be reactive with extracts or homogenates of the patient's own tumor. Lewis et al. [149] reported a case of simultaneous MGN and bronchogenic carcinoma in which immunoglobulin eluted from the kidney reacted with the surface plasma membrane of the tumor. Antibody with identical specificity against a crude tumor extract was present in the patient's serum. DaCosta et al. [50] reported that renal eluates from a patient with MGN and lung cancer reacted with homogenates of the lung tumor and normal human lung, but not with normal kidney. Wakashin et al. [270] reported three patients with gastric cancer in whom the glomerular eluates reacted with the patient's own tumor and tissue from other human gastrointestinal tumors. Couser et al. [48] reported a patient with nephrotic syndrome, elevated CEA, and colonic adenocarcinoma who developed a serum antibody after the tumor was resected that reacted with the glomerular deposits. Although CEA was not present in the glomerular deposits, the serum antibody reacted with tumor-related antigens in tumor homogenates, and the glomerular reactivity of the serum was abolished by absorption with the tumor. Olson et al. [184] described a patient with melanoma who developed proteinuria 4 months after diagnosis of the tumor. At autopsy, glomerular eluates contained both melanoma antigen and antimelanoma antibody. Although this last case fulfills the requirements for an immune complex disease and documents tumor antigen and specific antibody in the glomeruli, the patient had neither MGN nor the nephrotic syndrome. Higgins et al. [102] reported a patient with oat-cell carcinoma of the lung and MGN who had feulgen-positive material in the glomeruli in addition to deposits of IgG and C3. The renal eluate had weak antinuclear activity, and the authors postulated that tumor necrosis was responsible for the development of a DNA–anti-DNA glomerular immune complex disease.

Ozawa et al. [187] suggested that patients with renal-cell carcinoma may develop an autoimmune reaction against renal tubular epithelial antigen, the antigen implicated in the pathogenesis of the experimental model of MGN (Heymann nephritis). In support of this hypothesis, they reported three patients with renal-cell carcinoma who had renal tubular epithelial antigen-antibody complexes in serum cryoprecipitates and glomerular eluates. However, the pathogenetic significance of these results are difficult to interpret because the patients had no clinical evidence of glomerular disease, and although it is stated that immunoglobulins and complement components were present in the glomeruli, implying the presence of a subclinical nephritis, these vital morphologic features were not illustrated.

Eagen and Lewis [68] concluded from their review of the literature that the data quoted above support a pathogenetic role for tumor-related antigen-antibody systems in the immune complex glomerulopathy associated with carcinoma. However, Alpers and Cotran [8] reviewed essentially the same material and found that "the case for carcinoma-associated MGN may have been overstated." They were critical of the small number of immunopathologic studies and noted that in no case had the glomerular deposits been shown to contain both tumor-related antigen and antibody. They also pointed out that in reviews of the nephrotic syndrome, which included 1732 patients, there were only 7 associated malignancies [122]. However, the relationship in question is specifically between MGN and carcinoma, not the nephrotic syndrome in general and malignancy. Alpers and Cotran [8] also reviewed autopsy studies of cancer patients in which evidence of MGN was sought by electron and/or immunofluorescence microscopy; in 125 patients, not a single case of MGN was identified. They interpret these autopsy studies as negative evidence. However, when cancer cases are selected without regard to the presence of proteinuria, it is not surprising that such a common disease as cancer has a low associated incidence of a relatively uncommon disease such as MGN.

The critical question is why do only some patients with carcinoma get MGN? Since there is evidence that inherited immune-response genes play a role in the pathogenesis of idiopathic MGN, it is possible that carcinoma-associated MGN also requires genetic susceptibility in addition to a nephritogenic milieu. Thus cancer by itself may not be sufficient to cause MGN, but when it occurs in a susceptible individual, the host response to the tumor results in MGN. It seems fair to conclude from the available information that a variety of epithelial malignancies can cause MGN. Although admittedly incomplete, the data support an immune complex mechanism. In adults with MGN, the clinician should be aware of this relationship, and appropriate cancer screening tests should be performed as part of the diagnostic evaluation of the patient.

Sarcoidosis and Membranous Glomerulonephritis

Symptomatic renal involvement in sarcoidosis is most commonly due to an aberration of calcium metabolism presenting as nephrolithiasis or nephrocalcinosis [173,206]. Infiltration of the renal parenchyma by granulomas occurs in 15 to 40 percent of cases [140,152], but renal dysfunction due solely to granulomatous infiltration is rare [173]. Glomerulonephritis associated with sarcoidosis has been the subject of isolated cases reports, and Taylor et al. [252] found 33 cases up to 1982. At least three more cases have been described subsequently [13,118,268]. MGN is the most common lesion in sarcoid patients with glomerular disease, but other glomerular lesions have been described, including various types of proliferative glomerulonephritis, focal glomerulonephritis (including IgA nephritis), membranoproliferative glomerulonephritis, and chronic glomerulonephritis. When Taylor et al. [252] compared the glomerular pathology of patients with sarcoidosis and the nephrotic syndrome with a series of patients with the nephrotic syndrome, they found that the prevalence of MGN in biopsy-proven sarcoid glomerular disease (9 of 15) was significantly greater than the incidence of MGN in adults with the nephrotic syndrome (25 of 213). They interpreted these data to suggest that a causative relationship exists between sarcoidosis and MGN. In addition, they found a mixed temporal relationship between the diagnosis of sarcoidosis and MGN; sarcoidosis preceded the diagnosis of MGN in 10 cases by up to 18 years and followed the diagnosis of MGN in 4 cases by as much as 10 years. The clinical range of sarcoidosis described with MGN did not appear exceptional. Seventy-five percent of the patients with MGN and sarcoidosis reviewed by Taylor et al. presented with the nephrotic syndrome. Other reported presentations are asymptomatic proteinuria, frequently accompanied by hematuria [118, 162,268], and advanced renal insufficiency [13].

The glomerular pathology of MGN associated with sarcoidosis is identical to that of idiopathic MGN. By light microscopy, the cellularity is either normal or there is a slight increase of mesangial matrix and cellularity, and spikes are sometimes described in a generally thickened GBM [13,118,162,252,253,268]. Diffuse granular deposits of IgG and C3 along the GBM are seen by immunofluorescence microscopy [13,118,162, 253,268], and they are sometimes accompanied by IgM [162] and IgA [268]. Electron microscopy shows subepithelial electron-dense deposits [162, 252,253]. More aggressive forms of glomerulonephritis are reported in sarcoidosis, as exemplified by the following two cases. One, a 58-year-old man with a 10-year history of sarcoidosis, presented with edema, proteinuria, hematuria, decreased C3, and renal failure [253]. Renal biopsy showed segmental necrosis and epithelial crescents in 60 percent of the glomeruli in addition to MGN. Another patient presented with MGN in end-stage renal failure, and after receiving a transplant from an identical twin, he developed crescentic glomerulonephritis that progressed to end-stage failure in 2 years. In three biopsies of the transplanted kidney, there was no evidence of recurrence of the membranous lesion [13]. These two cases, in addition to the other forms of glomerulonephritis described with sarcoidosis [252], suggest that the altered immunologic milieu in sarcoidosis [115] (elevated circulating immune complexes and immunoglobulins, and increased antibodies to a variety of antigens) favors the development of glomerulonephritis in the patient with sarcoidosis. In that vein, it has been noted that as many as 70 percent of patients with sarcoidosis have circulating immune complexes [90, 101,120], but in two cases with glomerular involvement where circulating immune complexes were sought, they were not found [252,268]. Clinical activity of sarcoid and erythema nodosum have been associated with proteinuria in several cases [118,252].

In summary, MGN in particular and glomerulonephritis in general are rare occurrences in patients with sarcoidosis, and their pathogenetic relationship to altered immune status of patients with sarcoidosis is presently unknown. However, the patient with sarcoidosis who develops persistent proteinuria or the nephrotic syndrome is more likely to have a glomerular lesion than the more common forms of renal involvement in sarcoidosis, such as nephrolithiasis, nephrocalcinosis, or granulomatous infiltration of the kidneys.

Sjögren Syndrome and Membranous Glomerulonephritis

Renal involvement in Sjögren syndrome is unusual, and when it occurs, it usually presents with abnormalities of tubular function [248]. The most common finding in this setting is interstitial nephritis [265]. Sjögren syndrome is a chronic autoimmune inflammatory process that involves the salivary and lacrimal glands, and it may present either as a primary disease or as a component of another autoimmune disease such as rheumatoid arthritis or SLE [20]. Serologically, Sjögren syndrome is characterized by circulating immune complexes and multiple serum autoantibodies with immunologic specificity for a variety of cellular constituents [248]. There is some evidence that the tubulointerstitial nephritis is immunologically mediated [161]. Despite this apparently favorable immunologic milieu, glomerular involvement in Sjögren syndrome, in contrast with SLE, is unusual, and the relationship between the glomerular and tubular lesions is not known. Although there are reports of glomerular involvement in Sjögren syndrome, there are only a few well-documented cases of MGN [121,169,216, 223], and one of these is complicated by the presence of rheumatoid arthritis. The cases are too few in number to make any definitive comments about the glomerular pathology, but the morphologic findings are consistent with MGN. In a patient with Sjögren syndrome who develops proteinuria, especially with the nephrotic syndrome, it is likely to be the result of a glomerular lesion. Although membranoproliferative and nonspecific proliferative forms of glomerulonephritis have also been reported, the most common glomerular pathology is MGN.

REFERENCES

1. Abe, S., Amagasaki, Y., Konishi, K., Kato, E., Iyori, S., and Sakaguchi, H. Idiopathic membranous glomerulonephritis: Aspects of geographical differences. *J. Clin. Pathol.* 39:1193, 1986.
2. Abrass, C. K., Hall, C. L., Border, W. A., Brown, C. A., Glassock, R. J., Coggins, C. H., and the Collaborative Study of the Adult Idiopathic Nephrotic Syndrome. Circulating immune complexes in adults with idiopathic nephrotic syndrome. *Kidney Int.* 17:545, 1980.
3. Abreo, K., Abreo, F., Mitchell, B., and Schloemer, G. Idiopathic crescentic membranous glomerulonephritis. *Am. J. Kidney Dis.* 8:257, 1986.
4. Adu, D., Williams, D. G., Taube, D., Vilches, A. R., Turner, D. R., Cameron, J. S., and Ogg, C. S. Late onset systemic lupus erythematosus and lupus-like disease in patients with apparent idiopathic glomerulonephritis. *Q. J. Med.* 52:471, 1983.
5. Agodoa, L. C. Y., Striker, G. E., George, C. R. P., Glassock, R., and Quadracci, L. J. The appearance of nonlinear deposits of immunoglobulins in Goodpasture's syndrome. *Am. J. Med.* 61:407, 1976.
6. Ainsworth, S., Swain, R. P., Watabe, N., Brackett, N. C., Jr., Pilia, P., and Hennigar, G. R. Gold nephropathy: Ultrastructural, fluorescent, and energy-dispersive x-ray microanalysis study. *Arch. Pathol. Lab. Med.* 105:373, 1981.
7. Alexopoulos, E., Seron, D., Hartley, R. B., Nolasco, F., and Cameron, J. S. Immune mechanisms in idiopathic membranous nephropathy: The role of the interstitial infiltrates. *Am. J. Kidney Dis.* 13:404, 1989.
8. Alpers, C. E., and Cotran, R. S. Neoplasia and glomerular injury. *Kidney Int.* 30:465, 1986.
9. Bacon, P. A., Tribe, C. R., MacKenzie, J. C., Jones, J. V., Cumming, R. H., and Amer, B. Penicillamine nephropathy in rheumatoid arthritis: A clinical, pathological and immunopathological study. *Q. J. Med.* 45:661, 1976.

10. Banfi, G., Imbasciati, E., Guerra, L., Mihatsch, M. J., and Ponticelli, C. Extracapillary glomerulonephritis with necrotizing vasculitis in D-penicillamine-treated rheumatoid arthritis. *Nephron* 33:56, 1983.
11. Bannister, K. M., Howarth, G. S., Clarkson, A. R., and Woodroffe, A. J. Glomerular IgG subclass distribution in human glomerulonephritis. *Clin. Nephrol.* 19:161, 1983.
12. Bariéty, J., Druet, Ph. A., Lagrue, G., Samarcq, P., and Milliez, P. Les glomérulopathies "extramembraneuses" (G.E.M.). Étude morphologique en microscopie optique, électronique et en immunofluorescence. *Pathol. Biol. (Paris)* 18:3, 1970.
13. Beaufils, H., Gompel, A., Gubler, M. C., Lucsko, M., and Guedon, J. Pre- and posttransplant glomerulonephritis in a case of sarcoidosis. *Nephron* 35:124, 1983.
14. Bell, E. T. *Renal Diseases,* 2nd Ed. Philadelphia: Lea & Febiger, 1950.
15. Beregi, E., and Varga, I. Analysis of 260 cases of membranous glomerulonephritis in renal biopsy material. *Clin. Nephrol.* 2:215, 1974.
16. Berger, J., Yaneva, H., and Hinglais, N. Immunohistochemistry of Glomerulonephritis. In J. Hamburger, J. Crosnier, and M. H. Maxwell (Eds.), *Advances in Nephrology,* Vol. 1. Chicago: Year Book Medical, 1971. P. 11.
17. Bertani, T., Olesnicky, L., Abu-Regiaba, S., Glasberg, S., and Pirani, C. L. Concomitant presence of three different glomerular diseases in the same patient: Report of a case and review of the literature. *Nephron* 34:260, 1983.
18. Berthoux, F. C., Laurent, B., Le Petit, J.-C., Genin, C., Broutin, F., Touraine, F., Hassan, A. A., and Champailler, A. Immunogenetics and immunopathology of human primary membranous glomerulonephritis: HLA-A, B, DR antigens; functional activity of splenic macrophage Fc-receptors and peripheral blood T-Lymphocyte subpopulations. *Clin. Nephrol.* 22:15, 1984.
19. Black, D. A. K., Rose, G., and Brewer, D. B. Controlled trial of prednisone in adult patients with the nephrotic syndrome. *Br. Med. J.* 3:421, 1970.
20. Bloch, K. J., Buchanan, W. W., Wohl, M. J., and Bunim, J. J. Sjögren's syndrome: A clinical, pathological, and serological study of 62 cases. *Medicine (Baltimore)* 44:187, 1965.
21. Bolton, W. K., Atuk, N. O., Sturgill, B. C., and Westervelt, F. B., Jr. Therapy of the idiopathic nephrotic syndrome with alternate day steroids. *Am. J. Med.* 62:60, 1977.
22. Bonsib, S. M. Scanning electron microscopy of acellular glomeruli in human glomerulonephritis: Application of a technique. *Ultrastruct. Pathol.* 7:215, 1984.
23. Bonsib, S. M. Scanning electron microscopy of acellular glomeruli in nephrotic syndrome. *Kidney Int.* 27:678, 1985.
24. Border, W. A. Immune complex detection in glomerular diseases. *Nephron* 24:105, 1979.
25. Borochovitz, D., Kam, W. K., Nolte, M., Graner, S., and Kiss, J. Adenocarcinoma of the palate associated with nephrotic syndrome and epimembranous carcinoembryonic antigen deposits. *Cancer* 49:2097, 1982.
26. Brentjens, J. R., Sepulveda, M., Baliah, T., Bentzel, C., Erlanger, B. F., Elwood, C., Montes, M., Hsu, K. C., and Andres, G. A. Interstitial immune complex nephritis in patients with systemic lupus erythematosus. *Kidney Int.* 7:342, 1975.
27. Brueggemeyer, C. D., and Ramirez, G. Membranous nephropathy: A concern for malignancy. *Am. J. Kidney Dis.* 9:23, 1987.
28. Brun, C., Olsen, S., Raaschou, F., and Sorensen, A. W. S. The localization of gold in the human kidney following chrysotherapy. *Nephron* 1:265, 1964.
29. Cairns, S. A., London, R. A., and Mallick, N. P. The value of three immune complex assays in the management of systemic lupus erythematosus: An assessment of immune complex levels, size, and immunochemical properties in relation to disease activity and manifestations. *Clin. Exp. Immunol.* 40:273, 1980.
30. Cairns, S. A., London, R. A., and Mallick, N. P. Circulating immune complexes in idiopathic glomerular disease. *Kidney Int.* 21:507, 1982.
31. Cameron, J. S. Pathogenesis and treatment of membranous nephropathy. *Kidney Int.* 15:88, 1979.
32. Cameron, J. S. The Natural History of Glomerulonephritis. In D. Black and N. F. Jones (Eds.), *Renal Disease,* 4th Ed. Oxford: Blackwell, 1979.
33. Cameron, J. S. Treatment of membranous nephropathy. *N. Engl. J. Med.* 302:634, 1980.
34. Cameron, J. S., and Blandford, G. The simple assessment of selectivity in heavy proteinuria. *Lancet* 2:242, 1966.
34*a*. Cameron, J. S., Healy, M. J. R., and Adu, D. The Medical Research Council trial of short-term high-dose alternate-day prednisolone in idiopathic membranous nephropathy with nephrotic syndrome in adults. *Q. J. Med.* 74:133, 1990.
35. Cantrell, E. G. Nephrotic syndrome cured by removal of gastric carcinoma. *Br. Med. J.* 2:739, 1966.
36. Cattran, D. C., Delmore, T., Roscoe, J., Cole, E., Cardella, C., Charron, R., Ritchie, S., and the Toronto Glomerulonephritis Study Group.

A randomized controlled trial of prednisone in patients with idiopathic membranous nephropathy. *N. Engl. J. Med.* 320:210, 1989.

37. Chan, W. C., and Tsao, Y. C. Diffuse membranous glomerulonephritis in children. *J. Clin. Pathol.* 19:464, 1966.
38. Charpentier, B., and Levy, M. Cooperative study of de novo extramembranous glomerulonephritis in renal allografts in humans: Report of 19 new cases in 1550 renal transplant patients of the transplantation group of the Ile de France. *Nephrologie* 3:158, 1982.
39. Chavez, A., Mignon, F., and Morel-Maroger, L. Glomérulites extramembraneuses a propos de 92 observations. *Schweiz. Med. Wochenschr.* 107:899, 1977.
40. Cheong, I. K., Chong, S. M., Singh, N., and Suleiman, A. B. Extensive crescent formation in idiopathic membranous glomerulonephritis: A case report. *Med. J. Malaysia* 36:8, 1981.
41. Churg, J., and Grishman, E. Subacute and chronic glomerulonephritis: Histopathologic study by means of thin sections. *Am. J. Pathol.* 33:622, 1957.
42. Churg, J., Grishman, E., Goldstein, M. H., Yunis, S. L., and Porush, J. G. Idiopathic nephrotic syndrome in adults: A study and classification based on renal biopsies. *N. Engl. J. Med.* 272:165, 1965.
43. Collaborative Study of the Adult Idiopathic Nephrotic Syndrome. A controlled study of short-term prednisone treatment in adults with membranous nephropathy. *N. Engl. J. Med.* 301:1301, 1979.
44. Collins, A. B., Andres, G. A., and McCluskey, R. T. Lack of evidence for a role of renal tubular antigen in human membranous glomerulonephritis. *Nephron* 27:297, 1981.
45. Combes, B., Stastny, P., Shorey, J., Eigenbrodt, E. H., Barrera, A., Hull, A. R., and Carter, N. W. Glomerulonephritis with deposition of Australia antigen-antibody complexes in glomerular basement membrane. *Lancet* 2:234, 1971.
46. Costanza, M. E., Pinn, V., Schwartz, R. S., and Nathanson, L. Carcinoembryonic antigen-antibody complexes in a patient with colonic carcinoma and nephrotic syndrome. *N. Engl. J. Med.* 289:520, 1973.
47. Coupes, B. M., Short, C. D., O'Donoghue, D., Ballardie, F. W., Mallick, N. P., and Brenchley, P. E. C. Urinary MAC and C3d levels in human membranous nephropathy: Evidence for site of activation and clinical correlation. *Kidney Int.* 37:438, 1990.
48. Couser, W. G., Wagonfeld, J. B., Spargo, B. H., and Lewis, E. J. Glomerular deposition of tumor antigen in membranous nephropathy associated with colonic carcinoma. *Am. J. Med.* 57:962, 1974.
49. Couser, W. G. Mechanisms of glomerular injury in immune-complex disease (Nephrology Forum). *Kidney Int.* 28:569, 1985.
50. Da Costa, C. R., Dupont, E., Hamers, R., Hooghe, R., Dupuis, F., and Potuliege, R. Nephrotic syndrome in bronchogenic carcinoma: Report of two cases with immunochemical studies. *Clin. Nephrol.* 2:245, 1974.
51. Davies, D. J., Dowling, J., and Xipell, J. M. Gold nephropathy. *Pathology* 9:281, 1977.
52. Davis, J. A., Cohen, A. H., Weisbart, R., and Paulus, H. E. Glomerulonephritis in rheumatoid arthritis. *Arthritis Rheum.* 22:1018, 1979.
53. Davison, A. M., Cameron, J. S., Kerr, D. N. S., Ogg, C. S., and Wilkinson, R. W. The natural history of renal function in untreated idiopathic membranous glomerulonephritis in adults. *Clin. Nephrol.* 22:61, 1984.
54. Day, A. T., and Golding, J. R. Hazards of penicillamine therapy in the treatment of rheumatoid arthritis. *Postgrad. Med. J.* 50(Suppl. 2):71, 1974.
55. Demaine, A. G., Cameron, J. S., Taube, D. T., Vaughan, R. W., and Welsh, K. I. Immunoglobulin (Gm) allotype frequencies in idiopathic membranous nephropathy and minimal change nephropathy. *Transplantation* 37:507, 1984.
56. Demaine, A. G., Vaughan, R. W., Taube, D. H., and Welsh, K. I. Association of membranous nephropathy with T-cell receptor constant beta chain and immunoglobulin heavy chain switch region polymorphisms. *Immunogenetics* 27:19, 1988.
57. Denis, J., Mignon, F., Ramée, M.-P., Morel-Maroger, L., and Richet, G. Glomérulites extramembraneuses associées aux tumeurs viscérales. Etude clinique et histologique à propos de 10 cas et revue de la littérature. *Nouv. Presse Med.* 7:991, 1978.
58. Dérot, M., Kahn, J., Mazalton, A., and Peyrafort, J. Néphrite auriquë aigue mortelle après traitement aurique, chrysocyanose associée. *Bull. Mem. Soc. Med. Hop.* (*Paris*) 70:234, 1954.
59. Dische, F. E., Swinson, D. R., Hamilton, E. B., and Parsons, V. Immunopathology of penicillamine-induced glomerular disease. *J. Rheumatol.* 11:584, 1984.
60. Dixon, A. St. J., Davies, J., Dormandy, T. L., Hamilton, E. B. D., Holt, P. J. L., Mason, R. M., Thompson, M., Weber, J. C. P., and Zutshi, D. W. Synthetic D-penicillamine in rheumatoid arthritis: Double-blind study of a high and low dosage regimen. *Ann. Rheum. Dis.* 34:416, 1975.
61. Dixon, F. J., Feldman, J. D., and Vazquez, J. J. Experimental glomerulonephritis: The pathogen-

esis of a laboratory model resembling the spectrum of human glomerulonephritis. *J. Exp. Med.* 113:899, 1961.

62. Doi, T., Kanatsu, K., Nagai, H., Kohrogi, N., and Hamashima, Y. An overlapping syndrome of IgA nephropathy and membranous nephropathy? *Nephron* 35:24, 1983.
63. Doi, T., Mayumi, M., Kanatsu, K., Suehiro, F., and Hamashima, Y. Distribution of IgG subclasses in membranous nephropathy. *Clin. Exp. Immunol.* 58:57, 1984.
64. Donadio, J. V., Jr., Holley, K. E., Anderson, C. F., and Taylor, W. F. Controlled trial of cyclophosphamide in idiopathic membranous nephropathy. *Kidney Int.* 6:431, 1974.
65. Donadio, J. V., Jr., Torres, V. E., Velosa, J. A., Wagoner, R. D., Holley, K. E., Okamkura, M., Ilstrup, D. M., and Chu, C.-P. Idiopathic membranous nephropathy: The natural history of untreated patients. *Kidney Int.* 33:708, 1988.
66. Douglas, M. F. S., Rabideau, D. P., Schwartz, M. M., and Lewis, E. J. Evidence of autologous immune complex nephritis. *N. Engl. J. Med.* 305:1326, 1981.
67. Dyer, P. A., Klouda, P. T., Harris, R., and Mallick, N. P. Properdin factor B alleles in patients with idiopathic membranous nephropathy. *Tissue Antigens* 15:505, 1980.
68. Eagen, J. W., and Lewis, E. J. Glomerulopathies of neoplasia. *Kidney Int.* 11:297, 1977.
69. Edgington, T. S., Glassock, R. J., and Dixon, F. J. Autologous immune complex nephritis induced with renal tubular antigen: I. Identification and isolation of the pathogenic antigen. *J. Exp. Med.* 127:555, 1968.
70. Ehrenreich, T., and Churg, J. Pathology of Membranous Nephropathy. In S. C. Sommers (Ed.), *Pathology Annual 1968*, Vol. 3. New York: Appleton-Century-Crofts, 1968. P. 145.
71. Eknoyan, G., Gyorkey, F., Dichoso, C., Martinez-Maldonado, M., Suki, W. N., and Gyorkey, P. Renal morphological and immunological changes associated with acute viral hepatitis. *Kidney Int.* 1:413, 1972.
72. Ellis, D., Fisher, S. E., Smith, W. I., Jr., and Jaffe, R. Familial occurrence of renal and intestinal disease associated with tissue auto-antibodies. *Am. J. Dis. Child.* 136:323, 1982.
73. Erwin, D. T., Donadio, J. V., Jr., and Holley, K. E. The clinical course of idiopathic membranous nephropathy. *Mayo Clin. Proc.* 48:697, 1973.
74. Falck, H. M., Törnroth, T., Kock, B., and Wegelius, O. Fatal renal vasculitis and minimal change glomerulonephritis complicating treatment with penicillamine: Report on two cases. *Acta Med. Scand.* 205:133, 1979.
75. Falk, R. J., Dalmasso, A. P., Kim, Y., Tsai, C. H., Scheinman, J. I., Gewurz, H., and Michael, A. F. Neoantigen of the polymerized ninth component of complement: Characterization of a monoclonal antibody and immunohistochemical localization in renal disease. *J. Clin. Invest.* 72:560, 1983.
76. Forland, M., and Spargo, B. H. Clinicopathological correlations in idiopathic nephrotic syndrome with membranous nephropathy. *Nephron* 6:498, 1969.
77. Francis, K. L., Jenis, E. H., Jensen, G. E., and Calcagno, P. L. Gold-associated nephropathy. *Arch. Pathol. Lab. Med.* 108:234, 1984.
78. Franklin, W. A., Jennings, R. B., and Earle, D. P. Membranous glomerulonephritis: Long-term serial observations on clinical course and morphology. *Kidney Int.* 4:36, 1973.
79. Fukatsu, A., Matsuo, S., Killen, P. D., Martin, G. R., Andres, G. A., and Brentjens, J. R. The glomerular distribution of type IV collagen and laminin in human membranous glomerulonephritis. *Hum. Pathol.* 19:64, 1988.
80. Gaffney, E. F., and Panner, B. J. Membranous glomerulonephritis: Clinical significance of glomerular hypercellularity and parietal epithelial abnormalities. *Nephron* 29:209, 1981.
81. Ganote, C. E., Beaver, D. L., and Moses, H. L. Renal gold inclusions: A light and electron microscope study. *Arch. Pathol.* 81:429, 1966.
82. Gärtner, H.-V. Membranous glomerulonephritis: Prototype of an immune complex glomerulonephritis. *Veroff. Pathol.* 113:1, 1980.
83. Gärtner, H.-V., Fischbach, H., Wehner, H., Bohle, A., Edel, H. H., Kluthe, R., Scheler, F., and Schmülling, R. M. Comparison of clinical and morphological features of peri-(epi-extra) membranous glomerulonephritis. *Nephron* 13:288, 1974.
84. Germuth, F. G., Jr., Flanagan, C., and Montenegro, M. R. The relationships between the chemical nature of the antigen, antigen dosage, rate of antibody synthesis and the occurrence of arteritis and glomerulonephritis in experimental hypersensitivity. *Johns Hopkins Med. J.* 101:149, 1957.
85. Gluck, M. C., Gallo, G., Lowenstein, J., and Baldwin, D. S. Membranous glomerulonephritis: Evolution of clinical and pathologic features. *Ann. Intern. Med.* 78:1, 1973.
86. Graham, A. R., and Nagle, R. B. Quantitative electron microscopic study of membranous glomerulopathy. *Am. J. Clin. Pathol.* 80:816, 1983.
87. Griffel, B., and Bernheim, J. Glomerular deposits in idiopathic membranous glomerulopathy. *Arch. Pathol. Lab. Med.* 104:56, 1980.
88. Groggel, G. C., Adler, S., Rennke, H. G.,

Couser, W. G., and Salant, D. J. Role of the terminal complement pathway in experimental membranous nephropathy in the rabbit. *J. Clin. Invest.* 72:1048, 1983.

89. Grupe, W. E., and Kaplan, M. H. Demonstration of an antibody to proximal tubular antigen in the pathogenesis of experimental autoimmune nephrosis in rats. *J. Lab. Clin. Med.* 74:400, 1969.
90. Gupta, R. C., Kueppers, F., DeRemee, R. A., Huston, K. A., and McDuffie, F. C. Pulmonary and extrapulmonary sarcoidosis in relation to circulating immune complexes: A quantitation of immune complexes by two radioimmunoassays. *Am. Rev. Respir. Dis.* 116:261, 1977.
91. Habib, R., Antignac, C., Hinglais, N., Gagnadoux, M.-F., and Broyer, M. Glomerular lesions in the transplanted kidney in children. *Am. J. Kidney Dis.* 10:198, 1987.
92. Habib, R., and Kleinknecht, C. The Primary Nephrotic Syndrome of Childhood: Classification and Clinicopathologic Study of 406 Cases. In S. C. Sommers (Ed.), *Pathology Annual 1971*. New York: Appleton-Century-Crofts, 1971. P. 417.
93. Habib, R., Kleinknecht, C., and Gubler, M. C. Extramembranous glomerulonephritis in children: Report of 50 cases. *J. Pediatr.* 82:754, 1973.
94. Hall, C. L., Fothergill, N. J., Blackwell, M. M., Harrison, P. R., MacKenzie, J. C., and MacIver, A. G. The natural course of gold nephropathy: Long-term study of 21 patients. *Br. Med. J.* 295:745, 1987.
95. Hall, C. L., Jawad, S., Harrison, P. R., MacKenzie, J. C., Bacon, P. A., Klouda, P. T., and MacIver, A. G. Natural course of penicillamine nephropathy: A long-term study of 33 patients. *Br. Med. J.* 296:1083, 1988.
96. Hallauer, W., Gärtner, H. -V., Kronenberg, K. H., and Manz, G. Immunkomplex nephritis mit nephrotischem Syndrom unter Therapie mit D-Penizillamin. *Schweiz. Med. Wochenschr.* 104: 434, 1974.
97. Hardwicke, J., Blainey, J. D., Brewer, D. B., and Soothill, J. F. The Nephrotic Syndrome. In E. L. Becker (Ed.), *Clinical Nephrology: Proceedings of the Third International Congress of Nephrology*, Vol. 3. Basel: Karger, 1967.
98. Hartfall, S. J., Garland, H. G., and Goldie, W. Gold treatment of arthritis: A review of 900 cases. *Lancet* 2:838, 1937.
99. Hattori, S., Furuse, A., and Matsuda, I. Presence of HB_e antibody in glomerular deposits in membranous glomerulonephritis is associated with hepatitis B virus infection. *Am. J. Nephrol.* 8:384, 1988.
100. Hayslett, J. P., Bensch, K. G., Kashgarian, M., and Rosenberg, L. E. Focal glomerulitis due to penicillamine. *Lab. Invest.* 19:376, 1968.
101. Hedfors, E., and Norberg, R. Evidence for circulating immune complexes in sarcoidosis. *Clin. Exp. Immunol.* 16:493, 1974.
102. Higgins, M. R., Randall, R. E., Jr., and Still, W. J. S. Nephrotic syndrome with oat-cell carcinoma. *Br. Med. J.* 3:450, 1974.
103. Higuchi, A., Suzuki, Y., and Okada, T. Membranous glomerulonephritis in rheumatoid arthritis unassociated with gold or penicillamine treatment. *Ann. Rheum. Dis.* 46:488, 1987.
104. Hill, G. S., Robertson, J., Grossman, R., Perloff, L., and Barker, C. F. An unusual variant of membranous nephropathy with abundant crescent formation and recurrence in the transplanted kidney. *Clin. Nephrol.* 10:114, 1978.
105. Hirose, H., Udo, K., Kojima, M., Takahashi, Y., Mikakawa, Y., Miyamoto, K., Yoshizawa, H., and Mayumi, M. Deposition of hepatitis B e antigen in membranous glomerulonephritis: Identification by $F(ab')_2$ fragments of monoclonal antibody. *Kidney Int.* 26:338, 1984.
106. Honig, C., Mouradian, J. A., Montoliu, J., Susin, M., and Shkerman, R. L. Mesangial electron-dense deposits in membranous nephropathy. *Lab. Invest.* 42:427, 1980.
107. Honkanen, E. Survival in idiopathic membranous glomerulonephritis. *Clin. Nephrol.* 25:122, 1986.
108. Honkanen, E., Grönhagen-Riska, C., von Willebrand, E., Törnroth, T., and Laasonen, L. Renal mononuclear inflammatory cell populations in membranous glomerulonephritis: A fine-needle aspiration biopsy study. *Clin. Nephrol.* 28:232, 1987.
109. Honkanen, E., Törnroth, T., Pettersson, E., and Skrifvars, B. Membranous glomerulonephritis in rheumatoid arthritis not related to gold or D-penicillamine therapy: A report of four cases and review of the literature. *Clin. Nephrol.* 27:87, 1987.
110. Hoorntje, S. J., Kallenberg, C. G. M., Weening, J. J., Donker, A. J. M., The, T. H., and Hoedemaeker, P. J. Immune complex glomerulopathy in patients treated with captopril. *Lancet* 1:1212, 1980.
111. Hopper, J., Jr., Trew, P. A., and Biava, C. G. Membranous nephropathy: Its relative benignity in women. *Nephron* 29:18, 1981.
112. Hsu, H.-C., Wu, C.-Y., Lin, C.-Y., Lin, G.-J., Chen, C.-H., and Huang, F.-Y. Membranous nephropathy in 52 hepatitis B surface antigen (HB_sAg) carrier children in Taiwan. *Kidney Int.* 36:1103, 1989.
113. Hume, D. M., and Bryant, C. P. The development of recurrent glomerulonephritis. *Transplant. Proc.* 4:673, 1972.
114. Jaffe, I. A., Treser, G., Suzuki, Y., and Ehren-

reich, T. Nephropathy induced by D-penicillamine. *Ann. Intern. Med.* 69:549, 1968.
115. James, D. G., Neville, E., and Walker, A. Immunology of sarcoidosis. *Am. J. Med.* 59:388, 1975.
116. Jennette, J. C., Iskandar, S. S., and Dalldorf, F. G. Pathologic differentiation between lupus and nonlupus membranous glomerulopathy. *Kidney Int.* 24:377, 1983.
117. Jennette, J. C., Newman, W. J., and Diaz-Buxo, J. A. Overlapping IgA and membranous nephropathy. *Am. J. Clin. Pathol.* 88:74, 1987.
118. Jones, B., and Fowler, J. Membranous nephropathy associated with sarcoidosis. Response to prednisolone (Letter). *Nephron* 52:101, 1989.
119. Jones, D. B. Nephrotic Glomerulonephritis. *Am. J. Pathol.* 33:313, 1957.
120. Jones, J. V., Cumming, R. H., Asplin, C. M., Laszlo, G., and White, R. J. Evidence for circulating immune complexes in erythema nodosum and early sarcoidosis. *Ann. N.Y. Acad. Sci.* 278:212, 1976.
121. Kallen, R. J., and Spargo, B. Membranous Nephropathy in an Adolescent with Sjögren's Syndrome: Ultrastructural Evidence for an Immunopathologic Renal Lesion. In *Abstracts of the 4th Annual Meeting of the American Society of Nephrology.* 1970. P. 39.
122. Kaplan, B. S., Klassen, J., and Gault, M. H. Glomerular injury in patients with neoplasia. *Annu. Rev. Med.* 27:117, 1976.
123. Kapur, S., Salcedo, J., Chandra, R., and Antonovych, T. Evolution of membranous nephropathy from a proliferative and exudative glomerulonephritis: A report of three cases studied by serial biopsies. *Int. J. Pediatr. Nephrol.* 6:105, 1985.
124. Katz, A., and Little, A. H. Gold nephropathy: An immunopathologic study. *Arch. Pathol. Lab. Med.* 96:133, 1973.
125. Katz, W. A., Blodgett, R. C., Jr., and Pietrusko, R. G. Proteinuria in gold-treated rheumatoid arthritis. *Ann. Intern. Med.* 101:176, 1984.
126. Kida, H., Asamoto, T., Yokoyama, H., Tomosugi, N., and Hattori, N. Long-term prognosis of idiopathic membranous nephropathy. *Clin. Nephrol.* 25:64, 1986.
127. Klassen, J., Elwood, C., Grossberg, A. L., Milgrom, F., Montes, M., Sepulveda, M., and Andres, G. A. Evolution of membranous nephropathy into anti-glomerular-basement-membrane glomerulonephritis. *N. Engl. J. Med.* 290:1340, 1974.
128. Klouda, P. T., Acheson, E. J., Goldby, F. S., Lawler, W., Manos, J., Dyer, P. A., Harris, R., Mallick, N. P., and Williams, G. Strong association between idiopathic membranous nephropathy and HLA-DRw3. *Lancet* 2:770, 1979.
129. Knieser, M. R., Jenis, E. H., Lowenthal, D. T., Bancroft, W. H., Burns, W., and Shalhoub, R. Pathogenesis of renal disease associated with viral hepatitis. *Arch. Pathol.* 97:193, 1974.
130. Kobayashi, K., Harada, A., Onoyama, K., Shimamatsu, K., Maeda, T., Fujimi, S., and Omae, T. Idiopathic membranous glomerulonephritis associated with diabetes mellitus: Light, immunofluorescence and electron microscopic study. *Nephron* 28:163, 1981.
131. Kobayashi, Y., Fujii, K., Hiki, Y., and Chen, X. M. Coexistence of IgA nephropathy and membranous nephropathy. *Acta Pathol. Jpn.* 35:1293, 1985.
132. Kohler, P. F., Cronin, R. E., Hammond, W. S., Olin, D., and Carr, R. I. Chronic membranous glomerulonephritis caused by hepatitis B antigen-antibody immune complexes. *Ann. Intern. Med.* 81:448, 1974.
133. Korbet, S. M., Schwartz, M. M., Rosenberg, B. F., Sibley, R. K., and Lewis, E. J. Immunotactoid glomerulopathy. *Medicine (Baltimore)* 64:228, 1985.
134. Koutke, J. D., Gerig, J. S., Glickman, J. L., Sturgill, B. C., and Bolton, W. K. Progression of membranous nephropathy to acute crescentic rapidly progressive glomerulonephritis and response to pulse methylprednisolone. *Am. J. Nephrol.* 6:224, 1986.
135. Kurki, P., Helve, T., von Bonsdorff, M., Törnroth, T., Pettersson, E., Riska, H., and Miettinen, A. Transformation of membranous glomerulonephritis into crescentic glomerulonephritis with glomerular basement membrane antibodies: Serial determinations of anti-GBM before the transformation. *Nephron* 38:134, 1984.
136. Kusunoki, Y., Itami, N., Tochimaru, H., Takekoshi, Y., Nagasawa, S., and Yoshiki, T. Glomerular deposition of C4 cleavage fragment (C4d) and C4-binding protein in idiopathic membranous glomerulonephritis. *Nephron* 51:17, 1989.
137. Kuznetsky, K. A., Schwartz, M. M., Lohmann, L. A., and Lewis, E. J. Necrotizing glomerulonephritis in rheumatoid arthritis. *Clin. Nephrol.* 26:257, 1986.
138. Lachmann, P. J. Nephrotic syndrome from penicillamine. *Postgrad. Med. J. (Suppl.)* 44:235, 1968.
139. Lai, K. N., Lo, S. T. H., and Lai, F. M. Immunohistochemical study of the membrane attack complex of complement and S-protein in idiopathic and secondary membranous nephropathy. *Am. J. Pathol.* 135:469, 1989.
140. Lebacq, E., Verhaegen, H., and Desment, V.

Renal involvement in sarcoidosis. *Postgrad. Med. J.* 46:526, 1970.
141. Lee, H. S., Choi, Y., Yu, S. H., Koh, H. I., Kim, M. J., and Ko, K. W. A renal biopsy study of hepatitis B virus–associated nephropathy in Korea. *Kidney Int.* 34:537, 1988.
142. Lee, J. C., Dushkin, M., Eyring, E. J., Engleman, E. P., and Hopper, J., Jr. Renal lesions associated with gold therapy: Light and electron microscopic studies. *Arthritis Rheum.* 8:1, 1965.
143. Lee, J. C., Yamauchi, H., and Hopper, J., Jr. The association of cancer and the nephrotic syndrome. *Ann. Intern. Med.* 64:41, 1966.
144. Lehman, D. H., Wilson, C. B., and Dixon, F. J. Extraglomerular immunoglobulin deposits in human nephritis. *Am. J. Med.* 58:765, 1975.
145. Levy, M., Gagnadoux, M. F., Beziau, A., and Habib, R. Membranous glomerulonephritis associated with anti-tubular and anti-alveolar basement membrane antibodies. *Clin. Nephrol.* 10:158, 1978.
146. Levy, M., and Kleinknecht, C. Membranous glomerulonephritis and hepatitis B virus infection. *Nephron* 26:259, 1980.
147. Levy, M., Kleinknecht, C., and Peix, A. Membranous nephropathy and HB_sAg. *Lancet* 1:113, 1979.
148. Lewis, E. J. Management of the Nephrotic Syndrome in Adults. In J. S. Cameron and R. J. Glassock (Eds.), *The Nephrotic Syndrome.* New York: Marcel Dekker, 1988. P. 461.
149. Lewis, M. G., Loughbridge, L. W., and Phillips, T. M. Immunological studies in nephrotic syndrome associated with extrarenal malignancy. *Lancet* 2:134, 1971.
150. Libit, S. A., Burke, B., Michael, A. F., and Vernier, R. L. Extramembranous glomerulonephritis in childhood: Relationship to systemic lupus erythematosus. *J. Pediatr.* 88:394, 1976.
151. Lieberthal, W., Bernard, D. B., Donohoe, J. F., Stilmant, M. M., and Couser, W. G. Rapid recurrence of membranous nephropathy in a related renal allograft. *Clin. Nephrol.* 12:222, 1979.
152. Longcope, W. T., and Freiman, D. G. A study of sarcoidosis based on a combined investigation of 160 cases including 30 autopsies from the Johns Hopkins Hospital and Massachusetts General Hospital. *Medicine (Baltimore)* 3:1, 1952.
153. Maggiore, Q., Bartolomeo, F., L'Abbate, A., and Misefari, V. HB_sAg glomerular deposits in glomerulonephritis: Fact or artifact? *Kidney Int.* 19:579, 1981.
154. Magil, A., Webber, D., and Chow, V. Glomerulonephritis associated with hepatitis B surface antigenemia: Report of a case with features of both membranous and IgA nephropathy. *Nephron* 42: 335, 1986.
155. Makker, S. P. Brush border antibodies of Heymann nephritis of rats in normal human serum. *Proc. Soc. Exp. Biol. Med.* 154:9, 1977.
156. Makker, S. P., and Heymann, W. Demonstration of tubular basement membrane antibody in the pathogenesis of autoimmune nephrosis in rats. *Proc. Soc. Exp. Biol. Med.* 143:995, 1973.
157. Mallick, N. P., Short, C. D., and Manos, J. Clinical membranous nephropathy. *Nephron* 34: 209, 1983.
158. Manos, J., Short, C. D., Acheson, E. J., Dyer, P., Lawler, W., Mallick, N. P., and Williams, G. Relapsing idiopathic membranous nephropathy. *Clin. Nephrol.* 18:286, 1982.
159. Martini, A., Scotta, M. S., Notarangelo, L. D., Maggiore, G., Guarnaccia, S., and DeGiacomo, C. Membranous glomerulopathy and chronic small-intestinal enteropathy associated with autoantibodies directed against renal tubular basement membrane and the cytoplasm of intestinal epithelial cells. *Acta Paediatr. Scand.* 72:931, 1983.
160. Matsumoto, K., Okano, K., and Hatano, M. Defective in vitro T-cell colony formation in patients with membranous nephropathy. *Nephron* 42:91, 1986.
161. McCluskey, R. T. Immunologically Mediated Tubulointerstitial Nephritis. In R. S. Cotran (Ed.), *Tubulointerstitial Nephropathies.* New York: Churchill-Livingstone, 1982. P. 121.
162. McCoy, R. C., and Tisher, C. C. Glomerulonephritis associated with sarcoidosis. *Am. J. Pathol.* 68:339, 1972.
163. Medical Research Council Working Party. Controlled trial of azathioprin and prednisone in chronic renal disease. *Br. Med. J.* 2:239, 1971.
164. Merle, L. J., Reidenberg, M. M., Camacho, M. T., Jones, B. R., and Drayer, D. E. Renal injury in patients with rheumatoid arthritis treated with gold. *Clin. Pharmacol. Ther.* 28:216, 1980.
165. Meyboom, R. H. B. Metals. In M. N. G. Dukes (Ed.), *Meyler's Side Effects of Drugs,* Vol. 8. Amsterdam: Excerpta Medica, 1975. P. 504.
166. Milner, L. S., Dusheiko, G. M., Jacobs, D., Kala, U., Thomson, P. D., Ninin, D. T., and Murray, J. Biochemical and serological characteristics of children with membranous nephropathy due to hepatitis B virus infection: Correlation with hepatitis B e antigen, hepatitis B DNA and hepatitis D. *Nephron* 49:184, 1988.
167. Miyakawa, Y., Kitamura, K., Shibata, S., and Naruse, T. Demonstration of human nephritogenic tubular antigen in the serum and organs by radioimmunoassay. *J. Immunol.* 117:1203, 1976.
168. Morel-Maroger, L., Leathem, A., and Richet, G.

Glomerular abnormalities in nonsystemic diseases: Relationship between findings by light microscopy and immunofluorescence in 433 renal biopsy specimens. *Am. J. Med.* 53:170, 1972.
169. Moutsopoulos, H. M., Barlow, J. E., Lawley, T. J., Stahl, N. I., Antonovych, T. T., and Chused, T. M. Immune complex glomerulonephritis in sicca syndrome. *Am. J. Med.* 64:955, 1978.
170. Müller, G. A., Müller, C., Liebow, G., Kompf, J., Ising, H., and Bernet, P. Strong association of idiopathic membranous nephropathy (MN) with HLA-DR3 and MT-2 without involvement of HLA-B18 and no association to BfF1. *Tissue Antigens* 17:332, 1981.
171. Multicenter Trial Group. Controlled trial of D-penicillamine in severe rheumatoid arthritis. *Lancet* 1:275, 1973.
172. Murphy, B. F., Fairley, K. F., and Kincaid-Smith, P. S. Idiopathic membranous glomerulonephritis: Long-term follow-up in 139 cases. *Clin. Nephrol.* 30:175, 1988.
173. Muther, R. S., McCarron, D. A., and Bennett, W. M. Renal manifestation of sarcoidosis. *Arch. Intern. Med.* 141:643, 1981.
174. Nagi, A. H., Alexander, F., and Barabas, A. Z. Gold nephropathy in rats: Light and electron microscopic studies. *Exp. Mol. Pathol.* 15:354, 1971.
175. Nagy, J., Bajtai, G., Brasch, H., Süle, T., Ambrus, M., Deák, G., and Hámori, A. The role of hepatitis B surface antigen in the pathogenesis of glomerulopathies. *Clin. Nephrol.* 12:109, 1979.
176. Naruse, T., Kitamura, K., Miyakawa, Y., and Shibata, S. Deposition of renal tubular epithelial antigen along the glomerular capillary walls of patients with membranous glomerulonephritis. *J. Immunol.* 110:1163, 1973.
177. Naruse, T., Miyakawa, Y., Kitamura, K., and Shibata, S. Membranous glomerulonephritis mediated by renal tubular epithelial antigen-antibody complex. *J. Allergy Clin. Immunol.* 54:311, 1974.
178. Nguyen, B. P., Reisin, E., and Rodriguez, F. H., Jr. Idiopathic membranous glomerulopathy complicated by crescentic glomerulonephritis and renal vein thrombosis. *Am. J. Kidney Dis.* 12:326, 1988.
179. Nöel, L.-H., Aucouturier, P., Monteiro, R. C., Preud'Homme, J.-L., and LeSavre, P. Glomerular and serum immunoglobulin G subclasses in membranous nephropathy and anti-GBM nephritis. *Clin. Immunol. Immunopathol.* 46:186, 1988.
180. Nöel, L. H., Zanetti, M., Droz, D., and Barbanel, C. Long-term prognosis of idiopathic membranous glomerulonephritis. *Am. J. Med.* 66:82, 1979.
181. Okada, K., Kawakami, K., Miyao, M., and Oite, T. Ultrastructural alterations of glomerular anionic sites in idiopathic membranous glomerulonephritis. *Clin. Nephrol.* 26:7, 1986.
182. Olbing, H., Greifer, I., Bennett, B. P., Bernstein, J., and Spitzer, A. Idiopathic membranous nephropathy in children. *Kidney Int.* 3:381, 1973.
183. Olesnicky, L., Doty, S. B., Bertani, T., and Pirani, C. L. Tubular microfibrils in the glomeruli of membranous nephropathy. *Arch. Pathol. Lab. Med.* 108:902, 1984.
184. Olson, J. L., Philips, T. M., Lewis, M. G., and Solez, K. Malignant melanoma with renal dense deposits containing tumor antigens. *Clin. Nephrol.* 12:74, 1979.
185. Ooi, B. S., Ooi, Y. M., Hsu, A., and Hurtubise, P. E. Diminished synthesis of immunoglobulin by peripheral lymphocytes of patients with idiopathic membranous glomerulonephropathy. *J. Clin. Invest.* 65:789, 1980.
186. Ooi, B. S., Ooi, Y. M., and Pollak, V. E. Identification of circulating immune complexes in a subpopulation of patients with membranous glomerulonephropathy. *Clin. Immunol. Immunopathol.* 16:447, 1980.
187. Ozawa, T., Pluss, R., Lacher, J., Boedecker, E., Guggenheim, S., Hammond, W., and McIntosh, R. Endogenous immune complex nephropathy associated with malignancy: I. Studies on the nature and immunopathogenic significance of glomerular bound antigen and antibody, isolation and characterization of tumor specific antigen and antibody and circulating immune complexes. *Q. J. Med.* 44:523, 1975.
188. Papiha, S. S., Pareek, S. K., Rodger, R. S., Morley, A. R., Wilkinson, R., Roberts, D. F., and Kerr, D. N. S. HLA-A, B, DR, and Bf allotypes in patients with idiopathic membranous nephropathy. *Kidney Int.* 31:130, 1987.
189. Passerini, P., Pasquali, S., Cesana, B., Zucchelli, P., and Ponticelli, C. Long-term outcome of patients with membranous nephropathy after complete remission of proteinuria. *Nephrol. Dial. Transplant.* 4:525, 1989.
190. Pasternack, A., Törnroth, T., and Linder, E. Evidence of both anti-glomerular basement membrane and immune complex–mediated pathogenesis in the initial phase of Goodpasture's syndrome. *Clin. Nephrol.* 9:77, 1978.
191. Pearl, M. A., Burch, R. R., Carvajal, E., McCracken, B. H., Woody, H. B., and Sternberg, W. H. Nephrotic syndrome: A clinical and pathological study. *Arch. Intern. Med.* 112:130, 1963.
192. Pettersson, E., Törnroth, T., and Miettinen, A. Simultaneous anti-glomerular basement membrane and membranous glomerulonephritis: Case report and literature review. *Clin. Immunol. Immunopathol.* 3:171, 1984.
193. Pierides, A. M., Malasit, P., Morley, A. R., Wil-

kinson, R., Uldall, P. R., and Kerr, D. N. S. Idiopathic membranous nephropathy. *Q. J. Med.* 46:163, 1977.
194. Pollak, V. E., Rosen, S., Pirani, C. L., Muehrcke, R. C., and Kark, R. M. Natural history of lipoid nephrosis and of membranous glomerulonephritis. *Ann. Intern. Med.* 69:1171, 1968.
195. Ponticelli, C., Zucchelli, P., Imbasciati, E., Cagnoli, L., Pozzi, C., Passerini, P., Grassi, C., Limido, D., Pasquali, S., Volpini, T., Sasdelli, M., and Locatelli, F. Controlled trial of methylprednisolone and chlorambucil in idiopathic membranous nephropathy. *N. Engl. J. Med.* 310:946, 1984.
196. Ponticelli, C., Zucchelli, P., Passerini, P., Cagnoli, L., Cesana, B., Pozzi, C., Pasquali, S., Imbasciati, E., Grassi, C., Redaelli, B., Sasdelli, M., and Locatelli, F. A randomized trial of methylprednisolone and chlorambucil in idiopathic membranous nephropathy. *N. Engl. J. Med.* 320:8, 1989.
197. Portch, P. A., and Williams, G. Mesangial cells in membranous glomerulonephritis. *J. Clin. Pathol.* 26:660, 1973.
198. Prins, E. J. L., Hoorntje, S. J., Weening, J. J., and Donker, A. J. M. Nephrotic syndrome in a patient on captopril. *Lancet* 2:306, 1979.
199. Pruchno, C. J., Burns, M. W., Schulze, M., Johnson, R. J., Baker, P. J., and Couser, W. G. Urinary excretion of C5b-9 reflects disease activity in passive Heymann nephritis. *Kidney Int.* 36:65, 1989.
200. Ramirez, F., Brouhard, B. H., Travis, L. B., and Ellis, E. N. Idiopathic membranous nephropathy in children. *J. Pediatr.* 5:677, 1982.
201. Ramzy, M. H., Cameron, J. S., Turner, D. R., Neild, G. H., Ogg, C. S., and Hicks, J. The long-term outcome of idiopathic membranous nephropathy. *Clin. Nephrol.* 16:13, 1981.
202. Rastogi, S. P.. Hart-Mercer, J., and Kerr, D. N. S. Idiopathic membranous glomerulonephritis in adults: Remission following steroid therapy. *Q. J. Med.* 38:335, 1969.
203. Relman, A. S. What have we learned about the treatment of idiopathic membranous nephropathy with steroids? *N. Engl. J. Med.* 320:248, 1989.
204. Richet, G., Fillastre, J. P., Morel-Maroger, L., and Bariety, J. Change from diffuse proliferative to membranous glomerulonephritis: Serial biopsies in four cases. *Kidney Int.* 5:57, 1974.
205. Richman, A. V., Rifkin, S. I., and McAllister, C. J. Rapidly progressive glomerulonephritis: Combined antiglomerular basement membrane antibody and immune complex pathogenesis. *Hum. Pathol.* 12:597, 1981.
206. Richmond, J. M., Chambers, B., D'Apice, A. J. F., Whitworth, J. H., and Kincaid-Smith, P. Renal disease and sarcoidosis. *Med. J. Aust.* 2:36, 1981.
207. Ricker, W., and Clark, M. Sarcoidosis: A clinicopathologic review of three hundred cases, including twenty-two autopsies. *Am. J. Clin. Pathol.* 9:715, 1949.
208. Riemenschneider, T., Mackensen-Haen, S., Christ, H., and Bohle, A. Correlation between endogenous creatinine clearance and relative interstitial volume of the renal cortex in patients with diffuse membranous glomerulonephritis having a normal serum creatinine concentration. *Lab. Invest.* 43:145, 1980.
209. Roberts, J. L., Wyatt, R. J., Schwartz, M. M., and Lewis, E. J. Differential diagnosis of immune-bound antibodies in diffuse proliferative and membranous forms of lupus glomerulonephritis. *Clin. Immunol. Immunopathol.* 29:223, 1983.
210. Rocatello, D., Coppo, R., Amoroso, A., Curtoni, E. S., Martina, G., Basolo, B., Amore, A., Rollino, C., Picciotto, G., and Cordonnier, D. Failure to relate mononuclear phagocyte system function to HLA-A, B, C, DR, DQ antigens in membranous nephropathy. *Am. J. Kidney Dis.* 9:470, 1987.
211. Rosen, S. Membranous glomerulonephritis: Current status. *Hum. Pathol.* 2:209, 1971.
212. Rosendorff, C., Milne, F. J., Levy, H., Ninin, D. T., and Lewin, J. R. Nephrotic syndrome during captopril therapy. *S. Afr. Med. J.* 58:172, 1980.
213. Rosenman, E., Brisson, M. L., Bercovitch, D. D., and Rosenberg, A. Atypical membranous glomerulonephritis with fibrillar subepithelial deposits in a patient with malignant lymphoma. *Nephron* 48:226, 1988.
214. Rossen, R. D., Reisberg, M. A., Hersh, E. M., and Gutterman, J. U. Measurement of soluble immune complexes: A guide to prognosis in cancer patients. (Abstract) *Clin. Res.* 24:462A, 1976.
215. Row, P. G., Cameron, J. S., Turner, D. R., Evans, D. J., White, R. H. R., Ogg, C. S., Chantler, C., and Brown, C. B. Membranous nephropathy: Long-term follow-up and association with neoplasia. *Q. J. Med.* 44:207, 1975.
216. Safar, M., Bariéty, J., Lagrue, G., Samarcq, P., and Milliez, P. Association d'un syndrome néphrotique et d'un syndrome de Gougerot-Sjögren. *Sem. Hop. Paris* 40:1423, 1964.
217. Salant, D. J., Belok, S., Madaio, M. P., and Couser, W. G. A new role for complement in experimental membranous nephropathy in rats. *J. Clin. Invest.* 66:1339, 1980.
218. Samuels, B., Lee, J. C., Engleman, E. P., and Hopper, J., Jr. Membranous nephropathy in patients with rheumatoid arthritis: Relationship to gold therapy. *Medicine (Baltimore)* 57:319, 1978.
219. Sato, K., Oguchi, H., Hora, K., Furukawa, T.,

Furuta, S., Shigematsu, H., and Yoshizawa, S. Idiopathic membranous nephropathy in two brothers. *Nephron* 46:174, 1987.
220. Schulze, M., Baker, P. J., Johnson, R. J., Pruchno, C. J., Donadio, J. V., and Couser, W. G. Urinary complement C5b-9 excretion in membranous nephropathy. *Kidney Int.* 33:331, 1988.
221. Schwartz, M. M., and Korbet, S. M. Crescentic Glomerulonephritis. In I. Damjanov, A. H. Cohen, S. E. Mills, and R. H. Young (Eds.), *Progress in Reproductive and Urinary Tract Pathology,* Vol. 1. New York: Field and Wood, 1989. P. 163.
222. Schwartz, M. M., Roberts, J. L., Humes, C., Kawala, K., and Lewis, E. J. Clinical and pathological features of membranous glomerulonephritis of systemic lupus erythematosus. *Am. J. Nephrol.* 4:301, 1984.
223. Schwartzberg, M., Burnstein, S. L., Calabro, J. J., and Jacobs, J. B. The development of membranous glomerulonephritis in a patient with rheumatoid arthritis and Sjögren's syndrome. *J. Rheumatol.* 6:65, 1979.
224. Sharon, Z., Rohde, R. D., and Lewis, E. J. Report of a case of Goodpasture's syndrome with unusual immunohistology and antibody reactivity. *Clin. Immunol. Immunopathol.* 18:402, 1981.
225. Sharon, Z., Schwartz, M. M., Pauli, B. U., and Lewis, E. J. Impairment of glomerular clearance of foreign macroaggregates in chronic autologous immune complex nephritis. *Kidney Int.* 22:3, 1982.
226. Shearn, M. A., Biava, C., and Hopper, J., Jr. Mesangial deposits (by electron microscopy) in idiopathic membranous glomerulonephritis. *N. Engl. J. Med.* 301:212, 1979.
227. Shemesh, O., Ross, J. C., Deen, W. M., Grant, G. W., and Myers, B. D. Nature of the glomerular capillary injury in human membranous glomerulopathy. *J. Clin. Invest.* 77:868, 1986.
228. Short, C. D., Dyer, P. A., Cairns, S. A., Manos, J., Walton, C., Harris, R., and Mallick, N. A major histocompatibility system haplotype associated with poor prognosis in idiopathic membranous nephropathy. *Dis. Markers* 1:189, 1983.
229. Short, C. D., Feehally, J., Gokal, R., and Mallick, N. P. Familial membranous nephropathy. *Br. Med. J.* 289:1500, 1984.
230. Silverberg, D. S., Kidd, E. G., Shnitka, T. K., and Ulan, R. A. Gold nephropathy: A clinical and pathologic study. *Arthritis. Rheum.* 13:812, 1970.
231. Singh, A. K., and Makker, S. P. The distribution and molecular presentation of the brush border antigen of Heymann nephritis in various rat tissues. *Clin. Exp. Immunol.* 60:579, 1985.
232. Skrifvars, B. V., Törnroth, T. S., and Falck, H. M. Granulomatous glomerulonephritis in a patient with rheumatoid arthritis treated with gold salts. *Scand. J. Rheumatol.* 8:234, 1979.
233. Skrifvars, B. V., Törnroth, T. S., and Tallqvist, G. N. Gold-induced immune complex nephritis in seronegative rheumatoid arthritis. *Ann. Rheum. Dis.* 36:549, 1977.
234. Slusarczyk, J., Michalak, T., Nazarewicz-de Mezer, T., Krawczynski, K., and Nowoslawski, A. Membranous glomerulopathy associated with hepatitis B core antigen immune complexes in children. *Am. J. Pathol.* 98:29, 1980.
235. Sol, J. B., Planas, J. T., Pinel, B., Artal, E. M., and Carrera, M. Sindrome de Sjögren y glomerulonefritis membranosa. *Rev. Clin. Esp.* 177:191, 1985.
236. Southwest Pediatric Nephrology Study Group. Hepatitis B surface antigenemia in North American children with membranous glomerulonephropathy. *J. Pediatr.* 106:571, 1985.
237. Southwest Pediatric Nephrology Study Group. Comparison of idiopathic and systemic lupus erythematosus–associated membranous glomerulonephropathy in children. *Am. J. Kidney Dis.* 7:115, 1986.
238. Spargo, B., and Arnold, J. D. Glomerular extrinsic membranous deposit with the nephrotic syndrome. *Ann. N.Y. Acad. Sci.* 86:1043, 1960.
239. Stachura, I., Si, L., Madan, E., and Whiteside, T. Mononuclear cell subsets in human renal disease: Enumeration in tissue sections with monoclonal antibodies. *Clin. Immunol. Immunopathol.* 30:362, 1984.
240. Steinmuller, D. R., Stilmant, M. M., Idelson, B. A., Monaco, A. P., Sahyoun, A. I., Lewis, E. J., Davis, R. C., and Couser, W. G. De novo development of membranous nephropathy in cadaver renal allografts. *Clin. Nephrol.* 9:210, 1978.
241. Sternlieb, I. Penicillamine and the nephrotic syndrome: Results in patients with hepatolenticular degeneration. *JAMA* 198:1311, 1966.
242. Sternlieb, I., Bennett, B., and Scheinberg, I. H. D-Penicillamine induced Goodpasture's syndrome in Wilson's disease. *Ann. Intern. Med.* 82:673, 1975.
243. Stockman, A., Richter, D., Barraclough, D., Muirden, K. D., MacDonald, I., and Kincaid-Smith, P. Difficulties in the use of D-penicillamine in the treatment of rheumatoid arthritis. *Aust. N.Z. J. Med.* 9:495, 1979.
244. Stuve, J., and Galle, P. Role of mitochondria in the handling of gold by the kidney: A study by electron microscopy and electron probe microanalysis. *J. Cell Biol.* 44:667, 1970.
245. Strunk, S. W., and Ziff, M. Ultrastructural stud-

ies of the passage of gold thiomalate across the renal glomerular capillary wall. *Arthritis Rheum.* 13:39, 1970.
246. Sugisaki, T., Yoshida, T., McCluskey, R. T., Andres, G. A., and Klassen, J. Autoimmune cell-mediated tubulointerstitial nephritis induced in Lewis rats by renal antigens. *Clin. Immunol. Immunopathol.* 15:33, 1980.
247. Takekoshi, Y., Tanaka, M., Shida, N., Satake, Y., Saheki, Y., and Matsumoto, S. Strong association between membranous nephropathy and hepatitis-B surface antigenaemia in Japanese children. *Lancet* 2:1075, 1978.
248. Talal, N., Zisman, E., and Schur, P. H. Renal tubular acidosis, glomerulonephritis, and immunologic factors in Sjögren's syndrome. *Arthritis Rheum.* 11:774, 1968.
249. Tallqvist, G., Törnroth, T., Vanttinen, T., and Pasternack, A. Vacuolization of the glomerular basement membrane. *Acta Pathol. Microbiol. Scand.* [A]. 87:411, 1979.
250. Tateno, S., Sakai, T., Kobayashi, Y., and Shigematsu, H. Idiopathic membranous glomerulonephritis with crescents. *Acta Pathol. Jpn.* 31:211, 1981.
251. Taube, D., Brown, Z., and Williams, D. G. Impaired lymphocyte and suppressor cell function in minimal change nephropathy, membranous nephropathy and focal glomerulosclerosis. *Clin. Nephrol.* 22:176, 1984.
252. Taylor, R. G., Fisher, C., and Hoffbrand, B. I. Sarcoidosis and membranous glomerulonephritis: A significant association. *Br. Med. J.* 284:1297, 1982.
253. Taylor, T. K., Senekjian, H. O., Knight, T. F., Gyorkey, F., and Weinman, E. J. Membranous nephropathy with epithelial crescents in a patient with pulmonary sarcoidosis. *Arch. Intern. Med.* 139:1183, 1979.
254. The Captopril Collaborative Study Group. Does captopril cause renal damage in hypertensive patients? *Lancet* 1:988, 1982.
255. Thorpe, L. W., and Cavallo, T. Renal tubule brush border antigens: Failure to confirm a pathogenetic role in human membranous glomerulonephritis. *J. Clin. Lab. Immunol.* 3:125, 1980.
256. Tomaszewski, M. M., Hassell, L. H., Moore, J., Jr., and Antonovych, T. T. Goodpasture's syndrome: Local and diffuse deposition of antibody in glomerular basement membrane. Case report. *Clin. Nephrol.* 20:44, 1983.
257. Tomura, S., Kashiwabara, H., Tuchida, H., Shishido, H., Sakurai, S., Miyajima, T., Tsuji, K., and Takeuchi, J. Strong association of idiopathic membranous nephropathy with HLA-DR2 and MT1 in Japanese. *Nephron* 36:242, 1984.
258. Törnroth, T. Membranous Glomerulonephritis. In S. Rosen (Ed.), *Pathology of Glomerular Disease.* New York: Churchill-Livingstone, 1983.
259. Törnroth, T., and Skrifvars, B. Gold nephropathy prototype of membranous glomerulonephritis. *Am. J. Pathol.* 75:573, 1974.
260. Törnroth, T., and Skrifvars, B. The development and resolution of glomerular basement membrane changes associated with subepithelial immune deposits. *Am. J. Pathol.* 79:219, 1975.
261. Törnroth, T., Tallqvist, G., Pasternack, A., and Linder, E. Nonprogressive histologically mild membranous glomerulonephritis appearing in all evolutionary phases as histologically "early" membranous glomerulonephritis. *Kidney Int.* 14:511, 1978.
262. Truong, L., Gelfand, J., D'Agati, V., Tomaszewski, J., Appel, G., Hardy, M., and Pirani, C. L. De novo membranous glomerulonephropathy in renal allografts: A report of ten cases. *Am. J. Kidney Dis.* 14:131, 1989.
263. Tsao, Y. C., Chan, W. C., and Gibson, J. B. Persistent proteinuria in children. *Arch. Dis. Child.* 44:443, 1969.
264. Tubbs, R. R., Valenzuela, R., McCormack, L. J., Pohl, M. A., and Barenberg, S. Gold nephropathy. *N. Engl. J. Med.* 296:1413, 1977.
265. Tue, W. H., Shearn, M. A., Lee, J. C., and Hopper, J., Jr. Interstitial nephritis in Sjögren's syndrome. *Ann. Intern. Med.* 69:1163, 1968.
266. Tung, K. S. K., and Black, W. C. Association of renal glomerular and tubular immune complex disease and antitubular basement membrane antibody. *Lab. Invest.* 32:696, 1975.
267. Vaamonde, C. A., and Hunt, F. R. The nephrotic syndrome as a complication of gold therapy. *Arthritis Rheum.* 13:826, 1970.
268. Vidal, F., Oliver, J. A., Campanya, E., Baguer, A., Carrera, M., and Richart, C. Sarcoidosis presenting as multiple pulmonary nodules and nephrotic syndrome. *Postgrad. Med. J.* 62:1147, 1986.
269. Viol, G. W., Minielly, J. A., and Bistricki, T. Gold nephropathy: Tissue analysis by x-ray fluorescent spectroscopy. *Arch. Pathol. Lab. Med.* 101:635, 1977.
270. Wakashin, M., Wakashin, Y., Iesato, K., Ueda, S., Mori, Y., Tsuchida, H., Shigematsu, H., and Okuida, K. Association of gastric cancer and nephrotic syndrome: An immunologic study in three patients. *Gastroenterology* 78:749, 1980.
271. Ward, H. J., and Koyle, M. A. Immunopathologic features of de novo membranous nephropathy in renal allografts. *Transplantation* 45:524, 1988.
272. Warwick, G., and Boulton-Jones, J. M. Immu-

nosuppression for membranous nephropathy. *Lancet* 2:1361, 1988.
273. Watanabe, I., Whittier, F. C., Jr., Moore, J., and Cuppage, F. E. Gold nephropathy: Ultrastructural, fluorescence, and microanalytic studies of two patients. *Arch. Pathol. Lab. Med.* 100:632, 1976.
274. Wehrmann, M., Bohle, A., Bogenschütz, O., Eissele, R., Freislederer, A., Öhlschlegel, C., Schumm, G., Batz, C., and Gärtner, H.-V. Long-term prognosis of chronic idiopathic membranous glomerulonephritis: An analysis of 334 cases with particular regard to tubulointerstitial changes. *Clin. Nephrol.* 3:67, 1989.
275. Weksler, M. E., Carey, T., Day, N., Susin, M., Sherman, R., and Becker, C. Nephrotic syndrome in malignant melanoma: Demonstration of melanoma antigen-antibody complexes in kidney. (Abstract) *Kidney Int.* 6:112A, 1974.
276. Whitworth, J. A., Leibowitz, S., Kennedy, M. C., Cameron, J. S., Evans, D. J., Glassock, R. J., and Schoenfeld, L. S. Absence of glomerular renal tubular epithelial antigen in membranous glomerulonephritis. *Clin. Nephrol.* 5:159, 1976.
277. Wiggelinkhuizen, J., Sinclair-Smith, C., Stannard, L. M., and Smuts, H. Hepatitis B virus associated membranous glomerulonephritis. *Arch. Dis. Child.* 58:488, 1983.
278. Yamauchi, H., Linsey, M. S., Biava, C. G., and Hopper, J., Jr. Cure of membranous nephropathy after resection of carcinoma. *Arch. Intern. Med.* 145:2061, 1985.
279. Yaremko, M. L., Koukoulis, G., and Schwartz, M. M. Unpublished data, 1989.
280. Yarom, R., Stein, H., Peters, P. D., Slavin, S., and Hall, T. A. Nephrotoxic effect of parenteral and intraarticular gold. *Arch. Pathol. Lab. Med.* 99:36, 1975.
281. Yoshikawa, N., Ito, H., Yamada, Y., Hashimoto, H., Katayama, Y., Matsuyama, S., Hasegawa, O., Okada, S., Hajikano, H., Yoshizawa, H., Mayumi, M., and Matsuo, T. Membranous glomerulonephritis associated with hepatitis B antigen in children: A comparison with idiopathic membranous glomerulonephritis. *Clin. Nephrol.* 23:28, 1985.
282. Zager, R. A., Couser, W. G., Andrews, B. S., Bolton, W. K., and Pohl, M. A. Membranous nephropathy: A radioimmunologic search for anti-renal tubular epithelial antibodies and circulating immune complexes. *Nephron* 24:10, 1979.
283. Zanetti, M., Mandet, C., Duboust, A., Bedrossian, J., and Bariéty, J. Demonstration of a passive Heymann nephritis-like mechanism in a human kidney transplant. *Clin. Nephrol.* 15:272, 1981.

Robert H. Heptinstall

9

Crescentic Glomerulonephritis

BACKGROUND AND TERMINOLOGY

This chapter is devoted to a form of glomerulonephritis in which glomeruli show crescent formation in addition to changes in the capillary tuft. Clinically, severe renal failure is present at the outset or develops quickly, and various terms such as *subacute* [131], *stormy course* [80], *acute anuric* or *acute oliguric* [4,16,30,61,75], and *rapidly progressive type I* [46] have been used to describe this form of glomerulonephritis. For many years, *subacute glomerulonephritis* was the most favored name, but this was confusing in that certain clinicians used the same term to describe a slowly progressing disease with a nephrotic syndrome. In the first edition of this book in 1966, I suggested dropping the type I from Ellis's term [46] and simply calling the condition *rapidly progressive glomerulonephritis.* While this portrays the clinical picture, it conveys little idea of the pathologic features, and the terms *extracapillary* [132] and *crescentic glomerulonephritis* are more appropriate for the pathologist. Since this is a book about pathology, I shall use the name *crescentic glomerulonephritis* for this chapter.

It must be appreciated that crescents are found in many seemingly diverse conditions. Sometimes they are of little moment and are found in only occasional glomeruli, such as in malignant hypertension and around the periphery of infarcts. On other occasions they may materially alter the clinical picture and the outlook because they affect large numbers of glomeruli. This occurs in anti-glomerular basement membrane (anti-GBM) antibody disease and specific, well-defined forms of glomerulonephritis such as membranous, membranoproliferative, IgA, hereditary (Alport's syndrome), and poststreptococcal glomerulonephritis, and those complicating endocarditis and deep abscesses. Crescents are also of consequence in mixed essential cryoglobulinemia, systemic lupus erythematosus (SLE), Schönlein-Henoch syndrome, polyarteritis nodosa with glomerulonephritis, Wegener's syndrome, and rheumatoid arthritis. They also may be found in relapsing polychondritis and rarely in several other conditions. Table 9-1 lists these conditions and provides an index of their location in the book.

The immediate problem is to find a suitable name for that form of crescentic glomerulonephritis which remains when the above-mentioned conditions are excluded. Usually it shows segmental necrotizing and/or diffuse or segmental proliferative changes in the tuft, accompanied by variable numbers of crescents. Using immunofluorescence techniques on the glomeruli, three main groups are identified according to the pattern seen; the first is a linear distribution of IgG, with or without C3, along the capillary wall; the second is a granular pattern for immunoglobulins and C3 along the capillary wall or in the mesangium; whereas the third shows either no or only an irregular, often faint distribution of immunoglobulins and complement. From these observations it is considered that some cases are caused by anti-GBM antibodies (group 1), others by an immune complex mechanism (group 2), whereas the pathogenesis of the remainder is unknown (group 3). The most favored names at the present time are *idiopathic crescentic* or *idiopathic rapidly progressive glomerulonephritis,* and cases with all three immunofluorescence groups are included [38,39,57,79]. I have certain reservations about including all three groups under the heading of idiopathic, which in modern-day usage means that the cause is unknown [124]. The first group, that with linear fluorescence, is *caused* by anti-GBM antibodies, even though we do not know what initiates the formation of the antibodies. It therefore seems illogical to include this particular group under the heading of idiopathic. This was the attitude of Heilman et al. [63], who used the term *idiopathic rapidly progressive glomerulonephritis* to include only two groups and discussed anti-GBM antibody disease separately. Similarly, the propriety of including the group with granular deposits—regarded as immune complexes—under the heading of idiopathic is open to question when it is well recognized that immune complexes cause glomerular damage. Conventional nomenclature rarely ever precedes the various forms of immune complex glomerulonephritis with idiopathic, so why should crescentic glomerulonephritis caused by immune

Table 9-1. *Principal conditions with significant numbers of crescents*

I. Primary (so-called idiopathic) crescentic glomerulonephritis	This chapter
II. Anti-GBM antibody disease	
A. With lung and kidney involvement	Chap. 10
B. Restricted to kidney	Chap. 10
III. Complicating various forms of glomerulonephritis	
A. Postinfectious or infectious	Chap. 5
1. Poststreptococcal	
2. Visceral abscesses	
3. Endocarditis	
B. Membranoproliferative	Chap. 7
C. Membranous	Chap. 8
D. IgA	Chap. 6
E. Hereditary (Alport's syndrome)	Chap. 30
IV. Systemic diseases	
A. Systemic lupus erythematosus	Chap. 13
B. Schönlein-Henoch syndrome	Chap. 6
C. Essential mixed cryoglobulinemia	Chap. 24
D. Polyarteritis nodosa	Chap. 16
E. Wegener's syndrome	Chap. 16
F. Rheumatoid arthritis	Chap. 16
G. Relapsing polychondritis	Chap. 16
H. Takayasu's disease	Chap. 16
I. Temporal (giant-cell) arteritis	Chap. 16
V. Miscellaneous rare conditions	This chapter

complexes be singled out in this way? If this group, too, were to be excluded, the one with no, or scanty, deposits would be the sole representative of the idiopathic group.

The names *primary crescentic* and *primary rapidly progressive glomerulonephritis* are viable alternatives and overcome the objections just raised. *Primary* implies that the underlying lesion is primarily in the glomeruli and restricted to the kidney, thereby excluding systemic diseases. The use of the prefix *primary* is open to the criticism that various clearly defined forms of primary glomerulonephritis such as poststreptococcal, membranous, membranoproliferative, and IgA may, from time to time, assume a crescentic form. Since the object is to define a unique group divorced from these identifiable conditions, the prefix *primary* would not accomplish this unless these forms were deliberately excluded. Ideally, this is what should be done, with the identifiable forms retaining their unique name but being qualified by the addition of the prefix *crescentic* or *crescentic forms of*. Thus membranous glomerulonephritis complicated by crescents would be *crescentic membranous glomerulonephritis* or *crescentic form of membranous glomerulonephritis*. Unfortunately, some of these specific forms are not always clearly identifiable, and these will inevitably be included under primary crescentic glomerulonephritis.

In order to determine the extent to which specific forms of glomerulonephritis contribute to the pool of crescentic glomerulonephritis, from which patients with vasculitis and systemic diseases such as SLE, Schönlein-Henoch syndrome, and others, listed in Table 9-1, are excluded, we studied such a pool seen on our renal biopsy service. The ease with which these specific forms could be identified was addressed, and the features of the cases that remained after removal of the specific forms were noted. These represent cases of primary crescentic glomerulonephritis that would satisfy even the severest critics.

LOCAL STUDY OF CRESCENTIC GLOMERULONEPHRITIS

Material

The biopsies were mainly from patients seen at The Johns Hopkins Hospital but were supplemented with some from nephrologists in Baltimore and other parts of Maryland who regularly send us their material for interpretation. Cases were restricted to those in which there were no stigmata of generalized vasculitis either on clinical, angiographic, or histologic grounds, and also excluded were patients with SLE, Schönlein-Henoch syndrome, essential mixed cryoglobulinemia, and other systemic diseases listed in Table 9-1. There were 38 cases; all had immunofluorescence microscopy performed, and electron microscopy was available in all but 3. All had at least 30 percent of glomeruli containing crescents, and most had over 60 percent involved. They were allocated to three groups according to the immunofluorescence picture: group 1, with linear fluorescence for IgG with or without C3; group 2, with granular fluorescence for immunoglobulins and complement along the glomerular capillary walls and/or in the mesangium; and group 3, with negative or only localized positive fluorescence for immunoglobulins and/or complement.

Table 9-2 gives the numbers of cases, sex, and age according to group. Group 2 is presented in two different ways: first, before the specific forms of glomerulonephritis are identified—referred to as group 2 (initial)—and second, after identifiable specific forms are withdrawn—referred to as group 2 (corrected). It was found that group 1 was the smallest (4 cases). Group 2 is larger than group 3 before identifiable specific forms of glomerulonephritis are withdrawn (19 compared with 15) but smaller (12 compared with 15) after withdrawal. The only group with a pronounced sex difference was group 3, which was predominantly male; this is similar to the findings of others [88,118]. The mean and median ages in group 1 were high, which is consistent with the emergence of a group of older patients with anti-GBM antibody disease, usually without lung hemorrhage [112*a*]. The mean and median ages were higher in group 3 than in group 2, but this is barely appreciable when the identifiable specific forms are removed from group 2. The relatively high mean and median ages in group 3 is similar to that reported by Stilmant et al. [118].

Immunofluorescence and Electron Microscopic Findings

The results are given in Tables 9-3, 9-4, and 9-5. In order to avoid congestion, only immunoglobulins and complement are recorded. Fibrin/fibrinogen was present more or less constantly in cellular crescents and also was seen in the glomeruli corresponding to areas of necrosis, particularly in group 3.

GROUP 1

Little more need be said of group 1, since the immunofluorescence pattern is identical to that accepted as indicating anti-GBM antibody disease. Three of the four biopsies showed linear IgG (Fig.

TABLE 9-2. *Number of cases with sex and age distribution of three groups*

	Group 1	Group 2 (initial)*	Group 2 (corrected)†	Group 3
Number of cases	4	19	12	15
Sex	M, 2; F, 2	M, 12; F, 7	M, 8; F, 4	M, 12; F, 3
Age (years):				
Range	60–76	6–69	21–69	22–72
Mean	68	44	53	59
Median	68	49	59	64

*Group 2 (initial) includes all cases with immunoglobulins and complement.
†Group 2 (corrected) excludes cases with specific identifiable forms of glomerulonephritis.

Table 9-3. *Group 1: Immunofluorescence for immunoglobulins and complement*

Case number	GCW*	TBM†	Pulmonary hemorrhage
1	G++.L. C3+.Gr.‡	0	0
2	G++.L.	0	0
3	G+++.L.	G++.L. M+.L. C3+.L.	0
4	G++.L.	0	+

*GCW = glomerular capillary wall.
†TBM = tubular basement membrane.
‡L = linear; Gr = granular; other abbreviations as in Table 9-4.

9-1) without C3 along glomerular capillary walls (see Table 9-3), and a granular pattern for C3 in addition to linear IgG was recorded in one patient. No deposits were reported by electron microscopy in any case.

GROUP 2

In group 2 (see Table 9-4) there were significant amounts of immunoglobulins and complement in 16 cases, IgG alone in two, and C3 alone in one. The immune deposits were invariably granular and present in either the capillary wall or the mesangium or both. Electron microscopy confirmed these deposits except in two cases in which it was not performed and in one in which the glomeruli studied were sclerotic. Specific forms of immune complex glomerulonephritis were clearly identifiable in several instances. Two cases (cases 1 and 2 in Table 9-4), in conjunction with clinical and laboratory findings, were found to have a post-streptococcal form, and both were children. Three cases (cases 3, 4, and 5) had changes consistent with IgA nephritis, and electron microscopy revealed mesangial deposits in all three (Figs. 9-2 and 9-3). Case 10 was an example of membranous glomerulonephritis with crescents; both immunofluorescence and electron microscopy supported the diagnosis (Fig. 9-4). In one other patient (case 16), IgM was the dominant immunoglobulin in the mesangium and was accompanied by a mild mesangial hypercellularity and mesangial electron-dense deposits. This fits the description of IgM nephropathy (nephritis). Three others (cases 7, 8, and 9) had an immunofluorescence pattern in which IgA and either IgG or IgM stained with equal intensity in the mesangium. In two of these there were plentiful electron-dense deposits in the mesangium, but in the other they were sparse. All three showed mild mesangial hypercellularity by light microscopy and may well represent IgA nephritis, but because we cannot be certain of this, they are placed in the unidentifiable group. It is not possible from the biopsies or the clinical data available to identify a specific form of glomerulonephritis in the remaining 9 cases, but on the basis of concordance of immunofluorescence and electron microscopy in most, and the demonstration of deposits by one or other of these techniques in the others, a good case can be made for an immune complex background. Thus 7 cases can be allocated to a specific form of immune complex glomerulonephritis, leaving 12 unidentifiable.

GROUP 3

Table 9-5 presents data on the 15 biopsies in group 3. Cases 1 through 5 showed negative glomerular immunofluorescence and absence of electron-dense deposits. Only four cases displayed immunoglobulins. In three (cases 10, 11, and 13) there was an irregular mesangial pattern that never exceeded 1+ in intensity; electron-dense deposits were absent in two and scattered and scanty in one (case 13). The fourth case (case 12) had a linear pattern of low intensity along the glomerular capillaries for IgG and a stronger one for albumin; there were no circulating anti-GBM antibodies by

TABLE 9-4. *Group 2: results*

Case number	Glomerular immunofluorescence for immunoglobulins and complement*		Glomerular electron microscopic deposits†	
	Capillary wall	Mesangium	Capillary wall	Mesangium
1	G++. C3++.	0	N.D.	
2	G++. C3++.	0	S-ep Intra-m S-end	0
3	A+. C3+.	A+++.G++. C3++.	S-end (sparse)	+
4	0	A++. G+. C3++.	0	+
5	0	A+++.G++. C3+.	S-end (sparse)	+
6	G+. A+. C3+.	G++.A+. C3++.	Intra-m (sparse)	+
7	A+. C3+.	G+. A+. C3+.	Intra-m (sparse)	+
8	0	G+. A+. C3+.	0	sparse
9	0	A+.M+. C3+.	0	+
10	G++.C3++.	0	S-ep Intra-m	0
11	G++.C3+.	0	Intra-m	0
12	G+.	0	Sclerosis of glomeruli examined	
13	G+.	0	S-ep	0
14	M++.C3+.	0	Intra-m	0
15	C3++.	G+.M+.	N.D.	
16	0	M++.G+. C3++.	S-ep (sparse)	+
17	0	C3++.	S-ep (sparse) S-end (sparse)	+
18	0	G++.A+. C3++.	S-end	+
19	0	M++.C3+ Irregular	0	+

*Immunofluorescence: staining intensity + to +++; G = IgG; A = IgA; M = IgM; all deposits were granular; irregular = present only in scattered mesangia or along short lengths of capillary wall
†Electron-dense deposits: S-ep = subepithelial; S-end = subendothelial; Intra-m = intramembranous.
Mesangial: 0 = absent; + = present; N.D. = not done.

Table 9-5. *Group 3: results*

Case number	Glomerular immunofluorescence for immunoglobulins and complement* — Capillary wall	Mesangium	Glomerular electron microscopic deposits
1 to 5	0	0	0
6	0	C3+; irregular	0
7	0	C3 and C1q; faint, irregular	0
8	C3++; irregular	C3++; irregular	0
9	C1q+; irregular	C1q+; irregular	0
10	0	A.M. C3; faint, and irregular	0
11	0	M+.C3++; irregular	0
12	G+.L.† Alb++.L.	0	N.D.
13	0	M+; irregular	Occasional in mesangium
14	0	0	Occasional S-ep in capillary wall
15	0	0	Occasional S-ep and Intra-m in capillary wall

*All immunofluorescence deposits were granular unless followed by L (linear); Alb = albumin.
†Circulating anti-GBM antibodies negative.

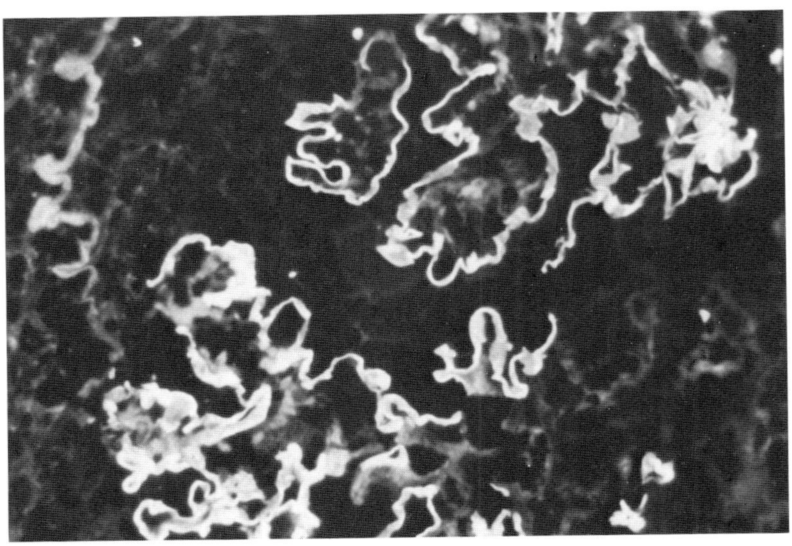

Fig. 9-1. *Linear fluorescence for IgG in a patient with crescentic glomerulonephritis of anti-GBM antibody pathogenesis.*

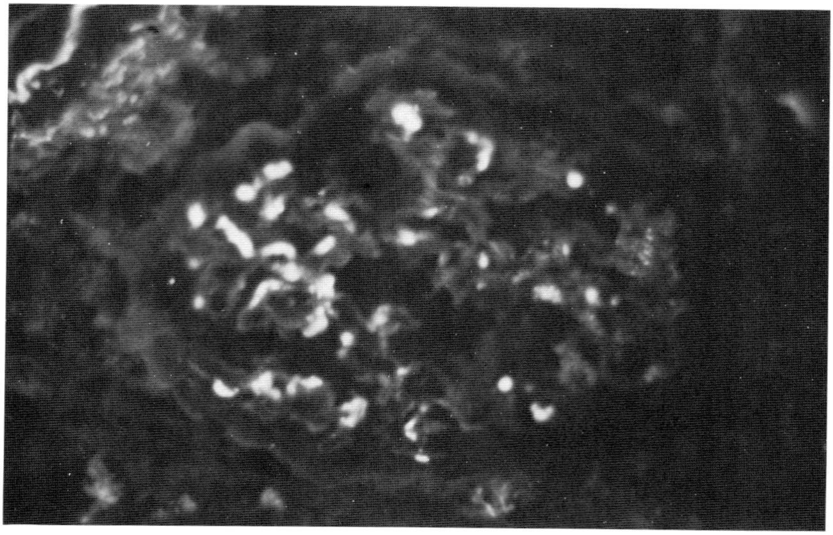

Fig. 9-2. *Mesangial deposition of IgA in a patient with crescentic glomerulonephritis superimposed on IgA nephritis.*

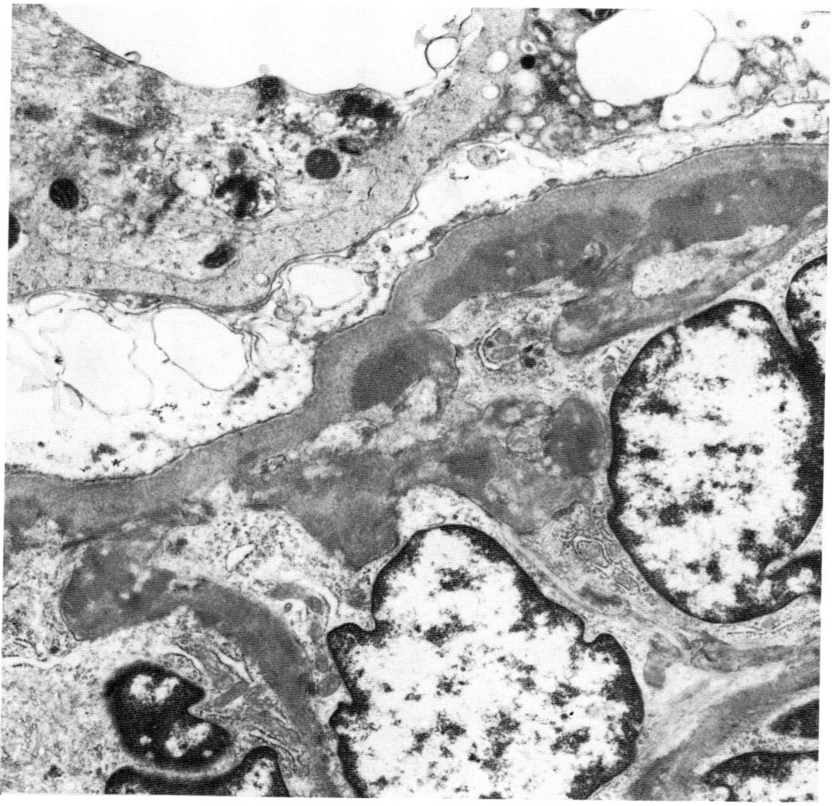

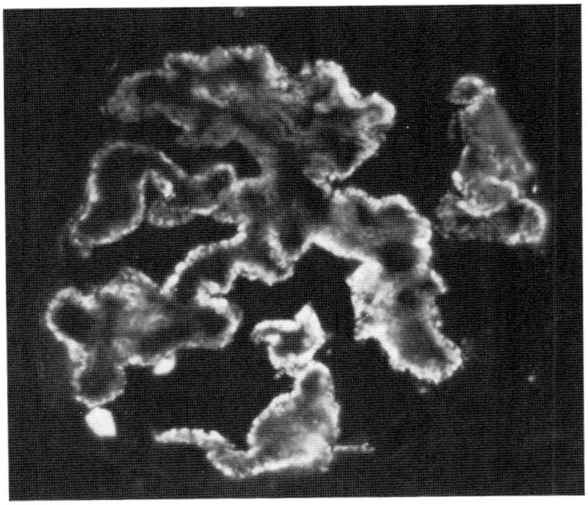

Fig. 9-4. *Granular deposition of IgG along capillary loops of a patient with crescentic glomerulonephritis superimposed on membranous glomerulonephritis.*

radioimmunoassay. Complement alone was present either in the mesangium or in the mesangium and the capillary walls (cases 6, 7, 8, and 9), but electron-dense deposits were absent in all. The remaining two cases (cases 14 and 15) were negative by immunofluorescence, but one showed occasional subepithelial electron-dense deposits in the capillary walls and the other occasional subepithelial and intramembranous deposits. Combining the immunofluorescence and electron microscopic observations, it appears that immune complexes can be excluded in all but three cases (cases 13, 14, and 15), and even in these three the evidence is far from compelling.

Light Microscopy

All cases showed at least 30 percent glomerular involvement by crescents, and the tufts showed hypercellularity or necrosis or mixtures of these. Glomerular sclerosis was widespread in some, and the morphology of the tuft was severely distorted.

Examples of the specific, identifiable forms are provided in the accompanying illustrations. Figures 9-5 and 9-6 are two of the cases of IgA nephritis. Figure 9-5 shows a large crescent compressing the glomerular tuft and is from the same case as in Figures 9-2 and 9-3; Figure 9-6 is from another case—with crescents in over half the glomeruli—and shows one of the less severely affected glomeruli in which generalized mesangial hypercellularity and a localized solidified area can be identified. Figure 9-7 illustrates a crescent undergoing fibrosis in a patient with membranous glomerulonephritis; Figure 9-8 shows the widespread crescent formation in a 10-year-old child with poststreptococcal glomerulonephritis; and Figure 9-9 shows an organizing crescent in a patient with predominantly IgM deposition in the mesangia.

Certain points are worth mentioning, but since the various features will be incorporated into the general pathology section later in the chapter, only the briefest comments will be made at this stage. First, the number of glomeruli accompanied by crescents varied little according to the groups, and all three showed over 90 percent of glomeruli affected in some of the cases. Second, hypercellularity of the tuft was more common in group 2 than in either group 1 or group 3. This is not surprising when it is considered that the initial group 2 included 2 cases of poststreptococcal glomerulonephritis, 3 of IgA nephritis with mesangial hypercellularity, and 1 of IgM nephropathy (nephritis). However, even when these were withdrawn, the remaining 12 cases showed greater degrees of either generalized or segmental hypercellularity of the tufts than were found in groups 1 and 3 (Fig. 9-10). Third, necrotizing changes in the glomerular tufts were more common in groups 1 and 3 than in group 2 (Figs. 9-11 and 9-12). In fact, a necrotizing form of glomerulonephritis was predominant in groups 1 and 3, whereas tuft necroses were present in only 4 of 19 cases in group 2. There was a particular paucity of necroses in those of poststreptococcal and IgA types. Fourth, the interstitial cellular reaction varied greatly from case

Fig. 9-3. *Electron-dense deposits in the mesangium in a patient whose immunofluorescence picture is shown in Fig. 9-2.* × *11,000.*

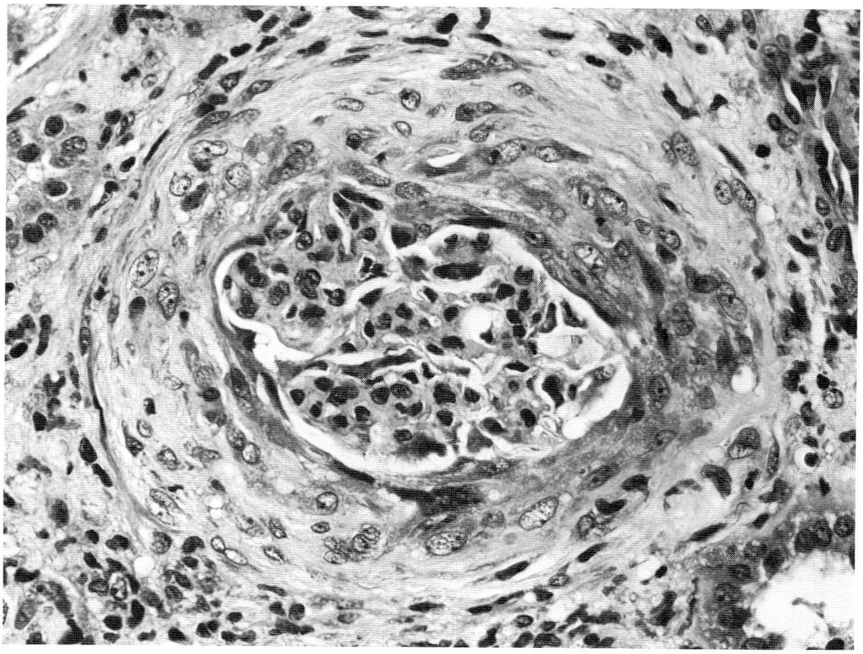

FIG. 9-5. *Large crescent in IgA nephritis. The glomerular tuft is considerably compressed, but IgA was detected in mesangial areas and was the predominant immunoglobulin present. H&E; ×400.*

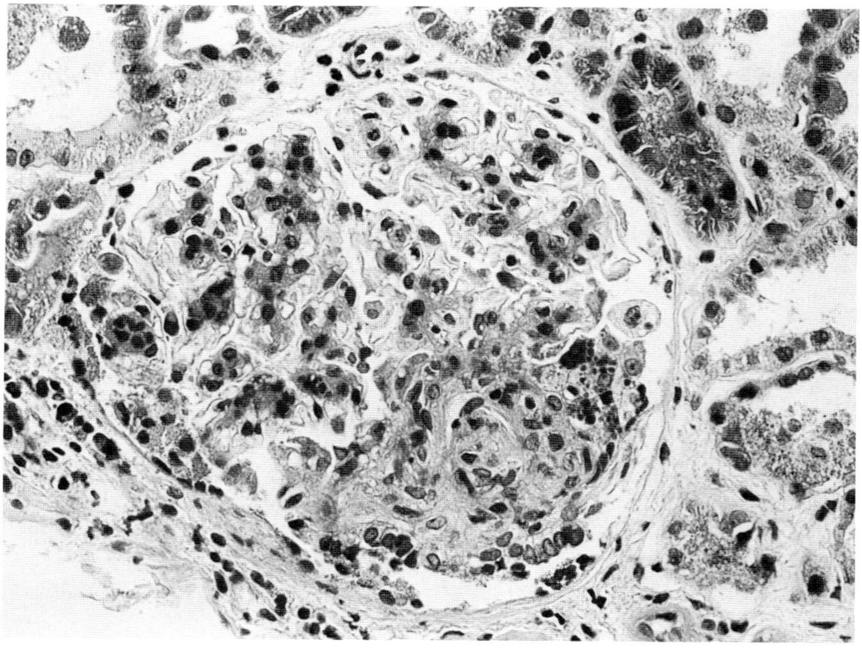

FIG. 9-6. *Generalized mesangial hypercellularity and a segmental area of solidification in IgA nephritis. Crescents were present in over half the glomeruli. H&E; ×325.*

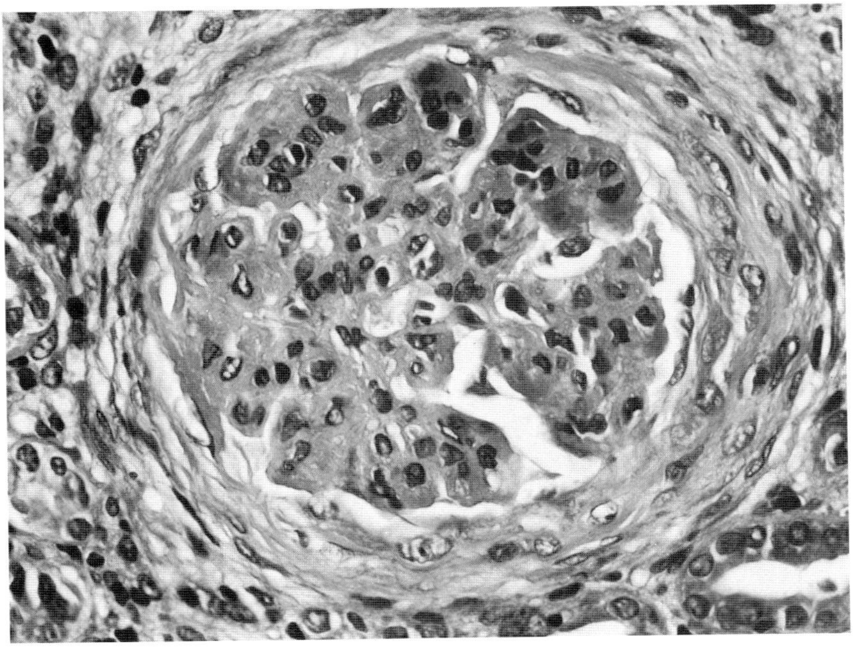

Fig. 9-7. *Glomerulus with fibrosing crescent in association with membranous glomerulonephritis. From same biopsy as in Fig. 9-4. H&E; ×500.*

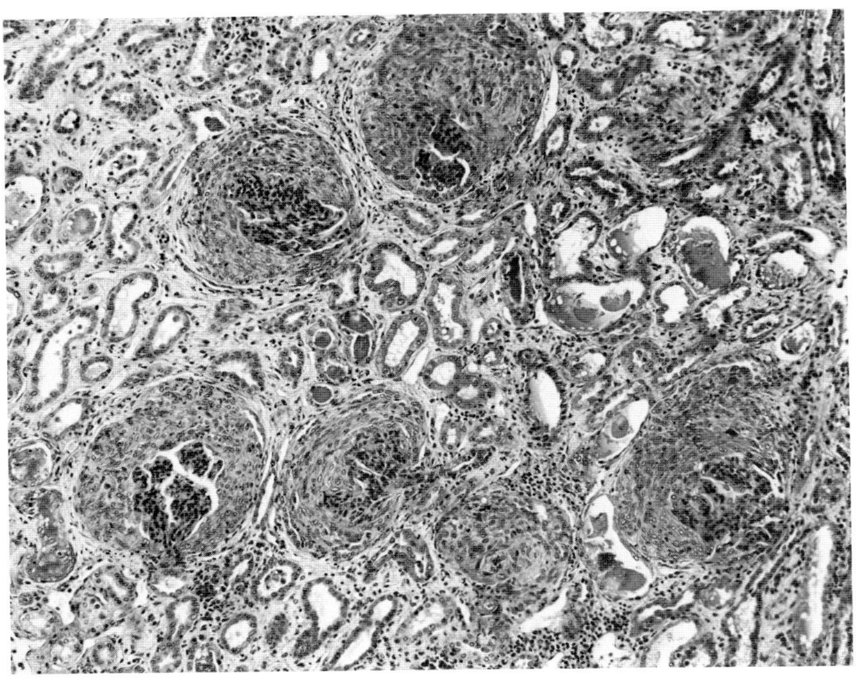

Fig. 9-8. *Extensive exuberant crescents in a 10-year-old child with poststreptococcal glomerulonephritis. The clinical story of this child is recounted in the section entitled Clinical Outcome and Factors Determining Prognosis. H&E; ×100.*

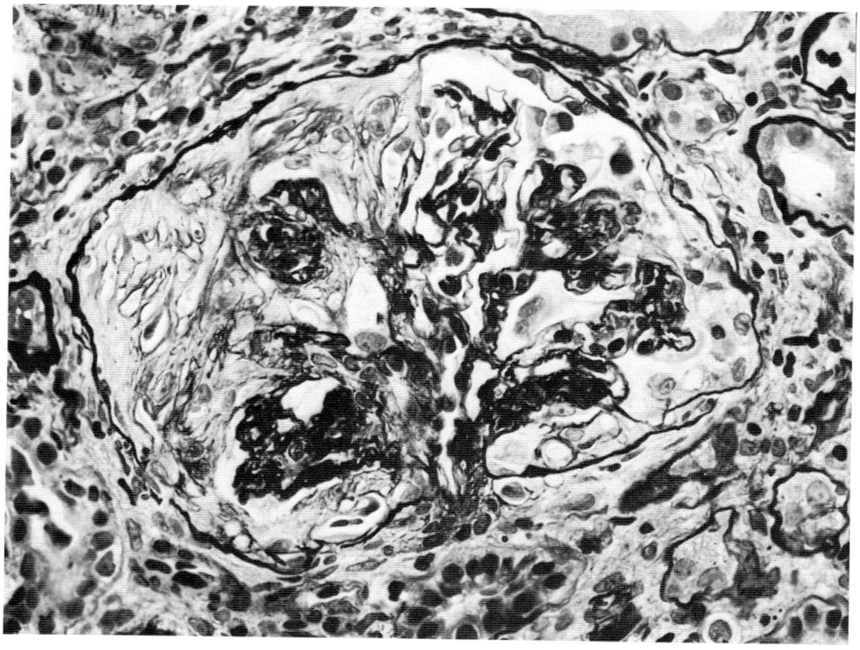

FIG. 9-9. *Crescent undergoing fibrosis in a patient with predominant IgM in generalized mesangial distribution. There is prominence of the mesangium in the glomerular tuft. Silver impregnation;* ×*400.*

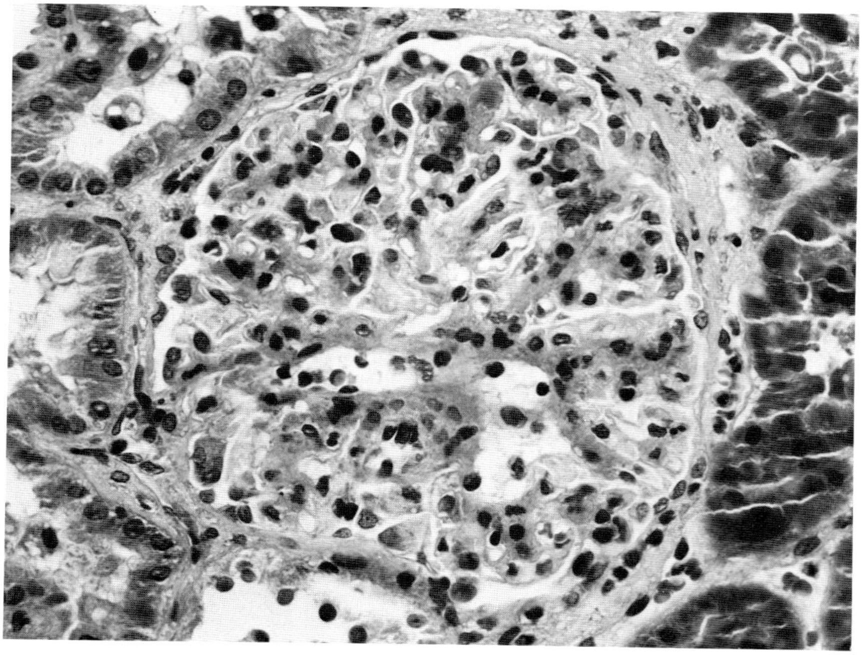

FIG. 9-10. *Diffuse glomerular hypercellularity in a patient from group 2 with no specific, identifiable form of glomerulonephritis. H&E;* ×*450.*

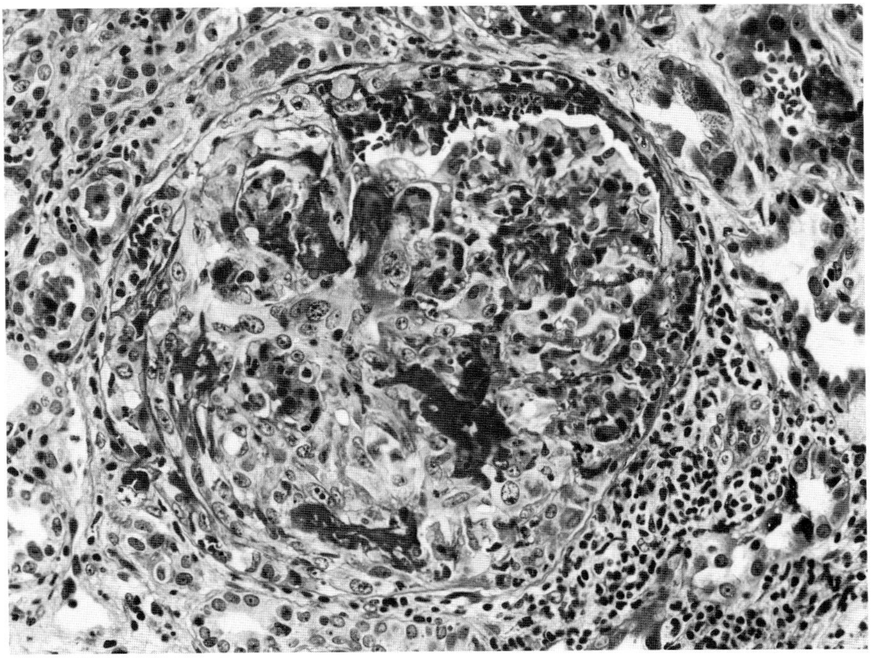

Fig. 9-11. *Glomerulus in anti-GBM antibody disease to show crescent formation, fibrin formation, and necrotizing changes in tuft. H&E; ×350.*

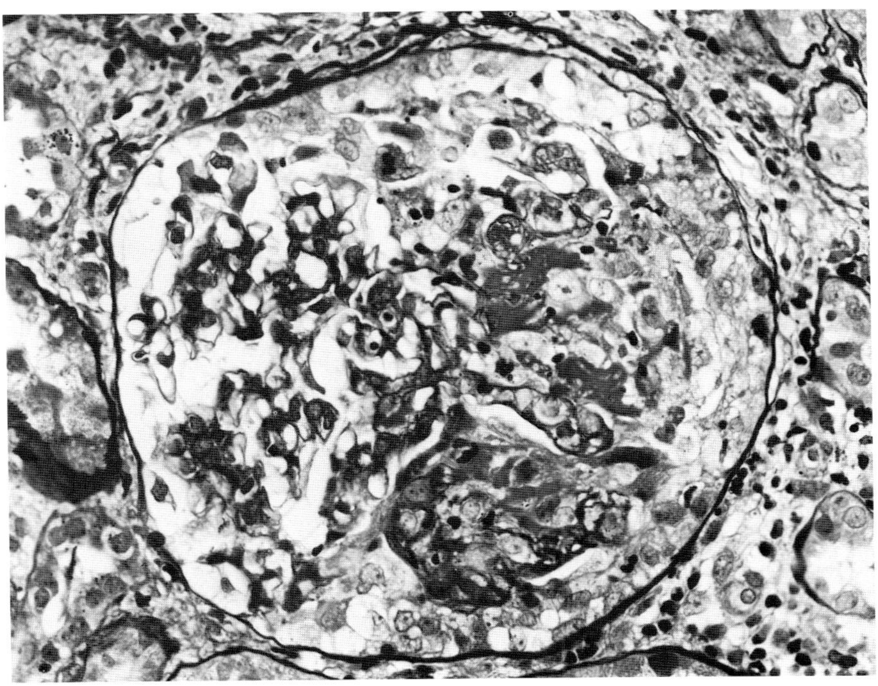

Fig. 9-12. *Glomerulus from a patient with group 3 crescentic glomerulonephritis to show thrombonecrosis in tuft and crescent formation. Periodic acid–methenamine silver; ×400.*

to case within the groups, and all three groups could display a considerable reaction.

Summary of Findings

The extent to which specific conditions contribute is as follows: All four cases in group 1 were examples of anti-GBM antibody disease on the basis of the immunofluorescence pattern and the presence of circulating antibodies. Among the 19 cases initially in group 2, it was possible to identify 2 cases of poststreptococcal glomerulonephritis, 3 of IgA nephritis, 1 of membranous glomerulonephritis, and 1 of IgM nephropathy (nephritis). Three others (cases 7, 8, and 9) had many of the stigmata of IgA nephritis, but 2 were accompanied by equal staining intensity for IgG and the other for IgM. The remaining 9 cases had the features of immune complex disease, but the immunofluorescence and electron microscopic findings—even together with the relevant clinical and laboratory data—were not sufficiently distinctive to allow them to be labeled as specific forms of glomerulonephritis. It should be added that 2 of the 9 had mildly hypercellular tufts, IgG along the glomerular capillary walls, and either intramembranous (case 11) or subepithelial (case 13) electron-dense deposits, but the supporting evidence for a postinfectious etiology is incomplete. Thus, when identifiable forms of glomerulonephritis are excluded, group 2 is reduced to either 12 cases or even to 7 if cases 7, 8, and 9 are accepted as IgA nephritis and cases 11 and 13 are accepted as postinfectious or even membranous glomerulonephritis. Group 3 (15 cases) remains singular in containing none of the specific forms of glomerulonephritis seen in the other two groups. The possibility must remain that some of them are examples of generalized vasculitis in which the biopsy failed to sample an inflamed vessel, but the clinical data gave no support to this.

The study reveals that specific forms of glomerulonephritis can be identified even when complicated by extensive crescent formation. The specific forms recognized are those known to be associated with crescents, but the relatively large number with IgA nephritis was surprising. No instances of membranoproliferative glomerulonephritis were encountered in the series, although, as described in Chapter 7, it is known that crescentic forms do occur.

Removal of the specific forms leaves a set of patients with primary crescentic glomerulonephritis whose numbers and breakdown will depend on the retention or not of group 1 (anti-GBM antibody type). Since this is a specific and identifiable group, I prefer to exclude it. This would mean that we are left with 27 cases, 12 of immune complex pathogenesis and 15 of unknown type. If group 1 is retained under the heading of *primary crescentic glomerulonephritis,* which is presently the convention, the final breakdown is 31 cases, 4 with anti-GBM antibody disease (group 1), 12 with immune complex pathogenesis (group 2), and 15 unknown (group 3).

PRIMARY CRESCENTIC GLOMERULONEPHRITIS

Despite my preference for excluding anti-GBM antibody disease from primary crescentic glomerulonephritis, I shall bow to convention and use the three immunofluorescence groupings in the descriptions that follow. However, since anti-GBM antibody glomerulonephritis is the subject of a separate chapter, I shall bring it into this one only in so far as comparisons with groups 2 and 3 are needed. It also should be noted at this point that the various authorities to be quoted use many different approaches to the topic, and obtaining clinical details that fit neatly into the three groupings is often difficult and sometimes impossible. In particular, some series include specific entities, particularly poststreptococcal glomerulonephritis. For convenience and economy of space, our own series is included in the references under Johns Hopkins Study of Primary Crescentic Glomerulonephritis [72].

Clinical Features

In most series, males are affected more commonly than females [63,96,101,137], and this is particularly true when no attempt is made to break the series down into the three pathogenetic groups.

When this is done, group 1 shows little difference in sex [37,63], except when cases with both pulmonary hemorrhage and glomerulonephritis (Goodpasture's syndrome) are included in the analysis [13,88]; in this instance, males predominated. Group 2 showed more males in one series [37] but more females in another [88], and group 3 had an excess of males [72,88,118], comparable with the situation in polyarteritis nodosa with glomerulonephritis, which resembles it very closely. Primary crescentic glomerulonephritis may occur at all ages, with means of 38 to 55 years being recorded in series including all cases [96,137] and 44 to 58 years when groups 2 and 3 are considered together [13,41,63,101] or singly [37,88,118]. Mean ages of 54 years [88], 53 years [72], and 58 years [37] were found in group 2, and 44 years [88], 58 years [118], and 59 years [72] in group 3. In group 1, the mean ages were from 43 to 68 years [13,37,63,72,101], but when those cases with pulmonary hemorrhage in addition to glomerulonephritis were included, the mean age was lower, 31 years in one study [88] and 33 years in another [13]. Patients in the eighth and ninth decades are cited in all groups, and several series reporting primary crescentic glomerulonephritis in children have been published [5,43,116]. It should be noted that the series in children contain appreciable numbers of cases of poststreptococcal glomerulonephritis.

Many patients present with oliguria or even anuria, and this is responsible for the older names of *acute oliguric* or *acute anuric glomerulonephritis* [4, 16,30,51,61,75,77,100]. Oligoanuria was present in 35 percent [137] and 69 percent [96] of two series without breakdown into groups; in 38 percent [63], 38 percent [88], and 100 percent [101] of patients in group 1; in 54 percent [88] of those in group 2; in 56 percent [118] of those in group 3; and in 27 percent [63] and 62 percent [101] of those in groups 2 and 3 combined. Regardless of the pathogenetic mechanism, this serious manifestation of renal failure occurs with great frequency. Raised serum levels of creatinine or urea nitrogen are common in all three groups, with marginally higher levels in group 1 compared with the other two groups [13,63,88]. Hematuria of the microscopic type, with or without red-cell casts, is present in virtually every case in all series, and gross hematuria is reported in some patients, particularly those in group 1 [101]. Proteinuria is frequently detected and is often in the nephrotic range [13,63,88,96,101,137]. It is present more often in those cases with proliferative changes in the glomerular tuft [96,101] and in group 2 [88], which as will be seen is more likely to have hypercellularity of the tuft than the other two groups. Hypertension may be present from the outset or develop as the disease progresses; it occurs in all three groups [5,13,101,118]. Various general features such as fever, increased ESR, anemia, fatigue, and dyspnea are common to all groups. Of considerable interest is the finding of lung hemorrhage with hemoptysis in all three groups [76], and this aspect will be discussed later in the chapter.

Serum complement levels were reduced in certain patients whose histologic picture revealed tuft hypercellularity [96,101], in 33 percent of patients in group 2 [88], in 17 percent of those in group 3 [88], and in those with poststreptococcal glomerulonephritis which are included in some series [4,43]. There was no reduction in complement levels in either group 1 [13,29,78,88] or in group 3 [118]. Similarly, cryoglobulins have been described in cases of presumed immune complex pathogenesis [3,12,87] but neither in group 1 [29] nor in group 3 [118]. Circulating immune complexes have been described in some patients [12,26] but were absent in group 3 [118]. Fibrin degradation products are sometimes found in the serum [35,36,98] and correlate well with the severity of the glomerular lesion [35].

The presence of antineutrophil cytoplasmic antibodies (ANCA) in the serum has been described [37*a*,48,71*a*,101*a*,134], and they are widely prevalent in group 3, or the pauci-immune group as it is sometimes called. In this group of primary crescentic glomerulonephritis it has been found that P-ANCA (anti-myeloperoxidase) occurs more commonly than C-ANCA (anti–29-kD serine protease) [37*a*,71*a*,101*b*], which is the reverse of the finding in Wegener's syndrome, in which C-ANCA is more common. In contrast, it is exceptional to find ANCA of any type in patients with group 2 (immune complex type) primary crescentic glomerulonephritis [37*a*,71*a*,101*a*]. More is said about ANCA in Chapters 3 and 16.

Pathologic Changes

GROSS APPEARANCE

The kidneys are usually enlarged, with a smooth subcapsular surface. The total renal mass in personally studied cases ranged from 240 to 470 g, with a mean of 360 g. The kidneys are often pale, but some are rather congested, and petechial hemorrhages may occur, as in malignant hypertension. The cortex is normal or expanded in width. This is one of the few conditions in which glomeruli can be seen convincingly; they stand out as gray, translucent dots. The medulla is often dark in contrast to the pale cortex.

MICROSCOPIC FINDINGS

Glomeruli

The most arresting change is the presence of crescents on the inside of Bowman's capsule. These are collections of pale-staining, often clear polygonal cells that commonly tend to be elongated (Figs. 9-13 and 9-14). In particularly large crescents the cytoplasm may have a basophilic tinge. The nuclei in general are vesicular, but some may be hyperchromatic, and mitotic figures are sometimes seen (Fig. 9-15). Crescents vary considerably in size, ranging from small collections of cells that occupy only part of the circumference of Bowman's capsule to enormous aggregations that occupy most of the capsular space. Large crescents may completely obliterate the lumen of the proximal convoluted tubule at its point of origin [31]

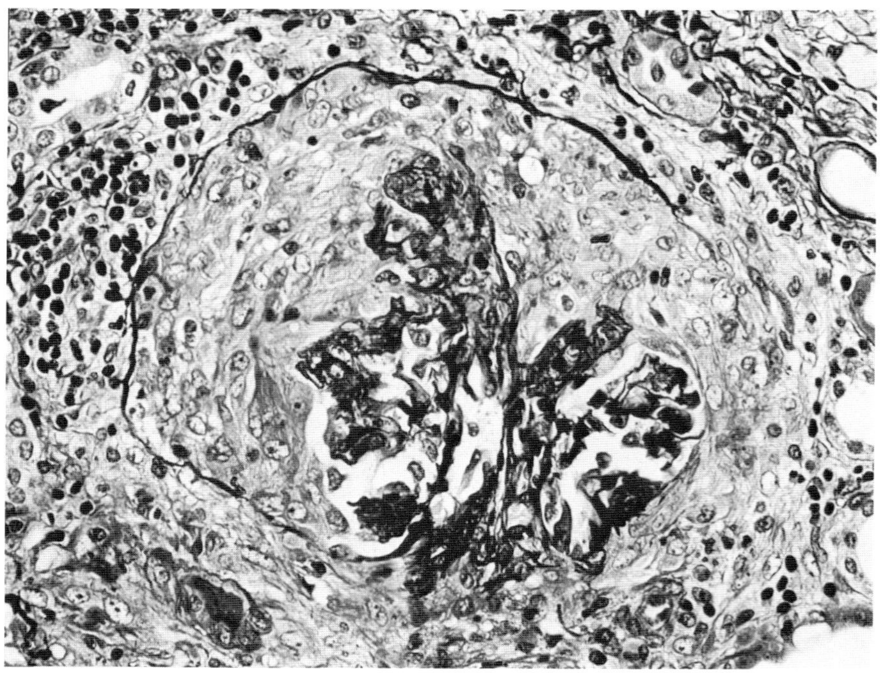

FIG. 9-13. *Large cellular crescent with shrunken tuft in anti-GBM antibody disease. Bowman's capsule is fractured in the lower right-hand corner so that the crescent is in continuity with the interstitium. Periodic acid–methenamine silver;* ×350.

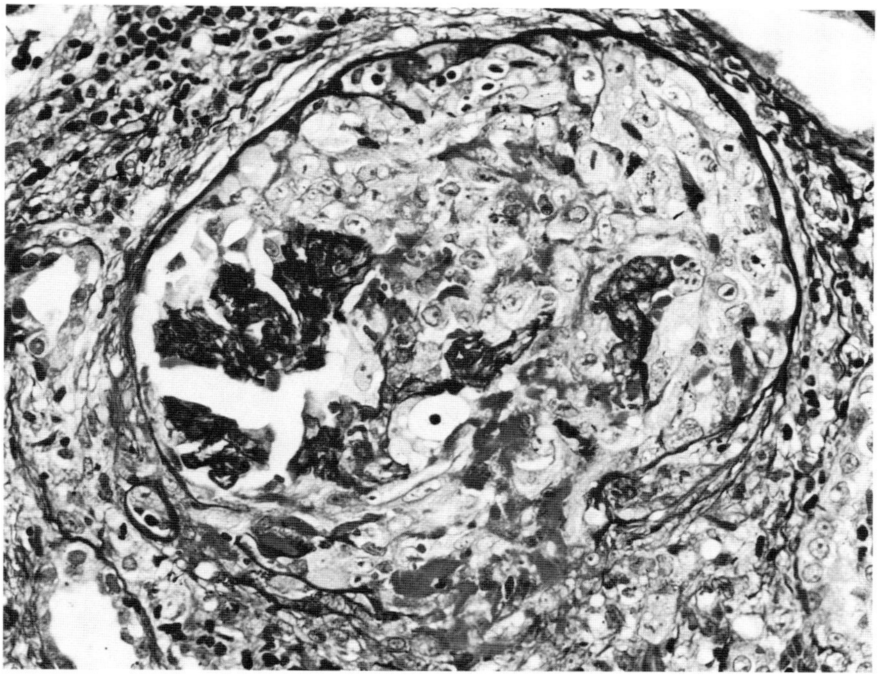

Fig. 9-14. *Crescent made up of large clear cells with considerable attenuation of tuft in a patient with group 3 crescentic glomerulonephritis. Periodic acid–methenamine silver;* ×*325.*

and clearly interfere with urine formation. They are often made up entirely of cells—the *cellular crescent*—whereas others contain connective tissue and are referred to as *fibrocellular crescents* (Fig. 9-16). The latter are almost certainly a later stage of the cellular crescent and are seen with increasing frequency as the duration of the illness increases. A later stage is the *fibrous crescent* (Fig. 9-17), and this is the type seen if the clinical course is long or if life is extended by dialysis. There is good evidence to show that crescents may actually disappear, and Figure 9-18 is from an autopsy on a patient whose biopsy 3 months earlier had shown exuberant crescents in over two-thirds of the glomeruli present. Life had been prolonged by dialysis, and at autopsy there were no cellular crescents and only a few of the fibrosed variety; the great majority of the glomeruli were solidified and devoid of any sort of crescent, as shown in the figure. Evidence for the disappearance of crescents has been provided by others [47,84]. Cellular crescents also may contain monocytes, T cells, red blood cells, and neutrophils, and fibrin can often be demonstrated by conventional techniques and almost invariably by immunofluorescence methods. No more will be said at this stage because a separate section is devoted to these aspects later in the chapter.

The number of crescents required to justify the diagnosis of crescentic glomerulonephritis varies from author to author; some use 30 percent or more of glomeruli showing crescents [37,63], while others use 50 percent or more [88,96,137]. It is important to remember that the number of glomeruli with crescents will vary according to the time at which the kidney is sampled; a very early

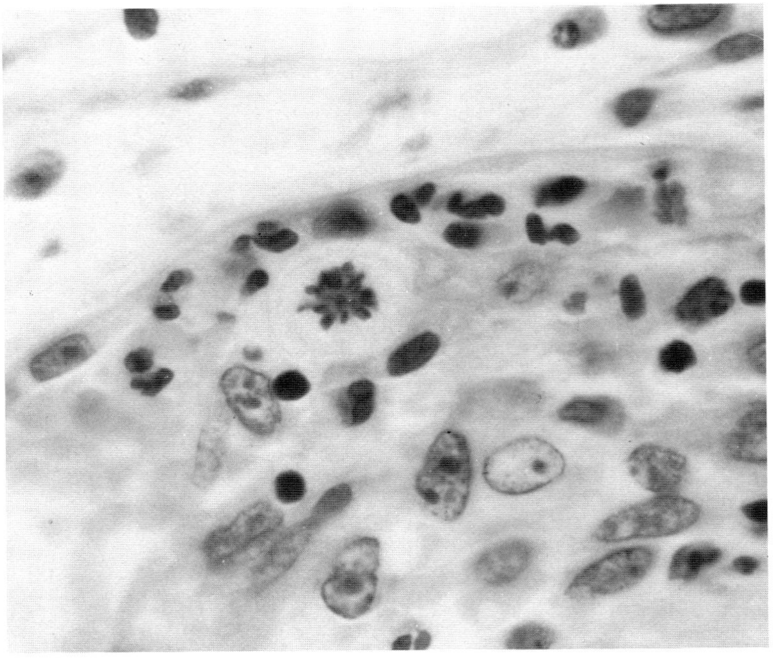

FIG. 9-15. *Mitotic figure in crescent from a patient with crescentic glomerulonephritis of anti-GBM pathogenesis. H&E; ×1700.*

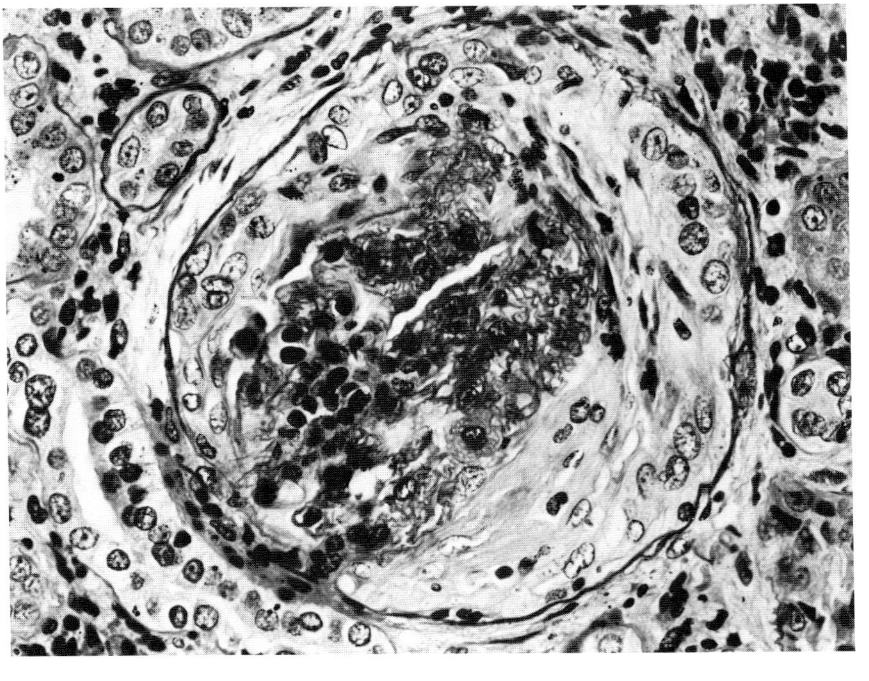

FIG. 9-16. *Group 3 crescentic glomerulonephritis with fibrocellular crescent. Fibrosis is clearly discernible on right-hand side, particularly near the bottom. Tuft is compressed and solidified. Periodic acid–methenamine silver; ×400.*

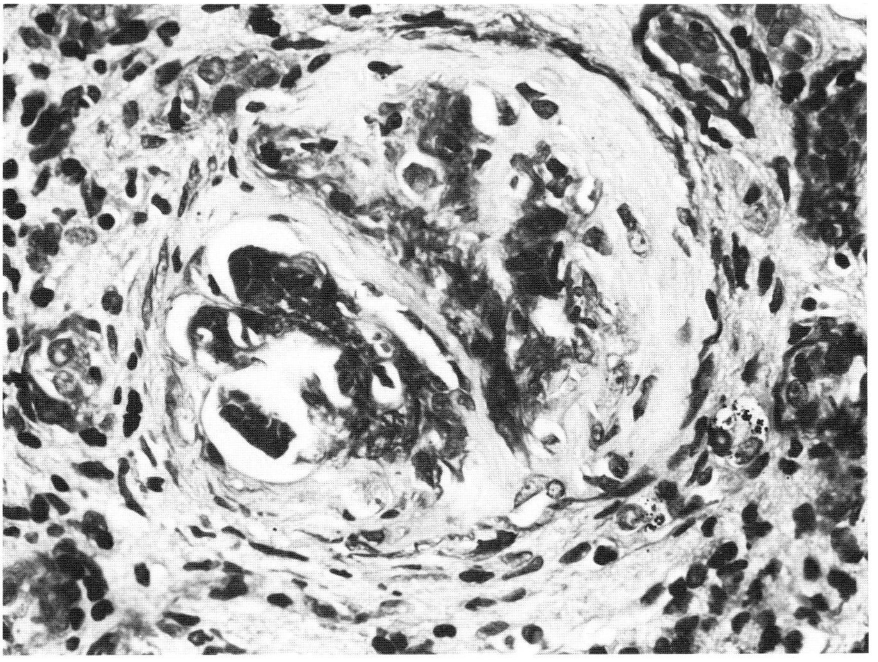

FIG. 9-17. *Glomerulus from another patient with group 3 crescentic glomerulonephritis showing fibrous crescent. The dark-staining tuft is considerably damaged. Periodic acid–methenamine silver; ×500.*

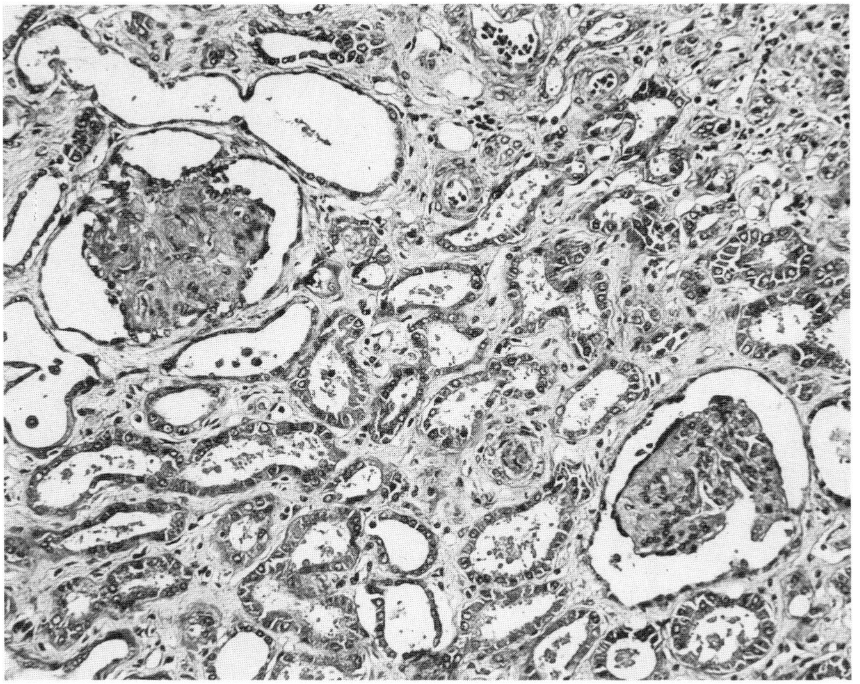

FIG. 9-18. *Severely scarred glomeruli and tubular loss in case referred to in text. No crescents, either fresh or fibrosed, are seen in the two glomeruli illustrated. H&E; ×150.*

biopsy would be expected to show fewer crescents than one performed at a later time when the pathologic process is more fully developed. This is best exemplified by certain cases of anti-GBM antibody pathogenesis [29,103,123], in which a relatively mild focal glomerulonephritis rapidly becomes transformed into a diffuse picture with crescents over a matter of weeks. In general, those cases with the greatest number of crescents have the worst outlook [96,137], particularly when the crescents are very large [116]. This, of course, is not absolute, and even when over 80 percent of glomeruli show crescents, improvement or stabilization of renal function has been reported [137]. More will be said of the various factors determining prognosis under Clinical Outcome and Factors Determining Prognosis.

Crescents, of course, do not occur in isolation and are invariably accompanied by changes in the glomerular tuft. Indeed, it is the changes in the tuft that initiate crescent formation. A common finding is *focal and segmental necrotizing glomerulonephritis,* a condition described in Chapter 4. This is the lesion that predominates in groups 1 and 3. It consists of variable numbers of lobules within the tuft showing fibrinoid necrosis, fibrin thrombi within capillary loops, or areas where capillary walls are disrupted, best seen with silver stains (Figs. 9-11, 9-12, and 9-19). These changes may be accompanied by localized hypercellularity of the tuft, with neutrophils present in some of them. In some instances a single lobule might be affected, whereas in others the entire tuft is involved. Fibrin is commonly seen in the capsular space in relation to these necrotic foci, and localized or more extensive extracapillary cellular proliferation is the common sequel. These areas of extracapillary cellular proliferation are, of course,

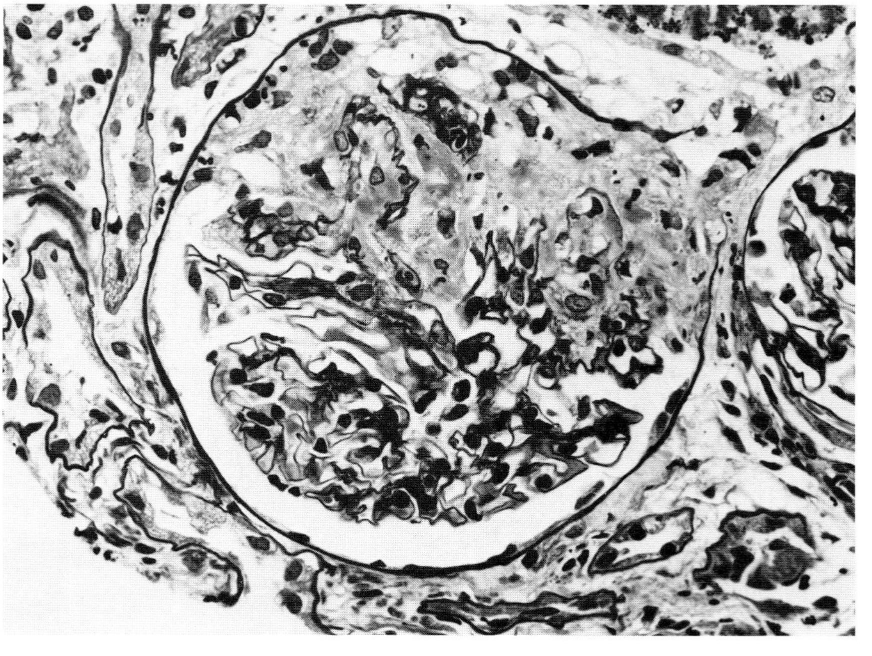

FIG. 9-19. *Glomerulus from group 3 crescentic glomerulonephritis to show discontinuities in capillary wall of tuft and appearance of fibrin-like material in relation to them in capsular space. Periodic acid–methenamine silver;* $\times 400$.

the crescents referred to earlier. Using sections stained with hematoxylin and eosin, it is often difficult to judge whether the hypercellularity is in the tuft or in an extracapillary position, so blurred may the area of demarcation be (Fig. 9-20). A silver impregnation or a periodic acid–Schiff preparation, by staining the capillary walls of the tuft and Bowman's capsule, will often, but not always, resolve this question. Exceptionally, multinucleated giant cells may be seen either in the crescents or in the outer part of the tuft [73,78,104]; their origin is not clear, and they have been regarded as derived from monocytes [73] or epithelial cells [104]. In my own experience, these have been encountered mainly in cases of anti-GBM antibody type (Fig. 9-21). A further change is that of mesangiolysis, best detected by electron microscopy [25], but also diagnosable by light microscopy, especially in the presence of capillary aneurysms [104].

In some patients with primary crescentic glomerulonephritis—most commonly those in group 2—there is a significant hypercellularity of the tuft, commonly called a *proliferative reaction* despite increasing evidence that infiltrating marrow-derived monocytes make a significant contribution to the cellular content. This may take the form of a focal and segmental hypercellular reaction (see Fig. 9-20A), or the hypercellularity may be diffuse and affect the whole tuft (see Fig. 9-10). While hypercellularity is a feature of group 2 cases when various specific forms of glomerulonephritis are included, it is also commonly present when they are excluded [72]. These hypercellular forms, particularly the focal and segmental type, may be accompanied by necrotizing changes in the tuft, but regardless of this, they may be associated with large numbers of crescents. Probably the best example of crescent formation in the absence of overt tuft necroses is poststreptococcal glomerulonephritis, about which more will be said later. We also noted a paucity of necrotizing changes in the tufts in cases of IgA nephritis with crescents [72].

In many cases there are more chronic lesions in the glomeruli, such as segmental or total sclerosis of the tuft, and a greater proportion of fibrous crescents (Fig. 9-22). Sclerosis of the tuft is more likely to occur in those cases with a slower tempo [10] or in those whose life has been prolonged by dialysis, but it may be seen in some of the more florid cases even at an apparently early stage [9,13,137]. A further change of note is the occurrence of ruptures of Bowman's capsule through which crescents are in continuity with the interstitium (see Fig. 9-13). Such ruptures are clearly of importance in the genesis and organization of crescents, as will be described later. Rarely, the breaks in Bowman's capsule are accompanied by granuloma formation, a situation referred to as *granulomatous glomerulonephritis.* In my own experience, granulomatous glomerulonephritis is more or less confined to group 1 patients when found in the setting of primary crescentic glomerulonephritis. It was noteworthy that it was not present in any of the 15 patients in group 3 in our series [72]. This was surprising in view of the many similarities of this group to polyarteritis with glomerulonephritis, in which granulomatous glomerular involvement is not uncommon (see Chap. 16). Since granulomatous glomerulonephritis is seen most often in Wegener's syndrome and in the form of glomerulonephritis accompanying polyarteritis nodosa, it is described in Chapter 16.

Before closing this section on the glomerulus, mention should be made of the cells contributing to the proliferative lesions in the tuft. Clearly, many of these are indigenous to the tuft, and mesangial cells make up most of them. On the other hand, there is now considerable evidence to show that mononuclear cells of bone marrow origin and T-lymphocytes make a significant contribution, thus belying the term *proliferative.* Monocytes have been demonstrated using nonspecific esterase as a histochemical marker [49,83] and by immunohistologic methods using monoclonal antibodies [22,102,117]. This observation supports the idea of a cell-mediated immunologic mechanism in some forms of crescentic glomerulonephritis. In two of these studies [22,117], monocytes and T cells were found in the glomerular tuft in all three pathogenetic groups of primary crescentic glomerulonephritis. In one study [22], there were differences in phenotypes, but they were insufficient to enable distinctions to be made among the three pathogenetic groups. More will be said of mono-

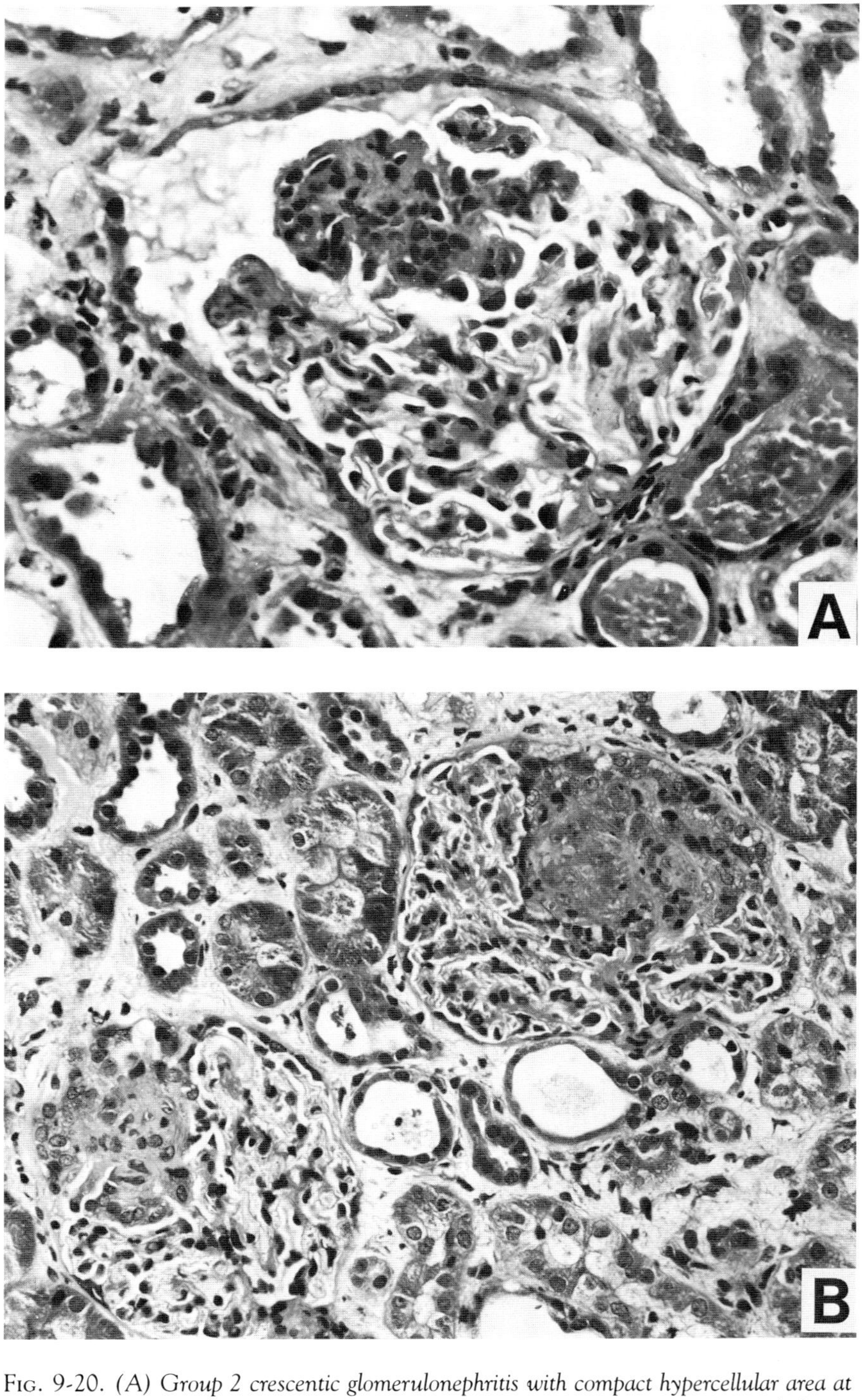

FIG. 9-20. (A) Group 2 crescentic glomerulonephritis with compact hypercellular area at top suggestive of lobular hyperplasia of the tuft. H&E; ×400. (B) Two glomeruli from a case of group 3 crescentic glomerulonephritis showing large hypercellular solid areas between tuft and Bowman's capsule suggestive of an extracapillary lesion. H&E; ×250. Both (A) and (B) illustrate the limitations of H&E staining in determining the precise location of hypercellular lesions.

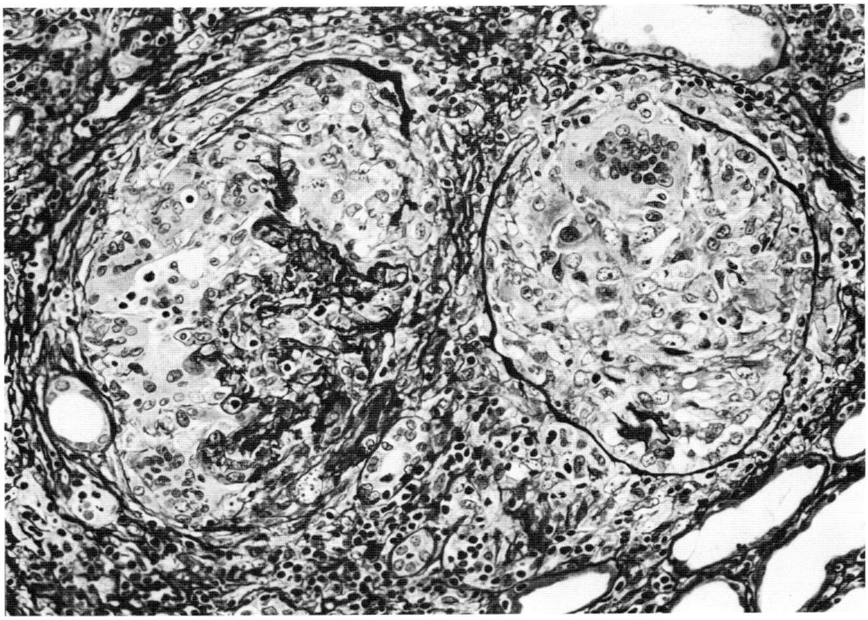

Fig. 9-21. *Multinucleated giant cells are present in these two large crescents. Anti-GBM antibody disease. Periodic acid–methenamine silver;* ×*240.*

cytes and lymphocytes under Etiology and Pathogenesis.

Tubules

Patchy tubular atrophy or loss is common and in some cases may be considerable. Hyalin droplet change is often a conspicuous feature in the tubules, and proliferative activity in the epithelium of the proximal convoluted tubules is sometimes seen and may be accompanied by mitoses [54]. Casts, red blood cells, neutrophils, and fibrin are commonly found in the tubular lumens. Necrosis of the tubular epithelium with damage to the basement membrane may be present [16], and this is particularly likely in the those cases in group 1 in which antitubular basement membrane antibody is present [6].

Interstitium

The interstitium usually contains chronic inflammatory cells, which in some cases are very plentiful and amount to a veritable interstitial nephritis (Fig. 9-23). The cells are usually mononuclear cells and lymphocytes with various admixtures of plasma cells. They may be arranged around the periphery of tubules or around Bowman's capsule. In particular, large numbers of cells may surround sclerotic glomeruli. Large numbers of T-lymphocytes have been identified in the interstitium using immunohistologic techniques [22,117]. In situations where there are breaks in Bowman's capsule, there may be continuity between the interstitial cellular reaction and crescents, and giant cells may be present as part of the interstitial exudate [73,104]. Giant cells are particularly likely in those cases with a granulomatous glomerular reaction. Edema is common, and fibrosis takes place as tubules disappear. The importance of the extent of interstitial fibrosis with regard to clinical outcome has been emphasized [119].

Blood Vessels

Since many of the patients are in the upper age group, it is not uncommon to see aging or hyper-

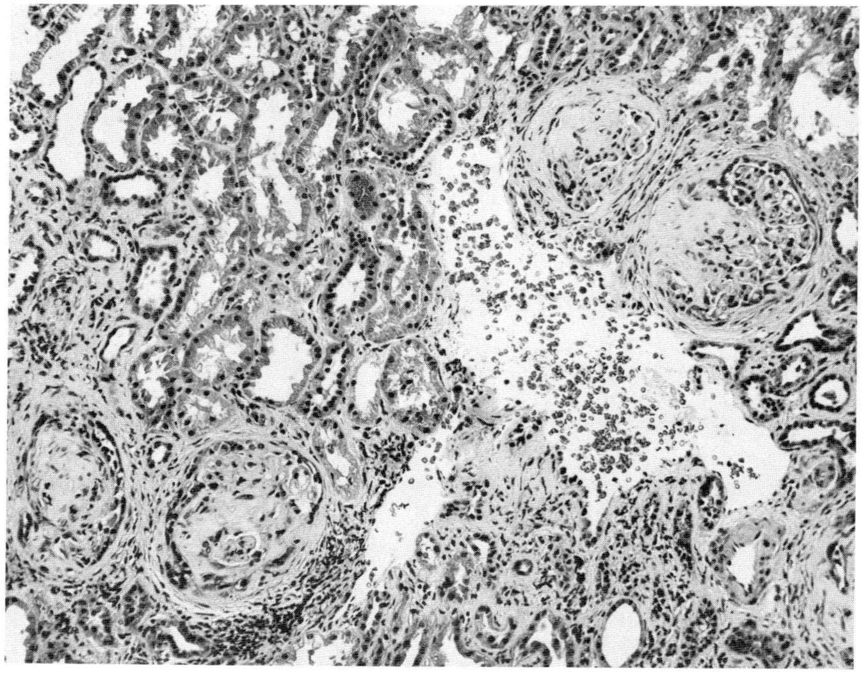

FIG. 9-22. *Section from a renal biopsy of a 33-year-old woman with severe oliguric form of glomerulonephritis. Glomeruli show considerable scarring that involves all or part of the tuft. H&E; ×125.*

tensive changes in arterioles (hyalinization) and arteries (intimal thickening). Actual arteritis is uncommon because, by definition, this would take the case out of the primary glomerulonephritis category. However, arteritis of small vessels may be seen in occasional patients of group 1 (anti-GBM antibody disease) [54,78,140] and in a small number of patients with poststreptococcal crescentic glomerulonephritis [71] when these cases are included in group 2, as they are in some series. Figure 9-24 demonstrates acute arteritis in a patient with poststreptococcal crescentic glomerulonephritis.

ELECTRON MICROSCOPIC FINDINGS

In patients with granular deposits by immunofluorescence (group 2), electron-dense deposits also may be present. These may be epimembranous [13,21,7,88,115], intramembranous [13,21,88], subendothelial [13,88,96], and mesangial [37,88,116]. In patients in groups 1 and 3, there are no deposits as a rule [13,14,29,52,72,73,88,117]. When poststreptococcal cases are deliberately included in group 2, there are epimembranous deposits [108, 111,116], which may be of the usual hump type or flatter and more extensive (Figs. 9-25 and 9-26). They may sometimes assume an intramembranous position. In the various series quoted, it is not possible to determine how assiduous the authors were in excluding specific forms of immune complex glomerulonephritis, and the findings quoted may well represent the intrusion of such cases. So far as our own study [72] was concerned, group 2 showed both capillary wall and mesangial deposits even when specific forms of glomerulonephritis known to assume crescentic forms were excluded (see Table 9-4).

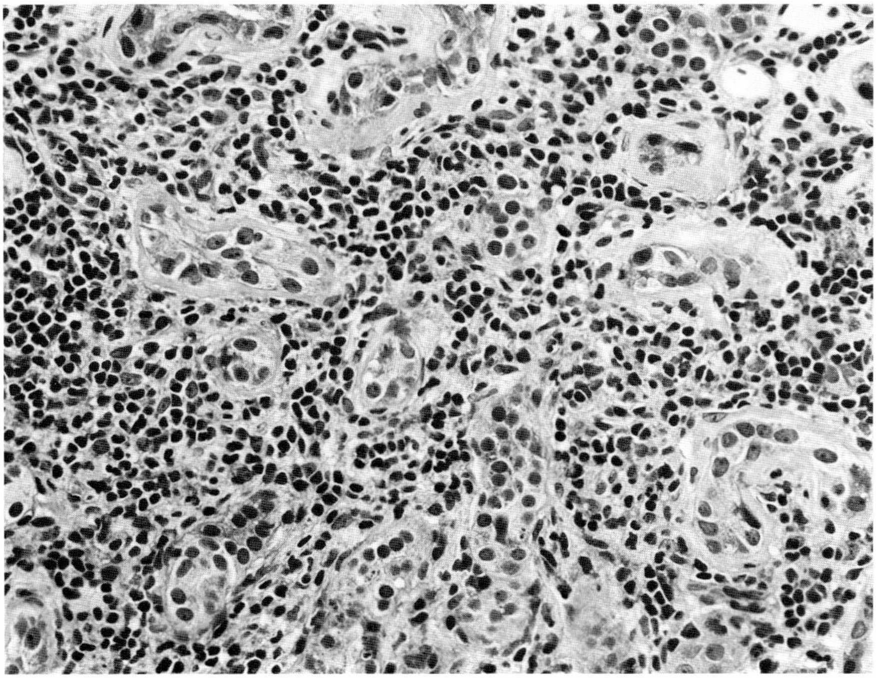

Fig. 9-23. *Extensive interstitial cellular infiltrate and tubular atrophy from a case of group 3 crescentic glomerulonephritis. H&E; ×250.*

Regardless of the presence or absence of deposits, there are certain changes common to all three groups [9,14,21,25,88,95,96,115,122]. Collapse and wrinkling of the capillary wall are frequently observed, and these are accompanied by a dense staining of the wall. Necrosis of cells in the tuft, intracapillary and extracapillary fibrin deposition, focal fusion of foot processes, mesangiolysis, and actual ruptures of the glomerular capillary walls are commonly described (Fig. 9-27). The last change is one mentioned by most authors and may be of importance in the development of crescents [25,90], a topic that will be taken up later. Bonsib [24] has described a technique in which scanning electron microscopy is utilized following selective removal of the podocytes. This permits a dramatic three-dimensional visualization of the breaches in the capillary wall (Fig. 9-28).

Increased numbers of cells are described, and it is of note that proliferation of visceral epithelial cells is recorded [21,90] with the likelihood that they contribute to the crescent. Basement-membrane–like material (mesangial matrix) is increased in glomeruli with sclerotic changes by light microscopy, and fine collagen fibers may make their appearance [13]. In virtually all accounts, the presence of fibrin is recorded in the capsular space or in relation to crescents (Fig. 9-29). Features of the crescents themselves are described in a separate section.

IMMUNOFLUORESCENCE FINDINGS

As described earlier, the immunofluorescence findings in primary crescentic glomerulonephritis fall into three main groups. These will be described in order.

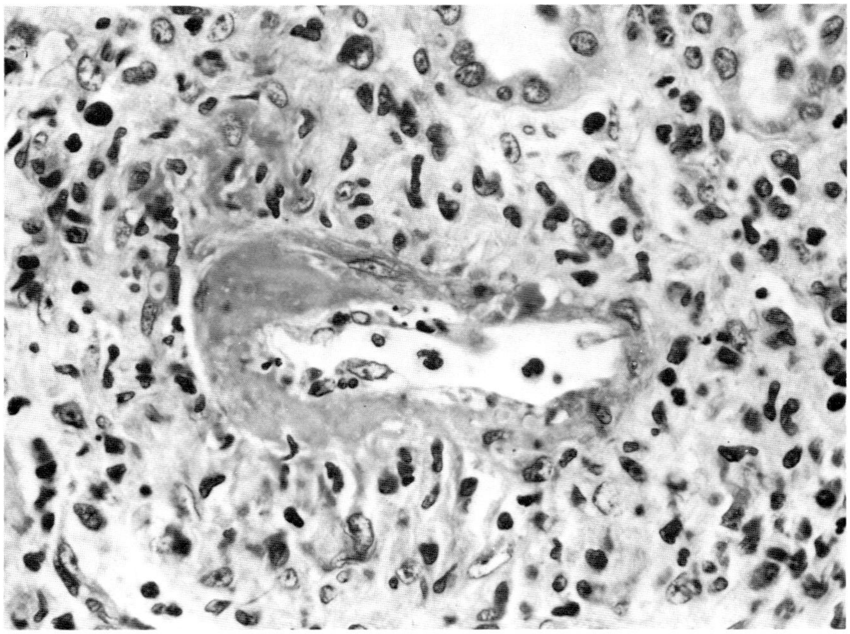

FIG. 9-24. *Arteritis in a small vessel from a 10-year-old girl with crescentic glomerulonephritis of poststreptococcal etiology. Arterial wall shows fibrinoid changes with accompanying cellular inflammatory reaction. H&E; ×500.*

Group 1

In this group there is linear fluorescence for IgG (see Fig. 9-1), usually accompanied by C3 in either a linear or granular pattern. It represents anti-GBM antibody disease, and since this is described separately in Chapter 10, all that will be done at this stage is to quote the frequency with which this group occurs in the larger series of primary crescentic glomerulonephritis. In six series [13,37,63,88,101,137] totaling 171 patients in whom immunofluorescence studies were performed, this pattern was encountered in 66 (39 percent). However, one of these series [13] differed from all the others in containing an unduly large number of patients with linear immunofluorescence (29 of 40). When this series is excluded from the calculation, it is found that anti-GBM antibody disease accounted for 37 of 131 patients (28 percent). It is therefore a significant contributor to the total group in these series, although in our own series [72] there were only 4 cases out of 31 (13 percent).

Group 2

A granular pattern for immunoglobulins and complement along the capillary walls or in the mesangium is commonly described [13,15,37,55,63, 88,94,96,101,105,115,137]. IgG is the most frequently found immunoglobulin (Fig. 9-30), but IgM and IgA also may be present. In some cases C3 is found without immunoglobulins [43,88,94, 137], and in others IgA is the predominant immunoglobulin [37,88,96,137]. A granular pattern for immunoglobulins and complement along glomerular capillary walls is particularly prominent in series involving children [5,31,43,111,116,129], largely because of the inclusion of poststreptococcal glomerulonephritis, which is still apparently a potent cause of crescentic glomerulonephritis in the young (Fig. 9-31). Doubtless other conditions,

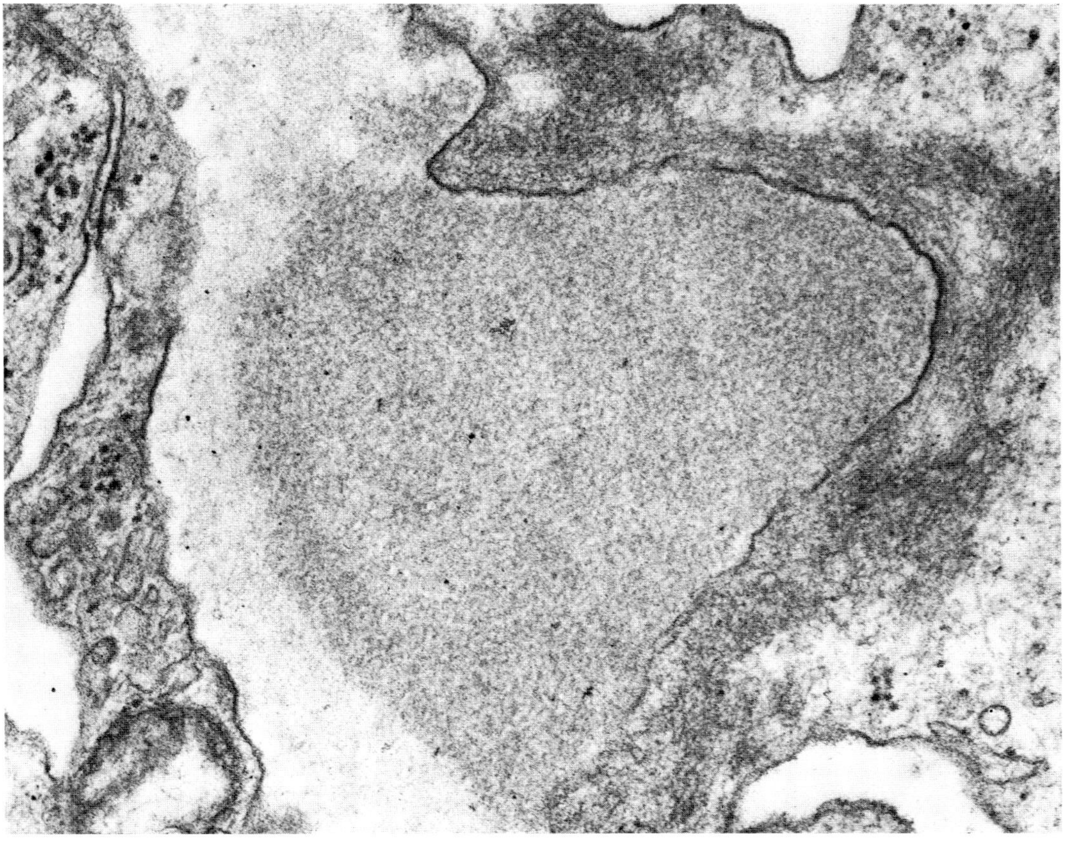

Fig. 9-25. *Typical hump of electron-dense material on epithelial side of glomerular capillary from a patient with crescentic poststreptococcal glomerulonephritis.* ×70,000. *(Courtesy of Dr. George Bannayan.)*

particularly IgA nephritis, are included in many series.

In many studies it is difficult to determine the contribution of group 2 to the general pool of primary crescentic glomerulonephritis. When the relatively few series that permit this evaluation are examined, it accounts for 33 percent [101], 39 percent [137], 48 percent [88], and 65 percent [37]. Even in these few series I encountered difficulty in assigning cases to the correct groups, and others may come to different conclusions. The only series that I can truly vouch for is our own [72], and in this, group 2 accounted for 12 of 31 cases (39 percent) when specific, identifiable forms of immune complex glomerulonephritis were excluded.

Group 3

This third group shows either negative glomerular immunofluorescence or only trivial, faintly staining, patchy collections of immunoglobulins or complement [13,52,63,88,93,101,105,118,134*a*,137, 138*a*]. Stilmant et al. [118] identified 16 patients with the group 3 pattern out of 46 with crescentic glomerulonephritis of various forms, including SLE, IgA nephritis, membranoproliferative glomerulonephritis, anti-GMB antibody disease, and

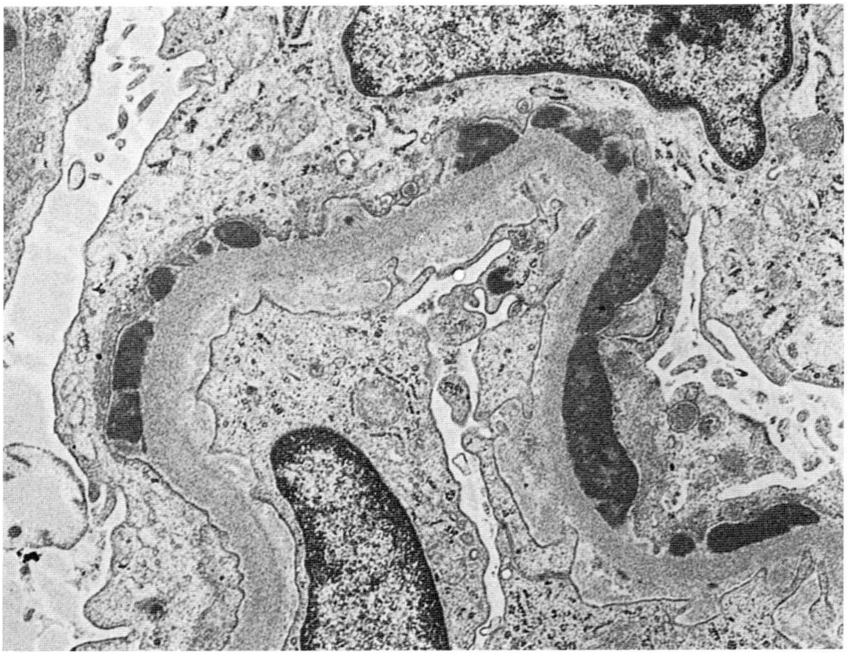

FIG. 9-26. *Extensive, flat, electron-dense deposits on epithelial side of glomerular capillary wall from a 10-year-old girl with crescentic glomerulonephritis of poststreptococcal type.* $\times 13,760$. *(Courtesy of Dr. E. Rappaport.)*

so on. In three other series of apparent primary crescentic glomerulonephritis, the group 3 pattern was found in 22 percent [88], 45 percent [137], and 47 percent [101] of cases in so far as they could be identified from the details supplied. In our own series of the primary crescentic form, 48 percent of cases were of this type [72].

The pathogenesis of group 3 is not known, but a cell-mediated type of immunity [85] and a pathogenic role for ANCA [71*a*] have been considered. As will be seen in Chapter 16, an identical histologic and immunofluorescence picture is seen in the glomerulonephritis that accompanies both polyarteritis and Wegener's syndrome. Since renal biopsies in both conditions often fail to reveal the underlying arteritis, it may be impossible to distinguish them from primary crescentic glomerulonephritis.

In addition to these immunofluorescence changes in the glomerular tuft, there is positive staining with antibody against fibrin/fibrinogen in the crescents in all three groups of primary crescentic glomerulonephritis (Fig. 9-32). Fibrin/fibrinogen is also demonstrable in the areas of thrombosis or necrosis in the glomerular tufts.

Formation of Crescents

Until comparatively recently, it had been considered that the crescents arose from the cells lining Bowman's capsule, with an added possibility that the visceral epithelial cells made a contribution. So strong was this belief that the term *epithelial crescent* was commonly used. Early ideas were developed from light microscopy, but better definition of cell types became possible with the intro-

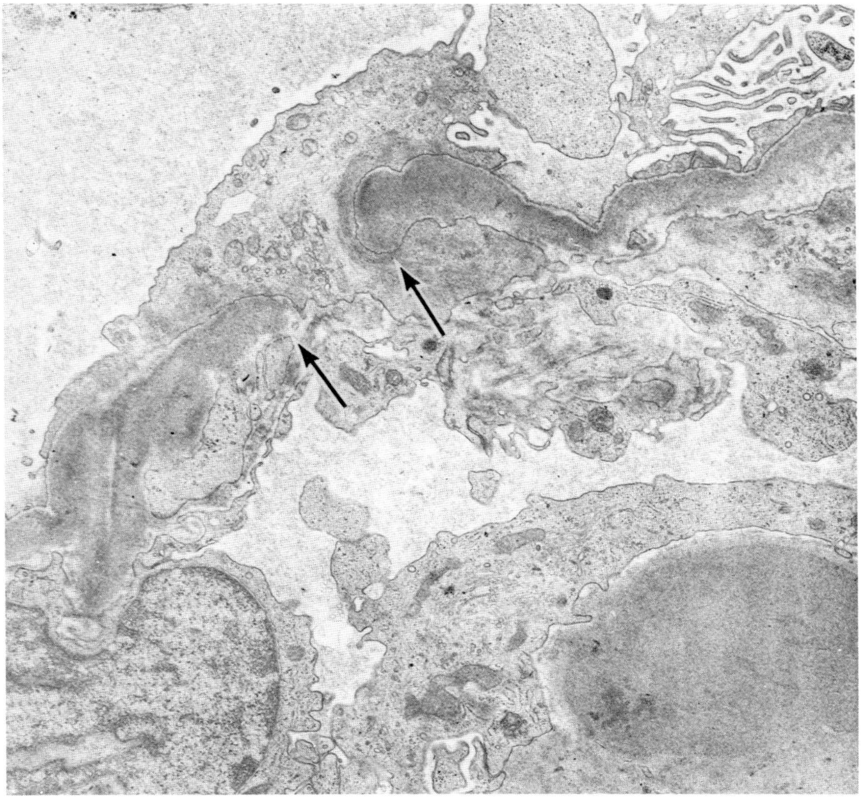

Fig. 9-27. *Electron micrograph to show break (arrow) in continuity of* GBM *in a patient with crescentic glomerulonephritis. Break is filled by cytoplasm of an epithelial cell. ×7100. (From Churg, J., Morita, T., and Suzuki, Y. In P. Kincaid-Smith, T. H. Mathew, and E. L. Becker (Eds.),* Glomerulonephritis: Morphology, Natural History, and Treatment. *New York: Wiley, 1973; used by permission.)*

duction of electron microscopy. Bacani et al. [9] regarded hyperplasia of both parietal and visceral epithelial cells as the origin of the crescent. This view was shared by others [21,90,95]. Morita et al. [95] described light and dark cells which they felt could arise from hyperplasia of both parietal and visceral cells. They also described the phagocytic nature of some of the crescentic cells, and although favoring epithelial cells as the main cellular constituent of the crescent, they were unable to exclude participation of wandering macrophages. Bohman et al. [21] observed a continuous spectrum of cell ultrastructure in the crescent and considered that both parietal and visceral epithelial cells were capable of transformation into the various cell types present. They, too, were careful to state that they could not exclude the participation of such cells as monocytes or fibroblasts.

Other evidence for an epithelial-cell origin of crescents is provided by the following observations: First, cells were seen in crescents that possessed certain characteristics of visceral epithelial cells, such as the presence of secretory bodies in the enlarged cisternae of the rough endoplasmic

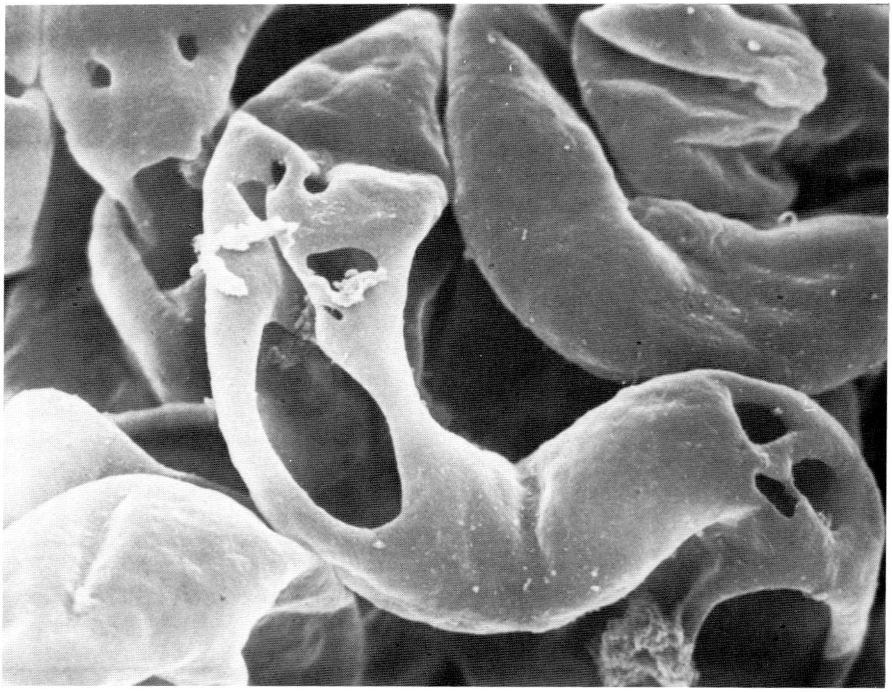

FIG. 9-28. *Scanning electron micrograph of focal necrotizing glomerulonephritis of nonimmune complex type after digestion of cellular elements. A large gap and several smaller ones are present in the capillary wall. From Bonsib, S. M.* Am. J. Pathol. *119:* 357, *1985, by permission of J. B. Lippincott.*

reticulum and the ability to produce basement membrane [53]. Second, no C3b receptors were found in proliferating crescentic cells, an observation interpreted to support the derivation of crescents from parietal epithelial cells [92]. It was pointed out, however, that the possibility of blockade of receptors by amounts of C3 not detectable by immunofluorescence could not be excluded. Third, experimental studies in the rabbit have supported the epithelial origin of crescents [34]. Fourth, studies on human crescents using immunohistologic techniques and monoclonal antibodies have demonstrated cytokeratin [62,81,141] and vimentin [141] in the crescentic cells. The first of these intermediate filaments is a constituent of parietal epithelial cells, and the second, of visceral epithelium.

In contrast to these observations, claims have been made that invading mononuclear cells are a major constituent of crescents. Kondo et al. [74] produced glomerulonephritis in rabbits by injecting duck nephrotoxic serum and observed the accumulation of clear monocytic cells in the glomerular tufts. Destructive changes ensued in the glomerular basement membranes, with migration of the monocytic cells through the ruptured membranes into the capsular space, accompanied by proliferation of epithelial cells at the damaged sites. These infiltrating clear monocytic cells were considered to be the principal constituent of the crescent, with proliferating epithelial cells also making a contribution. Cattell and Arlidge [33] also have shown in a nephrotoxic nephritis model in the rabbit that most dividing cells in glomeruli

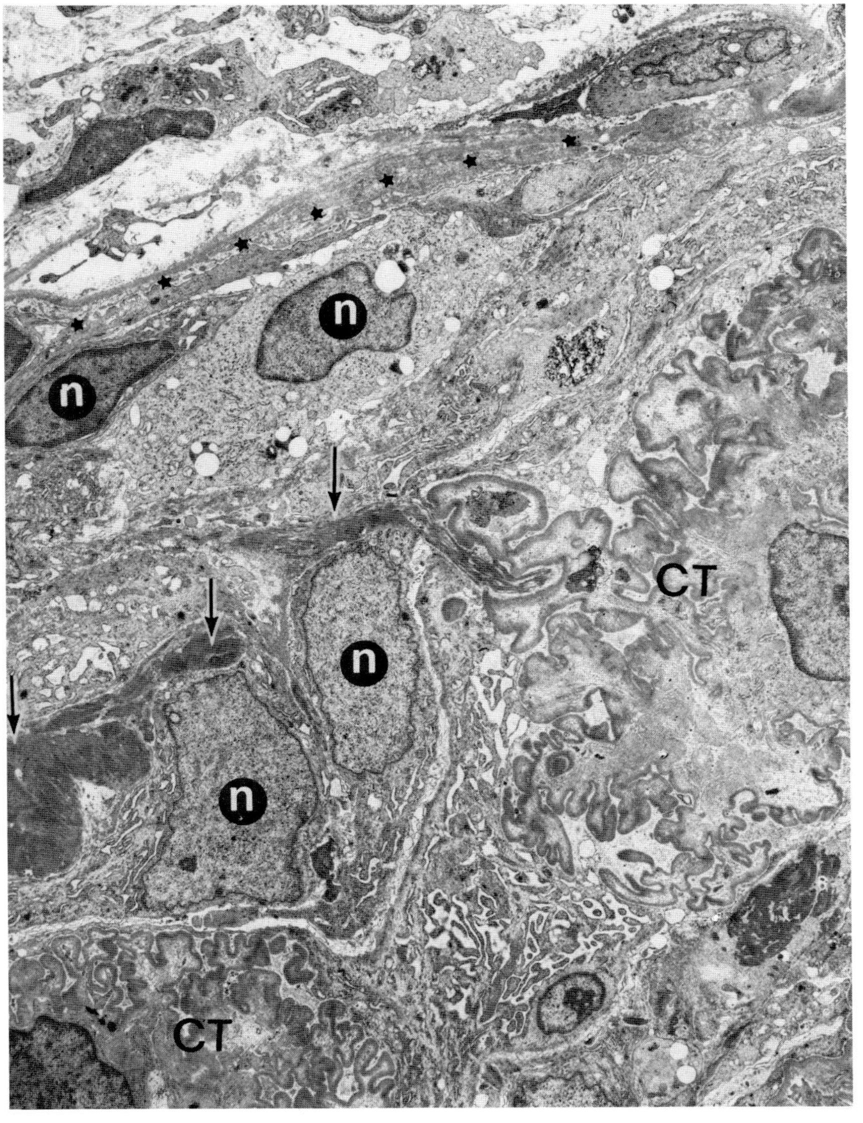

Fig. 9-29. *Electron micrograph to show fibrin (arrow) in cellular crescent from a patient with rapidly progressive glomerulonephritis. Bowman's capsule is marked by small stars. The nuclei of cells making up the crescents are labeled n. The collapsed and damaged capillary tuft is marked CT. ×3000. (Courtesy of Dr. T. Antonovych and the Director of the Armed Forces Institute of Pathology.)*

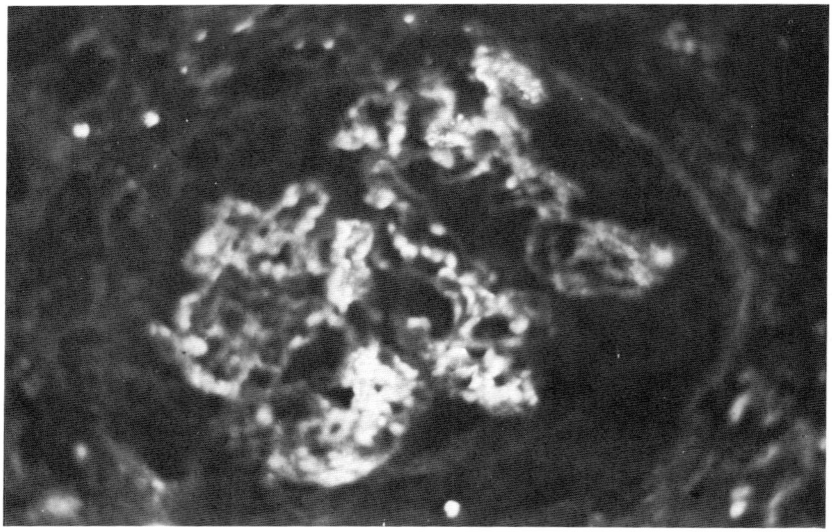

FIG. 9-30. *Granular immunofluorescence pattern along capillary walls for IgG in a case of group 2 crescentic glomerulonephritis of nonspecific type.*

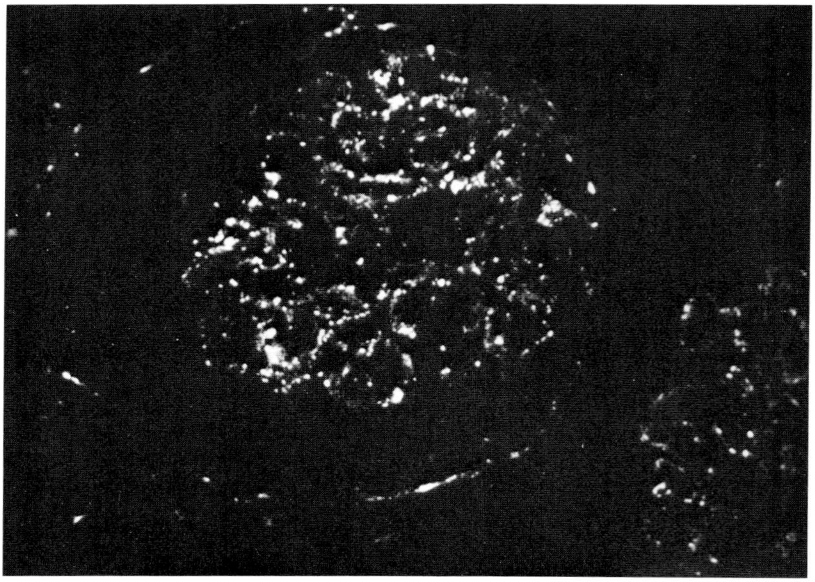

FIG. 9-31. *Fine granular fluorescence for C3 along glomerular capillary loops from a patient with crescentic glomerulonephritis of poststreptococcal type. (Courtesy of Dr. George Bannayan.)*

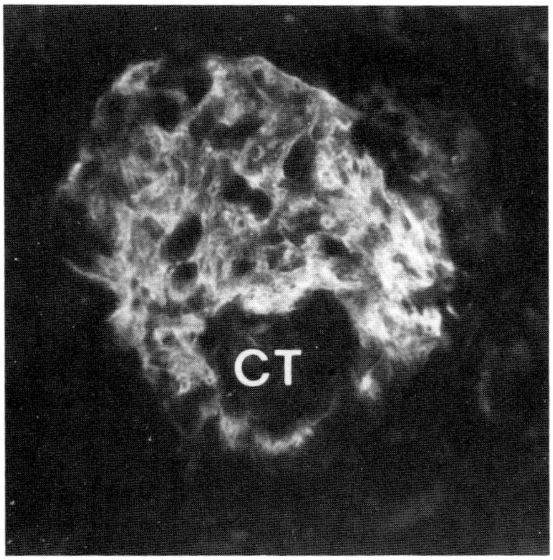

Fig. 9-32. *Glomerulus with large crescent stained with antifibrinogen antiserum. There is much positive fluorescence in the crescent, which occupies most of Bowman's space. The capillary tuft (CT) is collapsed and shows no fluorescence. (Courtesy of Dr. Heinz Bauer.)*

and Bowman's space are monocytes. They considered that these cells contribute significantly to crescents. Tissue-culture studies both in man [7,8] and in sheep and rabbits with experimentally induced glomerulonephritis [67] have supported the role of infiltrating mononuclear cells in crescent formation and have suggested that crescents consist of accumulated macrophages (monocytes) rather than proliferating epithelial cells. Monocytes have been demonstrated in human crescents using either histochemical [49] or immunohistologic methods [22,60,117]. Both T- and B-lymphocytes also were present in one of these studies [22]. Another study using histochemical markers and electron microscopy [82] revealed that monocytes and epithelial cells contributed to crescent formation in anti-GBM disease in contrast to a mainly epithelial constitution in immune complex–mediated crescentic glomerulonephritis. The participation of monocytes in crescent formation was found to be related to breaks in Bowman's capsule [27], whereas monocytes and T-lymphocytes predominated when there were breaks; epithelial cells were the principal constituent when the capsule was intact. An increasingly strong case is therefore being made for the role of circulating mononuclear cells in crescent formation.

The stimulus for crescent formation is thought to be the presence of fibrin in the capsular space, and both immunofluorescence techniques and electron microscopy have consistently revealed the presence of fibrinogen/fibrin in relation to the crescent in renal biopsy material. The early experimental work of Vassalli and McCluskey [130] gave considerable impetus, when it was shown that dicoumarol reduced the number of crescents in nephrotoxic serum nephritis in the rabbit. This was supported by experiments utilizing ancrod, a defibrinating agent obtained from the venom of the Malayan pit viper. When this substance was used in the rabbit, in both an anti-GBM antibody model [99] and an immune complex model [126], there was a considerable reduction in the number of crescents produced. This reduction was noted even when administration of ancrod was delayed until well into the course of the disease [125].

As noted earlier when dealing with electron microscopic appearances, the presence of fractures of the glomerular capillary basement membrane is a very common finding, and Min et al. [90] have suggested the following sequence. The inflammatory process in the glomerular tuft causes fractures of the capillary basement membrane through which intravascular contents escape with precipitation of fibrin in the capsular space. Proliferation of both visceral and parietal epithelium ensues with the initiation of crescent formation. The breaks in the capillary basement membrane also may be the means by which mononuclear cells gain access to the urinary space, as suggested by Kondo et al. [74]. Fibrinogen deposition in crescents is most common in those which are freshly formed; it tends to diminish or disappear as the crescents become fibrosed [97]. It has been recorded that antihemophilic factor (AHF, factor VIII), which is found along with fibrinogen in many pathologic processes, is not present in crescents [69]. Since AHF is an essential component of the intrinsic coagulation pathway, its absence in crescents suggested that this pathway is not involved in the process. Experimental studies in both the rat and rabbit, however, have demonstrated factor VIII–related antigens in crescents [114,127], implying that the intrinsic pathway cannot be completely excluded. Much attention has been paid to the extrinsic coagulation pathway and the procoagulant activity of macrophages and endothelium within the glomerulus [17,28,68, 127,138]. As a result of these experimental studies, a role for macrophage procoagulant activity has been suggested in the initiation of fibrin deposition in the glomeruli, but the mechanisms by which fibrin is formed in the capsular space are poorly understood. These aspects have been discussed by Salant [112], who raised the question of the source of procoagulant activity responsible for activating the extrinsic coagulation pathway components that leak into the capsular space. The alternatives are the macrophages that gain access to the space or tissue factor that is released from injured glomerular cells.

The importance of breaks in Bowman's capsule has been described by Olsen [104], who raised the possibility that the stimulus for crescent formation might come from the periglomerular tissue. This receives support from the observations of Boucher et al. [27] referred to earlier, which showed that monocytes are much more common in crescents associated with capsular breaks than in those without breaks. The chemotactic property of thrombin for monocytes [11] could well play a part in the migration of these cells.

Although the early crescents are cellular, they become fibrous with the passage of time. Their organization has been studied in man [25,95,120] and in the rat with anti-GBM antibody nephritis [114]. The origin of the collagen that appears and eventually replaces the original cellular crescent is not clear. There is evidence to suggest that in certain situations the collagen is the product of glomerular cells in so far as some of it is type IV and is found along with laminin; both of these are biosynthetic products of epithelial cells [120,141]. In human cases, type III collagen is present [120, 142], particularly when there are breaks in Bowman's capsule [120]. Since this type is not produced by glomerular epithelial cells, it is considered that interstitial cells have grown into the crescent. Cells with the characteristics of fibroblasts have been described both in the experimental model [114] and in man [95] and may well have originated from the interstitium. Morita et al. [95], however, have entertained the possibility that they are derived from epithelial cells. Fibronectin also has been described in crescents [106, 120,135,141], and it is likely that by binding to fibrin, to collagen, and to the cells of the crescent, it may play a part in the development of the fibrous crescent.

Clinical Outcome and Factors Determining Prognosis

This section gives an account of the outlook for patients with primary crescentic glomerulonephritis. An attempt will be made to do this according to the three groupings on the basis of glomerular immunofluorescence findings, but this is not always possible because of the different ways in which authors handle their data. I shall also discuss various features of the disease that might help in judging prognosis.

OLDER SERIES

Before passing on to more recent publications, a few words will be said about some of the older series that antedated chronic dialysis and many of the therapeutic agents used today. The prognosis was invariably dismal in those with the oliguric or anuric forms, and almost invariably the patients died in renal failure [16,20,30,61]. Whereas death usually occurred in a matter of weeks, 8 of 21 patients reported by Harrison et al. [61] fared differently. Two recovered completely, 5 recovered but had residual renal damage, and 1 survived for 3 years before succumbing to renal failure.

POSTSTREPTOCOCCAL AND OTHER POSTINFECTIOUS FORMS

It is of interest in the preceding series [61] that those who survived had the highest incidence of an infective background, with sore throat or otitis media being diagnosed in seven of the eight. This was an early example of the now well accepted belief that crescentic glomerulonephritis of postinfectious origin—mainly poststreptococcal—seems to have a better prognosis than most other forms of crescentic glomerulonephritis. Thus Nakamoto et al. [100] found that the prognosis was better in those cases of oliguric glomerulonephritis with proven streptococcal etiology, and a similar experience was described by Leonard et al. [77]. In an analysis of 29 patients with acute oliguric glomerulonephritis, the latter found 10 with raised ASO titers and 19 without. Of the 10 with raised levels, there were 7 who survived without the aid of chronic dialysis, whereas of the 19 without raised levels, only 2 survived without artificial aid.

In a study of children, Anand et al. [5] noted that of their 10 poststreptococcal cases, 5 developed terminal renal failure and as many as 5 recovered, apparently completely. The follow-up period for these 5 was 18 to 57 months. Of 7 with no streptococcal background, 4 developed terminal renal failure, while 3 improved but showed evidence of residual damage. In another study of 10 children with poststreptococcal crescentic glomerulonephritis, only 1 died, and the other 9 were alive with normal creatinine clearances after 8 months to 5 years [111]. In contrast, Forland et al. [51] described 5 patients with poststreptococcal oliguric glomerulonephritis, of whom 3 died and the 2 others required chronic dialysis or transplantation. Richardson et al. [108] also observed 2 such patients who required transplantation.

The length of follow-up is clearly of importance in assessing prognosis, and this is well brought out in the case from which Figure 9-8 was prepared. This 10-year-old girl, who was a patient of Dr. James Carey, had at the time of biopsy a serum creatinine level of 12 mg/100 ml, blood pressure of up to 140/100 mmHg, and heavy proteinuria; she had an ASO titer of over 800 units. Wedge biopsy showed over 95 percent of the glomeruli to contain crescents with proliferative changes in the tufts, arteritis in several small blood vessels (see Fig. 9-24), and an intense interstitial infiltration with plasma cells. The immunofluorescence pattern was granular for IgG and C3 along the capillary loops, and electron microscopy showed deposits in the glomerular capillary basement membranes and in a subendothelial position. Following a short course of steroids, the patient made a good recovery, and 4 years later she was well with a BUN of 19 mg/100 ml, blood pressure of 110/80 mmHg, and urine free of protein. However, over the next 7 years there was deterioration of renal function necessitating chronic dialysis and eventual transplantation. The case is salutary in that end-stage renal disease occurred, despite apparent recovery maintained for several years and emphasizes that long-term observation is required before claims of cure are made.

A good prognosis also has been described in certain patients with other forms of postinfectious glomerulonephritis, and Beaufils et al. [12] have shown in patients with visceral abscesses and glomerular disease sufficient to cause acute renal failure that cure of the infection leads to recovery. Whitworth et al. [137] also have described patients with crescentic glomerulitis associated with bacterial endocarditis or pulmonary abscesses who recovered.

PROGNOSIS ACCORDING TO IMMUNOFLUORESCENCE GROUPINGS

When the prognosis for primary crescentic glomerulonephritis is analyzed according to glomerular immunofluorescence grouping, the poorest outlook is in *group 1*, namely that with an anti-GBM antibody pathogenesis. In seven cases of this type studied by Briggs et al. [29], six required transplantation or died and one required dialysis. Of the patients of McLeish et al. [88], seven of eight required dialysis, but one survived and had a plasma creatinine level of 2.0 mg/100 ml. Of the 12 cases described by Beirne et al. [13] with glomerulonephritis but with no pulmonary hemorrhage, 6 survived, but 4 of these required hemodialysis to sustain life; the remaining 2, although not requiring hemodialysis, had decreased renal function. Others describe the onset of renal failure within weeks of the onset of disease with no remission [14,37,63,64,73,101,139]. More will be said of this group in Chapter 10, and this brief account is given for comparison with the other two groups.

When the *group with a diffuse granular pattern on immunofluorescence microscopy (group 2)* is considered, the results are variable. McLeish et al. [88] experienced a uniformly poor prognosis in this group, and of the 13 cases studied, 9 were on hemodialysis at follow-up. Two had died during the acute phase, and 2 were alive without the help of dialysis. Both of the latter had raised serum creatinine levels. Cohen et al. [37] reported that 72 percent of their 11 patients required chronic dialysis, and the remainder died within several months of presentation. Whitworth et al. [137] divided their patients into two groups on the basis of the numbers of glomeruli showing crescents; the first had over 80 percent involved, and the second had 50 to 80 percent involved. Of the 17 with a diffuse granular pattern, there were 6 in the first group; at follow-up, 2 had died, 1 was on chronic dialysis, 2 were alive without dialysis but with some functional impairment, and 1 had recovered completely. In their second group, there were 11 patients; 3 had died, 4 were on chronic dialysis, 1 had a decreased creatinine clearance without dialysis, but 3 had recovered, apparently completely. Thus of 17 patients studied, 4 recovered completely. It should be recorded that 2 of these had glomerulonephritis related to infections, 1 of them having bacterial endocarditis and the other a pulmonary abscess. The overall prognosis for those with a granular pattern is bad, but certain patients will recover, particularly those with postinfectious glomerulonephritis.

The group with no immunoglobulins or only patchy deposits in the glomeruli (group 3) shows the best overall prognosis, with the possible exception of postinfectious cases. In the series of Stilmant et al. [118], of 16 patients, 6 were on chronic dialysis at follow-up, but 10 survived without external help. Of this group of 10, 7 had elevated levels of serum creatinine and 3 had normal levels. Three of the six reported by McLeish et al. [88] were alive and required no dialysis, with serum creatinine levels of 2.0, 2.5, and 2.7 mg/100 ml. Beirne et al. [13] had 11 patients in this category, of whom 3 died, 2 were on chronic dialysis, and 6 survived with what was described as adequate native kidney function, which in 3 of them was normal. The worst prognosis was in the series studied by Whitworth et al. [137]. Of 18 patients available for follow-up, 6 had died, 7 were on dialysis, and 5 recovered, of whom 1 had normal function.

HISTOLOGIC FEATURES IN PROGNOSIS

Histologic features have been sought to try to assess the outcome, but very few of these have proved completely satisfactory. In general terms, the number of glomeruli showing crescents is useful; that is, the greater the number involved, the poorer is the prognosis. Morrin et al. [96] found value in assessing the number of glomeruli with crescents. It was found that no patient recovered function who had crescents in all glomeruli, that only 39 percent of patients recovered who had over 80 percent of glomeruli involved, but that 90 percent of patients who had fewer than 80 percent of glomeruli involved had some degree of remission. Even this criterion is not infallible, however, and certain patients with a high percentage of glomeruli with crescents may show remarkable degrees of recovery, while those with smaller numbers may pursue a rapid course. This is well brought out in the studies of Hind et al. [64] and Furlong et al. [52]. A more convincing case for the prognostic implication of crescents can be made in group 1 (anti-GBM antibody disease), and Walker et al. [133] found a significant correlation between renal deterioration and number of crescents in this condition. With regard to the implication of crescents, the observations of Whitworth et al. [137] are of interest. Setting out to determine whether the histologic picture was related to clinical features, they found that only half the patients with more than 80 percent of glomeruli with crescents had "rapidly progressive glomerulonephritis" from a clinical point of view. This is important because it is usually assumed that crescentic glomerulonephritis and rapidly progressive glomerulonephritis are synonymous.

The study of Neild et al. [101] allows comparisons to be made between those with necrotizing changes in the tuft and those with proliferative changes. In the necrotizing group of 11 patients, 5 died, 3 were on chronic dialysis, 2 had decreased creatinine clearance, and 1 had a clearance of 96 ml/min. Follow-up of the group with proliferation in the tuft (8 patients) revealed that 1 had died, 1 had end-stage renal failure, 3 had decreased clearance, but 3 had clearance in excess of 60 ml/min. In a somewhat comparable study, Morrin et al. [96] sought to see if there were differences from a prognostic point of view between those patients with crescents and no proliferative changes in the tuft, on the one hand, and those with both crescents and proliferative changes in the tuft, on the other. They found that recovery occurred in only 30 percent of the former compared with 50 percent of the latter, an observation previously made by Sonsino et al. [115] and Striker et al. [119]. While this does not enable predictions to be made on an individual case, there are several points of interest in this observation. First, it is likely that the group with tuft proliferation would include more cases of postinfectious glomerulonephritis with the better prognosis referred to earlier. The same applies to the proliferative group of Neild et al. [101]. Second, the crescents in the group with proliferation were usually less compact, and necroses in the tuft were less obvious.

It is important to realize that patients with predominant crescent formation and few proliferative changes in the tuft do show necroses and destructive changes. I stress this point because there is a belief that the predominantly crescentic type simply shows compressed tufts. This is not so; they almost invariably show damage. In fact, insufficient attention has been paid to the degree of glomerular tuft damage, and I have seen cases pursuing a rapid azotemic course with relatively few crescents but extensive damage to the tuft. Analogy can be drawn with the form of glomerulonephritis accompanying polyarteritis in this respect; in that condition, crescents may be scanty in the face of rapidly deteriorating renal function. The important changes are in the glomerular tuft.

Interstitial changes have been viewed as important prognostic indicators, and Striker et al. [119] have addressed this issue. In a group of patients with cellular proliferation in the tuft and crescent formation, they found that those with interstitial fibrosis involving more than 30 percent of the tissue were either anuric or had a serum creatinine over 3.5 mg/100 ml at the last follow-up. Interstitial fibrosis and tubular atrophy were both considered to be significant factors in determining prognosis in the report of the Southwest Pediatric Nephrology Study Group [116], which included 50 children with crescentic glomerulonephritis. Other features associated with a poor prognosis were the predominance of large crescents or fibrous crescents, global glomerular sclerosis, and gaps in Bowman's capsule. Tubulointerstitial inflammatory-cell infiltration also was regarded as a factor in causing renal death by another group [63], who also were impressed by the poorer prognosis in older patients.

OTHER PROGNOSTIC FEATURES

Clinically, anuria and impaired renal function at presentation are likely to be associated with a poor prognosis, but as with histologic features, many exceptions occur.

Finally, although the ultimate prognosis was poor in both, two distinct clinicopathologic groups of patients were identified by Baldwin et al. [10]. The first consisted of 10 patients with severe renal failure (6 with oliguria) at outset, all of whom very quickly developed end-stage renal failure. Biopsy showed very large numbers of circumferential crescents, with most patients having necrosis but little proliferation in the tufts. The second group was made up of 16 patients with an insidious presentation, mild to moderate renal failure (none had oliguria), hematuria, proteinuria (nephrotic syndrome in 8), and hypertension in an appreciable number. Although 11 progressed to end-stage renal failure and 3 more had deteriorating renal function, the clinical course was measured in years. Biopsy at outset revealed crescents in over 50 percent of glomeruli in 8 patients, but in general they were smaller than in the first group. The glomerular tufts showed greater cellularity but fewer necroses than the first group. This study is important in identifying a group of patients with crescentic glomerulonephritis who pursue an indolent course, once again emphasizing that the terms *crescentic* and *rapidly progressive* are not synonymous.

Etiology and Pathogenesis

This discussion is restricted to cases of primary crescentic glomerulonephritis, with the exception that reference will be made to poststreptococcal glomerulonephritis with crescents. This will be done because many authors deliberately include it, and others, while professing to exclude it, almost certainly include undiagnosed cases. Anti-GBM disease will be referred to because it is a significant contributor, although a more detailed account of its pathogenesis will be given in Chapter 10.

ETIOLOGY

Remarkably little is known about this aspect. As will be discussed in Chapter 10, it is suspected that volatile hydrocarbons and viruses may play a role in initiating the group with anti-GBM antibodies (group 1). It is surprising that apart from group A streptococci and occasional bacterial species isolated from cases with endocarditis and abscesses, no common responsible agent has been identified in the group with immune complexes (group 2). The group A streptococcus is still a potent factor in producing crescentic glomerulonephritis [5,56,61, 77,91,93,104,111,116], particularly in childhood. There is no good explanation why certain patients with poststreptococcal glomerulonephritis should develop a crescentic picture while the majority do not. Strictly speaking, cases with poststreptococcal glomerulonephritis are not true primary crescentic glomerulonephritis and should not be described here, but it is highly likely that unrecognized cases make their way into group 2.

It is always tempting to suggest that viruses might be implicated, and a study by Graham et al. [58] in which type IV nuclear bodies were identified suggested that this might be so. Type IV nuclear bodies are spherical intranuclear structures consisting of a dense central core surrounded by a clear halo as seen in plastic-embedded sections stained with toluidine blue. Under the electron microscope, they consist of 20-nm particles surrounded by microfibrillar material. They are frequently associated with virus-induced disease, and this was the basis for the claim made by the authors [58]. Davies et al. [42] suggested an arbovirus (Ross River virus) etiology in eight patients with segmental necrotizing glomerulonephritis with crescents. This was based on clinical grounds and the demonstration of serum antibodies to this virus. Since the virus in question is mosquito transmitted and apparently described only in Australia and the Southwest Pacific area, it is unlikely to be the cause of many cases of crescentic glomerulonephritis worldwide.

PATHOGENESIS

Group 1 patients have an anti-GBM antibody pathogenesis, which will be discussed in Chapter 10. Group 2 is regarded as having an immune complex pathogenesis mainly on the basis of a granular immunofluorescence pattern for immunoglobulins and complement either along the capillary walls or in the mesangium. Further evidence is provided by decreased serum complement levels in the serum [5,50,96,137], the demonstration of circulating immune complexes [12,26], the presence of cryoglobulinemia [3,12,87,137], and the finding of electron-dense deposits in relation to the glomerular capillary basement membrane or in the mesangium. It must be added that in all probability many of the cases on which these observations were made were postinfectious in origin, since there is a poverty of series in which this type of case was specifically excluded. It is also clear that certain cases with IgA nephritis make their way into group 2, and we were particularly struck by the numbers in our own series [72]. The pathogenesis of this condition is described in Chapter 6.

Group 3 remains enigmatic from a pathogenetic point of view, and there are few clues available owing to the dearth of publications in which significant numbers of cases in this group have been identified. Stilmant et al. [118] found that there was no decrease in serum complement levels, no circulating immune complexes, no cryoglobulinemia, no demonstration of rheumatoid factor, and normal levels of anti-DNA antibody. Couser [39] has drawn comparison with the form of glomerulonephritis that accompanies polyarteritis nodosa (so-called microscopic polyarteritis) and has pointed out the many points of similarity. Since we are also ignorant of the pathogenesis of polyarteritis and its glomerulonephritis, this is of little help. However, over the past several years, considerable attention has been paid to the role of ANCA [48] in both conditions, which may provide some clue to common mechanisms. The matter is addressed later under Antineutrophil Cytoplasmic Antibodies (ANCA).

Mechanisms of Glomerular Damage

A considerable amount of information now exists as to the ways in which glomeruli are damaged and crescents are formed in several forms of glomerulonephritis. Much of this information is derived from experimental studies on both anti-GBM antibody and immune complex models, supplemented by studies in human cases. Excellent reviews are available [39,79,112], and the matter is well covered in Chapter 3. Only the salient points will be mentioned here.

Central to the issue is damage to the glomerular capillary wall. Mediation of this damage can be effected by neutrophils, macrophages, and complement. Neutrophils damage the capillary wall by secreting proteases and toxic oxygen products, their localization in the capillaries being determined by complement-mediated chemotaxis, immune adherence, or increased adhesivity of endothelial cells induced by cytokines. Neutrophils are certainly seen in some cases of crescentic glomerulonephritis, but in others they are inconspicuous. Macrophages (monocytes) have received considerable attention over recent years, and their presence in human crescentic glomerulonephritis was alluded to earlier in the section dealing with the pathology of the glomerulus. Macrophages, like neutrophils, produce proteases and toxic oxygen products, but they have other important functions. These include expression of procoagulant activity, which is of consequence in fibrin formation both in the capillary lumen and in the capsular space; production of various cytokines, which induce endothelial cells to express procoagulant activity; increased adhesivity for various cells, including neutrophils; and elaboration of PAF, thromboxane A_2, and leukotrienes. Their role in the genesis of crescents has already been referred to, and this will be returned to later under Cell-Mediated Mechanisms. The damaging effects of the terminal components of complement, C5b-9 (membrane attack complex), occurring independently of inflammatory cells also have received attention [40]. While the membrane attack complex has been studied mainly in laboratory animals, there is at least one report of it being present in cases of human crescentic glomerulonephritis [65].

Role of Fibrin

The role of fibrin is clearly important in the pathogenesis of the lesions of crescentic glomerulonephritis. Fibrin is intimately related to the development of the crescent, as was described in the section dealing with that structure, and observations on procoagulant activity by macrophages in experimental glomerulonephritis [68,127,128,138] underline its importance. Observations in man also support its role. It was shown by Robson et al. [109] that six children with crescentic glomerulonephritis had persistent evidence of intravascular coagulation. Long-term anticoagulation resulted in remarkable improvement, presumably by interfering with glomerular fibrin deposition. Particularly striking were the changes seen in repeat renal biopsies. In these there was virtually no glomerular sclerosis despite an initial histologic picture of large crescents in most glomeruli and concomitant severe changes in the tufts. There are also studies that relate the level of fibrin degradation products in the urine to both the presence and site of fibrin in the glomerulus, as well as to the presence of crescents. Naish et al. [98] showed that disproportionately high titers of fibrin degradation products were found in the urine of patients with fibrin in an extracapillary position, namely those with crescents. Mesangial fibrin, however, was not associated with such high titers. Urinary fibrin degradation products have been shown to represent fibrinolysis of glomerular fibrin [36,45], and good correlations have been shown between the presence of fibrin in glomeruli, glomerular fibrinolytic activity as assessed by a slide technique on biopsy material, and urinary fibrin degradation products.

Cell-Mediated Mechanisms

There is a growing interest in the possibility that cell-mediated immune mechanisms play a role in crescentic glomerulonephritis, particularly in those cases in group 3. Although such a suggestion was made in 1970 by Rocklin et al. [110] on the basis of the ability of lymphocytes from certain patients with anti-GBM antibody glomerulonephritis to exhibit in vitro activity against preparations of GBM, it had to await the demonstration that monocytes (macrophages) participate to a significant degree in glomerular inflammation to gain respectability. Monocytes have now been described in various experimental models of glomerulonephritis, and a pathogenic role has been demonstrated [66,70,74,113]. They have also been described in human crescentic glomerulonephritis [22,49,83,102,117], as have T cells [22,102,117], thus providing the constituents for a cell-mediated mechanism. While the presence of macrophages and lymphocytes supports this mechanism, more direct evidence is needed. This was provided by the studies of Bhan et al. [18,19], who "planted" small amounts of rabbit anti-rat GBM IgG or immune complexes containing rabbit anti-BSA IgG in the glomeruli of rats. Glomerular abnormalities in the form of hypercellularity and necroses only occurred after rats received T cells passively transferred from donor rats that were specifically sensitized to rabbit IgG. Salant [112] has described this aspect and, quoting from other investigators, feels that these various studies suggest that sensitized T cells in glomeruli might direct the influx of macrophages. One of the most convincing studies on the role of cell-mediated mechanisms is that of Bolton et al. [23], who demonstrated an antibody-independent role for T cells in the induction of proliferative glomerulonephritis. This experiment utilized chickens whose humorally mediated immunity was depressed by bursectomy. It revealed that proliferative glomerular lesions—often with crescents—could occur following immunization with bovine GBM despite the absence of demonstrable anti-GBM antibodies. Moreover, labeled lymphocytes from immunized chickens with a deficiency of B cells migrated to the glomeruli of normal chickens after passive transfer. Thus there is increasing evidence for cell-mediated immunity playing a part in certain forms of glomerulonephritis, and this may well account for cases of group 3 primary crescentic glomerulonephritis.

Antineutrophil Cytoplasmic Antibodies (ANCA)

As mentioned earlier, ANCA are commonly present in the serum of patients with group 3 primary crescentic glomerulonephritis (pauci-immune type) [37*a*, 48, 71*a*, 101*a*, 134], whereas they are seldom found in patients with group 2 (immune complex type) [37*a*, 71*a*, 101*a*]. Although the association with ANCA is undoubted—as it also is in patients with crescentic glomerulonephritis accompanied by vasculitis—there is no compelling evidence for a pathogenic role for ANCA at the present time. In vitro studies (48*a*] have shown that both C-ANCA and myeloperoxidase-specific ANCA are able to induce neutrophil activation with release of reactive oxygen species, thereby suggesting their pathogenic potential. However, there is as yet no in vivo evidence for the ability of ANCA to cause damage comparable with that available for glomerular injury by anti-GBM antibodies (see Chap. 10).

MISCELLANEOUS CONDITIONS IN WHICH CRESCENTS MAY BE FOUND

Table 9-1 gave a list of these conditions and directed the reader to their positions in the book. A few conditions in which crescentic glomerulonephritis is found on rare occasions will be mentioned here.

Malignant Tumors

Alpers and Cotran [3a] have reviewed the association of malignant tumors (carcinoma and lymphoma) and crescentic glomerulonephritis. They cautioned against the ready assertion that the malignancy caused the glomerular lesion in several of the series reviewed, pointing out that the consequences of tumor therapy, altered host response to infection, and cryoglobulinemia complicating the clinical picture could all be factors in producing glomerular changes. They regarded three cases of lymphoma and glomerulonephritis [107,111*a*] as providing the best evidence for a cause-and-effect relationship. In the two cases described by Petzel et al. [107], immunohistology revealed granular IgG and C3 confined to the mesangium in one and the mesangium and capillary loops in the other; small deposits in the mesangium and capillary walls were demonstrated by electron microscopy. A case published since the review of Alpers and Cotran provides the best evidence to date of lymphoma causing severe glomerulonephritis with crescent formation [107*a*]. The patient, a 48-year-old man, presented with the simultaneous onset of non-Hodgkin's lymphoma and renal failure. Renal biopsy revealed focal necrotizing glomerulonephritis with crescent formation, absence of immunoglobulins but the presence of C3 in the mesangium and occasional capillary loops, and the presence of plentiful mesangial deposits with scattered small intramembranous deposits by electron microscopy. Treatment of the lymphoma resulted in its resolution and a return of renal function to normal. A second renal biopsy revealed only patchy mild mesangial hypercellularity, trace amounts of glomerular IgG and C3, and sparse, small, mesangial electron-dense deposits. Immune complex deposition related to the lymphoma was suggested as the mechanism for the glomerular changes.

It therefore appears that the best evidence for crescentic forms of glomerulonephritis being caused by malignant tumors is provided by lymphomas. The pathogenesis is not altogether clear, but there is some suggestion that immune complexes are involved.

Chronic Relapsing Pancreatitis

Chronic relapsing pancreatitis was accompanied by crescents in 70 percent of glomeruli in a case in which episodes of acute glomerulonephritis followed exacerbations of chronic relapsing pancreatitis [44]. On the basis of electron and immunofluorescence microscopy, it was felt that the renal changes were of immune complex pathogenesis.

Idiopathic Retroperitoneal Fibrosis

Idiopathic retroperitoneal fibrosis has been accompanied by crescentic glomerulonephritis [143] of apparent immune complex type. One of the points of interest is the support this gives to the idea that retroperitoneal fibrosis is a local manifestation of an immunologically mediated systemic disease (see also Chap. 23).

GENERAL DISCUSSION ON PRIMARY CRESCENTIC GLOMERULONEPHRITIS

As defined earlier, *primary crescentic glomerulonephritis* refers to that group of patients which remains when generalized vasculitis, certain forms of systemic diseases, and specific forms of glomerulonephritis are excluded. Exclusion of these various conditions is usually possible using clinical, laboratory, and pathologic findings. Even when this has been accomplished, however, we are still left with a far from homogeneous entity, and biopsies can be allocated to three immunohistologic groupings, which in a general way reflect different pathogenetic mechanisms.

As discussed earlier, the first of these patterns suggests anti-GBM-antibody disease, and this is confirmed by the demonstration of circulating antibodies. Since this is a highly specific and clearly defined entity that can stand on its own, a strong case can be made for removing it from the category of primary crescentic glomerulonephritis.

In a similar way, it is necessary to remove specific forms of glomerulonephritis from group 2, the group in which an immune complex pathogenesis is suggested by the immunofluorescence pattern. As pointed out earlier, it is well known that poststreptococcal glomerulonephritis gives rise to a crescentic form [4,5,43,51,91,108,111,116], and the same is true of glomerulonephritis of IgA [1, 2,136], membranoproliferative [32,59,86,89,121], membranous (discussed in Chap. 8) and various other types. As we have shown [72], it is possible to identify certain of these specific crescentic forms among group 2 patients. When these are removed, we are still left with appreciable numbers of cases with demonstrable immunoglobulins and electron-dense deposits in the glomeruli that do not conform to recognizable types. Some of these may be variants of specific forms or specific forms whose characteristic appearances have been altered or rendered unrecognizable by the intensity of the pathologic process. Supportive of this is the finding in our own material, mentioned earlier, of several cases with immunofluorescence and electron microscopic findings differing very little from known entities. However, certain cases remained that bore little resemblance to known conditions, suggesting that they were indeed primary crescentic forms of likely immune complex pathogenesis.

There are also problems in assigning cases to group 3 with complete certainty. The difficulties fall into two main categories: first, that of clearly excluding cases with systemic vasculitis, and second, that of eliminating cases of immune complex pathogenesis (group 2).

The first of these arises because group 3 primary crescentic glomerulonephritis is virtually identical to the type of glomerulonephritis that accompanies polyarteritis nodosa, sometimes referred to as the *microscopic* form. Some authors have discussed both under the general heading of *focal necrotizing glomerulonephritis*, which is the basic glomerular lesion [52,105*a*,134*a*]. In both conditions, males are more commonly affected—a 4 : 1 ratio in our group 3 patients—and the age incidence is surprisingly similar. The mean and median ages of our group 3 patients were 59 and 64 years, respectively, virtually identical to the 60 and 64 years observed in 13 biopsies that we studied in patients who had polyarteritis nodosa with glomerulonephritis. There is a great resemblance from the point of view of light, immunofluorescence, and electron microscopy; in fact, the difference is indistinguishable on renal biopsy if the tissue sampled does not show arteritis. Since arteritis is absent from biopsies of polyarteritis nodosa just as often as it is present (owing mainly to the small size of the sample), it is clear that other means must be sought in order to distinguish the two conditions. Biopsy of extrarenal sites is employed to detect vasculitis, and angiography is employed to demonstrate aneurysms, which are features of arteritis. Although many clinical and laboratory features are similar [38], constitutional symptoms such as fever, myalgia, arthralgia, mononeuritis multiplex, and so on are heavily relied on to make the diagnosis of polyarteritis, especially when biopsy is negative for vasculitis and angiography is unrevealing. Although P-ANCA has been described as occurring more frequently than C-ANCA in patients with primary (renal-restricted) crescentic glomerulonephritis of group 3 or pauci-immune type [37*a*,71*a*,101*b*], this distinction is not absolute and cannot be used to exclude the vasculitis group. The idea that group 3 primary crescentic glomerulonephritis represents vasculitis localized to the glomerular capillaries is very much in vogue and has been discussed by several authors [39,41, 79,138*a*]. The flurry of activity with ANCA has strengthened the notion of a pathologic continuum of ANCA-associated glomerulonephritis that would include primary crescentic glomerulonephritis (group 3 or pauci-immune type), polyarteritis nodosa, and Wegener's syndrome [71*a*]. It is also of note that in a prospective study assessing the effects of steroids and cytoxan on patients with ANCA-associated glomerulonephritis, there were no differences in either patient or renal survival when the renal-limited group was compared with those with systemic vasculitis [47*a*].

The other problem in assigning cases to group 3 is the distinction between groups 2 and 3. Some authors [37] consider that even sparse deposits of immunoglobulins and/or complement justify placing cases with this pattern in group 2 with an immune complex pathogenesis. As a consequence, no group 3 cases appeared in these authors' series of 11 patients. It should be added that electron microscopy in this series revealed deposits in the great majority of cases, supporting the idea of an immune complex pathogenesis. The interpretation of immunofluorescence preparations is often arbitrary, and confirmation of immune deposits by electron microscopy is highly desirable. In the review of our own cases of crescentic glomerulonephritis, electron microscopy was the final arbiter on several occasions. Yet with three exceptions we had little trouble in allocating cases to either group 2 or group 3. These were cases 13, 14, and 15 in Table 9-5; in these, scanty capillary wall or mesangial electron-dense deposits were noted, whereas immunofluorescence microscopy revealed only irregular mesangial deposition of IgM or none at all. Since the classification is based on immunofluorescence patterns, and since the electron-dense deposits were so scanty, we chose to include them in group 3. The problem of distinguishing between group 2 (immune complex) and group 3 (pauci-immune) primary crescentic glomerulonephritis has been partially resolved by the introduction of serum assays for ANCA. As described earlier, it is exceptional to find ANCA in patients with immune complex forms of the crescentic glomerulonephritis compared with the great frequency with which ANCA are found in the pauci-immune group [37*a*, 71*a*, 101*a*]. Further studies will be needed to determine the accuracy of this means of separation.

In summary, primary crescentic glomerulonephritis is characterized by crescent formation with a variety of changes in the tuft that may be necrotizing, proliferative, and/or sclerosing. Before it can be diagnosed, generalized vasculitis, systemic diseases, and specific forms of glomerulonephritis must be excluded. On the basis of immunofluorescence microscopy, three groups are identified: group 1 with a linear pattern for immunoglobulins, indicating anti-GBM antibody pathogenesis; group 2 with a granular pattern along the glomerular capillary walls or in the mesangium for immunoglobulins and complement, signifying an immune complex mechanism; and group 3, in which there are negative findings or only scant, irregular deposition of immunoglobulins and/or complement. Since group 1 represents a discrete entity, a powerful case can be made for excluding it from primary crescentic glomerulonephritis, leaving only groups 2 and 3. Group 2 probably contains specific forms of glomerulonephritis rendered unrecognizable or modified by the severity of the process giving rise to crescent formation. It is therefore a group that will probably account for decreasing numbers of cases as ways are developed to recognize these modified specific forms. Group 3 (pauci-immune type) is unique, and the etiology and pathogenesis are not understood. Cell-mediated mechanisms are appealing, and ANCA may well turn out to be pathogenic. At the present time, it is a group fully deserving of either prefix, *primary* or *idiopathic.*

REFERENCES

1. Abe, T., Kida, H., Yoshimura, M., Yokoyama, H., Koshino, Y., Tomosugi, N., and Hattori, N. Participation of extracapillary lesions (ECL) in progression of IgA nephropathy. *Clin. Nephrol.* 25:37, 1986.
2. Abuelo, J. G., Esparza, A. R., Matarese, R. A., Endreny, R. G., Carvalho, J. S., and Allegra, S. R. Crescentic IgA nephropathy. *Medicine (Baltimore)* 63:396, 1984.
3. Adam, C., Morel-Maroger, L., and Richet, G. Cryoglobulins in glomerulonephritis not related to systemic disease. *Kidney Int.* 3:334, 1973.
3*a*. Alpers, C. E., and Cotran, R. S. Neoplasia and glomerular injury. *Kidney Int.* 30:465, 1986.
4. Alwall, N., Erlanson, P., Tornberg, A., Fajers, C. M., and Moëll, H. Two cases of acute glomerular nephritis with severe oliguria for 75 days: Clinical course, roentgenological studies on kidney size, and postmortem findings. *Acta Med. Scand.* 161:85, 1958.
5. Anand, S. K., Trygstad, C. W., Sharma, H. M., and Northway, J. D. Extracapillary proliferative glomerulonephritis in children. *Pediatrics* 56:434, 1975.
6. Andres, G., Brentjens, J., Kohli, R., Anthone, R., Anthone, S., Baliah, T., Montes, M., Mookerjee, B. K., Prezyna, A., Sepulveda, M., Venuto, R., and Elwood, C. Histology of human tubulointerstitial nephritis associated with antibodies to renal basement membranes. *Kidney Int.* 13:480, 1978.
7. Atkins, R. C., Glasgow, E. F., Holdsworth, S. R., Thomson, N. M., and Hancock, W. W. Tissue culture of isolated glomeruli from patients with glomerulonephritis. *Kidney Int.* 17:515, 1980.
8. Atkins, R. C., Holdsworth, S. R., Glasgow, E. F., and Matthews, F. E. The macrophage in human rapidly progressive glomerulonephritis. *Lancet* 1:830, 1976.
9. Bacani, R. A., Velasquez, F., Kanter, A., Pirani, C. L., and Pollak, V. E. Rapidly progressive (nonstreptococcal) glomerulonephritis. *Ann. Intern. Med.* 69:463, 1968.
10. Baldwin, D. S., Neugarten, J., Feiner, H. D., Gluck, M., and Spinowitz, B. The existence of a protracted course in crescentic glomerulonephritis. *Kidney Int.* 31:790, 1987.
11. Bar-Shavit, R., Kahn, A., and Wilner, G. D. Monocyte chemotaxis: Stimulation by specific exosite region in thrombin. *Science* 220:728, 1983.
12. Beaufils, M., Morel-Maroger, L., Sraer, J. D., Kanfer, A., Kourilsky, O., and Richet, G. Acute renal failure of glomerular origin during visceral abscesses. *N. Engl. J. Med.* 295:185, 1976.
13. Beirne, G. J., Wagnild, J. P., Zimmerman, S. W., Macken, P. D., and Burkholder, P. M. Idiopathic crescentic glomerulonephritis. *Medicine (Baltimore)* 56:349, 1977.
14. Berg, R., Bergstrand, A., Bergström, J., Cunningham, R., Tagesson, C., and Wasserman, J. Rapidly progressive glomerulonephritis with antibodies against glomerular basement membranes in serum and kidneys. *Clin. Nephrol.* 5:37, 1976.
15. Berger, J., Yaneva, H., and Hinglais, N. Im-

munohistochemistry of Glomerulonephritis. In J. Hamburger, J., Crosnier, and M. H. Maxwell (Eds.), *Advances in Nephrology*, Vol. 1. Chicago: Year Book Medical. 1971. P. 11.
16. Berlyne, G. M., and Baker, S. B., de C. Acute anuric glomerulonephritis. *Q. J. Med.* 33:105, 1964.
17. Bevilacqua, M. P., Pober, J. S., Wheeler, M. E., Cotran, R. S., and Gimbrone, M. A., Jr. Interleukin-1 activation of vascular endothelium: Effects on procoagulant activity and leukocyte adhesion. *Am. J. Pathol.* 121:393, 1985.
18. Bhan, A. K., Collins, A. B., Schneeberger, E. E., and McCluskey, R. T. A cell-mediated reaction against glomerular-bound immune complexes. *J. Exp. Med.* 150:1410, 1979.
19. Bhan, A. K., Schneeberger, E. E., Collins, A. B., and McCluskey, R. T. Evidence for a pathogenic role of a cell-mediated immune mechanism in experimental glomerulonephritis. *J. Exp. Med.* 148: 246, 1978.
20. Bialestock, D., and Tange, J. D. Acute necrotizing glomerulitis: The clinical features and pathology in nine cases. *Australas. Ann. Med.* 8:281, 1959.
21. Bohman, S. O., Olsen, S., and Petersen, V. P. Glomerular ultrastructure in extracapillary glomerulonephritis. *Acta Pathol. Microbiol. Scand.* [A] 82(Suppl. 249):29, 1974.
22. Bolton, W. K., Innes, D. J., Jr., Sturgill, B. C., and Kaiser, D. L. T-cells and macrophages in rapidly progressive glomerulonephritis: Clinicopathologic correlations. *Kidney Int.* 32:869, 1987.
23. Bolton, W. K., Tucker, F. L., and Sturgill, B. C. New avian model of experimental glomerulonephritis consistent with mediation by cellular immunity: Nonhumorally mediated glomerulonephritis in chickens. *J. Clin. Invest.* 73:1263, 1984.
24. Bonsib, S. M. Glomerular basement membrane discontinuities: Scanning electron microscopic study of acellular glomeruli. *Am. J. Pathol.* 119: 357, 1985.
25. Bonsib, S. M. Glomerular basement membrane necrosis and crescent organization. *Kidney Int.* 33:966, 1988.
26. Border, W. A. Immune complex detection in glomerular diseases. *Nephron* 24:105, 1979.
27. Boucher, A., Droz, D., Adafer, E., and Noël, L.-H. Relationship between the integrity of Bowman's capsule and the composition of cellular crescents in human crescentic glomerulonephritis. *Lab. Invest.* 56:526, 1987.
28. Brentjens, J. R. Editorial: Glomerular procoagulant activity and glomerulonephritis. *Lab. Invest.* 57:107, 1987.
29. Briggs, W. A., Johnson, J. P., Teichman, S., Yeager, H. C., and Wilson, C. B. Antiglomerular basement membrane antibody–mediated gomerulonephritis and Goodpasture's syndrome. *Medicine (Baltimore)* 58:348, 1979.
30. Brun, C., Gormsen, H., Hilden, T., Iversen, P., and Raaschou, F. Kidney biopsy in acute glomerulonephritis. *Acta Med. Scand.* 160:155, 1958.
31. Burkholder, P. M., and Bradford, W. D. Proliferative glomerulonephritis in children: A correlation of varied clinical and pathologic patterns utilizing light, immunofluorescence, and electron microscopy. *Am. J. Pathol.* 56:423, 1969.
32. Cameron, J. S., Turner, D. R., Heaton, J., Williams, D. G., Ogg, C. S., Chantler, C., Haycock, G. B., and Hicks, J. Idiopathic mesangiocapillary glomerulonephritis: Comparison of types I and II in children and adults and long-term prognosis. *Am. J. Med.* 74:175, 1983.
33. Cattell, V., and Arlidge, S. The origin of proliferating cells in the glomerulus and Bowman's capsule in nephrotoxic serum nephritis: Effects of unilateral renal irradiation. *Br. J. Exp. Pathol.* 62:669, 1981.
34. Cattell, V., and Jamieson, S. W. The origin of glomerular crescents in experimental nephrotoxic serum nephritis in the rabbit. *Lab. Invest.* 39:584, 1978.
35. Chirawong, P., Nanra, R. S., and Kincaid-Smith, P. Fibrin degradation products and the role of coagulation in "persistent" glomerulonephritis. *Ann. Intern. Med.* 74:853, 1971.
36. Clarkson, A. R., MacDonald, M. K., Petrie, J. J. B., Cash, J. D., and Robson, J. S. Serum and urinary fibrin/fibrinogen degradation products in glomerulonephritis. *Br. Med. J.* 3:447, 1971.
37. Cohen, A. H., Border, W. A., Shankel, E., and Glassock, R. J. Crescentic glomerulonephritis: Immune vs. nonimmune mechanisms. *Am. J. Nephrol.* 1:78, 1981.
37*a*. Cohen Tervaert, J. W., Goldschmeding, R., Elema, J. D., van der Giessen, M., Huitema, M. G., van der Hem, G. K., The, T. H., von dem Borne, A. E. G., Kr., and Kallenberg, C. G. M. Autoantibodies against myeloid lysosomal enzymes in crescentic glomerulonephritis. *Kidney Int.* 37:799, 1990.
38. Couser, W. G. Idiopathic rapidly progressive glomerulonephritis. *Am. J. Nephrol.* 2:57, 1982.
39. Couser, W. G. Rapidly progressive glomerulonephritis: Classification, pathogenetic mechanisms, and therapy. *Am. J. Kidney Dis.* 11:449, 1988.
40. Couser, W. G., Baker, P. J., and Adler, S. Complement and the direct mediation of immune glomerular injury: A new perspective. *Kidney Int.* 28:879, 1985.
41. Croker, B. P., Lee, T., and Gunnells, J. C. Clinical and pathologic features of polyarteritis nodosa

and its renal-limited variant: Primary crescentic and necrotizing glomerulonephritis. *Hum. Pathol.* 18:38, 1987.
42. Davies, D. J., Moran, J. E., Niall, J. F., and Ryan, G. B. Segmental necrotising glomerulonephritis with antineutrophil antibody: Possible arbovirus aetiology? *Br. Med. J.* 285:606, 1982.
43. Davis, C. A., McEnery, P. T., Maby, S., McAdams, A. J., and West, C. D. Observations on the evolution of idiopathic rapidly progressive glomerulonephritis. *Clin. Nephrol.* 9:91, 1978.
44. Dickmeyer, J. P., Wolfson, W., Kowell, A., and Dornfeld, L. Reversible crescentic glomerulonephritis following an acute exacerbation of chronic relapsing pancreatitis. *Arch. Intern. Med.* 137:1065, 1977.
45. Ekberg, M., and Pandolfi, M. Origin of urinary fibrin/fibrinogen degradation products in glomerulonephritis. *Br. Med. J.* 2:17, 1975.
46. Ellis, A. Natural history of Bright's disease: Clinical, histological and experimental observations. *Lancet* 1:1, 1942.
47. Faarup, P., Norgaard, T., Elling, F., and Jensen, H. Structural changes in kidneys of patients with oliguric extracapillary glomerulonephritis during immunosuppressive therapy. *Acta Pathol. Microbiol. Scand.* [A] 86:409, 1978.
47a. Falk, R. J., Hogan, L. S., Jennette, J. C., and the North Carolina Glomerular Disease Collaborative Network. A prospective cohort study of 70 patients with antineutrophil cytoplasmic autoantibody (ANCA)–associated glomerulonephritis (GN) (Abstract). *Kidney Int.* 37:256, 1990.
48. Falk, R. J., and Jennette, J. C. Antineutrophil cytoplasmic autoantibodies with specificity for myeloperoxidase in patients with systemic vasculitis and idiopathic necrotizing and crescentic glomerulonephritis. *N. Engl. J. Med.* 318:1651, 1988.
48*a*. Falk, R. J., Terrell, R. S., Charles, L. A., and Jennette, J. C. Antineutrophil cytoplasmic autoantibodies induce neutrophils to degranulate and produce oxygen radicals in vitro. *Proc. Natl. Acad. Sci. USA* 87:4115, 1990.
49. Ferrario, F., Castiglione, A., Colasanti, G., Barbiano Di Belgioioso, G., Bertoli, S., and D'Amico, G. The detection of monocytes in human glomerulonephritis. *Kidney Int.* 28:513, 1985.
50. Fischel, E. E., and Gajdusek, D. C. Serum complement in acute glomerulonephritis and other renal diseases. *Am. J. Med.* 12:190, 1952.
51. Forland, M., Jones, R. E., Easterling, R. E., and Forrester, R. H. Clinical and renal biopsy observations in oliguric glomerulonephritis. *J. Chronic Dis.* 19:163, 1966.
52. Furlong, T. J., Ibels, L. S., and Eckstein, R. P. The clinical spectrum of necrotizing glomerulonephritis. *Medicine (Baltimore)* 66:192, 1987.
53. Gabbert, H., and Thoenes, W. Formation of basement membrane in extracapillary proliferates in rapidly progressive glomerulonephritis. *Virchows Arch.* [B] 25:265, 1977.
54. Garcia-Cáceres, U. Histologic aspects of subacute glomerulonephritis, with special reference to proliferative alterations in the epithelium of renal tubules. *Am. J. Pathol.* 35:755, 1959.
55. Gärtner, H. V., Wehner, H., and Bohle, A. The immunohistological findings in various forms of glomerulonephritis: A comparative investigation based on 335 renal biopsies: II. Minimal proliferating intercapillary glomerulonephritis (with nephrotic syndrome), focal sclerosing, epi-extra-perimembranous, membranoproliferative and extracapillary (rapidly progressive) glomerulonephritis. *Pathol. Res. Pract.* 162:198, 1978.
56. Gill, D. G., Turner, D. R., Chantler, C., and Cameron, J. S. The progression of acute proliferative poststreptococcal glomerulonephritis to severe epithelial crescent formation. *Clin. Nephrol.* 8:449, 1977.
57. Glassock, R. J. Natural history and treatment of primary proliferative glomerulonephritis: A review. *Kidney Int.* 28(Suppl. 17):S136, 1985.
58. Graham, A. R., Payne, C. M., and Nagle, R. B. A quantitative light- and electron microscopic study of type IV nuclear bodies in crescentic glomerulonephritis. *Am. J. Pathol.* 102:359, 1981.
59. Habib, R., Kleinknecht, C., Gubler, M. C., and Levy, M. Idiopathic membranoproliferative glomerulonephritis in children: Report of 105 cases. *Clin. Nephrol.* 1:194, 1973.
60. Hancock, W. W., and Atkins, R. C. Cellular composition of crescents in human rapidly progressive glomerulonephritis identified using monoclonal antibodies. *Am. J. Nephrol.* 4:177, 1984.
61. Harrison, C. V., Loughridge, L. W., and Milne, M. D. Acute oliguric renal failure in acute glomerulonephritis and polyarteritis nodosa. *Q. J. Med.* 33:39, 1964.
62. Harrison, D. J., and MacDonald, M. K. The origin of cells in the glomerular crescent investigated by the use of monoclonal antibodies. *Histopathology* 10:945, 1986.
63. Heilman, R. L., Offord, K. P., Holley, K. E., and Velosa, J. A. Analysis of risk factors for patient and renal survival in crescentic glomerulonephritis. *Am. J. Kidney Dis.* 9:98, 1987.
64. Hind, C. R. K., Paraskevakou, H., Lockwood, C. M., Evans, D. J., Peters, D. K., and Rees, A. J. Prognosis after immunosuppression of patients with crescentic nephritis requiring dialysis. *Lancet* 1:263, 1983.
65. Hinglais, N., Kazatchkine, M. D., Bhakdi, S.,

Appay, M.-D., Mandet, C., Grossetete, J., and Bariety, J. Immunohistochemical study of the C5b-9 complex of complement in human kidneys. *Kidney Int.* 30:399, 1986.
66. Holdsworth, S. R., Neale, T. J., and Wilson, C. B. Abrogation of macrophage-dependent injury in experimental glomerulonephritis in the rabbit: Use of an antimacrophage serum. *J. Clin. Invest.* 68:686, 1981.
67. Holdsworth, S. R., Thomson, N. M., Glasgow, E. F., Dowling, J. P., and Atkins, R. C. Tissue culture of isolated glomeruli in experimental crescentic glomerulonephritis. *J. Exp. Med.* 147:98, 1978.
68. Holdsworth, S. R., and Tipping, P. G. Macrophage-induced glomerular fibrin deposition in experimental glomerulonephritis in the rabbit. *J. Clin. Invest.* 76:1387, 1985.
69. Hoyer, J. R., Michael, A. F., and Hoyer, L. W. Immunofluorescent localization of antihemophilic factor antigen and fibrinogen in human renal diseases. *J. Clin. Invest.* 53:1375, 1974.
70. Hunsicker, L. G., Shearer, T. P., Plattner, S. B., and Weisenburger, D. The role of monocytes in serum sickness nephritis. *J. Exp. Med.* 150:413, 1979.
71. Ingelfinger, J. R., McCluskey, R. T., Schneeberger, E. E., and Grupe, W. E. Necrotizing arteritis in acute poststreptococcal glomerulonephritis: Report of a recovered case. *J. Pediatr.* 91:228, 1977.
71*a*. Jennette, J. C., Wilkman, A. S., and Falk, R. J. Antineutrophil cytoplasmic autoantibody–associated glomerulonephritis and vasculitis. *Am. J. Pathol.* 135:921, 1989.
72. Johns Hopkins Study of Primary Crescentic Glomerulonephritis. Unpublished observations.
73. Kalowski, S., McKay, D. G., Howes, E. L., Jr., Csavossy, I., and Wolfson, M. Multinucleated giant cells in antiglomerular basement membrane antibody-induced glomerulonephritis. *Nephron* 16:415, 1976.
74. Kondo, Y., Shigematsu, H., and Kobayashi, Y. Cellular aspects of rabbit Masugi nephritis: II. Progressive glomerular injuries with crescent formation. *Lab. Invest.* 27:620, 1972.
75. Lanari, A., Paz, R. A., and Rodo, Y. J. E. Glomerulonephritis aguda oligoanurica. Evolución pronóstico de los sobrevivientes. *Medicina (B. Aires)* 27:1, 1967.
76. Leatherman, J. W., Davies, S. F., and Hoidal, J. R. Alveolar hemorrhage syndromes: Diffuse microvascular lung hemorrhage in immune and idiopathic disorders. *Medicine (Baltimore)* 63:343, 1984.
77. Leonard, C. D., Nagle, R. B., Striker, G. E., Cutler, R. E., and Scribner, B. H. Acute glomerulonephritis with prolonged oliguria: An analysis of 29 cases. *Ann. Intern. Med.* 73:703, 1970.
78. Lewis, E. J., Cavallo, T., Harrington, J. T., and Cotran, R. S. An immunopathologic study of rapidly progressive glomerulonephritis in the adult. *Hum. Pathol.* 2:185, 1971.
79. Lewis, E. J., and Schwartz, M. M. Idiopathic crescentic glomerulonephritis. *Semin. Nephrol.* 2:193, 1982.
80. Löhlein, M. Über Nephritis nach dem heutigen Stande der pathologischanatomischen Forschung. *Ergeb. Inn. Med. Kinderheilkd.* 5:411, 1910.
81. Magil, A. B. Histogenesis of glomerular crescents: Immunohistochemical demonstration of cytokeratin in crescent cells. *Am. J. Pathol.* 120:222, 1985.
82. Magil, A. B., and Wadsworth, L. D. Monocyte involvement in glomerular crescents: A histochemical and ultrastructural study. *Lab. Invest.* 47:160, 1982.
83. Magil, A. B., Wadsworth, L. D., and Loewen, M. Monocytes and human renal glomerular disease: A quantitative evaluation. *Lab. Invest.* 44:27, 1981.
84. McCluskey, R. T., and Baldwin, D. S. Natural history of acute glomerulonephritis. *Am. J. Med.* 35:213, 1963.
85. McCluskey, R. T., and Bhan, A. K. Cell-mediated mechanisms in renal diseases. *Kidney Int.* 21(Suppl. 11):S6, 1982.
86. McCoy, R. C., Clapp, J., and Seigler, H. F. Membranoproliferative glomerulonephritis: Progression from the pure form to the crescentic form with recurrence after transplantation. *Am. J. Med.* 59:288, 1975.
87. McIntosh, R. M., Griswold, W. R., Chernack, W. B., Williams, G., Strauss, J., Kaufman, D. B., Koss, M. N., McIntosh, J. R., Cohen, R., and Weil, R., III. Cryoglobulins: III. Further studies of the nature, incidence, clinical, diagnostic, prognostic, and immunopathologic significance of cryoproteins in renal disease. *Q. J. Med.* 44:285, 1975.
88. McLeish, K. R., Yum, M. N., and Luft, F. C. Rapidly progressive glomerulonephritis in adults: Clinical and histologic correlations. *Clin. Nephrol.* 10:43, 1978.
89. Miller, M. N., Baumal, R., Poucell, S., and Steele, B. T. Incidence and prognostic importance of glomerular crescents in renal diseases of childhood. *Am. J. Nephrol.* 4:244, 1984.
90. Min, K. W., Györkey, G., Györkey, P., Yium, J. J., and Eknoyan, G. The morphogenesis of glomerular crescents in rapidly progressive glomerulonephritis. *Kidney Int.* 5:47, 1974.
91. Modai, D., Pik, A., Behar, M., Eidelman, A.,

Averbukh, Z., Weissgarten, J., Gabizon, D., and Rosenmann, E. Biopsy proven evolution of post-streptococcal glomerulonephritis to rapidly progressive glomerulonephritis of a postinfectious type. *Clin. Nephrol.* 23:198, 1985.

92. Moran, J., Colasanti, G., Amos, N., and Peters, D. K. C3b receptors in glomerular disease. *Clin. Exp. Immunol.* 28:212, 1977.
93. Morel-Maroger, L., Kourilsky, O., Mignon, F., and Richet, G. Antitubular basement membrane antibodies in rapidly progressive poststreptococcal glomerulonephritis: Report of a case. *Clin. Immunol. Immunopathol.* 2:185, 1974.
94. Morel-Maroger, L., Leathem, A., and Richet, G. Glomerular abnormalities in nonsystemic diseases: Relationship between findings by light microscopy and immunofluorescence in 433 renal biopsy specimens. *Am. J. Med.* 53:170, 1972.
95. Morita, T., Suzuki, Y., and Churg, J. Structure and development of the glomerular crescent. *Am. J. Pathol.* 72:349, 1973.
96. Morrin, P. A. F., Hinglais, N., Nabarra, B., and Kreis, H. Rapidly progressive glomerulonephritis: A clinical and pathologic study. *Am. J. Med.* 65:446, 1978.
97. Nagai, T., Tamura, T., and Kawai, C. Immunohistologic findings in the glomerular crescents in various renal diseases. *Jpn. Circ. J.* 43:83, 1979.
98. Naish, P., Evans, D. J., and Peters, D. K. Urinary fibrinogen derivative excretion and intraglomerular fibrin deposition in glomerulonephritis. *Br. Med. J.* 1:544, 1974.
99. Naish, P., Penn, G. B., Evans, D. J., and Peters, D. K. The effect of defibrination on nephrotoxic serum nephritis in rabbits. *Clin. Sci.* 42:643, 1972.
100. Nakamoto, S., Dunea, G., Kolff, W. J., and McCormack, L. J. Treatment of oliguric glomerulonephritis with dialysis and steroids. *Ann. Intern. Med.* 63:359, 1965.
101. Neild, G. H., Cameron, J. S., Ogg, C. S., Turner, D. R., Williams, D. G., Brown, C. B., Chantler, C., and Hicks, J. Rapidly progressive glomerulonephritis with extensive glomerular crescent formation. *Q. J. Med.* 52:395, 1983.

101*a*. Niles, J. L., Pan, G.-L., Collins, A. B., Shannon, T., Skates, S., Fienberg, R., Arnaout, M. A., and McCluskey, R. T. Value of antigen-specific radioimmunoassays for antineutrophil cytoplasmic antibodies (ANCA) in the diagnosis of rapidly progressive glomerulonephritis. *JASN* (*in press*).

101*b*. Noël, L. H., Chen, N., Nusbaum, P., Lesavre, J. P., and Grünfeld, J. P. Characterization of antineutrophil cytoplasm antibodies (ANCA) in different forms of vasculitis and in rapidly progressive glomerulonephritis (Abstract). *Kidney Int.* 37:444, 1990.

102. Nolasco, F. E. B., Cameron, J. S., Hartley, B., Coelho, A., Hildreth, G., and Reuben, R. Intraglomerular T cells and monocytes in nephritis: Study with monoclonal antibodies. *Kidney Int.* 31:1160, 1987.
103. Nowakowski, A., Grove, R. B., King, L. H., Jr., Antonovych, T. T., Fortner, R. W., Knieser, M. R., Carter, C. B., and Knepshield, J. H. Goodpasture's syndrome: Recovery from severe pulmonary hemorrhage after bilateral nephrectomy. *Ann. Intern. Med.* 75:243, 1971.
104. Olsen, S. Extracapillary glomerulonephritis: A semiquantitative light microscopical study of 59 patients. *Acta Pathol. Microbiol. Scand.* [A] 82 (Suppl. 249):7, 1974.
105. Olsen, S., Petersen, V. P., and Hansen, E. S. Immunofluorescence studies of extracapillary glomerulonephritis. *Acta Pathol. Microbiol. Scand* [A] 82(Suppl. 249):20, 1974.

105*a*. Parfrey, P. S., Hutchinson, T. A., Jothy, S., Cramer, B. C., Martin, J., Hanley, J. A., and Seely, J. F. The spectrum of diseases associated with necrotizing glomerulonephritis and its prognosis. *Am. J. Kidney Dis.* 6:387, 1985.

106. Pettersson, E. E., and Colvin, R. B. Cold-insoluble globulin (fibronectin, LETS protein) in normal and diseased human glomeruli: Papain-sensitive attachment to normal glomeruli and deposition in crescents. *Clin. Immunol. Immunopathol.* 11:425, 1978.
107. Petzel, R. A., Brown, D. C., Staley, N. A., McMillen, J. J., Sibley, R. K., and Kjellstrand, C. M. Crescentic glomerulonephritis and renal failure associated with malignant lymphoma. *Am. J. Clin. Pathol.* 71:728, 1979.

107*a*. Pollock, C. A., Ibels, L. S., Levi, J. A., Eckstein, R. P., and Wakeford, P. Acute renal failure due to focal necrotizing glomerulonephritis in a patient with non-Hodgkin's lymphoma. *Nephron* 48:197, 1988.

108. Richardson, J. A., Rosenau, W., Lee, J. C., and Hopper, J., Jr. Kidney transplantation for rapidly progressive glomerulonephritis. *Lancet* 2:180, 1970.
109. Robson, A. M., Cole, B. R., Kienstra, R. A., Kissane, J. M., Alkjaersig, N., and Fletcher, A. P. Severe glomerulonephritis complicated by coagulopathy: Treatment with anticoagulant and immunosuppressive drugs. *J. Pediatr.* 90:881, 1977.
110. Rocklin, R. E., Lewis, E. J., and David, J. R. In vitro evidence for cellular hypersensitivity to glomerular-basement-membrane antigens in human glomerulonephritis. *N. Engl. J. Med.* 283:497, 1970.

111. Roy, S., III., Murphy, W. M., and Arant, B. S., Jr. Poststreptococcal crescenteric glomerulonephritis in children: Comparison of quintuple therapy versus supportive care. *J. Pediatr.* 98:403, 1981.
111*a*. Sagel, J., Muller, H., and Logan, E. Lymphoma and the nephrotic syndrome. *S. Afr. Med. J.* 45:79, 1971.
112. Salant, D. J. Immunopathogenesis of crescentic glomerulonephritis and lung purpura. *Kidney Int.* 32:408, 1987.
112*a*. Savage, C. O. S., Pusey, C. D., Bowman, C., Rees, A. J., and Lockwood, C. M. Antiglomerular basement membrane antibody–mediated disease in the British Isles 1980–4. *Br. Med. J.* 292:301, 1986.
113. Schreiner, G. F., Cotran, R. S., Pardo, V., and Unanue, E. R. A mononuclear cell component in experimental immunological glomerulonephritis. *J. Exp. Med.* 147:369, 1978.
114. Silva, F. G., Hoyer, J. R., and Pirani, C. L. Sequential studies of glomerular crescent formation in rats with antiglomerular basement membrane–induced glomerulonephritis and the role of coagulation factors. *Lab. Invest.* 51:404, 1984.
115. Sonsino, E., Nabarra, B., Kazatchkine, M., Hinglais, N., and Kreis, H. Extracapillary Proliferative Glomerulonephritis: So-Called Malignant Glomerulonephritis. In J. Hamburger, J. Crosnier, and M. H. Maxwell (Eds.), *Advances in Nephrology,* Vol. 2. Chicago: Year Book Medical, 1972. P. 121.
116. Southwest Pediatric Nephrology Study Group. A clinicopathologic study of crescentic glomerulonephritis in 50 children: A report of the Southwest Pediatric Nephrology Study Group. *Kidney Int.* 27:450, 1985.
117. Stachura, I., Si., L., and Whiteside, T. L. Mononuclear-cell subsets in human idiopathic crescentic glomerulonephritis (ICGN): Analysis in tissue sections with monoclonal antibodies. *J. Clin. Immunol.* 4:202, 1984.
118. Stilmant, M. M., Bolton, W. K., Sturgill, B. C., Schmitt, G. W., and Couser, W. G. Crescentic glomerulonephritis without immune deposits: Clinicopathologic features. *Kidney Int.* 15:184, 1979.
119. Striker, G. E., Cutler, R. E., Huang, T. W., and Benditt, E. P. Renal Failure, Glomerulonephritis and Glomerular Epithelial Cell Hyperplasia. In P. Kincaid-Smith, T. H. Mathew, and E. L. Becker (Eds.), *Glomerulonephritis: Morphology, Natural History, and Treatment.* New York: Wiley, 1973. P. 657.
120. Striker, L. M.-M., Killen, P. D., Chi, E., and Striker, G. E. The composition of glomerulosclerosis: I. Studies in focal sclerosis, crescentic glomerulonephritis, and membranoproliferative glomerulonephritis. *Lab. Invest.* 51:181, 1984.
121. Swainson, C. P., Robson, J. S., Thomson, D., and MacDonald, M. K. Mesangiocapillary glomerulonephritis: A long-term study of 40 cases. *J. Pathol.* 141:449, 1983.
122. Suc, J. M., Durand, D., Conte, J., Mignon-Conte, M., Orfila, C., That, H. T., and Duchet, J. P. The use of heparin in the treatment of idiopathic rapidly progressive glomerulonephritis. *Clin. Nephrol.* 5:9, 1976.
123. Teague, C. A., Doak, P. B., Simpson, I. J., Rainer, S. P., and Herdson, P. B. Goodpasture's syndrome: An analysis of 29 cases. *Kidney Int.* 13:492, 1978.
124. Thomas, L. *The Medusa and the Snail.* New York: Viking Press, 1979. P. 113.
125. Thomson, N. M., Moran, J., Simpson, I. J., and Peters, D. K. Defibrination with ancrod in nephrotoxic nephritis in rabbits. *Kidney Int.* 10:343, 1976.
126. Thomson, N. M., Simpson, I. J., Evans, D. J., and Peters, D. K. Defibrination with ancrod in experimental chronic immune complex nephritis. *Clin. Exp. Immunol.* 20:527, 1975.
127. Tipping, P. G., and Holdsworth, S. R. The participation of macrophages, glomerular procoagulant activity, and factor VIII in glomerular fibrin deposition: Studies on anti-GBM antibody-induced glomerulonephritis in rabbits. *Am. J. Pathol.* 124:10, 1986.
128. Tipping, P. G., Lowe, M. G., and Holdsworth, S. R. Glomerular macrophages express augmented procoagulant activity in experimental fibrin-related glomerulonephritis in rabbits. *J. Clin. Invest.* 82:1253, 1988.
129. Urizar, R. E., Tinglof, B., McIntosh, R., Litman, N., Barnett, E., Wilkerson, J., Smith, F., Jr., and Vernier, R. L. Immunosuppressive therapy of proliferative glomerulonephritis in children. *Am. J. Dis. Child.* 118:411, 1969.
130. Vassalli, P., and McCluskey, R. T. The pathogenic role of the coagulation process in rabbit Masugi nephritis. *Am. J. Pathol.* 45:653, 1964.
131. Volhard, F. Die doppelseitigen hämatogenen Nierenerkrankungen (Bright'sche Krankheit). In L. Mohr and R. Staehelin (Eds.), *Handbuch der Inneren Medizin,* Vol. 3, Part 2. Berlin: Springer, 1918. P. 1149.
132. Volhard, F., and Fahr, T. *Die Brightsche Nierenkrankheit.* Berlin: Springer, 1914.
133. Walker, R. G., Scheinkestel, C., Becker, G. J., Owen, J. E., Dowling, J. P., and Kincaid-Smith, P. Clinical and morphological aspects of the management of crescentic anti-glomerular basement membrane antibody (anti-GBM) nephritis/Goodpasture's syndrome. *Q. J. Med.* 54:75, 1985.
134. Walters, M. D. S., Savage, C. O. S., Dillon, M.

J., Lockwood, C. M., and Barratt, T. M. Anti-neutrophil cytoplasm antibody in crescentic glomerulonephritis. *Arch. Dis. Child.* 63:814, 1988.

134*a*. Weiss, M. A., and Crissman, J. D. Segmental necrotizing glomerulonephritis: Diagnostic, prognostic, and therapeutic significance. *Am. J. Kidney Dis.* 6:199, 1985.

135. Weiss, M. A., Ooi, B. S., Ooi, Y. M., Engvall, E., and Ruoslahti, E. Immunofluorescent localization of fibronectin in the human kidney. *Lab. Invest.* 41:340, 1979.

136. Welch, T. R., McAdams, A. J., and Berry, A. Rapidly progressive IgA nephropathy. *Am. J. Dis. Child.* 142:789, 1988.

137. Whitworth, J. A., Morel-Maroger, L., Mignon, F., and Richet, G. The significance of extracapillary proliferation: Clinicopathological review of 60 patients. *Nephron* 16:1, 1976.

138. Wiggins, R. C., Glatfelter, A., and Brukman, J. Procoagulant activity in glomeruli and urine of rabbits with nephrotoxic nephritis. *Lab. Invest.* 53:156, 1985.

138*a*. Wilkowski, M. J., Velosa, J. A., Holley, K. E., Offord, K. P., Chu, C.-P., Torres, V. E., McCarthy, J. T., Donadio, J. V., Jr., and Wagoner, R. D. Risk factors in idiopathic renal vasculitis and glomerulonephritis. *Kidney Int.* 36:1133, 1989.

139. Wilson, C. B., and Dixon, F. J. Antiglomerular basement membrane antibody–induced glomerulonephritis. *Kidney Int.* 3:74, 1973.

140. Wu, M. J., Rajaram, R., Shelp, W. D., Beirne, G. J., and Burkholder, P. M. Vasculitis in Goodpasture's syndrome. *Arch. Pathol. Lab. Med.* 104:300, 1980.

141. Yoshioka, K., Takemura, T., Akano, N., Miyamoto, H., Iseki, T., and Maki, S. Cellular and noncellular compositions of crescents in human glomerulonephritis. *Kidney Int.* 32:284, 1987.

142. Yoshioka, K., Takemura, T., Tohda, M., Akano, N., Miyamoto, H., Ooshima, A., and Maki, S. Glomerular localization of type III collagen in human kidney disease. *Kidney Int.* 35:1203, 1989.

143. Zabetakis, P. M., Novich, R. K., Matarese, R. A., and Michelis, M. F. Idiopathic retroperitoneal fibrosis: A systemic connective tissue disease? *J. Urol.* 122:100, 1979.

Robert H. Heptinstall

10

Antiglomerular Basement Membrane Antibody Disease

HISTORICAL ASPECTS AND TERMINOLOGY

Antiglomerular basement membrane (anti-GBM) antibody disease is manifest either as a combination of glomerulonephritis and pulmonary hemorrhage or as glomerulonephritis occurring on its own. The glomerulonephritis is usually a severe crescentic form, as described in Chapter 9, but less severe forms are becoming increasingly identified, largely owing to the widespread application of immunofluorescence techniques to renal biopsies and the availability of methods to detect anti-GBM antibodies in the circulation. Exceptionally, pulmonary hemorrhage may occur in anti-GBM antibody disease in the absence of renal damage [151,154,160].

The combination of lung hemorrhage and glomerulonephritis has attracted considerable attention over the past three decades. Although relatively uncommon, it is of considerable importance because many of the cases described are caused by anti-GBM antibodies, and much of our knowledge of this mechanism has been derived from patients with this clinical combination. Attention was called to such an association by Parkin et al. [102] in a paper entitled Hemorrhagic and Interstitial Pneumonitis with Nephritis. Seven patients were described in whom the alveoli of the lung contained red blood cells and hemosiderin-containing macrophages in association with a necrotizing alveolitis with inflammatory cells in the septa. The kidneys showed severe glomerular proliferative and necrotizing changes. Four of the patients showed evidence of polyarteritis. Stanton and Tange [129] described a similar combination of lung hemorrhage and glomerulonephritis and directed attention to Goodpasture's paper [45] on influenza, in which the author described an 18-year-old man who developed hemoptysis and died shortly after an attack of influenza. On postmortem examination, cellular proliferation in the glomeruli, fibrinous exudate in the capsular space, and red blood cells in tubules were found in the kidneys; pulmonary hemorrhages were prominent features, and there was evidence of vascular necrosis in the spleen and gut. Stanton and Tange suggested the name *Goodpasture's syndrome* for the entity of pulmonary hemorrhage and glomerulonephritis, and this eponymous term is now in general use. Certain points should be made concerning the term *Goodpasture's syndrome.* Some prefer to include only those cases in which an anti-GBM antibody pathogenesis is demonstrated, and others will not accept cases with vasculitis. This is nonsense, because on both counts Goodpasture's original case would be excluded; no anti-GBM antibodies were demonstrated because they were unheard of at that time, and vasculitis was present. Moreover, vasculitis has been shown to occur in patients with anti-GBM antibody disease [73,157], further demonstrating the futility of these restrictions.

Fortunately, this chapter is mainly concerned with anti-GBM antibody disease, and contentious matters of nomenclature are not likely to be an issue, except in the section dealing with various other conditions in which lung hemorrhage and glomerulonephritis occur together. In this instance, the simple descriptive term will be used, qualified by the presumed pathogenetic mechanism or associated condition.

ANTIGLOMERULAR BASEMENT MEMBRANE (ANTI-GBM) ANTIBODY DISEASE

Clinical Features

When patients with anti-GBM antibody disease are divided into those with a combination of lung hemorrhage and glomerulonephritis and those with glomerulonephritis alone, it is found that the former predominate [11,20,48,143,151,153]. Among 400 patients whose serum or tissue was referred for anti-GBM antibody assay and judged to be positive, Wilson [151] recorded that two-thirds had the combination, with a third having only glomerulonephritis. The disease was confined to the lung in approximately 2 percent.

In the same series [151], over two-thirds of those with lung hemorrhage and glomerulonephritis were male, and two-thirds of both males and females were under 30 years of age. In contrast, when glomerulonephritis occurred alone, the sex distribution was more nearly equal, with males showing a slight predominance. While half the male subjects were under 30 years of age, it was observed that half the women were in the sixth and seventh decades. In a comparable group of 71 patients in the British Isles whose serum was referred for assay and found to contain anti-GBM antibodies, Savage et al. [119] also recorded that both sexes were affected equally when glomerulonephritis was the sole manifestation and that two-thirds of the females were over 50 years of age. Males predominated among those patients with both lung hemorrhage and glomerulonephritis; they were mainly in the third decade, but as in most other series, a certain number were over the age of 60 years. Similar age and sex patterns relative to anti-GBM antibody glomerulonephritis with and without pulmonary hemorrhage were found in the various series dealing with primary crescentic glomerulonephritis [11,25,48,88,96] and were quoted in Chapter 9. In most accounts, Caucasians predominate [119,151], although other racial groups may be affected. The condition has been described in identical twins [30,126], and there is a significant association with HLA-DR2 [110,113], suggesting an inherited predisposition.

Hemoptysis may be the first symptom in those with pulmonary involvement. It is usually of small amount and is repeated at intervals of varying duration, although large amounts of blood are occasionally produced. Anemia soon develops, and this very constant feature seems out of proportion to the amount of blood expectorated. The anemia, which is of a microcytic, hypochromic type, is caused mainly by the extensive bleeding into the alveoli and may be very profound. Dyspnea develops and may become severe. Bilateral alveolar infiltrates are seen on chest radiographs, and pulmonary function tests are severely deranged in certain patients. Increasing numbers of patients with evidence of anti-GBM antibodies are now being described in whom pulmonary changes predominate over those in the kidney [1,6,38,60,83, 118,137,160].

In those patients with both lung hemorrhage and glomerulonephritis, it is usual for pulmonary symptoms to appear first, and renal problems may be appreciated only when the patient is thoroughly examined. At this time, such features as hematuria, abnormal urinary sediment, proteinuria, and elevated serum creatinine levels may be detected. Severe renal manifestations such as oliguria or anuria frequently develop with great speed following the onset of hemoptysis or dyspnea and are often the presenting feature in those with disease localized to the kidney [40,48,57,88,96,104, 119,143]. Hematuria is constantly present when the kidney is involved and may cause discoloration of the urine when profuse. Red-cell casts frequently accompany hematuria. Proteinuria is common, and the mean 24-hour excretion was 2.4 g in one substantial series [153]; nephrotic-range proteinuria has been recorded on numerous occasions [11,20,48,52,57,143]. Hypertension may be present [11,40,48,57], but the mechanism is not clear.

Apart from the demonstration of circulating anti-GBM antibodies, detected either by indirect immunofluorescence methods, ELISA, or radioimmunoassay, there are very few specific laboratory abnormalities. Anemia is a common feature, particularly of those with pulmonary hemorrhage, and microangiopathic hemolytic anemia has been recorded [130]. Serum creatinine levels rise commensurate with the severity of the renal damage; serum complement levels are not usually depressed; antinuclear antibodies are hardly ever demonstrated; and for inexplicable reasons, circulating immune complexes are occasionally detected [52,141,142].

Antineutrophil cytoplasmic antibodies (ANCA) —described more fully in Chapters 3 and 16— have been found in certain patients with anti-GBM antibody disease [53*a*, 75,96*a*]. In one study [53*a*, 75], sera from 889 patients with rapidly progressive glomerulonephritis were assayed for the two autoantibodies; 47 (5 percent) were positive for anti-GBM antibody, 246 (28 percent) for ANCA, and 20 (2 percent) for both. It was considered that the 20 patients with both types of autoantibodies had coexisting anti-GBM antibody disease and systemic vasculitis. This was based on the authors' belief that a positive ANCA assay is indicative of systemic vasculitis. Niles et al. [96*a*] detected ANCA in 8 of 18 patients who had necrotizing and crescentic glomerulonephritis and evidence of anti-GBM antibodies. They speculated that anti-GBM antibodies were produced secondarily in these 8 patients in response to glomerular damage resulting from ANCA-associated glomerulonephritis. There is also a case report [142*a*] of the coexistence of Wegener's granulomatosis and anti-GBM antibody disease. ANCA were not sought in this patient, but as discussed in Chapters 3 and 16, it is common to find them in Wegener's granulomatosis.

Other relevant features are the apparent seasonal incidence with maximal occurrence in the spring and early summer [119] and the history that might be elicited of exposure to volatile hydrocarbons [8,62] or sniffing of hydrocarbon-containing glue [16]. Cigarette smoking has been noted to be particularly common among those patients who have lung hemorrhage [31].

Pathologic Changes in the Kidney

GROSS APPEARANCE

In those patients with the florid crescentic form of glomerulonephritis, both kidneys are increased in size with small subcapsular hemorrhages and a mottled, widened cortex. There may be petechial hemorrhages on the pelvic lining. Kidneys obtained from patients who have been on dialysis are smaller and show fewer hemorrhages.

MICROSCOPIC FINDINGS

The findings by light microscopy vary according to the stage at which the disease is seen and to factors that we do not presently understand. For example, some cases are seen in which the glomeruli are not severely injured—usually those with predominant lung involvement—while others show extensive glomerular damage with crescent formation. Yet even those cases with mild glomerular abnormalities display a generalized fixation of immunoglobulin along the glomerular capillary walls. Again, for reasons not understood, some of those cases with mild glomerular involvement appear to show little progression of the lesion, whereas others proceed with great speed to develop a diffuse crescentic form of glomerulonephritis. It is tempting to suggest that the intensity of the renal disease might be related to the titer of anti-GBM antibody. In addressing this problem, Briggs et al. [20] pointed out the difficulties in making such comparisons. Chief of these was the different intervals between onset of symptoms and the time of performing the initial assays so that the titer obtained may not have represented the maximum level. These authors felt that in certain of their cases there might have been a relation between a high absolute titer and a rapidly progressive course. Peters et al. [104] noted that the highest titers were generally seen in patients with the severest lesions—those requiring dialysis—but overall there was a poor correlation between antibody level and renal function.

Glomeruli

Glomeruli in the early stages and in the milder cases often show a focal involvement [6,17,20, 26,34,98,130,136]. This consists of certain glomeruli showing localized areas of cellular proliferation or necrosis and the other glomeruli exhibiting no apparent change (Figs. 10-1 and 10-2). Some glomeruli may show localized solidified areas, presumably the sequel to necrosis. Small crescents may be found in the affected glomeruli, and red cells are occasionally present in the capsular space. A variant of this change is a mild increase in mesangium in all glomeruli, with localized areas of proliferation or necrosis present in a certain number of them [4,20,137]. Still other mild or early cases simply show an increase in mesangial cellularity or mesangial substance in all glomeruli, none of them having localized or segmental areas of proliferation or necrosis [20,38,83]. There are a few cases recorded in which there are no changes in the glomeruli by light microscopy in the presence of circulating anti-GBM antibody and diffuse linear fluorescence for IgG [1,118, 137,160]. There were no urinary abnormalities or simply the finding of microhematuria in this last group. The evolution of these changes will be described later.

The changes seen in the glomeruli in cases with a more serious clinical picture, particularly those with oliguria or anuria, are much more severe and

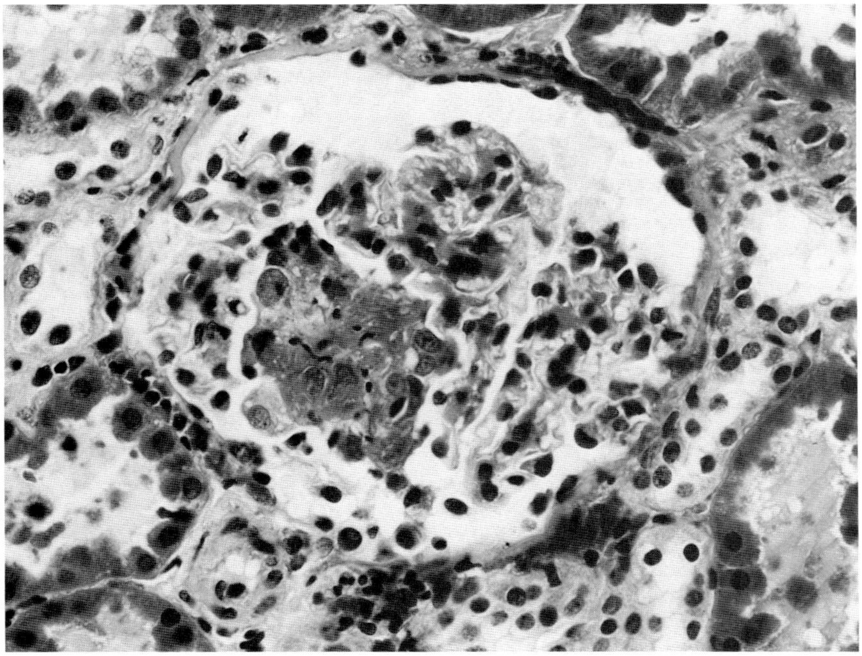

Fig. 10-1. *Glomerulus with localized area of necrosis from a 28-year-old women referred to in section Clinical Course and Outcome who presented with hemoptysis and was found to have microscopic hematuria. Fewer than 10 percent of the glomeruli showed the type of lesion illustrated here. H&E;* ×500.

extensive. Most of the glomeruli are involved in a necrotizing process that may be segmental or may affect the whole of the tuft and is often associated with crescent formation (Fig. 10-3). The lesions are sometimes accompanied by increased numbers of cells, many of which are monocytes [13,36, 97,128]. T-lymphocytes also have been demonstrated [13,97,128], and in some instances there is a considerable influx of neutrophils (Fig. 10-4). Multinucleated giant cells are sometimes seen in the more peripheral parts of the tuft, merging with crescents (Figs. 10-5 and 9-21); the origin of these cells is not clear, but some have regarded them as derived from monocytes [59] and others from epithelial cells [99]. Crescents are plentiful and are often so large as to fill Bowman's space (Fig. 10-6). These and their mode of formation were adequately described and illustrated in the preceding chapter (see Figs. 9-13 and 9-15), but it should be noted that monocytes are particularly plentiful in the crescents of anti-GBM antibody glomerulonephritis [79]. Fibrin is frequently present in the capsular space and is usually surrounded by the cells of the crescent. Red blood cells and neutrophils also may be seen in the capsular space, presumably having gained access by the disruptive changes in the tuft. Segmental areas of sclerosis are also seen in the tuft, and particularly in those patients supported by dialysis, the entire tuft may be sclerotic. While most of the crescents are of the cellular type, fibrocellular and fibrous forms may be seen in the more long-standing cases. Bowman's capsule may be disrupted either wholly or in part so that the crescent merges with the cellular interstitium (see Figs. 10-3 and 9-13). In those cases in which giant cells are present, this se-

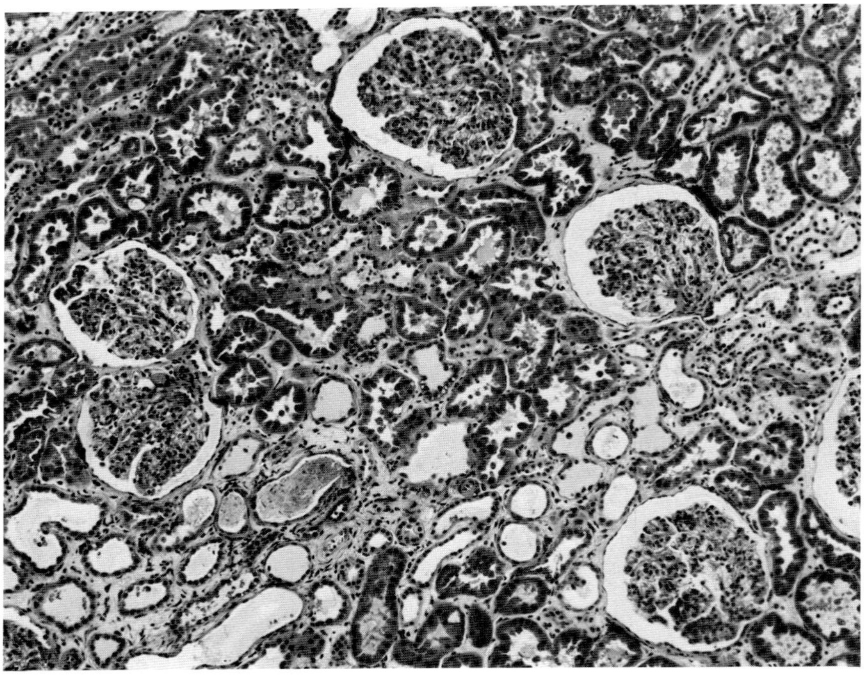

FIG. 10-2. *Five glomeruli with no, or only trivial, abnormalities from same patient as in Fig. 10-1. H&E; × 100.*

quence of changes may give rise to a picture justifying the term *granulomatous glomerulonephritis.* As described in Chapter 9, it is likely that interstitial cells contribute to the formation and subsequent organization of crescents through gaps in Bowman's capsule [19]. Even in these widespread forms of glomerulonephritis, it is not unusual to find glomeruli that appear normal or show only exquisitely localized necrotizing or proliferative lesions. The impression is given that the changes in this severe form represent a massive form of focal and segmental glomerulonephritis.

Tubules

Tubules show little change when the early focal and segmental glomerulonephritic process is present, but even at this stage, some may contain red blood cells and some may appear atrophic. In the florid stage, there is widespread loss and atrophy, and eosinophilic cast-like material, neutrophils, and red cells are frequently found in the tubular lumens. Iron pigment is sometimes seen in the tubular epithelium. In some cases, actual tubular necroses may be present, and regenerative activity may be demonstrated in the epithelium (Fig. 10-7). As will be described later, a linear fluorescence pattern for IgG along the tubular basement membranes is sometimes found in anti-GBM antibody disease. This is regarded as indicating the presence of antitubular basement membrane (anti-TBM) antibodies. Andres et al. [5] showed a greater degree of tubulointerstitial reaction in patients demonstrating anti-TBM antibodies and attributed a pathogenic role to them. Breaks were demonstrated in the TBMs with migration of neutrophils, lymphocytes, and monocytes from the interstitium into the tubular lumens.

Interstitium

Interstitial changes consist of edema and infiltration by chronic inflammatory cells of several types. Using monoclonal antibodies and immu-

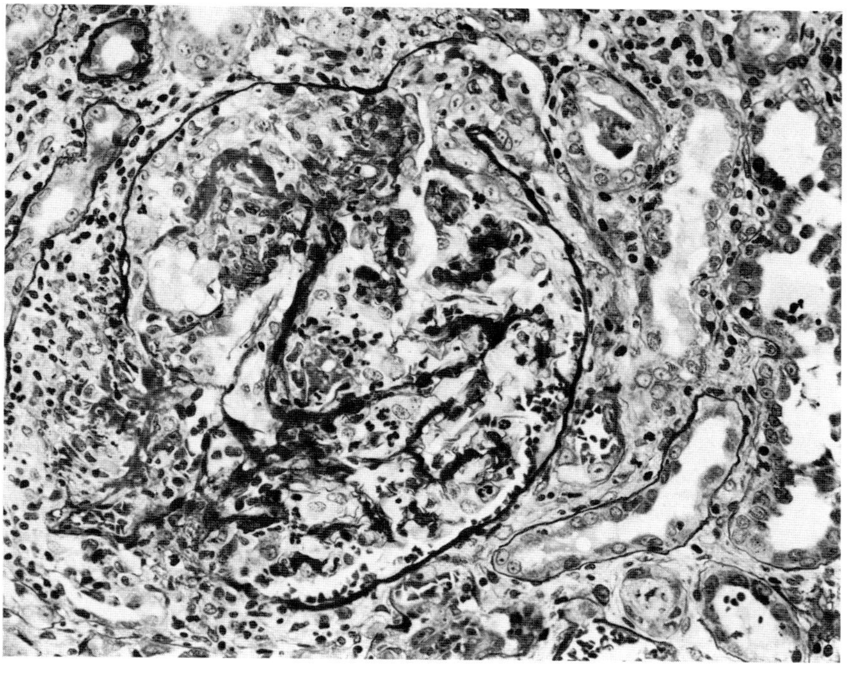

FIG. 10-3. *Glomerulus from florid anti-GBM antibody disease with completely disorganized tuft, fibrin in capsular space, and crescent formation that can be seen occluding the origin of the proximal convoluted tubule (top). Bowman's capsule is fractured in lower left corner with continuity of changes between interstitium and Bowman's space. Periodic acid–methenamine silver;* × *300.*

nohistologic techniques, it has been shown that many of these cells are monocytes and T-lymphocytes [13,128]. In the study on anti-TBM antibodies referred to earlier [5], particularly dense interstitial inflammatory exudates were found in patients with these antibodies, and interstitial giant cells were reported in relation to damaged tubules. Interstitial giant cells were present in one of our own cases in which there was linear staining for IgG along TBMs (Fig. 10-8). Fibrosis is present in patients who have been maintained on dialysis and in those who have survived a longer time without external aid.

Blood Vessels

Blood vessels usually show inconspicuous changes, although interlobular arteries may have varying degrees of intimal thickening. In certain patients, necrotizing changes with infiltrating inflammatory cells are present in arterioles and small arteries [73,157]. This is a rare change, but it undoubtedly does occur as part of anti-GBM antibody–mediated disease. Fibrinoid change, extravasation of red cells into the media, and fibrin plugs in the lumen also have been described in arterioles [130].

ELECTRON MICROSCOPIC FINDINGS

The electron microscopic picture has been described on a number of occasions [4,20,35,43,98,103,107,136,137,140]. Endothelial and epithelial cells of the tuft are increased and swollen, and there is patchy fusion of foot processes. There is increase in basement membrane–like material, especially in areas that appear sclerotic by light microscopy. The capillaries are frequently oc-

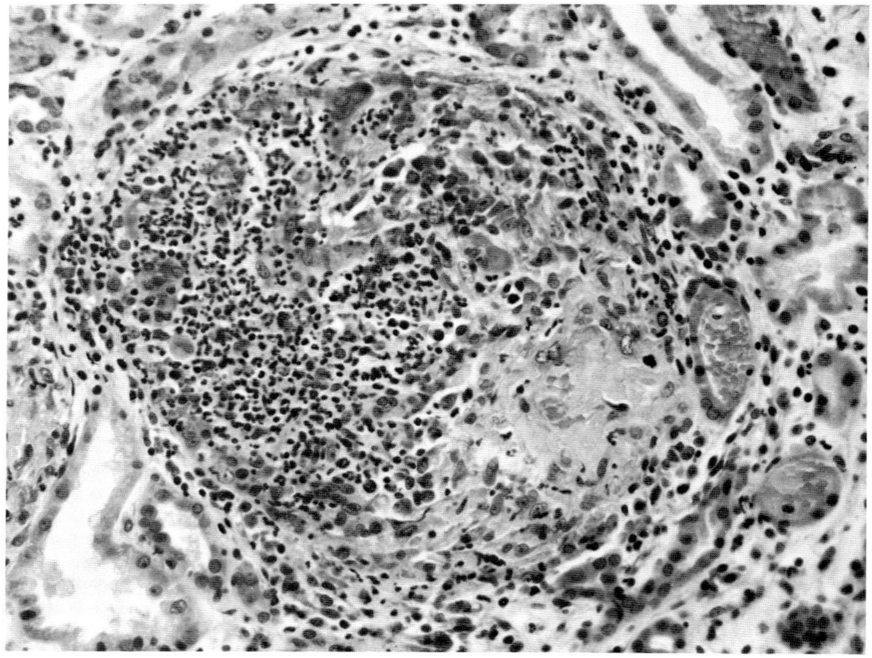

FIG. 10-4. *This glomerulus is completely disrupted and shows considerable numbers of neutrophils. From a case with widespread crescent formation. H&E; ×270.*

cluded by swollen endothelial cells, and fibrin may be present either in the lumen or under the endothelium. The basement membrane is sometimes modestly thickened, with finely nodular irregularities of the endothelial aspect. A rarefied zone may be seen between the basement membrane and the endothelium, and this feature has been observed very frequently (Fig. 10-9). Fractures of the basement membrane have been described [15,43,136] (Fig. 10-10), and these can be particularly well demonstrated by scanning electron microscopy following selective removal of the podocytes by chemical methods [14,15]. There is often localized collapse of the capillary wall, which has a rather granular appearance.

Of interest are a variety of virus-like particles seen by various observers [4,98,140]. They have been described in the epithelial cells of the tuft and considered to resemble a paramyxovirus [140]. They also have been noted in endothelial cells [4,98] and likened to a myxovirus [4].

Electron-dense deposits of the type seen in immune complex disease are not usually recorded, but as noted in the description under Immunofluorescence Findings, deposits may be seen in cases of proven anti-GBM antibody type with anomolous immunofluorescence patterns [4,103,114]. The deposits were usually on the epithelial side of the GBM (as in membranous glomerulonephritis) but in one case were on both sides. There are also cases recorded in which anti-GBM antibody disease has clearly developed in patients with existing membranous glomerulonephritis characterized by typical electron-dense deposits [61,94]. There are also others with demonstrable circulating anti-GBM antibodies in which at the time of biopsy a linear fluorescence for IgG along the glomerular capillary wall coexisted with subepithelial electron-dense deposits [105,139]. In one of them [139] there was a granular rather than a linear pattern for C3 along the glomerular capillary walls. I have seen a case in which renal biopsy showed

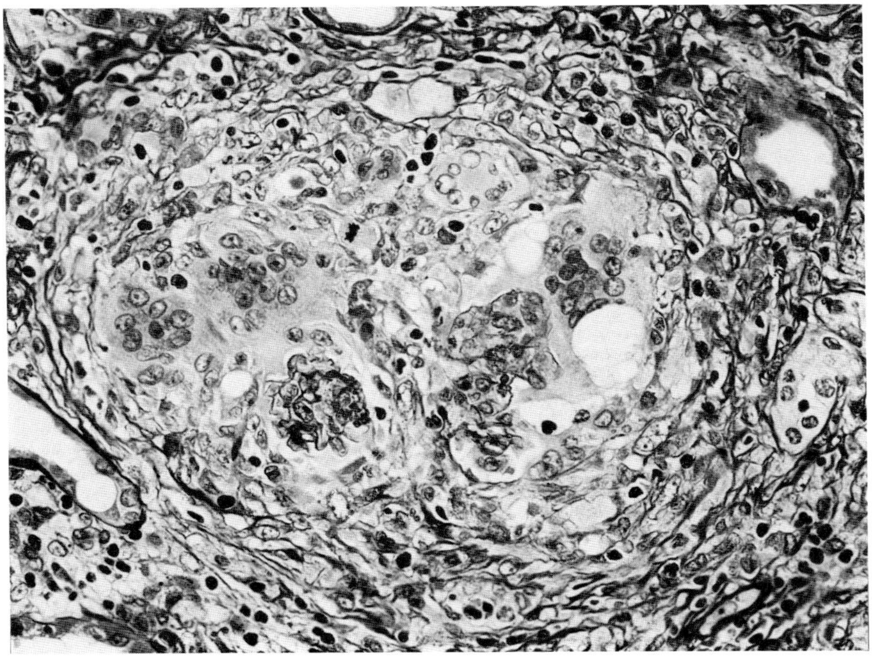

Fig. 10-5. *Enlarged glomerulus from anti-GBM antibody disease with crescent formation among which are several multinucleated giant cells. There are only a few remnants of the tuft shown by their argyrophilia. Bowman's capsule has been severely damaged. Periodic acid–methenamine silver;* ×350.

mild glomerular hypercellularity, crescents in 10 percent of glomeruli, linear glomerular capillary wall fluorescence for IgG and C3, patchy linear fluorescence for IgG along TBMs, and small subepithelial electron-dense deposits along the glomerular capillary walls. This was a 60-year-old patient of Dr. Ted Lewers who presented with swelling of her legs and was found to have a 24-hour protein excretion of 3.4 g. Her serum creatinine level was 1.2 mg/100 ml, serum complement levels were within normal limits, and anti-GBM antibodies were present in the circulation. Although uncommon, these cases with electron-dense deposits in the capillary wall may prove important in the pathogenesis of anti-GBM antibody disease, since by damaging the GBM they may well release antigen to initiate the formation of antibodies. This is especially so in those cases where the membranous glomerulonephritis convincingly antedates the anti-GBM antibody disease.

IMMUNOFLUORESCENCE FINDINGS

A continuous linear pattern of IgG along the glomerular capillary walls is the finding that is characteristic of the glomerulonephritis of anti-GBM antibody pathogenesis (Figs. 10-11, 10-12, and 9-1). Immunoelectron microscopy has shown that the IgG is localized to the lamina rara interna [127]. A combination of IgG and C3 is most commonly encountered [20,25,72,90,98,119,136,153], but C3 often stains less intensely than IgG [20,136,153]. In certain patients, IgG is found without C3 [20,82,90,119,136,153]. It is of historical interest that a linear pattern for gamma globulin, with equivocal staining for complement, was described before the concept of anti-GBM an-

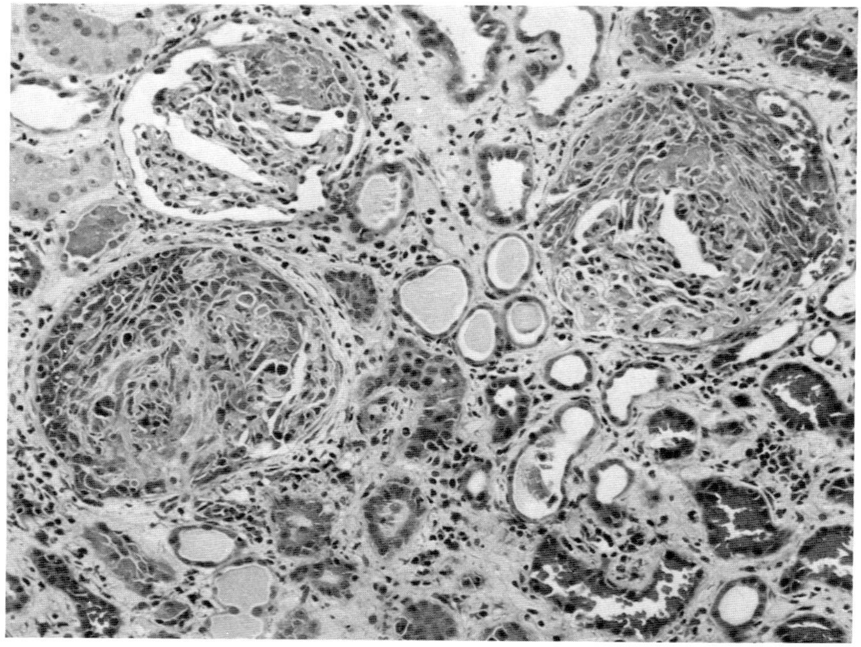

FIG. 10-6. *Section shows three glomeruli, two with very large crescents. One (upper left) has either a segmental lesion of the tuft or a small crescent; without the benefit of a silver stain, it may not be possible to tell the two apart. The patient was a young man with hemoptysis and rapidly progressive azotemic glomerulonephritis. There was glomerular linear fluorescence for IgG and C3. H&E; ×165.*

tibody was formulated [122]. In order to appreciate the frequency with which these patterns occur, Wilson and Dixon [153] recorded their findings in 22 specimens; they found staining of equal intensity in 6, C3 less intense than IgG in 12, and IgG in only 4. The staining pattern with C3 is linear along the glomerular capillary wall and usually affects all the loops (Fig. 10-13), although it has been noted to be segmental and irregular in some instances [153]. It also has been recorded as granular [20,43,157] (Fig. 10-14). A granular pattern for C4 has been described in the absence of C3 [160]. The frequency with which IgM is found in the glomeruli varies; in three series it was demonstrated in 13 of 25 [136], 3 of 20 [153], and 1 of 16 specimens [20]. It occurred in linear, granular, and segmental patterns. Of interest is a case of Border et al. [17] in which a linear pattern for IgA and a nonlinear pattern for IgM and C3 were found in the glomeruli; IgG was negative. Similar cases have been described in which IgA in a linear distribution was the predominant immunoglobulin. In one instance [119] it was accompanied by C3, and in another it was accompanied by IgM and C3 [35]. IgM and C3 occurring together in a linear pattern also have been described [119]. Fibrinogen is found in relation to the crescents and sometimes in the tufts, as is the case with other forms of necrotizing crescentic glomerulonephritis.

Immunoglobulins with or without C3 also may be found in a linear pattern along TBMs

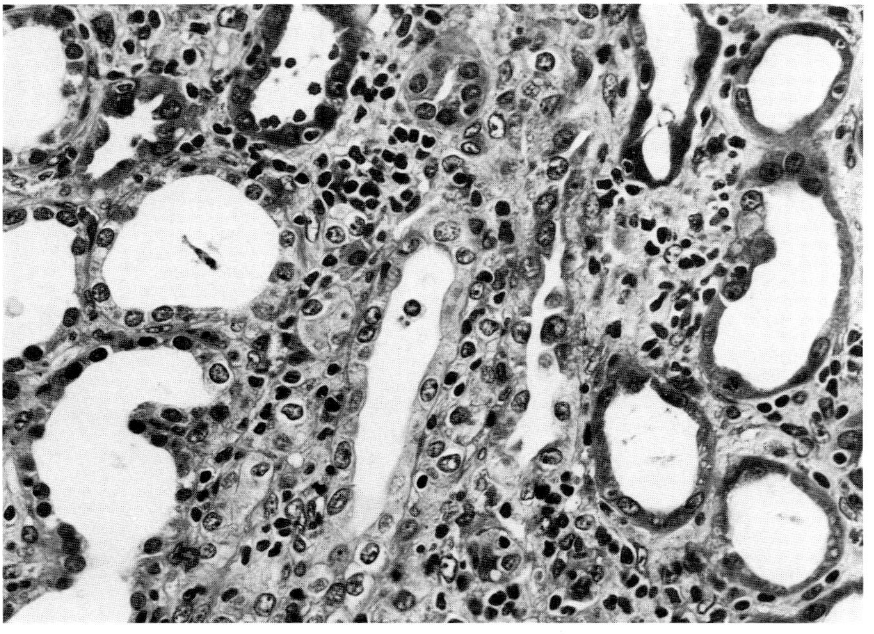

Fig. 10-7. *Section from anti-GBM antibody crescentic glomerulonephritis to show regenerating tubular epithelium to right side of picture. Several chronic inflammatory cells are scattered throughout the interstitium. H&E;* ×*400.*

[5,17,70,136,153] (Figs. 10-11 and 10-15). In the large series of Lehman et al. [70], 37 of 47 patients (79 percent) demonstrated linear immunoglobulin along TBMs; IgG was present in all, but IgA and IgM were each found once, and C3 was detected in 22 patients. Staining was less intense than in the glomeruli and was often very focal with involvement of no more than 10 percent of tubules in a cross section. Exceptionally, up to 90 percent of tubules were stained. When immunoglobulin was eluted from kidney tissue, the eluates bound to TBM in over 80 percent of cases; usually the binding was to less than 20 percent of tubules, but a minority of eluates bound more or less diffusely. This varied reactivity suggested that more than one tubular antigen might be involved in the process [152]. The case of Border et al. [17], referred to earlier in this section, is unique in that IgA was the predominant immunoglobulin and was present in a strongly reacting, continuous linear pattern along TBMs; IgM and C3 were present in a weakly staining nonlinear pattern. Bowman's capsule occasionally contains immunoglobulins [17,136, 153].

Of considerable interest are the immunofluorescence findings in the cases referred to under Microscopic Findings in which focal glomerulonephritis, mesangial increase, or normal glomeruli were found on biopsy [1,4,6,17,20,26,38,83, 118,136,137,160]. In all of these, a linear fluorescence for immunoglobulin, with or without C3, was apparently present on a widespread scale in the glomeruli. Such a case is demonstrated in Figure 10-16, which is from the same biopsy as illustrated in Figures 10-1 and 10-2. Why these cases remain comparatively tranquil in the presence of antibody on the GBMs is not understood.

In certain cases of proven anti-GBM antibody pathogenesis, anomalous immunofluorescence patterns have been described [4,103,114]. In one of

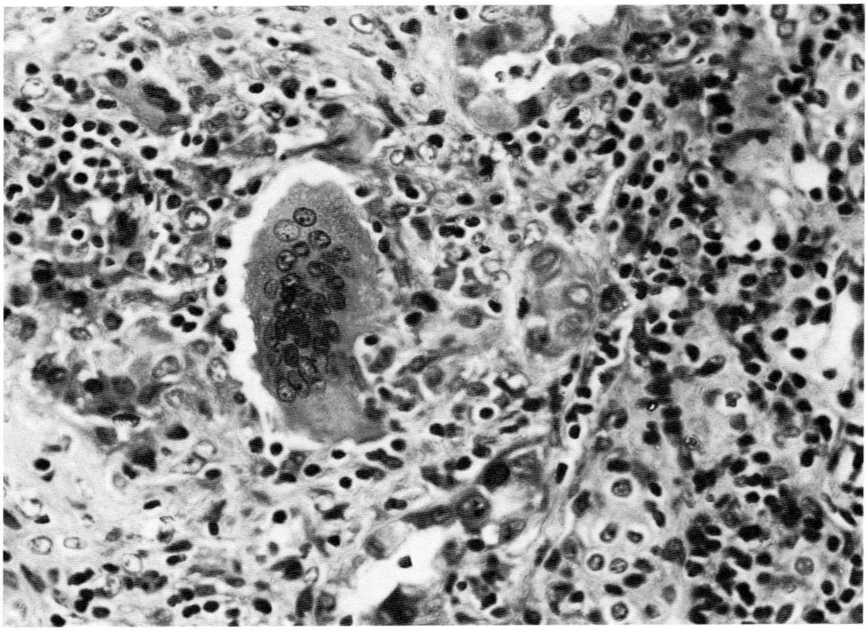

FIG. 10-8. *Multinucleated giant cell in interstitium accompanied by chronic inflammatory cells from patient with positive fluorescence for IgG along TBMs. H&E; ×400.*

these [4], serial biopsies revealed a transformation from a linear pattern for IgG and C3 to one with both linear and granular deposits of IgG. This coincided with a decrease in anti-GBM antibody levels in the serum. Electron microscopy revealed the appearance of electron-dense deposits on the epithelial side of the GBM. Another case [103] exhibited two continuous lines of fluorescence for IgG in the glomeruli, and one of these was considered to be caused by the small dense deposits on the epithelial side of the GBM seen by electron microscopy. The closeness of the deposits was regarded as being responsible for a linear rather than a granular pattern. Two other cases with demonstrable circulating anti-GBM antibodies showed a linear fluorescence for IgG with a suggestion that in certain stretches of the capillary wall there was a finely granular pattern [114]. C3 was revealed with a diffusely granular distribution. Electron microscopy revealed subepithelial deposits in one and subendothelial and subepithelial deposits in the other.

Pathologic Changes in the Lung

Space does not permit an extensive account of the pulmonary aspects, and only a brief description will be given. The introduction of transbronchial biopsy has allowed studies to be carried out during life, whereas at one time the only material available was that obtained at autopsy or by open biopsy.

The lungs are almost invariably enlarged and firm, keeping their shape when removed at autopsy. They have purplish areas of various sizes on the pleural aspect that signify the presence of blood in alveoli. Histologically, the alveoli contain large numbers of red blood cells, iron pigment in macrophages (siderophages), and fibrin (Fig. 10-17). The relative and absolute amounts of

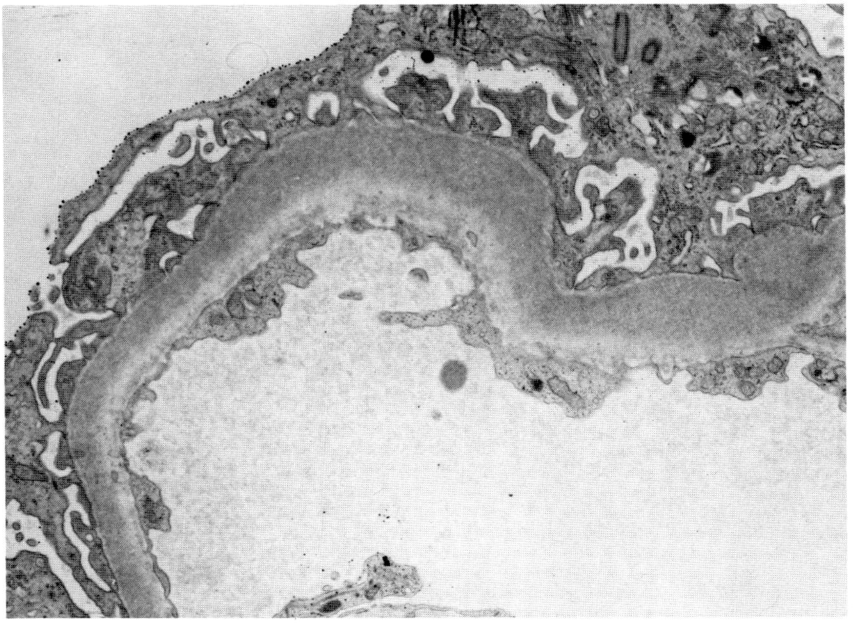

FIG. 10-9. *Electron micrograph from a patient with lung hemorrhage and glomerulonephritis of anti-GBM antibody pathogenesis. No immune deposits are seen, but there is an electron-lucent zone on the endothelial side of the GBM.* × *10,000. (Courtesy of Dr. T. Antonovych and the Director of the Armed Forces Institute of Pathology.)*

these constituents depend on the duration and severity of the clinical disease, although usually the lungs contain more blood than would be anticipated from the amount expectorated during life. The alveolar septa may show congested capillaries and be thickened with elastic fragmentation; however, in most cases the reticulin and elastic patterns are little altered. Siderophages may be seen in relation to the septa, and inflammatory cells and necroses have been described. In personally studied cases, I have never been impressed by necrotizing or inflammatory septal changes and have always regarded any changes in the septa as being a reaction to, rather than a cause of, the hemorrhage. Edema fluid also may be present, but this is not usually pronounced. Scattered areas of bronchopneumonia may be found, and infection with *Pneumocystis carinii* has been noted [136].

When direct immunofluorescence techniques have been used on lung tissue, linear fluorescence has been described along the alveolar septa for both IgG and C3 [7,10,29,66,81,90,118,136], as well as for IgG but not C3 [1,20,57,90,137] (Fig. 10-18). Positive fluorescence for IgG or anti-human gamma globulin has been obtained in a linear or focal globular distribution by others [67,82, 135], who did not study complement. Negative results for immunoglobulins and complement were obtained by other investigators [32,34,122]. A linear distribution for IgA alone has been described in one case; in this, an IgA antibody was eluted from the lung that reacted with normal GBM, TBM, Bowman's capsule, and pulmonary alveolar septa [17]. Fibrin is also demonstrable in the alveoli by immunofluorescence techniques.

Electron microscopy has revealed a variety of

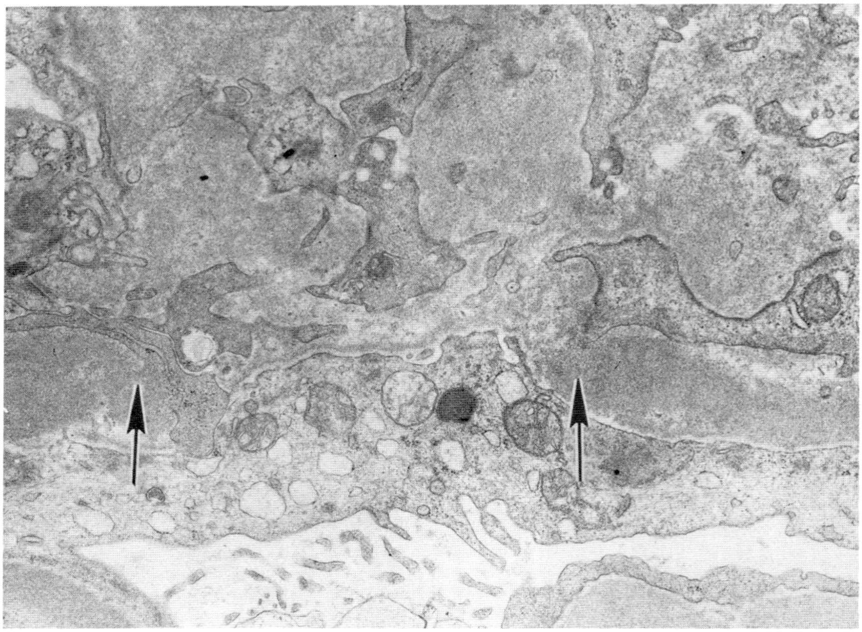

Fig. 10-10. *GBM from a patient with lung hemorrhage and glomerulonephritis of anti-GBM pathogenesis showing break in continuity between two arrows.* ×10,000. *(Courtesy of Dr. T. Antonovych and the Director of the Armed Forces Institute of Pathology.)*

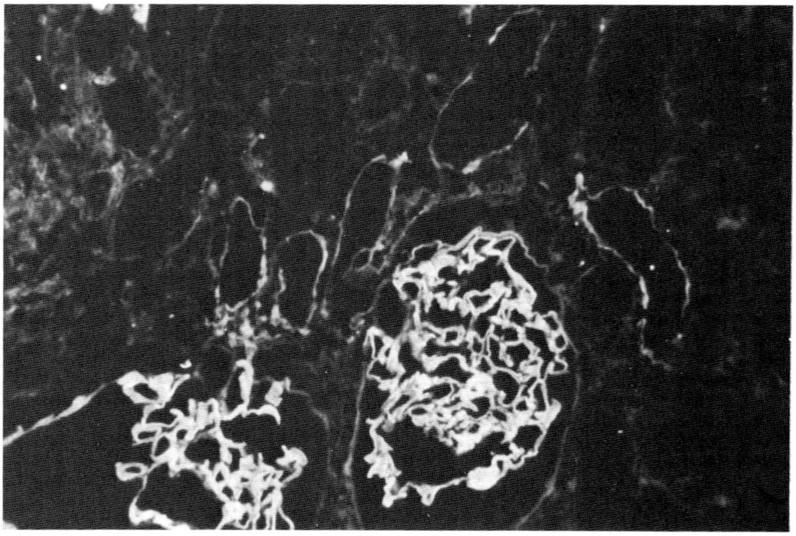

Fig. 10-11. *Two glomeruli at the bottom of the picture show linear fluorescence for IgG along capillary walls with, in addition, fainter positive fluorescence along several TBMs. From a 60-year-old man with crescentic glomerulonephritis.*

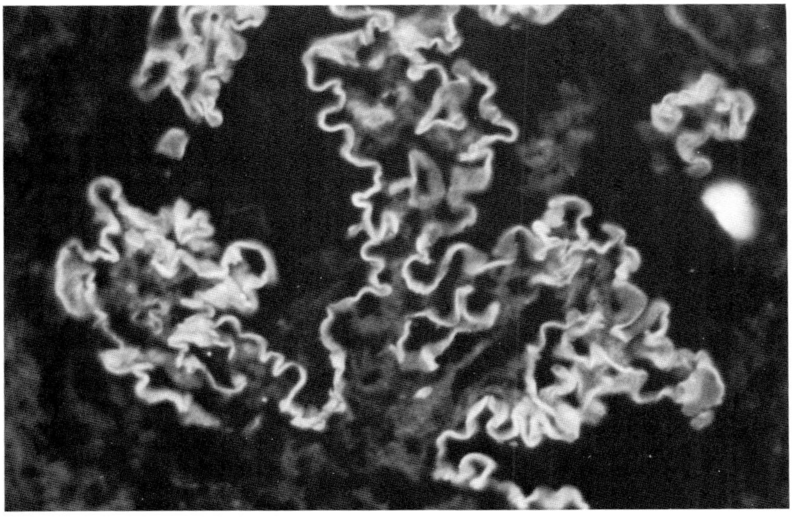

Fig. 10-12. *Higher-power view from the same patient as illustrated in Fig. 10-11 to show linear deposition of IgG along glomerular capillary walls.*

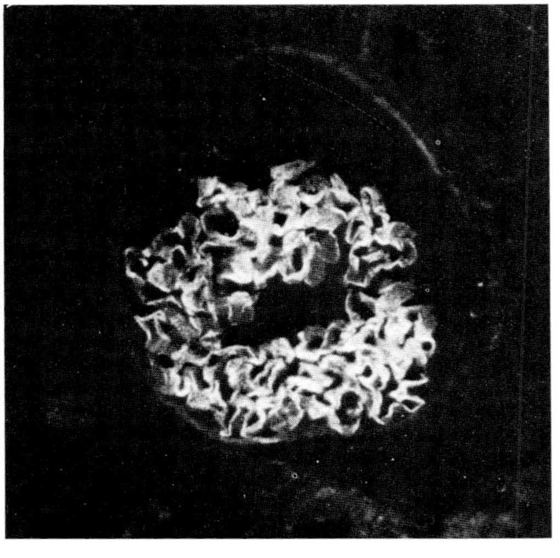

Fig. 10-13. *Linear fluorescence along glomerular capillary walls for C3 from a patient with lung hemorrhage and crescentic glomerulonephritis of anti-GBM antibody pathogenesis.*

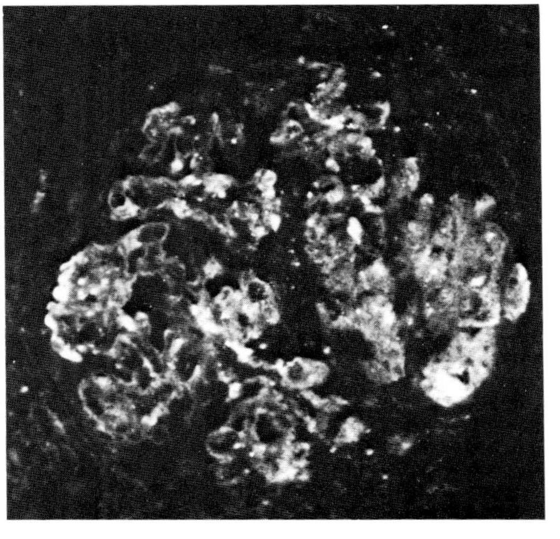

Fig. 10-14. *Granular fluorescence for C3 along glomerular capillary walls in a patient with anti-GBM antibody disease.*

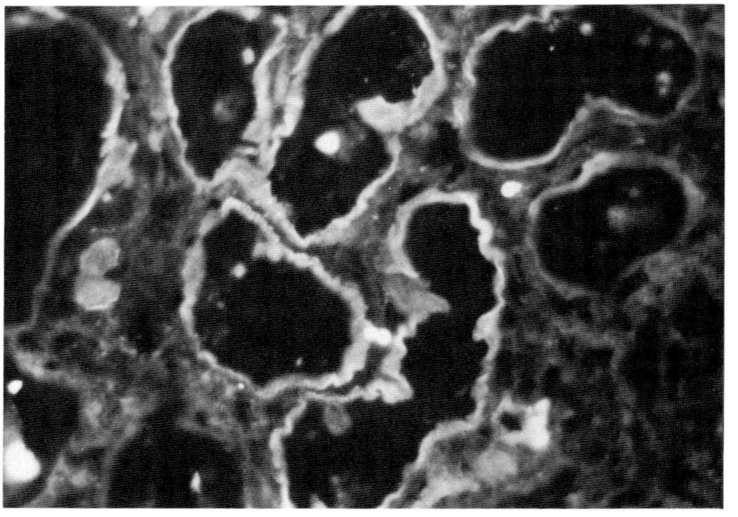

FIG. 10-15. *Positive linear fluorescence for IgG along TBMs from same patient shown in Figs. 10-11 and 10-12.*

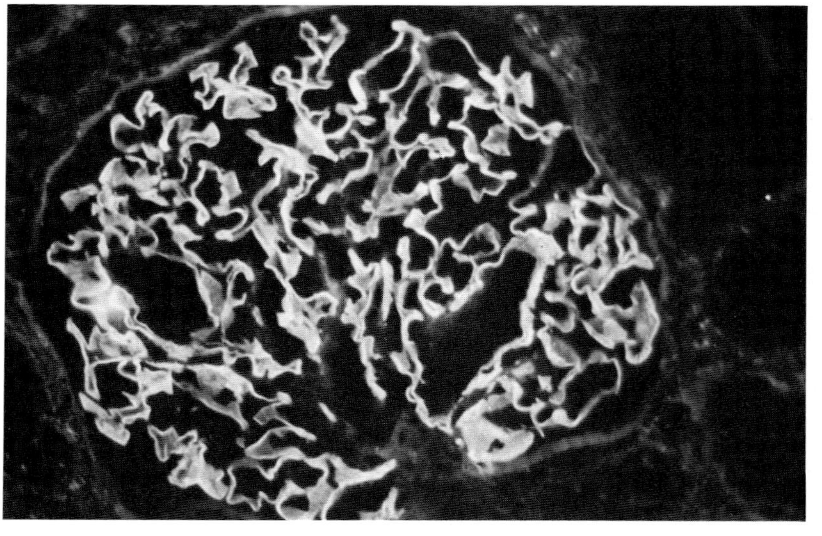

FIG. 10-16. *Linear fluorescence for IgG along glomerular capillary walls from the patient depicted in Figs. 10-1 and 10-2. The glomerular shape is preserved because 90 percent of the glomeruli were devoid of significant lesions.*

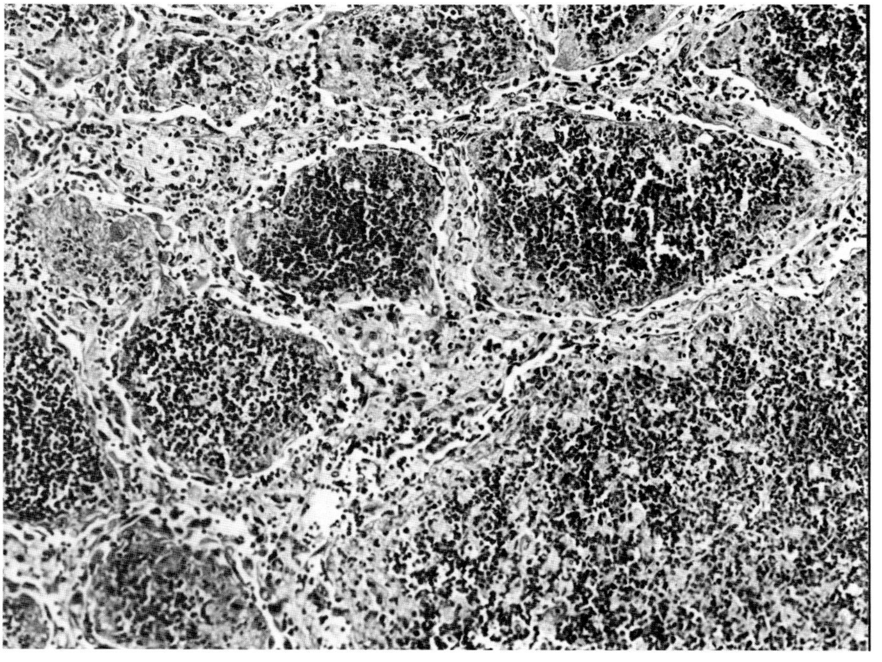

Fig. 10-17. *Section of lung obtained at autopsy from a patient with pulmonary hemorrhage and glomerulonephritis of anti-GBM antibody pathogenesis. The alveoli are stuffed with red blood cells. H&E;* $\times 215$.

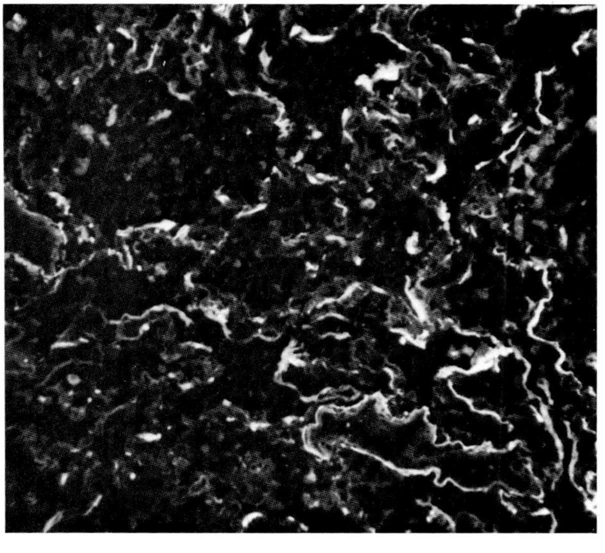

Fig. 10-18. *Positive fluorescence for IgG along alveolar walls from a patient with anti-GBM antibody disease. (From Germuth, F. G., Jr., and Rodriguez, E.* Immunopathology of the Renal Glomerulus. *Boston: Little, Brown, 1973.)*

changes [18,32,136]; these include hyperplasia of type I and type II alveolar epithelial cells, diffuse vascular injury with wide endothelial gaps through which migration of red cells and monocytes occurs, diffusely fragmented basement membranes, and an electron-dense layer on the basement membrane.

Clinical Course and Outcome

In those patients in whom there are only mild focal glomerular changes—referred to under Microscopic Findings—there may be no worsening of renal function over prolonged periods of observation [1,4,6,20,73,118,136,160]. As noted earlier, these are often patients in whom pulmonary symptoms are predominant. Such a clinical picture was seen in a patient whose renal biopsy was seen on our service. This was a 28-year-old woman with hemoptysis and evidence of pulmonary hemorrhage by transbronchial biopsy. She was found to have microscopic hematuria, some red-cell casts, and a serum creatinine level that ranged between 1.0 and 1.5 mg/100 ml. Renal biopsy (see Figs. 10-1 and 10-2) revealed a focal glomerulonephritis involving less than 10 percent of glomeruli, with small crescents in some of those with lesions. There was a 3+ linear fluorescence for IgG along the glomerular capillary walls (see Fig. 10-16), and circulating anti-GBM antibodies were demonstrated by radioimmunoassay. After successful treatment with immunosuppressive agents and plasmapheresis, the patient was well 2½ years later with a serum creatinine level of 1.2 mg/100 ml and no circulating anti-GBM antibodies.

In certain instances, however, these mild renal changes may develop into a more widespread crescentic form of glomerulonephritis with rapid deterioration in renal function. Good documentation of this is provided by Briggs et al. [20], who in two patients demonstrated a transformation from a focal glomerulonephritis on the first biopsy to a necrotizing proliferative form with crescent formation within a span of 4 weeks. Rapidly progressive renal failure developed over this period that was sufficient to warrant dialysis in both, and subsequent transplantation in one of them. Teague et al. [136] described a patient with minor focal glomerulonephritis who developed a florid necrotizing crescentic type of lesion and died within 15 weeks, while a case is recorded of a similar transformation over a period of 1 week [98]. These rapid transformations were well documented in patients with lung hemorrhage before the introduction of immunologic techniques [12,58,78,115], and it is highly likely that some of these were of anti-GBM antibody type.

The outlook as far as severe derangement or death of the kidney is concerned is still dismal in most of the severe crescentic forms of anti-GBM antibody glomerulonephritis [11,20,25,40,48,51, 52,57,88,104,108,112,119,136,153]. This is so in both the type with concomitant lung hemorrhage and in that without it, even in spite of modern therapy. Certain clinical features are particularly sinister, and those patients with oliguria or anuria seldom recover renal function [40,48,51,80, 104,143]. Similarly, those requiring dialysis early in the course of the disease fare badly, and of 21 such patients in one study, none recovered renal function despite vigorous therapy using plasmapheresis, steroids, and cytotoxic drugs [51]. So poor is the outlook for renal recovery with oligoanuria that some believe aggressive therapy (immunosuppression and plasmapheresis) in this group should be reserved for those with pulmonary hemorrhage (which is more responsive to treatment), deteriorating renal function in those who are not dialysis-dependent, and in preparation for transplantation [40,104]. High levels of serum creatinine at the onset of illness also have been shown to augur badly [57,119], and exclusive of patients who were dialysis-dependent, renal functional improvement took place in only 1 of 12 with a level above 6.8 mg/100 ml compared with improvement in 21 of 27 with levels below this mark [119]. All patients in the first group and most in the second received immunosuppressive therapy and plasmapheresis.

The most useful prognostic indicator using renal biopsy is the number of glomeruli affected by crescents [57,80,143]. This was very convincingly brought out in the study of Walker et al. [143], in which patients with more than 85 percent of glomeruli bearing crescents had a significantly worse outlook than those with lesser involvement. As was noted in Chapter 9, the prognostic implications of numbers of crescents are not so convincing when primary crescentic glomerulonephritis is considered as a whole [41,51].

While we have seen that those patients with florid renal lesions and large numbers of crescents almost invariably develop renal insufficiency and that many of those with minor lesions do not suffer serious damage, there is little information available on the intermediate group with appreciable numbers of crescents, say on the order of 15 to 50 percent involvement. Some of these will undoubtedly develop more extensive lesions because it must be remembered that the appearance in a biopsy is partly a function of the time at which it is performed, and as noted before, the pathologic process in anti-GBM antibody glomerulonephritis can progress very rapidly. Such cases with appreciable numbers of crescents are described in various series in which immunosuppression and plasmapheresis are employed, and stabilization of renal function is reported in some of them [2,57,143]. Serum creatinine levels are elevated in many of these patients at follow-up, and when repeat renal biopsies are performed, increased numbers of sclerotic glomeruli and a less hectic picture are recorded.

Progressive glomerular scarring independent of the original immunologic insult has been considered to account for the increase in serum creatinine that may occur over time in certain patients who made a good initial recovery from their acute disease [104].

Pulmonary failure and life-threatening hemorrhage from the lung are additional hazards for patients with anti-GBM antibody disease [112,153]. Ever since the demonstration of the pathogenic effects of these antibodies on the lung, attempts have been made to lower their level in the circulation in the hope of reducing pulmonary hemorrhage. One of the earliest forms of treatment was bilateral nephrectomy, the rationale being that the suspected source of the antigen would be eliminated. Successes in controlling pulmonary hemorrhage were reported with this technique [20, 28,98,103,125,153], although a rare patient showed deterioration [82]. Considerable success in reducing anti-GBM levels is now achieved using immunosuppressive drugs coupled with plasmapheresis [20,35,57,76,104,119,143], and this is reflected in the lowering of pulmonary complications. So successful may this treatment be that control of pulmonary hemorrhage was achieved in 29 of 33 patients in one series [104]. Despite these good results, a fatal pulmonary hemorrhage still takes place in certain patients [20,51,52,119, 143]. Sepsis may occur as a serious complication, and it figures as a cause of death in several series [11,40,51,52]. The effects of immunosuppression and plasmapheresis on the renal lesions were alluded to earlier, and the only additional point that needs to be made is the use of this form of treatment in preparation for renal transplantation. Presumably by lowering the level of circulating antibody the procedure minimizes the risk of the original glomerular disease developing in the grafted kidney; beneficial effects are reported [27].

Clinical relapses occur during plasmapheresis and immunosuppressive treatment and are manifest by fever and deterioration in pulmonary and renal function. Rees et al. [111] observed that these early relapses were more related to intercurrent bacterial infections than to a rise in level of anti-GBM antibody. Relapses may occur at a later time [2,29,60], and in this situation, the reappearance of anti-GBM antibodies may be the explanation. A good example is provided by a case in which a young man with pulmonary hemorrhage went into remission under treatment, and circulating antibodies disappeared [60]. After 5 uneventful years he developed severe pulmonary hemorrhage and hematuria that coincided with the reappearance of circulating anti-GBM antibodies. Treatment with immunosuppressive agents and plasmapheresis resulted in clearing of the chest radiographs and virtual restoration of pulmonary function to normal; hematuria abated and antibodies to GBM disappeared. In another case, exacerbation of pulmonary hemorrhage coincided with a high level of circulating immune complexes with no change in anti-GBM antibodies at that time [142]. The explanation for this is not patent.

PULMONARY HEMORRHAGE AND GLOMERULONEPHRITIS NOT ASSOCIATED WITH ANTI-GBM ANTIBODIES

It must not be imagined that pulmonary hemorrhage with glomerulonephritis is restricted to patients with anti-GBM antibody disease. It may be found in a variety of conditions, and in the great majority the hemorrhage appears at the alveolar level as in anti-GBM antibody disease.

Polyarteritis Nodosa

Pulmonary hemorrhage is remarkably common in this condition. As described in the introductory section, the original paper by Parkin et al. [102] describing seven patients with lung hemorrhage and glomerulonephritis contained four with polyarteritis nodosa. In three substantial series of patients dealing with polyarteritis accompanied by glomerulonephritis (so-called microscopic form), lung hemorrhage occurred in 9 percent [3], 19 percent [123], and 32 percent [121] of patients. Viewing the matter from a different aspect, polyarteritis—or systemic vasculitis, as the authors chose to call it—accounted for 6 of 26 cases (23 percent) of diffuse alveolar hemorrhage [69]. For purposes of comparison, anti-GBM antibody disease accounted for 10 (38 percent) of these cases. When autopsies have been performed and the lungs examined, there has been little evidence of arteritis as a source of the bleeding in the lungs despite widespread arteritic changes elsewhere [50,78, 138]. The hemorrhage is presumed to come from the alveolar capillaries as in anti-GBM antibody disease, and in a series of patients with pulmonary hemorrhage and systemic vasculitis described by Mark and Ramirez [80*a*], there was evidence of capillaritis causing disruption of the interalveolar septa in the lung. A similar alveolitis was described in two patients with pulmonary hemorrhage complicating polyarteritis accompanied by crescentic glomerulonephritis [15*a*]. One of these patients had antineutrophil cytoplasmic antibodies (ANCA). Since the study of Mark and Ramirez antedated the current interest in ANCA, these autoantibodies were not sought, but as will be discussed in a later section (p. 697), they may well relate to the pulmonary capillaritis and ensuing hemorrhage.

Wegener's Syndrome

Lung hemorrhage occurs in this condition [47, 106], and Haworth et al. [47] consider that the prevalence of hemorrhage is underestimated. They found it to be present in 22 of their 53 cases of Wegener's syndrome (42 percent). To assess pulmonary hemorrhage, they measured the diffusing capacity of carbon monoxide and corrected for alveolar volume. The resultant transfer coefficient was regarded as a sensitive index of pulmonary hemorrhage. In some cases, the pulmonary hemorrhage in Wegener's syndrome comes from the nodular granulomas and the arteritic lesions that are commonly found (see Chap. 16). In other cases, however, there is a more generalized form of *alveolar* hemorrhage [49,69,95], and in their review of alveolar hemorrhage syndromes in 1984, Leatherman et al. [69] related that 11 examples of this were on record in Wegener's syndrome. They described how the patients differ from those with typical Wegener's syndrome; lung involvement is initially manifest as alveolar hemorrhage rather than as nodules or localized infiltrates, and upper airway disease is exceptional. They also pointed out that the renal involvement in these cases is particularly severe. The mechanism by which the bleeding takes place is not clear, but capillaritis (alveolitis) has been claimed as a likely candidate [80*a*, 95]. As will be described in Chapter 16, alveolitis has been demonstrated as a not infrequent feature of Wegener's syndrome [157*a*]. The possible pathogenic role of ANCA will be discussed later (p. 697).

In exceptional cases, concomitant anti-GBM antibody disease may be present [142*a*], and a case of Wegener's syndrome with lung hemorrhage has been described in which linear glomerular staining for IgG was present in a crescentic glomerulonephritis [101]. Only when lung biopsy was performed was the diagnosis of Wegener's syndrome made. Circulating anti-GBM antibodies were sought but were not demonstrated.

Glomerulonephritis

Crescentic glomerulonephritis of apparent primary type (see Chap. 9) may be complicated by lung hemorrhage. Group 2 (immune complexes in the glomeruli) and group 3, or the pauci-immune group (no or trivial glomerular deposition of immunoglobulins and/or complement), have both been implicated. Lung hemorrhage in group 2 was described in children in two reports [9,77], and adult cases were cited by Leatherman et al. [69] in their review. Group 3 has been implicated on several occasions [11,15*a*,69,134], but it must be remembered that it is often difficult to differentiate this form of primary crescentic glomerulonephritis from crescentic glomerulonephritis accompanying generalized vasculitis, because in both the glomerulonephritis is of the type with no or trivial immunoglobulin deposition. The importance of ANCA as the pathogenetic mechanism of pulmonary hemorrhage is again apparent in light of the high prevalence of these autoantibodies in patients with crescentic glomerulonephritis—with or without vasculitis—of the type with scanty or no immunoglobulin deposition.

Cases of glomerulonephritis with immune complex deposition in the glomeruli other than severe crescentic forms also may have pulmonary hemorrhage [74,77,116], and it is of note that in one patient with chronic glomerulonephritis induced by immune complexes [77], a lung biopsy revealed no complexes along the alveolar walls. An absence of immune complexes in the lung also was recorded in a case of IgA nephritis in which there was lung hemorrhage [159]. Other conditions associated with lung hemorrhage include necrotizing glomerulonephritis of undetermined type [101] and rheumatoid arthritis associated with vasculitis and crescentic glomerulonephritis [69].

Antineutrophil Cytoplasmic Antibodies (ANCA) and Pulmonary Hemorrhage

In the preceding sections it was described how alveolar hemorrhage can occur in the three conditions of polyarteritis, Wegener's syndrome, and primary crescentic glomerulonephritis, principally of the type with no or scant immunoglobulins in the glomeruli. It was also pointed out that capillaritis or alveolitis was a common feature and a likely cause of the alveolar hemorrhage. Although little had been written about ANCA at the time most of these papers were published, it is now known that all three conditions may be accompanied by these autoantibodies. Furthermore, in two recent studies [54*a*, 96*a*] in which lung tissue was examined and serum assayed for ANCA in patients with necrotizing crescentic glomerulonephritis of the type with no or scanty immunoglobulin deposition, capillaritis was found in association with ANCA in some instances. In one series [54*a*], capillaritis was found in 9 of 15 lung specimens from patients positive for ANCA and in 5 of 13 in the other [96*a*]. While it would be premature to accept the idea that ANCA are pathogenic and responsible for the capillaritis, it is worthy of further study.

Following Treatment with Penicillamine

Several instances have been recorded of patients with Wilson's disease, rheumatoid arthritis, or primary biliary cirrhosis who developed lung hemorrhage and glomerulonephritis while undergoing treatment with penicillamine [44,69,84,133]. In the three patients with Wilson's disease described by Sternlieb et al. [133], penicillamine had been administered for 2 to 3½ years before fatal pulmonary hemorrhages and rapidly progressive glomerulonephritis supervened. Autopsy in two of them revealed large numbers of red blood cells and hemosiderin in the lungs, together with crescentic glomerulonephritis. Immunofluorescence microscopy was performed in only one of these cases, and a patchy, interrupted staining for IgG and C3 (referred to in one place in the text as "granular") was found in the glomeruli; similar studies in the lung were negative. Circulating anti-GBM antibodies were not sought. Gibson et al. [44] described a 51-year-old man with rhematoid arthritis treated with penicillamine for 2 years. He presented with dyspnea, chest pain, hemoptysis, and oliguria. Extensive bilateral pulmonary shadows were seen in radiographs of the lung, and renal biopsy revealed a severe glomerulonephritis with crescents. Immunofluorescence findings in the glomeruli were negative. The patient's renal function deteriorated, and he was placed on chronic dialysis. Matloff and Kaplan's case [84[occurred during penicillamine treatment for primary biliary cirrhosis. Pulmonary failure with severe hemoptysis predominated, but urinary changes consisting of protein, red blood cells, and red-cell casts were present. No renal biopsy was done, but cryoglobulins were detected in the blood; there was absence of C1q binding, and serum complement levels were normal. Anti-GBM antibodies were absent from the serum using an immunofluorescence technique. Leatherman et al. [69] mentioned three more cases in their review. Crescentic glomerulonephritis without vasculitis was described either with granular deposits of IgG and C3 in the glomeruli or with negative glomerular immunofluorescence. It appears as though the mechanism of lung hemorrhage is independent of anti-GBM antibodies, but its precise nature is unknown.

Systemic Lupus Erythematosus

Although there are many pulmonary complications of SLE [92], diffuse alveolar hemorrhage is one of the more serious. In a review of 23 well-authenticated cases of this complication of SLE, Leatherman et al. [69] related how 16 of them (70 percent) died, often within a few days. Granular immunodeposits along the alveolar septa were reported in some of these cases, and it is tempting to suggest that they had a role in the causation of the bleeding.

Source of Hemorrhage in Lung

It is apparent from these various reports that there is a strong association of glomerulonephritis—usually a severe form—and lung hemorrhage. Unfortunately, few ideas are expressed as to the pathogenesis of the pulmonary bleeding. Anti-GBM antibody pathogenesis was excluded in virtually all cases described, and there was little evidence of immune complexes in the alveolar septa except in the case of SLE. In some of the conditions with blood vessel inflammation, it would be possible for the hemorrhage to come from ruptured vessels, but with the exception of Wegener's syndrome, the cases described showed no pulmonary vascular involvement. Even in Wegener's syndrome it was noted that the hemorrhage was often of a diffuse alveolar type, which suggested that it came from alveolar capillaries rather than from cavitating nodules or ruptured arteries or veins.

USE OF TERM GOODPASTURE'S SYNDROME

The ubiquity of lung hemorrhage with glomerulonephritis and the different conditions in which it is found once again puts into question the wisdom of using the term *Goodpasture's syndrome.* If it is used simply to describe any condition in which there is lung hemorrhage and glomerulonephritis, it will embrace a large number of conditions, and any particular case will need to be qualified by adding the condition responsible for it. This offers no advantage over the simple descriptive term of *lung hemorrhage and glomerulonephritis,* qualified by adding the associated condition or mechanism, if known. Furthermore, it can be downright confusing when some use the eponym to describe any case of lung hemorrhage and glomerulonephritis, while others use it solely for those of anti-GBM antibody pathogenesis. It was probably a useful term at a time when the various conditions contributing to it were not identified, but now it seems to have outlived its usefulness.

IDIOPATHIC PULMONARY HEMOSIDEROSIS AND OTHER CONDITIONS WITH DIFFUSE ALVEOLAR HEMORRHAGE

The pulmonary lesion in anti-GBM antibody disease resembles very closely the condition of idiopathic pulmonary hemosiderosis, and a few words will be said about this condition. It was originally described in children by Ceelen [23] almost 60 years ago but is now known to occur in adults as well as children. Clinically, it is characterized by hemoptysis, lung infiltrates, dyspnea, disturbed pulmonary function, and anemia. It gets its name from the large number of hemosiderin-laden macrophages in the alveoli and is in most respects identical to the picture described earlier in anti-GBM antibody lung disease. Hemorrhage appears to come from alveolar capillaries. Changes by electron microscopy are those of nonspecific injury [33,53], although sparse focal fractures of alveolar capillary basement membranes have been described [32]. Immunofluorescence studies, however, differ from those in anti-GBM antibody disease, and no immunoglobulin deposition is recorded in the alveolar walls [32,33,53]. It should be remarked, however, that there must be a considerable overlap between idiopathic pulmonary hemosiderosis and those cases of anti-GBM antibody disease with changes apparently localized to the lung. It is therefore likely that certain patients designated as having idiopathic pulmonary hemosiderosis in the days before anti-GBM antibody disease was appreciated were indeed suffering from the latter condition. The same argument would hold even today in patients inadequately investigated.

In their comprehensive review of diffuse alveolar hemorrhage, Leatherman et al. [69] have described various other causes. These include Schönlein-Henoch syndrome (in which is quoted a case with IgA occurring in a granular pattern in the lung), Behçet's disease, rheumatoid arthritis, following lymphangiography, and in patients who have inhaled trimellitic anhydride, a chemical used in the plastics industry and in paints.

RECURRENCE OF ANTI-GBM ANTIBODY DISEASE IN RENAL TRANSPLANTS

Transplantation in patients with anti-GBM antibody disease presents special problems because of the danger of the disease developing in the graft. The matter will be described in Chapter 27, and all that needs to be said at this stage is that it is considered imprudent to perform transplantation in the presence of circulating antibody because this is the situation in which glomerulonephritis is likely to develop in the donor kidney [20,153].

ETIOLOGY AND PATHOGENESIS OF ANTI-GBM ANTIBODY DISEASE

The experimental basis of anti-GBM antibody disease and certain basic immunologic observations in man are discussed in Chapter 3, and only those aspects which relate directly to the clinical and pathologic features of human disease will be recounted here.

Anti-GBM Antibody and the Kidney

There is good evidence for believing that anti-GBM antibodies are pathogenic for glomerular capillaries. First, there are numerous observations in biopsy material to indicate the fixation of IgG and C3 to the capillary wall in a characteristic linear pattern. These were described in an earlier section dealing with immunofluorescence findings. Second, Lerner et al. [72] demonstrated that antibodies with an affinity for GBM could be eluted from the kidneys of patients with lung hemorrhage and glomerulonephritis in which this linear pattern had been noted. This was accomplished by applying the eluates to frozen sections of normal human kidney and incubating with fluorescein-labeled anti-human IgG after washing the sections. Linear fluorescence was obtained along the glomerular capillary walls. These observations have been repeated on several occasions [20,66,82,107,153]. Third, the nephritogenic potential of the eluted antibody was shown by the ability of renal-eluate IgG to produce a severe progressive glomerulonephritis on injection into squirrel monkeys [72]. Fourth, antibody obtained from the sera of certain patients with lung hemorrhage and glomerulonephritis also gives a linear glomerular pattern when applied to normal kidney [82,90, 153]. Fifth, antibody to GBM can be demonstrated in the sera by radioimmunoassay [91, 155].

Of interest are those cases in which positive linear fluorescence in the glomeruli is present for IgG but not for C3. Many of these are of proven anti-GBM antibody type [20,82,90,119,136,153]. The reason for the absence of C3 is not apparent, but it has been shown that it is not due to the presence of IgG subtypes that lack the ability to fix complement [90]. On the other hand, however, it has been shown that patients with IgG but no C3 need not have anti-GBM antibody–mediated disease. For example, Koffler et al. [65] have shown this pattern in patients with SLE in whom they were unable to elute anti-GBM antibodies, and Gallo [42] had the same experience in four patients, two of whom were diabetics. In addition, nonspecific linear deposits also may be seen in kidneys obtained at autopsy and in those perfused in preparation for transplantation; in these there seems to be an unusual nonimmunologic affinity of the GBM for IgG [153]. Because linear fluorescence for IgG can be seen in these various conditions, Wilson and Dixon [154] suggested that linear fluorescence be regarded as only the first stage in diagnosing anti-GBM antibody–mediated disease and that the diagnosis be confirmed by demonstrating antibody in the serum or kidney eluates. A similar nonpathogenic linear staining for IgA without C3 also has been described [39].

Anti-GBM Antibody and the Lung

Immunofluorescence studies also have been carried out on the lung, because any mechanism suggested should be able to explain the pulmonary picture. Direct immunofluorescence studies of lungs from patients with anti-GBM antibody disease have shown positive staining of the alveolar walls for IgG, with or without C3, as described earlier under Pathologic Changes in the Lung. Elution studies have revealed the following: Eluates of kidneys showed an affinity for alveolar walls of normal human lung in some studies [66,107] but not in others [72,82]. Eluates of lungs gave a linear staining pattern with normal human glomeruli and with normal human lung [66]. A variant on the usual type of case has been described in which there was IgA anti-GBM antibody instead of the usual IgG type [17]. Eluates from both the lung and kidney in this instance contained an IgA antibody that bound in a linear fashion to GBM, TBM, and Bowman's capsule of normal kidney, as well as to the alveolar capillary basement membrane of normal human lung.

The antigenic similarity between basement membranes in the lung and in kidney has long been recognized [46,132,150]. Steblay and Rudofsky [132] were able to produce a progressive glomerulonephritis in sheep by immunization with human lung and Freund's adjuvant; sheep IgG and C3 were demonstrated in a linear pattern along the glomerular capillary walls. Except that the source of the antigen is different, this appears to be identical to the model developed by Steblay [131], in which sheep were injected with heterologous glomerular basement membranes and Freund's adjuvant (Fig. 10-19). In the model using lung as antigen, eluate from the nephritic kidney contained antibody that reacted with the alveolar walls of human lung (Fig. 10-20). The similarities to human anti-GBM antibody are apparent. Further relevant experiments are those in which pulmonary hemorrhage and glomerulonephritis were produced in rats following intravenous injection of rabbit anti–rat lung basement membrane antibody [46,150]. Anti–rat lung antibodies could be demonstrated in alveoli and GBMs. A model developed in the mouse using antigen derived from the globular domain of type IV collagen is of great interest [145]. It will be seen in the next section that the antigen thought to be involved in anti-GBM antibody disease—the so-called Goodpasture antigen—resides in this globular domain. Immunization of mice with the globular domain of type IV collagen derived from the mouse Engelbreth-Holm-Swarm tumor resulted in pulmonary hemorrhage and a mild form of glomerulonephritis. Tissue-bound antibodies, along with C3, were detected by immunofluorescence in a linear pattern along alveolar walls and GBMs. An undue amount of pulmonary fibrosis was an anomalous feature.

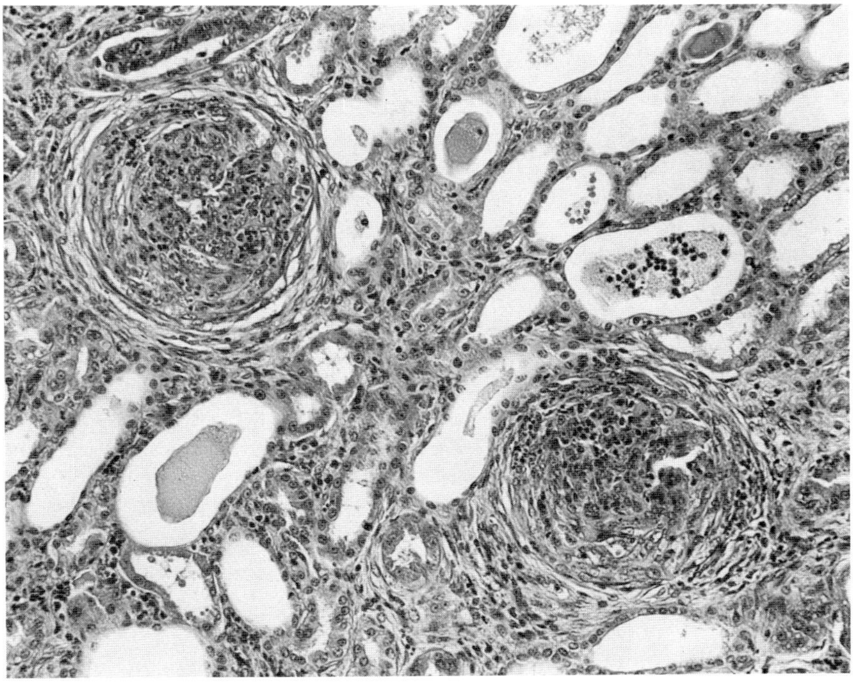

Fig. 10-19. *Two glomeruli from sheep given injections of GBM and Freund's adjuvant. Crescents are seen in both. H&E; ×175. (Courtesy of Dr. Raymond Steblay.)*

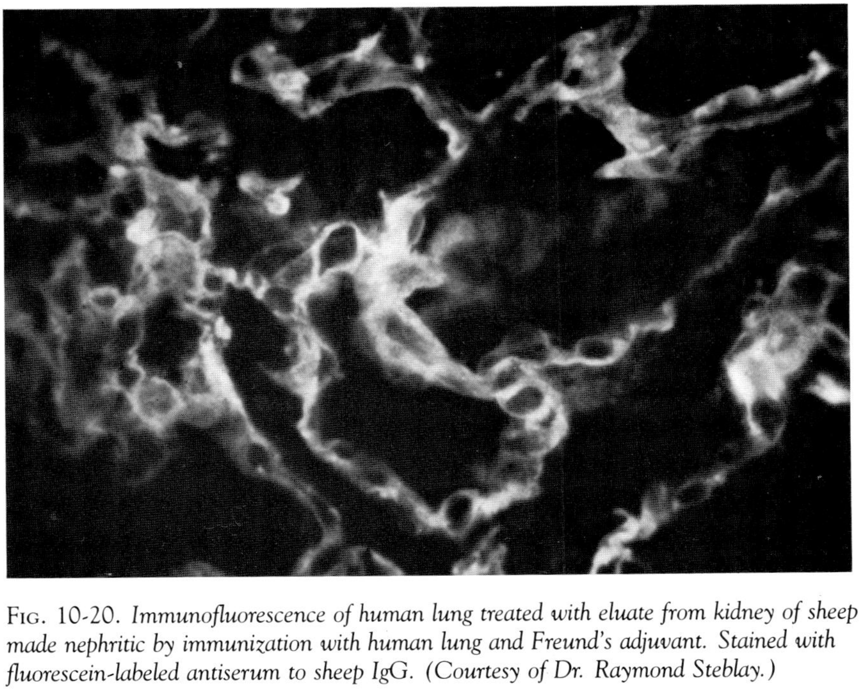

Fig. 10-20. *Immunofluorescence of human lung treated with eluate from kidney of sheep made nephritic by immunization with human lung and Freund's adjuvant. Stained with fluorescein-labeled antiserum to sheep IgG. (Courtesy of Dr. Raymond Steblay.)*

Location of the Goodpasture Antigen

A considerable amount of work has been done to identify the antigen responsible for the production of anti-GBM antibodies, the so-called Goodpasture antigen. From studies on bovine and human GBMs, it appears that the antigen is present in collagenase-resistant domains, specifically the globular domain of type IV collagen [146,147]. The globular domain—also called the NC1 domain—is the area where two molecules of type IV collagen are linked together at their carboxy-terminal ends and exists in a hexameric form with monomeric and dimeric units [144]; the Goodpasture antigen is considered to be localized to monomeric M2 and dimeric D2 [21,148]. M2 was subsequently designated as the NC1 domain of the α_3 chain of type IV collagen [118a]. This complex and rapidly moving subject has been well reviewed by Hudson et al. [52*a*].

The widespread distribution of the Goodpasture antigen was revealed in a study using a monoclonal antibody (P1) to the autoantigenic component of human GBM [109]. There was linear binding to GBM, Bowman's capsule, TBM, and basement membranes in lung and choroid plexus. In addition, there was binding to membranes of the lens capsule, choroid and retina of the eye, and cochlea, all of which are structures that may be involved in Alport's syndrome (hereditary nephritis); the significance of this will be discussed later. Also, the staining pattern of the monoclonal antibody P1 has been compared with that of an antibody to type IV collagen [22]. With P1, the same reactive sites were found as listed earlier, but there were sites in certain structures where there was reactivity to the type IV collagen not shared by P1. Two possible explanations are that type IV collagen is heterogeneous and need not carry the Goodpasture antigen and that the cryptic nature of the antigen prevents its demonstration in certain locations.

With regard to the latter explanation, it has been demonstrated that the epitope of the Goodpasture antigen is sequestered in the hexamer of the globular domain [149] but becomes exposed and binds with antibody obtained from patients with anti-GBM antibody disease when the hexamer dissociates into its subunits after suitable chemical treatment of in vitro GBM preparations. This is shown diagrammatically in Figure 10-21, which is a slightly modified illustration from the discussion of Hudson et al. [52*a*]. This inaccessibility of the antigen may explain why there is an inconstant reactivity of anti-GBM antibodies with other basement membranes, such as in the lung, and absent reactivity in various other organs tested [89]. Yoshioka et al. [158] addressed this matter and showed that anti-GBM antibodies were able to react with lung, placenta, and skin basement membranes when tissue sections were treated with acid urea, whereas they were unable to react in their native state. This was explained by an unmasking of hidden antigenic determinants. The importance of this is apparent, particularly to explain why some patients with anti-GBM antibody disease develop lung hemorrhage while others do not. The possibility arises that such stimuli as viral infections [156], cigarette smoking [31], and exposure to hydrocarbons [8,16,62] could unmask the antigenic sites in a similar way so that antibody could gain access to them with consequent damage.

There are other reasons, however, why anti-GBM antibody may have difficulty in reaching antigenic sites and exerting a pathogenic effect. Salant [117] has discussed this with regard to the lung. He pointed out that whereas the endothelium of the glomerular capillary wall is fenestrated, alveolar endothelium is not, so there is an effective barrier to the passage of anti-GBM antibodies. The experiment of Jennings et al. [55] was cited, in which rabbits were exposed to the gamma globulin fraction of an antiserum directed against alveolar basement membrane prepared in the goat. Whereas goat IgG became fixed to the GBM, it could not be detected in alveolar basement membrane until the rabbits were exposed to 100% oxygen. Following this there was a linear deposition of goat IgG along the rabbit alveoli with death of the animals from pulmonary edema and hemorrhagic pneumonitis. It was concluded that the inhalation of oxygen had increased endothelial permeability to antibodies, allowing them to fix to, and damage, the alveolar basement membrane.

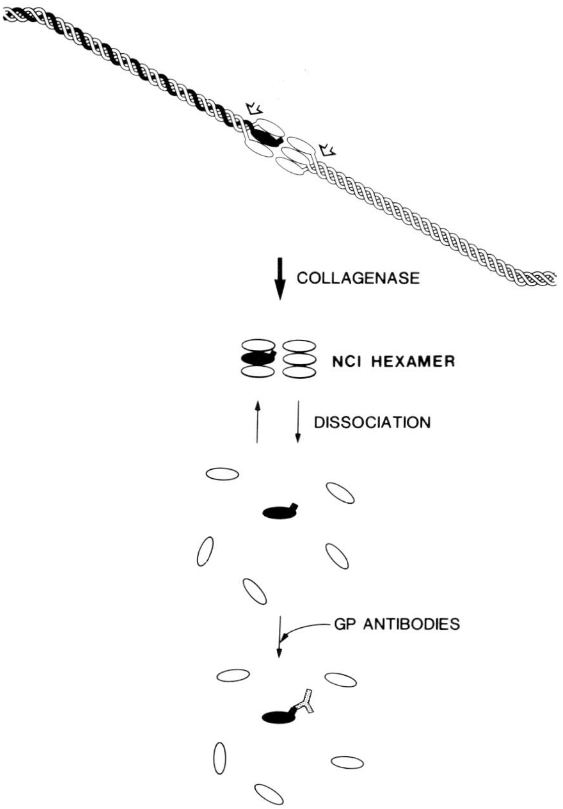

Fig. 10-21. *Diagram showing release of the NC1 hexamer from GBM and mechanism of unmasking Goodpasture determinant(s). NC1 hexamer is released from collagen IV matrix upon collagenase digestion. It is derived from NC1 domains of two adjoining protomers and consists of six subunits (three from each protomer) that are derived from carboxyl-terminal regions (NC1) of respective chains. The Goodpasture antigen (α_3 chain) is shown in black, and Goodpasture determinant(s) are represented by small black projecting square. Antibody is cross-hatched inverted Y. (Supplied by Dr. Billy G. Hudson. Adapted from Hudson, B. G., et al. Biology of disease: Goodpasture syndrome.* Lab. Invest. *61: 256, 1989, Fig. 10. Copyright by U.S.–Canadian Academy of Pathology.)*

Again, analogy could be drawn with cigarette smoking, viral infections, and volatile hydrocarbons (mentioned earlier) as agents that might cause increased permeability of pulmonary capillaries in man and so expose the alveoli to potentially damaging antibodies.

Alport's syndrome (hereditary nephritis) was referred to earlier, and its relevance to anti-GBM antibody disease will now be mentioned, although the matter will be taken up again in Chapter 30. On the basis of failure of the GBM in this condition to react with anti-GBM antibodies, it has been suggested that it lacks the Goodpasture antigen [54,56,86,100]. This has received support from two later studies. First, when immunochemical and biochemical studies were made on the NC1 domain of type IV collagen obtained from the GBMs of three patients with Alport's syndrome [63], it was found that there was an absence of the normally occurring 28-kD monomers, regarded by these authors as the probable target in anti-GBM antibody disease [64]. Second, using the monoclonal antibody P1 directed against the Goodpasture antigen, Savage et al. [120] noted reduced or absent binding in renal biopsies from 10 patients with Alport's syndrome.

Transplantation in patients with end-stage renal disease caused by Alport's syndrome might therefore be expected to result in the development of anti-GBM antibody disease in the grafted kidney, and this has been described [86,93,124]. However, it appears in relatively few patients (see Chap. 30) and may be related to the immunosuppressive therapy accompanying transplantation. The glomerulonephritis that occurs in the grafted kidney is of crescentic type with linear immunofluorescence for IgG, again providing good evidence for anti-GBM antibodies being pathogenic.

Factors Responsible for Antibody Production

Despite the many observations made on anti-GBM glomerulonephritis, we are still largely ignorant of the factors that initiate antibody production. The kidney and the lung are the chief candidates for providing the antigen against which antibody is made. While there are occasional cases recorded that provide appropriate circumstances for the production of antibodies against antigen residing in the GBM, these are highly unique and far removed from the usual case. For example, as described earlier, several cases are on record in which membranous glomerulonephritis has apparently caused conversion to an anti-GBM antibody–induced type [61,68,94,114], presumably by damaging the GBM. Normal urine has been shown to contain GBM antigen, and the possibility has been raised that under certain circumstances these urinary antigens might be the immunogens in glomerulonephritis [71]. The role of viruses has been considered [125] with a virus-antivirus immune complex sparking off the release of GBM antigen, but this is purely speculative, although virus-like structures have been noted in the glomeruli by electron microscopy [4,98,140].

Viruses are potentially likely to cause damage to alveolar basement membrane in the lung, which is the other principal potential source of antigen. Benoit et al. [12] noted the appearance of a large number of cases of lung hemorrhage and glomerulonephritis following an influenza epidemic, and the seasonal incidence of anti-GBM antibody disease reported in the British Isles [119] could be consistent with a viral background, although there is no proof that this is so. Influenza A2 titers have been reported elevated in two patients with anti-GBM antibody disease [29,156]. Inhalation of volatile hydrocarbons [8,37,62] and sniffing of hydrocarbon-containing glue [15] have been invoked as agents that might damage the alveolar basement membrane. The various studies making claims for hydrocarbons have been assessed [24], and the opinion has been reached that additional evidence is needed before a causal relationship with anti-GBM antibody disease can be accepted. The effects of cigarette smoking have been studied [31], and in a group of 47 patients with anti-GBM antibody disease, it was found that all 37 who were cigarette smokers developed pulmonary hemorrhage, whereas only 2 of the 10 nonsmokers had this feature. While this study does not address the issue of production of anti-GBM antibodies, it does offer an explanation for the occurrence of pulmonary hemorrhage in the presence of such antibodies by suggesting that there is increased permeability of the lung capillaries that allows antibody to reach antigenic sites in the alveolar basement membrane.

Various observations such as the occurrence of the disease in identical twins [30,126] and a significant association with HLA-DR2 [110,113] suggest an inherited susceptibility to anti-GBM antibody disease. A weaker association with HLA-B7 was found, and it was noted that patients inheriting HLA-B7 together with DR2 had significantly higher plasma creatinine levels, greater numbers of crescents, and a worse prognosis than those inheriting HLA-DR2 alone [110].

Choroid Plexus and Tubular Basement Membranes (TBM)

In studies using the monoclonal antibody P1, choroid plexus and TBMs have been shown to contain the Goodpasture antigen [22,109]. The implication is that either of these two structures could be a site of injury in anti-GBM antibody disease or, alternatively, a source of antigen to initiate antibody formation.

The choroid plexus has been shown to display linear fluorescence for IgG in patients with anti-GBM antibody disease [22,87], but it is seldom reported as a source of intraventricular hemorrhage. I have seen this only once in a patient with proven anti-GBM antibodies. This was a 65-year-old woman whose intraventricular hemorrhage was not detected during life and was diagnosed only at postmortem examination. Immunofluorescence studies were precluded because the brain had been fixed for 2 weeks according to the usual routine. McIntosh et al. [87] have suggested that choroid plexus could serve as a source of antigen to trigger antibody formation, but little evidence is advanced to support this.

Fixation of antibody to TBMs is common in anti-GBM antibody disease, and the various immunofluorescence patterns, together with the damaging effects on the tubules, were related earlier in the chapter. Since the matter of anti-TBM antibodies is discussed in Chapter 3 and is the subject of a recent review by Wilson [152], no more will be said except that there is little to suggest that TBMs are the source of antigen in anti-GBM antibody disease.

Cell-Mediated Mechanisms

Although there is abundant evidence for anti-GBM antibodies being responsible for glomerular damage, the possibility has been raised that cell-mediated mechanisms also may play a part in patients with anti-GBM antibody disease. McCluskey and Bhan [85] raised this issue, recalling previous observations that lymphocytes from patients with anti-GBM antibody disease show in vitro activity against basement-membrane preparations and quoting their own experiments, which showed that cell-mediated mechanisms can induce glomerular injury. Studies in human anti-GBM antibody glomerulonephritis have revealed large numbers of monocytes and T cells in glomeruli and interstitium [13,97,128] that are consistent with the idea of a cell-mediated mechanism. Experimental aspects of this are described in Chapter 3.

SPECIFICITY OF RENAL LESION IN ANTI-GBM ANTIBODY DISEASE

The histologic picture, as judged by light microscopy, is far from specific regardless of its stage. The early stages are indistinguishable from other forms of focal and segmental necrotizing glomerulonephritis, and the fully developed diffuse crescentic type cannot be distinguished from group 3 primary crescentic glomerulonephritis or the glomerulonephritis of polyarteritis nodosa, Wegener's syndrome, relapsing polychondritis, and rheumatoid arthritis unless arteritis is present in the biopsy in those cases in which it is a feature. The situation is compounded by the fact that arteritis may be present in the occasional case of anti-GBM antibody disease [73,157]. Even the additional clinical information of pulmonary hemorrhage is of little help, since it may be found in other forms of crescentic glomerulonephritis, as related earlier.

Immunofluorescence microscopy coupled with the finding of circulating anti-GBM antibodies enables all the above-mentioned conditions to be excluded. The presence of a linear fluorescence for IgG with or without C3 along the glomerular capillary wall is highly suggestive of anti-GBM antibody disease. As described earlier, however, this should be supported by the demonstration of circulating anti-GBM antibodies or of antibodies eluted from renal tissue. This is necessary because from time to time a linear glomerular fluorescence for IgG is encountered in the absence of anti-GBM antibody disease. The demonstration of a more intense linear glomerular pattern for albumin is a feature of those cases in which linear IgG is detected in the absence of anti-GBM antibody disease, and this is exemplified by case 12 in our series of biopsies of primary crescentic glomerulonephritis referred to in Table 9-5 in Chapter 9. Even though this patient had a florid crescentic glomerulonephritis, it was clearly of group 3 primary type because of the more intense linear glomerular staining with albumin coupled with the absence of circulating antibodies to GBM.

It is also important to recall that even the less severe or early forms of anti-GBM antibody disease show the linear glomerular pattern for IgG, which provides the initial information for making the correct diagnosis.

REFERENCES

1. Abboud, R. T., Chase, W. H., Ballon, H. S., Grzybowski, S., and Magil, A. Goodpasture's syndrome: Diagnosis by transbronchial lung biopsy. *Ann. Intern. Med.* 89:635, 1978.
2. Adler, S., Bruns, F. J., Fraley, D. S., and Segel, D. P. Rapid progressive glomerulonephritis: Relapse after prolonged remission. *Arch. Intern. Med.* 141:852, 1981.
3. Adu, D., Howie, A. J., Scott, D. G. I., Bacon, P. A., McGonigle, R. J. S., and Michael, J. Polyarteritis and the kidney. *Q. J. Med.* 62:221, 1987.
4. Agodoa, L. C. Y., Striker, G. E., George, C. R. P., Glassock, R., and Quadracci, L. J. The appearance of nonlinear deposits of immunoglobulins in Goodpasture's syndrome. *Am. J. Med.* 61:407, 1976.

5. Andres, G., Brentjens, J., Kohli, R., Anthone, R., Anthone, S., Baliah, T., Montes, M., Mookerjee, B. K., Prezyna, A., Sepulveda, M., Venuto, R., and Elwood, C. Histology of human tubulointerstitial nephritis associated with antibodies to renal basement membranes. *Kidney Int.* 13:480, 1978.
6. Bailey, R. R., Simpson, I. J., Lynn, K. L., Neale, T. J., Doak, P. B., and McGiven, A. R. Goodpasture's syndrome with normal renal function. *Clin. Nephrol.* 15:211, 1981.
7. Beechler, C. R., Enquist, R. W., Hunt, K. K., Ward, G. W., and Knieser, M. R. Immunofluorescence of transbronchial biopsies in Goodpasture's syndrome. *Am. Rev. Respir. Dis.* 121:869, 1980.
8. Beirne, G. J., and Brennan, J. T. Glomerulonephritis associated with hydrocarbon solvents mediated by antiglomerular basement membrane antibody. *Arch. Environ. Health* 25:365, 1972.
9. Beirne, G. J., Kopp, W. L., and Zimmerman, S. W. Goodpasture syndrome: Dissociation from antibodies to glomerular basement membrane. *Arch. Intern. Med.* 132:261, 1973.
10. Beirne, G. J., Octaviano, G. N., Kopp, W. L., and Burns, R. O. Immunohistology of the lung in Goodpasture's syndrome. *Ann. Intern. Med.* 69:1207, 1968.
11. Beirne, G. J., Wagnild, J. P., Zimmerman, S. W., Macken, P. D., and Burkholder, P. M. Idiopathic crescentic glomerulonephritis. *Medicine (Baltimore)* 56:349, 1977.
12. Benoit, F. L., Rulon, D. B., Theil, G. B., Doolan, P. D., and Watten, R. H. Goodpasture's syndrome: A clinicopathologic entity. *Am. J. Med.* 37:424, 1964.
13. Bolton, W. K., Innes, D. J., Jr., Sturgill, B. C., and Kaiser, D. L. T-cells and macrophages in rapidly progressive glomerulonephritis: Clinicopathologic correlations. *Kidney Int.* 32:869, 1987.
14. Bonsib, S. M. Glomerular basement membrane discontinuities: Scanning electron microscopic study of acellular glomeruli. *Am. J. Pathol.* 119:357, 1985.
15. Bonsib, S. M. Glomerular basement membrane necrosis and crescent organization. *Kidney Int.* 33:966, 1988.
15*a*. Bonsib, S. M., and Walker, W. P. Pulmonary-renal syndrome: Clinical similarity amidst etiologic diversity. *Mod. Pathol.* 2:129, 1989.
16. Bonzel, K.-E., Müller-Wiefel, D. E., Ruder, H., Wingen, A.-M., Waldherr, R., and Weber, M. Antiglomerular basement membrane antibody–mediated glomerulonephritis due to glue sniffing. *Eur. J. Pediatr.* 146:296, 1987.
17. Border, W. A., Baehler, R. W., Bhathena, D., and Glassock, R. J. IgA anti-basement membrane nephritis with pulmonary hemorrhage. *Ann. Intern. Med.* 91:21, 1979.
18. Botting, A. J., Brown, A. L., Jr., and Divertie, M. B. The pulmonary lesion in a patient with Goodpasture's syndrome: As studied with the electron microscope. *Am. J. Clin. Pathol.* 42:387, 1964.
19. Boucher, A., Droz, D., Adafer, E., and Noël, L. H. Relationship between the integrity of Bowman's capsule and the composition of cellular crescents in human crescentic glomerulonephritis. *Lab. Invest.* 56:526, 1987.
20. Briggs, W. A., Johnson, J. P., Teichman, S., Yeager, H. C., and Wilson, C. B. Antiglomerular basement membrane antibody–mediated glomerulonephritis and Goodpasture's syndrome. *Medicine (Baltimore)* 58:348, 1979.
21. Butkowski, R. J., Wieslander, J., Wisdom, B. J., Barr, J. F., Noelken, M. E., and Hudson, B. G. Properties of the globular domain of type IV collagen and its relationship to the Goodpasture antigen. *J. Biol. Chem.* 260:3739, 1985.
22. Cashman, S. J., Pusey, C. D., and Evans, D. J. Extraglomerular distribution of immunoreactive Goodpasture antigen. *J. Pathol.* 155:61, 1988.
23. Ceelen, W. Die Kreislaufstörungen der Lunge. In F. Henke and O. Lubarsch (Eds.), *Handbuch der Speziellen Pathologischen Anatomie und Histologie,* Vol. 3, Part 3. Berlin: Springer, 1931. P. 1.
24. Churchill, D. N., Fine, A., and Gault, M. H. Association between hydrocarbon exposure and glomerulonephritis: An appraisal of the evidence. *Nephron* 33:169, 1983.
25. Cohen, A. H., Border, W. A., Shankel, E., and Glassock, R. J. Crescentic glomerulonephritis: Immune vs. nonimmune mechanisms. *Am. J. Nephrol.* 1:78, 1981.
26. Cohen, L. H., Wilson, C. B., and Freeman, R. M. Goodpasture syndrome: Recovery after severe renal insufficiency. *Arch. Intern. Med.* 136:835, 1976.
27. Cove-Smith, J. R., McLeod, A. A., Blamey, R. W., Knapp, M. S., Reeves, W. G., and Wilson, C. B. Transplantation, immunosuppression and plasmapheresis in Goodpasture's syndrome. *Clin. Nephrol.* 9:126, 1978.
28. Curtis, J. J., Bhathena, D., Leach, R. P., Galla, J. H., Lucas, B. A., and Luke, R. G. Goodpasture's syndrome in a patient with the nail-patella syndrome. *Am. J. Med.* 61:401, 1976.
29. Dahlberg, P. J., Kurtz, S. B., Donadio, J. V., Jr., Holley, K. E., Velosa, J. A., Williams, D. E., and Wilson, C. B. Recurrent Goodpasture's syndrome. *Mayo Clin. Proc.* 53:533, 1978.
30. D'Apice, A. J. F., Kincaid-Smith, P., Becker, G.

J., Loughhead, M. G., Freeman, J. W., and Sands, J. M. Goodpasture's syndrome in identical twins. *Ann. Intern. Med.* 88:61, 1978.
31. Donaghy, M., and Rees, A. J. Cigarette smoking and lung haemorrhage in glomerulonephritis caused by autoantibodies to glomerular basement membrane. *Lancet* 2:1390, 1983.
32. Donald, K. J., Edwards, R. L., and McEvoy, J. D. S. Alveolar capillary basement membrane lesions in Goodpasture's syndrome and idiopathic pulmonary hemosiderosis. *Am. J. Med.* 59:642, 1975.
33. Donlan, C. J., Jr., Srodes, C. H., and Duffy, F. D. Idiopathic pulmonary hemosiderosis: Electron microscopic, immunofluorescent, and iron kinetic studies. *Chest* 68:577, 1975.
34. Duncan, D. A., Drummond, K. N., Michael, A. F., and Vernier, R. L. Pulmonary hemorrhage and glomerulonephritis: Report of six cases and study of the renal lesion by the fluorescent antibody technique and electron microscopy. *Ann. Intern. Med.* 62:920, 1965.
35. Espinosa-Meléndez, E., Forbes, R. D. C., Hollomby, D. J., Ahuja, J., and Katz, M. G. Goodpasture's syndrome treated with plasmapheresis: Report of a case. *Arch. Intern. Med.* 140:542, 1980.
36. Ferrario, F., Castiglione, A., Colasanti, G., Barbiano Di Belgioioso, G., Bertoli, S., and D'Amico, G. The detection of monocytes in human glomerulonephritis. *Kidney Int.* 28:513, 1985.
37. Finn, R., Fennerty, A. G., and Ahmad, R. Hydrocarbon exposure and glomerulonephritis. *Clin. Nephrol.* 14:173, 1980.
38. Fitzcharles, M. A., and Benatar, S. R. Goodpasture's syndrome: Case report of a survivor. *S. Afr. Med. J.* 53:63, 1978.
39. Fivush, B., Melvin, T., Solez, K., and McLean, R. H. Idiopathic linear glomerular IgA deposition. *Arch. Pathol. Lab. Med.* 110:1189, 1986.
40. Flores, J. C., Taube, D., Savage, C. O. S., Cameron, J. S., Lockwood, C. M., Williams, D. G., and Ogg, C. S. Clinical and immunological evolution of oligoanuric anti-GBM nephritis treated by haemodialysis. *Lancet* 1:5, 1986.
41. Furlong, T. J., Ibels, L. S., and Eckstein, R. P. The clinical spectrum of necrotizing glomerulonephritis. *Medicine (Baltimore)* 66:192, 1987.
42. Gallo, G. Elution studies in kidneys with linear deposition of immunoglobulin in glomeruli. *Am. J. Pathol.* 61:377, 1970.
43. Germuth, F. G., Jr., Choi, I. J., Taylor, J. J., and Rodriguez, E. Anti-basement membrane disease: I. The glomerular lesions of Goodpasture's disease and experimental disease in sheep. *Johns Hopkins Med. J.* 131:367, 1972.
44. Gibson, T., Burry, H. C., and Ogg, C. Goodpasture syndrome and D-penicillamine. *Ann. Intern. Med.* 84:100, 1976.
45. Goodpasture, E. W. The significance of certain pulmonary lesions in relation to the etiology of influenza. *Am. J. Med. Sci.* 158:863, 1919.
46. Hagadorn, J. E., Vazquez, J. J., and Kinney, T. R. Immunologic studies of an experimental model resembling Goodpasture's syndrome. *Am. J. Pathol.* 57:17, 1969.
47. Haworth, S. J., Savage, C. O. S., Carr, D., Hughes, J. M. B., and Rees, A. J. Pulmonary haemorrhage complicating Wegener's granulomatosis and microscopic polyarteritis. *Br. Med. J.* 290:1775, 1985.
48. Heilman, R. L., Offord, K. P., Holley, K. E., and Velosa, J. A. Analysis of risk factors for patient and renal survival in crescentic glomerulonephritis. *Am. J. Kidney Dis.* 9:98, 1987.
49. Hensley, M. J., Feldman, N. T., Lazarus, J. M., and Galvanek, E. G. Diffuse pulmonary hemorrhage and rapidly progressive renal failure: An uncommon presentation of Wegener's granulomatosis. *Am. J. Med.* 66:894, 1979.
50. Heptinstall, R. H., and Salmon, M. V. Pulmonary haemorrhage with extensive glomerular disease of the kidney. *J. Clin. Pathol.* 12:272, 1959.
51. Hind, C. R. K., Paraskevakou, H., Lockwood, C. M., Evans, D. J., Peters, D. K., and Rees, A. J. Prognosis after immunosuppression of patients with crescentic nephritis requiring dialysis. *Lancet* 1:263, 1983.
52. Holdsworth, S., Boyce, N., Thomson, N. M., and Atkins, R. C. The clinical spectrum of acute glomerulonephritis and lung haemorrhage (Goodpasture's syndrome). *Q. J. Med.* 55:75, 1985.
52*a*. Hudson, B. G., Wieslander, J., Wisdom, B. J., Jr., and Noelken, M. E. Biology of disease: Goodpasture syndrome: Molecular architecture and function of basement membrane antigen. *Lab. Invest.* 61:256,1989.
53. Irwin, R. S., Cottrell, T. S., Hsu, K. C., Griswold, W. R., and Thomas, H. M., III. Idiopathic pulmonary hemosiderosis: An electron microscopic and immunofluorescent study. *Chest* 65:41, 1974.
53*a*. Jayne, D. R. W., Marshall, P. D., Jones, S. J., and Lockwood, C. M. Autoantibodies to GBM and neutrophil cytoplasm in rapidly progressive glomerulonephritis. *Kidney Int.* 37:965, 1990.
54. Jenis, E. H., Valeski, J. E., and Calcagno, P. L. Variability of anti-GBM binding in hereditary nephritis. *Clin. Nephrol.* 15:111, 1981.
54*a*. Jennette, J. C., Wilkman, A. S., and Falk, R. J. Antineutrophil cytoplasmic autoantibody–associ-

ated glomerulonephritis and vasculitis. *Am. J. Pathol.* 135:921, 1989.

55. Jennings, L., Roholt, O. A., Pressman, D., Blau, M., Andres, G. A., and Brentjens, J. R. Experimental anti-alveolar basement membrane antibody–mediated pneumonitis: I. The role of increased permeability of the alveolar capillary wall induced by oxygen. *J. Immunol.* 127:129, 1981.
56. Jeraj, K., Kim, Y., Vernier, R. L., Fish, A. J., and Michael, A. F. Absence of Goodpasture's antigen in male patients with familial nephritis. *Am. J. Kidney Dis.* 2:626, 1983.
57. Johnson, J. P., Moore, J., Jr., Austin, H. A., III, Balow, J. E., Antonovych, T. T., and Wilson, C. B. Therapy of anti-glomerular basement membrane antibody disease: Analysis of prognostic significance of clinical, pathologic and treatment factors. *Medicine (Baltimore)* 64:219, 1985.
58. Johnson, J. R., and McGovern, V. J. Goodpasture's syndrome and Wegener's granulomatosis. *Aust. Ann. Med.* 11:250, 1962.
59. Kalowski, S., McKay, D. G., Howes, E. L., Jr., Csavossy, I., and Wolfson, M. Multinucleated giant cells in antiglomerular basement membrane antibody–induced glomerulonephritis. *Nephron* 16:415, 1976.
60. Klaska, R. J., Abboud, R. T., Ballon, H. S., and Grossman, L. Goodpasture's syndrome: Recurrence after a five-year remission. Case report and review of the literature. *Am. J. Med.* 84:751, 1988.
61. Klassen, J., Elwood, C., Grossberg, A. L., Milgrom, F., Montes, M., Sepulveda, M., and Andres, G. A. Evolution of membranous nephropathy into antiglomerular-basement-membrane glomerulonephritis. *N. Engl. J. Med.* 290:1340, 1974.
62. Kleinknecht, D., Morel-Maroger, L., Callard, P., Adhémar, J.-P., and Mahieu, P. Antiglomerular basement membrane nephritis after solvent exposure. *Arch. Intern. Med.* 140:230, 1980.
63. Kleppel, M. M., Kashtan, C. E., Butkowski, R. J., Fish, A. J., and Michael, A. F. Alport familial nephritis: Absence of 28-kilodalton non-collagenous monomers of type IV collagen in glomerular basement membrane. *J. Clin. Invest.* 80:263, 1987.
64. Kleppel, M. M., Michael, A. F., and Fish, A. J. Antibody specificity of human glomerular basement membrane type IV collagen NC1 subunits: Species variation in subunit composition. *J Biol. Chem.* 261:16547, 1986.
65. Koffler, D., Agnello, V., Carr, R. I., and Kunkel, H. G. Variable patterns of immunoglobulin and complement deposition in the kidneys of patients with systemic lupus erythematosus. *Am. J. Pathol.* 56:305, 1969.
66. Koffler, D., Sandson, J., Carr, R., and Kunkel, H. G. Immunologic studies concerning the pulmonary lesions in Goodpasture's syndrome. *Am. J. Pathol.* 54:293, 1969.
67. Kroe, D. J., and Pitcock, J. A. Goodpasture's syndrome: An immunofluorescent study of the pulmonary and renal lesions. *South. Med. J.* 61:183, 1968.
68. Kurki, P., Helve, T., von Bonsdorff, M., Törnroth, T., Pettersson, E., Riska, H., and Miettinen, A. Transformation of membranous glomerulonephritis into crescentic glomerulonephritis with glomerular basement membrane antibodies: Serial determinations of anti-GBM before the transformation. *Nephron* 38:134, 1984.
69. Leatherman, J. W., Davies, S. F., and Hoidal, J. R. Alveolar hemorrhage syndromes: Diffuse microvascular lung hemorrhage in immune and idiopathic disorders. *Medicine (Baltimore)* 63:343, 1984.
70. Lehman, D. H., Wilson, C. B., and Dixon, F. J. Extraglomerular immunoglobulin deposits in human nephritis. *Am. J. Med.* 58:765, 1975.
71. Lerner, R. A., and Dixon, F. J. The induction of acute glomerulonephritis in rabbits with soluble antigens isolated from normal homologous and autologous urine. *J. Immunol.* 100:1277, 1968.
72. Lerner, R. A., Glassock, R. J., and Dixon, F. J. The role of anti-glomerular basement membrane antibody in the pathogenesis of human glomerulonephritis. *J. Exp. Med.* 126:989, 1967.
73. Lewis, E. J., Cavallo, T., Harrington, J. T., and Cotran, R. S. An immunopathologic study of rapidly progressive glomerulonephritis in the adult. *Hum. Pathol.* 2:185, 1971.
74. Lewis, E. J., Schur, P. H., Busch, G. J., Galvanek, E., and Merrill, J. P. Immunopathologic features of a patient with glomerulonephritis and pulmonary hemorrhage. *Am. J. Med.* 54:507, 1973.
75. Lockwood, C. M., Jayne, D. R., Marshall, P., Jones, S., and Savage, C. O. S. A prospective study of the incidence of anti-GBM and anti-neutrophil cytoplasm antibodies in patients with rapidly progressive nephritis (Abstract). *Kidney Int.* 33:329, 1988.
76. Lockwood, C. M., Rees, A. J., Pearson, T. A., Evans, D. J., Peters, D. K., and Wilson, C. B. Immunosuppression and plasma-exchange in the treatment of Goodpasture's syndrome. *Lancet* 1:711, 1976.
77. Loughlin, G. M., Taussig, L. M., Murphy, S. A., Strunk, R. C., and Kohnen, P. W. Immune-complex-mediated glomerulonephritis and pulmonary hemorrhage simulating Goodpasture syndrome. *J. Pediatr.* 93:181, 1978.

78. Maddock, R. K., Jr., Stevens, L. E., Reemtsma, K., and Bloomer, H. A. Goodpasture's syndrome: Cessation of pulmonary hemorrhage after bilateral nephrectomy. *Ann. Intern. Med.* 67: 1258, 1967.
79. Magil, A. B., and Wadsworth, L. D. Monoctye involvement in glomerular crescents: A histochemical and ultrastructural study. *Lab. Invest.* 47:160, 1982.
80. Marcandoro, J., and Sobel, A. Syndrome de Goodpasture: Evolution du pronostic de 1955 à 1982. *Presse Med.* 12:1483, 1983.
80*a*. Mark, E. J., and Ramirez, J. F. Pulmonary capillaritis and hemorrhage in patients with systemic vasculitis. *Arch. Pathol. Lab. Med.* 109:413, 1985.
81. Markowitz, A. S., Battifora, H. A., Schwartz, F., and Aseron, C. Immunological aspects of Goodpasture's syndrome. *Clin. Exp. Immunol.* 3:585, 1968.
82. Martinez, J. S., and Kohler, P. F. Variant "Goodpasture's syndrome?" The need for immunologic criteria in rapidly progressive glomerulonephritis and hemorrhagic pneumonitis. *Ann. Intern. Med.* 75:67, 1971.
83. Mathew, T. H., Hobbs, J. B., Kalowski, S., Sutherland, P. W., and Kincaid-Smith, P. Goodpasture's syndrome: Normal renal diagnostic findings. *Ann. Intern. Med.* 82:215, 1975.
84. Matloff, D. S., and Kaplan, M. M. D-Penicillamine-induced Goodpasture's-like syndrome in primary biliary cirrhosis: Successful treatment with plasmapheresis and immunosuppressives. *Gastroenterology* 78:1046, 1980.
85. McCluskey, R. T., and Bhan, A. K. Cell-mediated mechanisms in renal diseases. *Kidney Int.* 21(Suppl. 11):S6, 1982.
86. McCoy, R. C., Johnson, H. K., Stone, W. J., and Wilson, C. B. Absence of nephritogenic GBM antigen(s) in some patients with hereditary nephritis. *Kidney Int.* 21:642, 1982.
87. McIntosh, R. M., Copack, P., Chernack, W. B., Griswold, W. R., Weil, R., and Koss, M. N. The human choroid plexus and autoimmune nephritis. *Arch. Pathol.* 99:48, 1975.
88. McLeish, K. R., Yum, M. N., and Luft, F. C. Rapidly progressive glomerulonephritis in adults: Clinical and histologic correlations. *Clin. Nephrol.* 10:43, 1978.
89. McPhaul, J. J., Jr., and Dixon, F. J. Characterization of human anti-glomerular basement membrane antibodies eluted from glomerulonephritic kidneys. *J. Clin. Invest.* 49:308, 1970.
90. McPhaul, J. J., Jr., and Dixon, F. J. Characterization of immunoglobulin G anti-glomerular basement membrane antibodies eluted from kidneys of patients with glomerulonephritis: II. IgG subtypes and in vitro complement fixation. *J. Immunol.* 107:678, 1971.
91. McPhaul, J. J., Jr., and Mullins, J. D. Glomerulonephritis mediated by antibody to glomerular basement membrane: Immunological, clinical, and histopathological characteristics. *J. Clin. Invest.* 57:351, 1976.
92. Meyers, O. L. Pulmonary involvement in systemic lupus erythematosus. *Scand. J. Rheumatol. (Suppl.)* 54:19, 1984.
93. Milliner, D. S., Pierides, A. M., and Holley, K. E. Renal transplantation in Alport's syndrome: Antiglomerular basement membrane glomerulonephritis in the allograft. *Mayo Clin. Proc.* 57:35, 1982.
94. Moorthy, A. V., Zimmerman, S. W., Burkholder, P. M., and Harrington, A. R. Association of crescentic glomerulonephritis with membranous glomerulonephropathy: A report of 3 cases. *Clin. Nephrol.* 6:319, 1976.
95. Myers, J. L., and Katzenstein, A.-L. A. Wegener's granulomatosis presenting with massive pulmonary hemorrhage and capillaritis. *Am. J. Surg. Pathol.* 11:895, 1987.
96. Neild, G. H., Cameron, J. S., Ogg, C. S., Turner, D. R., Williams, D. G., Brown, C. B., Chantler, C., and Hicks, J. Rapidly progressive glomerulonephritis with extensive glomerular crescent formation. *Q. J. Med.* 52:395, 1983.
96*a*. Niles, J. L., Pan, G., Collins, A. B., Shannon, T., Skates, S., Fienberg, R., Arnaout, M. A., and McCluskey, R. T. Value of antigen-specific radioimmunoassays for anti-neutrophil cytoplasmic antibodies (ANCA) in the diagnosis of rapidly progressive glomerulonephritis. *JASN* (*in press*).
97. Nolasco, F. E. B., Cameron, J. S., Hartley, B., Coelho, A., Hildreth, G., and Reuben, R. Intraglomerular T cells and monoctyes in nephritis: Study with monoclonal antibodies. *Kidney Int.* 31:1160, 1987.
98. Nowakowski, A., Grove, R. B., King, L. H., Jr., Antonovych, T. T., Fortner, R. W., Knieser, M. R., Carter, C. B., and Knepshield, J. H. Goodpasture's syndrome: Recovery from severe pulmonary hemorrhage after bilateral nephrectomy. *Ann. Intern. Med.* 75:243, 1971.
99. Olsen, S. Extracapillary glomerulonephritis: A semiquantitative lightmicroscopical study of 59 patients. *Acta Pathol. Microbiol. Scand.* [A] 82 (Suppl. 249):7, 1974.
100. Olson, D. L., Anand, S. K., Landing, B. H., Heuser, E., Grushkin, C. M., and Lieberman, E. Diagnosis of hereditary nephritis by failure of glomeruli to bind anti-glomerular basement membrane antibodies. *J. Pediatr.* 96:697, 1980.

101. Parfrey, P. S., Hutchinson, T. A., Jothy, S., Cramer, B. C., Martin, J., Hanley, J. A., and Seely, J. F. The spectrum of diseases associated with necrotizing glomerulonephritis and its prognosis. *Am. J. Kidney Dis.* 6:387, 1985.
102. Parkin, T. W., Rusted, I. E., Burchell, H. B., and Edwards, J. E. Hemorrhagic and interstitial pneumonitis with nephritis. *Am. J. Med.* 18:220, 1955.
103. Pasternack, A., Törnroth, T., and Linder, E. Evidence of both anti-GBM and immune complex mediated pathogenesis in the initial phase of Goodpasture's syndrome. *Clin. Nephrol.* 9:77, 1978.
104. Peters, D. K., Rees, A. J., Lockwood, C. M., and Pusey, C. D. Treatment and prognosis in antibasement membrane antibody–mediated nephritis. *Transplant. Proc.* 14:513, 1982.
105. Pettersson, E., Törnroth, T., and Miettinen, A. Simultaneous anti-glomerular basement membrane and membranous glomerulonephritis: Case report and literature review. *Clin. Immunol. Immunopathol.* 31:171, 1984.
106. Pinching, A. J., Lockwood, C. M., Pussell, B. A., Rees, A. J., Sweny, P., Evans, D. J., Bowley, N., and Peters, D. K. Wegener's granulomatosis: Observations on 18 patients with severe renal disease. *Q. J. Med.* 52:435, 1983.
107. Poskitt, T. R. Immunologic and electron microscopic studies in Goodpasture's syndrome. *Am. J. Med.* 49:250, 1970.
108. Proskey, A. J., Weatherbee, L., Easterling, R. E., Greene, J. A., and Weller, J. M. Goodpasture's syndrome: A report of five cases and review of the literature. *Am. J. Med.* 48:162, 1970.
109. Pusey, C. D., Dash, A., Kershaw, M. J., Morgan, A., Reilly, A., Rees, A. J., and Lockwood, C. M. A single autoantigen in Goodpasture's syndrome identified by a monoclonal antibody to human glomerular basement membrane. *Lab. Invest.* 56:23, 1987.
110. Rees, A. J. The HLA complex and susceptibility to glomerulonephritis. *Plasma Ther. Transfus. Technol.* 5:455, 1984.
111. Rees, A. J., Lockwood, C. M., and Peters, D. K. Enhanced allergic tissue injury in Goodpasture's syndrome by intercurrent bacterial infection. *Br. Med. J.* 2:723, 1977.
112. Rees, A. J., Lockwood, C. M., and Peters, D. K. Nephritis Due to Antibodies to GBM. In P. Kincaid-Smith, A. J. F. d'Apice, and R. C. Atkins (Eds.), *Progress in Glomerulonephritis.* New York: Wiley, 1979. P. 347.
113. Rees, A. J., Peters, D. K., Compston, D. A. S., and Batchelor, J. R. Strong association between HLA-DRw2 and antibody-mediated Goodpasture's syndrome. *Lancet* 1:966, 1978.
114. Richman, A. V., Rifkin, S. I., and McAllister, C. J. Rapidly progressive glomerulonephritis: Combined antiglomerular basement antibody and immune complex pathogenesis. *Hum. Pathol.* 12: 597, 1981.
115. Rusby, N. L., and Wilson, C. Lung purpura with nephritis. *Q. J. Med.* 29:501, 1960.
116. Saint-Hillier, Y., Mahieu, P., Charnaux, Y., Colomb, H., Hory, B., Pageau, G., and Pérol, C. Glomérulonéphrites extra-capillaires et hémorragies pulmonaires: Syndrome de Goodpasture a immuns complexes. A propos de deux observations. *J. Urol. Nephrol. (Paris)* 85:341, 1979.
117. Salant, D. J. Immunopathogenesis of crescentic glomerulonephritis and lung purpura. *Kidney Int.* 32:408, 1987.
118. Saraf, P., Berger, H. W., and Thung, S. N. Goodpasture's syndrome with no overt renal disease. *Mt. Sinai J. Med.* 45:451, 1978.
118*a*. Saus, J., Wieslander, J., Langeveld, J. P. M., Quinones, S., and Hudson, B. G. Identification of the Goodpasture antigen as the α_3(IV) chain of collagen IV. *J. Biol. Chem.* 263:13374, 1988.
119. Savage, C. O. S., Pusey, C. D., Bowman, C., Rees, A. J., and Lockwood, C. M. Antiglomerular basement membrane antibody mediated disease in the British Isles 1980–4. *Br. Med. J.* 292:301, 1986.
120. Savage, C. O. S., Pusey, C. D., Kershaw, M. J., Cashman, S. J., Harrison, P., Hartley, B., Turner, D. R., Cameron, J. S., Evans, D. J., and Lockwood, C. M. The Goodpasture antigen in Alport's syndrome: Studies with a monoclonal antibody. *Kidney Int.* 30:107, 1986.
121. Savage, C. O. S., Winearls, C. G., Evans, D. J., Rees, A. J., and Lockwood, C. M. Microscopic polyarteritis: Presentation, pathology and prognosis. *Q. J. Med.* 56:467, 1985.
122. Scheer, R. L., and Grossman, M. A. Immune aspects of the glomerulonephritis associated with pulmonary hemorrhage. *Ann. Intern. Med.* 60: 1009, 1964.
123. Serra, A., Cameron, J. S., Turner, D. R., Hartley, B., Ogg, C. S., Neild, G. H., Williams, D. G., Taube, D., Brown, C. B., and Hicks, J. A. Vasculitis affecting the kidney: Presentation, histopathology and long-term outcome. *Q. J. Med.* 53:181, 1984.
124. Shah, B., First, M. R., Mendoza, N. C., Clyne, D. H., Alexander, J. W., and Weiss, M. A. Alport's syndrome: Risk of glomerulonephritis induced by antiglomerular-basement-membrane antibody after renal transplantation. *Nephron* 50:34, 1988.
125. Siegel, R. R. The basis of pulmonary disease resolution after nephrectomy in Goodpasture's syndrome. *Am. J. Med. Sci.* 259:201, 1970.

126. Simonsen, H., Brun, C., Thomsen, O. F., Larsen, S., and Ladefoged, J. Goodpasture's syndrome in twins. *Acta Med. Scand.* 212:425, 1982.
127. Sisson, S., Dysart, N. K., Jr., Fish, A. J., and Vernier, R. L. Localization of the Goodpasture antigen by immunoelectron microscopy. *Clin. Immunol. Immunopathol.* 23:414, 1982.
128. Stachura, I., Si, L., and Whiteside, T. L. Mononuclear-cell subsets in human idiopathic crescentic glomerulonephritis (ICGN): Analysis in tissue sections with monoclonal antibodies. *J. Clin. Immunol.* 4:202, 1984.
129. Stanton, M. C., and Tange, J. D. Goodpasture's syndrome: Pulmonary haemorrhage associated with glomerulonephritis. *Australas. Ann. Med.* 7:132, 1958.
130. Stave, G. M., and Croker, B. P. Thrombotic microangiopathy in anti-glomerular basement membrane glomerulonephritis. *Arch. Pathol. Lab. Med.* 108:747, 1984.
131. Steblay, R. W. Glomerulonephritis induced in sheep by injections of heterologous glomerular basement membrane and Freund's complete adjuvant. *J. Exp. Med.* 116:253, 1962.
132. Steblay, R. W., and Rudofsky, U. Autoimmune glomerulonephritis induced in sheep by injections of human lung and Freund's adjuvant. *Science* 160:204, 1968.
133. Sternlieb, I., Bennett, B., and Scheinberg, I. H. D-Penicillamine-induced Goodpasture's syndrome in Wilson's disease. *Ann. Intern. Med.* 82:673, 1975.
134. Stilmant, M. M., Bolton, W. K., Sturgill, B. C., Schmitt, G. W., and Couser, W. G. Crescentic glomerulonephritis without immune deposits: Clinicopathologic features. *Kidney Int.* 15:184, 1979.
135. Sturgill, B. C., and Westervelt, F. B. Immunofluorescence studies in a case of Goodpasture's syndrome. *JAMA* 194:914, 1965.
136. Teague, C. A., Doak, P. B., Simpson, I. J., Rainer, S. P., and Herdson, P. B. Goodpasture's syndrome: An analysis of 29 cases. *Kidney Int.* 13:492, 1978.
137. Teichman, S., Briggs, W. A., Knieser, M. R., and Enquist, R. W. Goodpasture's syndrome: Two cases with contrasting early course and management. *Am. Rev. Respir. Dis.* 113:223, 1976.
138. Thomashow, B. M., Felton, C. P., and Navarro, C. Diffuse intrapulmonary hemorrhage, renal failure and a systemic vasculitis: A case report and review of the literature. *Am. J. Med.* 68:299, 1980.
139. Tomaszewski, M.-M., Hassell, L. H., Moore, J., Jr., and Antonovych, T. T. Goodpasture's syndrome: Local and diffuse deposition of antibody in glomerular basement membrane. Case report. *Clin. Nephrol.* 20:44, 1983.
140. Tsai, C. C., Kissane, J. M., and Germuth, F. G., Jr. Paramyxovirus-like structures in Goodpasture's syndrome. *Lancet* 2:601, 1974.
141. Tung, K. S. K., Woodroffe, A. J., Ahlin, T. D., Williams, R. C., Jr., and Wilson, C. B. Application of the solid phase C1q and Raji cell radioimmune assays for the detection of circulating immune complexes in glomerulonephritis. *J. Clin. Invest.* 62:61, 1978.
142. Vanhille, P., Raviart, B., Morel-Maroger, L., Mahieu, P., and Santoro, F. Circulating immune complexes appearing in Goodpasture's syndrome. *Br. Med. J.* 1:1166, 1980.
142*a*. Wahls, T. L., Bonsib, S. M., and Schuster, V. L. Coexistent Wegener's granulomatosis and anti-glomerular basement membrane disease. *Hum. Pathol.* 18:202, 1987.
143. Walker, R. G., Scheinkestel, C., Becker, G. J., Owen, J. E., Dowling, J. P., and Kincaid-Smith, P. Clinical and morphological aspects of the management of crescentic anti-glomerular basement membrane antibody (anti-GBM) nephritis/Goodpasture's syndrome. *Q. J. Med.* 54:75, 1985.
144. Weber, S., Engel, J., Wiedemann, H., Glanville, R. W., and Timpl, R. Subunit structure and assembly of the globular domain of basement-membrane collagen type IV. *Eur. J. Biochem.* 139:401, 1984.
145. Wick, G., von der Mark, H., Dietrich, H., and Timpl, R. Globular domain of basement membrane collagen induces autoimmune pulmonary lesions in mice resembling human Goodpasture disease. *Lab. Invest.* 55:308, 1986.
146. Wieslander, J., Barr, J. F., Butkowski, R. J., Edwards, S. J., Bygren, P., Heinegård, D., and Hudson, B. G. Goodpasture antigen of the glomerular basement membrane: Localization to noncollagenous regions of type IV collagen. *Proc. Natl. Acad. Sci. USA* 81:3838, 1984.
147. Wieslander, J., Bygren, P., and Heinegård, D. Isolation of the specific glomerular basement membrane antigen involved in Goodpasture syndrome. *Proc. Natl. Acad. Sci. USA* 81:1544, 1984.
148. Wieslander, J., Kataja, M., and Hudson, B. G. Characterization of the human Goodpasture antigen. *Clin. Exp. Immunol.* 69:332, 1987.
149. Wieslander, J., Langeveld, J., Butkowski, R., Jodlowski, M., Noelken, M., and Hudson, B. G. Physical and immunochemical studies of the globular domain of type IV collagen: Cryptic properties of the Goodpasture antigen. *J. Biol. Chem.* 260:8564, 1985.
150. Willoughby, W. F., and Dixon, F. J. Experimental hemorrhagic pneumonitis produced by heterologous antilung antibody. *J. Immunol.* 104:28, 1970.
151. Wilson, C. B. Nephritogenic antibody mecha-

nisms involving antigens within the glomerulus. *Immunol. Rev.* 55:257, 1981.

152. Wilson, C. B. Study of the immunopathogenesis of tubulointerstitial nephritis using model systems. *Kidney Int.* 35:938, 1989.
153. Wilson, C. B., and Dixon, F. J. Anti-glomerular basement membrane antibody-induced glomerulonephritis. *Kidney Int.* 3:74, 1973.
154. Wilson, C. B., and Dixon, F. J. Diagnosis of immunopathologic renal disease. *Kidney Int.* 5:389, 1974.
155. Wilson, C. B., Marquardt, H., and Dixon, F. J. Radioimmunoassay (RIA) for circulating anti-glomerular basement membrane (GBM) antibodies. (Abstract) *Kidney Int.* 6:114A, 1974.
156. Wilson, C. B., and Smith, R. C. Goodpasture's syndrome associated with influenza A2 virus infection. *Ann. Intern. Med.* 76:91, 1972.

157*a*. Yoshikawa, Y., and Watanabe, T. Pulmonary lesions in Wegener's granulomatosis: A clinicopathologic study of 22 autopsy cases. *Hum. Pathol.* 17:401, 1986.

158. Yoshioka, K., Michael, A. F., Velosa, J., and Fish, A. J. Detection of hidden nephritogenic antigen determinants in human renal and nonrenal basement membranes. *Am. J. Pathol.* 121:156, 1985.
159. Yum, M. N., Lampton, L. M., Bloom, P. M., and Edwards, J. L. Asymptomatic IgA nephropathy associated with pulmonary hemosiderosis. *Am. J. Med.* 64:1056, 1978.
160. Zimmerman, S. W., Varanasi, U. R., and Hoff, B. Goodpasture's syndrome with normal renal function. *Am. J. Med.* 66:163, 1979.

Index